Marks'
Basic Medical Biochemistry
A Clinical Approach

SECOND EDITION

Colleen Smith, PhD (deceased)

Professor of Biochemistry
Division of Basic Sciences
Mercer University School of Medicine
Macon, Georgia

Allan Marks, MD

Associate Professor of Internal Medicine
Department of Internal Medicine
Temple University School of Medicine
Philadelphia, Pennsylvania

Michael Lieberman, PhD

Distinguished Teaching Professor
Department of Molecular Genetics
University of Cincinnati College of Medicine
Cincinnati, Ohio

Illustrations by Matthew Chansky

Marks'
Basic Medical Biochemistry

A Clinical Approach

SECOND EDITION

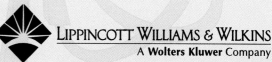

LIPPINCOTT WILLIAMS & WILKINS
A **Wolters Kluwer** Company
Philadelphia • Baltimore • New York • London
Buenos Aires • Hong Kong • Sydney • Tokyo

Editor: Betty Sun
Managing Editor: Kathleen H. Scogna
Marketing Manager: Joe Schott
Production Editor: Christina Remsberg
Compositor: Techbooks Inc.
Printer: Quebecor-Dubuque

351 West Camden Street
Baltimore, Maryland 21201-2436 USA

530 Walnut Street
Philadelphia, PA 19106

Printed in the United States of America

First Edition, 1996

Library of Congress Cataloging-in-Publication Data

Smith, Colleen M.
Marks' basic medical biochemistry / Colleen Smith, Allan Marks, Michael Lieberman.—2nd ed.
p. ; cm.
Rev. Ed. of: Basic medical biochemistry / Dawn B. Marks. c1996.
Includes bibliographical references and index.
ISBN 0-7817-2145-8
1. Biochemistry. 2. Clinical biochemistry. I. Title: Basic medical biochemistry. II. Marks, Allan D. III. Lieberman, M. A. (Michael A.) IV. Marks, Dawn B. V. Marks, Dawn B. Basic medical biochemistry. VI. Title.
[DNLM: 1. Biochemistry. 2. Clinical Medicine. QU 4 S6439m 2005]
QP514.2.S574 2005
612.1'111—dc22

2004046571

To purchase additional copies of this book, call our customer service department at **(800) 638-3030** or fax orders to **(301) 824-7390**. International customers should call **(301) 714-2324.**

Visit Lippincott Williams & Wilkins on the Internet: http://www.LWW.com. Lippincott Williams & Wilkins customer service representatives are available from 8:30 am to 6:00 pm, EST.

05 06 07 08 09
1 2 3 4 5 6 7 8 9 10

Dedication

We dedicate this edition to two coauthors of the original book, entitled *Basic Medical Biochemistry: A Clinical Approach*: Dr. Dawn Marks and Dr. Colleen Smith. Their vision, their unflagging enthusiasm, and their ability to simplify the complex were recognized repeatedly throughout their careers with the awarding of the highest accolades for excellence in teaching offered by the University and by the School of Medicine at their respective institutions. These qualities and their strong conviction that one learns and retains medically related information more effectively when it is reinforced with clinical correlation were the principle forces that drove the design and purpose of the first edition.

Their untimely deaths (Dawn in 2000 and Colleen in 2002) cut short their work on revising the book. Yet their hopes and plans for this second edition were our hopes and plans as well. We have attempted to remain true to their vision and, in so doing, to honor their memory.

Allan D. Marks, MD
Michael A. Lieberman, PhD

Preface to the Second Edition

Marks' Basic Medical Biochemistry: A Clinical Approach, second edition, is intended to cover human biochemistry in a comprehensive fashion but without excessive detail. The aim of the book is to help students learn to use biochemistry in the process of clinical problem solving. The text not only provides students with a comprehensive, cohesive base of information; it also encourages students to use the basic information within a clinical context.

The clinical material is presented in the form of "patients." These patients are composites of the patients seen by one of the authors (Allan D. Marks, MD) in his internal medicine practice. The patients have names intended to serve as mnemonics that help students remember the case histories. As the chapters evolve, the patients appear and reappear as their problems are examined in light of the biochemical concepts covered in the text. Many of the patients are seen repeatedly throughout the book with exacerbations or new facets of their original problem or with totally unrelated problems that require medical attention. The patients are people with personalities and quirks that must be considered in their treatment. Some patients comply with their treatment plan, and some do not. Some are cured, some get progressively worse despite appropriate treatment, and, as in real life, some die.

NEW TO THIS EDITION

There has been a long lag between the first and second editions (8 years). This is due, in part, to the deaths of two authors from the first edition, Dawn Marks and Colleen Smith. In honor of Dawn Marks' vision for the first edition of this book, as well as her notes concerning the second edition, the book has been renamed *Marks' Basic Medical Biochemistry: A Clinical Approach.*

The goal in revising the book was to retain the straightforward nature of the biochemistry and to continue to integrate medical applications. A major change made in the second edition is the complete overhaul of the end-of- chapter questions: they now more resemble USMLE-type questions, and complete explanations for all questions are available. Another significant change is the inclusion of a "Tissue" section at the end of the book that deals with the application of biochemistry to the physiology of different organs and tissues. The inclusion of this new section has necessitated a restructuring of earlier chapters so that tissue-specific biochemistry could be discussed in this last section of the book. The specific changes that have been made in the book's organization and content are as follows:

1. All chapters have been updated, where necessary.
2. A new electronic product, available on a CD-ROM included in the back of the book, provides animations of key biochemical processes, additional USMLE-formatted review questions, web links, and "medical files" on each of the patients presented in the book.
3. Nucleotide metabolism has been given its own chapter (Chapter 41), because of its importance in understanding various types of drugs that interfere with DNA synthesis
4. The section on Molecular Endocrinology (Chapters 43–47, first edition) has been eliminated, as it overlaps considerably with what is taught in many medical

school physiology courses. The material that remains has been assigned to other chapters (i.e., the biosynthesis of steroid hormones has been moved to Chapter 34 [the chapter on cholesterol metabolism]; the mechanism of action of steroid hormones is presented in Chapter 11 [the chapter on biochemistry and cell biology]; and the mechanism of action of hormones, other than insulin and glucagon, which regulate fuel metabolism, is presented in Chapter 43).

5. A new chapter has been added concerning ethanol metabolism (Chapter 25).

6. Chapters 5 and 6 from the first edition (relationship of organic chemistry to biochemistry, and structures of the major compounds of the body) have been combined (both topics are covered in Chapter 5 of the second edition).

7. Chapter 9 of the first edition, entitled Enzymes, has been split into two chapters in the second edition (Chapter 8, enzymes as catalysts, and Chapter 9, regulation of enzymes).

8. Chapter 24 of the first edition (basic concepts in the regulation of fuel metabolism by insulin, glucagon, and other hormones) has its material split between Chapter 11 of the second edition (cell signaling by chemicals), and Chapter 26 (regulation of fuel metabolism by insulin and glucagon).

9. Material from first edition Chapters 28 and 29 (pentose phosphate pathway and pathways for the interconversion of sugars) have been combined, with material relating to red blood cells being moved to Chapter 44 in the new tissue section.

10. Chapter 30 of the second edition does not contain information concerning proteoglycans, which has been moved to the connective tissue section, Chapter 49.

11. Chapter 31 of the second edition, gluconeogenesis and maintenance of blood glucose during fasting, contains material from both Chapters 27 and 31 from the first edition.

12. The tissue section contains chapters on hormones that regulate fuel metabolism (Chapter 43), the components of blood (Chapter 44), the reactions of blood (Chapter 45), liver metabolism (Chapter 46), muscle metabolism (Chapter 47), nervous system metabolism (Chapter 48), and connective tissue metabolism (Chapter 49). Material from the first edition, which has now been moved to the tissue section, includes heme biosynthesis and oxygen binding to hemoglobin (Chapter 44), the blood coagulation cascade (Chapter 45), proteoglycan metabolism (Chapter 49), collagen biosynthesis (Chapter 49), and neurotransmitter biosynthesis (Chapter 48). New material in this section includes xenobiotic metabolism (Chapter 46), blood cell differentiation (Chapter 44), regulation of energy use by the muscle (Chapter 47), and a more detailed explanation of connective tissue proteins (Chapter 49).

HOW TO USE THIS BOOK

Icons identify the various components of the book: the patients who are presented at the start of each chapter; the clinical notes, biochemical notes, questions, and answers that appear in the margins; and the clinical and biochemical comments that are found at the end of each chapter.

Each chapter starts with an abstract that summarizes the information so that students can recognize the key words and concepts they are expected to learn. The next component of each chapter is the "Waiting Room" containing patients with complaints and a description of the events that led them to seek medical help.

 indicates a female patient

indicates a male patient

 indicates a patient who is a baby or young child

As each chapter unfolds, icons appear in the margin, identifying information related to the material presented in the text:

 indicates a clinical note, usually related to the patients in the waiting room for that chapter. These notes explain signs or symptoms of a patient or give some other clinical information relevant to the text.

 indicates a book note, which elaborates on some aspect of the basic biochemistry presented in the text. These notes provide tidbits, pearls, or just reemphasize a major point of the text.

Questions and answers also appear in the margin and should help to keep students thinking as they read the text:

 indicates a question

 indicates the answer to the question. The answer to a question is always located on the next page. If two questions appear on one page, the answers are given in order on the next page.

Each chapter ends with "Clinical Comments" and "Biochemical Comments":

 indicates clinical comments that give additional clinical information, often describing the treatment plan and the outcome

 indicates biochemical comments that add biochemical information not covered in the text or that explore some facet of biochemistry in more detail or from another angle

"Suggested References" are listed at the end of the chapter for students who would like to pursue a particular topic in more depth. We have added comments about the references to help steer readers to those that would be most helpful for their particular purpose or interest.

Finally, "Review Questions" are presented. These questions are written in a USMLE-like format, and many of them take a clinical slant. Answers to the review questions, along with detailed explanations, are provided in an appendix.

ACKNOWLEDGMENTS

The authors would like to thank Dr. Wayne Glasgow for the initial draft of Chapter 35; Dr. Kris Detmer for the initial drafts of Chapters 44 and 45; Dr. Bruce Giffin for substantially revising and improving Chapters 47 and 48; and Dr. Winston Kao for his help with Chapter 49. In addition, the authors would like to acknowledge Dr. Anna Walker, who read preliminary drafts of Chapters 44 and 45; Angela Thompson, who proofread many of the early chapters for Dr. Smith; and Cullen Scott, a medical student who did library research for the second edition. We would also like to thank all of the reviewers who worked hard to review the chapters and who made excellent suggestions for revisions. Matt Chansky, the illustrator, deserves a tremendous amount of credit for interpreting our stick drawings and creating the excellent illustrations in the text. Matt also used his extraordinary talents to create the animations available on the CD. Kathleen Scogna, the developmental editor, displayed immense patience with the authors, and she also deserves much praise.

Any errors in the text are the authors' responsibility, and Dr. Lieberman would appreciate being informed of such errors. And finally, Dr. Lieberman would like to thank the past 20 years of first-year medical students at the University Of Cincinnati College of Medicine, who have put up with his various attempts at teaching biochemistry, while always keeping in the back of his mind "how is this relevant to medicine"? The comments these students have made have greatly influenced the manner in which he teaches this material.

Table of Contents

Fuel Metabolism

I n order to survive, humans must meet two basic metabolic requirements: we must be able to synthesize everything our cells need that is not supplied by our diet, and we must be able to protect our internal environment from toxins and changing conditions in our external environment. In order to meet these requirements, we metabolize our dietary components through four basic types of pathways: fuel oxidative pathways, fuel storage and mobilization pathways, biosynthetic pathways, and detoxification or waste disposal pathways. Cooperation between tissues and responses to changes in our external environment are communicated though transport pathways and intercellular signaling pathways (Fig. I.1).

The foods in our diet are the fuels that supply us with energy in the form of calories. This energy is used for carrying out diverse functions such as moving, thinking, and reproducing. Thus, a number of our metabolic pathways are *fuel oxidative pathways* that convert fuels into energy that can be used for biosynthetic and mechanical work. But what is the source of energy when we are not eating— between meals, and while we sleep? How does the hunger striker in the morning headlines survive so long? We have other metabolic pathways that are *fuel storage pathways*. The fuels that we store can be molibized during periods when we are not eating or when we need increased energy for exercise.

Our diet also must contain the compounds we cannot synthesize, as well as all the basic building blocks for compounds we do synthesize in our *biosynthetic pathways*. For example we have dietary requirements for some amino acids, but we can synthesize other amino acids from our fuels and a dietary nitrogen precursor. The compounds required in our diet for biosynthetic pathways include certain amino acids, vitamins, and essential fatty acids.

Detoxification pathways and *waste disposal pathways* are metabolic pathways devoted to removing toxins that can be present in our diets or in the air we breathe, introduced into our bodies as drugs, or generated internally from the metabolism of dietary components. Dietary components that have no value to the body, and must be disposed of, are called xenobiotics.

In general, biosynthetic pathways (including fuel storage) are referred to as *anabolic pathways,* that is, pathways that synthesize larger molecules from smaller components. The synthesis of proteins from amino acids is an example of an anabolic pathway. *Catabolic* pathways are those pathways that break down larger molecules into smaller components. Fuel oxidative pathways are examples of catabolic pathways.

In the human, the need for different cells to carry out different functions has resulted in cell and tissue specialization in metabolism. For example, our adipose tissue is a specialized site for the storage of fat and contains the metabolic pathways that allow it to carry out this function. However, adipose tissue is lacking many of the pathways that synthesize required compounds from dietary precursors. To enable our cells to cooperate in meeting our metabolic needs during changing conditions of diet, sleep, activity, and health, we need *transport pathways* into the blood and between tissues and *intercellular signaling pathways*. One means of communication is for *hormones* to carry signals to tissues about our dietary state. For example, a message that we have just had a meal, carried by the hormone insulin, signals adipose tissue to store fat.

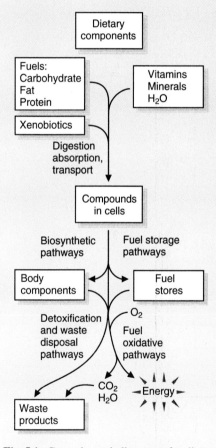

Fig. I.1. General metabolic routes for dietary components in the body. The types of Pathways are named in blue.

1

In the following section, we will provide an overview of various types of dietary components and examples of the pathways involved in utilizing these components. We will describe the fuels in our diet, the compounds produced by their digestion, and the basic patterns of fuel metabolism in the tissues of our bodies. We will describe how these patterns change when we eat, when we fast for a short time, and when we starve for prolonged periods. Patients with medical problems that involve an inability to deal normally with fuels will be introduced. These patients will appear repeatedly throughout the book and will be joined by other patients as we delve deeper into biochemistry.

1 Metabolic Fuels and Dietary Components

*Fuel Metabolism. We obtain our fuel primarily from **carbohydrates, fats**, and **proteins** in our diet. As we eat, our foodstuffs are **digested** and **absorbed**. The products of digestion circulate in the blood, enter various tissues, and are eventually taken up by cells and **oxidized** to produce **energy**. To completely convert our fuels to carbon dioxide (CO_2) and water (H_2O), molecular **oxygen** (O_2) is required. We breathe to obtain this oxygen and to eliminate the **carbon dioxide** (CO_2) that is produced by the oxidation of our foodstuffs.*

*Fuel Stores. Any dietary fuel that exceeds the body's immediate energy needs is stored, mainly as **triacylglycerol** (fat) in adipose tissue, as **glycogen** (a carbohydrate) in muscle, liver, and other cells, and, to some extent, as **protein** in muscle. When we are fasting, between meals and overnight while we sleep, fuel is drawn from these stores and is oxidized to provide energy (Fig. 1.1).*

*Fuel Requirements. We require enough energy each day to drive the **basic functions** of our bodies and to support our **physical activity**. If we do not consume enough food each day to supply that much energy, the body's fuel stores supply the remainder, and we lose weight. Conversely, if we consume more food than required for the energy we expend, our body's fuel stores enlarge, and we gain weight.*

*Other Dietary Requirements. In addition to providing energy, the diet provides **precursors** for the **biosynthesis** of compounds necessary for cellular and tissue structure, function, and survival. Among these precursors are the **essential fatty acids** and essential **amino acids** (those that the body needs but cannot synthesize). The diet must also supply **vitamins**, **minerals**, and **water**.*

*Waste Disposal. Dietary components that we can utilize are referred to as nutrients. However, both the diet and the air we breathe contain **xenobiotic compounds**, compounds that have no use or value in the human body and may be toxic. These compounds are excreted in the urine and feces together with metabolic waste products.*

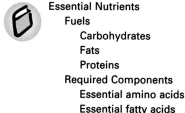

Essential Nutrients
    Fuels
        Carbohydrates
        Fats
        Proteins
    Required Components
        Essential amino acids
        Essential fatty acids
        Vitamins
        Minerals
        Water

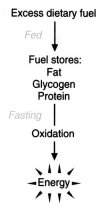

Excess dietary fuel

Fed ↓

Fuel stores:
Fat
Glycogen
Protein

Fasting ↓

Oxidation

↓

←Energy→

Fig. 1.1. Fate of excess dietary fuel in fed and fasting states.

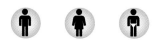

Percy Veere is a 59-year-old school teacher who was in good health until his wife died suddenly. Since that time, he has experienced an increasing degree of fatigue and has lost interest in many of the activities he previously enjoyed. Shortly after his wife's death, one of his married children moved far from home. Since then, Mr. Veere has had little appetite for food. When a

Percy Veere has a strong will. He is enduring a severe reactive depression after the loss of his wife. In addition, he must put up with the sometimes life-threatening antics of his hyperactive grandson, Dennis (the Menace) Veere. Yet through all of this, he will "persevere."

3

neighbor found Mr. Veere sleeping in his clothes, unkempt, and somewhat confused, she called an ambulance. Mr. Veere was admitted to the hospital psychiatry unit with a diagnosis of mental depression associated with dehydration and malnutrition.

Otto Shape is a 25-year-old medical student who was very athletic during high school and college, and is now "out-of-shape." Since he started medical school, he has been gaining weight (at 5 feet 10 inches tall, he currently weighs 187 lb). He has decided to consult a physician at the student health service before the problem gets worse.

Ivan Applebod is a 56-year-old accountant who has been morbidly obese for a number of years. He exhibits a pattern of central obesity, called an "apple shape," which is caused by excess adipose tissue deposited in the abdominal area. His major recreational activities are watching TV while drinking scotch and soda and doing occasional gardening. At a company picnic, he became very "winded" while playing baseball and decided it was time for a general physical examination. At the examination, he weighed 264 lb at 5 feet 10 inches tall. His blood pressure was slightly elevated, 155 mm Hg systolic (normal = 140 mm Hg or less) and 95 mm Hg diastolic (normal = 90 mm Hg or less).

Ann O'Rexia is a 23-year-old buyer for a woman's clothing store. Despite the fact that she is 5 feet 7 inches tall and weighs 99 lb, she is convinced she is overweight. Two months ago, she started a daily exercise program that consists of 1 hour of jogging every morning and 1 hour of walking every evening. She also decided to consult a physician about a weight reduction diet.

I. DIETARY FUELS

The major fuels we obtain from our diet are carbohydrates, proteins, and fats. When these fuels are oxidized to CO_2 and H_2O in our cells, energy is released by the transfer of electrons to O_2. The energy from this oxidation process generates heat and adenosine triphosphate (ATP) (Fig 1.2). Carbon dioxide travels in the blood to the lungs, where it is expired, and water is excreted in urine, sweat, and other secretions. Although the heat that is generated by fuel oxidation is used to maintain body temperature, the main purpose of fuel oxidation is to generate ATP. ATP provides the energy that drives most of the energy-consuming processes in the cell, including biosynthetic reactions, muscle contraction, and active transport across membranes. As these processes use energy, ATP is converted back to adenosine diphosphate (ADP) and inorganic phosphate (P_i). The generation and utilization of ATP is referred to as the ATP–ADP cycle.

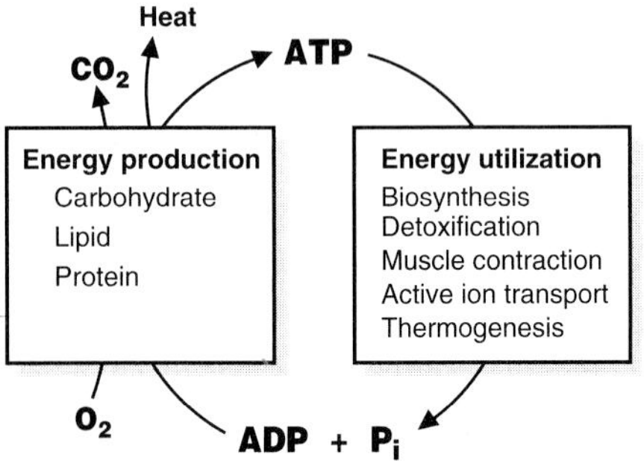

The oxidation of fuels to generate ATP is called respiration (Fig. 1.3). Before oxidation, carbohydrates are converted principally to glucose, fat to fatty acids, and protein to amino acids. The pathways for oxidizing glucose, fatty acids, and amino acids have many features in common. They first oxidize the fuels to acetyl CoA, a precursor of the tricarboxylic acid (TCA) cycle. The TCA cycle is a series of reactions that completes the oxidation of fuels to CO_2 (see Chapter 19). Electrons lost from the fuels during oxidative reactions are transferred to O_2 by a series of proteins in the electron transport chain (see Chapter 20). The energy of electron transfer is used to convert ADP and P_i to ATP by a process known as oxidative phosphorylation.

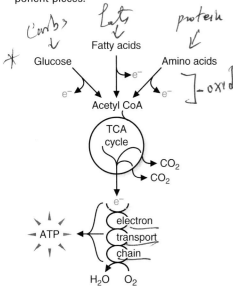

Fig. 1.2. The ATP–ADP cycle.

Oxidative pathways are catabolic; that is, they break molecules down. In contrast, anabolic pathways build molecules up from component pieces.

Fig. 1.3. Generation of ATP from fuel components during respiration. Glucose, fatty acids, and amino acids are oxidized to acetyl CoA, a substrate for the TCA cycle. In the TCA cycle, they are completely oxidized to CO_2. As fuels are oxidized, electrons (e^-) are transferred to O_2 by the electron transport chain, and the energy is used to generate ATP.

In discussions of metabolism and nutrition, energy is often expressed in units of calories. "Calorie" in this context really means kilocalorie (kcal). Energy is also expressed in joules. One kilocalorie equals 4.18 kilojoules (kJ). Physicians tend to use units of calories, in part because that is what their patients use and understand.

A. Carbohydrates

The major carbohydrates in the human diet are starch, sucrose, lactose, fructose, and glucose. The polysaccharide starch is the storage form of carbohydrates in plants. Sucrose (table sugar) and lactose (milk sugar) are disaccharides, and fructose and glucose are monosaccharides. Digestion converts the larger carbohydrates to monosaccharides, which can be absorbed into the bloodstream. Glucose, a monosaccharide, is the predominant sugar in human blood (Fig. 1.4).

Oxidation of carbohydrates to CO_2 and H_2O in the body produces approximately 4 kcal/g (Table 1.1). In other words, every gram of carbohydrate we eat yields approximately 4 kcal of energy. Note that carbohydrate molecules contain a significant amount of oxygen and are already partially oxidized before they enter our bodies (see Fig. 1.4).

B. Proteins

Proteins are composed of amino acids that are joined to form linear chains (Fig. 1.5). In addition to carbon, hydrogen, and oxygen, proteins contain approximately 16% nitrogen by weight. The digestive process breaks down proteins to their constituent amino acids, which enter the blood. The complete oxidation of proteins to CO_2, H_2O, and NH_4^+ in the body yields approximately 4 kcal/g.

C. Fats

Fats are lipids composed of triacylglycerols (also called triglycerides). A triacylglycerol molecule contains 3 fatty acids esterified to one glycerol moiety (Fig. 1.6).

Fats contain much less oxygen than is contained in carbohydrates or proteins. Therefore, fats are more reduced and yield more energy when oxidized. The complete oxidation of triacylglycerols to CO_2 and H_2O in the body releases approximately 9 kcal/g, more than twice the energy yield from an equivalent amount of carbohydrate or protein.

The food "calories" used in everyday speech are really "Calories," which = kilocalories. "Calorie," meaning kilocalorie, was originally spelled with a capital C, but the capitalization was dropped as the term became popular. Thus, a 1-calorie soft drink actually has 1 Cal (1 kcal) of energy.

Table 1.1. Caloric Content of Fuels

	kcal/g
Carbohydrate	4
Fat	9
Protein	4
Alcohol	7

Q: An analysis of **Ann O'Rexia's** diet showed she ate 100 g carbohydrate, 20 g protein, and 15 g fat each day. Approximately how many calories did she consume per day?

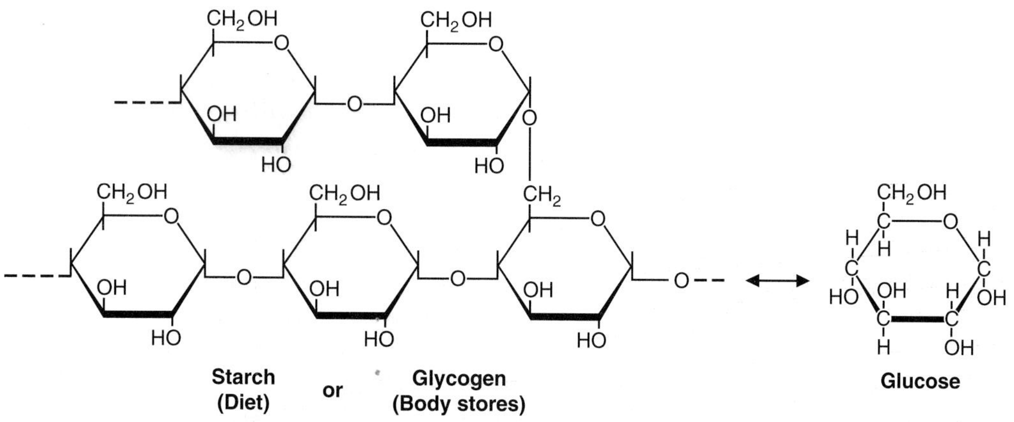

Starch   or   **Glycogen**
(Diet)   **(Body stores)**

Glucose

Fig. 1.4. Structure of starch and glycogen. Starch, our major dietary carbohydrate, and glycogen, the body's storage form of glucose, have similar structures. They are polysaccharides (many sugar units) composed of glucose, which is a monosaccharide (one sugar unit). Dietary disaccharides are composed of two sugar units.

Miss O'Rexia consumed

$100 \times 4 = 400$ kcal as carbohydrate
$20 \times 4 = 80$ kcal as protein
$15 \times 9 = 135$ kcal as fat

for a total of 615 kcal/day.

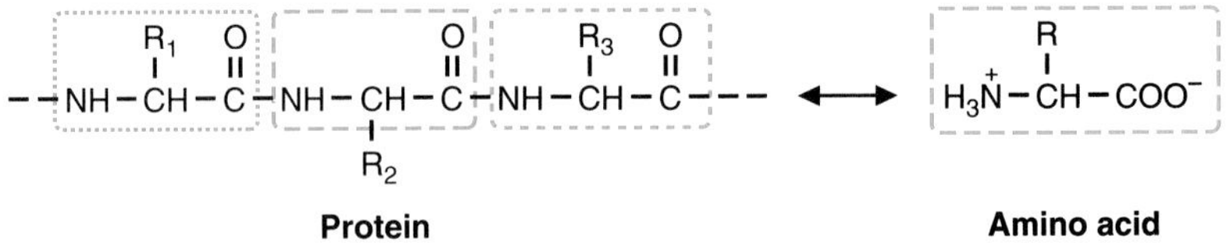

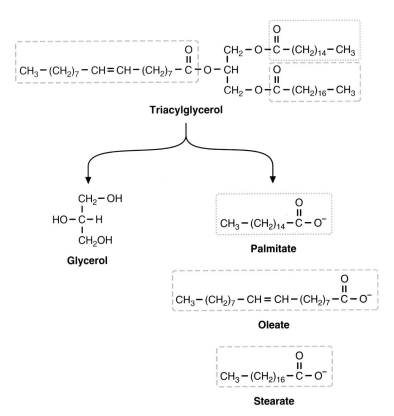

Fig. 1.5. General structure of proteins and amino acids. R = side chain. Different amino acids have different side chains. For example, R_1 might be $-CH_3$; R_2, ⊚ ; R_3, $-CH_2-COO^-$.

Fig. 1.6. Structure of a triacylglycerol. Palmitate and stearate are saturated fatty acids, i.e., they have no double bonds. Oleate is monounsaturated (one double bond). Polyunsaturated fatty acids have more than one double bond.

Ivan Applebod ate 585 g carbohydrate, 150 g protein, and 95 g fat each day. In addition, he drank 45 g alcohol. How many calories did he consume per day?

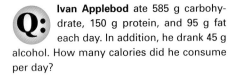

It is not surprising that our body fuel stores consist of the same kinds of compounds found in our diet, because the plants and animals we eat also store fuels in the form of starch or glycogen, triacylglycerols, and proteins.

D. Alcohol

Many people used to believe that alcohol (ethanol, in the context of the diet) has no caloric content. In fact, ethanol (CH_3CH_2OH) is oxidized to CO_2 and H_2O in the body and yields approximately 7 kcal/g—that is, more than carbohydrate but less than fat.

II. BODY FUEL STORES

Although some of us may try, it is virtually impossible to eat constantly. Fortunately, we carry supplies of fuel within our bodies (Fig. 1.7). These fuel stores are light in weight, large in quantity, and readily converted into oxidizable substances. Most of us are familiar with fat, our major fuel store, which is located in adipose tissue. Although fat is distributed throughout our bodies, it tends to increase in quantity in our hips and thighs and in our abdomens as we advance into middle age. In addition to our fat stores, we also have important, although much smaller, stores of carbohydrate in the form of glycogen located primarily in our liver and muscles. Glycogen

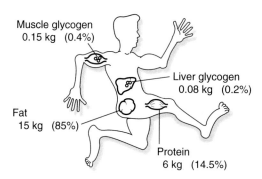

Muscle glycogen
0.15 kg (0.4%)

Liver glycogen
0.08 kg (0.2%)

Fat
15 kg (85%)

Protein
6 kg (14.5%)

Fig. 1.7. Fuel composition of the average 70-kg man after an overnight fast (in kilograms and as percentage of total stored calories).

Mr. Applebod consumed
$585 \times 4 = 2,340$ kcal as carbohydrate
$150 \times 4 = 600$ kcal as protein
$95 \times 9 = 855$ kcal as fat
$45 \times 7 = 315$ kcal as alcohol

for a total of 4,110 kcal/day.

consists of glucose residues joined together to form a large, branched polysaccharide (see Fig. 1.4). Body protein, particularly the protein of our large muscle masses, also serves to some extent as a fuel store, and we draw on it for energy when we fast.

A. Fat

Our major fuel store is adipose triacylglycerol (triglyceride), a lipid more commonly known as fat. The average 70-kg man has approximately 15 kg stored triacylglycerol, which accounts for approximately 85% of his total stored calories (see Fig. 1.7).

Two characteristics make adipose triacylglycerol a very efficient fuel store: the fact that triacylglycerol contains more calories per gram than carbohydrate or protein (9 kcal/g versus 4 kcal/g) and the fact that adipose tissue does not contain much water. Adipose tissue contains only about 15% water, compared to tissues such as muscle that contain about 80%. Thus, the 70-kg man with 15 kg stored triacylglycerol has only about 18 kg adipose tissue.

B. Glycogen

Our stores of glycogen in liver, muscle, and other cells are relatively small in quantity but are nevertheless important. Liver glycogen is used to maintain blood glucose levels between meals. Thus, the size of this glycogen store fluctuates during the day; an average 70-kg man might have 200 g or more of liver glycogen after a meal but only 80 g after an overnight fast. Muscle glycogen supplies energy for muscle contraction during exercise. At rest, the 70-kg man has approximately 150 g of muscle glycogen. Almost all cells, including neurons, maintain a small emergency supply of glucose as glycogen.

C. Protein

Protein serves many important roles in the body; unlike fat and glycogen, it is not solely a fuel store. Muscle protein is essential for body movement. Other proteins serve as enzymes (catalysts of biochemical reactions) or as structural components of cells and tissues. Only a limited amount of body protein can be degraded, approximately 6 kg in the average 70-kg man, before our body functions are compromised.

III. DAILY ENERGY EXPENDITURE

If we want to stay in energy balance, neither gaining nor losing weight, we must, on average, consume an amount of food equal to our daily energy expenditure. The daily energy expenditure (DEE) includes the energy to support our basal metabolism (basal metabolic rate or resting metabolic rate) and our physical activity, plus the energy required to process the food we eat (diet-induced thermogenesis).

In biochemistry and nutrition, the standard reference is often the 70-kg (154-lb) man. This standard probably was chosen because in the first half of the 20th century, when many nutritional studies were performed, young healthy medical and graduate students (who were mostly men) volunteered to serve as subjects for these experiments.

What would happen to a 70-kg man if the 135,000 kcal stored as triacylglycerols in his 18 kg of adipose tissue were stored instead as skeletal muscle glycogen? It would take approximately 34 kg glycogen to store as many calories. Glycogen, because it is a polar molecule with –OH groups, binds approximately 4 times its weight in water, or 136 kg. Thus, his fuel stores would weigh 170 kg.

Daily energy expenditure =
RMR + Physical Activity + DIT
where RMR is the resting metabolic rate and DIT is diet-induced thermogenesis. BMR (basal metabolic rate) is used interchangeably with RMR in this equation.

A. Resting Metabolic Rate

The resting metabolic rate (RMR) is a measure of the energy required to maintain life: the functioning of the lungs, kidneys and brain, the pumping of the heart, the maintenance of ionic gradients across membranes, the reactions of biochemical pathways, and so forth. Another term used to describe basal metabolism is the basal metabolic rate (BMR). The BMR was originally defined as the energy expenditure of a person mentally and bodily at rest in a thermoneutral environment 12 to 18 hours after a meal. However, when a person is awakened and their heat production or oxygen consumption is measured, they are no longer sleeping or totally at mental rest, and their metabolic rate is called the resting metabolic rate (RMR). It is also sometimes called the resting energy expenditure (REE). The RMR and BMR differ very little in value.

The BMR, which is usually expressed in kcal/day, is affected by body size, age, sex, and other factors (Table 1.2). It is proportional to the amount of metabolically active tissue (including the major organs) and to the lean (or fat-free) body mass. Obviously, the amount of energy required for basal functions in a large person is greater than the amount required in a small person. However, the BMR is usually lower for women than for men of the same weight because women usually have more metabolically inactive adipose tissue. Body temperature also affects the BMR, which increases by 12% with each degree centigrade increase in body temperature (i.e., "feed a fever; starve a cold"). The ambient temperature affects the BMR, which increases slightly in colder climates as thermogenesis is activated. Excessive secretion of thyroid hormone (hyperthyroidism) causes the BMR to increase, whereas diminished secretion (hypothyroidism) causes it to decrease. The BMR increases during pregnancy and lactation. Growing children have a higher BMR per kilogram body weight than adults, because a greater proportion of their bodies is composed of brain, muscle, and other more metabolically active tissues. The BMR declines in aging individuals because their metabolically active tissue is shrinking and body fat is increasing. In addition, large variations exist in BMR from one adult to another, determined by genetic factors.

A rough estimate of the BMR may be obtained by assuming it is 24 kcal/day/kg body weight and multiplying by the body weight. An easy way to remember this is 1 kcal/kg/hr. This estimate works best for young individuals who are near their ideal weight. More accurate methods for calculating the BMR use empirically derived equations for different gender and age groups (Table 1.3). Even these calculations do not take into account variation among individuals.

B. Physical Activity

In addition to the RMR, the energy required for physical activity contributes to the DEE. The difference in physical activity between a student and a lumberjack is enormous, and a student who is relatively sedentary during the week may be much

Table 1.2. Factors Affecting BMR Expressed per kg Body Weight

Gender (males higher than females)
Body temperature (increased with fever)
Environmental temperature (increased in cold)
Thyroid status (increased in hyperthyroidism)
Pregnancy and lactation (increased)
Age (decreases with age)

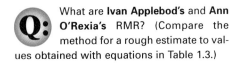

Q: What are **Ivan Applebod's** and **Ann O'Rexia's** RMR? (Compare the method for a rough estimate to values obtained with equations in Table 1.3.)

Registered dieticians use extensive tables for calculating energy requirements, based on height, weight, age, and activity level. A more accurate calculation is based on the fat-free mass (FFM), which is equal to the total body mass minus the mass of the person's adipose tissue. With FFM, the BMR is calculated using the equation $BMR = 186 + FFM \times 23.6$ kcal/kg per day. This formula eliminates differences between sexes and between aged versus young individuals that are attributable to differences in relative adiposity. However, determining FFM is relatively cumbersome—it requires weighing the patient underwater and measuring the residual lung volume.

Indirect calorimetry, a technique that measures O_2 consumption and CO_2 production, can be used when more accurate determinations are required for hospitalized patients. A portable indirect calorimeter is used to measure oxygen consumption and the respiratory quotient (RQ), which is the ratio of O_2 consumed to CO_2 produced. The RQ is 1.00 for individuals oxidizing carbohydrates, 0.83 for protein, and 0.71 for fat. From these values, the daily energy expenditure (DEE) can be determined.

Table 1.3. Equation for Predicting BMR from Body Weight (W) in kg

Males		Females	
Age Range (years)	BMR kcal/day	Age Range (years)	BMR kcal/day
0–3	60.9W − 54	0–3	61.0W − 51
3–10	22.7W + 495	3–10	22.5W + 499
10–18	17.5W + 651	10–18	12.2W + 746
18–30	15.3W + 679	18–30	14.7W + 496
30–60	11.6W + 879	30–60	8.7W + 829
>60	13.5W + 487	>60	10.5W + 596

From Energy and protein requirements: report of a Joint FAO/WHO/UNU Expert Consultation. Technical report series no. 724. Geneva World Health Organization, 1987;71. See also Schofield et al. Hum Nutr Clin Nutr 1985;39 (suppl).

Table 1.4. Typical Activities with Corresponding Hourly Activity Factors

ACTIVITY CATEGORY	Hourly Activity Factor (for Time in Activity)
Resting: sleeping, reclining	1.0
Very light: seated and standing activities, driving, laboratory work, typing, sewing, ironing, cooking, playing cards, playing a musical instrument	1.5
Light: walking on a level surface at 2.5–3 mph, garage work, electrical trades, carpentry, restaurant trades, house cleaning, golf, sailing, table tennis	2.5
Moderate: walking 3.5–4 mph, weeding and hoeing, carrying loads, cycling, skiing, tennis, dancing	5.0
Heavy: walking uphill with a load, tree felling, heavy manual digging, mountain climbing, basketball, football, soccer	7.0

Reprinted with permission from Recommended Dietary Allowances, 10th Ed. Washington, DC: National Academy Press, 1989.

The hourly activity factor is multiplied by the BMR (RMR) per hour times the number of hours engaged in the activity to give the caloric expenditure for that activity. If this is done for all of the hours in a day, the sum over 24 hours will approximately equal the daily energy expenditure.

Mr. **Applebod** weighs 264 lb or 120 kg (264 lb divided by 2.2 lb/kg). His estimated RMR = 24 kcal/kg/day × 120 = 2,880 kcal/day. His RMR calculated from Table 1.3 is only 2,271 kcal (11.6 W + 879 = (11.6 × 120) + 879). **Miss O'Rexia** weighs 99 lb or 45 kg (99/2.2 lb/kg). Her estimated RMR = (24 kcal/kg/day) × (45 kg) = 1,080 kcal/day. Her RMR from Table 1.3 is very close to this value (14.7 W + 496 = 1,157 kcal/day). Thus, the rough estimate does not work well for obese patients because a disproportionately larger proportion of their body weight is metabolically inactive adipose tissue.

more active during the weekend. Table 1.4 gives factors for calculating the approximate energy expenditures associated with typical activities.

A rough estimate of the energy required per day for physical activity can be made by using a value of 30% of the RMR (per day) for a very sedentary person (such as a medical student who does little but study) and a value of 60 to 70% of the RMR (per day) for a person who engages in about 2 hours of moderate exercise per day (see Table 1.4). A value of 100% or more of the RMR is used for a person who does several hours of heavy exercise per day.

Based on the activities listed in Table 1.4, the average U.S. citizen is rather sedentary. Sedentary habits correlate strongly with risk for cardiovascular disease, so it is not surprising that cardiovascular disease is the major cause of death in this country.

C. Diet-Induced Thermogenesis

Our DEE includes a component related to the intake of food known as diet-induced thermogenesis (DIT) or the thermic effect of food (TEF). DIT was formerly called the specific dynamic action (SDA). After the ingestion of food, our metabolic rate increases because energy is required to digest, absorb, distribute, and store nutrients.

The energy required to process the types and quantities of food in the typical American diet is probably equal to approximately 10% of the kilocalories ingested. This amount is roughly equivalent to the error involved in rounding off the caloric content of carbohydrate, fat, and protein to 4, 9, and 4, respectively. Therefore, DIT is often ignored and calculations are based simply on the RMR and the energy required for physical activity.

D. Calculations of Daily Energy Expenditure

The total daily energy expenditure is usually calculated as the sum of the RMR (in kcal/day) plus the energy required for the amount of time spent in each of the various types of physical activity (see Table 1.4). An approximate value for the daily energy expenditure can be determined from the RMR and the appropriate percentage of the RMR required for physical activity (given above). For example, a very sedentary medical student would have a DEE equal to the RMR plus 30% of the RMR (or 1.3 × RMR) and an active person's daily expenditure could be 2 times the RMR.

E. Healthy Body Weight

Ideally, we should strive to maintain a weight consistent with good health. Overweight people are frequently defined as more than 20% above their ideal weight. But what is the ideal weight? The body mass index (BMI), calculated as

What are reasonable estimates for **Ivan Applebod's** and **Ann O'Rexia's** daily energy expenditure?

BMI equals:

Weight/height^2 (kg/m^2)

or

$$\frac{\text{Weight (lbs)} \times 704}{\text{height}^2 \text{ (in}^2)}$$

Where the height is measured without shoes and the weight is measured with minimal clothing.
BMI values of:

$$18.5 - 24.9 = \text{desirable}$$
$$<18.5 = \text{underweight}$$
$$25 - 29.9 = \text{overweight}$$
$$\geq 30 = \text{obese}$$

Q: Are **Ivan Applebod** and **Ann O'Rexia** in a healthy weight range?

A: Mr. **Applebod's** BMR is 2,271 kcal/day. He is sedentary, so he only requires approximately 30% more calories for his physical activity. Therefore, his daily expenditure is approximately 2,271 + (0.3 × 2,271) or 1.3 × 2,271 or 2,952 kcal/day. **Miss O'Rexia's** BMR is 1,157 kcal/day. She performs 2 hours of moderate exercise per day (jogging and walking), so she requires approximately 65% more calories for her physical activity. Therefore, her daily expenditure is approximately 1,157 + (0.65 × 1157) or 1.65 × 1,157 or 1,909 kcal/day.

weight/height^2 (kg/m^2), is currently the preferred method for determining whether a person's weight is in the healthy range.

In general, adults with BMI values below 18.5 are considered underweight. Those with BMIs between 18.5 and 24.9 are considered to be in the healthy weight range, between 25 and 29.9 are in the overweight or preobese range, and above 30 are in the obese range.

F. Weight Gain and Loss

To maintain our body weight, we must stay in caloric balance. We are in caloric balance if the kilocalories in the food we eat equal our DEE. If we eat less food than we require for our DEE, our body fuel stores supply the additional calories,

To evaluate a patient's weight, physicians need standards of obesity applicable in a genetically heterogeneous population. Life insurance industry statistics have been used to develop tables giving the weight ranges, based on gender, height, and body frame size, that are associated with the greatest longevity, such as the Metropolitan Height and Weight Tables. However, these tables are considered inadequate for a number of reasons (e.g., they reflect data from upper-middle-class white groups). The BMI is the classification that is currently used clinically. It is based on two simple measurements, height without shoes and weight with minimal clothing. Patients can be shown their BMI in a nomogram and need not use calculations. The healthy weight range coincides with the mortality data derived from life insurance tables. The BMI also shows a good correlation with independent measures of body fat. The major weakness of the use of the BMI is that some very muscular individuals may be classified as obese when they are not. Other measurements to estimate body fat and other body compartments, such as weighing individuals underwater, are more difficult, expensive, and time consuming and have generally been confined to research purposes.

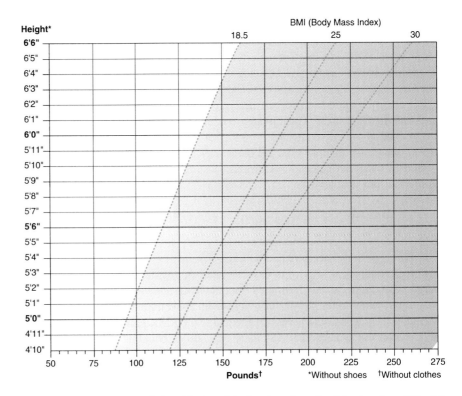

If patients are above or below ideal weight (such as **Ivan Applebod** or **Ann O'Rexia**), the physician, often in consultation with a registered dietician, prescribes a diet designed to bring the weight into the ideal range.

and we lose weight. Conversely, if we eat more food than we require for our energy needs, the excess fuel is stored (mainly in our adipose tissue), and we gain weight (Fig. 1.8).

When we draw on our adipose tissue to meet our energy needs, we lose approximately 1 lb whenever we expend approximately 3,500 calories more than we consume. In other words, if we eat 1,000 calories less than we expend per day, we will lose about 2 lb/week. Because the average individual's food intake is only about 2,000 to 3,000 calories/day, eating one-third to one-half the normal amount will cause a person to lose weight rather slowly. Fad diets that promise a loss of weight much more rapid than this have no scientific merit. In fact, the rapid initial weight loss the fad dieter typically experiences is attributable largely to loss of body water. This loss of water occurs in part because muscle tissue protein and liver glycogen are degraded rapidly to supply energy during the early phase of the diet. When muscle tissue (which is approximately 80% water) and glycogen (approximately 70% water) are broken down, this water is excreted from the body.

IV. DIETARY REQUIREMENTS

In addition to supplying us with fuel and with general-purpose building blocks for biosynthesis, our diet also provides us with specific nutrients that we need to remain healthy. We must have a regular supply of vitamins and minerals and of the essential fatty acids and essential amino acids. "Essential" means that they are essential in the diet; the body cannot synthesize these compounds from other molecules and therefore must obtain them from the diet. Nutrients that the body requires in the diet only under certain conditions are called "conditionally essential."

The Recommended Dietary Allowance (RDA) and the Adequate Intake (AI) provide quantitative estimates of nutrient requirements. The RDA for a nutrient is the average daily dietary intake level necessary to meet the requirement of nearly all (97–98%) healthy individuals in a particular gender and life stage group. Life stage group is a certain age range or physiologic status (i.e., pregnancy or lactation). The RDA is intended to serve as a goal for intake by individuals. The AI is a recommended intake value that is used when not enough data are available to establish an RDA.

A. Carbohydrates

No specific carbohydrates have been identified as dietary requirements. Carbohydrates can be synthesized from amino acids, and we can convert one type

 Malnutrition, the absence of an adequate intake of nutrients, occurs in the United States principally among children of families with incomes below the poverty level, the elderly, individuals whose diet is influenced by alcohol and drug usage, and those who make poor food choices. More than 13 million children in the United States live in families with incomes below the poverty level. Of these, approximately 10% have clinical malnutrition, most often anemia resulting from inadequate iron intake. A larger percentage have mild protein and energy malnutrition and exhibit growth retardation, sometimes as a result of parental neglect. Childhood malnutrition may also lead to learning failure and chronic illness later in life. A weight for age measurement is one of the best indicators of childhood malnourishment because it is easy to measure, and weight is one of the first parameters to change during malnutrition.

The term *kwashiorkor* refers to a disease originally seen in African children suffering from a protein deficiency. It is characterized by marked hypoalbuminemia, anemia, edema, pot belly, loss of hair, and other signs of tissue injury. The term *marasmus* is used for prolonged protein–calorie malnutrition, particularly in young children.

 Q: Are **Ivan Applebod** and **Ann O'Rexia** gaining or losing weight?

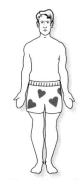
Positive caloric balance
Consumption > Expenditure

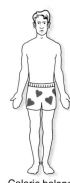
Caloric balance
Consumption = Expenditure

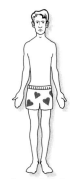
Negative caloric balance
Consumption < Expenditure

Fig. 1.8. Caloric balance.

A: **Ivan Applebod**'s weight is classified as obese. His BMI is 264 lb × 704/70 in² = 37.9. **Ann O'Rexia** is underweight. Her BMI is 99 lb × 704/67 in² = 15.5.

Mr. Applebod expends about 2,952 kcal/day and consumes 4,110. By this calculation, he consumes 1,158 more kcal than he expends each day and is gaining weight. **Miss O'Rexia** expends 1,909 kcal/day while she consumes only 615. Therefore, she expends 1,294 more kcal/day than she consumes, so she is losing weight.

of carbohydrate to another. However, health problems are associated with the complete elimination of carbohydrate from the diet, partly because a low-carbohydrate diet must contain higher amounts of fat to provide us with the energy we need. High-fat diets are associated with obesity, atherosclerosis, and other health problems.

B. Essential Fatty Acids

Although most lipids required for cell structure, fuel storage, or hormone synthesis can be synthesized from carbohydrates or proteins, we need a minimal level of certain dietary lipids for optimal health. These lipids, known as essential fatty acids, are required in our diet because we cannot synthesize fatty acids with these particular arrangements of double bonds. The essential fatty acids α-linoleic and α-linolenic acid are supplied by dietary plant oils, and eicosapentaenoic acid (EPA) and docosahexaenoic acid (DHA) are supplied in fish oils. They are the precursors of the eicosanoids (a set of hormone-like molecules that are secreted by cells in small quantities and have numerous important effects on neighboring cells). The eicosanoids include the prostaglandins, thromboxanes, leukotrienes, and other related compounds.

C. Protein

The RDA for protein is approximately 0.8 g high-quality protein per kilogram of ideal body weight, or approximately 60 g/day for men and 50 g/day for women. "High-quality" protein contains all of the essential amino acids in adequate amounts. Proteins of animal origin (milk, egg, and meat proteins) are high quality. The proteins in plant foods are generally of lower quality, which means they are low in one or more of the essential amino acids. Vegetarians may obtain adequate amounts of the essential amino acids by eating mixtures of vegetables that complement each other in terms of their amino acid composition.

1.   ESSENTIAL AMINO ACIDS

Different amino acids are used in the body as precursors for the synthesis of proteins and other nitrogen-containing compounds. Of the 20 amino acids commonly required in the body for synthesis of protein and other compounds, nine amino acids are essential in the diet of an adult human because they cannot be synthesized in the body. These are lysine, isoleucine, leucine, threonine, valine, tryptophan, phenylalanine, methionine, and histidine.

Certain amino acids are conditionally essential, that is, required in the diet only under certain conditions. Children and pregnant women have a high rate of protein synthesis to support growth, and require some arginine in the diet, although it can be synthesized in the body. Histidine is essential in the diet of the adult in very small quantities because adults efficiently recycle histidine. The increased requirement of children and pregnant women for histidine is therefore much larger than their increased requirement of other essential amino acids. Tyrosine and cysteine are considered conditionally essential. Tyrosine is synthesized from phenylalanine, and it is required in the diet if phenylalanine intake is inadequate, or if an individual is congenitally deficient in an enzyme required to convert phenylalanine to tyrosine (the congenital disease phenylketonuria). Cysteine is synthesized by using sulfur from methionine, and it also may be required in the diet under certain conditions.

Students often use mnemonics to remember the essential amino acids. One common mnemonic is "Little TV tonight. Ha!" or **LIL** (<u>l</u>ysine-<u>i</u>soleucine-<u>l</u>eucine) **TV** (<u>t</u>hreonine-<u>v</u>aline) **To** (<u>t</u>ryptophan) **PM** (<u>p</u>henyl- alanine-<u>m</u>ethionine). **(HA)** (<u>h</u>istidine-<u>a</u>rginine)!

2.   NITROGEN BALANCE

The proteins in the body undergo constant turnover; that is, they are constantly being degraded to amino acids and resynthesized. When a protein is degraded, its amino acids are released into the pool of free amino acids in the body. The amino acids from dietary proteins also enter this pool. Free amino acids can have one of three fates: they are used to make proteins, they serve as precursors for synthesis of essential nitrogen-containing compounds (e.g., heme, DNA, RNA), or they are oxidized as fuel to yield energy. When amino acids are oxidized, their nitrogen atoms are excreted in the urine principally in the form of urea. The urine also contains smaller amounts of other nitrogenous excretory products (uric acid, creatinine, and NH_4^+) derived from the degradation of amino acids and compounds synthesized from amino acids (Table 1.5). Some nitrogen is also lost in sweat, feces, and cells that slough off.

Nitrogen balance is the difference between the amount of nitrogen taken into the body each day (mainly in the form of dietary protein) and the amount of nitrogen in compounds lost (Table 1.6). If more nitrogen is ingested than excreted, a person is said to be in positive nitrogen balance. Positive nitrogen balance occurs in growing individuals (e.g., children, adolescents, and pregnant women), who are synthesizing more protein than they are breaking down. Conversely, if less nitrogen is ingested than excreted, a person is said to be in negative nitrogen balance. A negative nitrogen balance develops in a person who is eating either too little protein or protein that is deficient in one or more of the essential amino acids. Amino acids are continuously being mobilized from body proteins. If the diet is lacking an essential amino acid or if the intake of protein is too low, new protein cannot be synthesized, and the unused amino acids will be degraded, with the nitrogen appearing in the urine. If a negative nitrogen balance persists for too long, bodily function will be impaired by the net loss of critical proteins. In contrast, healthy adults are in nitrogen balance (neither positive nor negative), and the amount of nitrogen consumed in the diet equals its loss in urine, sweat, feces, and other excretions.

D. Vitamins

Vitamins are a diverse group of organic molecules required in very small quantities in the diet for health, growth, and survival (Latin *vita*, life). The absence of a vitamin from the diet or an inadequate intake results in characteristic deficiency signs and, ultimately, death. Table 1.7 lists the signs or symptoms of deficiency for each vitamin, its RDA or AI for young adults, and common food sources. The amount of each vitamin required in the diet is small (in the microgram or milligram range), compared with essential amino acid requirements (in the gram range). The vitamins are often divided into two classes, water-soluble vitamins and fat-soluble vitamins. This classification has little relationship to their function but is related to the absorption and transport of fat-soluble vitamins with lipids.

Most vitamins are used for the synthesis of coenzymes, complex organic molecules that assist enzymes in catalyzing biochemical reactions, and the deficiency symptoms reflect an inability of cells to carry out certain reactions. However, some vitamins also act as hormones. We will consider the roles played by individual vitamins as we progress through the subsequent chapters of this text.

Although the RDA or AI for each vitamin varies with age and sex, the difference is usually not very large once adolescence is reached. For example, the RDA for

Table 1.5. Major Nitrogenous Excretion Products

Urea
Creatinine
Uric acid
NH_4^+

Multiple vitamin deficiencies accompanying malnutrition are far more common in the United States than the characteristic deficiency diseases associated with diets lacking just one vitamin, because we generally eat a variety of foods. The characteristic deficiency diseases arising from single vitamin deficiencies were often identified and described in humans through observations of populations consuming a restricted diet because that was all that was available. For example, thiamine deficiency was discovered by a physician in Java, who related the symptoms of beri-beri to diets composed principally of polished rice. Today, single vitamin deficiencies usually occur as a result of conditions that interfere with the uptake or utilization of a vitamin or as a result of poor food choices or a lack of variety in the diet. For example, peripheral neuropathy associated with vitamin E deficiency can occur in children with fat malabsorption, and alcohol consumption can result in beri-beri. Vegans, individuals who consume diets lacking all animal products, can develop deficiencies in vitamin B_{12}.

In the hospital, it was learned that **Mr. Percy Veere** had lost 32 lb in the 8 months since his last visit to his family physician. On admission, his hemoglobin (the iron-containing compound in the blood, which carries O_2 from the lungs to the tissues) was 10.7 g/dL (reference range, males = 12 – 15.5), his serum iron was 38 μg/dL (reference range, males = 42 – 135), and other hematologic indices were also abnormal. These values are indicative of an iron deficiency anemia. His serum folic acid level was 0.9 ng/mL (reference range = 3 – 20), indicating a low intake of this vitamin. His vitamin B_{12} level was 190 pg/mL (reference range = 180 – 914). A low blood vitamin B_{12} level can be caused by decreased intake, absorption, or transport, but it takes a long time to develop. His serum albumin was 3.2 g/dL (reference range = 3.5 – 5.0), which is an indicator of protein malnutrition or liver disease.

Table 1.6. Nitrogen Balance

Positive Nitrogen Balance	Growth (e.g., childhood, pregnancy)	Dietary N > Excreted N
Nitrogen Balance	Normal healthy adult	Dietary N = Excreted N
Negative Nitrogen Balance	Dietary deficiency of total protein or amino acids; catabolic stress	Dietary N < Excreted N

Table 1.7. VITAMINS [a]

Vitamin	Dietary Reference Intakes (DRI) Females (F) Males (M) (18–30 yrs old)	Some Common Food Sources	Consequences of Deficiency (Names of deficiency diseases are in bold)
Water-soluble vitamins			
Vitamin C	**RDA** F: 75 mg M: 90 mg **UL:** 2 g	Citrus fruits; potatoes; peppers, broccoli, spinach; strawberries	**Scurvy:** defective collagen formation leading to subcutaneous hemorrhage, aching bones, joints, and muscle in adults, rigid position and pain in infants.
Thiamin	**RDA** F: 1.1 mg M: 1.2 mg	Enriched cereals and breads; unrefined grains; pork; legumes, seeds, nuts	**Beri-beri:** (wet) Edema; anorexia, weight loss; apathy, decrease in short-term memory, confusion; irritability; muscle weakness; an enlarged heart
Riboflavin	**RDA** F: 1.1 mg M: 1.3 mg	Dairy products; fortified cereals; meats, poultry, fish; legumes	**Ariboflavinosis:** Sore throat, hyperemia, edema of oral mucusal membranes; cheilosis, angular stomatis; glossitis, magenta tongue; seborrheic dermatitis; normochromic normocylic anemia
Niacin[b]	**RDA** F: 14 mg NEQ M: 16 mg NEQ **UL:** 35 mg	Meat: chicken, beef, fish; enriched cereals or whole grains; most foods	**Pellagra:** Pigmented rash in areas exposed to sunlight; vomiting; constipation or diarrhea; bright red tongue; neurologic symptoms
Vitamin B$_6$ (pyridoxine)	**RDA** F: 1.3 mg M: 1.3 mg **UL:** 100 mg	Chicken, fish, pork; eggs; fortified cereals, unmilled rice, oats; starchy vegetables; noncitrus fruits; peanuts, walnuts	Seborrheic dermatitis; microcytic anemia; epileptiform convulsions; depression and confusion
Folate	**RDA** F: 400 μg M: 400 μg	Citrus fruits; dark green vegetables; fortified cereals and breads; legumes	Impaired cell division and growth; **megaloblastic anemia**; neural tube defects
Vitamin B$_{12}$	**RDA** F: 2.4 μg M: 2.4 μg	Animal products[c]	**Megaloblastic anemia** Neurologic symptoms
Biotin	**AI** F: 30 μg M: 30 μg	Liver Egg yolk	Conjunctivitis; central nervous system abnormalities; glossitis; alopecia; dry, scaly dermatitis
Pantothenic acid	**AI** F: 5 mg M: 5 mg	Wide distribution in foods, especially animal tissues; whole grain cereals; legumes	Irritability and restlessness; fatigue, apathy, malaise; gastiointestinal symptoms; neurological symptoms
Choline	**AI** F: 550 mg M: 425 mg **UL:** 3.5 g	Milk; liver; eggs; peanuts	Liver damage
Fat-soluble vitamins			
Vitamin A	**RDA** F: 700 μg M: 900 μg **UL:** 3000 μg	Carrots; Dark green and leafy vegetables; sweet potatoes and squash; broccoli	Night blindness; **xerophthalmia;** keratinization of epithelium in GI, respiratory and genitourinary tract, skin becomes dry and scaly
Vitamin K	**RDA** Γ: 90 μg M: 120 μg	Green leafy vegetables; cabbage family (brassica); Bacterial flora of intestine	Defective blood coagulation; hemorrhagic anemia of the newborn
Vitamin D	**AI**[d] F: 5 μg M: 5 μg **UL:** 50 μg	Fortified milk; Exposure of skin to sunlight	**Rickets** (in children); inadequate bone mineralization (osteomalacia)
Vitamin E	**RDA** F: 15 mg M: 15 mg **UL:** 1 g	Vegetable oils, margarine; wheat germ; nuts; green leafy vegetables	Muscular dystrophy, neurologic abnormalities.

Dietary Reference Intakes (DRI): Recommended Dietary Allowance (RDA); Adequate Intake (AI); Tolerable Upper Intake Level (UL)
[a]Information for this table is from Dietary Reference Intakes for Thiamin, Riboflavin, Niacin, Vitamin B$_6$, Folate, Vitamin B$_{12}$, Pantothenic Acid, Biotin, and Choline (1998); Dietary Reference Intakes for Vitamin C, Vitamin E, Selenium, and Carotenoids (2000); Dietary Reference Intakes for Calcium, Phosphorus, Magnesium, Vitamin D, and Fluoride (1997), Dietary Reference Intakes for Vitamin A, Vitamin K, Arsenic, Boron, Chromium, Copper, Iodine, Iron, Manganese, Molybdenum, Nickel, Silicon, Vanadium, and Zinc (2001). Washington, DC: Food and Nutrition Board, Institute of Medicine, National Academy Press.
[b]neq = niacin equivalents. Niacin can be synthesized in the human from tryptophan, and this term takes into account a conversion factor for dietary tryptophan.
[c]Vitamin B$_{12}$ is found only in animal products.
[d]Dietary requirement assumes the absence of sunlight.

riboflavin is 0.9 mg/day for males between 9 and 13 years of age, 1.3 mg/day for males 19 to 30 years of age, still 1.3 mg/day for males older than 70 years, and 1.1 mg/day for females aged 19 to 30 years. The largest requirements occur during lactation (1.6 mg/day).

Vitamins, by definition, cannot be synthesized in the body, or are synthesized from a very specific dietary precursor in insufficient amounts. For example, we can synthesize the vitamin niacin from the essential amino acid tryptophan, but not in sufficient quantities to meet our needs. Niacin is therefore still classified as a vitamin.

Excessive intake of many vitamins, both fat-soluble and water-soluble, may cause deleterious effects. For example, high doses of vitamin A, a fat-soluble vitamin, can cause desquamation of the skin and birth defects. High doses of vitamin C cause diarrhea and gastrointestinal disturbances. One of the Reference Dietary Intakes is the Tolerable Upper Intake Level (UL), which is the highest level of daily nutrient intake that is likely to pose no risk of adverse effects to almost all individuals in the general population. As intake increases above the UL, the risk of adverse effects increases. Table 1.7 includes the UL for vitamins known to pose a risk at high levels. Intake above the UL occurs most often with dietary or pharmacologic supplements of single vitamins, and not from foods.

E. Minerals

Many minerals are required in the diet. They are generally divided into the classifications of electrolytes (inorganic ions that are dissolved in the fluid compartments of the body), minerals (required in relatively large quantities), trace minerals (required in smaller quantities), and ultratrace minerals (Table 1.8).

Sodium (Na^+), potassium (K^+), and chloride (Cl^-) are the major electrolytes (ions) in the body. They establish ion gradients across membranes, maintain water balance, and neutralize positive and negative charges on proteins and other molecules.

Calcium and phosphorus serve as structural components of bones and teeth and are thus required in relatively large quantities. Calcium (Ca^{2+}) plays many other roles in the body; for example, it is involved in hormone action and blood clotting. Phosphorus is required for the formation of ATP and of phosphorylated intermediates in metabolism. Magnesium activates many enzymes and also forms a complex with ATP. Iron is a particularly important mineral because it functions as a component of hemoglobin (the oxygen-carrying protein in the blood) and is part of many enzymes. Other minerals, such as zinc or molybdenum, are required in very small quantities (trace or ultra-trace amounts).

Sulfur is ingested principally in the amino acids cysteine and methionine. It is found in connective tissue, particularly in cartilage and skin. It has important functions in metabolism, which we will describe when we consider the action of coenzyme A, a compound used to activate carboxylic acids. Sulfur is excreted in the urine as sulfate.

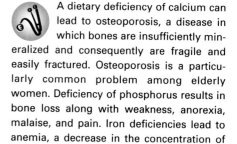

A dietary deficiency of calcium can lead to osteoporosis, a disease in which bones are insufficiently mineralized and consequently are fragile and easily fractured. Osteoporosis is a particularly common problem among elderly women. Deficiency of phosphorus results in bone loss along with weakness, anorexia, malaise, and pain. Iron deficiencies lead to anemia, a decrease in the concentration of hemoglobin in the blood.

 Which foods would provide Percy Veere with good sources of folate and vitamin B_{12}?

Table 1.8. Minerals Required in the Diet

Electrolytes	Minerals	Trace Minerals	Ultratrace or Trace Minerals[a]
Sodium	Calcium	Iodine	Manganese
Potassium	Phosphorus	Selenium	Fluoride
Chloride	Magnesium	Copper	Chromium
	Iron	Zinc	Molybdenum
	Sulfur		Others?

[a] These minerals are classified as trace or as ultratrace.

Folate is found in fruits and vegetables: citrus fruits (e.g., oranges), green leafy vegetables (e.g., spinach and broccoli), fortified cereals, and legumes (e.g., peas) (see Table 1.7). Conversely, vitamin B_{12} is found only in foods of animal origin, including meats, eggs, and milk.

Minerals, like vitamins, have adverse effects if ingested in excessive amounts. Problems associated with dietary excesses or deficiencies of minerals are described in subsequent chapters in conjunction with their normal metabolic functions.

F. Water

Water constitutes one half to four fifths of the weight of the human body. The intake of water required per day depends on the balance between the amount produced by body metabolism and the amount lost through the skin, through expired air, and in the urine and feces.

V. DIETARY GUIDELINES

Dietary guidelines or goals are recommendations for food choices that can reduce the risk of developing chronic or degenerative diseases while maintaining an adequate intake of nutrients. Many studies have shown an association between diet and exercise and decreased risk of certain diseases, including hypertension, atherosclerosis, stroke, diabetes, certain types of cancer, and osteoarthritis. Thus, the American Heart Institute and the American Cancer Institute, as well as several other groups, have developed dietary and exercise recommendations to decrease the risk of these diseases. The "Dietary Guidelines for Americans (2000)", prepared under the joint authority of the US Department of Agriculture and the US Department of Health and Human Services, merges many of these recommendations. Recommended servings of different food groups are displayed as the food pyramid (Fig. 1.9). Issues of special concern for physicians who advise patients include the following:

A. General Recommendations

- Aim for a healthy weight and be physically active each day. For maintenance of a healthy weight, caloric intake should balance caloric expenditure. Accumulate at least 30 minutes of moderate physical activity (such as walking 2 miles) daily. A regular exercise program helps in achieving and maintaining ideal weight, cardiovascular fitness, and strength.
- Choose foods in the proportions recommended in the food pyramid, including a variety of grains and a variety of fruits and vegetables daily.
- Keep food safe to eat. For example, refrigerate leftovers promptly.

B. Vegetables, Fruits, and Grains

- Diets rich in vegetables, fruits, and grain products should be chosen. Five or more servings of vegetables and fruits should be eaten each day, particularly green and yellow vegetables and citrus fruits. Six or more daily servings of grains should be eaten (starches and other complex carbohydrates, in the form of breads, fortified cereals, rice, and pasta). In addition to energy, vegetables, fruits, and grains supply vitamins, minerals, protective substances (such as carotenoids), and fiber. Fiber, the indigestible part of plant food, has various beneficial effects, including relief of constipation.
- The consumption of refined sugar in foods and beverages should be reduced to below the American norm. Refined sugar has no nutritional value other than its caloric content, and it promotes tooth decay.

C. Fats

- Fat intake should be reduced. For those at risk of heart attacks or strokes, fat should account for no more than 30% of total dietary calories, and saturated fatty acids

Food Guide Pyramid

A Guide to Daily Food choices

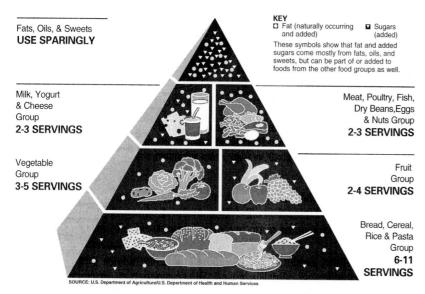

Fats, Oils, & Sweets
USE SPARINGLY

KEY
☐ Fat (naturally occurring and added)   ☑ Sugars (added)
These symbols show that fat and added sugars come mostly from fats, oils, and sweets, but can be part of or added to foods from the other food groups as well.

Milk, Yogurt & Cheese Group
2-3 SERVINGS

Meat, Poultry, Fish, Dry Beans, Eggs & Nuts Group
2-3 SERVINGS

Vegetable Group
3-5 SERVINGS

Fruit Group
2-4 SERVINGS

Bread, Cereal, Rice & Pasta Group
6-11 SERVINGS

SOURCE: U.S. Department of Agriculture/U.S. Department of Health and Human Services

Fig. 1.9. The Food Guide Pyramid. The pyramid shows the number of servings that should be eaten each day from each food group. Within each group, a variety of foods should be eaten. Some examples of serving size: Grain products—1 slice of white bread or ½ cup of cooked rice; Vegetable group—½ cup cooked vegetables; Fruit group—1 apple or banana; Milk Group—1 cup of milk or 2 oz processed cheese; Meat and Beans Group—2–3 oz cooked lean meat or fish or 1 egg or 2 tbsp peanut butter. Nutrition and Your Health: Dietary Guidelines for Americans, 2000. Washington, DC: Dietary Guidelines Committee: The U.S. Department of Agriculture and the U.S. Department of Health and Human Services.

should account for 10% or less. Foods high in saturated fat include cheese, whole milk, butter, regular ice cream, and many cuts of beef. Trans fatty acids, such as the partially hydrogenated vegetable oils used in margarine, should also be avoided.

- Cholesterol intake should be less than 300 mg/day in subjects without atherosclerotic disease and less than 200 mg/day in those with established atherosclerosis.

D. Proteins

- Protein intake for adults should be approximately 0.8 g/kg ideal body weight per day. The protein should be of high quality and should be obtained from sources low in saturated fat (e.g., fish, lean poultry, and dry beans). Vegetarians should eat a mixture of vegetable proteins that ensures the intake of adequate amounts of the essential amino acids.

E. Alcohol

- Alcohol consumption should not exceed moderate drinking. Moderation is defined as no more than one drink per day for women and no more than two drinks per day for men. A drink is defined as 1 regular beer, 5 ounces of wine (a little over ½ cup), or 1.5 ounces of an 80-proof liquor, such as whiskey. Pregnant women should drink no alcohol.

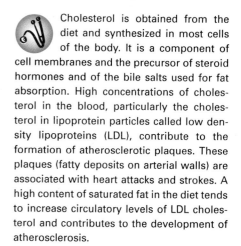

Cholesterol is obtained from the diet and synthesized in most cells of the body. It is a component of cell membranes and the precursor of steroid hormones and of the bile salts used for fat absorption. High concentrations of cholesterol in the blood, particularly the cholesterol in lipoprotein particles called low density lipoproteins (LDL), contribute to the formation of atherosclerotic plaques. These plaques (fatty deposits on arterial walls) are associated with heart attacks and strokes. A high content of saturated fat in the diet tends to increase circulatory levels of LDL cholesterol and contributes to the development of atherosclerosis.

The ingestion of alcohol by pregnant women can result in fetal alcohol syndrome (FAS), which is marked by prenatal and postnatal growth deficiency, developmental delay, and craniofacial, limb, and cardiovascular defects.

The high intake of sodium and chloride (in table salt) of the average American diet appears to be related to the development of hypertension (high blood pressure) in individuals who are genetically predisposed to this disorder.

F.   Vitamins and Minerals

- Sodium intake should be decreased in most individuals. Sodium is usually consumed as salt, NaCl. Individuals prone to salt-sensitive hypertension should eat less than 3 g sodium per day (approximately 6 g NaCl).
- Many of the required vitamins and minerals can be obtained from eating a variety of fruits, vegetables, and grains (particularly whole grains). However, calcium and iron are required in relatively high amounts. Low-fat or nonfat dairy products and dark green leafy vegetables provide good sources of calcium. Lean meats, shellfish, poultry, dark meat, cooked dry beans, and some leafy green vegetables provide good sources of iron. Vitamin B_{12} is found only in animal sources.
- Dietary supplementation in excess of the recommended amounts (for example, megavitamin regimens) should be avoided.
- Fluoride should be present in the diet, at least during the years of tooth formation, as a protection against dental caries.

VI. XENOBIOTICS

In addition to nutrients, our diet also contains a large number of chemicals called xenobiotics, which have no nutritional value, are of no use in the body, and can be harmful if consumed in excessive amounts. These compounds occur naturally in foods, can enter the food chain as contaminants, or can be deliberately introduced as food additives.

Dietary guidelines of the American Cancer Society and the American Institute for Cancer Research make recommendations relevant to the ingestion of xenobiotic compounds, particularly carcinogens. The dietary advice that we eat a variety of food helps to protect us against the ingestion of a toxic level of any one xenobiotic compound. It is also suggested that we reduce consumption of salt-cured, smoked, and charred foods, which contain chemicals that can contribute to the development of cancer. Other guidelines encourage the ingestion of fruits and vegetables that contain protective chemicals called antioxidants.

CLINICAL COMMENTS

Otto Shape. Otto Shape sought help in reducing his weight of 187 lb (BMI of 27) to his previous level of 154 lb (BMI of 22, in the middle of the healthy range). Otto Shape was 5 feet 10 inches tall, and he calculated that his maximum healthy weight was 173 lbs. He planned on becoming a family physician, and he knew that he would be better able to counsel patients in healthy behaviors involving diet and exercise if he practiced them himself. With this information and assurances from the physician that he was otherwise in good health, Otto embarked on a weight loss program. One of his strategies involved recording all the food he ate and the portions. To analyze his diet for calories, saturated fat, and nutrients, he used the Interactive Healthy Eating Index, available online from the USDA Food and Nutrition Information Center.

Physicians have an average lifespan that is longer than the general population, and generally practice healthier behaviors, especially with regard to fat consumption, exercise, alcohol consumption, and smoking. Physicians who practice healthy behaviors are more likely to counsel patients with respect to these behaviors and are better able to motivate their patients.

Ivan Applebod. Ivan Applebod weighed 264 lb and was 70 inches tall with a heavy skeletal frame. For a male of these proportions, a BMI of 18.5 to 24.9 would correspond to a weight between 129 and 173 lb. He is currently almost 100 lb overweight, and his BMI of 37.9 is in the obese range.

Mr. Applebod's physician cautioned him that exogenous obesity (caused by overeating) represents a risk factor for atherosclerotic vascular disease, particularly when the distribution of fat is primarily "central" or in the abdominal region (apple shape, in contrast to the pear shape, which results from adipose tissue deposited in the buttocks and hips). In addition, obesity may lead to other cardiovascular risk factors such as hypertension (high blood pressure), hyperlipidemia (high blood lipid levels), and type 2 diabetes mellitus (characterized by hyperglycemia). He already has a mild elevation in both systolic and diastolic blood pressure. Furthermore, his total serum cholesterol level was 296 mg/dL, well above the desired normal value (200 mg/dL).

Mr. Applebod was referred to the hospital's weight reduction center, where a team of physicians, dieticians, and psychologists could assist him in reaching his ideal weight range.

Ann O'Rexia. Because of her history and physical examination, Ann O'Rexia was diagnosed as having early anorexia nervosa, a behavioral disorder that involves both emotional and nutritional disturbances. Miss O'Rexia was referred to a psychiatrist with special interest in anorexia nervosa, and a program of psychotherapy and behavior modification was initiated.

Percy Veere. Percy Veere weighed 125 lb and was 71 inches tall (without shoes) with a medium frame. His BMI was 17.5, which is significantly underweight. At the time his wife died, he weighed 147 lbs. For his height, a BMI in the healthy weight range corresponds to weights between 132 and 178 lb.

Mr. Veere's malnourished state was reflected in his admission laboratory profile. The results of hematologic studies were consistent with an iron deficiency anemia complicated by low levels of folic acid and vitamin B_{12}, two vitamins that can affect the development of normal red blood cells. His low serum albumin level was caused by insufficient protein intake and a shortage of essential amino acids, which result in a reduced ability to synthesize body proteins. The psychiatrist requested a consultation with a hospital dietician to evaluate the extent of Mr. Veere's marasmus (malnutrition caused by a deficiency of both protein and total calories) as well as his vitamin and mineral deficiencies.

The prevalence of obesity in the U.S. population is increasing. In 1962, 12.8% of the population had a BMI equal to or greater than 30 and therefore were clinically obese. That number increased to 14.5% by 1980 and to 22.5% by 1998. An additional 30% were pre-obese in 1998 (BMI = 25.0 − 29.9). Therefore, more than 50% of the population is currently overweight, that is, obese or pre-obese.

Increased weight increases cardiovascular risk factors, including hypertension, diabetes, and alterations in blood lipid levels. It also increases the risk for respiratory problems, gallbladder disease, and certain types of cancer.

BIOCHEMICAL COMMENTS

Dietary Reference Intakes. Dietary Reference Intakes (DRIs) are quantitative estimates of nutrient intakes that can be used in evaluating and planning diets for healthy people. They are prepared by the Standing Committee on the Scientific Evaluation of Dietary Reference Intakes (DRI) of the Food and Nutrition Board, Institute of Medicine, and the National Academy of Science, with active input of Health Canada. The four reference intake values are the Recommended Dietary Allowance (RDA), the Estimated Average Requirement (EAR), the Adequate Intake (AI), and the Tolerable Upper Intake Level (UL). For each vitamin, the Committee has reviewed available literature on studies with humans and established criteria for adequate intake, such as prevention of certain deficiency symptoms, prevention of developmental abnormalities, or decreased risk of chronic degenerative disease. The criteria are not always the same for each life stage group. A requirement is defined as the lowest continuing intake level of a nutrient able to satisfy these criteria. The EAR is the daily intake value that is estimated to meet the requirement in half of the apparently healthy individuals in a life stage or gender group. The RDA is the EAR plus 2 standard deviations of the mean, which is the amount that should satisfy the requirement in 97 to 98% of the population. The AI level instead of an RDA is set for nutrients when there is not enough data to determine the EAR.

The Tolerable Upper Intake Level (UL) refers to the highest level of daily nutrient intake consumed over time that is likely to pose no risks of adverse effects for almost all healthy individuals in the general population. Adverse effects are defined as any significant alteration in the structure or function of the human organism. The

An example of the difference between the AI and the EAR is provided by riboflavin. Very few data exist on the nutrient requirements of very young infants. However, human milk is the sole recommended food for the first 4 to 6 months, so the AI of the vitamin riboflavin for this life stage group is based on the amount in breast milk consumed by healthy full-term infants. Conversely, the riboflavin EAR for adults is based on a number of studies in humans relating dietary intake of riboflavin to biochemical markers of riboflavin status and development of clinical deficiency symptoms.

UL does not mean that most individuals who consume more than the UL will suffer adverse health effects, but that the risk of adverse effects increases as intake increases above the UL.

Suggested References

A good, comprehensive textbook on nutrition is Shils ME, Olson JA, Shike M, Ross, AC. Modern nutrition in health and disease. Baltimore: Williams & Wilkins, 1999. Extensive nutrition tables, including Metropolitan Height and Weight Tables, are available in the appendices.

Recent Dietary References Intakes prepared by the Food and Nutrition Board of the National Academy of Science (1997–2001) are available in several volumes published by the National Academy Press (see Table 1.7) and may be consulted online at http://books.nap.edu/.

To analyze diets for calories and nutrient contents, consult food databases and resource lists made available by the USDA. The site www.nal.usda.gov/fnic provides lists of resources on food composition, such as the database U.S. Department of Agriculture, Agricultural Research Service. 2001. USDA Nutrient Database for Standard Reference, Release 14. Nutrient Data Laboratory Homepage, http://www.nal.usda.gov/fnic/foodcomp. This site also provides lists of resources for diet analysis, and links to the Interactive Healthy Eating Index, which is a program students can use to analyze their diets (http://147.208.9.133). A useful computer program for evaluating the diet of individuals, the MSU Nutriguide, can be obtained from Department of Nutrition, Michigan State University.

Dietary recommendations change frequently as new data become available. Current Dietary Recommendations are available from the following sources: Food and Nutrition Information Center, National Agricultural Library, USDA (www.fns.usda.gov); National Heart, Lung, and Blood Institute Information Center (www.nhlbi.nih.gov); American Heart Association (www.Americanheart.org); American Institute for Cancer Research (www.aicr.org); and the American Diabetes Association (www.diabetes.org). Another reliable source for nutrition information on the internet is www.navigator.tufts.edu.

A number of medical schools in the United States have received Nutrition Academic Awards from the National Institute of Heart, Blood and Lung, National Institutes of Health (www.nhlbi.nih.gov/funding/naa). These schools are developing products for medical nutrition education.

REVIEW QUESTIONS—CHAPTER 1

Directions: For each question below, select the single best answer.

1. In the process of respiration, fuels

    (A) are stored as triacylglycerols.
    (B) are oxidized to generate ATP.
    (C) release energy principally as heat.
    (D) combine with CO_2 and H_2O.
    (E) combine with other dietary components in anabolic pathways.

2. The caloric content per gram of fuel

    (A) is higher for carbohydrates than triacylglycerols.
    (B) is higher for protein than for fat.
    (C) is proportionate to the amount of oxygen in a fuel.
    (D) is the amount of energy that can be obtained from oxidation of the fuel.
    (E) is higher for children than adults.

3. The resting metabolic rate is

    (A) equivalent to the caloric requirement of our major organs and resting muscle.
    (B) generally higher per kilogram body weight in women than in men.
    (C) generally lower per kilogram body weight in children than adults.
    (D) decreased in a cold environment.
    (E) approximately equivalent to the daily energy expenditure.

4. The RDA is

   (A) the average amount of a nutrient required each day to maintain normal function in 50% of the U.S. population.
   (B) the average amount of a nutrient ingested daily by 50% of the U.S. population.
   (C) the minimum amount of a nutrient ingested daily that prevents deficiency symptoms.
   (D) a reasonable dietary goal for the intake of a nutrient by a healthy individual.
   (E) based principally on data obtained with laboratory animals.

5. A 35-year old sedentary male patient weighing 120 kg was experiencing angina (chest pain) and other signs of coronary artery disease. His physician, in consultation with a registered dietician, conducted a 3-day dietary recall. The patient consumed an average of 585 g carbohydrate, 150 g protein, and 95 g fat each day. In addition, he drank 45 g alcohol. The patient

   (A) consumed between 2,500 and 3,000 kcal per day.
   (B) had a fat intake within the range recommended in current dietary guidelines (i.e., year 2000).
   (C) consumed 50% of his calories as alcohol.
   (D) was deficient in protein intake.
   (E) was in negative caloric balance.

2 The Fed or Absorptive State

The Fed State. *During a **meal**, we ingest carbohydrates, lipids, and proteins, which are subsequently **digested** and **absorbed**. Some of this food is **oxidized** to meet the immediate **energy** needs of the body. The amount consumed in **excess** of the body's energy needs is transported to the **fuel depots**, where it is stored. During the period from the start of absorption until absorption is completed, we are in the **fed**, or absorptive, state. Whether a fuel is oxidized or stored in the fed state is determined principally by the concentration of two **endocrine hormones** in the blood, **insulin** and **glucagon**.*

Fate of Carbohydrates. *Dietary carbohydrates are digested to monosaccharides, which are absorbed into the blood. The major monosaccharide in the blood is **glucose** (Fig 2.1). After a meal, glucose is **oxidized** by various tissues for energy, enters biosynthetic pathways, and is **stored** as **glycogen**, mainly in liver and muscle. Glucose is the major biosynthetic precursor in the body, and the carbon skeletons of most of the compounds we synthesize can be synthesized from glucose. Glucose is also converted to **triacylglycerols**. The liver packages triacylglycerols, made from glucose or from fatty acids obtained from the blood, into very low-density lipoproteins (VLDL) and releases them into the blood. The fatty acids of the VLDL are mainly stored as triacylglycerols in adipose tissue, but some may be used to meet the energy needs of cells.*

Fate of Proteins. *Dietary proteins are digested to **amino acids**, which are absorbed into the blood. In cells, the amino acids are converted to **proteins** or used to make various **nitrogen-containing compounds** such as neurotransmitters and heme. The carbon skeleton may also be **oxidized** for energy directly, or converted to glucose.*

Fate of Fats. *Triacylglycerols are the major lipids in the diet. They are digested to fatty acids and 2-monoacylglycerols, which are resynthesized into **triacylglycerols** in intestinal epithelial cells, packaged in **chylomicrons**, and secreted by way of the lymph into the blood. The **fatty acids** of the chylomicron triacylglycerols are stored mainly as triacylglycerols in **adipose** cells. They are subsequently oxidized for energy or used in biosynthetic pathways, such as synthesis of membrane lipids.*

Hormones are compounds that are synthesized by the endocrine glands of the body. They are secreted into the bloodstream and carry messages to different tissues concerning changes in the overall physiologic state of the body or the needs of tissues.

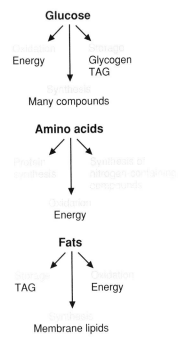

Fig. 2.1. Major fates of fuels in the fed state.

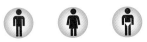

THE WAITING ROOM

Ivan Applebod returned to his doctor for a second visit. His initial efforts to lose weight had failed dismally. In fact, he now weighed 270 lb, an increase of 6 lb since his first visit 2 months ago (see Chapter 1). He reported that the recent death of his 45-year-old brother of a heart attack had made him realize that he must pay more attention to his health. Because

Mr. Applebod's brother had a history of hypercholesterolemia and because Mr. Applebod's serum total cholesterol had been significantly elevated (296 mg/dL) at his first visit, his blood lipid profile was determined, his blood glucose level was measured, and a number of other blood tests were ordered. (The blood lipid profile is a test that measures the content of the various triacylglycerol- and cholesterol-containing particles in the blood.) His blood pressure was 162 mm Hg systolic and 98 mm Hg diastolic or 162/98 mm Hg (normal = 140/90 mm Hg or less). His waist circumference was 48 inches (healthy values for men, less than 40; for women, less than 35).

The body can make fatty acids from a caloric excess of carbohydrate and protein. These fatty acids, together with the fatty acids of chylomicrons (derived from dietary fat), are deposited in adipose tissue as triacylglycerols. Thus, **Ivan Applebod's** increased adipose tissue is coming from his intake of all fuels in excess of his caloric need.

I. DIGESTION AND ABSORPTION

After a meal is consumed, foods are digested (broken down into simpler components) by a series of enzymes in the mouth, stomach, and small intestine. The products of digestion eventually are absorbed into the blood. The period during which digestion and absorption occur constitutes the fed state (Fig. 2.2)

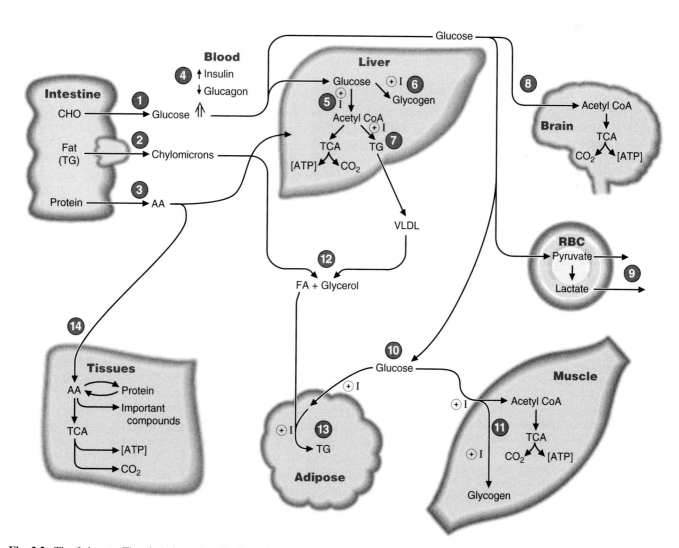

Fig. 2.2. The fed state. The circled numbers indicate the approximate order in which the processes occur. TG = triacylglycerols; FA = fatty acid; AA = amino acid; RBC = red blood cell; VLDL = very-low-density lipoprotein; I = insulin; $\oplus$ = stimulated by.

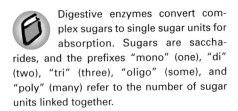

Digestive enzymes convert complex sugars to single sugar units for absorption. Sugars are saccharides, and the prefixes "mono" (one), "di" (two), "tri" (three), "oligo" (some), and "poly" (many) refer to the number of sugar units linked together.

Enzymes are proteins that catalyze biochemical reactions; in other words, they increase the speed at which reactions occur. Their names usually end in "ase."

Proteins are amino acids linked through peptide bonds. Dipeptides have two amino acids, tripeptides have three amino acids, and so on. Digestive proteases are enzymes that cleave the peptide bonds between the amino acids (see Chap.1, Fig. 1.5).

Fats must be transported in the blood bound to protein or in lipoprotein complexes because they are insoluble in water. Thus, both triacylglycerols and cholesterol are found in lipoprotein complexes.

The laboratory studies ordered at the time of his second office visit show that **Ivan Applebod** has hyperglycemia, an elevation of blood glucose above normal values. At the time of this visit, his 2-hour postprandial blood glucose level was 205 mg/dL. (Two-hour postprandial refers to the glucose level measured 2 hours after a meal, when glucose should have been taken up by tissues and blood glucose returned to the fasting level, approximately 80–100 mg/dL.) His blood glucose determined after an overnight fast was 162 mg/dL. Because both of these blood glucose measurements were significantly above normal, a diagnosis of type 2 diabetes mellitus, formerly known as non–insulin-dependent diabetes mellitus (NIDDM), was made. In this disease, liver, muscle, and adipose tissue are relatively resistant to the action of insulin in promoting glucose uptake into cells and storage as glycogen and triacylglycerols. Therefore, more glucose remains in his blood.

A. Carbohydrates

Dietary carbohydrates are converted to monosaccharides. Starch, a polymer of glucose, is the major carbohydrate of the diet. It is digested by salivary α-amylase, and then by pancreatic α-amylase, which acts in the small intestine. Di-, tri-, and oligosaccharides produced by these α-amylases are cleaved to glucose by digestive enzymes located on the surface of the brush border of the intestinal epithelial cells. Dietary disaccharides also are cleaved by enzymes in this brush border. Sucrase converts the disaccharide sucrose (table sugar) to glucose and fructose, and lactase converts the disaccharide lactose (milk sugar) to glucose and galactose. Monosaccharides produced by digestion and dietary monosaccharides are absorbed by the intestinal epithelial cells and released into the hepatic portal vein, which carries them to the liver.

B. Proteins

Dietary proteins are cleaved to amino acids by proteases (see Fig. 2.2, circle 3). Pepsin acts in the stomach, and the proteolytic enzymes produced by the pancreas (trypsin, chymotrypsin, elastase, and the carboxypeptidases) act in the lumen of the small intestine. Aminopeptidases and di- and tripeptidases associated with the intestinal epithelial cells complete the conversion of dietary proteins to amino acids, which are absorbed into the intestinal epithelial cells and released into the hepatic portal vein.

C. Fats

The digestion of fats is more complex than that of carbohydrates or proteins because they are not very soluble in water. The triacylglycerols of the diet are emulsified in the intestine by bile salts, which are synthesized in the liver and stored in the gallbladder . Pancreatic lipase converts the triacylglycerols in the lumen of the intestine to fatty acids and 2-monoacylglycerols (glycerol with a fatty acid esterified at carbon 2), which interact with bile salts to form tiny microdroplets called micelles. The fatty acids and 2-monoacylglycerols are absorbed from these micelles into the intestinal epithelial cells, where they are resynthesized into triacylglycerols. The triacylglycerols are packaged with proteins, phospholipids, cholesterol, and other compounds into the lipoprotein complexes known as chylomicrons, which are secreted into the lymph and ultimately enter the bloodstream (see Fig. 2.2, circle 2).

II.   CHANGES IN HORMONE LEVELS AFTER A MEAL

After a typical high carbohydrate meal, the pancreas is stimulated to release the hormone insulin, and release of the hormone glucagon is inhibited (see Fig. 2.2, circle 4). Endocrine hormones are released from endocrine glands, such as the pancreas, in response to a specific stimulus. They travel in the blood, carrying messages between tissues concerning the overall physiologic state of the body. At their target tissues, they adjust the rate of various metabolic pathways to meet the changing conditions. The endocrine hormone insulin, which is secreted from the pancreas in response to a high-carbohydrate meal, carries the message that dietary glucose is available and can be used and stored. The release of another hormone, glucagon, is suppressed by glucose and insulin. Glucagon carries the message that glucose must be generated from endogenous fuel stores. The subsequent changes in circulating hormone levels cause changes in the body's metabolic patterns, involving a number of different tissues and metabolic pathways.

III. FATE OF GLUCOSE AFTER A MEAL

A. Conversion to Glycogen, Triacylglycerols, and CO₂ in the Liver

Because glucose leaves the intestine via the hepatic portal vein, the liver is the first tissue it passes through. The liver extracts a portion of this glucose from the blood. Some of the glucose that enters hepatocytes (liver cells) is oxidized in adenosine triphosphate (ATP)-generating pathways to meet the immediate energy needs of these cells and the remainder is converted to glycogen and triacylglycerols or used for biosynthetic reactions. In the liver, insulin promotes the uptake of glucose by increasing its use as a fuel and its storage as glycogen and triacylglycerols (see Fig. 2.2, circles 5, 6, and 7).

As glucose is being oxidized to CO_2, it is first oxidized to pyruvate in the pathway of glycolysis. Pyruvate is then oxidized to acetyl CoA. The acetyl group enters the tricarboxylic acid (TCA) cycle, where it is completely oxidized to CO_2. Energy from the oxidative reactions is used to generate ATP.

Liver glycogen stores reach a maximum of approximately 200 to 300 g after a high-carbohydrate meal, whereas the body's fat stores are relatively limitless. As the glycogen stores begin to fill, the liver also begins converting some of the excess glucose it receives to triacylglycerols. Both the glycerol and the fatty acid moieties of the triacylglycerols can be synthesized from glucose. The fatty acids are also obtained preformed from the blood. The liver does not store triacylglycerols, however, but packages them along with proteins, phospholipids, and cholesterol into the lipoprotein complexes known as very-low-density lipoproteins (VLDL), which are secreted into the bloodstream. Some of the fatty acids from the VLDL are taken up by tissues for their immediate energy needs, but most are stored in adipose tissue as triacylglycerols.

 In the liver and most other tissues, glucose, fats, and other fuels are oxidized to the 2-carbon acetyl group

$$(CH_3-\overset{\overset{\displaystyle O}{\|}}{C}-)$$ of acetyl CoA. CoA, which makes the acetyl group more reactive, is a cofactor (coenzyme A) derived from the vitamin pantothenate. The acetyl group of acetyl CoA is completely oxidized to CO_2 in the TCA cycle (see Fig 1.4). Adenosine triphosphate (ATP) is the final product of these oxidative pathways. It contains energy derived from the catabolic energy-producing oxidation reactions and transfers that energy to anabolic and other energy-requiring processes in the cell.

B. Glucose Metabolism In Other Tissues

The glucose from the intestine that is not metabolized by the liver travels in the blood to peripheral tissues (most other tissues), where it can be oxidized for energy. Glucose is the one fuel that can be used by all tissues. Many tissues store small amounts of glucose as glycogen. Muscle has relatively large glycogen stores.

Insulin greatly stimulates the transport of glucose into the two tissues that have the largest mass in the body, muscle and adipose tissue. It has much smaller effects on the transport of glucose into other tissues.

Fuel metabolism is often discussed as though the body consisted only of brain, skeletal and cardiac muscle, liver, adipose tissue, red blood cells, kidney, and intestinal epithelial cells ("the gut"). These are the dominant tissues in terms of overall fuel economy, and they are the tissues we describe most often. Of course, all tissues require fuels for energy, and many have very specific fuel requirements.

1. BRAIN AND OTHER NEURAL TISSUES

The brain and other neural tissues are very dependent on glucose for their energy needs. They generally oxidize glucose via glycolysis and the TCA cycle completely to CO_2 and H_2O, generating ATP (see Fig. 2.2, circle 8). Except under conditions of starvation, glucose is their only major fuel. Glucose is also a major precursor of neurotransmitters, the chemicals that convey electrical impulses (as ion gradients) between neurons. If our blood glucose drops much below normal levels, we become dizzy and light-headed. If blood glucose continues to drop, we become comatose and ultimately die. Under normal, nonstarving conditions, the brain and the rest of the nervous system require roughly 150 g glucose each day.

2. RED BLOOD CELLS

Glucose is the only fuel used by red blood cells, because they lack mitochondria. Fatty acid oxidation, amino acid oxidation, the TCA cycle, the electron transport chain, and oxidative phosphorylation (ATP generation that is dependent on oxygen

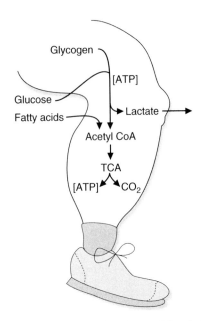

Fig. 2.3 Oxidation of fuels in exercising skeletal muscle. Exercising muscle uses more energy than resting muscle, and, therefore fuel utilization is increased to supply more ATP.

and the electron transport chain) occur principally in mitochondria. Glucose, in contrast, generates ATP from anaerobic glycolysis in the cytosol and, thus, red blood cells obtain all their energy by this process. In anaerobic glycolysis, the pyruvate formed from glucose is converted to lactate and then released into the blood (see Fig. 2.2, circle 9).

Without glucose, red blood cells could not survive. Red blood cells carry O_2 from the lungs to the tissues. Without red blood cells, most of the tissues of the body would suffer from a lack of energy because they require O_2 to completely convert their fuels to CO_2 and H_2O.

3.   MUSCLE

Exercising skeletal muscles can use glucose from the blood or from their own glycogen stores, converting glucose to lactate through glycolysis or oxidizing it completely to CO_2 and H_2O. Muscle also uses other fuels from the blood, such as fatty acids (Fig. 2.3). After a meal, glucose is used by muscle to replenish the glycogen stores that were depleted during exercise. Glucose is transported into muscle cells and converted to glycogen by processes that are stimulated by insulin.

4.   ADIPOSE TISSUE

Insulin stimulates the transport of glucose into adipose cells as well as into muscle cells. Adipocytes oxidize glucose for energy, and they also use glucose as the source of the glycerol moiety of the triacylglycerols they store (see Fig. 2.2, circle 10).

IV. FATE OF LIPOPROTEINS IN THE FED STATE

Two types of lipoproteins, chylomicrons and VLDL, are produced in the fed state. The major function of these lipoproteins is to provide a blood transport system for triacylglycerols, which are very insoluble in water. However, these lipoproteins also contain the lipid cholesterol, which is also somewhat insoluble in water. The triacylglycerols of chylomicrons are formed in intestinal epithelial cells from the products of digestion of dietary triacylglycerols. The triacylglycerols of VLDL are synthesized in the liver.

When these lipoproteins pass through blood vessels in adipose tissue, their triacylglycerols are degraded to fatty acids and glycerol (see Fig. 2.2, circle 12). The fatty acids enter the adipose cells and combine with a glycerol moiety that is produced from blood glucose. The resulting triacylglycerols are stored as large fat droplets in the adipose cells. The remnants of the chylomicrons are cleared from the blood by the liver. The remnants of the VLDL can be cleared by the liver, or they can form low-density lipoprotein (LDL), which is cleared by the liver or by peripheral cells.

Most of us have not even begun to reach the limits of our capacity to store triacylglycerols in adipose tissue. The ability of humans to store fat appears to be limited only by the amount of tissue we can carry without overloading the heart.

V. FATE OF AMINO ACIDS IN THE FED STATE

The amino acids derived from dietary proteins travel from the intestine to the liver in the hepatic portal vein (see Fig. 2.2, circle 3). The liver uses amino acids for the synthesis of serum proteins as well as its own proteins, and for the biosynthesis of nitrogen-containing compounds that need amino acid presursors, such as the

Ivan Applebod's total cholesterol level is now 315 mg/dL, slightly higher than his previous level of 296. (The currently recommended level for total serum cholesterol is 200 mg/dL or less.) His triacylglycerol level is 250 mg/dL (normal is between 60 and 160 mg/dL). These lipid levels clearly indicate that Mr. Applebod has a hyperlipidemia (high level of lipoproteins in the blood) and therefore is at risk for the future development of atherosclerosis and its consequences, such as heart attacks and strokes.

nonessential amino acids, heme, hormones, neurotransmitters, and purine and pyrimidine bases (e.g., adenine and cytosine in DNA). The liver also may oxidize the amino acids or convert them to glucose or ketone bodies and dispose of the nitrogen as the nontoxic compound urea.

Many of the amino acids will go into the peripheral circulation, where they can be used by other tissues for protein synthesis and various biosynthetic pathways, or oxidized for energy (see Fig. 2.2, circle 14). Proteins undergo turnover; they are constantly being synthesized and degraded. The amino acids released by protein breakdown enter the same pool of free amino acids in the blood as the amino acids from the diet. This free amino acid pool in the blood can be used by all cells to provide the right ratio of amino acids for protein synthesis or for biosynthesis of other compounds. In general, each individual biosynthetic pathway using an amino acid precursor is found in only a few tissues in the body.

VI. SUMMARY OF THE FED (ABSORPTIVE) STATE

After a meal, the fuels that we eat are oxidized to meet our immediate energy needs. Glucose is the major fuel for most tissues. Excess glucose and other fuels are stored, as glycogen mainly in muscle and liver, and as triacylglycerols in adipose tissue. Amino acids from dietary proteins are converted to body proteins or oxidized as fuels.

CLINICAL COMMENTS

Ivan Applebod. Mr. Applebod was advised that his obesity represents a risk factor for future heart attacks and strokes. He was told that his body has to maintain a larger volume of circulating blood to service his extra fat tissue. This expanded blood volume not only contributes to his elevated blood pressure (itself a risk factor for vascular disease) but also puts an increased workload on his heart. This increased load will cause his heart muscle to thicken and eventually to fail.

Mr. Applebod's increasing adipose mass has also contributed to his development of type 2 diabetes mellitus, characterized by hyperglycemia (high blood glucose levels). The mechanism behind this breakdown in his ability to maintain normal levels of blood glucose is, at least in part, a resistance by his triacylglycerol-rich adipose cells to the action of insulin.

In addition to diabetes mellitus, Mr. Applebod has a hyperlipidemia (high blood lipid level—elevated cholesterol and triacylglycerols), another risk factor for cardiovascular disease. A genetic basis for Mr. Applebod's disorder is inferred from a positive family history of hypercholesterolemia and premature coronary artery disease in a brother.

At this point, the first therapeutic steps should be nonpharmacologic. Mr. Applebod's obesity should be treated with caloric restriction and a carefully monitored program of exercise. A reduction of dietary fat and sodium would be advised in an effort to correct his hyperlipidemia and his hypertension, respectively.

BIOCHEMICAL COMMENTS

Anthropometric Measurements. Anthropometry uses measurements of body parameters to monitor normal growth and nutritional health in well-nourished individuals and to detect nutritional inadequacies or excesses. In adults, the measurements most commonly used are: height, weight,

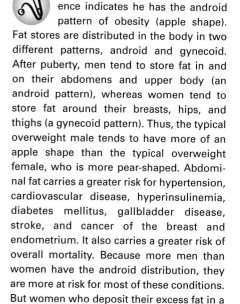

Ivan Applebod's waist circumference indicates he has the android pattern of obesity (apple shape). Fat stores are distributed in the body in two different patterns, android and gynecoid. After puberty, men tend to store fat in and on their abdomens and upper body (an android pattern), whereas women tend to store fat around their breasts, hips, and thighs (a gynecoid pattern). Thus, the typical overweight male tends to have more of an apple shape than the typical overweight female, who is more pear-shaped. Abdominal fat carries a greater risk for hypertension, cardiovascular disease, hyperinsulinemia, diabetes mellitus, gallbladder disease, stroke, and cancer of the breast and endometrium. It also carries a greater risk of overall mortality. Because more men than women have the android distribution, they are more at risk for most of these conditions. But women who deposit their excess fat in a more android manner have a greater risk than women whose fat distribution is more gynecoid.

Upper body fat deposition tends to occur more by hypertrophy of the existing cells, whereas lower body fat deposition is by differentiation of new fat cells (hyperplasia). This may partly explain why many women with lower body obesity have difficulty losing weight.

triceps skinfold thickness, arm muscle circumference, and waist circumference. In infants and young children, length and head circumference are also measured.

Weight and height. Weight should be measured by using a calibrated beam or lever balance-type scale, and the patient should be in a gown or in underwear. Height for adults should be measured while the patient stands against a straight surface, without shoes, with the heels together, and with the head erect and level. The weight and height are used in calculation of the body mass index (BMI).

To obtain reliable measures of skinfold thickness, procedures are carefully defined. For example, in the triceps measurement, a fold of skin in the posterior aspect of the nondominant arm midway between shoulder and elbow is grasped gently and pulled away from the underlying muscle. The skinfold thickness reading is taken at a precise time, 2 to 3 seconds after applying the caliper, because the caliper compresses the skin. Even when these procedures are performed by trained dieticians, reliable measurements are difficult to obtain.

Skinfold thickness. Over half of the fat in the body is deposited in subcutaneous tissue under the skin, and the percentage increases with increasing weight. To provide an estimate of the amount of body fat, a standardized calipers is used to pinch a fold of the skin, usually at more than one site (e.g., the biceps, triceps, subscapular, and suprailiac areas). Obesity by this physical anthropometric technique is defined as a fatfold thickness greater than the 85th percentile for young adults; that is, 18.6 mm for males and 25.1 mm for females.

Mid-Arm Anthropometry. The arm muscle circumference (AMC), also called the mid upper arm muscle circumference (MUAMC), reflects both caloric adequacy and muscle mass and can serve as a general index of marasmic-type malnutrition. The arm circumference is measured at the midpoint of the left upper arm by a fiberglass flexible-type tape. The arm muscle circumference can be calculated from a formula that subtracts a factor related to the skinfold thickness (SFT) from the arm circumference:

$$\text{MUAMC (cm)} = \text{arm circumference (cm)} - (3.14 \times \text{SFT mm})/10$$

Where MUAMC is the mid upper arm muscle circumference in cm and SFT is the skinfold thickness, expressed in millimeters.

MUAMC values can be compared with reference graphs available for both sexes and all ages. Protein–calorie malnutrition and negative nitrogen balance induce muscle wasting and decrease muscle circumference.

The **waist-to-hip ratio** has been used instead of the waist circumference as a measure of abdominal obesity in an attempt to correct for differences between individuals with respect to body type or bone structure. In this measurement, the waist circumference is divided by the hip circumference (measured at the iliac crest). The average waist-to-hip ratio for men is 0.93 (with a range of 0.75–1.10), and the average for women was 0.83 (with a range of 0.70–1.00). However, the waist circumference may actually correlate better with intraabdominal fat and the associated risk factors than the waist-to-hip ratio.

Waist Circumference. The waist circumference is another anthropometric measurement that serves as an indicator of body composition but is used as a measure of obesity and body fat distribution (the "apple shape"), not malnutrition. It is the distance around the natural waist of a standing individual (at the umbilicus). A high-risk waistline is more than 35 inches (88 cm) for women and more than 40 inches (102 cm) for men.

Suggested References

Garrow JS. Obesity. In: Cohen RD, Lewis B, Alberti KGMM, Denman AM, eds. The metabolic and molecular basis of acquired disease. London: Bailliere Tindall, 1990.

A group of articles about obesity and regulation of body weight appeared in Science 1998;280:1363–1390.

REVIEW QUESTIONS—CHAPTER 2

1. During digestion of a mixed meal,

    (A) starch and other polysaccharides are transported to the liver.
    (B) proteins are converted to dipeptides, which enter the blood.
    (C) dietary triacylglycerols are transported in the portal vein to the liver.
    (D) monosaccharides are transported to adipose tissue via the lymphatic system.
    (E) glucose levels increase in the blood.

2. After digestion of a high carbohydrate meal,

    (A) glucagon is released from the pancreas.
    (B) insulin stimulates the transport of glucose into the brain.
    (C) liver and skeletal muscle use glucose as their major fuel.
    (D) skeletal muscles convert glucose to fatty acids.
    (E) red blood cells oxidize glucose to CO_2.

3. Amino acids derived from digestion of dietary protein

    (A) provide nitrogen for synthesis of nonessential amino acids in the liver.
    (B) can be converted to glucose in most tissues.
    (C) cannot be converted to adipose tissue fat.
    (D) release nitrogen that is converted to urea in skeletal muscle.
    (E) are generally converted to body proteins or excreted in the urine.

4. Elevated levels of chylomicrons were measured in the blood of a patient. What dietary therapy would be most helpful in lowering chylomicron levels?

    (A) Decreased intake of calories
    (B) Decreased intake of fat
    (C) Decreased intake of cholesterol
    (D) Decreased intake of starch
    (E) Decreased intake of sugar

5. A male patient exhibited a BMI of 33 kg/m^2 and a waist circumference of 47 inches. What dietary therapy would you consider most helpful?

    (A) Decreased intake of total calories, because all fuels can be converted to adipose tissue triacylglycerols
    (B) The same amount of total calories, but substitution of carbohydrate calories for fat calories
    (C) The same amount of total calories, but substitution of protein calories for fat calories
    (D) A pure-fat diet, because only fatty acids synthesized by the liver can be deposited as adipose triacylglycerols
    (E) A limited food diet, such as the ice cream and sherry diet

3 Fasting

Pathways named with the suffix "lysis" are those in which complex molecules are broken down or "lysed" into smaller units. For instance, in glycogenolysis, glycogen is lysed into glucose subunits; in glycolysis, glucose is lysed into two pyruvate molecules; in lipolysis, triacylglycerols are lysed into fatty acids and glycerol; in proteolysis, proteins are lysed into their constituent amino acids.

Gluconeogenesis means formation (genesis) of new (neo) glucose, and by definition, converts new (noncarbohydrate) precursors to glucose.

Degrees of protein–energy malnutrition (marasmus) are classified according to BMI.

Protein–energy Malnutrition	BMI (kg/cm^2)
I	17.0–18.4
II	16.0–16.9
III	<16.0

Percy Veere has grade I protein–energy malnutrition. At his height of 71 inches, his body weight would have to be above 132 lb to achieve a BMI greater than 18.5. **Ann O'Rexia** has grade III malnutrition. At 66 inches, she needs a body weight greater than 114 lb to achieve a BMI of 18.5.

The Fasting State. Fasting begins approximately 2 to 4 hours after a meal, when blood glucose levels return to basal levels, and continues until blood glucose levels begin to rise after the start of the next meal. Within about 1 hour after a meal, blood glucose levels begin to fall. Consequently, **insulin** *levels decline, and* **glucagon** *levels rise. These changes in hormone levels trigger the* **release of fuels** *from the body stores.* **Liver glycogen** *is* **degraded** *by the process of* **glycogenolysis**, *which supplies glucose to the blood.* **Adipose triacylglycerols** *are* **mobilized** *by the process of* **lipolysis**, *which releases fatty acids and glycerol into the blood. Use of* **fatty acids** *as a fuel increases with the length of the fast; they are the* **major fuel** *oxidized during overnight fasting.*

Fuel Oxidation. During fasting, **glucose** *continues to be* **oxidized** *by* **glucose-dependent tissues** *such as the brain and red blood cells, and* **fatty acids** *are oxidized by tissues such as muscle and liver. Muscle and most other tissues oxidize fatty acids completely to CO_2 and H_2O. However, the* **liver** *partially oxidizes fatty acids to smaller molecules called* **ketone bodies**, *which are released into the blood. Muscle, kidney, and certain other tissues derive energy from completely oxidizing ketone bodies in the tricarboxylic acid (TCA) cycle.*

Maintenance of Blood Glucose. As fasting progresses, the **liver produces glucose** *not only by* **glycogenolysis** *(the release of glucose from glycogen), but also by a second process called* **gluconeogenesis** *(the synthesis of glucose from noncarbohydrate compounds. The major* **sources of carbon** *for gluconeogenesis are* **lactate**, **glycerol**, *and* **amino acids**. *When the carbons of the amino acids are converted to glucose by the liver, their* **nitrogen** *is converted to* **urea**.

Starvation. When we fast for 3 or more days, we are in the starved state. **Muscle** *continues to burn fatty acids but* **decreases** *its use of* **ketone bodies**. *As a result, the concentration of ketone bodies rises in the blood to a level at which the* **brain** *begins to* **oxidize** *them for energy. The brain then needs less glucose, so the liver decreases its rate of gluconeogenesis. Consequently, less* **protein** *in muscle and other tissues is degraded to supply amino acids for gluconeogenesis, Protein sparing preserves vital functions for as long as possible. Because of these changes in the fuel utilization patterns of various tissues, humans can survive for extended periods without ingesting food.*

THE WAITING ROOM

Percy Veere had been admitted to the hospital with a diagnosis of mental depression associated with malnutrition (see Chap. 1). At the time of admission, his body weight of 125 lb gave him a body mass index (BMI) of 17.5 (healthy range, 18.5–24.9). His serum albumin was 10% below the low end of the normal range, and he exhibited signs of iron and vitamin deficiencies.

Additional tests were made to help evaluate Mr. Veere's degree of malnutrition and his progress toward recovery. His arm circumference and triceps skinfold were measured, and his mid upper arm muscle circumference was calculated (see Chap. 2, Anthropometric Measurements). His serum transferrin, as well as his serum albumin, were measured. Fasting blood glucose and serum ketone body concentration were determined on blood samples drawn the next day before breakfast. A 24-hour urine specimen was collected to determine ketone body excretion and creatinine excretion for calculation of the creatinine–height index, a measure of protein depletion from skeletal muscle.

Ann O'Rexia was receiving psychological counseling for anorexia nervosa, but with little success (see Chap. 1). She saw her gynecologist because she had not had a menstrual period for 5 months. She also complained of becoming easily fatigued. The physician recognized that Ann's body weight of 85 lb was now less than 65% of her ideal weight. (Her BMI was now 13.7.) The physician recommended immediate hospitalization. The admission diagnosis was severe malnutrition secondary to anorexia nervosa. Clinical findings included decreased body core temperature, blood pressure, and pulse (adaptive responses to malnutrition). Her physician ordered measurements of blood glucose and ketone body levels and made a spot check for ketone bodies in the urine as well as ordering tests to assess the functioning of her heart and kidneys.

I. THE FASTING STATE

Blood glucose levels peak approximately 1 hour after eating and then decrease as tissues oxidize glucose or convert it to storage forms of fuel. By 2 hours after a meal, the level returns to the fasting range (between 80 and 100 mg/dL). This decrease in blood glucose causes the pancreas to decrease its secretion of insulin, and the serum insulin level decreases. The liver responds to this hormonal signal by starting to degrade its glycogen stores and release glucose into the blood.

If we eat another meal within a few hours, we return to the fed state. However, if we continue to fast for a 12-hour period, we enter the basal state (also known as the postabsorptive state). A person is generally considered to be in the basal state after an overnight fast, when no food has been eaten since dinner the previous evening. By this time, the serum insulin level is low and glucagon is rising. Figure 3.1 illustrates the main features of the basal state.

A. Blood Glucose and the Role of the Liver during Fasting

The liver maintains blood glucose levels during fasting, and its role is thus critical. Glucose is the major fuel for tissues such as the brain and neural tissue, and the sole fuel for red blood cells. Most neurons lack enzymes required for oxidation of fatty acids, but can use ketone bodies to a limited extent. Red blood cells lack mitochondria, which contain the enzymes of fatty acid and ketone body oxidation, and can use only glucose as a fuel. Therefore, it is imperative that blood glucose not decrease too rapidly nor fall too low.

Initially, liver glycogen stores are degraded to supply glucose to the blood, but these stores are limited. Although liver glycogen levels may increase to 200 to 300 g after a meal, only approximately 80 g remain after an overnight fast. Fortunately, the liver has another mechanism for producing blood glucose, known as gluconeogenesis. In gluconeogenesis, lactate, glycerol, and amino acids are used as carbon sources to synthesize glucose. As fasting continues, gluconeogenesis progressively adds to the glucose produced by glycogenolysis in the liver.

Percy Veere had not eaten much on his first day of hospitalization. His fasting blood glucose determined on the morning of his second day of hospitalization was 72 mg/dL (normal, overnight fasting = 80–100 mg/dL). Thus, in spite of his malnutrition and his overnight fast, his blood glucose was being maintained at nearly normal levels through gluconeogenesis using amino acid precursors. If his blood glucose had decreased below 50 to 60 mg/dL during fasting, his brain would have been unable to absorb glucose fast enough to obtain the glucose needed for energy and neurotransmitter synthesis, resulting in coma and eventual death. Although many other tissues, such as the red blood cell, are also totally or partially dependent on glucose for energy, they are able to function at lower concentrations of blood glucose than the brain.

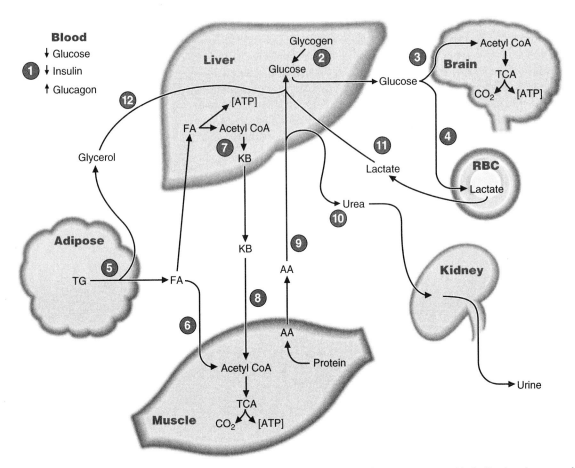

Fig. 3.1. Basal state. This state occurs after an overnight (12-hour) fast. The circled numbers serve as a guide indicating the approximate order in which the processes begin to occur. KB = ketone bodies. Other abbreviations are defined in Figure 2.1.

Lactate is a product of glycolysis in red blood cells and exercising muscle, glycerol is obtained from lipolysis of adipose triacylglycerols, and amino acids are generated by the breakdown of protein. Because our muscle mass is so large, most of the amino acid is supplied from degradation of muscle protein. These compounds travel in the blood to the liver, where they are converted to glucose by gluconeogenesis. Because the nitrogen of the amino acids can form ammonia, which is toxic to the body, the liver converts this nitrogen to urea. Urea has two amino groups for just one carbon (NH_2-CO-NH_2). It is a very soluble, nontoxic compound that can be readily excreted by the kidneys and thus is an efficient means for disposing of excess ammonia.

As fasting progresses, gluconeogenesis becomes increasingly more important as a source of blood glucose. After a day or so of fasting, liver glycogen stores are depleted and gluconeogenesis is the only source of blood glucose.

B. Role of Adipose Tissue During Fasting

Adipose triacylglycerols are the major source of energy during fasting. They supply fatty acids, which are quantitatively the major fuel for the human body. Fatty acids are not only oxidized directly by various tissues of the body; they are also partially oxidized in the liver to 4-carbon products called ketone bodies. Ketone bodies are subsequently oxidized as a fuel by other tissues.

As blood insulin levels decrease and blood glucagon levels rise, adipose triacylglycerols are mobilized by a process known as lipolysis. They are converted to fatty acids and glycerol, which enter the blood.

On the second day of hospitalization, **Percy Veere's** serum ketone body level was 110 μM. (Normal valve after a 12-hour fast, is approximately 70 μM.) No ketone bodies were detectable in his urine. At this stage of protein–energy malnutrition, Mr. Veere still has remaining fat stores. After 12 hours of fasting, most of his tissues are using fatty acids as a major fuel, and the liver is beginning to produce ketone bodies from fatty acids. As these ketone bodies increase in the blood, their use as a fuel will increase.

It is important to realize that most fatty acids cannot provide carbon for gluconeogenesis. Thus, of the vast store of food energy in adipose tissue triacylglycerols, only the small glycerol portion travels to the liver to enter the gluconeogenic pathway.

Fatty acids serve as a fuel for muscle, kidney, and most other tissues. They are oxidized to acetyl CoA, and subsequently to CO_2 and H_2O in the TCA cycle, producing energy in the form of adenosine triphosphate (ATP). In addition to the ATP required to maintain cellular integrity, muscle uses ATP for contraction, and the kidney uses it for urinary transport processes.

Most of the fatty acids that enter the liver are converted to ketone bodies rather than being completely oxidized to CO_2. The process of conversion of fatty acids to acetyl CoA produces a considerable amount of energy (ATP), which drives the reactions of the liver under these conditions. The acetyl CoA is converted to the ketone bodies acetoacetate and β-hydroxybutyrate, which are released into the blood (Fig. 3.2).

The liver lacks an enzyme required for ketone body oxidation. However, ketone bodies can be further oxidized by most other cells with mitochondria, such as muscle and kidney. In these tissues, acetoacetate and β-hydroxybutyrate are converted to acetyl CoA and then oxidized in the TCA cycle, with subsequent generation of ATP.

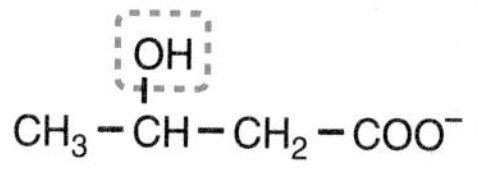

C. Summary of the Metabolic Changes during a Brief Fast

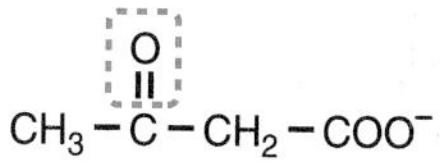

In the initial stages of fasting, stored fuels are used for energy (see Fig. 3.1). The liver plays a key role by maintaining blood glucose levels in the range of 80 to 100 mg/dL, first by glycogenolysis and subsequently by gluconeogenesis. Lactate, glycerol, and amino acids serve as carbon sources for gluconeogenesis. Amino acids are supplied by muscle. Their nitrogen is converted in the liver to urea, which is excreted by the kidneys.

Fatty acids, which are released from adipose tissue by the process of lipolysis, serve as the body's major fuel during fasting. The liver oxidizes most of its fatty acids only partially, converting them to ketone bodies, which are released into the blood. Thus, during the initial stages of fasting, blood levels of fatty acids and ketone bodies begin to increase. Muscle uses fatty acids, ketone bodies, and (when exercising and while supplies last) glucose from muscle glycogen. Many other tissues use either fatty acids or ketone bodies. However, red blood cells, the brain, and other neural tissues use mainly glucose. The metabolic capacities of different tissues with respect to pathways of fuel metabolism are summarized in Table 3.1.

II. METABOLIC CHANGES DURING PROLONGED FASTING

If the pattern of fuel utilization that occurs during a brief fast were to persist for an extended period, the body's protein would be quite rapidly consumed to the point at which critical functions would be compromised. Fortunately, metabolic changes occur during prolonged fasting that conserve (spare) muscle protein by causing muscle protein turnover to decrease. Figure 3.3 shows the main features of metabolism during prolonged fasting (starvation).

B. Role of Liver During Prolonged Fasting

After 3 to 5 days of fasting, when the body enters the starved state, muscle decreases its use of ketone bodies and depends mainly on fatty acids for its fuel. The

Fig. 3.2. β-Hydroxybutyrate and acetoacetate. These compounds are ketone bodies formed in the liver. A third ketone body, acetone (CH_3-CO-CH_3), is produced by nonenzymatic decarboxylation of acetoacetate. However, acetone is expired in the breath and not metabolized to a significant extent in the body.

The liver synthesizes a number of serum proteins and releases them into the blood. These proteins decrease in the blood during protein malnutrition. Two of these serum proteins, albumin and transferrin (an iron-binding transport protein), are often measured to assess the state of protein malnutrition. Serum albumin is the traditional standard of protein malnutrition. Neither measurement is specific for protein malnutrition. Serum albumin and transferrin levels decrease with hepatic disease, certain renal diseases, surgery, and a number of other conditions, in addition to protein malnutrition. Serum transferrin levels also decrease in iron deficiency. **Percy Veere's** values were below the normal range for both of these proteins, indicating that his muscle mass is unable to supply sufficient amino acids to sustain both synthesis of serum proteins by the liver and gluconeogenesis.

Table 3.1. Metabolic Capacities of Various Tissues

Process	Liver	Adipose Tissue	Kidney Cortex	Muscle	Brain	RBC
TCA cycle (acetyl CoA → CO_2 + H_2O)	+++	++	+++	+++	+++	−−
β-Oxidation of fatty acids	+++	−−	++	+++	−−	−−
Ketone body formation	+++	−−	+	−−	−−	−−
Ketone body utilization	−−	+	+	+++	+++ (prolonged starvation)	−−
Glycolysis (glucose → CO_2 + H_2O)	+++	++	++	+++	+++	−−
Lactate production (glucose → lactate)	+	+	−−−	+++ exercise	+	+++
Glycogen metabolism (synthesis and degradation)	+++	+	+	+++	+	−−
Gluconeogenesis (lactate, amino acids, glycerol → glucose)	+++	−−	+	−−	−−	−−
Urea cycle (ammonia → urea)	+++	−−	−−	−−	−−	−−
Lipogenesis (glucose → fatty acids)	+++	+	−−	−−	−−	−−

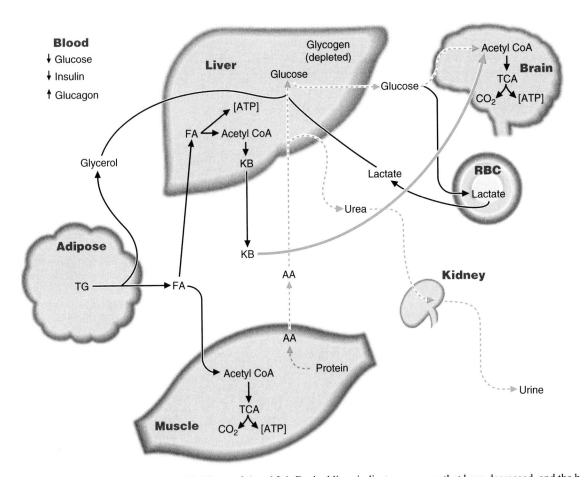

Fig. 3.3. Starved state. Abbreviations are defined in Figures 2.1 and 3.1. Dashed lines indicate processes that have decreased, and the heavy solid line indicates a process that has increased relative to the fasting state.

liver, however, continues to convert fatty acids to ketone bodies. The result is that the concentration of ketone bodies rises in the blood (Fig. 3.4). The brain begins to take up these ketone bodies from the blood and to oxidize them for energy. Therefore, the brain needs less glucose than it did after an overnight fast (Table 3.2).

Glucose is still required, however, as an energy source for red blood cells, and the brain continues to use a limited amount of glucose, which it oxidizes for energy and uses as a source of carbon for the synthesis of neurotransmitters. Overall, however, glucose is "spared" (conserved). Less glucose is used by the body, and, therefore, the liver needs to produce less glucose per hour during prolonged fasting than during shorter periods of fasting.

Because the stores of glycogen in the liver are depleted by approximately 30 hours of fasting, gluconeogenesis is the only process by which the liver can supply glucose to the blood if fasting continues. The amino acid pool, produced by the breakdown of protein, continues to serve as a major source of carbon for gluconeogenesis. A fraction of this amino acid pool is also being used for biosynthetic functions (e.g., synthesis of heme and neurotransmitters) and new protein synthesis, processes that must continue during fasting. However, as a result of the decreased rate of gluconeogenesis during prolonged fasting, protein is "spared"; less protein is degraded to supply amino acids for gluconeogenesis.

While converting amino acid carbon to glucose in gluconeogenesis, the liver also converts the nitrogen of these amino acids to urea. Consequently, because glucose production decreases during prolonged fasting compared with early fasting, urea production also decreases (Fig. 3.5).

B. Role of Adipose Tissue During Prolonged Fasting

During prolonged fasting, adipose tissue continues to break down its triacylglycerol stores, providing fatty acids and glycerol to the blood. These fatty acids serve as the major source of fuel for the body. The glycerol is converted to glucose, whereas the fatty acids are oxidized to CO_2 and H_2O by tissues such as muscle. In the liver, fatty acids are converted to ketone bodies that are oxidized by many tissues, including the brain.

A number of factors determine how long we can fast and still survive. The amount of adipose tissue is one factor, because adipose tissue supplies the body with its major source of fuel. However, body protein levels can also determine the length of time we can fast. Glucose is still used during prolonged fasting (starvation), but in greatly reduced amounts. Although we degrade protein to supply amino acids for gluconeogenesis at a slower rate during starvation than during the first days of a fast, we are still losing protein that serves vital functions for our tissues. Protein can become so depleted that the heart, kidney, and other vital tissues stop functioning, or we can develop an infection and not have adequate reserves to mount an immune response. In addition to fuel problems, we are also deprived of the vitamin and mineral precursors of coenzymes and other compounds necessary for tissue function. Because of either a lack of ATP or a decreased intake of electrolytes, the electrolyte composition of the blood or cells could become incompatible with life. Ultimately, we die of starvation.

Table 3.2. Metabolic Changes during Prolonged Fasting Compared with Fasting 24 Hours

Muscle	↓	Use of ketone bodies
Brain	↑	Use of ketone bodies
Liver	↓	Gluconeogenesis
Muscle	↓	Protein degradation
Liver	↓	Production of urea

 Ann O'Rexia's admission laboratory studies showed a blood glucose level of 65 mg/dL (normal fasting blood glucose = 80 – 100 mg/dL). Her serum ketone body concentration was 4,200 μM (normal = ~70 μM). The Ketostix (Bayer Diagnostics, Mishawaha, IN) urine test was moderately positive, indicating that ketone bodies were present in the urine. In her starved state, ketone body use by her brain is helping to conserve protein in her muscles and vital organs.

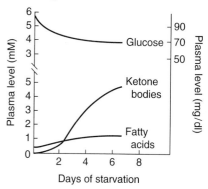

Fig. 3.4. Changes in the concentration of fuels in the blood during prolonged fasting.

 Death by starvation occurs with loss of roughly 40% of body weight, when approximately 30 to 50% of body protein has been lost, or 70 to 95% of body fat stores. Generally, this occurs at BMIs of approximately 13 for men, and 11 for women.

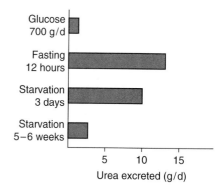

Fig. 3.5. Changes in urea excretion during fasting. Urea production is very low in a person consuming only glucose. It increases during fasting as muscle protein is broken down to supply amino acids for gluconeogenesis. However, as fasting progresses, urea synthesis decreases. Because the brain meets some of its energy needs by oxidizing ketone bodies after 3 to 5 days of fasting, gluconeogenesis decreases, sparing protein in muscle and other tissues.

Creatinine–Height Index. The most widely used biochemical marker for estimating body muscle mass is the 24-hour urinary creatinine excretion. Creatinine is a degradation product formed in active muscle at a constant rate, in proportion to the amount of muscle tissue present in a patient. In a protein-malnourished individual, urinary creatinine will decrease in proportion to the decrease in muscle mass. To assess depletion of muscle mass, creatinine excreted is expressed relative to the height, the creatinine–height index (CHI). The amount of creatinine (in milligrams) excreted by the subject in 24 hours is divided by the amount of creatinine excreted by a normal, healthy subject of the same height and sex. The resulting ratio is multiplied by 100 to express it as a percentage. **Percy Veere**'s CHI was 85% (80–90% of normal indicates a mild deficit; 60–80% indicates a moderate deficit; less than 60% of normal indicates a severe deficit of muscle mass).

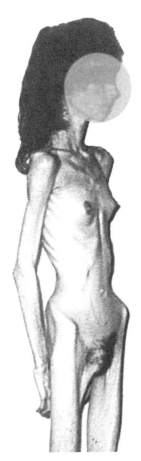

Fig. 3.6. Photograph of a patient with anorexia nervosa. From a MedCom slide, 1970.

CLINICAL COMMENTS

Percy Veere. As a result of his severely suppressed appetite for food, Percy Veere has developed a mild degree of protein–calorie malnutrition. When prolonged, this type of protein malnutrition can cause changes in the villi of the small intestine that reduce its absorptive capacity for what little food is ingested.

Despite his insufficient intake of dietary carbohydrates, Mr. Veere's blood glucose level is 72 mg/dL, close to the lower limit (80 mg/dL) of the normal range for a well-nourished, healthy person after a 12-hour fast. This is the finding you would expect; it reflects the liver's capacity to maintain adequate levels of blood glucose by means of gluconeogenesis, even during prolonged and moderately severe caloric restriction. Amino acids from degradation of protein, principally in skeletal muscle, supply most of the precursors for gluconeogenesis.

Percy Veere has several indicators of his protein malnutrition: his serum albumin and transferrin levels are below normal, his mid-upper-arm muscle circumference (MUAMC) is at the 12th percentile, and his creatinine–height index (CHI) was at 85%. The low levels of serum proteins reflect a low dietary protein intake, and possibly diminished capacity to absorb dietary amino acids. Consequently, amino acids are being mobilized from degradation of protein in muscle and other tissues to supply precursors for new protein synthesis as well as gluconeogenesis. The result is a loss of muscle mass, indicated by the MUAMC and the CHI, and decreased levels of serum proteins.

Fatty acids mobilized from adipose tissue are the major source of energy for most tissues. Because he is eating, and not in total starvation, his ketone bodies were only moderately elevated in the blood (110 μM vs. normal of 70 μM) and did not appear in the urine.

After several psychological counseling sessions, and the promise of an extended visit from his grandchild, Mr. Veere resumed his normal eating pattern.

Ann O'Rexia. Ann O'Rexia has anorexia nervosa, a chronic disabling disease in which poorly understood psychological and biologic factors lead to disturbances in the patient's body image. These patients typically pursue thinness in spite of the presence of severe emaciation and a "skeletal appearance" (Fig. 3.6). They generally have an intense fear of being overweight and deny the seriousness of their low body weight.

Amenorrhea (lack of menses) usually develops during anorexia nervosa and other conditions when a woman's body fat content falls to approximately 22% of her total body weight. The immediate cause of amenorrhea is a reduced production of the gonadotropic protein hormones (luteinizing hormone and follicle-stimulating hormone) by the anterior pituitary; the connection between this hormonal change and body fat content is not yet understood.

Ms. O'Rexia is suffering from the consequences of prolonged and severe protein and caloric restriction. Fatty acids, released from adipose tissue by lipolysis, are being converted to ketone bodies in the liver, and the level of ketone bodies in the blood is extremely elevated (4,200 μM vs. normal of 70 μM). The fact that her kidneys are excreting ketone bodies is reflected in the moderately positive urine test for ketone bodies noted on admission.

Although Ms. O'Rexia's blood glucose is below the normal fasting range (65 mg/dL vs. normal of 80 mg/dL), she is experiencing only a moderate degree of hypoglycemia (low blood glucose) despite her severe, near starvation diet. Her blood glucose level reflects the ability of the brain to use ketone bodies as a fuel when they are elevated in the blood, thereby decreasing the amount of glucose that must be synthesized from amino acids provided by protein degradation.

Ms. O'Rexia's BMI showed that she was close to death through starvation. She was therefore hospitalized and placed on enteral nutrition (nutrients provided through tube feeding). The general therapeutic plan, outlined in Chapter 1, of nutritional restitution and identification and treatment of those emotional factors leading to the patient's anorectic behavior was continued. She was coaxed into eating small amounts of food while hospitalized.

BIOCHEMICAL COMMENTS

Clinical Use of Metabolite Measurements in Blood and Urine. When a patient develops a metabolic problem, it is difficult to examine cells to determine the cause. To obtain tissue for metabolic studies, biopsies must be performed. These procedures can be difficult, dangerous, or even impossible, depending on the tissue. Cost is an additional problem. However, both blood and urine can be obtained readily from patients, and measurements of substances in the blood and urine can help in diagnosing a patient's problem. Concentrations of substances that are higher or lower than normal indicate which tissues are malfunctioning. For example, if blood urea nitrogen (BUN) levels are low, a problem centered in the liver might be suspected because urea is produced in the liver. Conversely, high blood levels of urea suggest that the kidney is not excreting this compound normally. Decreased urinary and blood levels of creatinine indicate diminished production of creatinine by skeletal muscle. However, high blood creatinine levels could indicate an inability of the kidney to excrete creatinine, resulting from renal disease. If high levels of ketone bodies are found in the blood or urine, the patient's metabolic pattern is that of the starved state. If the high levels of ketone bodies are coupled with elevated levels of blood glucose, the problem is most likely a deficiency of insulin; that is, the patient probably has type 1, formerly called insulin-dependent, diabetes mellitus. Without insulin, fuels are mobilized from tissues rather than being stored.

These relatively easy and inexpensive tests on blood and urine can be used to determine which tissues need to be studied more extensively to diagnose and treat the patient's problem. A solid understanding of fuel metabolism helps in the interpretation of these simple tests.

Suggested References

Owen OE, Tappy L, Mozzoli MA, Smalley KJ. Acute starvation. In: Cohen RD, Lewis B, Alberti KGMM, Denman AM (eds). The Metabolic and Molecular Basis of Acquired Disease. London: Bailliere Tindall, 1990.

Walsh BT, Devlin MJ. Eating disorders: progress and problems. Science 1998;280:1387–1390.

 REVIEW QUESTIONS—CHAPTER 3

You will need some information from Chapters 1 and 2, as well as Chapter 3, to answer these questions.

1. By 24 hours after a meal,

    (A) gluconeogenesis in the liver is the major source of blood glucose.
    (B) muscle glycogenolysis provides glucose to the blood.
    (C) muscles convert amino acids to blood glucose.
    (D) fatty acids released from adipose tissue provide carbon for synthesis of glucose.
    (E) ketone bodies provide carbon for gluconeogenesis.

2.   The liver is the only tissue that

    (A) contains significant glycogen stores.
    (B) oxidizes fatty acids during overnight fasting.
    (C) oxidizes ketone bodies during overnight fasting.
    (D) converts ammonia to urea.
    (E) converts glucose to lactate.

3.   In a well-nourished individual, as the length of fasting increases from overnight to 1 week,

    (A) blood glucose levels decrease by approximately 50%.
    (B) red blood cells switch to using ketone bodies.
    (C) muscles decrease their use of ketone bodies, which increase in the blood.
    (D) the brain begins to use fatty acids as a major fuel.
    (E) adipose tissue triacylglycerols are nearly depleted.

4.   A hospitalized patient had low levels of serum albumin and high levels of blood ammonia. His CHI was 98%. His BMI was 20.5. Blood urea nitrogen was not elevated, consistent with normal kidney function. The diagnosis most consistent with these finding is

    (A) loss of hepatic function (e.g., alcohol-induced cirrhosis).
    (B) anorexia nervosa.
    (C) kwashiorkor (protein malnutrition).
    (D) marasmus (protein–energy malnutrition).
    (E) decreased absorption of amino acids by intestinal epithelial cells (e.g., celiac disease).

5.   Otto Shape, an overweight medical student (see Chapter 1), discovered that he could not exercise enough during his summer clerkship rotations to lose 2 to 3 lb per week. He decided to lose weight by eating only 300 kcal/day of a dietary supplement that provided half the calories as carbohydrate and half as protein. In addition, he consumed a multivitamin supplement. During the first 3 days on this diet,

    (A) his protein intake met the RDA for protein.
    (B) his carbohydrate intake met the fuel needs of his brain.
    (C) both his adipose mass and his muscle mass decreased.
    (D) he remained in nitrogen balance.
    (E) he developed severe hypoglycemia.

Chemical and Biological Foundations of Biochemistry

The discipline of biochemistry developed as chemists began to study the molecules of cells, tissues, and body fluids and physicians began to look for the molecular basis of various diseases. Today, the practice of medicine depends on understanding the roles and interactions of the enormous number of different chemicals enabling our bodies to function. The task is less overwhelming if one knows the properties, nomenclature and function of classes of compounds, such as carbohydrates and enzymes. The intent of this section is to review some of this information in a context relevant to medicine. Students enter medical school with different scientific backgrounds and some of the information in this section will, therefore, be familiar to many students.

We begin by discussing the relationship of metabolic acids and buffers to blood pH in Chapter 4. Chapter 5 focuses on the nomenclature, structure, and some of the properties of the major classes of compounds found in the human body. The structure of a molecule determines its function and its fate, and the common name of a compound can often tell you something about its structure.

Proteins are linear chains of amino acids that fold into complex 3-dimensional structures. They function in the maintenance of cellular and tissue structure and the transport and movement of molecules. Some proteins are enzymes, which are catalysts that enormously increase the rate of chemical reactions in the body. Chapters 6 and 7 describe the amino acids and their interactions within proteins that provide proteins with a flexible and functional 3-dimensional structure. Chapters 8 and 9 describe the properties, functions, and regulation of enzymes.

Our proteins and other compounds function within a specialized environment defined by their location in cells or body fluids. Their ability to function is partially dependent on membranes that restrict the free movement of molecules. Chapter 10 includes a brief review of the components of cells, their organization into subcellular organelles, and the manner in which various types of molecules move into cells and between compartments within a cell.

In a complex organism like the human, different cell types carry out different functions. This specialization of function requires cells to communicate with each other. One of the ways they communicate is through secretion of chemical messengers that carry a signal to another cell. In Chapter 11, we consider some of the principles of cell signaling and describe some of the chemical messenger systems.

Both in this book and in medical practice, you will need to interconvert different units used for the weight and size of compounds and for their concentration in blood and other fluids. Table 1 provides definitions of some of the units used for these interconversions.

The nomenclature used to describe patients may include the name of a class of compounds. For example a patient with diabetes mellitus who has hyperglycemia has hyper (high) concentrations of carbohydrates (glyc) in her blood (emia).

From a biochemist's point of view, most metabolic diseases are caused by enzymes and other proteins that malfunction and the pharmacological drugs used to treat these diseases correct that malfunction. For example, individuals with atherosclerosis, who have elevated blood cholesterol levels, are treated with a drug that inhibits an enzyme in the pathway for cholesterol synthesis. Even a bacterial infection can be considered a disease of protein function, if one considers the bacterial toxins that are proteins, the enzymes in our cells affected by these toxins, and the proteins involved in the immune response when we try to destroy these bacteria.

Q: Di Abietes had an elevated blood glucose level of 684 mg/dL. What is the molar concentration of glucose in Di's blood? (Hint: the molecular weight of glucose ($C_6H_{12}O_6$) is 180 grams per mole.)

A: mg/dL is the common way clinicians in the United States express blood glucose concentration. A concentration of 684 mg/dL is 684 mg per 100 mL of blood, or 6,480 mg per one liter (L), or 6.48 g/L. If 6.84 g/L is divided by 180 grams per mole, one obtains a value of 0.038 mol/L, which is 0.038 M, or 38 mM.

Table 1 Common Units Expressed in Equivalent Ways

1 M	1 mol/L	molecular weight in g/L
1 mM	1 millimol/L	10^{-3} mol/L
1 mM	1 micromol/L	10^{-6} mol/L
1 μM	1 nanomol/L	10^{-9} mol/L
1 mL	1 milliliter	10^{-3} L
1 mg%	1 mg/100 mL	10^{-3} g/100 mL
1 mg/dL	1 mg/100 mL	10^{-3} g/100 mL
1 mEq/L	1 milliequivalent/L	mM X valence of ion
1 kg	1000 g	2.2 lbs (pounds)
1 cm	10^{-2} m	0.394 inches

4   Water, Acids, Bases, and Buffers

Approximately 60% of our body is water. It acts as a solvent for the substances we need, such as K^+, glucose, adenosine triphosphate (ATP), and proteins. It is important for the transport of molecules and heat. Many of the compounds produced in the body and dissolved in water contain chemical groups that act as acids or bases, releasing or accepting hydrogen ions. The hydrogen ion content and the amount of body water are controlled to maintain a constant environment for the cells called homeostasis (same state) (Fig. 4.1). Significant deviations from a constant environment, such as acidosis or dehydration, may be life-threatening. This chapter describes the role of water in the body and the buffer systems used by the body to protect itself from acids and bases produced from metabolism.

Water. *Water is distributed between intracellular and extracellular compartments, the latter comprising interstitial fluids, blood, and lymph. Because water is a **dipolar molecule** with an uneven distribution of electrons between the hydrogen and oxygen atoms, it forms hydrogen bonds with other polar molecules and acts as a **solvent**.*

The pH of water. *Water dissociates to a slight extent **to form hydrogen (H^+) and hydroxyl (OH^-) ions**. The concentration of hydrogen ions determines the acidity of the solution, which is expressed in terms of **pH**. The pH of a solution is the negative log of its hydrogen ion concentration.*

Acids and Bases. *An **acid** is a substance that can **release hydrogen ions** (protons), and a **base** is a substance that can **accept hydrogen ions**. When dissolved in water, almost all the molecules of a **strong acid** dissociate and release their hydrogen ions, but only a small percentage of the total molecules of a weak acid dissociate. A **weak acid** has a characteristic **dissociation constant, K_a**. The relationship between the pH of a solution, the K_a of an acid, and the extent of its dissociation are given by the **Henderson-Hasselbalch equation**.*

Buffers. *A buffer is a mixture of an **undissociated acid** and its **conjugate base** (the form of the acid having lost its proton). It causes a solution to resist changes in pH when either H^+ or OH^- is added. A buffer has its greatest buffering capacity in the pH range near its **pK_a** (the negative log of its K_a). Two factors determine the effectiveness of a buffer, its pK_a relative to the pH of the solution and its concentration.*

Metabolic Acids and Bases. *Normal metabolism generates CO_2, **metabolic acids** (e.g., **lactic acid** and **ketone bodies**) and **inorganic acids** (e.g., **sulfuric acid**). The major source of acid is CO_2, which reacts with water to produce **carbonic acid**. To maintain the pH of body fluids in a range compatible with life, the body has **buffers** such as **bicarbonate, phosphate,** and **hemoglobin** (see Fig 4.1). Ultimately, **respiratory mechanisms** remove carbonic acid through the **expiration of CO_2**, and the **kidneys excrete acid** as **ammonium ion (NH_4^+)** and other ions.*

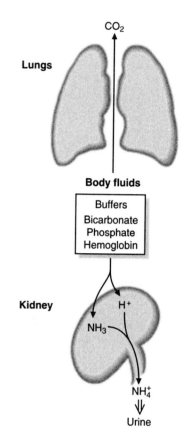

Fig. 4.1. Maintenance of body pH. The body produces approximately 13 to 22 moles of acid per day from normal metabolism. The body protects itself against this acidity by buffers that maintain a neutral pH and by the expiration of CO_2 through the lungs and the excretion of NH_4^+ and other ions through the kidney.

Di Abietes has a ketoacidosis. When the amount of insulin she injects is inadequate, she remains in a condition similar to a fasting state even though she ingests food (see Chapters 2 and 3). Her liver continues to metabolize fatty acids to the ketone bodies acetoacetic acid and β-hydroxybutyric acid. These compounds are weak acids that dissociate to produce anions (acetoacetate and β–hydroxybutyrate, respectively) and hydrogen ions, thereby lowering her blood and cellular pH below the normal range.

THE WAITING ROOM

Dianne (Di) Abietes is a 26-year-old woman who was diagnosed with type 1 diabetes mellitus at the age of 12 years. She has an absolute insulin deficiency resulting from autoimmune destruction of the β-cells of her pancreas. As a result, she depends on daily injections of insulin to prevent severe elevations of glucose and ketone bodies in her blood.

When **Di Abietes** could not be aroused from an afternoon nap, her roommate called an ambulance, and Di was brought to the emergency room of the hospital in a coma. Her roommate reported that Di had been feeling nauseated and drowsy and had been vomiting for 24 hours. Di is clinically dehydrated, and her blood pressure is low. Her respirations are deep and rapid, and her pulse rate is rapid. Her breath has the "fruity" odor of acetone.

Blood samples are drawn for measurement of her arterial blood pH, arterial partial pressure of carbon dioxide ($PaCO_2$), serum glucose, and serum bicarbonate (HCO_3^-). In addition, serum and urine are tested for the presence of ketone bodies, and Di is treated with intravenous normal saline and insulin. The laboratory reports that her blood pH is 7.08 (reference range $= 7.36 - 7.44$) and that ketone bodies are present in both blood and urine. Her blood glucose level is 648 mg/dL (reference range $= 80 - 110$ after an overnight fast, and no higher than 200 in a casual glucose sample taken without regard to the time of a last meal).

Percy Veere is a 59-year-old schoolteacher who persevered through a period of malnutrition associated with mental depression precipitated by the death of his wife (see Chapters 1 and 3). Since his recovery, he has been looking forward to an extended visit from his grandson.

Dennis "the Menace" Veere, age 3 years, was brought to the emergency department by his grandfather, **Percy Veere.** While Dennis was visiting his grandfather, he climbed up on a chair and took a half-full 500-tablet bottle of 325-mg aspirin (acetylsalicylic acid) tablets from the kitchen counter. Mr. Veere discovered Dennis with a mouthful of aspirin, which he removed, but he could not tell how many tablets Dennis had already swallowed. When they arrived at the emergency room, the child appeared bright and alert, but Mr. Veere was hyperventilating.

I. WATER

Water is the solvent of life. It bathes our cells, dissolves and transports compounds in the blood, provides a medium for movement of molecules into and throughout cellular compartments, separates charged molecules, dissipates heat, and participates in chemical reactions. Most compounds in the body, including proteins, must interact with an aqueous medium function. In spite of the variation in the amount of water we ingest each day and produce from metabolism, our body maintains a nearly constant amount of water that is approximately 60% of our body weight (Fig. 4.2).

A. Fluid Compartments in the Body

Total body water is roughly 50 to 60% of body weight in adults and 75% of body weight in children. Because fat has relatively little water associated with it, obese people tend to have a lower percentage of body water than thin people, women tend to have a lower percentage than men, and older people have a lower percentage than younger people.

Approximately 40% of the total body water is intracellular and 60% extracellular. The extracellular water includes the fluid in plasma (blood after the cells have been removed) and interstitial water (the fluid in the tissue spaces, lying between

A. Total body water

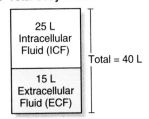

B. Extracellular fluid

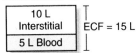

Fig. 4.2. Fluid compartments in the body based on an average 70-kg man.

cells). Transcellular water is a small, specialized portion of extracellular water that includes gastrointestinal secretions, urine, sweat, and fluid that has leaked through capillary walls because of such processes as increased hydrostatic pressure or inflammation.

B. Hydrogen Bonds in Water

The dipolar nature of the water (H_2O) molecule allows it to form hydrogen bonds, a property that is responsible for the role of water as a solvent. In H_2O, the oxygen atom has two unshared electrons that form an electron dense cloud around it. This cloud lies above and below the plane formed by the water molecule (Fig. 4.3). In the covalent bond formed between the hydrogen and oxygen atoms, the shared electrons are attracted toward the oxygen atom, thus giving the oxygen atom a partial negative charge and the hydrogen atom a partial positive charge. As a result, the oxygen side of the molecule is much more electronegative than the hydrogen side, and the molecule is dipolar.

Both the hydrogen and oxygen atoms of the water molecule form hydrogen bonds and participate in hydration shells. A hydrogen bond is a weak noncovalent interaction between the hydrogen of one molecule and the more electronegative atom of an acceptor molecule. The oxygen of water can form hydrogen bonds with two other water molecules, so that each water molecule is hydrogen-bonded to approximately four close neighboring water molecules in a fluid three-dimensional lattice (see Fig. 4.3).

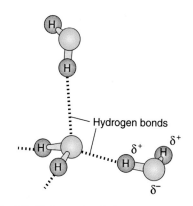

Fig. 4.3. Hydrogen bonds between water molecules. The oxygen atoms are shown in blue.

1. WATER AS A SOLVENT

Polar organic molecules and inorganic salts can readily dissolve in water because water also forms hydrogen bonds and electrostatic interactions with these molecules. Organic molecules containing a high proportion of electronegative atoms (generally oxygen or nitrogen) are soluble in water because these atoms participate in hydrogen bonding with water molecules (Fig. 4.4). Chloride (Cl^-), bicarbonate (HCO_3^-), and other anions are surrounded by a hydration shell of water molecules arranged with their hydrogen atoms closest to the anion. In a similar fashion, the oxygen atom of water molecules interacts with inorganic cations such as Na^+ and K^+ to surround them with a hydration shell.

Although hydrogen bonds are strong enough to dissolve polar molecules in water and to separate charges, they are weak enough to allow movement of water and solutes. The strength of the hydrogen bond between two water molecules is only approximately 4 kcal, roughly 1/20th of the strength of the covalent O–H bond in the water molecule. Thus, the extensive water lattice is dynamic and has many strained bonds that are continuously breaking and reforming. The average hydrogen bond between water molecules lasts only about 10 psec (1 picosecond is 10^{-12} sec), and each water molecule in the hydration shell of an ion stays only 2.4 nsec (1 nanosecond = 10^{-9} sec). As a result, hydrogen bonds between water molecules and polar solutes continuously dissociate and reform, thereby permitting solutes to move through water and water to pass through channels in cellular membranes.

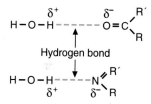

Fig. 4.4. Hydrogen bonds between water and polar molecules. R denotes additional atoms.

2. WATER AND THERMAL REGULATION

The structure of water also allows it to resist temperature change. Its heat of fusion is high, so a large drop in temperature is needed to convert liquid water to the solid state of ice. The thermal conductivity of water is also high, thereby facilitating heat dissipation from high energy-using areas such as the brain into the blood and the total body water pool. Its heat capacity and heat of vaporization are remarkably high; as liquid water is converted to a gas and evaporates from the

Table 4.1. Distribution of ions in body fluids.

	ECF* mmol/L	ICF
Cations		
Na^+	145	12
K^+	4	150
Anions		
Cl^-	105	5
HCO_3^-	25	12
Inorganic Phosphate	2	100

*The content of inorganic ions is very similar in plasma and interstitial fluid, the two components of the extracellular fluid. (ECF, extracellular fluid; ICF, intracellular fluid).

In the emergency room, **Di Abietes** was rehydrated with intravenous saline, which is a solution of 0.9% NaCl. Why was saline used instead of water?

Di Abietes has an osmotic diuresis. Because her blood levels of glucose and ketone bodies are so high, these compounds are passing from the blood into the glomerular filtrate in the kidneys and then into the urine. As a consequence of the high osmolality of the glomerular filtrate, much more water is being excreted in the urine than usual. Thus, Di has polyuria (increased urine volume). As a result of water lost from the blood into the urine, water passes from inside cells into the interstitial space and into the blood, resulting in an intracellular dehydration. The dehydrated cells in the brain are unable to carry out their normal functions. As a result, Di is in a coma.

$$H_2O \; \rightleftharpoons \; H^+ + OH^-$$

Fig. 4.5. The dissociation of water.

The laboratory reported that **Di Abietes'** blood pH was 7.08 (reference range = 7.37 – 7.43) What was the [H^+] in her blood compared with the concentration at a normal pH of 7.4?

Equation 4.1. Definition of pH.

$$pH = -\log [H^+]$$

skin, we feel a cooling effect. Water responds to the input of heat by decreasing the extent of hydrogen bonding and to cooling by increasing the bonding between water molecules.

C. Electrolytes

Both extracellular fluid (ECF) and intracellular fluid (ICF) contain electrolytes, a general term applied to bicarbonate and inorganic anions and cations. The electrolytes are unevenly distributed between compartments; Na^+ and Cl^- are the major electrolytes in the ECF (plasma and interstitial fluid), and K^+ and phosphates such as HPO_4^{-2} are the major electrolytes in cells (Table 4.1) This distribution is maintained principally by energy-requiring transporters that pump Na^+ out of cells in exchange for K^+ (see Chapter 10).

D. Osmolality and Water Movement

Water distributes between the different fluid compartments according to the concentration of solutes, or osmolality, of each compartment. The osmolality of a fluid is proportionate to the total concentration of all dissolved molecules, including ions, organic metabolites, and proteins (usually expressed as milliosmoles (mOsm)/kg water). The semipermeable cellular membrane that separates the extracellular and intracellular compartments contains a number of ion channels through which water can freely move, but other molecules cannot. Likewise, water can freely move through the capillaries separating the interstitial fluid and the plasma. As a result, water will move from a compartment with a low concentration of solutes (lower osmolality) to one with a higher concentration to achieve an equal osmolality on both sides of the membrane. The force it would take to keep the same amount of water on both sides of the membrane is called the osmotic pressure.

As water is lost from one fluid compartment, it is replaced with water from another to maintain a nearly constant osmolality. The blood contains a high content of dissolved negatively charged proteins and the electrolytes needed to balance these charges. As water is passed from the blood into the urine to balance the excretion of ions, the blood volume is repleted with water from interstitial fluid. When the osmolality of the blood and interstitial fluid is too high, water moves out of the cells. The loss of cellular water also can occur in hyperglycemia, because the high concentration of glucose increases the osmolality of the blood.

II. ACIDS AND BASES

Acids are compounds that donate a hydrogen ion (H^+) to a solution, and bases are compounds (such as the OH^- ion) that accept hydrogen ions. Water itself dissociates to a slight extent, generating hydrogen ions (H^+), which are also called protons, and hydroxide ions (OH^-)(Fig. 4.5). The hydrogen ions are extensively hydrated in water to form species such as H_3O^+, but nevertheless are usually represented as simply H^+. Water itself is neutral, neither acidic nor basic.

A. The pH of Water

The extent of dissociation by water molecules into H^+ and OH^- is very slight, and the hydrogen ion concentration of pure water is only 0.0000001 M, or 10^{-7} mol/L. The concentration of hydrogen ions in a solution is usually denoted by the term *pH*, which is the negative $\log_{10}$ of the hydrogen ion concentration expressed in mol/L (Equation 4.1). Therefore, the pH of pure water is 7.

The dissociation constant for water, K_d, expresses the relationship between the hydrogen ion concentration [H^+], the hydroxide ion concentration [OH^-], and the concentration of water $[H_2O]$ at equilibrium (Equation 4.2). Because water dissociates to such a small extent, $[H_2O]$ is essentially constant at 55.5 M. Multiplication of the K_d for water (approximately 1.8×10^{-16} M) by 55.5 M gives a value of approximately 10^{-14} $(M)^2$, which is called the ion product of water (K_w) (Equation 4.3). Because K_w, the product of $[H^+]$ and $[OH^-]$, is always constant, a decrease of $[H^+]$ must be accompanied by a proportionate increase of $[OH^-]$.

A pH of 7 is termed neutral because $[H^+]$ and $[OH^-]$ are equal. Acidic solutions have a greater hydrogen ion concentration and a lower hydroxide ion concentration than pure water (pH < 7.0), and basic solutions have a lower hydrogen ion concentration and a greater hydroxide ion concentration (pH > 7.0).

B. Strong and Weak Acids

During metabolism, the body produces a number of acids that increase the hydrogen ion concentration of the blood or other body fluids and tend to lower the pH (Table 4.2). These metabolically important acids can be classified as weak acids or strong acids by their degree of dissociation into a hydrogen ion and a base (the anion component). Inorganic acids such as sulfuric acid (H_2SO_4) and hydrochloric acid (HCl) are strong acids that dissociate completely in solution (Fig. 4.6). Organic acids containing carboxylic acid groups (e.g., the ketone bodies acetoacetic acid and β-hydroxybutyric acid) are weak acids that dissociate only to a limited extent in water. In general, a weak acid (HA), called the conjugate acid, dissociates into a hydrogen ion and an anionic component (A^-), called the conjugate base. The name of an undissociated acid usually ends in "ic acid" (e.g., acetoacetic acid) and the name of the dissociated anionic component ends in "ate" (e.g., acetoacetate).

The tendency of the acid (HA) to dissociate and donate a hydrogen ion to solution is denoted by its K_a, the equilibrium constant for dissociation of a weak acid (Equation 4.4). The higher the K_a, the greater is the tendency to dissociate a proton.

In the Henderson-Hasselbalch equation, the formula for the dissociation constant of a weak acid is converted to a convenient logarithmic equation (Equation 4.5). The term pK_a represents the negative log of K_a. If the pK_a for a weak acid is known, this

Dennis Veere has ingested an unknown number of acetylsalicylic acid (aspirin) tablets. Acetylsalicylic acid is rapidly converted to salicylic acid in the body. The initial effect of aspirin is to produce a respiratory alkalosis caused by a stimulation of the "metabolic" central respiratory control center in the hypothalamus. This increases the rate of breathing and the expiration of CO_2. This is followed by a complex metabolic acidosis caused partly by the dissociation of salicylic acid (salicylic acid ↔ salicylate$^-$ + H^+, pK_a = ~3.5).

Acetylsalicylate

Salicylate also interferes with mitochondrial ATP production, resulting in increased generation of CO_2 and accumulation of lactate and other organic acids in the blood. Subsequently, salicylate may impair renal function, resulting in the accumulation of strong acids of metabolic origin, such as sulfuric acid and phosphoric acid. Usually, children who ingest toxic amounts of aspirin are acidotic by the time they arrive in the emergency room.

Equation 4.2. Dissociation of water.

$$Kd = \frac{[H^+]\,[OH^-]}{[H_2O]}$$

Equation 4.3. The ion product of water.

$$K_w = [H^+]\,[OH^-] = 1 \times 10^{-14}$$

Equation 4.4. The K acid

For the reaction
$$HA \leftrightarrow A^- + H^+$$

$$K_a = \frac{[H^+]\,[A^-]}{[HA]}$$

 0.9% NaCl is 0.9 g NaCl/100 mL, equivalent to 9 g/L. NaCl has a molecular weight of 58 g/mole, so the concentration of NaCl in isotonic saline is 0.155 M, or 155 mM. If all of the NaCl were dissociated into Na^+ and Cl^- ions, the osmolality would be 310 mOsm/kg water. Because NaCl is not completely dissociated and some of the hydration shells surround undissociated NaCl molecules, the osmolality of isotonic saline is approximately 290 mOsm/kg H_2O. The osmolality of plasma, interstitial fluids, and ICF is also approximately 290 mOsm/kg water, so that no large shifts of water or swelling occur when isotonic saline is given intravenously.

Equation 4.5. The Henderson-Hasselbalch equation

$$pH = pK_a + \log \frac{[A^-]}{[HA]}$$

From inspection, you can tell that her $[H^+]$ is greater than normal, but less than 10 times higher. A 10-fold change in $[H^+]$ changes the pH by 1 unit. For Di, the pH of 7.08 = -log $[H^+]$, and therefore her $[H^+]$ is $1 \times 10^{-7.08}$. To calculate her $[H^+]$, express -7.08 as $-8 + 0.92$. The antilog to the base 10 of 0.92 is 8.3. Thus, her $[H^+]$ is 8.3×10^{-8} compared to 4.0×10^{-8} at pH 7.4, or slightly more than double the normal value.

Table 4.2. Acids in the Blood of a Healthy Individual.

Acid	Anion	pK$_a$	Major Sources
Strong acid			
Sulfuric acid (H$_2$SO$_4$)	Sulfate SO$_4$$^{-2}$	Completely Dissociated	Dietary sulfate and S-containing amino acids
Weak acid			
Carbonic acid (R-COOH)	Bicarbonate (R-COO$^-$)	3.80	CO$_2$ from TCA cycle
Lactic acid (R-COOH)	Lactate (R-COO$^-$)	3.73	Anaerobic glycolysis
Pyruvic acid (R-COOH)	Pyruvate (R-COO$^-$)	2.39	Glycolysis
Citric acid (R-3COOH)	Citrate (R-3COO$^-$)	3.13; 4.76; 6.40	TCA cycle and diet (e.g., citrus fruits)
Acetoacetic acid (R-COOH)	Acetoacetate (R-COO$^-$)	3.62	Fatty acid oxidation to ketone bodies
β-Hydroxybutyric acid (R-COOH)	β-Hydroxybutyrate (R-COO$^-$)	4.41	Fatty acid oxidation to ketone bodies
Acetic acid (R-COOH)	Acetate (R-COO$^-$)	4.76	Ethanol metabolism
Dihydrogen phosphate (H$_2$PO$_4$$^-$)	Monohydrogen phosphate (HPO$_4$$^{-2}$)	6.8	Dietary organic phosphates
Ammonium ion (NH$_4$$^+$)	Ammonia (NH$_3$)	9.25	Dietary nitrogen-containing compounds

equation can be used to calculate the ratio of the unprotonated to the protonated form at any pH. From this equation, you can see that a weak acid is 50% dissociated at a pH equal to its pK$_a$.

Most of the metabolic carboxylic acids have pK$_a$s between 2 and 5, depending on the other groups on the molecule (see Table 4.2). The pK$_a$ reflects the strength of an acid. Acids with a pK$_a$ of 2 are stronger acids than those with a pK$_a$ of 5 because, at any pH, a greater proportion is dissociated.

III. BUFFERS

Buffers, which consist of a weak acid and its conjugate base, cause a solution to resist changes in pH when hydrogen ions or hydroxide ions are added. In Figure 4.7, the pH of a solution of the weak acid acetic acid is graphed as a function of the

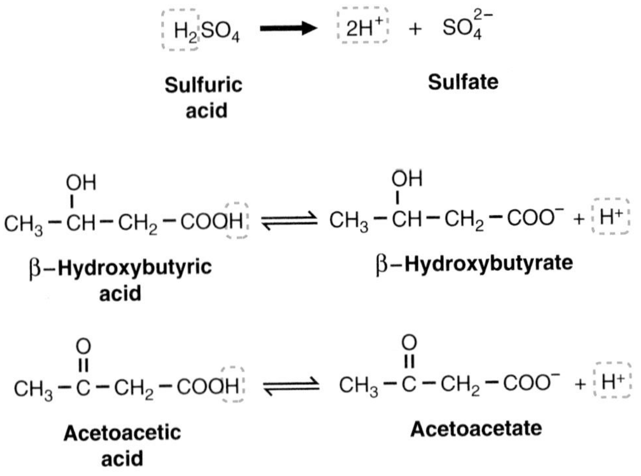

Fig. 4.6. Dissociation of acids. Sulfuric acid is a strong acid that dissociates into H$^+$ ions and sulfate. The ketone bodies acetoacetic acid and β-hydroxybutyric acid are weak acids that partially dissociate into H$^+$ and their conjugate bases.

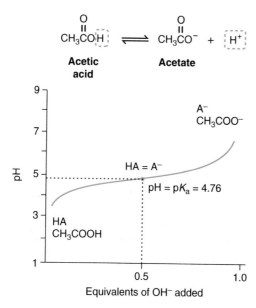

Fig. 4.7. The titration curve for acetic acid.

amount of OH^- that has been added. The OH^- is expressed as equivalents of total acetic acid present in the dissociated and undissociated forms. At the midpoint of this curve, 0.5 equivalents of OH^- have been added, and half of the conjugate acid has dissociated so that $[A^-]$ equals $[HA]$. This midpoint is expressed in the Henderson-Hasselbalch equation as the pK_a, defined as the pH at which 50% dissociation occurs. As you add more OH^- ions and move to the right on the curve, more of the conjugate acid molecules (HA) dissociate to generate H^+ ions, which combine with the added OH^- ions to form water. Consequently, only a small increase in pH results. If you add hydrogen ions to the buffer at its pK_a (moving to the left of the midpoint in Fig. 4.7), conjugate base molecules (A^-) combine with the added hydrogen ions to form HA, and almost no decrease in pH occurs.

As can be seen from Figure 4.7, a buffer can only compensate for an influx or removal of hydrogen ions within approximately 1 pH unit of its pK_a. As the pH of a buffered solution changes from the pK_a to one pH unit below the pK_a, the ratio of $[A^-]$ to HA changes from 1:1 to 1:10. If more hydrogen ions were added, the pH would fall rapidly because relatively little conjugate base remains. Likewise, at 1 pH unit above the pK_a of a buffer, relatively little undissociated acid remains. More concentrated buffers are more effective simply because they contain a greater total number of buffer molecules per unit volume that can dissociate or recombine with hydrogen ions.

IV. METABOLIC ACIDS AND BUFFERS

An average rate of metabolic activity produces roughly 22,000 mEq acid per day. If all of this acid were dissolved at one time in unbuffered body fluids, their pH would be less than 1. However, the pH of the blood is normally maintained between 7.36 and 7.44, and intracellular pH at approximately 7.1 (between 6.9 and 7.4). The widest range of extracellular pH over which the metabolic functions of the liver, the beating of the heart, and conduction of neural impulses can be maintained is 6.8 to 7.8. Thus, until the acid produced from metabolism can be excreted as CO_2 in expired air and as ions in the urine, it needs to be buffered in the body fluids. The major buffer systems in the body are: the bicarbonate–carbonic acid buffer system, which operates principally in extracellular fluid; the hemoglobin buffer system in red blood cells; the phosphate buffer system in all types of cells; and the protein buffer system of cells and plasma.

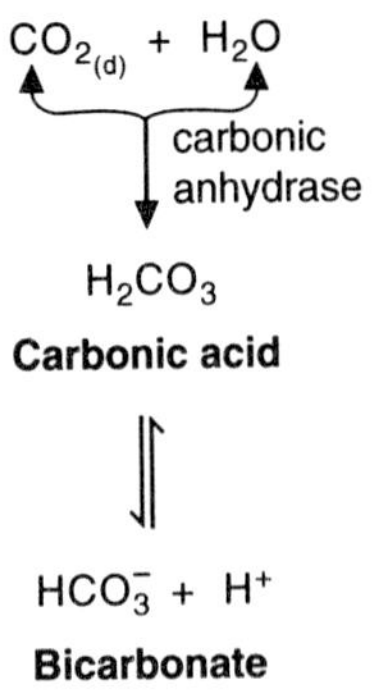

$$CO_{2(d)} + H_2O$$

carbonic anhydrase

$$H_2CO_3$$

Carbonic acid

$$HCO_3^- + H^+$$

Bicarbonate

Fig. 4.8. The bicarbonate buffer system.

The pK_a for dissociation of bicarbonate anion (HCO_3^-) into H^+ and carbonate (CO_3^{-2}) is 9.8; therefore, only trace amounts of carbonate exist in body fluids.

Equation 4.6: The Henderson-Hasselbalch equation for the bicarbonate buffer system

$$pH = pK_a + \log \frac{[A^-]}{[HA]}$$

$$pH = 6.1 + \log \frac{[HCO_3^-]}{[H_2CO_3] + [CO_2(d)]}$$

$$pH = 6.1 + \log \frac{[HCO_3^-]}{0.03 Paco_2}$$

where $[CO_2(d)]$ is the concentration of dissolved CO_2, the $[HCO_3^-]$ is expressed as mEq/mL, and $Paco_2$ as mm Hg. The constant of 0.03 is a solubility constant that also corrects for the use of different units.

A. The Bicarbonate Buffer System

The major source of metabolic acid in the body is the gas CO_2, produced principally from fuel oxidation in the TCA cycle. Under normal metabolic conditions, the body generates more than 13 moles of CO_2 per day (approximately 0.5 – 1 kg). CO_2 dissolves in water and reacts with water to produce carbonic acid, H_2CO_3, a reaction accelerated by the enzyme carbonic anhydrase (Fig. 4.8). Carbonic acid is a weak acid that partially dissociates into H^+ and bicarbonate anion, HCO_3^-.

Carbonic acid is both the major acid produced by the body, and its own buffer. The pK_a of carbonic acid itself is only 3.8, so at the blood pH of 7.4 it is almost completely dissociated and theoretically unable to buffer and generate bicarbonate. However, carbonic acid can be replenished from CO_2 in body fluids and air because the concentration of dissolved CO_2 in body fluids is approximately 500 times greater than that of carbonic acid. As base is added and H^+ is removed, H_2CO_3 dissociates into hydrogen and bicarbonate ions, and dissolved CO_2 reacts with H_2O to replenish the H_2CO_3 (see Fig. 4.8). Dissolved CO_2 is in equilibrium with the CO_2 in air in the alveoli of the lungs, and thus the availability of CO_2 can be increased or decreased by an adjustment in the rate of breathing and the amount of CO_2 expired. The pK_a for the bicarbonate buffer system in the body thus combines K_h (the hydration constant for the reaction of water and CO_2 to form H_2CO_3) with the chemical pK_a to obtain the value of 6.1 used in the Henderson-Hasselbalch equation (Equation 4.6). To use the terms for blood components measured in the emergency room, the dissolved CO_2 is expressed as a fraction of the partial pressure of CO_2 in arterial blood, $Paco_2$.

B. Bicarbonate and Hemoglobin in the Red Blood Cell

The bicarbonate buffer system and hemoglobin in red blood cells cooperate in buffering the blood and transporting CO_2 to the lungs. Most of the CO_2 produced from tissue metabolism in the TCA cycle diffuses into the interstitial fluid and the blood plasma and then into red blood cells (Fig. 4.9, circle 1). Although no carbonic anhydrase can be found in blood plasma or interstitial fluid, the red blood cells contain high amounts of this enzyme, and CO_2 is rapidly converted to carbonic acid (H_2CO_3) within these cells (circle 2). As the carbonic acid dissociates (circle 3), the H^+ released is also buffered by combination with hemoglobin (Hb, circle 4). The side chain of the amino acid histidine in hemoglobin has a pK_a of 6.7 and is thus able to accept a proton. The bicarbonate anion is transported out of the red blood cell into the blood in exchange for chloride anion, and thus bicarbonate is relatively high in the plasma (circle 5) (see Table 4.1).

As the red blood cell approaches the lungs, the direction of the equilibrium reverses. CO_2 is released from the red blood cell, causing more carbonic acid to dissociate into

The partial pressure of CO_2 ($Paco_2$) in **Di Abietes'** arterial blood was 28 mm Hg (reference range = 37 – 43), and her serum bicarbonate level was 8 mEq/L (reference range = 24 – 28). Elevated levels of ketone bodies had produced a ketoacidosis, and **Di Abietes** was exhaling increased amounts of CO_2 by breathing deeply and frequently (Kussmaul's breathing) to compensate. Why does this occur? Ketone bodies are weak acids that partially dissociate, increasing H^+ levels in the blood and the interstitial fluid surrounding the "metabolic" respiratory center in the hypothalamus that controls the rate of breathing. As a result of the decrease in pH, her respiratory rate increased, causing a fall in the partial pressure of arterial CO_2 ($Paco_2$). As bicarbonate and increased protons combined to form carbonic acid and produce more CO_2, her bicarbonate concentration decreased ($HCO_3^- + H^+ \rightarrow H_2CO_3 \rightarrow CO_2 + H_2O$). As shown by Di's low arterial blood pH of 7.08, the Kussmaul's breathing was unable to fully compensate for the high rate of acidic ketone body production.

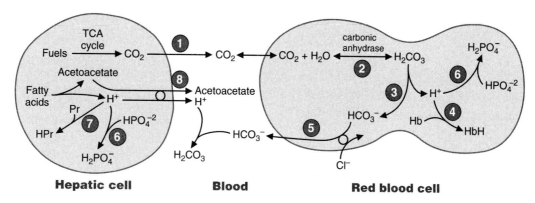

Fig. 4.9. Buffering systems of the body. CO_2 produced from cellular metabolism is converted to bicarbonate and H^+ in the red blood cells. Within the red blood cell, the H^+ is buffered by hemoglobin (Hb) and phosphate (HPO_4^{-2}). The bicarbonate is transported into the blood to buffer H^+ generated by the production of other metabolic acids, such as the ketone body acetoacetic acid. Other proteins (Pr) also serve as intracellular buffers.

CO_2 and water and more hydrogen ions to combine with bicarbonate. Hemoglobin loses some it of its hydrogen ions, a feature that allows it to bind oxygen more readily (see Chapter 7). Thus, the bicarbonate buffer system is intimately linked to the delivery of oxygen to tissues.

The respiratory center within the hypothalamus, which controls the rate of breathing, is sensitive to changes in pH. As the pH falls, individuals breathe more rapidly and expire more CO_2. As the pH rises, they breathe more shallowly. Thus, the rate of breathing contributes to regulation of pH through its effects on the dissolved CO_2 content of the blood.

Bicarbonate and carbonic acid, which diffuse through the capillary wall from the blood into interstitial fluid, provide a major buffer for both plasma and interstitial fluid. However, blood differs from interstitial fluid in that the blood contains a high content of extracellular proteins, such as albumin, which contribute to its buffering capacity through amino acid side chains that are able to accept and release protons. The protein content of interstitial fluid is too low to serve as an effective buffer.

C. Intracellular pH

Phosphate anions and proteins are the major buffers involved in maintaining a constant pH of intracellular fluids. The inorganic phosphate anion $H_2PO_4^-$ dissociates to generate H^+ and the conjugate base, HPO_4^{-2} with a pK_a of 7.2 (see Fig. 4.9, circle 6). Thus, phosphate anions play a major role as an intracellular buffer in the red blood cell and in other types of cells, where their concentration is much higher than in blood and interstitial fluid (See Table 4.1, extracellular fluid). Organic phosphate anions, such as glucose 6-phosphate and ATP, also act as buffers. Intracellular fluid contains a high content of proteins that contain histidine and other amino acids that can accept protons, in a fashion similar to hemoglobin (see Fig. 4.9, circle 7).

The transport of hydrogen ions out of the cell is also important for maintenance of a constant intracellular pH. Metabolism produces a number of other acids in addition to CO_2. For example, the metabolic acids acetoacetic acid and β-hydroxybutyric acid are produced from fatty acid oxidation to ketone bodies in the liver, and lactic acid is produced by glycolysis in muscle and other tissues. The pK_a for most metabolic carboxylic acids is below 5, so these acids are completely dissociated at the pH of blood and cellular fluid. Metabolic anions are transported out of the cell together with H^+ (see Fig. 4.9, circle 8). If the cell becomes too acidic, more H^+ is transported out in exchange for Na^+ ions by a different transporter. If the cell becomes too alkaline, more bicarbonate is transported out in exchange for Cl^- ions.

Both **Di Abietes** and **Percy Veere** were hyperventilating when they arrived at the emergency room: Ms. Abietes in response to her primary metabolic acidosis and Mr. Veere in response to anxiety. Hyperventilation raised blood pH in both cases: In Ms. Abietes case it partially countered the acidosis and in Mr. Veere's case it produced a respiratory alkalosis (abnormally high arterial blood pH).

Phosphoric acid (H_3PO_4) dissociates into H^+ ions and dihydrogen phosphate ($H_2PO_4^-$) with a pK_a of 2.15. The dissociation of $H_2PO_4^-$ into H^+ and monohydrogen ions (HPO_4^{-2}) occurs with a pK_a of 7.20. Monohydrogen phosphate dissociates into H^+ and phosphate anions (PO_4^{-3}) with a pK_a of 12.4.

D. Urinary Hydrogen, Ammonium, and Phosphate Ions

The nonvolatile acid that is produced from body metabolism cannot be excreted as expired CO_2 and is excreted in the urine. Most of the nonvolatile acid hydrogen ion is excreted as undissociated acid that generally buffers the urinary pH between 5.5 and 7.0. A pH of 5.0 is the minimum urinary pH. The acid secretion includes inorganic acids such as phosphate and ammonium ions, as well as uric acid, dicarboxylic acids, and tricarboxylic acids such as citric acid (see Table 4.2). One of the major sources of nonvolatile acid in the body is sulfuric acid (H_2SO_4). Sulfuric acid is generated from the sulfate-containing compounds ingested in foods and from metabolism of the sulfur-containing amino acids, cysteine and methionine. It is a strong acid that is dissociated into H^+ and sulfate anion (SO_4^{-2}) in the blood and urine (see Fig. 4.6). Urinary excretion of $H_2PO_4^-$ helps to remove acid. To maintain metabolic homeostasis, we must excrete the same amount of phosphate in the urine that we ingest with food as phosphate anions or organic phosphates such as phospholipids. Whether the phosphate is present in the urine as $H_2PO_4^-$ or HPO_4^{-2} depends on the urinary pH and the pH of blood.

Ammonium ions are major contributors to buffering urinary pH, but not blood pH. Ammonia (NH_3) is a base that combines with protons to produce ammonium (NH_4^+) ions ($NH_3 + H^+ \leftrightarrow NH_4^+$), a reaction that occurs with a pK_a of 9.25. Ammonia is produced from amino acid catabolism or absorbed through the intestine, and kept at very low concentrations in the blood because it is toxic to neural tissues. Cells in the kidney generate NH_4^+ and excrete it into the urine in proportion to the acidity (proton concentration) of the blood. As the renal tubular cells transport H^+ into the urine, they return bicarbonate anions to the blood.

E. Hydrochloric Acid

Hydrochloric acid (HCl), also called gastric acid, is secreted by parietal cells of the stomach into the stomach lumen, where the strong acidity denatures ingested proteins so they can be degraded by digestive enzymes. When the stomach contents are released into the lumen of the small intestine, gastric acid is neutralized by bicarbonate secreted from pancreatic cells and by cells in the intestinal lining.

Q: Ammonium ions are acids that dissociate to form the conjugate base, ammonia, and hydrogen ions. What is the form present in blood? In urine?

 Diabetes mellitus is diagnosed by the concentration of plasma glucose (plasma is blood from which the red blood cells have been removed by centrifugation). Because plasma glucose normally increases after a meal, the normal reference ranges and the diagnostic level are defined relative to the time of consumption of food, or to consumption of a specified amount of glucose during an oral glucose tolerance test. After an overnight fast, values for the fasting plasma glucose below 110 mg/dL are considered normal and above 126 mg/dL define diabetes mellitus. Fasting plasma glucose values greater or equal to 110 and less than 126 mg/dL define an intermediate condition termed impaired fasting glucose. Normal casual plasma glucose levels (casual is defined as any time of day without regard to the time since a last meal) should not be above 200 mg/dL. A 2-hour postprandial (after a meal or after an oral glucose load) plasma glucose level between 140 and 199 mg/dL defines a condition known as impaired glucose tolerance. A level above 200 mg/dL defines "overt" diabetes mellitus.

CLINICAL COMMENTS

Dianne Abietes. Di Abietes has type 1 diabetes mellitus (formerly called juvenile or insulin-dependent diabetes mellitus, IDDM). She maintains her insulin level through two daily subcutaneous (under the skin) injections of insulin. If her blood insulin levels fall too low, free fatty acids leave her adipocytes (fat cells) and are converted by the liver to the ketone bodies acetoacetic acid and β-hydroxybutyric acid. As these acids accumulate in the blood, a metabolic acidosis known as diabetic ketoacidosis (DKA) develops. Until insulin is administered to reverse this trend, several compensatory mechanisms operate to minimize the extent of the acidosis. One of these mechanisms is a stimulation of the respiratory center in the hypothalamus induced by the acidosis, which leads to deeper and more frequent respiration (Kussmaul's respiration). CO_2 is expired more rapidly than normal, and the blood pH rises. The results of the laboratory studies performed on **Di Abietes** in the emergency room were consistent with a moderately severe DKA. Her arterial blood pH and serum bicarbonate were low, and ketone bodies were present in her blood and urine (normally, ketone bodies are not present in the urine). In addition, her serum glucose level was 648 mg/dL (reference range = 80 − 110 fasting and no higher than 200 in a random glucose sample). Her hyperglycemia, which induces an osmotic diuresis, contributed to her dehydration and the hyperosmolality of her body fluids.

Treatment was initiated with intravenous saline solutions to replace fluids lost with the osmotic diuresis and hyperventilation. The osmotic diuresis resulted from increased urinary water volume to dilute the large amounts of glucose and ketone bodies excreted in the urine. Hyperventilation increased the water of respiration lost with expired air. A loading dose of regular insulin was given as an intravenous bolus followed by additional insulin each hour as needed. The patient's metabolic response to the treatment was monitored closely.

Dennis Veere. Dennis remained alert in the emergency room. While awaiting the report of his initial serum salicylate level, his stomach was lavaged, and several white tablets were found in the stomach aspirate. He was examined repeatedly and showed none of the early symptoms of salicylate toxicity, such as respiratory stimulation, upper abdominal distress, nausea, or headache.

His serum salicylate level was reported as 92 μg/mL (the usual level in an adult receiving a therapeutic dosage of 4−5 g/day is 120−350 μg/mL, and a level of 800 μg/mL is considered potentially lethal). He was admitted for overnight observation and continued to do well. A serum salicylate level the following morning was 24 μg/mL. He was discharged later that day.

Percy Veere. At the emergency room, Mr. Veere complained of light-headedness and "pins and needles" (paresthesias) in his hands and around his lips. These symptoms resulted from an increase in respiratory drive mediated in this case through the "behavioral" rather than the "metabolic" central respiratory control system (as seen in **Di Abietes** when she was in diabetic ketoacidosis). The behavioral system was activated in Mr. Veere's case by his anxiety over his grandson's potential poisoning. His alveolar hyperventilation caused Mr. Veere's $Paco_2$ to decrease below the normal range of 37 to 43 mm Hg. The alkalemia caused his neurologic symptoms. After being reassured that his grandson would be fine, Mr. Veere was asked to breathe slowly into a small paper bag placed around his nose and mouth, allowing him to reinhale the CO_2 being exhaled through hyperventilation. Within 20 minutes, his symptoms disappeared.

BIOCHEMICAL COMMENTS

Body water and dehydration. Dehydration, or loss of water, occurs when salt and water intake is less than the combined rates of renal plus extrarenal volume loss (Fig. 4.10). In a true hypovolemic state, total body water, functional ECF volume, and ICF volume are decreased. One of the causes of hypovolemia is an intake of water that is inadequate to resupply the daily excretion volume (maintenance of fluid homeostasis). The amount of water lost by the kidneys is determined by the amount of water necessary to dilute the ions, acids, and other solutes excreted. Both urinary solute excretion and water loss in expired air, which amount to almost 400 mL/day, occur during fasting as well as during periods of normal food intake. Thus, people who are lost in the desert or shipwrecked continue to lose water in air and urine, in addition to their water loss through the skin and sweat glands. Comatose patients and patients who are debilitated and unable to swallow also continue to lose water and become dehydrated. Dysphagia (loss of appetite), such as **Percy Veere** experienced during his depression (see Chapters 1 and 3), can result in dehydration because food intake is normally a source of fluid. Cerebral injuries that cause a loss of thirst also can lead to dehydration.

Dehydration also can occur secondary to excessive water loss through the kidneys, lungs, and skin. Excessive renal loss could be the result of impaired kidney function, or impaired response by the hormones that regulate water balance (e.g.,

A: The pK_a for dissociation of ammonium ions is 9.25. Thus, the undissociated conjugate acid form, NH_4^+, predominates at the physiologic pH of 7.4 and urinary pH of 5.5 to 7.0. Ammonia is an unusual conjugate base because it is not an anion.

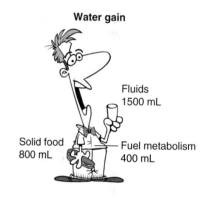

Water gain

Fluids 1500 mL

Solid food 800 mL

Fuel metabolism 400 mL

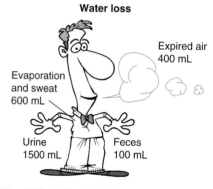

Water loss

Expired air 400 mL

Evaporation and sweat 600 mL

Urine 1500 mL

Feces 100 mL

Fig. 4.10. Body fluid homeostasis (constant body water balance). Intake is influenced by availability of fluids and food, thirst, hunger, and the ability to swallow. The rates of breathing and evaporation and urinary volume influence water loss. The body adjusts the volume of urinary excretion to compensate for variations in other types of water loss and for variations in intake. The hormones aldosterone and antidiuretic hormone (ADH) help to monitor blood volume and osmolality through mechanisms regulating thirst and sodium and water balance.

antidiuretic hormone [ADH] and aldosterone). However, in individuals such as **Di Abietes** with normal kidney function, dehydration can occur as a response to water dilution of the high concentrations of ketone bodies, glucose, and other solutes excreted in the urine (osmotic diuresis). If the urinary water loss is associated with an acidosis, hyperventilation occurs, increasing the amount of water lost in expired air. Water loss in expired air (pulmonary water loss) could occur also as a result of a tracheotomy or cerebral injury. An excessive loss of water and electrolytes through the skin can result from extensive burns.

Gastrointestinal water losses also can result in dehydration. We secrete approximately 8 to 10 L fluid per day into our intestinal lumen. Normally, more than 90% of this fluid is reabsorbed in the intestines. The percentage reabsorbed can be decreased by vomiting, diarrhea, tube drainage of gastric contents, or loss of water into tissues around the gut via bowel fistulas.

Suggested References

Many physiology textbooks have good in-depth descriptions of acid-base balance. A very useful reference for medical students is: Brensilver J, Goldberger, E. A Primer of Water, Electrolyte, and Acid-Base Syndromes. 8th Ed. Philadelphia: F.A. Davis, 1996 .

For additional information on toxic effects of aspirin, see Roberts LJ II, Morrow JD. Analgesic-antipyretic and antiinflammatory agents and drugs employed in the treatment of gout. In: Hardman JG, Limbird LE, Goodman AG, eds. Goodman and Gilman's The Pharmacological Basis of Therapeutics. New York: McGraw-Hill, 2001:697−701.

 REVIEW QUESTIONS—CHAPTER 4

1. A decrease of blood pH from 7.5 to 6.5 would be accompanied by which of the following changes in ion concentration?

   (A) A 10-fold increase in hydrogen ion concentration.
   (B) A 10-fold increase in hydroxyl ion concentration.
   (C) An increase in hydrogen ion concentration by a factor of 7.5/6.5.
   (D) A decrease in hydrogen ion concentration by a factor of 6.5/7.5.
   (E) A shift in concentration of buffer anions, with no change in hydrogen ion concentration.

2. Which of the following describes a universal property of buffers?

   (A) Buffers are usually composed of a mixture of strong acids and strong bases.
   (B) Buffers work best at the pH at which they are completely dissociated.
   (C) Buffers work best at the pH at which they are 50% dissociated.
   (D) Buffers work best at one pH unit lower than the pK_a.
   (E) Buffers work equally well at all concentrations.

3. A patient with an enteropathy (intestinal disease) produced large amounts of ammonia (NH_3) from bacterial overgrowth in the intestine. The ammonia was absorbed through the intestine into the portal vein and entered the circulation. Which of the following is a likely consequence of his ammonia absorption?

   (A) A decrease of blood pH
   (B) Conversion of ammonia to ammonium ion in the blood
   (C) A decreased concentration of bicarbonate in the blood
   (D) Kussmaul's respiration
   (E) Increased expiration of CO_2

4. Which of the following physiologic/pathologic conditions is most likely to result in an alkalosis, provided that the body could not fully compensate?

   (A) Production of lactic acid by muscles during exercise
   (B) Production of ketone bodies by a patient with diabetes mellitus
   (C) Repeated vomiting of stomach contents, including HCl
   (D) Diarrhea with loss of the bicarbonate anions secreted into the intestine
   (E) An infection resulting in a fever and hypercatabolism

5. Laboratory tests on the urine of a patient identified the presence of methylmalonate ($^-OOC\text{-}CH(CH_3)\text{-}COO^-$). Methylmalonate

   (A) is a strong acid.
   (B) is the conjugate base of a weak acid.
   (C) is 100% dissociated at its pK_a.
   (D) is 50% dissociated at the pH of the blood.
   (E) is a major intracellular buffer.

5 Structures of the Major Compounds of the Body

The body contains compounds of great structural diversity, ranging from relatively simple sugars and amino acids to enormously complex polymers such as proteins and nucleic acids. Many of these compounds have common structural features related to their names, their solubility in water, the pathways in which they participate, or their physiologic function. Thus, learning the terminology used to describe individual compounds and classes of compounds can greatly facilitate learning biochemistry.

In this chapter, we describe the major classes of carbohydrates and lipids and some of the classes of nitrogen-containing compounds. The structures of amino acids, proteins, the nucleic acids, and vitamins are covered in more detail in subsequent chapters.

Functional Groups on Molecules. *Organic molecules are composed principally of carbon and hydrogen. However, their unique characteristics are related to structures termed functional groups involving* **oxygen, nitrogen, phosphorus,** *or* **sulfur***.*

Carbohydrates*. Carbohydrates, commonly known as sugars, can be classified by their carbonyl group (****aldo-*** *or* ***ketosugars****), the number of carbons they contain (e.g., pentoses, hexoses), or the positions of the hydroxyl groups on their asymmetric carbon atoms (****D- or L-sugars, stereoisomers,*** *or* ***epimers****). They can also be categorized according to their substitutents (e.g.,* ***amino sugars****), or the number of monosaccharides (such as glucose) joined through* ***glycosidic bonds*** *(****disaccharides, oligosaccharides****, and* ***polysaccharides****.).* ***Glycoproteins*** *and* ***proteoglycans*** *have sugars attached to their protein components.*

Lipids*. Lipids are a group of structurally diverse compounds defined by their* ***hydrophobicity****; they are not very soluble in water. The major lipids of the human body are the* ***fatty acids****, which are esterified to* ***glycerol*** *to form* ***triacylglycerols*** *(triglycerides) or* ***phosphoacylglycerols*** *(phosphoglycerides). In the* ***sphingolipids****, a fatty acid is attached to sphingosine, which is derived from serine and another fatty acid.* ***Glycolipids*** *contain sugars attached to a lipid hydroxyl group. Specific* ***polyunsaturated fatty acids*** *are precursors of* ***eicosanoids****. The lipid* ***cholesterol*** *is a component of membranes, and the precursor of other compounds that contain the steroid nucleus, such as the* ***bile salts*** *and* ***steroid hormones****. Cholesterol is one of the compounds synthesized from a 5-carbon precursor called the* ***isoprene*** *unit.*

Nitrogen-containing compounds*. Nitrogen in* ***amino groups*** *or* ***heterocyclic ring*** *structures often carries a positive charge at neutral pH.* ***Amino acids*** *contain a carboxyl group, an amino group, and one or more additional carbons.* ***Purines, pyrimidines****, and* ***pyridines*** *have heterocyclic nitrogen-containing ring structures.* ***Nucleosides*** *comprise one of these ring structures attached to a sugar. The addition of a phosphate produces a* ***nucleotide****.*

CH_3CH_2OH **Ethanol**
CH_3OH **Methanol**

The names of chemical groups are often incorporated into the common name of a compound, and denote important differences in chemical structure. For example, in the name *ethanol*, the "eth" denotes the ethyl group (CH_3CH_2-), the "ol" denotes the alcohol group (OH), and the "an" denotes the single bonds between the carbon atoms. Methanol contains a methyl group (CH_3) instead of the ethyl group. Methanol (also called wood alcohol) is much more toxic to humans than ethanol, the alcohol in alcoholic beverages. Ingestion of methanol results in visual disturbances, bradycardia, coma, and seizures.

Hydrophobic molecules are transported in the blood bound to carrier proteins or incorporated into lipoprotein complexes that have a hydrophobic lipid core and a more polar surface.

THE WAITING ROOM

 Di Abietes recovered from her bout of diabetic ketoacidosis and was discharged from the hospital (see Chapter 4). She has returned for a follow-up visit as an outpatient. She reports that she has been compliant with her recommended diet and that she faithfully gives herself insulin by subcutaneous injection twice daily. Her serum glucose levels are monitored in the hospital laboratory approximately every 2 weeks, and she self-monitors her blood glucose levels every other day.

Lotta Topaigne is a 47-year-old woman who came to the physician's office complaining of a severe throbbing pain in the right great toe that began 8 hours earlier. The toe has suffered no trauma but appears red and swollen. It is warmer than the surrounding tissue and is exquisitely tender to even light pressure. Ms. Topaigne is unable to voluntarily flex or extend the joints of the digit, and passive motion of the joints causes great pain.

I. FUNCTIONAL GROUPS ON BIOLOGIC COMPOUNDS

A. Biologic Compounds

The organic molecules of the body consist principally of carbon, hydrogen, oxygen, nitrogen, sulfur, and phosphorus joined by covalent bonds. The key element is carbon, which forms four covalent bonds with other atoms. Carbon atoms are joined through double or single bonds to form the carbon backbone for structures of varying size and complexity (Fig. 5.1). Groups containing 1, 2, 3, 4, and 5 carbons plus hydrogen are referred to as methyl, ethyl, propionyl, butyl, and pentanyl groups, respectively. If the carbon chain is branched, the prefix "iso" is used. If the compound contains a double bond, "ene" is sometimes incorporated into the name. Carbon structures that are straight or branched with single or double bonds, but do not contain a ring, are called aliphatic.

Carbon-containing rings are found in a number of biologic compounds. One of the most common is the six-membered carbon-containing benzene ring, sometimes called a phenyl group (see Fig. 5.1). This ring has three double bonds, but the electrons are shared equally by all six carbons and delocalized in planes above and below the ring. Compounds containing the benzene ring, or a similar ring structure with benzene-like properties, are called aromatic.

B. Functional Groups

Biochemical molecules are defined both by their carbon skeleton and by structures called functional groups that usually involve bonds between carbon and oxygen, carbon and nitrogen, carbon and sulfur, and carbon and phosphate groups (Fig. 5.2). In carbon–carbon and carbon–hydrogen bonds, the electrons are shared equally between atoms, and the bonds are nonpolar and relatively unreactive. In carbon–oxygen and carbon–nitrogen bonds, the electrons are shared unequally, and the bonds are polar and more reactive. Thus, the properties of the functional groups usually determine the types of reactions that occur and the physiologic role of the molecule.

Functional group names are often incorporated into the common name of a compound. For example, a ke**tone** might have a name that ends in "one" like ace**tone**, and the name of a compound that contains a hydroxyl (alco**hol** or OH group) might end in "ol" (e.g., ethan**ol**). The acyl group is the portion of the molecule that provides

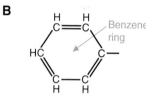 **Di Abietes** had a metabolic acidosis resulting from an increased hepatic production of ketone bodies. Her response to therapy was followed with screening tests for ketone bodies in her urine that employed a paper strip containing nitroprusside, a compound that reacts with keto groups. Her blood glucose was measured with an enzymatic assay that is specific for the sugar D-glucose and will not react with other sugars.

A

Single bond   Double bond

CH_3
     $CH - CH = CH -$
CH_3

Aliphatic isopentenyl group

B

Benzene ring

Aromatic phenyl group

Fig. 5.1. Examples of aliphatic and aromatic compounds. **A.** An *isoprene* group, which is an aliphatic group. The "iso" prefix denotes branching, and the "ene" denotes a double bond. **B.** A benzene ring (or phenyl group), which is an aromatic group.

Q: The ketone bodies synthesized in the liver are β-hydroxybutyrate and acetoacetate. A third ketone body, acetone, is formed by the nonenzymatic decarboxylation of acetoacetate.

$$\begin{array}{c} OH \\ | \\ CH_3 - CH - CH_2 - COO^- \end{array}$$

β-Hydroxybutyrate

$$CH_3 - \overset{O}{\underset{||}{C}} - CH_2 - \overset{O}{\underset{||}{C}} - O^- \rightarrow CH_3 - \overset{O}{\underset{||}{C}} - CH_3 + CO_2$$

Acetoacetate   **Acetone**

Acetone is volatile and accounts for the sweet mousy odor in the breath of patients such as **Di Abietes** when they have a ketoacidosis. What functional groups are present in each of these ketone bodies?

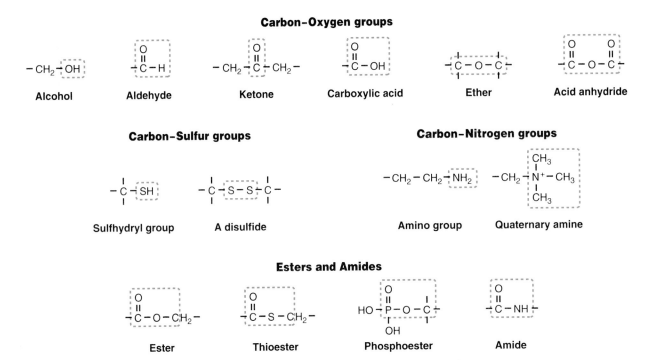

Fig. 5.2. Major types of functional groups found in biochemical compounds of the human body.

Q:

CH₂OH   H−C
| ‖
H−C−OH   O
| H−C−OH
CH₂OH |
         CH₂OH

A   **B**

Which compound is glycer**ol**, and which is glycer**aldehyde**?

Q: Judging from the structures shown in the question on page 55 which compound is more oxidized, β-hydroxybutyrate or acetoacetate? Which is more reduced?

A: β-hydroxybutyr**ate** and acetoacet**ate** are carboxyl**ates** (dissociated carboxylic acids). Acet**o**acetate and acet**one** contain keto/ket**one** groups. Because β-**hydroxy**butyrate contains an alcohol (**hydroxyl**) group and not a keto group, the general name of ketone bodies for these compounds is really a misnomer.

the carbonyl (–C=O) group in an ester or amide linkage. It is denoted in a name by an "yl" ending. For example, the fat stores of the body are tri**acyl**glycer**ols**. Three acyl (fatty acid) groups are esterified to glycer**ol**, a compound containing three alcohol groups. In the remainder of this chapter, we will bold the portions of names of compounds that refer to a class of compounds or a structural feature.

1. OXIDIZED AND REDUCED GROUPS

The carbon–carbon and carbon–oxygen groups are described as "oxidized" or "reduced" according to the number of electrons around the carbon atom. Oxidation is the loss of electrons and results in the loss of hydrogen atoms together with one or two electrons, or the gain of an oxygen atom or hydroxyl group. Reduction is the gain of electrons and results in the gain of hydrogen atoms or loss of an oxygen atom. Thus, the carbon becomes progressively more oxidized (and less reduced) as we go from an alcohol to an aldehyde or a ketone to a carboxyl group (see Fig. 5.2). Carbon–carbon double bonds are more oxidized (and less reduced) than carbon–carbon single bonds.

2. GROUPS THAT CARRY A CHARGE

Acidic groups contain a proton that can dissociate, usually leaving the remainder of the molecule as an anion with a negative charge (see Chapter 4). In biomolecules, the major anionic substituents are carboxyl**ate** groups, phosph**ate** groups, or sulf**ate** groups (the "ate" suffix denotes a negative charge) (Fig. 5.3). Phosphate groups attached to metabolites are often abbreviated as P with a circle around it, or just as "P", as in glucose-6-**P**.

Compounds containing nitrogen are usually basic and can acquire a positive charge (Fig. 5.4). Nitrogen has five electrons in its valence shell. If only three of these electrons form covalent bonds with other atoms, the nitrogen has no charge. If the remaining two electrons form a bond with a hydrogen ion or a carbon atom, the nitrogen carries a positive charge. Amines consist of nitrogen attached through single bonds to hydrogen atoms and to one or more carbon atoms. Primary amines, such as dop**amine**, have one carbon–nitrogen bond. These amines are weak acids with a pK_a of approximately 9, so that at pH 7.4 they carry a positive charge. Secondary, tertiary, and quarternary amines have 2, 3, and 4 nitrogen–carbon bonds, respectively (see Fig. 5.4).

C. Polarity of Bonds and Partial Charges

Polar bonds are covalent bonds in which the electron cloud is denser around one atom (the atom with the greater electronegativity) than the other. Oxygen is more electronegative than carbon, and a carbon–oxygen bond is therefore polar, with the oxygen atom carrying a partial negative charge and the carbon atom carrying a partial positive charge (Fig. 5.5). In nonpolar carbon–carbon bonds and carbon–hydrogen bonds, the two electrons in the covalent bond are shared almost equally. Nitrogen, when it has only three covalent bonds, also carries a partial negative charge relative to carbon, and the carbon–nitrogen bond is polarized. Sulfur can carry a slight partial negative charge.

1. SOLUBILITY

Water is a dipolar molecule in which the oxygen atom carries a partial negative charge and the hydrogen atoms carry partial positive charges (see Chapter 4). For molecules to be soluble in water, they must contain charged or polar groups that can associate with the partial positive and negative charges of water. Thus, the solubility of organic molecules in water is determined by both the proportion of polar to nonpolar groups attached to the carbon–hydrogen skeleton and to their relative positions in the molecule. Polar groups or molecules are called hydrophilic (water-loving), and nonpolar groups or molecules are hydrophobic (water-fearing). Sugars such as glucose 6-phosphate, for example, contain so many polar groups that they are very hydrophilic and almost infinitely water-soluble (Fig. 5.6). The water molecules interacting with a polar or ionic compound form a hydration shell around the compound.

Compounds that have large nonpolar regions are relatively water insoluble. They tend to cluster together in an aqueous environment and form weak associations through van der Waals forces, often termed hydrophobic bonds. Hydrophobic compounds are essentially pushed together as the water molecules maximize the number of energetically favorable hydrogen bonds they can form with each other in the water lattice. Thus, lipids form droplets or separate layers in an aqueous environment (e.g., vegetable oils in a salad dressing).

2. REACTIVITY

Another consequence of bond polarity is that atoms that carry a partial (or full) negative charge are attracted to atoms that carry a partial (or full) positive charge and vice versa. These partial or full charges dictate the course of biochemical reactions—which follow the same principles of electrophilic and nucleophilic attack characteristic of organic reactions in general. The partial positive charge on the carboxyl carbon attracts more negatively charged groups and accounts for many of the reactions of carboxylic acids. An ester is formed when a carboxylic acid and an alcohol combine, splitting out water (Fig. 5.7). Similarly, a thioester is formed when an acid combines with a sulfhydryl group, and an amide is formed when an acid combines with an amine. Similar reactions result in the formation of a phosphoester from phosphoric acid and an alcohol and in the formation of an anhydride from two acids.

D. Nomenclature

Biochemists use two systems for the identification of the carbons in a chain. In the first system, the carbons in a compound are numbered, starting with the carbon in

Carboxylate group

Phosphate group

Sulfate group

Fig. 5.3. Examples of anions formed by dissociation of acidic groups. At physiologic pH, carboxylic acids, phosphoric acid, and sulfuric acid are dissociated into hydrogen ions and negatively charged anions.

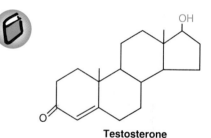

Testosterone

In medicine and biochemistry, the common or trivial names of compounds are used rather than the systematic nomenclature favored by chemists. Sometimes such names reflect functional groups, classes of compounds or the source from which the compound was first isolated. The compound testosterone provides an example. It was first isolated from monkey testis, the "ster" in its name denotes the steroid ring structure, and the "one" denotes a ketone group.

A: "A" contains three **alcohol** groups and is called glycer**ol**. Compound B contains an **aldehyde group**, and is called glycer**aldehyde**.

A: Acetoacetate is more oxidized than β-hydroxybutyrate. The carbon in the keto group contains one less hydrogen than the carbon to which the OH group is attached. It has lost an electron.

the most oxidized group (e.g., the carboxyl group). In the second system, the carbons are given Greek letters, starting with the carbon next to the most oxidized group. Hence, the compound shown in Figure 5.8 is known as 3-hydroxybutyrate or β-hydroxybutyrate.

II. CARBOHYDRATES

A. Monosaccharides

Simple monosaccharides consist of a linear chain of three or more carbon atoms, one of which forms a carbonyl group through a double bond with oxygen (Fig. 5.9). The other carbons of an unmodified monosaccharide contain hydroxyl groups, resulting in the general formula for an unmodified sugar of $C_nH_{2n}O_n$. The suffix "ose" is used for the names of sugars. If the carbonyl group is an aldehyde, the sugar is an aldose; if the carbonyl group is a ketone, the sugar is a ketose. Monosaccharides are also classified according to their number of carbons: Sugars containing 3, 4, 5, 6, and 7 carbons are called trioses, tetroses, pentoses, hexoses, and heptoses, respectively. Fructose is therefore a ketohexose (see Fig. 5.9), and glucose is an aldohexose (see Fig. 5.6).

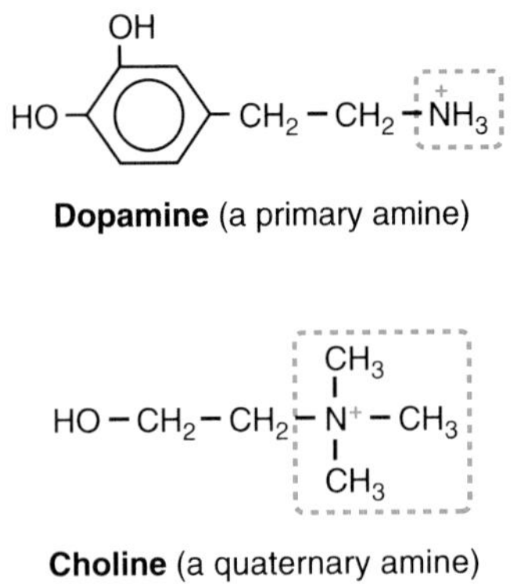

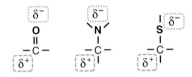

Dopamine (a primary amine)

Choline (a quaternary amine)

Fig. 5.4. Examples of amines. At physiologic pH, many amines carry positive charges.

Fig. 5.5. Partial charges on carbon–oxygen, carbon–nitrogen, and carbon–sulfur bonds.

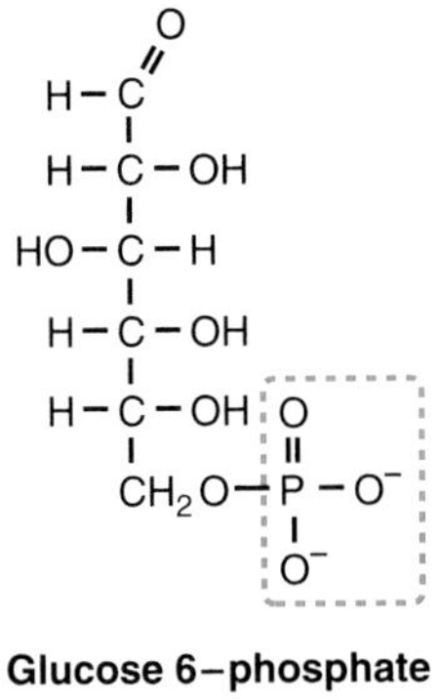

Glucose 6–phosphate

Fig. 5.6. Glucose 6-phosphate, a very polar and water-soluble molecule.

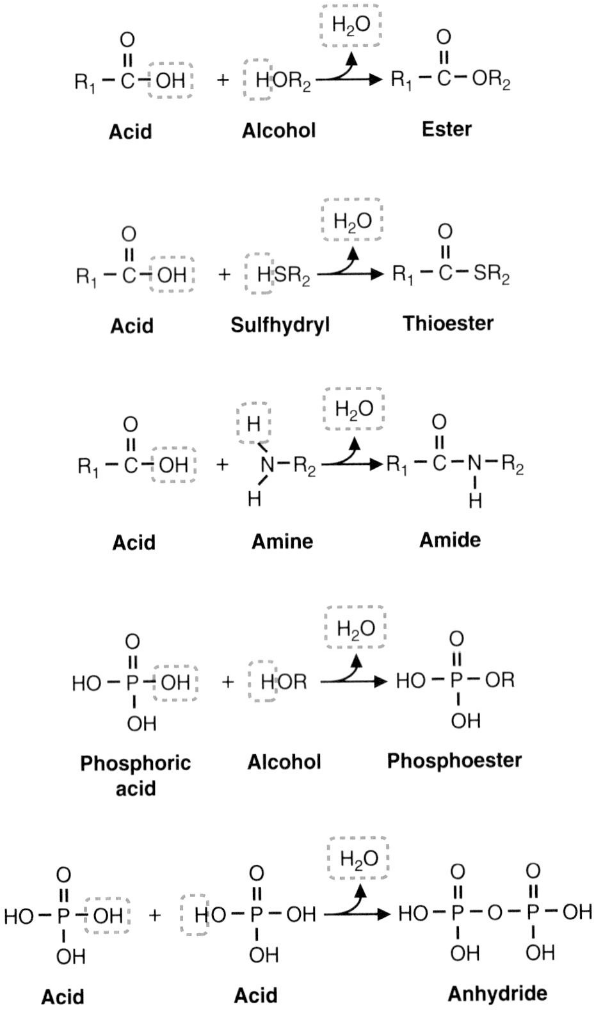

Fig. 5.7. Formation of esters, thioesters, amides, phosphoesters and anhydrides.

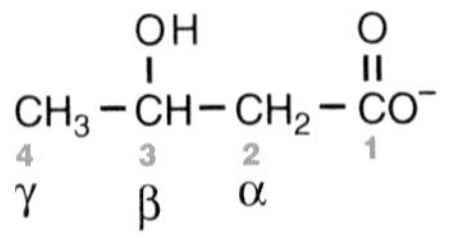

Acid   Alcohol   Ester

Acid   Sulfhydryl   Thioester

Acid   Amine   Amide

Phosphoric acid   Alcohol   Phosphoester

Acid   Acid   Anhydride

Fig. 5.8. Two systems for identifying the carbon atoms in a compound. This compound is called 3-hydroxybutyrate or β-hydroxybutyrate.

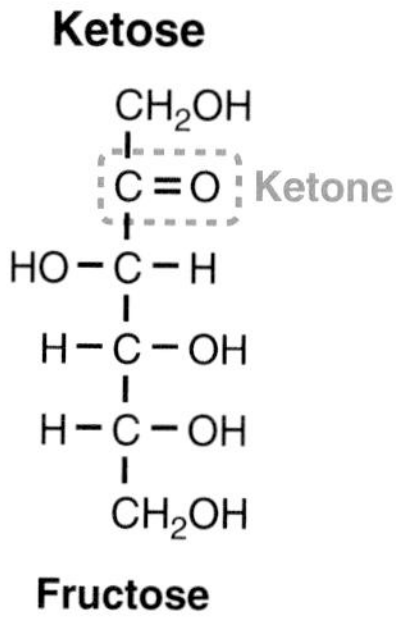

Ketose

$$CH_2OH$$
$$C = O \quad \text{Ketone}$$
$$HO - C - H$$
$$H - C - OH$$
$$H - C - OH$$
$$CH_2OH$$

Fructose

Fig. 5.9. Fructose is a ketohexose.

 The stereospecificity of D-glucose is still frequently denoted in medicine by the use of its old name, dextrose. A solution used for intravenous infusions in patients is a 5% (5 g/100 mL) solution of dextrose.

Q: Are D-mannose and D-galactose stereoisomers? Are they epimers of each other? (see Fig. 5.12)

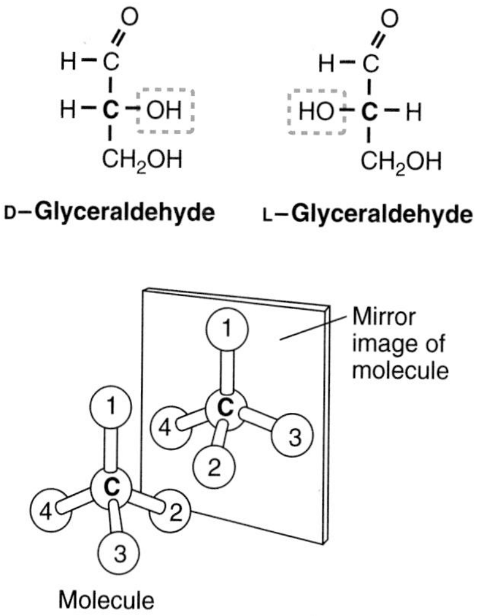

$$H - C \nearrow^{O}$$
$$H - C - OH$$
$$CH_2OH$$

$$H - C \nearrow^{O}$$
$$HO - C - H$$
$$CH_2OH$$

D–Glyceraldehyde   **L–Glyceraldehyde**

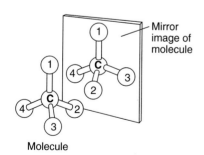

Molecule

Fig. 5.10. D- and L-Glyceraldehyde. The carbon in the center contains four different substituent groups arranged around it in a tetrahedron. A different arrangement creates an isomer that is a nonsuperimposable mirror image. If you rotate the mirror image structure so that groups 1 and 2 align, group 3 will be in the position of group 4, and group 4 will be in position 3.

1.   D- AND L-SUGARS

A carbon atom that contains four different chemical groups forms an asymmetric (or chiral) center (Fig. 5.10). The groups attached to the asymmetric carbon atom can be arranged to form two different isomers that are mirror images of each other and not superimposable. Monosaccharide stereoisomers are designated D or L based on whether the position of the hydroxyl group furthest from the carbonyl carbon matches D or L glyceraldehyde (Fig. 5.11). Although a more sophisticated system of nomenclature using the designations of (R) and (S) is generally used to describe the positions of groups on complex molecules such as drugs, the D and L designation is still used in medicine for describing sugars and amino acids. Because glucose (the major sugar in human blood) and most other sugars in human tissues belong to the D series, sugars are assumed to be D unless L is specifically added to the name.

2.   STEREOISOMERS AND EPIMERS

Stereoisomers have the same chemical formula but differ in the position of the hydroxyl group on one or more of their asymmetric carbons (Fig. 5.12). A sugar with n asymmetric centers has 2^n stereoisomers unless it has a plane of symmetry. Epimers are stereoisomers that differ in the position of the hydroxyl group at only one of their asymmetric carbons. D-glucose and D-galactose are epimers of each other, differing only at position 4, and can be interconverted in human cells by enzymes called epimerases. D-mannose and D-glucose are also epimers of each other.

3.   RING STRUCTURES

Monosaccharides exist in solution mainly as ring structures in which the carbonyl (aldehyde or ketone) group has reacted with a hydroxyl group in the same molecule to form a five- or six-membered ring (Fig. 5.13). The oxygen that was on the hydroxyl group is now part of the ring, and the original carbonyl carbon, which now contains a –OH group, has become the anomeric carbon atom. An hydroxyl group on the anomeric carbon drawn down below the ring is in the α-position; drawn up above the ring, it is in the β position. In the actual three-dimensional structure, the ring is not planar but usually takes a "chair" conformation in which the hydroxyl groups are located at a maximal distance from each other.

In solution, the hydroxyl group on the anomeric carbon spontaneously (nonenzymatically) changes from the α to the β position through a process called mutarotation. When the ring opens, the straight chain aldehyde or ketone is formed. When the ring closes, the hydroxyl group may be in either the α or the β position (Fig. 5.14). This process occurs more rapidly in the presence of cellular enzymes called mutarotases. However, if the anomeric carbon forms a bond with another molecule, that bond is fixed in the α or β position, and the sugar cannot mutarotate. Enzymes are specific for α or β bonds between sugars and other molecules, and react with only one type.

4.   SUBSTITUTED SUGARS

Sugars frequently contain phosphate groups, amino groups, sulfate groups or N-acetyl groups. Most of the free monosaccharides within cells are phosphorylated at their terminal carbons, which prevents their transport out of the cell (see glucose 6-phosphate in Fig. 5.6). Amino sugars such as galacto**samine** and gluco**samine** contain an amino group instead of a hydroxyl group on one of the carbon atoms, usually carbon 2 (Fig. 5.15). Frequently this amino group has been acetylated to form an N-acetylated sugar. In complex molecules termed proteoglycans, many of

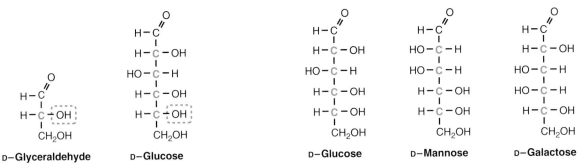

Fig. 5.11. D-Glyceraldehyde and D-glucose. These sugars have the same configuration at the asymmetric carbon atom farthest from the carbonyl group. Both belong to the D series. Asymmetric carbons are shown in blue.

Fig. 5.12. Examples of stereoisomers. These compounds have the same chemical formula ($C_6H_{12}O_6$) but differ in the positions of the hydroxyl groups on their asymmetric carbons (in blue).

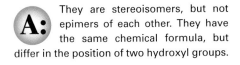

A: They are stereoisomers, but not epimers of each other. They have the same chemical formula, but differ in the position of two hydroxyl groups.

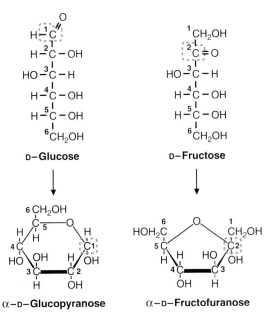

Fig. 5.13. Pyranose and furanose rings formed from glucose and fructose. The anomeric carbons are highlighted.

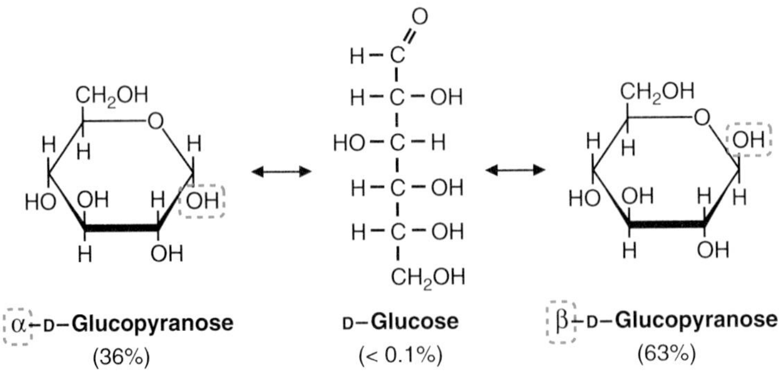

Fig. 5.14. Mutarotation of glucose in solution, with percentages of each form at equilibrium.

the *N*-acetylated sugars also contain negatively charged sulfate groups attached to a hydroxyl group on the sugar.

5. OXIDIZED AND REDUCED SUGARS

Sugars can be oxidized at the aldehyde carbon to form an acid. Technically the compound is no longer a sugar, and the ending on its name is changed from "-ose" to "onic acid" or "onate" (e.g., gluc**onic** acid, Fig. 5.16). If the carbon containing the terminal hydroxyl group is oxidized, the sugar is called a uronic acid (e.g., glu**curonic** acid).

If the aldehyde of a sugar is reduced, all of the carbon atoms contain alcohol (hydroxyl) groups, and the sugar is a poly**ol** (e.g., sorbit**ol**)(see Fig. 5.16). If one of

Oxidized sugars

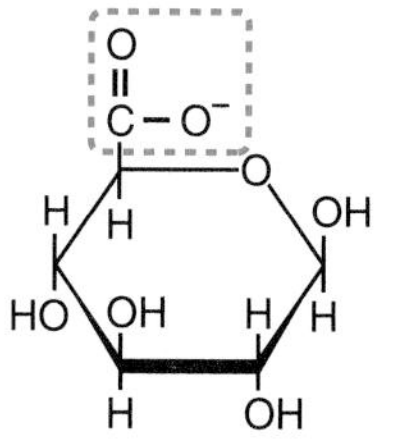

β–D–Glucuronate

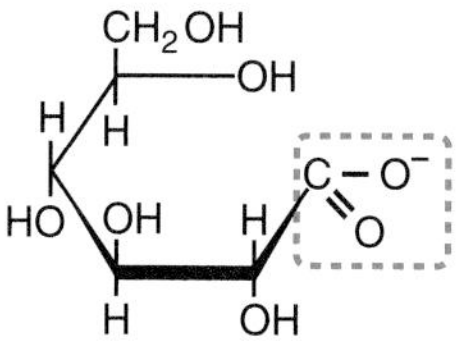

D–Gluconate

Reduced sugars

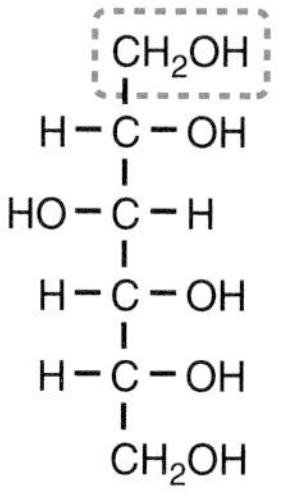

D–Sorbitol

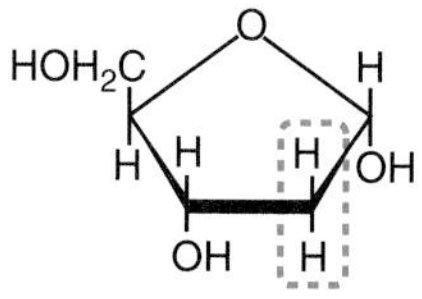

Deoxyribose

Fig. 5.16. Oxidized and reduced sugars. The affected group is shown in blue. Gluconic acid (D-gluconate) is formed by oxidation of the glucose aldehyde carbon. Glucuronic acid is formed by oxidation of the glucose terminal OH group. Sorbitol, a sugar alcohol, is formed by reduction of the glucose aldehyde group. Deoxyribose is formed by reduction of ribose.

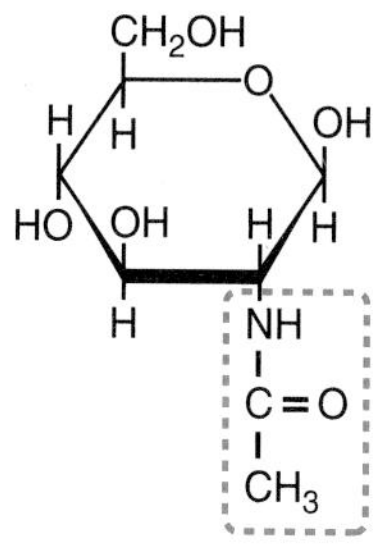

N–Acetyl–β–D–glucosamine

Fig. 5.15. An *N*-acetylated amino sugar. The *N*-denotes the amino group to which the acetyl group is attached, shown in the blue box.

Proteoglycans contain many long unbranched polysaccharide chains attached to a core protein. The polysaccharide chains, called glycosaminoglycans, are composed of repeating disaccharide units containing oxidized acid sugars (such as glucuronic acid), sulfated sugars, and N-acetylated amino sugars. The large number of negative charges causes the glycosaminoglycan chains to radiate out from the protein so that the overall structure resembles a bottlebrush. The proteoglycans are essential parts of the extracellular matrix, the aqueous humor of the eye, secretions of mucus-producing cells, and cartilage.

the hydroxyl groups of a sugar is reduced so that the carbon contains only hydrogen, the sugar is a deoxysugar, such as the **deoxy**ribose in DNA.

B. Glycosides

1. N- AND O-GLYCOSIDIC BONDS

The hydroxyl group on the anomeric carbon of a monosaccharide can react with an –OH or an –NH group of another compound to form a glyc**osidic** bond. The linkage may be either α or β, depending on the position of the atom attached to the anomeric carbon of the sugar. *N*-glycosidic bonds are found in nucle**osides** and nucle**otides**. For example, in the adenosine moiety of ATP, the nitrogenous base adenine is linked to the sugar ribose through a β-*N*-glycosidic bond (Fig. 5.17). In contrast, *O*-glycosidic bonds, such as those found in lactose, join sugars to each other or attach sugars to the hydroxyl group of an amino acid on a protein.

2. DISACCHARIDES, OLIGOSACCHARIDES, AND POLYSACCHARIDES

A disaccharide contains two monosaccharides joined by an *O*-glycosidic bond. Lactose, which is the sugar in milk, consists of galactose and glucose linked through a β(1→4) bond formed between the β –OH group of the anomeric carbon of galactose and the hydroxyl group on carbon 4 of glucose (see Fig. 5.17). Oligosaccharides contain from 3 to roughly 12 monosaccharides linked together. They are often found

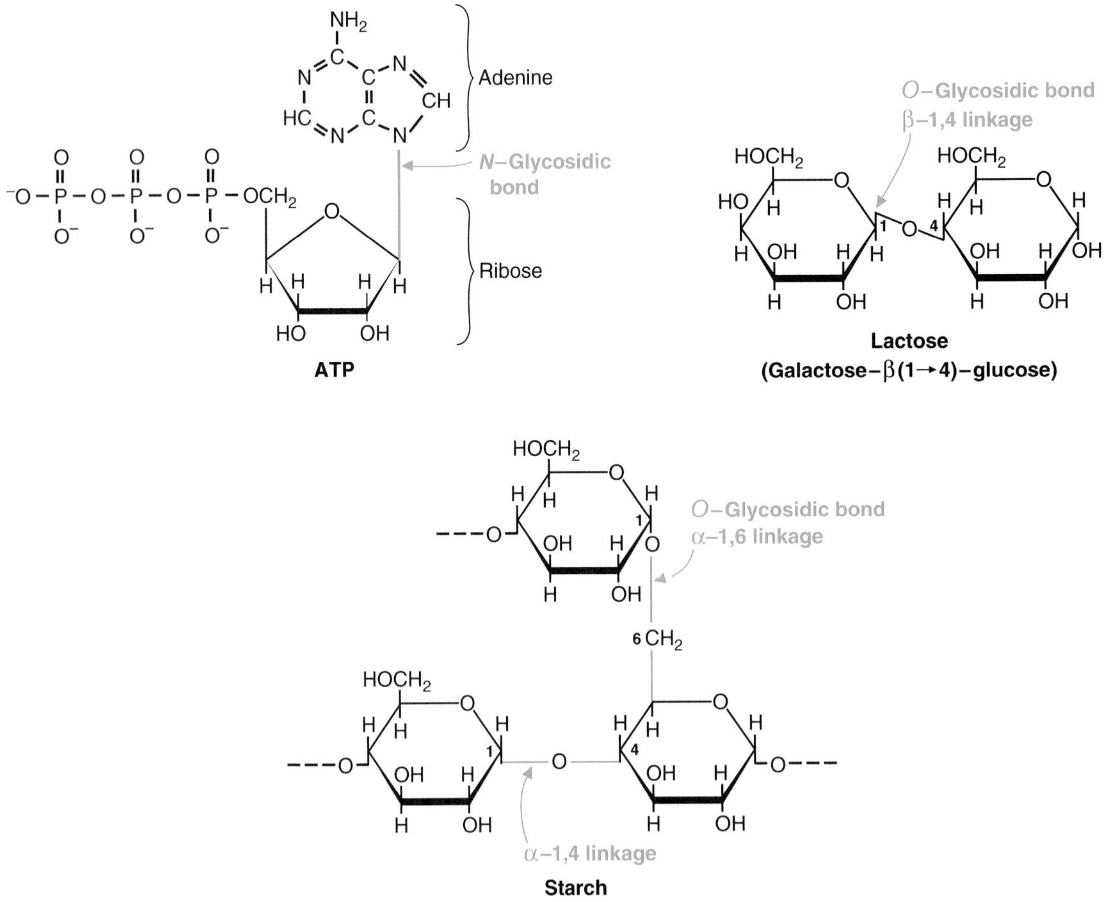

Fig. 5.17. *N*- and *O*-glycosidic bonds. Adenosine triphosphate (ATP) contains a β, *N*-glycosidic bond. Lactose contains an *O*-glycosidic β(1 → 4) bond. Glycogen contains α-1,4 and α-1,6 *O*-glycosidic bonds.

attached through *N-* or *O*-glycosidic bonds to proteins to form **glyco**proteins (see Chapter 6). Polysaccharides contain tens to thousands of monosaccharides joined by glycosidic bonds to form linear chains or branched structures. Amylopectin (a form of starch) and glycogen (the storage form of glucose in human cells) are branched polymers of glucosyl residues linked through $\alpha(1 \rightarrow 4)$ and $\alpha(1 \rightarrow 6)$ bonds.

III. LIPIDS

A. Fatty Acids

Fatty acids are usually straight aliphatic chains with a methyl group at one end (called the ω-carbon) and a carboxyl group at the other end (Fig. 5.18). Most fatty acids in the human have an even number of carbon atoms, usually between 16 and 20. Saturated fatty acids have single bonds between the carbons in the chain, and unsaturated fatty acids contain one or more double bonds. The most common saturated fatty acids present in the cell are palmitic acid (C16) and stearic acid (C18). Although these two fatty acids are generally called by their common names, shorter fatty acids are often called by the Latin word for the number of carbons, such as octanoic acid (8 carbons) and decanoic acid (10 carbons).

Monounsaturated fatty acids contain one double bond, and polyunsaturated fatty acids contain two or more double bonds (see Fig. 5.18). The position of a double bond is designated by the number of the carbon in the double bond that is closest to the carboxyl group. For example, oleic acid, which contains 18 carbons and a double bond between position 9 and 10, is designated 18:1, Δ^9. The number 18 denotes the number of carbon atoms, 1 (one) denotes the number of double bonds, and Δ^9

The melting point of a fatty acid increases with chain length and decreases with the degree of saturation. Thus, fatty acids with many double bonds, such as those in vegetable oils, are liquid at room temperature and saturated fatty acids, such as those in butterfat, are solids. Lipids with lower melting points are more fluid at body temperature and contribute to the fluidity of our cellular membranes.

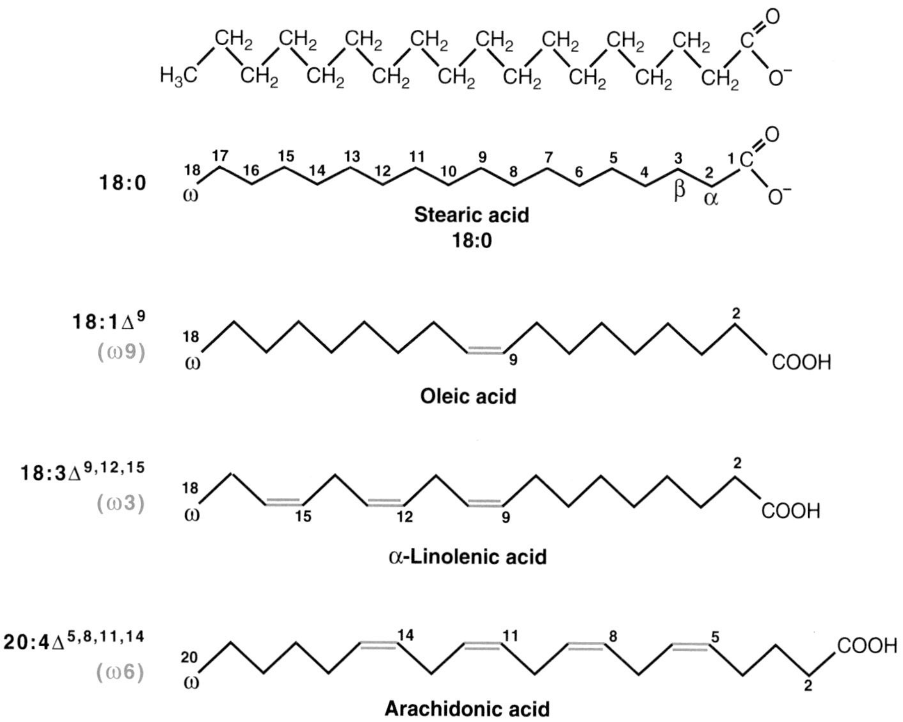

Fig. 5.18. Saturated fatty acids and unsaturated fatty acids. In stearic acid, the saturated fatty acid at the top of the figure, all the atoms are shown. A more common way of depicting the same structure is shown below. The carbons are either numbered starting with the carboxyl group or given Greek letters starting with the carbon next to the carboxyl group. The methyl (or ω) carbon at the end of the chain is always called the ω-carbon regardless of the chain length. 18:0 refers to the number of carbon atoms (18) and the number of double bonds (0). In the unsaturated fatty acids shown, not all of the carbons are numbered, but note that the double bonds are *cis* and spaced at three-carbon intervals. Both ω3 and ω6 fatty acids are required in the diet.

The eicosanoids are a group of hormone-like compounds produced by many cells in the body. They are derived from polyunsaturated fatty acids such as arachidonic acid that contain 20 carbons (eicosa) and have 3, 4, or 5 double bonds. The prostaglandins, thromboxanes, and leukotrienes belong to this group of compounds.

Palmitoleic acid, oleic acid, and arachidonic acid are the most common unsaturated fatty acids in the cell. Palmitoleic acid is a 16:1, Δ^9 fatty acid. How would you name it as an ω fatty acid?

denotes the position of the double bond between the 9th and 10th carbon atoms. Oleic acid can also be designated 18:1(9), without the Δ. Fatty acids are also classified by the distance of the double bond closest to the ω end (the methyl group at the end farthest from the carboxyl group). Thus oleic acid is an ω9 fatty acid, and linolenic acid is an ω3 fatty acid. Arachidonic acid, a polyunsaturated fatty acid with 20 carbons and 4 double bonds, is an ω6 fatty acid that is completely described as 20:4, $\Delta^{5,8,11,14}$.

The double bonds in most naturally occurring fatty acids are in the *cis* configuration (Fig. 5.19). The designation *cis* means that the hydrogens are on the same side of the double bond and the acyl chains on the other side. In *trans* fatty acids, the acyl chains are on opposite sides of the double bond. Margarine and the fat used in preparing French fries are probably the major sources of *trans* fatty acids found in humans. Trans fatty acids are produced by the chemical hydrogenation of polyunsaturated fatty acids in vegetable oils and are not a natural food product.

C. Acylglycerols

An **acyl**glycerol comprises glycerol with one or more fatty acids (the **acyl** group) attached through ester linkages (Fig. 5.20). Monoacylglycerols, diacylglycerols, and triacylglycerols contain 1, 2, or 3 fatty acids esterified to glycerol, respectively. Tri**acyl**glycerols rarely contain the same fatty acid at all three positions and are therefore called mixed triacylglycerols. Unsaturated fatty acids, when present, are most often esterified to carbon 2. In the three-dimensional configuration of glycerol, carbons 1 and 3 are not identical, and enzymes are specific for one or the other carbon.

D. Phosphoacylglycerols

Phosphoacylglycerols contain fatty acids esterified to position 1 and 2 of glycerol and a phosphate (alone or with a substituent) attached to carbon 3. If only a phosphate group is attached to carbon 3, the compound is **phospha**tidic acid (see Fig. 5.21). Phosphatidic acid is a precursor for the synthesis of the other phosphoacylglycerols.

Phosphatidylchol**ine** is one of the major phosphoacylglycerols found in membranes (see Fig. 5.21). The am**ine** is positively charged at neutral pH, and the phosphate negatively charged. Thus, the molecule is amphipathic; it contains large polar and nonpolar regions. Phosphatidylcholine is also called lecithin. Removal of a fatty acyl group from a phosphoacyl glycerol leads to a lyso-lipid. For example, removing the fatty acyl group from lecithin forms lysolecithin.

E. Sphingolipids

Sphingolipids do not have a glycerol backbone; they are formed from sphingosine. (Fig. 5.22). Shingos**ine** is derived from ser**ine** and a specific fatty acid, palmitate. Cer**amides** are **amides** formed from sphingosine by attaching a fatty acid to the

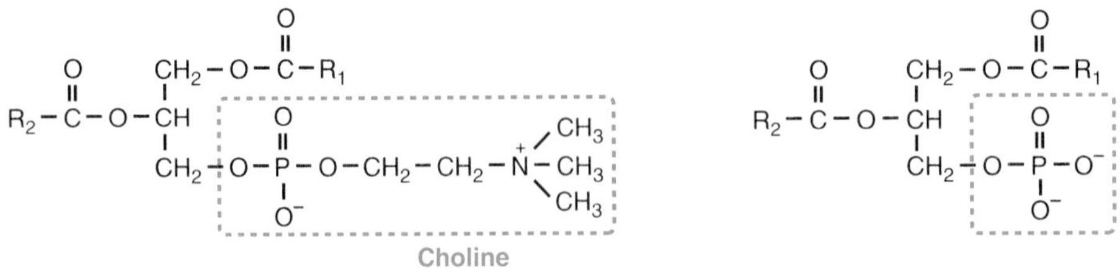

Trans

Cis

Fig. 5.19. *Cis* and *trans* double bonds in fatty acid side chains. Note that the *cis* double bond causes the chain to bend.

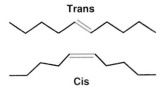

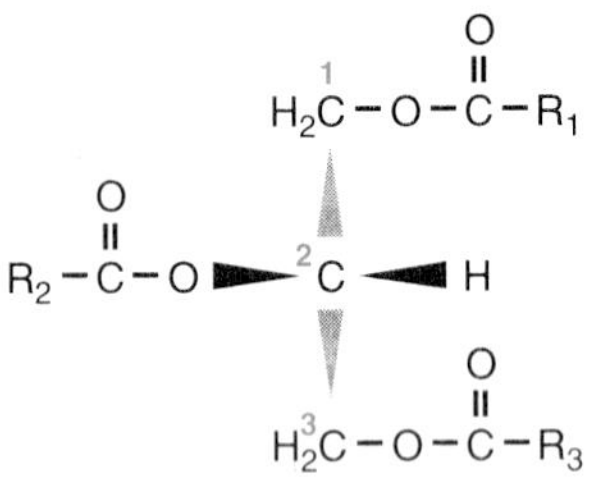

Triacyl–*sn*–glycerol

Fig. 5.20. A triacylglycerol. Note that carbons 1 and 3 of the glycerol moiety are not identical. The broad end of each arrowhead is closer to the reader than the narrow, pointed end.

Phosphatidylcholine

Phosphatidic acid

Fig. 5.21. Phosphoacylglycerols. Phospholipids found in membranes, such as phosphatidylcholine, have a polar group attached to the phosphate.

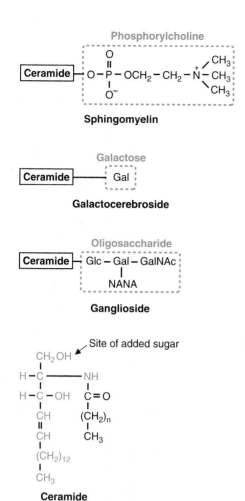

A: Palmitoleic acid is an ω7 fatty acid. It has one double bond between the 9th and 10th carbons. It has 16 carbons, like palmitic acid, so the double bond must be at the 7th carbon from the ω end.

Fig. 5.22. Sphingolipids, derivatives of ceramide. The structure of ceramide is shown at the bottom of the figure. The portion of ceramide shown in blue is sphingosine. The NH and OH were contributed by serine. Different groups are added to the hydroxyl group of ceramide to form sphingomyelin, galactocerebrosides, and gangliosides. NANA = N-acetylneuraminic acid, also called sialic acid; Glc = glucose; Gal = galactose; GalNAc = N-acetylgalactosamine.

amino group. Various sphingolipids are then formed by attaching different groups to the hydroxyl group on ceramide. As reflected in the names for cerebro**sides** and gangli**osides**, these sphingolipids contain sugars attached to the hydroxyl group of ceramide through glycosidic bonds. They are glycolipids (more specifically, glycosphingolipids). Sphingomyelin, which contains a phophorylcholine group attached to ceramide, is a component of cell membranes and the myelin sheath around neurons.

F. Steroids

Steroids contain a four-ring structure called the steroid nucleus (Fig. 5.23). Cholesterol is the steroid precursor in human cells from which all of the steroid hormones are synthesized by modifications to the ring or C20 side chain. Although cholesterol is not very water soluble, it is converted to amphipathic water-soluble bile salts such as cholic acid. Bile salts line the surfaces of lipid droplets called micelles in the lumen of the intestine, where they keep the droplets emulsified in the aqueous environment.

Cholesterol is one of the compounds synthesized in the human from branched 5-carbon units with one double bond called an isoprenyl unit (see Fig. 5.1A). Isoprenyl

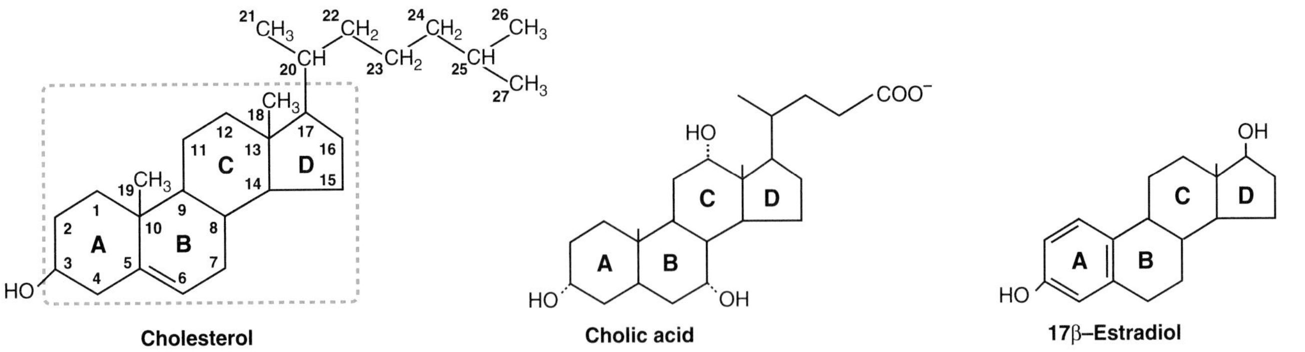

Fig. 5.23. Cholesterol and its derivatives. The steroid nucleus is shown in blue. The bile salt, cholic acid, and the steroid hormone 17β-estradiol are derived from cholesterol and contain the steroid ring structure.

Q: What structural features account for the differences in the solubility of cholesterol, estradiol and cholic acid in the body? (see Fig. 5.23)

units are combined in long chains to form other structures, such as the side chains of coenzyme Q in humans and vitamin A in plants.

IV. NITROGEN-CONTAINING COMPOUNDS

Nitrogen, as described in Section IB2, is an electronegative atom with two unshared electrons in its outer valence shell. At neutral pH, the nitrogen in amino groups is usually bonded to four other atoms and carries a positive charge. However, the presence of nitrogen atom in an organic compound will increase its solubility in water, whether the nitrogen is charged or uncharged.

A. Amino Acids

Amino acids are compounds that contain an amino group and a carboxylic acid group. In proteins, the amino acids are always L-α amino acids (the amino group is attached to the α carbon in the L-configuration) (Fig. 5.24). These same amino acids also serve as precursors of nitrogen-containing compounds in the body, such as phosphatidylcholine (see Fig. 5.21) and are the basis of most human amino acid metabolism. However, our metabolic reactions occasionally produce an amino acid that has a β or γ amino group, such as the neurotransmitter γ-aminobutyric acid (see Fig. 5.24). However, only α amino acids are incorporated into proteins.

Although D-amino acids are not usually incorporated into proteins in living organisms, they serve many other functions in bacteria, such as synthesis of cross-links in cell walls.

B. Nitrogen-Containing Ring Structures

1.   PURINES, PYRIMIDINES AND PYRIDINES

Nitrogen is also a component of ring structures referred to as heterocyclic rings or nitrogenous bases. The three most common types of nitrogen-containing rings in the

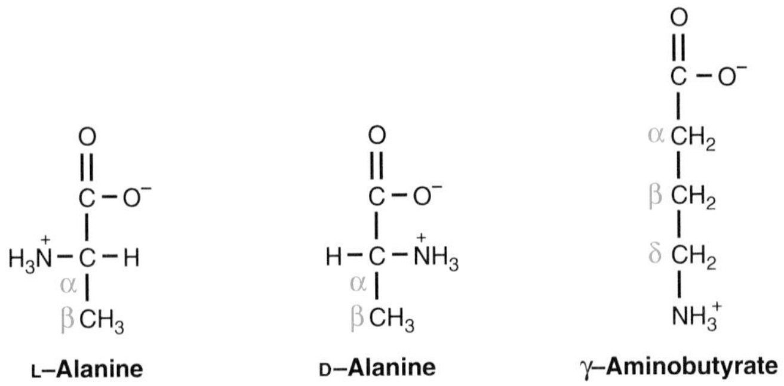

Fig. 5.24. The structure of amino acids.

body are pur**ines** (e.g., aden**ine**), pyrimid**ines** (e.g., thym**ine**), and pyrid**ines** (e.g., the vitamins nicot**in**ic acid, also called niacin, and pyridox**ine**, also called vitamin B$_6$) (Fig.5.25). The suffix "**ine**" denotes the presence of nitrogen (am**ine**) in the ring. The pyrimidine uracil is an exception to this general type of nomenclature. The utility of these nitrogen-containing ring structures lies in the ability of the nitrogen to form hydrogen bonds and to accept and donate electrons while still part of the ring. In contrast, the unsubstituted aromatic benzene ring, in which electrons are distributed equally among all six carbons (see Fig. 5.1), is nonpolar, hydrophobic, and relatively unreactive.

2. NUCLEOSIDES AND NUCLEOTIDES

Nitrogenous bases form nucleosides and nucleotides. A nucleoside consists of a nitrogenous base joined to a sugar, usually ribose or deoxyribose, through an *N*-glycosidic bond (see Fig. 5.17). If phosphate groups are attached to the sugar, the compound becomes a nucleotide. In the name of the nucleotide adenosine triphosphate (ATP), the addition of the ribose is indicated by the name change from adenine to aden**osine** (for the glyc**osidic** bond). Monophosphate, diphosphate, or triphosphate are added to the name to indicate the presence of 1, 2, or 3 phosphate groups in the nucleotide. The structures of the nucleotides that serve as precursors of DNA and RNA are discussed in more detail in Section Three, Chapter 12.

3. TAUTOMERS

In many of the nitrogen-containing rings, the hydrogen can shift to produce a tautomer, a compound in which the hydrogen and double bonds have changed position (i.e., –N=C–OH → –NH–C=O) (Fig. 5.26). Tautomers are considered the same compound, and the structure may be represented either way. Generally one tautomeric form is more reactive than the other. For example, in the two tautomeric forms of uric acid, a proton can dissociate from the enol form to produce urate.

V. FREE RADICALS

Radicals are compounds that have a single electron, usually in an outer orbital. Free radicals are radicals that exist independently in solution or in a lipid environment.

Q: Compounds that cannot be oxidized as fuels in the human are often excreted in the urine. Chemical modifications often occur in the liver, kidney, or other tissues that inactivate or detoxify the chemicals, make them more water-soluble, or otherwise target such molecules for excretion. Uric acid, the basis of **Lotta Topaigne**'s pain, is excreted in the urine (see Fig. 5.26). Judging from the similarity in structure, do you think it is derived from the degradation of purines, pyrimidines, or pyridines?

A: Cholesterol is composed almost entirely of CH_2 groups and is therefore water-insoluble. Estradiol is likewise relatively water-insoluble. However, cholic acid contains a hydrophilic carboxyl group, and three hydroxyl groups. As shown by the dashed lines, the three hydroxyl groups all lie on one side of the molecule, thus creating a hydrophilic surface.

Lotta Topaigne's gout is caused by depositions of monosodium urate crystals in the joint of her big toe. At a blood pH of 7.4, all of the uric acid has dissociated a proton to form urate, which is not very water-soluble and forms crystals of the Na^+ salt. In the more acidic urine generated by the kidney, the acidic form, uric acid, may precipitate to form kidney stones.

Purines

Adenine (A)

Guanine (G)

Pyrimidine

Thymine (T)

Pyridine

Nicotinic acid

Fig. 5.25. The nitrogenous bases.

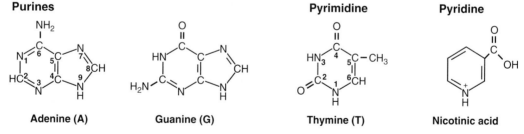

Uric acid
(Keto form)

Uric acid
(Enol form)

pK 5.4

Urate

Fig. 5.26. Tautomers of uric acid. The tautomeric form affects the reactivity. The enol form dissociates a proton to form urate.

Free radicals are not just esoteric reactants; they are the agents of cell death and destruction. They are involved in all chronic disease states (e.g., coronary artery disease, diabetes mellitus, arthritis, and emphysema) as well as acute injury (e.g., radiation, strokes, myocardial infarction, and spinal cord injury). Through free radical defense mechanisms in our cells, we can often restrict the damage attributed to the "normal" aging process.

A: Uric acid contains two rings and is similar to the purines adenine and guanine (adenine is shown in Fig. 5.25). In fact, it is the urinary excretion product formed from the oxidation of these two purine bases. It is not very soluble in water, particularly if the pH is near the pK_a of its acidic OH group. If present in excess amounts, Na^+ urate tends to precipitate in joints, causing the severe pain of gout experienced by **Ms. Topaigne**.

The reducing sugar test. The reducing sugar test was used for detection of sugar in the urine long before specific enzymatic assays for glucose and galactose became available. In this test, the aldehyde group of a sugar is oxidized as it donates electrons to copper; the copper becomes reduced and produces a blue color. In alkaline solution, keto sugars (e.g., fructose) also react in this test because they form tautomers that are aldehydes. Ring structures of sugars will also react, but only if the ring can open (i.e., it is not attached to another compound through a glycosidic bond). Until a specific test for fructose becomes available, a congenital disease resulting in the presence of fructose in the urine is indicated by a positive reducing sugar test and negative results in the specific enzymatic assays for glucose or galactose.

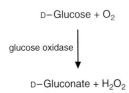

D−Glucose + O_2

glucose oxidase

D−Gluconate + H_2O_2

Fig. 5.27. Glucose oxidase.

Although many enzymes generate radicals as intermediates in reactions, these are not usually released into the cell to become free radicals.

Many of the compounds in the body are capable of being converted to free radicals by natural events that remove one of their electrons, or by radiation. Radiation, for example, dissociates water into the hydrogen atom and the hydroxyl radical:

$$H_2O \leftrightarrow H\bullet + OH\bullet$$

In contrast, water normally dissociates into a proton and the negatively charged hydroxyl ion. The hydroxyl radical forms organic radicals by taking one electron (as H•) from a compound such as an unsaturated membrane lipid, which then has a single unpaired electron and is a new radical.

Compounds that are radicals may be written with, or without, the radical showing. For example, nitrogen dioxide, a potent, reactive, toxic radical present in smog and cigarette smoke, may be designated in medical and lay literature as NO_2 rather than $NO_2\bullet$. Superoxide, a radical produced in the cell and that is the source of much destruction, is correctly written as the superoxide anion, O_2^-. However, to emphasize its free radical nature, the same compound is sometimes written as $O_2^-\bullet$. If a compound is designated as a radical in the medical literature, you can be certain that it is a reactive radical, and that its radical nature is important for the pathophysiology under discussion. (Reactive oxygen and nitrogen-containing free radicals are discussed in more detail in Chapter 24).

CLINICAL COMMENTS

Dianne Abietes. The severity of clinical signs and symptoms in patients with diabetic ketoacidosis (DKA), such as **Di Abietes**, is directly correlated with the concentration of ketone bodies in the blood. Direct quantitative methods for measuring acetoacetate and β-hydroxybutyrate are not routinely available. As a result, clinicians usually rely on semiquantitative reagent strips (Ketostix, Bayer Diagnostics, Mishawaha, IN) or tablets (Acetest, Bayer Diagnostics, Mishawaha, IN) to estimate the level of acetoacetate in the blood and the urine. The nitroprusside on the strips and in the tablets reacts with acetoacetate and to a lesser degree with acetone (both of which have ketone groups), but does not react with β-hydroxybutyrate (which does not have a ketone group). β-hydroxybutyrate is the predominant ketone body present in the blood of a patient in DKA, and its concentration could decline at a disproportionately rapid rate compared with that of acetoacetate and acetone. Therefore, tests employing the nitroprusside reaction to monitor the success of therapy in such a patient may be misleading.

In contrast to the difficulty of ketone body measurements, diabetic patients can self-monitor blood glucose levels at home, thereby markedly decreasing the time and expense of the many blood glucose determinations they need. Blood obtained from a finger prick is placed on the pad of a plastic strip. The strip has been impregnated with an enzyme (usually the bacterial enzyme glucose oxidase) that specifically converts the glucose in the blood to a compound (hydrogen peroxide, H_2O_2) that reacts with a dye to produce a color (Fig. 5.27). The intensity of the color, which is directly proportionate to the concentration of glucose in the patient's blood, is read on an instrument called a blood glucose monitor.

Lotta Topaigne. Ms. Topaigne has acute gouty arthritis (podagra) involving her right great toe. Polarized light microscopy of the fluid aspirated from the joint space showed crystals of monosodium urate phagocytosed by white blood cells. The presence of the relatively insoluble urate crystals within the joint space activates an inflammatory cascade leading to the classic components of joint inflammation (pain, redness, warmth, swelling, and limitation of joint motion).

BIOCHEMICAL COMMENTS

 Chlorinated Aromatic Hydrocarbon Environmental Toxins. As a result of human endeavor, toxic compounds containing chlorinated benzene rings have been widely distributed in the environment. The pesticide DDT and the class of chemicals called dioxins provide examples of chlorinated aromatic hydrocarbons and structurally related compounds that are very hydrophobic and poorly biodegraded (Fig. 5.28). As a consequence of their persistence and lipophilicity, these chemicals are concentrated in the adipose tissue of fish, fish-eating birds, and carnivorous mammals, including humans.

DDT, a chlorinated biphenyl, was widely used in the United States as an herbicide between the 1940s and 1960s (see Fig. 5.28). Although it has not been used in this country since 1972, the chlorinated benzene rings are resistant to biodegradation, and U.S. soil and water are still contaminated with small amounts. DDT is still used in other parts of the world. Because this highly lipophilic molecule is stored in the fat of animals, organisms accumulate progressively greater amounts of DDT at each successive stage of the food chain. Fish-eating birds, one of the organisms at the top of the food chain, have declined in population because of the effect of DDT on the thickness of their eggshells. DDT is not nearly as toxic in the human, although long-term exposure or exposure to high doses may cause reversible neurologic symptoms, hepatotoxic effects, or cancer.

Dioxins, specifically chlorinated dibenzo-p-dioxins (CDDs), constitute another class of environmental toxins that are currently of great concern (see Fig. 5.28). They have been measured at what is termed background levels in the blood, adipose tissue, and breast milk of all humans tested. CDDs are formed as a byproduct during the production of other chlorinated compounds and herbicides, and from the chlorine bleaching process used by pulp and paper mills. They are released during the incineration of industrial, municipal, and domestic waste, and during the combustion of fossil fuels, and are found in cigarette smoke and the exhaust from gasoline and diesel fuels. They can also be formed from the combustion of organic matter during forest fires. They enter the atmosphere as particulate matter, are vaporized, and can spread large distances to enter soil and water.

As humans at the top of the food chain, we have acquired our background levels of dioxins principally through the consumption of food, primarily meat, dairy products,

 Most of this chapter has dealt with the names and structures of compounds that are nutrients for the human or metabolites that can be produced from reactions in the human body. However, our health is also affected by naturally occurring and man-made xenobiotic compounds (compounds that have no nutrient value and are not produced in the human) that we ingest, inhale, or absorb through our skin. DDT and dioxins provide examples of chlorinated aromatic hydrocarbons, an important class of manmade chemicals present in the environment.

The accumulation of DDT in adipose tissue may be protective in the human because it decreases the amount of DDT available to pass through nonpolar lipid membranes to reach neurons in the brain, or pass through placental membranes to reach the fetus. Eventually we convert DDT to more polar metabolites that are excreted in the urine. However, some may pass with lipid into the breast milk of nursing mothers.

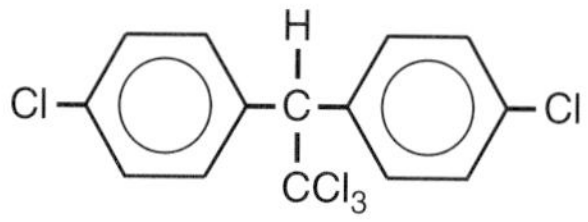

DDT

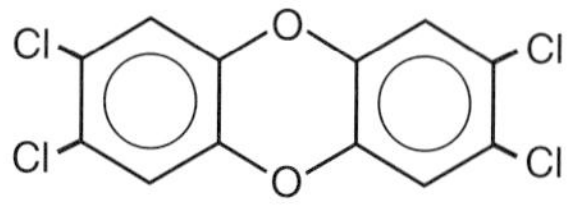

Chlorodibenzo-p-dioxin

Fig. 5.28. Environmental toxins. Dichlorodiphenyl trichlorethane (DDT) is a member of a class of aromatic hydrocarbons that contain two chlorinated benzene (phenyl) rings joined by a chlorinated ethane molecule. Chlorodibenzo-p-dioxin's (CDDs) are a related class of more than 75 chlorinated hydrocarbons that all contain a dibenzo-p-dioxin (DD) molecule comprising two benzene rings joined via two oxygen bridges at adjacent carbons on each of the benzene rings. 2,3,7,8 Tetrachlorodibenzo-p-dioxin, shown above, is one of the most toxic and the most extensively studied. Chlorinated dibenzofurans (CDF) are structurally and toxicologically related.

Most of what is known about the toxicity of dioxins in the human comes from individuals exposed incidentally or chronically to higher levels (e.g., industrial accidents or presence in areas sprayed with Agent Orange or other herbicides contaminated with dioxins.). The lowest dose effects are probably associated with thymic atrophy and decreased immune response, chloracne and related skin lesions, and neoplasia (cancer). Dioxins can cross into the placenta to cause developmental and reproductive effects, decreased prenatal growth, and prenatal mortality.

and fish. Once in the human body, dioxins are stored in human fat and adipose tissue, and have an average half-life of approximately 5 to 15 years. They are unreactive, poorly degraded, and not readily converted to more water-soluble compounds that can be excreted in the urine. They are slowly excreted in the bile and feces, and together with lipids enter the breast milk of nursing mothers.

Suggested References

Nomenclature of chemical compounds. Most undergraduate organic textbooks provide a more detailed account of the nomenclature used for organic molecules, including the R,S nomenclature for chiral centers.

Environmental toxins. Good literature reviews for many environmental toxins are published by the U.S. Department of Health and Human Services: Public Health Service Agency for Toxic Substances and Disease Registry, including: Toxicological Profile for Chlorinated Dibenzo-p-dioxins, 1998, and the Toxicological Profile for 4,4′-DDT, 4,4′-DDE, 4,4′-DDD (Update), 1994.

 REVIEW QUESTIONS—CHAPTER 5

Directions: Select the single best answer for each of the questions below. Base your answers on your knowledge of nomenclature. You need not recognize any of the structures shown to answer the questions.

1. Which of the following is a universal characteristic of water-soluble organic compounds?

    (A) They are composed of carbon and hydrogen atoms.
    (B) They must contain a group that has a full negative charge.
    (C) They must contain a group that has a full positive charge.
    (D) They contain polar groups that can hydrogen bond with water.
    (E) They contain aromatic groups.

2. $CH_2OH–CH_2–CH_2–COO^-$
    A patient was admitted to the hospital emergency room in a coma. Laboratory tests found high levels of the compound shown above in her blood. On the basis of its structure (and your knowledge of the nomenclature of functional groups), you identify the compound as

    (A) methanol (wood alcohol).
    (B) ethanol (alcohol).
    (C) ethylene glycol (antifreeze).
    (D) β-hydroxybutyrate (a ketone body).
    (E) γ-hydroxybutyrate (the "date rape" drug).

3. A patient was diagnosed with a deficiency of the lysosomal enzyme α-glycosidase. The name of the deficient enzyme suggests that it hydrolyzes a glycosidic bond, which is a bond formed

    (A) through multiple hydrogen bonds between two sugar molecules.
    (B) between the anomeric carbon of a sugar and an O–H (or N) of another molecule.
    (C) between two anomeric carbons in polysaccharides.
    (D) internally between the anomeric carbon of a monosaccharide and its own 5th carbon hydroxyl group.
    (E) between the carbon containing the aldol or keto group and the α carbon.

4. A patient was diagnosed with a hypertriglyceridemia. This condition is named for the high blood levels of lipids composed of

    (A) 3 fatty acyl groups attached to a glycerol backbone.
    (B) a glycerol lipid containing a phosporylcholine group.
    (C) a sphingolipid containing three fatty acyl groups.
    (D) three glycerol moieties attached to a fatty acid.
    (E) three glyceraldehyde moieties attached to a fatty acid.

5. A patient was diagnosed with a sphingolipidoses, which are congenital diseases involving the inability to degrade sphingolipids. All sphingolipids have in common

    (A) a glycerol backbone.
    (B) ceramide.
    (C) phosphorylcholine.
    (D) N-acetylneuraminic acid (NANA).
    (E) a steroid ring structure to which sphingosine is attached.

6 Amino Acids in Proteins

The genetic code is the sequence of three bases (nucleotides) in DNA containing the information for the linear sequence of amino acids in a polypeptide chain (its primary structure). A gene is the portion of DNA that encodes a functional product, such as a polypeptide chain. Mutations, which are changes in the nucleotides in a gene, result in a change in the products of that gene that may be inherited. The genetically inherited disease sickle cell anemia is, for example, caused by a mutation in the gene encoding one of the subunits of hemoglobin. Hemoglobin is the protein present in red blood cells that reversibly binds O_2 and transports it to tissues. The adult hemoglobin protein comprises four polypeptide chains, 2α and 2β. The α and β subunits differ in primary structure (i.e., they have different sequences of amino acids and are encoded by different genes). Sickle cell anemia is caused by a mutation in DNA that changes just one amino acid in the hemoglobin β chains from a glutamic acid to a valine.

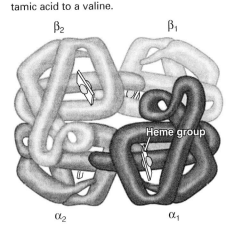

Proteins have many functions in the body. They serve as transporters of hydrophobic compounds in the blood, as cell adhesion molecules that attach cells to each other and to the extracellular matrix, as hormones that carry signals from one group of cells to another, as ion channels through lipid membranes, and as enzymes that increase the rate of biochemical reactions. The unique characteristics of a protein are dictated by its linear sequence of amino acids, termed its primary structure. The primary structure of a protein determines how it can fold and how it interacts with other molecules in the cell to perform its function. The primary structures of all of the diverse human proteins are synthesized from 20 amino acids arranged in a linear sequence determined by the genetic code.

General properties of amino acids. Each of the amino acids used for protein synthesis has the same general structure (Fig. 6.1). It contains a **carboxylic acid** group, an **amino group** attached to the **α-carbon** in an **L configuration**, a **hydrogen atom**, and a chemical group called **a side chain** that is different for each amino acid. In solution, the free amino acids exist as **zwitterions**, ions in which the amino group is positively charged and the carboxylate group is negatively charged. In proteins, these amino acids are joined into linear polymers called **polypeptide chains** through **peptide bonds** between the carboxylic acid group of one amino acid and the amino group of the next amino acid.

Classification of amino acids according to chemical properties of the side chains. The chemical properties of the side chain determine the types of bonds and interactions each amino acid in a polypeptide chain can make with other molecules. Thus, amino acids are often grouped by polarity of the side chain (**charged, nonpolar hydrophobic,** or **uncharged polar**) or by structural features (**aliphatic, cyclic,** or **aromatic**). The side chains of the **nonpolar hydrophobic** amino acids (alanine, valine, leucine, isoleucine, phenylalanine, and methionine) cluster together to exclude water in the **hydrophobic effect.** The **uncharged polar** amino acids (serine, threonine, tyrosine, asparagine, and glutamine) participate in **hydrogen bonding.** Cysteine, which contains a sulfhydryl group, forms **disulfide bonds.** The negatively charged **acidic** amino acids (aspartate and glutamate) form **ionic (electrostatic) bonds** with positively charged molecules, such as the **basic** amino acids (lysine, arginine, and histidine). The charge on the amino acid at a particular pH is determined by the pK_a of each group that has a dissociable proton.

Amino acid substitutions in the primary structure. Mutations in the genetic code result in proteins with an altered **primary structure.** Mutations resulting in single amino acid substitutions can affect the functioning of a protein or can confer an advantage specific to a tissue or a set of circumstances. Many proteins such as **hemoglobin** exist in the human population as **polymorphisms** (genetically determined variations in primary structure.)

Within the same individual, the primary structure of many proteins varies with the stage of development and is present in **fetal** and **adult isoforms,** such as fetal and adult hemoglobin. The primary structure of some proteins, such as **creatine kinase,** can also vary between tissues (**tissue-specific isozymes**) or between intracellular locations in the same tissue. **Electrophoretic separation** of tissue-specific isozymes has been useful in medicine as a means of identifying the tissue site of injury.

β_2 β_1

Heme group

α_2 α_1

*Modified amino acids. In addition to the amino acids encoded by DNA that form the primary structure of proteins, many proteins contain specific amino acids that have been modified by **phosphorylation, oxidation, carboxylation,** or other reactions. When these reactions are enzyme-catalyzed, they are referred to **as post-translational modifications**.*

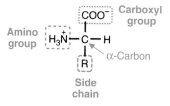

Fig. 6.1. General structure of the amino acids found in proteins.

THE WAITING ROOM

Will Sichel is a 17-year-old boy who came to the hospital emergency room with severe pain in his lower back, abdomen, and legs, which began after a 2-day history of nausea and vomiting caused by gastroenteritis. He was diagnosed as having sickle cell disease at age 3 years and has been admitted to the hospital on numerous occasions for similar vaso-occlusive sickle cell crises.

On admission, the patient's hemoglobin level in peripheral venous blood was 7.8 g/dL (reference range = 12–16 g/dL). The hematocrit or packed cell volume (the percentage of the total volume of blood made up by red blood cells) was 23.4% (reference range = 41–53%). His serum total bilirubin level (a pigment derived from hemoglobin degradation) was 2.3 mg/dL (reference range = 0.2−1.0 mg/dL). An x-ray of his abdomen showed radiopaque stones in his gallbladder. With chronic hemolysis (red blood cell destruction), the amount of heme degraded to bilirubin is increased. These stones are the result of the chronic excretion of excessive amounts of bilirubin from the liver into the bile, leading to bilirubinate crystal deposition in the gallbladder lumen.

Cal Kulis is an 18-year-old boy who was brought to the hospital by his mother because of the sudden onset of severe pain in the left flank radiating around his left side toward his pubic area. His urine was reddish-brown in color, and his urinalysis showed the presence of many red blood cells. When his urine was acidified with acetic acid, clusters of flat hexagonal transparent crystals of cystine were noted. An x-ray of his abdomen showed radiopaque calculi (stones) in both kidneys. There was no family history of kidney stone disease.

The term *calculus* is used to describe any abnormal concretion (concrete-like precipitate) of mineral salts. These almost always form within the cavity of a hollow organ, such as the kidney (kidney or renal stones) or the lumen of a duct (e.g., common bile duct stones).

Di Abietes, who has type 1 diabetes mellitus, was giving herself subcutaneous injections of insulin regular NPH beef insulin twice daily after her disease was first diagnosed (see Chapters 4 and 5). Subsequently, her physician switched her to synthetic human insulin. At this visit, her physician changed her insulin therapy and has written a prescription for Humalog mix 75/25 (Eli Lilly, Indianapolis, IN), a mixture of Humalog in protamine suspension and unbound Humalog insulin (25%).

Ann Jeina is a 54-year-old woman who is 68 inches tall and weighs 198 lb. She has a history of high blood pressure and elevated serum cholesterol levels. After a heated argument with a neighbor, Mrs. Jeina experienced a "tight pressure-like band of pain" across her chest, associated with shortness of breath, sweating, and a sense of light-headedness.

After 5 hours of intermittent chest pain, she went to the hospital emergency room, where her electrocardiogram showed changes consistent with an acute infarction of the anterior wall of her heart. She was admitted to the cardiac care unit. Blood was sent to the laboratory for various tests, including the total creatine kinase (CK) level and the MB ("muscle–brain") fraction of CK in the blood.

The term *angina* describes a crushing or compressive pain. The term *angina pectoris* is used when this pain is located in the center of the chest, often radiating to the neck or arms. The most common mechanism for the latter symptom is a decreased supply of oxygen to the heart muscle caused by atherosclerotic coronary artery disease, which results in obstruction of the vessels that supply aterial blood to cardiac muscle.

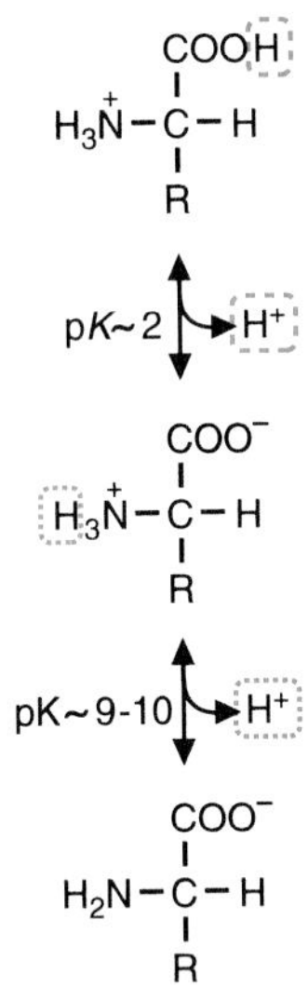

Fig. 6.2. Dissociation of the α-carboxyl and α-amino groups of amino acids. At physiologic pH (~7), a form in which both the α-carboxyl and α-amino groups are charged predominates. Some amino acids also have ionizable groups on their side chains.

The L-stereospecificity is often incorporated into the names of drugs derived from amino acids either as "L" or "levo" for the direction in which L amino acids rotate polarized light. For example, patients with Parkinson's disease are treated with L-DOPA (a derivative of the amino acid L-tyrosine), and hypothyroid patients are treated with levothyroxine (a different derivative of L-tyrosine)

I. GENERAL STRUCTURE OF THE AMINO ACIDS

Twenty different amino acids are commonly found in proteins. They are all α-amino acids, amino acids in which the amino group is attached to the α-carbon (the carbon atom next to the carboxylate group) (see Fig 6.1). The α-carbon has two additional substituents, a hydrogen atom and an additional chemical group called a side chain (-R). The side chain is different for each amino acid.

At a physiologic pH of 7.4, the amino group on these amino acids carries a positive charge, and the carboxylic acid group is negatively charged (Fig. 6.2). The pK_a of the primary carboxylic acid groups for all of the amino acids is approximately 2 (1.8–2.4). At pH values much lower than the pK_a (higher hydrogen ion concentrations), all of the carboxylic acid groups are protonated. At the pK_a, 50% of the molecules are dissociated into carboxylate anions and protons, and at a pH of 7.4, more than 99% of the molecules are dissociated (see Chapter 4). The pK_a for all of the α-amino groups is approximately 9.5 (8.8–11.0), so that at the lower pH of 7.4, most of the amino groups are fully protonated and carry a positive charge. The form of an amino acid that has both a positive and a negative charge is called a zwitterion. Because these charged chemical groups can form hydrogen bonds with water molecules, all of these amino acids are water-soluble at physiologic pH.

In all of the amino acids but glycine, the α-carbon is an asymmetric carbon atom that has four different substituents and can exist in either the D or L configuration (Fig. 6.3). The amino acids in mammalian proteins are all L-amino acids represented with the amino group to the left if the carboxyl group is at the top of the structure. These same amino acids serve as precursors of nitrogen-containing compounds synthesized in the body, and thus human amino acid metabolism is also centered on L-amino acids. The amino acid glycine is neither D nor L because the α-carbon atom contains two hydrogen atoms.

The chemical properties of the amino acids give each protein its unique characteristics. Proteins are composed of one or more linear polypeptide chains containing

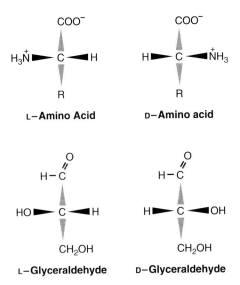

Fig. 6.3. L- and D-amino acids. The L forms are the only ones found in human proteins. Bonds coming out of the paper are shown by black arrows; those going in, by shaded arrows. The α-amino groups and H-atoms come toward the reader, and the α-carboxyl and side chains go away. The L and D forms are mirror images that cannot be superimposed by rotating the molecule. The reference for the L and D forms are the stereoisomers of glyceraldehyde.

hundreds of amino acids. The sequence of amino acids, termed the primary structure, is determined by the genetic code for the protein. In the polypeptide chains, amino acids are joined through peptide bonds between the carboxylic acid of one amino acid and the amino group of the adjacent amino acid (Fig. 6.4). Thus, the amino group, the α-carbon, and the carboxyl groups form the peptide backbone, and the side chains of the amino acids extend outward from this backbone. The side chains interact with the peptide backbone of other regions of the chain or with the side chains of other amino acids in the protein to form hydrophobic regions, electrostatic bonds, hydrogen bonds, or disulfide bonds. These interactions dictate the folding pattern of the molecule. The three-dimensional folding of the protein forms distinct regions called binding sites that are lined with amino acid side chains that interact specifically with another molecule termed a ligand (such as the heme in hemoglobin). Thus, the chemical properties of the side chains determine how the protein folds, how it binds specific ligands, and how it interacts with its environment (such as the aqueous medium of the cytoplasm).

The names of the different amino acids have been given three-letter and one-letter abbreviations (Table 6.1). The three-letter abbreviations use the first two letters in the name plus the third letter of the name or the letter of a characteristic sound, such as trp for tryptophan. The one-letter abbreviations use the first letter of the name of the most frequent amino acid in proteins (such as an "A" for alanine). If the first letter has already been assigned, the letter of a characteristic sound is used (such as an "R" for arginine). Single-letter abbreviations are usually used to denote the amino acids in a polypeptide sequence.

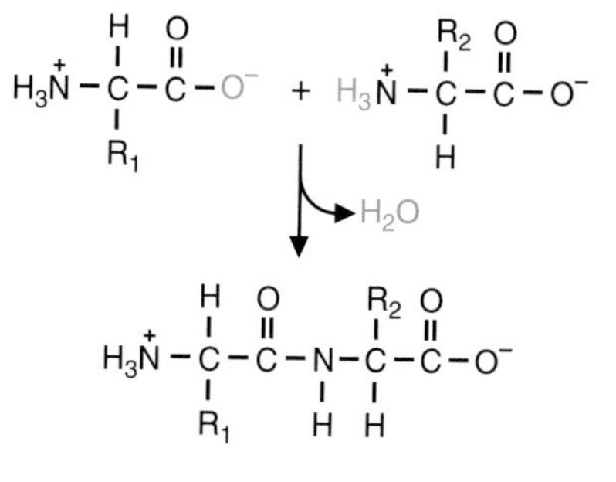

II. CLASSIFICATION OF AMINO ACID SIDE CHAINS

In Figure 6.5, the 20 amino acids used for protein synthesis are grouped into different classifications according to the polarity and structural features of the side chains. These groupings can be helpful in describing common functional roles or metabolic pathways of the amino acids. However, some amino acid side chains fit into a number of different classifications and are therefore grouped differently in different textbooks. Two of the characteristics of the side chain that are useful for classification are its pK_a and its hydropathic index, shown in Table 6.2 The hydropathic index is a scale used to denote the hydrophobicity of the side chain; the more positive the hydropathic index, the greater the tendency to cluster with other nonpolar molecules and exclude water in the hydrophobic effect. The more negative the hydropathic index of an amino acid, the more hydrophilic is its side chain.

A. Nonpolar, Aliphatic Amino Acids

Glycine is the simplest amino acid, and it really does not fit well into any classification because its side chain is only a hydrogen atom. Alanine and the branched chain amino acids (valine, leucine, and isoleucine) have bulky, nonpolar, aliphatic side chains. The high degree of hydrophobicitiy of the branched chain amino acid side chains is denoted by their high hydropathic index (see Table 6.2). Electrons are shared equally between the carbon and hydrogen atoms in these side chains, so that they cannot hydrogen bond with water. Within proteins, these amino acid side chains will cluster together to form hydrophobic cores. Their association is also promoted by van der Waals forces between the positively charged nucleus of one atom and the electron cloud of another. This force is effective over short distances when many atoms pack closely together.

The roles of proline and glycine in amino acid structure differ from those of the nonpolar amino acids. The amino acid proline contains a ring involving its α-carbon and its α-amino group, which are part of the peptide backbone. This rigid ring

Fig. 6.4. Peptide bonds. Amino acids in a polypeptide chain are joined through peptide bonds between the carboxyl group of one amino acid and the amino group of the next amino acid in the sequence.

According to some biochemists, "W" stands for the characteristic sound in "twyptophan" (see Table 6.1).

Table 6.1. Abbreviations for the Amino Acids

Name	Abbreviations*	
	Three-Letter	**One-Letter**
Alanine	Ala	A
Arginine	Arg	R
Asparagine	Asn	N
Aspartate	Asp	D
Cysteine	Cys	C
Glutamate	Glu	E
Glutamine	Gln	Q
Glycine	Gly	G
Histidine	His	H
Isoleucine	Ile	I
Leucine	Leu	L
Lysine	Lys	K
Methionine	Met	M
Phenylalanine	Phe	F
Proline	Pro	P
Serine	Ser	S
Threonine	Thr	T
Tryptophan	Trp	W
Tyrosine	Tyr	Y
Valine	Val	V

*Three-letter abbreviations are generally used. One-letter abbreviations are used mainly to list the amino acid sequences of long protein chains.

Q: The proteolytic digestive enzyme chymotrypsin cleaves the peptide bonds formed by the carboxyl groups of large, bulky uncharged amino acids. Which amino acids fall into this category?

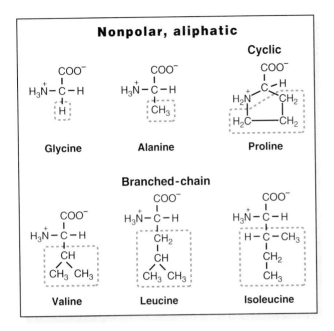

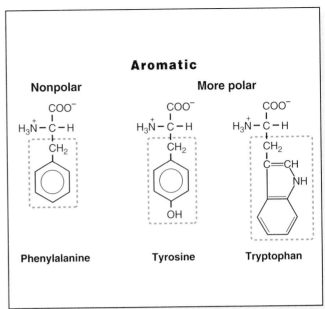

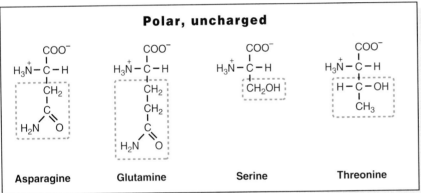

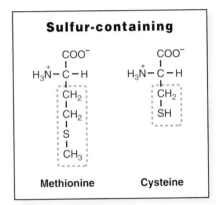

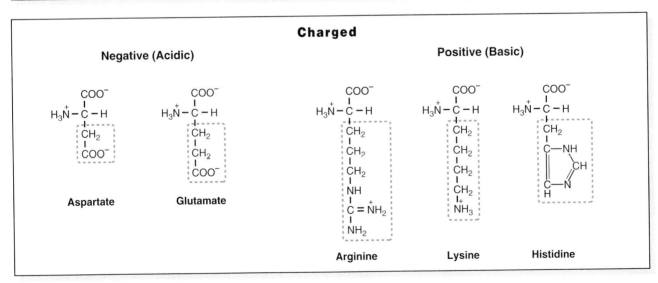

Fig. 6.5. The side chains of the amino acids. The side chains are highlighted. The amino acids are grouped by the polarity and structural features of their side chains. These groupings are not absolute, however. Tyrosine and tryptophan, often listed with the nonpolar amino acids, are more polar than other aromatic amino acids because of their phenolic and indole rings, respectively.

Table 6.2. Properties of the Common Amino Acids

Amino Acid	pK$_{a1}$* (Carboxyl)	pK$_{a2}$ (Amino)	pK$_{aR}$ (R Group)	Hydropathy Index**
Nonpolar aliphatic				
Glycine	2.4	9.8		−0.4
Proline	2.0	11.0		−1.6
Alanine	2.3	9.7		1.8
Leucine	2.4	9.6		3.8
Valine	2.3	9.6		4.2
Isoleucine	2.4	9.7		4.5
Aromatic				
Phenylalanine	1.8	9.1		2.8
Tyrosine	2.2	9.1	10.5	−1.3
Tryptophan	2.4	9.4		−0.9
Polar uncharged				
Threonine	2.1	9.6	13.6	−0.7
Serine	2.2	9.2	13.6	−0.8
Aspargine	2.0	8.8		−3.5
Glutamine	2.2	9.1		−3.5
Sulfur-containing				
Cysteine	2.0	10.3	8.4	2.5
Methionine	2.3	9.2		1.9
Charged negative				
Aspartate	1.9	9.6	3.9	−3.5
Glutamate	2.2	9.7	4.1	−3.5
Charged positive				
Histidine	1.8	9.3	6.0	−3.2
Lysine	2.2	9.0	10.5	−3.9
Arginine	2.2	9.0	12.5	−4.5
Average	2.2	9.5		

*When these amino acids reside in proteins, the pK$_a$ for the side chains may vary to some extent from the value for the free amino acid, depending on the local environment of the amino acid in the three-dimensional structure of the protein.
**The hydropathy index is a measure of the hydrophobicity of the amino acid (the higher the number, the more hydrophobic). Values based on Kyte J, Doolittle RF. J Mol Biol 1982;157:105B132.

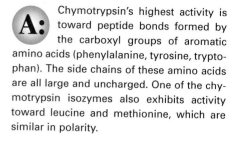

A: Chymotrypsin's highest activity is toward peptide bonds formed by the carboxyl groups of aromatic amino acids (phenylalanine, tyrosine, tryptophan). The side chains of these amino acids are all large and uncharged. One of the chymotrypsin isozymes also exhibits activity toward leucine and methionine, which are similar in polarity.

causes a kink in the peptide backbone that prevents it from forming its usual configuration. Because the side chain of glycine is so small compared with that of other amino acids, it causes the least amount of steric hindrance in a protein (i.e., it does not significantly impinge on the space occupied by other atoms or chemical groups). Therefore, glycine is often found in bends or in the tightly packed chains of fibrous proteins.

B. Aromatic Amino Acids

The aromatic amino acids have been grouped together because they all contain ring structures with similar properties, but their polarity differs a great deal. The aromatic ring is a six-membered carbon–hydrogen ring with three conjugated double bonds (the benzene ring or phenyl group). The substituents on this ring determine whether the amino acid side chain engages in polar or hydrophobic interactions. In the amino acid phenylalanine, the ring contains no substituents, and the electrons are shared equally between the carbons in the ring, resulting in a very nonpolar hydrophobic structure in which the rings can stack on each other (Fig. 6.6). In tyrosine, a hydroxyl group on the phenyl ring engages in hydrogen bonds, and the side chain is therefore more polar and more hydrophilic. The more complex ring structure in tryptophan is an indole ring with a nitrogen that can engage in hydrogen bonds. Tryptophan is therefore also more polar than phenylalanine.

C. Aliphatic, Polar, Uncharged Amino Acids

Amino acids with side chains that contain an amide group (asparagine and glutamine) or a hydroxyl group (serine and threonine) can be classified as aliphatic, polar, uncharged amino acids. Asparagine and glutamine are amides of the amino

A. Hydrophobic interaction

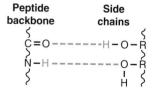

B. Hydrogen bonds

Fig. 6.6. Hydrophobic and hydrogen bonds. **A.** Strong hydrophobic interactions occur with the stacking of aromatic groups in phenylalanine side chains. **B.** Examples of hydrogen bonds in which a hydrogen atom is shared by a nitrogen in the peptide backbone and an oxygen atom in an amino acid side chain or between an oxygen in the peptide backbone and an oxygen in an amino acid side chain.

Cal Kulis passed a renal stone shortly after admission, with immediate relief of flank pain. Stone analysis showed its major component to be cystine. Normally, amino acids are filtered by the renal glomerular capillaries into the tubular urine but are almost entirely reabsorbed from this fluid back into the blood via transport proteins in the proximal tubular cells of the kidney. Cal Kulis has cystinuria, a genetically inherited amino acid substitution in the transport protein that normally reabsorbs cystine, arginine, and lysine from the kidney lumen back into the renal tubular cells. Therefore, his urine contained high amounts of these amino acids. Cystine, which is less soluble than other amino acids, precipitates in the urine to form renal stones (calculi).

 Will Sichel has sickle cell anemia caused by a point mutation in his DNA that changes the sixth amino acid in the β-globin chain of hemoglobin from glutamate to valine. What difference would you expect to find in the chemical bonds formed by these two amino acids?

acids aspartate and glutamate. The hydroxyl groups and the amide groups in the side chains allow these amino acids to form hydrogen bonds with water, with each other and the peptide backbone, or with other polar compounds in the binding sites of the proteins (see Fig. 6.6). As a consequence of their hydrophilicity, these amino acids are frequently found on the surface of water-soluble globular proteins. Cysteine, which is sometimes included in this class of amino acids, has been separated into the class of sulfur-containing amino acids.

D. Sulfur-Containing Amino Acids

Both cysteine and methionine contain sulfur. The side chain of cysteine contains a sulfhydryl group that has a pK_a of approximately 8.4 for dissociation of its hydrogen, so cysteine is predominantly undissociated and uncharged at the physiologic pH of 7.4. The free cysteine molecule in solution can form a covalent disulfide bond with another cysteine molecule through spontaneous (nonenzymatic) oxidation of their sulfhydryl groups. The resultant amino acid, cystine, is present in blood and tissues, and is not very water-soluble. In proteins, the formation of a cystine disulfide bond between two appropriately positioned cysteine sulfhydryl groups often plays an important role in holding two polypeptide chains or two different regions of a chain together (Fig. 6.7). Methionine, although it contains a sulfur group, is a nonpolar amino acid with a large bulky side chain that is hydrophobic. It does not contain a sulfhydryl group and cannot form disulfide bonds. Its important and central role in metabolism is related to its ability to transfer the methyl group attached to the sulfur atom to other compounds.

E. The Acidic and Basic Amino Acids

The amino acids aspartate and glutamate have carboxylic acid groups that carry a negative charge at physiologic pH (see Fig. 6.5). The basic amino acids histidine,

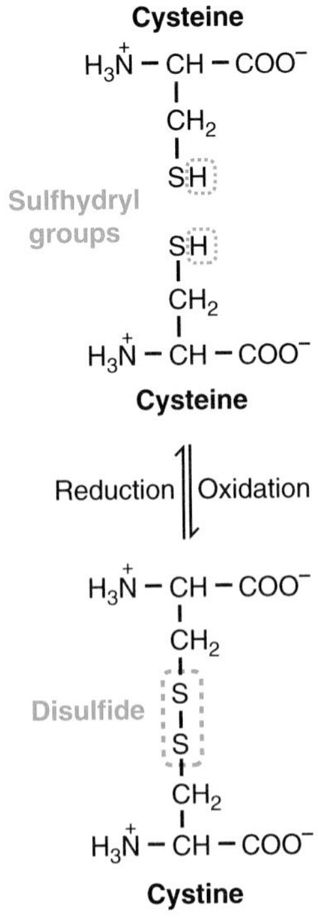

Cysteine

$$H_3\overset{+}{N} - CH - COO^-$$
$$|$$
$$CH_2$$
$$|$$
$$SH$$

Sulfhydryl groups

$$SH$$
$$|$$
$$CH_2$$
$$|$$
$$H_3\overset{+}{N} - CH - COO^-$$

Cysteine

Reduction ⇅ Oxidation

$$H_3\overset{+}{N} - CH - COO^-$$
$$|$$
$$CH_2$$
$$|$$
$$S$$
Disulfide $$|$$
$$S$$
$$|$$
$$CH_2$$
$$|$$
$$H_3\overset{+}{N} - CH - COO^-$$

Cystine

Fig. 6.7. A disulfide bond. Covalent disulfide bonds may be formed between two molecules of cysteine or between two cysteine residues in a protein. The disulfide compound is called cystine. The hydrogens of the cysteine sulfhydryl groups are removed during oxidation.

lysine, and arginine have side chains containing nitrogen that can be protonated and positively charged at physiologic and lower pH values. Histidine has a nitrogen-containing imidazole ring for a side chain, lysine has a primary amino group on the 6th or ε carbon (from the sequence α, β, γ, δ, ε), and arginine has a guanidinium group.

The positive charges on the basic amino acids enables them to form ionic bonds (electrostatic bonds) with negatively charged groups, such as the side chains of acidic amino acids or the phosphate groups of coenzymes (Fig. 6.8). In addition, lysine and arginine side chains often form ionic bonds with negatively charged compounds bound to the protein binding sites, such as the phosphate groups in ATP. The acidic and basic amino acid side chains also participate in hydrogen bonding and the formation of salt bridges (such as the binding of an inorganic ion such as Na^+ between two partially or fully negatively charged groups).

The charge on these amino acids at physiologic pH is a function of their pK_as for dissociation of protons from the α-carboxylic acid groups, the α-amino groups, and the side chains. The titration curve of histidine illlustrates the changes in amino acid structure occurring as the pH of the solution is changed from less than 1 to 14 by the addition of hydroxide ions (Fig. 6.9). At low pH, all groups carry protons; amino groups have a positive charge, and carboxylic acid groups have zero charge. As the pH is increased by the addition of alkali (OH^-), the proton dissociates from the carboxylic acid group, and its charge changes from zero to negative with a pK_a of approximately 2, the pH at which 50% of the protons have dissociated.

The histidine side chain is an imidazole ring with a pK_a of approximately 6 that changes from a predominantly protonated positively charged ring to an uncharged ring at this pH. The amino group on the α–carbon titrates at a much higher pH (between 9 and 10), and the charge changes from positive to zero as the pH rises. The pH at which the net charge on the molecules in solution is zero is called the isoelectric point (pI). At this pH, the molecules will not migrate in an electric field toward either a positive pole (cathode) or a negative pole (anode), because the number of negative charges on each molecule is equal to the number of positive charges.

Amino acid side chains change from uncharged to negatively charged, or positively charged to uncharged as they release protons (Fig. 6.10). The acidic amino acids lose a proton from their carboxylic acid side chains at a pH of roughly 4, and are thus negatively charged at pH 7.4. Cysteine and tyrosine lose protons at their pK_as (~ 8.4 and 10.5, respectively), so their side chains are uncharged at physiologic pH. Histidine, lysine, and arginine side chains change from positively charged to neutral at their pK_as. The side chains of the two basic amino acids, arginine and lysine, have pK_a values above 10, so that the positively charged form always predominates at physiologic pH. The side chain of histidine (pK_a ~ 6.0) dissociates near physiologic pH, so only a portion of the histidine side chains carry a positive charge (see Fig. 6.9).

In proteins, only the amino acid side chains and the amino group at the amino terminal and carboxyl group at the carboxyl terminal have dissociable protons. All of the other carboxylic acid and amino groups on the α-carbons are joined in peptide bonds that have no dissociable protons. The amino acid side chains might have very different pK_as than those of the free amino acids if they are involved in hydrogen or ionic bonds with other amino acid side chains. The pK_a of the imidazole group of histidine, for example, is often shifted to a higher value between 6 and 7 so that it adds and releases a proton in the physiologic pH range.

III. VARIATIONS IN PRIMARY STRUCTURE

Although almost every amino acid in the primary structure of a protein contributes to its conformation (three-dimensional structure), the primary structure of a protein

A: Glutamate carries a negative charge on its side chain at physiologic pH and thus can engage in ionic bonds or hydrogen bonds with water or other side chains. Valine is a hydrophobic amino acid and therefore tends to interact with other hydrophobic side chains to exclude water. (The effect of this substitution on hemoglobin structure is described in more detail in Chapter 7.)

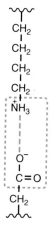

Fig. 6.8. Electrostatic interaction between the positively charged side chain of lysine and the negatively charged side chain of aspartate.

Electrophoresis is a technique used to separate proteins on the basis of charge that has been extremely useful in medicine to identify proteins with different amino acid composition. The net charge on a protein at a certain pH is a summation of all of the positive and negative charges on all of the ionizable amino acid side chains plus the N-terminal amino and C-terminal carboxyl groups. Theoretically, the net charge of a protein at any pH could be determined from its amino acid composition by calculating the concentration of positively and negatively charged groups from the Henderson-Hasselbalch equation (see Chapter 4). However, hydrogen bonds and ionic bonds between amino acid side chains in the protein make this calculation unrealistic.

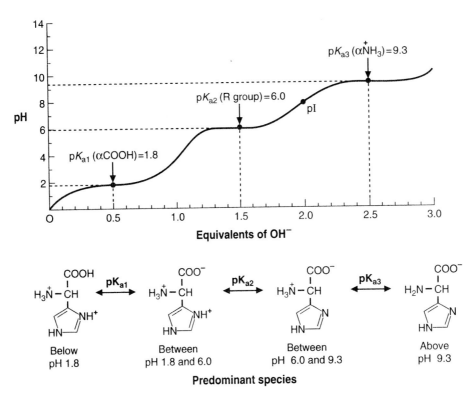

Fig. 6.9. Titration curve of histidine. The ionic species that predominates in each region is shown below the graph. pI is the isoelectric point (at which there is no net charge on the molecule).

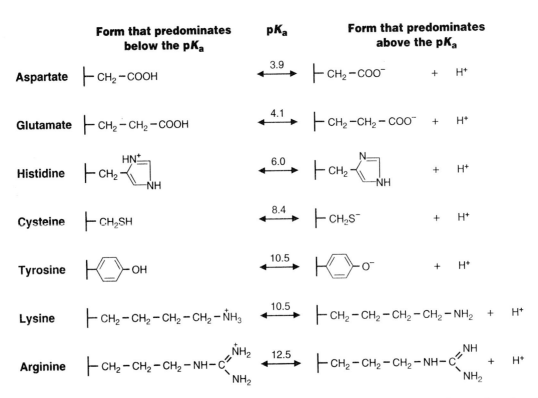

Fig. 6.10. Dissociation of the side chains of the amino acids. As the pH increases, the charge on the side chain goes from 0 to + or from + to 0. The pK$_a$ is the pH at which half the molecules of an amino acid in solution have side chains that are charged. Half are uncharged.

can vary to some degree between species. Even within the human species, the amino acid sequence of a normal functional protein can vary somewhat among individuals, tissues of the same individual, and the stage of development. These variations in the primary structure of a functional protein are tolerated if they are confined to noncritical regions (called variant regions), if they are conservative substitutions (replace one amino acid with one of similar structure), or if they confer an advantage. If many different amino acid residues are tolerated at a position, the region is called hypervariable. In contrast, the regions that form binding sites or are critical for forming a functional three-dimensional structure are usually invariant regions that have exactly the same amino acid sequence from individual to individual, tissue to tissue, or species to species.

A. Polymorphism in Protein Structure

Within the human population, the primary structure of a protein may vary slightly among individuals. The variations generally arise from mutations in DNA that are passed to the next generation. The mutations can result from the substitution of one base for another in the DNA sequence of nucleotides (a point mutation), from deletion or insertions of bases into DNA, or from larger changes (see Chap.14). For many alleles, the variation has a distinct phenotypic consequence that contributes to our individual characteristics, produces an obvious dysfunction (a congenital or genetically inherited disease), or increases susceptibility to certain diseases. A defective protein may differ from the most common allele by as little as a single amino acid that is a nonconservative substitution (replacement of one amino acid with another of a different polarity or very different size) in an invariant region. Such mutations might affect the ability of the protein to carry out its function, catalyze a particular reaction, reach the appropriate site in a cell, or be degraded. For other proteins, the variations appear to have no significance.

Variants of an allele that occur with a significant frequency in the population are referred to as polymorphisms. Thus far in studies of the human genome, almost one third of the genetic loci appear to be polymorphic. When a particular variation of an allele, or polymorphism, increases in the general population to a frequency of over

Q: Is the substitution of a glutamate for a valine in sickle cell hemoglobin a conservative replacement? What about the substitution of an aspartate for a glutamate?

For the most part, human chromosomes occur as homologous pairs, with each member of a pair containing the same genetic information. One member of the pair is inherited from the mother and one from the father. Genes are arranged linearly along each chromosome. A genetic locus is a specific position or location on a chromosome. Alleles are alternate versions of a gene at a given locus. For each locus (site), we have two alleles of each gene, one from our mother and one from our father. If both alleles of a gene are identical, the individual is homozygous for this gene; if the alleles are different, he is heterozygous for this gene. **Will Sichel** has two identical alleles for the sickle variant of the β-globin gene that results in substitution of a valine for a glutamate residue at the sixth position of the β-globin chain. He is, therefore, homozygous and has sickle cell anemia. Individuals with one normal gene and one sickle cell allele are heterozygous. They are carriers of the disease and have sickle cell trait.

Will Sichel's hemoglobin, HbS, comprises two normal α chains and 2 β-globin chains with the sickle cell variant ($\alpha_2\beta_2{}^S$). The change in amino acid composition from a glutamate to a valine in the β chain allows sickle hemoglobin to be separated from normal adult hemoglobin (HbA, or ($\alpha_2\beta_2{}^A$)) by electrophoresis. In electrophoresis, an aliquot of blood or other solution containing proteins is applied to a support, such as paper or a gel. When an electrical field is applied, proteins migrate a distance toward the anode (negative pole) or cathode (positive pole) that reflects small differences in their net charge. Electrophoresis of **Will Sichel's** blood shows that he is homozygous for the sickle cell variant, HbS, and has increased amounts of fetal hemoglobin, HbF. Individuals with sickle cell trait are heterozygous and have both HbA and HbS, plus small amounts of HbF ($\alpha_2\gamma_2$).

In heterozygous individuals with sickle cell trait, the sickle cell allele provides some protection against malaria. Malaria is caused by the parasite *Plasmodium fulciparum*, which spends part of its life cycle in red blood cells. The infected red blood cells of individuals with normal hemoglobin (HbA) develop protrusions that attach to the lining of capillaries. This attachment occludes the vessels and prevents oxygen from reaching cells in the affected region, resulting in cell death. In heterozygous individuals, HbS in infected cells aggregates into long fibers that cause the cell to become distorted. These distorted cells containing the parasite are preferentially recognized by the spleen and are rapidly destroyed, thus ending the life of the parasite.

In **Will Sichel** and other homozygous individuals with sickle cell anemia, the red blood cells sickle more frequently, especially under conditions of low oxygen tension (see Chapter 7). The result is a vaso-occlusive crisis in which the sickled cells clog capillaries and prevent oxygen from reaching cells (ischemia), thereby causing pain. The enhanced destruction of the sickled cells by the spleen results in anemia. Consequently, the sickle cell allele is of little advantage to homozygous individuals.

Because heterozygous individuals occur more frequently in a population than homozygous individuals, a selective advantage in a heterozygous state can outweigh a disadvantage in a homozygous state, causing the mutation to become a stable polymorphism in a population. As a consequence, the frequency of sickle cell anemia in parts of equatorial Africa in which malaria was endemic in the past is 1 in 25 births. Migration from Africa accounts for the high frequency of sickle cell anemia among blacks in the United States, which is approximately 1/400 at birth.

The substitution of a glutamate for a valine is a nonconservative replacement because a negatively charged amino acid is substituted for a hydrophobic branched chain aliphatic amino acid. However, the substitution of an aspartate for a glutamate is a conservative replacement because the two amino acids have the same polarity and nearly the same size.

1%, it is considered stable. The sickle cell allele is an example of a point mutation that is stable in the human population. Its persistence is probably attributable to selective pressure for the heterozygous mutant phenotype, which confers some protection against malaria.

B. Protein Families and Superfamilies.

A homologous family of proteins is composed of proteins related to the same ancestral protein. Groups of proteins with similar, but not identical, structure and function that have evolved from the same gene after the gene was duplicated are called paralogs and considered members of the same protein family. Once a gene has duplicated, one gene can continue to perform original function, and the second copy can mutate into a protein with another function or another type of regulation. This process is called divergent evolution. Very large families of homologous proteins are called a superfamily, which is subdivided by name into families of proteins with the most similarity in structure.

The paralogs of a protein family are considered different proteins and have different names because they have different functions. They are all present in the same individual. Myoglobin and the different chains of hemoglobin, for example, are paralogs and members of the same globin family that have similar, but not identical, structures and functions. Myoglobin, an intracellular heme protein present in most cells that stores and tranports O_2 to mitochondria, is a single polypeptide chain containing one heme oxygen-binding site. In contrast, hemoglobin is composed of four globin chains, each with a heme oxygen-binding site that is present in red blood cells and transports O_2 from the lungs to tissues. The gene for myoglobin is assumed to have evolved from gene duplication of the α-chain for hemoglobin, which evolved from duplication of the β-chain. Figure 6.11 compares a region of the structure of myoglobin and the α and β chains of hemoglobin. Among these three proteins, only 15 invariant (identical) residues are present, but many of the other amino acid residues are conservative substitutions.

Homologous families of proteins are proteins that have the same ancestral protein and arose from the same gene. The term *homologs* includes both orthologs and paralogs. Orthologs are genes from different species that have evolved from a common ancestral gene as different species developed (for example, human and pork insulin). By contrast, paralogs are genes related by duplication within the genome of a single species (e.g., myoglobin and hemoglobin). Normally, othologs retain the same function in the course of evolution, whereas paralogs evolve new functions that may, or may not, be related to the original one.

To compare the primary structure of two homologous polypeptide chains, the sequences are written left to right from the amino terminal to the carboxyl terminal. The sequences are aligned with computer programs that maximize the identity of amino acids and minimize the differences caused by segments that are present in one protein and not in the other.

The primary structure of human globin proteins

	1	5	10	15
Myoglobin	gly-----leu-ser-asp-gly-glu-trp-gln-leu-val-leu-asn-val-trp-gly-lys-val-
β chain Hemoglobin	val-his-leu-thr-pro-glu-glu-lys-ser-ala-val-thr-ala-leu-trp-gly-lys-val-
α chain hemoglobin	val-----leu-ser-pro-ala-asp-lys-thr-asn-val-lys-ala-ala-trp-gly-lys-val-
ζ chain Hemoglobin	met-ser-leu-thr-lys-thr-glu-arg-thr-ile-ile-val-ser-met-trp-ala-lys-ile-
γ chain Hemoglobin	met-gly-his-phe-thr-glu-glu-asp-lys-ala-thr-ile-thr-ser-leu-trp-gly-lys-val-

Fig 6.11. The primary structures of a region in human globin proteins. Gaps in the structure, indicated with dashes, are introduced to maximize the alignment between proteins in structure comparisons. They are assumed to coincide with mutations that caused a deletion. Regions of sequence similarity (identity and conservative substitution) are indicated in blue. Within these regions, there are smaller regions of invariant residues that are exactly the same from protein to protein. Myoglobin is a single polypeptide chain. The α and β chains are part of hemoglobin A ($\alpha_2\beta_2$). The ζ chain is part of embryonic hemoglobin ($\zeta_2\varepsilon_2$). The γ chain is part of fetal hemoglobin (HbF), $\alpha_2\gamma_2$.

C. Tissue and Developmental Variations in Protein Structure

Within the same individual, different isoforms or isozymes of a protein may be synthesized during different stages of fetal and embryonic development, may be present in different tissues, or may reside in different intracellular locations. Isoforms of a protein all have the same function. If they are isozymes (isoforms of enzymes), they catalyze the same reactions. However, isoforms have somewhat different properties and amino acid structure.

1. DEVELOPMENTAL VARIATION

Hemoglobin isoforms provide an example of variation during development. Hemoglobin is expressed as the fetal isozyme HbF during the last trimester of pregnancy until after birth, when it is replaced with HbA. HbF is composed of two hemoglobin α and 2 hemoglobin γ polypeptide chains, in contrast to the adult hemoglobin, hemoglobin A, which is 2 α and 2 β chains. During the embryonic stages of development, chains with a different amino acid composition, the embryonic ε and ζ chains, are produced (see Fig. 6.11). These differences are believed to arise evolutionarily from mutation of a duplicated α gene to produce ζ, and mutation of a duplicate α gene to produce ε. The fetal and embryonic forms of hemoglobin have a much higher affinity for O_2 than the adult forms, and thus confer an advantage at the low O_2 tensions to which the fetus is exposed. At different stages of development, the globin genes specific for that stage are expressed and translated.

2. TISSUE-SPECIFIC ISOFORMS

Proteins that differ somewhat in primary structure and properties from tissue to tissue, but retain essentially the same function, are called tissue-specific isoforms or isozymes. The enzyme creatine kinase is an example of a protein that exists as tissue-specific isozymes, each composed of two subunits with 60 to 72% sequence homology. Of the two creatine kinases that bind to the muscle sarcomere, the M form is produced in skeletal muscle, and the B polypeptide chains are produced in the brain. The protein comprises two subunits, and skeletal muscle therefore produces an MM creatine kinase, and the brain produces a BB form. The heart produces both types of chains and therefore forms a heterodimer, MB, as well as an MM dimer. Two more creatine kinase isozymes are found in mitochondria, a heart mitochondrial creatine kinase, and the "universal" isoform found in other tissues. (In general, most proteins present in both the mitochondria and cytosol will be present as different isoforms.) The advantage conferred on different tissues by having their own isoform of creatine kinase is unknown. However, tissue-specific isozymes such as MB creatine kinase are useful in diagnosing sites of tissue injury and cell death.

The structure of proteins involved in the response to hormones has been studied in greater depth than many other types of proteins, and most of these proteins are present as several tissue-specific isoforms that help different tissues respond differently to the same hormone. One of these proteins present in cell membranes is adenylyl cyclase, an enzyme that catalyzes the synthesis of intracellular 3′,5′ cyclic adenosine monophosphate (cAMP) (Fig. 6.12). In human tissues, at least nine different isoforms of adenylyl cyclase are coded by different genes in different tissues. Although they have an overall sequence homology of 50%, the two intracellular regions involved in the synthesis of cAMP are an invariant consensus sequence with a 93% identity. The different isoforms help cells respond differently to the same hormone.

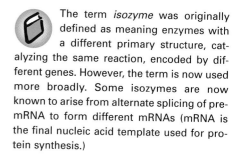

The term *isozyme* was originally defined as meaning enzymes with a different primary structure, catalyzing the same reaction, encoded by different genes. However, the term is now used more broadly. Some isozymes are now known to arise from alternate splicing of pre-mRNA to form different mRNAs (mRNA is the final nucleic acid template used for protein synthesis.)

A myocardial infarction (heart attack) is caused by an atheromatous obstruction or a severe spasm in a coronary artery that prevents the flow of blood to an area of heart muscle. Thus, heart cells in this region suffer from a lack of oxygen and blood-borne fuel. Because the cells cannot generate ATP, the membranes become damaged, and enzymes leak from the cells into the blood.

Creatine kinase (CK or CPK) is one of these enzymes. The protein is composed of two subunits, which may be either of the muscle (M) or the brain (B) type. The MB form, containing one M and one B subunit, is found primarily in cardiac muscle. It can be separated electrophoretically from other CK isozymes and the amount in the blood used to determine if a myocardial infarction has occurred. On admission to the hospital, **Ann Jeina's** total CK was 182 units/L (reference range 5 38–174 U/L). Her MB fraction was 6.8% (reference range 5% or less of the total CK). Although these values are only slightly elevated, they are typical of the phase immediately following a myocardial infarction. Additional information was provided by myoglobin and troponin T (Tn-T) measurements.

Extracellular side

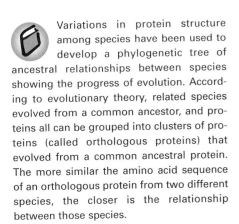

Intracellular side

Fig 6.12. Invariant regions in the isoforms of adenylyl cyclase. The invariant regions are on the cytosolic side of the membrane in the C1 and C2 loops shown in blue. These amino acid residues participate in the catalytic function of the enzyme, synthesis of 3′,5′-cyclic AMP. The protein also has several helical regions that span the membrane (M1 helices and M2 helices), represented as tubes. An oligosaccharide chain is attached to an extracellular domain. N is the amino terminus. (Copyrighted from Taussig R, Gilman AG. J Biol Chem Mammalian membrane-bound adenylyl cyclases 1995;270:1–4.)

🔖 Variations in protein structure among species have been used to develop a phylogenetic tree of ancestral relationships between species showing the progress of evolution. According to evolutionary theory, related species evolved from a common ancestor, and proteins all can be grouped into clusters of proteins (called orthologous proteins) that evolved from a common ancestral protein. The more similar the amino acid sequence of an orthologous protein from two different species, the closer is the relationship between those species.

🩺 Although bovine (beef) insulin is identical to human insulin in those amino acid residues essential for activity, the amino acid residues that are in the variable regions can act as antigens and stimulate the formation of antibodies against bovine insulin. Consequently, recombinant DNA techniques have been used for the synthesis of insulin, identical in structure to native insulin, such as Humulin (intermediate-acting insulin) (see Chapter 17 for information on recombinant DNA technology.) Although **Di Abietes** had not yet experienced an allergic response to her beef insulin, the cost of Humulin is now sufficiently low that most patients are being changed from beef insulin to the synthetic forms of human insulin.

🔖 The 20 DNA-encoded amino acids form the linear sequence of amino acids known as the primary structure of the protein, and determine the folding pattern for the three-dimensional conformation of the protein. Posttranslational modifications usually occur once the protein has already folded into its characteristic pattern. They are like accessories (jewelry, ties, etc.) that provide additional variations to your basic wardrobe.

D. Species Variations in the Primary Structure of Insulin

Species variations in primary structure are also important in medicine, as illustrated by the comparison of human, beef, and pork insulin. Insulin is one of the hormones that are highly conserved between species, with very few amino acid substitutions and none in the regions that affect activity. Insulin is a polypeptide hormone of 51 amino acids that is composed of two polypeptide chains (Fig. 6.13). It is synthesized as a single polypeptide chain, but is cleaved in three places before secretion to form the C peptide and the active insulin molecule containing the A and B chains. The folding of the A and B chains into the correct three-dimensional structure is promoted by the presence of one intrachain and two interchain disulfide bonds formed by cysteine residues. The invariant residues consist of the cysteine residues engaged in disulfide bonds and the residues that form the surface of the insulin molecule that binds to the insulin receptor. The amino acid substitutions in bovine and porcine insulin (shown in blue in Fig. 6.13.) are not in amino acids that affect its activity. Consequently, bovine and pork insulin were used for many years for the treatment of diabetes mellitus. However, even with only a few different amino acids, some patients developed an immune response to these insulins.

IV. MODIFIED AMINO ACIDS

After synthesis of a protein has been completed, a few amino acid residues in the primary sequence may be further modified in enzyme-catalyzed reactions that add a chemical group, oxidize, or otherwise modify specific amino acids in the protein. Because protein synthesis occurs by a process known as translation, these changes are called posttranslational modification. More than 100 different posttranslationally modified amino acid residues have been found in human proteins. These modifications change the structure of one or more specific amino acids on a protein in a way that may serve a regulatory function, target or anchor the protein in membranes, enhance a protein's association with other proteins, or target it for degradation (Fig. 6.14).

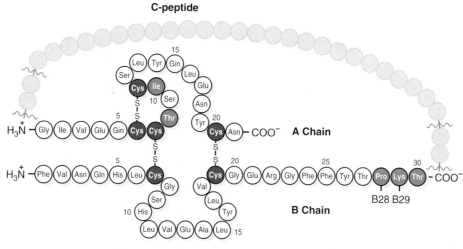

Structure of human insulin

Fig. 6.13. The primary structure of human insulin. The substituted amino acids in bovine (beef) and porcine (pork) insulin are shown in blue. Threonine 30 at the carboxy terminal of the B chain is replaced by alanine in both beef and pork insulin. In beef insulin, threonine 8 on the A chain is also replaced with alanine, and isoleucine 10 with valine. The cysteine residues, which form the disulfide bonds holding the chains together, are invariant. In the bioengineered insulin Humalog (lispro insulin), the position of proline at B28 and lysine at B29 is switched. Insulin is synthesized as a longer precursor molecule, proinsulin, which is one polpeptide chain. Proinsulin is converted to insulin by proteolytic cleavage of certain peptide bonds (squiggly lines in the figure). The cleavage removes a few amino acids and the 31–amino acid C-peptide that connects the A and B chains. The active insulin molecule, thus, has two nonidentical chains.

B. Glycosylation

Oligosaccharides (small carbohydrate chains) are bound to proteins by either *N*-linkages or *O*-linkages (see Fig. 6.14). *N*-linked oligosaccharides are found attached to cell surface proteins, where they protect the cell from proteolysis or an immune attack. In contrast, an *O*-glycosidic link is a common way of attaching oligosaccharides to the serine or threonine hydroxyl groups in secreted proteins. The intracellular polysaccharide glycogen is attached to a protein through an *O*-glycosidic linkage to a tyrosine.

C. Fatty Acylation or Prenylation

Many membrane proteins contain a covalently attached lipid group that interacts hydrophobically with lipids in the membrane. Palmitoyl groups (C16) are often attached to plasma membrane proteins, and the myristoyl group (C14) is often attached to proteins in the lipid membranes of intracellular vesicles (see Fig. 6.14). The farnesyl (C15) or geranylgeranyl group (C20) are synthesized from the five-carbon isoprene unit (isopentenyl pyrophosphate, see Fig. 5.1A) and are therefore called isoprenoids. These are attached in ether linkage to a specific cysteine residue of certain membrane proteins, particularly proteins involved in regulation.

Adenylyl cyclase is posttranslationally modified (see Fig. 6.12). It has an oligosaccharide chain attached to the external portion of the protein. Some of the isozymes contain serine residues on the intracellular portion of the chain that may be phosphorylated by a protein kinase.

D. Regulatory Modifications

Phosphorylation, acetylation, and adenosine diphosphate (ADP)-ribosylation of specific amino acid residues in a polypeptide can alter bonding by that residue and change the activity of the protein (see Fig. 6.14). Phosphorylation of an OH group on serine, threonine, or tyrosine by a protein kinase (an enzyme that transfers a phosphate group from ATP to a protein) introduces a large, bulky, negatively charged group that can alter the activity of a protein. Reversible acetylation occurring on lysine residues of histone proteins in the chromosome changes their

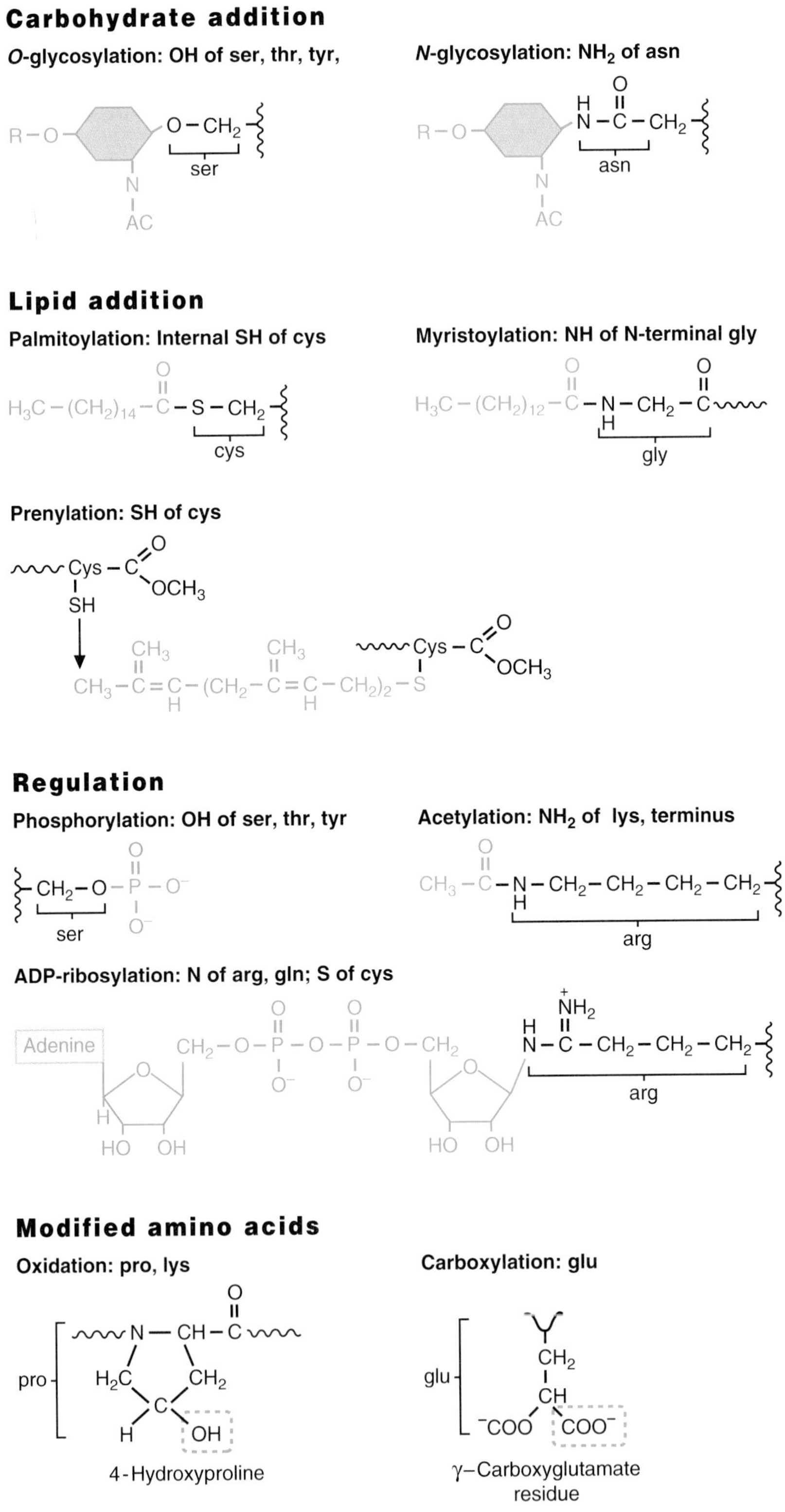
Carbohydrate addition
O-glycosylation: OH of ser, thr, tyr,
N-glycosylation: NH2 of asn
ser
asn
Lipid addition
Palmitoylation: Internal SH of cys
Myristoylation: NH of N-terminal gly
cys
gly
Prenylation: SH of cys
Regulation
Phosphorylation: OH of ser, thr, tyr
Acetylation: NH2 of lys, terminus
ser
arg
ADP-ribosylation: N of arg, gln; S of cys
Adenine
arg
Modified amino acids
Oxidation: pro, lys
Carboxylation: glu
pro
glu
4-Hydroxyproline
γ–Carboxyglutamate residue

Fig. 6.14. Posttranslational modifications of amino acids in proteins. Some of the common amino acid modifications and the sites of attachment are illustrated. The added group is shown in blue. Because these modifications are enzyme-catalyzed, only a specific amino acid in the primary sequence is altered. R-O-hexagon refers to an oligosaccharide. In *N*-glycosylation, the attached sugar is usually N-acetylglucosamine (N-Ac).

interaction with the negatively charged phosphate groups of DNA. ADP-ribosylation is the transfer of an ADP-ribose from NAD^+ to an arginine, glutamine, or a cysteine residue on a target protein in the membrane (primarily in leukocytes, skeletal muscles, brain, and testes). This modification may regulate the activity of these proteins

E. Other Amino Acid Posttranslational Modifications

A number of other posttranslational modifications of amino acid side chains alter the activity of the protein in the cell (see Fig 6.14). Carboxylation of the γ carbon of glutamate (carbon 4) in certain blood clotting proteins is important for attaching the clot to a surface. Calcium ions mediate this attachment by binding to the two negatively charged carboxyl groups of γ–glutamate and two additional negatively charged groups provided by phospholipids in the cell membrane. Collagen, an abundant fibrous extracellular protein, contains the oxidized amino acid hydroxyproline. The addition of the hydroxyl group to the proline side chain provides an extra polar group that can engage in hydrogen bonding between the polypeptide strands of the fibrous protein.

F. Selenocysteine

The unusual amino acid selenocysteine is found in a few enzymes and is required for their activity (Fig. 6.15). Its synthesis is not a posttranslational modification, however, but a modification to serine that occurs while serine is bound to a unique tRNA. The selenocysteine is then inserted into the protein as it is being synthesized.

A number of pathogenic bacteria produce bacterial toxins that are ADP-ribosyl transferases (NAD^+-glycohydrolases). These enzymes hydrolyze the N-glycosidic bond of NAD^+ and transfer the ADP-ribose portion to a specific amino acid residue on a protein in the affected human cell. Cholera A-B toxin, a pertussis toxin, and a diptheria toxin are all ADP-ribosyl transferases.

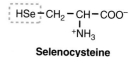

$$HSe-CH_2-CH-COO^-$$
$$^+NH_3$$

Selenocysteine

Fig. 6.15. Selenocysteine.

CLINICAL COMMENTS

Will Sichel. Will Sichel was treated for 3 days with parenteral (intravascular) narcotics, hydration, and nasal inhalation of oxygen for his vaso-occlusive crisis. The diffuse severe pains of sickle cell crises result from occlusion of small vessels in a variety of tissues, thereby causing damage to cells from ischemia (low blood flow) or hypoxia (low levels of oxygen). Vaso-occlusion occurs when HbS molecules in red blood cells polymerize in the capillaries, where the partial pressure of O_2 (pO_2) is low. This polymerization causes the red blood cells to change from a biconcave disc to a sickle shape that cannot deform to pass through the narrow capillary lumen. The cells aggregate in the capillaries and occlude blood flow.

In addition, **Will Sichel** was treated with hydroxyurea therapy, which increases the production of red blood cells containing fetal hemoglobin. HbF molecules cannot participate in sickling. **Will Sichel's** acute symptoms gradually subsided. Had his severe pain persisted, partial exchange blood transfusions would have been considered because no other effective therapy is currently available. Patients with sickle cell anemia periodically experience sickle cell crises, and Will's physician urged him to seek medical help whenever symptoms reappeared.

Cal Kulis. Mr. Kulis has cystinuria, a relatively rare disorder, with a prevalence that ranges between 1 in 2,500 to 1 in 15,000 births, depending on the population studied. It is a genetically determined disease with a complex recessive mode of inheritance resulting from allelic mutations. These mutations lead to a reduction in the activity of renal tubular cell transport proteins that normally carry cystine from the tubular lumen into the renal tubular cells. The transport of the basic amino acids (lysine, arginine, and ornithine, an amino acid found in the urea cycle but not in proteins) is also often compromised, and they appear in the urine.

Because cystine is produced by oxidation of cysteine, conservative treatment of cystinuria includes decreasing the amount of cysteine within the body and, hence, the amount of cystine eventually filtered by the kidneys. Reduction of cysteine levels is accomplished by restricting dietary methionine, which contributes its sulfur to the pathway for cysteine formation. To increase the amount of cystine that remains in solution, the volume of fluid ingested daily is increased. Crystallization of cystine is further prevented by chronically alkalinizing the urine. Finally, drugs may be administered to enhance the conversion of urinary cystine to more soluble compounds. If these conservative measures fail to prevent continued cystine stone formation, existing stones may be removed by a surgical technique that involves sonic fracture. The fragmented stones may then pass spontaneously or may be more easily extracted surgically because of their smaller size.

 The switch in position of amino acids in lispro does not affect the action of this synthetic insulin on cells because it is not in a critical invariant region, but it does affect the ability of insulin to bind zinc. Normally, human insulin is secreted from the pancreas as a zinc hexamer in which six insulin molecules are bound to the zinc atom. When zinc insulin is injected, the binding to zinc slows the absorption from the subcutaneous (under the skin) injection site. Lispro cannot bind zinc to form a hexamer, and thus it is absorbed much more quickly than other insulins.

 Di Abietes. Di Abietes' treatment was first changed to daily injections of Humulin instead of beef insulin. Humulin is now mass-produced by recombinant DNA techniques that insert the human DNA sequences for the insulin A and B chains into the *Escherichia coli* or yeast genome (see Chapter 17). The insulin chains that are produced are then extracted from the media and treated to form the appropriate disulfide bonds between the chains. As costs have fallen for production of the synthetic human insulins, they have replaced pork insulin and the highly antigenic beef insulin.

Di's physician then recommended that she take Humalog, an insulin preparation containing lispro, an ultra–fast-acting bioengineered insulin analog in which lysine at position B29 has been moved to B28 and proline at B28 has been moved to B29 (hence, lispro) (see Fig. 6.13). With lispro, Di will be able to time her injections minutes before her consumption of carbohydrate-containing meals, rather than having to remember to give herself an insulin injection 1 hour before a meal.

 Ann Jeina. Mrs. Jeina continued to be monitored in the cardiac care unit. At admission, her CK levels were elevated (182 units/L compared with a reference range of 38–174 U/L), and the MB fraction was high at 6.8% of the total (reference = <5% of the total). Her total CK continued to rise (228 units/L 12 hours after admission and 266 units/L at 24 hours), as did her MB fraction (8% at 12 hours and 10.8% at 24 hours). Within 2 hours of the onset of an acute myocardial infarction, the MB form of CK begins leaking from heart cells that were injured by the ischemic process. These rising serum levels of the MB fraction (and, therefore, of the total CK) reach their peak 12 to 36 hours later and usually return to normal within 3 to 5 days from the onset of the infarction (Fig. 6.16). In addition to the CK measurements, her blood levels were also analyzed for myoglobin and the heart isoform of troponin-T, a protein involved in muscle contraction (see Chapter 7).

BIOCHEMICAL COMMENTS

Enzyme and Protein Databases. Large databases of protein structure have been assembled to collate data from various laboratories around the world. The National Library of Medicine maintains a website, PubMed, which catalogues the medical literature, and a search engine that allows you to search for reference articles by topic or author

Creatine kinase isozymes in blood

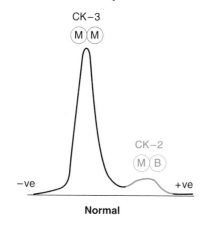

Normal

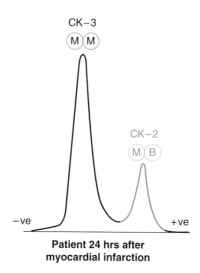

**Patient 24 hrs after
myocardial infarction**

Fig. 6.16. Electrophoretic separation of serum creatine kinase enzymes from a normal healthy adult and from a patient who had a myocardial infarction 24 hours previously. Creatine kinase catalyzes the reversible transfer of a phosphate from ATP to creatine to form phosphocreatine and ADP. The reaction is an important part of energy metabolism in heart muscle, skeletal muscle, and brain. Three different forms of the dimer exist: BB (or CK-1) found in brain, MB (or CK-2) found only in heart, and MM (or CK-3), found only in skeletal and heart muscle (cathode, −ve; anode, +ve).

(http://www.ncbi.nlm.nih.gov/pubmed). From the menu, you can directly enter a protein database or a structure database. These databases are linked, so that you can type in the name of a protein, such as human hemoglobin chain A, obtain a list of contributors to sequence data, and retrieve a complete amino acid sequence for many proteins. You can link to PubMed to find recent articles about the protein, or you can link to the structure database. A program called Cn3D can be downloaded from this site that allows you to view the three-dimensional versions of the protein structures.

These databases are only a few of more than 500 biologic databases that have been assembled to collate and exchange biologic information in the areas of DNA, RNA, genomics, gene mapping, and protein structure. The first issue of the *Journal of Nucleic Acid Research* each year provides a description of currently available biologic databases. Their goal is to provide information that can relate a particular DNA sequence or mutation to the protein involved, to its function, and to the pathologic consequences of a particular amino acid substitution, by comparing proteins that have similar functional elements.

Will these databases be of any use to the practicing physician or to the practice-oriented medical student? Very few students will ever want to do protein modeling. However, students and physicians may wish to use the literature search in PubMed as part of their approach to evidence-based medicine. They also may wish to use it to track definitions or fundamental knowledge about particular topics. Thus, a move has begun to link biomedical and basic science textbooks to PubMed.

Suggested Reference

Tatusov RL, Koonin EV, Lipman, DJ. A genomic perspective on protein families. Science 1997;278:631–637.

 REVIEW QUESTIONS—CHAPTER 6

1. In a polypeptide at physiologic pH, hydrogen bonding may occur between

    (A) the side chains of a leucine residue and a lysine residue.
    (B) the side chains of an aspartyl residue and a glutamyl residue.
    (C) the terminal α-amino group and the terminal α-carboxyl group.
    (D) the amide group in the peptide bond and an aspartyl side chain.
    (E) the SH groups of two cysteine residues.

2. Which of the following shows the linear sequence of atoms joined by covalent bonds in a peptide backbone?

    (A) –N–C–C–N–C–C–N–C–C
    (B) –N–C–O–N–C–O–N–C–O–
    (C) –N–C–C–O–N–C–C–O–N–C–C–O–
    (D) –N–H–C–C–N–H–C–C–N–H–C–C–
    (E) –N–H–C–O–H–N–H–C–O–H–N–H–C–C–

3. **Di Abietes'** different preparations of insulin contain some insulin complexed with protamine that is absorbed slowly after injection. Protamine is a protein preparation from rainbow trout sperm containing arginine-rich peptides that bind insulin. Which of the following provides the best explanation for complex formation between protamine and insulin?

    (A) Arginine is a basic amino acid that binds to negatively charged amino acid side chains in insulin.
    (B) Arginine is a basic amino acid that binds to the α-carboxylic acid groups at the N-terminals of insulin chains.
    (C) Arginine is a large bulky hydrophobic amino acid that complexes with leucine and phenylalanine in insulin.
    (D) Arginine forms disulfide bonds with the cysteine residues that hold the A and B chains together.
    (E) Arginine has a side chain that forms peptide bonds with the carboxyl terminals of the insulin chains.

4. Protein kinases phosphorylate proteins only at certain hydroxyl groups on amino acid side chains. Which of the following groups of amino acids all contain side chain hydroxyl groups?

    (A) aspartate, glutamate, and serine
    (B) serine, threonine, and tyrosine
    (C) threonine, phenylalanine, and arginine
    (D) lysine, arginine, and proline
    (E) alanine, asparagine, and serine

5. In a single individual, the primary structures of enzymes catalyzing the same reaction

    (A) are exactly the same from cell type to cell type, although the amount of enzyme may differ.
    (B) stay the same throughout the lifetime of that individual.
    (C) are identical if the enzymes are paralogs.
    (D) are identical to all members of the homologous family.
    (E) may differ between different cellular compartments of the same cell.

7 Structure–Function Relationships in Proteins

Diseases can be caused by changes in protein structure that affect the protein's ability to bind other molecules and carry out its function. They also can be caused by conformational changes in proteins that affect their solubility and degradability. In amyloidosis AL, immunoglobulin chains form an insoluble protein aggregate called amyloid in organs and tissues. Alzheimer's disease and familial amyloid polyneuropathy are neurodegenerative diseases characterized by the deposition of amyloid. Prion diseases result from misfolding and aggregation of a normal cellular protein. Even in sickle cell anemia, the mutation in hemoglobin principally affects the quarternary structure of hemoglobin and its solubility, and not its ability to bind oxygen.

A multitude of different proteins can be formed from only 20 common amino acids because these amino acids can be linked together in an enormous variety of sequences determined by the genetic code. The sequence of amino acids, its primary structure, determines the way a protein folds into a unique three-dimensional structure, which is its native conformation. Once folded, the three-dimensional structure of a protein forms binding sites for other molecules, thereby dictating the function of the protein in the body. In addition to creating binding sites, a protein must fold in such a way that it is flexible, stable, able to function in the correct site in the cell, and capable of being degraded by cellular enzymes.

Levels of protein structure. Protein structure is described in terms of four different levels: primary, secondary, tertiary, and quarternary (Fig. 7.1). The primary structure of a protein is the linear sequence of amino acids in the polypeptide chain. Secondary structure consists of local regions of polypeptide chains formed into structures generally stabilized by hydrogen bonds, such as the regular structures called α-helices and β-sheets. The rigidity of the peptide backbone determines the types of secondary structure that can occur. The tertiary structure involves folding of the secondary structural elements into an overall three-dimensional conformation. In globular proteins such as myoglobin, the tertiary structure generally forms a densely packed hydrophobic core with polar amino acid side chains on the outside. Some proteins exhibit quaternary structure, the combination of two or more subunits, each composed of a polypeptide chain.

Domains and folds. The tertiary structure of a globular protein is made up of structural domains, regions of structure that are recognized as separate and linked to other domains in a simple way. Within a domain, a combination of secondary

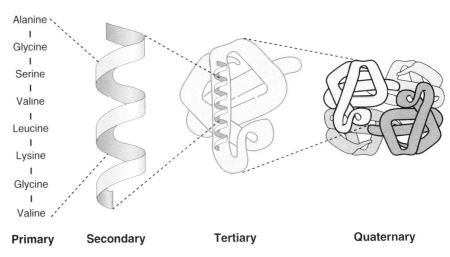

Alanine
|
Glycine
|
Serine
|
Valine
|
Leucine
|
Lysine
|
Glycine
|
Valine

Primary **Secondary** **Tertiary** **Quaternary**

Fig. 7.1. Levels of structure in a protein.

*structural elements forms a fold, such as the **nucleotide binding fold,** or an **actin fold.** Folds are defined by their similarity in a number of different proteins.*

*   **Quarternary structure.** Assembly of globular polypeptide subunits into a multisubunit complex can provide the opportunity for **cooperative binding** of ligands (e.g., O_2 binding to hemoglobin), form **binding sites** for complex molecules (e.g., antigen binding to immunoglobulin), and increase **stability** of the protein. The polypeptide chains of **fibrous proteins** such as **collagen** are aligned along an axis, have repeating elements, and are extensively linked to each other through hydrogen bonds.*

*   **Ligand binding.** Proteins form binding sites for a specific molecule, called a **ligand** (e.g., ATP or O_2) or for another protein. The affinity of a binding site for its ligand is quantitatively characterized by an **association** or **affinity constant, K_a,** (or its **dissociation constant, K_d**).*

*   **Folding of proteins.** The primary structure of a protein dictates the way that it folds into its tertiary structure, which is a **stable conformation** that is identical to the shape of other molecules of the same protein (that is, its **native conformation**.) **Chaperonins** act as templates to overcome the kinetic barrier to reaching a stable conformation. **Prion proteins** cause neurodegenerative diseases by acting as a template for misfolding. Heat, acid, and other agents cause proteins to **denature,** that is, to unfold or refold and lose their native three-dimensional conformation.*

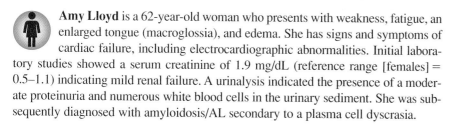

THE WAITING ROOM

 Will Sichel, who has sickle cell anemia, was readmitted to the hospital with symptoms indicating that he was experiencing another sickle cell crisis (see Chapter 6).

 Anne Jeina is a 54-year-old woman who arrived in the hospital 4 days ago, approximately 5 hours after she began to feel chest pain (see Chapter 6). In the emergency room, the physician had drawn blood for the measurement of myoglobin, CK-MB (creatine kinase, muscle-brain fraction) and cTN-T (cardiac troponin T subunit). The results from these tests had supported the diagnosis of an acute MI (myocardial infarction), and Mrs. Jeina was hospitalized.

 Amy Lloyd is a 62-year-old woman who presents with weakness, fatigue, an enlarged tongue (macroglossia), and edema. She has signs and symptoms of cardiac failure, including electrocardiographic abnormalities. Initial laboratory studies showed a serum creatinine of 1.9 mg/dL (reference range [females] = 0.5–1.1) indicating mild renal failure. A urinalysis indicated the presence of a moderate proteinuria and numerous white blood cells in the urinary sediment. She was subsequently diagnosed with amyloidosis/AL secondary to a plasma cell dyscrasia.

 Amyloidosis is a term encompassing many diseases that share a common feature—the extracellular deposition of pathologic insoluble fibrillar proteins called amyloid in organs and tissues. In **Amy Lloyd**'s disease, amyloidosis/AL, the amyloid is derived from immunoglobulin light chains (AL = **a**myloidosis, **l**ight-chain related).

Di Abietes returned to her physician's office for a routine visit to monitor her treatment (see Chapters 4, 5, and 6.) Her physician drew blood for an HbA_{1c} (pronounced hemoglobin A-1- c) determination. The laboratory reported a value of 8.5%, compared with to a normal reference range of 5.8 to 7.2%.

I. GENERAL CHARACTERISTICS OF THREE-DIMENSIONAL STRUCTURE

The overall conformation of a protein, the particular position of the amino acid side chains in three-dimensional space, gives a protein its function.

Globular

Fibrous

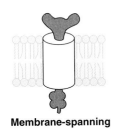

Membrane-spanning

Fig. 7.2. General shapes of proteins.

Requirements of a Protein Structure
Function
Binding specificity
Flexibility
Solubility or lipophilicity
Stability
Degradability

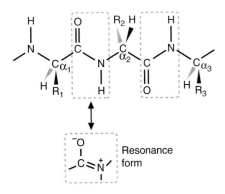

Resonance form

Fig. 7.3. The peptide backbone. Because of the resonance nature of the peptide bond, the C and N of the peptide bonds form a series of rigid planes. Rotation within allowed torsion angles can occur around the bonds attached to the α-carbon. The side chains are *trans* to each other, and alternate above and below the peptide chain. The actual peptide bond is a hybrid between the resonance forms shown, resulting in a partial negative charge on the carbonyl oxygen, a partial positive charge on the nitrogen, and partial double bond character for the peptide bond itself.

A. Descriptions of Protein Structure

Proteins are generally grouped into major structural classifications: globular proteins, fibrous proteins, transmembrane proteins, and DNA-binding proteins (Fig. 7.2). Globular proteins are usually soluble in aqueous medium and resemble irregular balls. The fibrous proteins are geometrically linear, arranged around a single axis, and have a repeating unit structure. Another general classification, transmembrane proteins, consists of proteins that have one or more regions aligned to cross the lipid membrane. DNA-binding proteins, usually classified separately, are considered in Chapter 16.

The structure of these proteins is often described according to levels called primary, secondary, tertiary, and quaternary structure (see Fig. 7.1). The primary structure is the linear sequence of amino acid residues joined through peptide bonds to form a polypeptide chain. The secondary structure refers to recurring structures (such as the regular structure of the α-helix) that form in short localized regions of the polypeptide chain. The overall three-dimensional conformation of a protein is its tertiary structure. The quarternary structure is the association of polypeptide subunits in a geometrically specific manner.

B. Requirements of the Three-Dimensional Structure

The overall three-dimensional structure of a protein must meet certain requirements to enable the protein to function in the cell or extracellular medium of the body. The first requirement is the creation of a binding site that is specific for just one molecule, or a group of molecules with similar structural properties. The specific binding sites of a protein usually define its role. The three-dimensional structure also must exhibit the degrees of flexibility and rigidity appropriate to its function. Some rigidity is essential for the creation of binding sites and for a stable structure (i.e., a protein that just flopped all over the place could not accomplish anything). However, flexibility and mobility in structure enables the protein to fold as it is synthesized, and to adapt as it binds other proteins and small molecules. The three-dimensional structure must have an external surface appropriate for its environment (e.g., cytoplasmic proteins need to keep polar amino acids on the surface to remain soluble in an aqueous environment). In addition, the conformation must also be stable, with little tendency to undergo refolding into a form that cannot fulfill its function or that precipitates in the cell. Finally, the protein must have a structure that can de degraded when it is damaged or no longer needed in the cell. Almost every region in the sequence of amino acids, the primary structure, participates in fulfilling one or more of these requirements through the chemical properties of the peptide bonds and the individual amino acid side chains.

II. THE THREE-DIMENSIONAL STRUCTURE OF THE PEPTIDE BACKBONE

The amino acids in a polypeptide chain are sequentially joined by peptide bonds between the carboxyl group of one amino acid and amide group of the next amino acid in the sequence (Fig. 7.3). Usually the peptide bond assumes a *trans* configuration in which successive α-carbons and their R groups are located on opposite sides of the peptide bond.

The polypeptide backbone can only bend in a very restricted way. The peptide bond itself is a hybrid of two resonance structures, one of which has double bond character, so that the carboxyl and amide groups that form the bond must, therefore, remain planar (see Fig. 7.3.). As a consequence, the peptide backbone consists of a sequence of rigid planes formed by the peptide groups (see Fig. 7.3). However, rotation within certain allowed angles (torsion angles) can occur around the bond between the α-carbon and the α-amino group and around the bond between the α-carbon and the carbonyl group. This rotation is subject to steric constraints that maximize the distance between atoms in the different amino acid side chains and forbid torsion (rotation) angles that place the side chain atoms too close to each other. These folding constraints, which depend on the specific amino acids present, limit the secondary and tertiary structures that can be formed from the polypeptide chain.

III. SECONDARY STRUCTURE

Regions within polypeptide chains form recurring, localized structures known as secondary structures. The two regular secondary structures called the α-helix and the α-sheet contain repeating elements formed by hydrogen bonding between atoms of the peptide bonds. Other regions of the polypeptide chain form nonregular nonrepetitive secondary structures, such as loops and coils.

A. The α-Helix

The α-helix is a common secondary structural element of globular proteins, membrane-spanning domains, and DNA-binding proteins. It has a stable rigid conformation that maximizes hydrogen bonding while staying within the allowed rotation angles of the polypeptide backbone. The peptide backbone of the α-helix is formed by strong hydrogen bonds between each carbonyl oxygen atom and the amide hydrogen (N-H) of an amino acid residue located four residues further down the chain (Fig. 7.4). Thus, each peptide bond is connected by hydrogen bonds to the peptide bond four amino acid residues ahead of it and four amino acid residues behind it in the amino acid sequence. The core of the helix is tightly packed, thereby maximizing association energies between atoms. The *trans* side chains of the amino acids project backward and outward from the helix, thereby avoiding steric hindrance with the polypeptide backbone and with each other (Fig. 7.5).

B. β-Sheets

β-Sheets are a second type of regular secondary structure that maximizes hydrogen bonding between the peptide backbones while maintaining the allowed torsion angles. In β-sheets, the hydrogen bonding usually occurs between regions of separate neighboring polypeptide strands aligned parallel to each other (Fig. 7.6). Thus, the carbonyl oxygen of one peptide bond is hydrogen-bonded to the nitrogen of a peptide bond on an adjacent strand. (This pattern contrasts with the α-helix in which the peptide backbone hydrogen bonds are within the same strand.) Optimal hydrogen bonding occurs when the sheet is bent (pleated) to form β-pleated sheets.

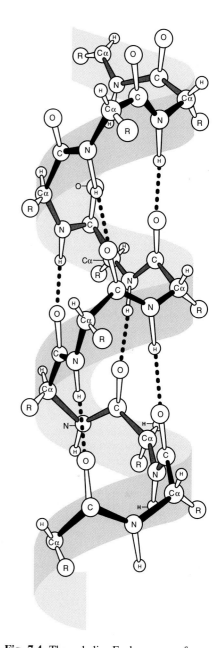

Fig. 7.4. The α-helix. Each oxygen of a carbonyl group of a peptide bond forms a hydrogen bond with the hydrogen atom attached to a nitrogen atom in a peptide bond four amino acids further along the chain. The result is a highly compact and rigid structure.

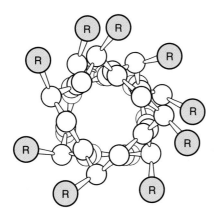

Fig. 7.5. A view down the axis of an α-helix. The side chains (R) jut out from the helix. Steric hindrance occurs if they come within their van der Waals radii of each other, and a stable helix cannot form.

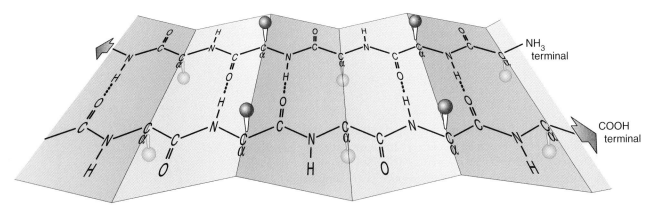

Fig. 7.6. A β-pleated sheet. In this case, the chains are oriented in opposite directions (antiparallel). The large arrows show the direction of the carboxy terminal. The amino acid side chains (R) in one strand are *trans* to each other, and alternate above and below the plane of the sheet, which can have a hydrophobic face and a polar face that engages in hydrogen bonding.

A renal biopsy used in the diagnosis of **Amy Lloyd**'s disease showed amorphous deposits in the glomeruli. When stained with Congo red dye, these deposits appeared red with ordinary light microscopy and exhibited apple green fluorescence when viewed in polarized light. This staining is characteristic of the amyloid fibril structure, which is composed of repeated β-sheets aligned orthogonally (perpendicular) to the axis of the fiber.

A number of diseases involve deposition of a characteristic amyloid fiber. However, in each of these diseases, the amyloid is derived from a different protein that has changed its conformation (three-dimensional structure) to that of the amyloid repeated β-sheet structure. Once amyloid deposition begins, it seems to proceed rapidly, as if the fibril itself were promoting formation and deposition of more fibrils (a phenomenon called "seeding"). The different clinical presentations in each of these diseases results from differences in the function of the native protein and the site of amyloid deposition.

The β-pleated sheet is described as parallel if the polypeptide strands run in the same direction (as defined by their amino and carboxy terminals) and anti-parallel if they run in opposite directions. Antiparallel strands are often the same polypeptide chain folded back on itself, with simple hairpin turns or long runs of polypeptide chain connecting the strands. The amino acid side chains of each polypeptide strand alternate between extending above and below the plane of the β-sheet (see Fig. 7.6). Parallel sheets tend to have hydrophobic residues on both sides of the sheets; antiparallel sheets usually have a hydrophobic side and a hydrophilic side. Frequently, sheets twist in one direction.

C. Nonrepetitive Secondary Structures

α-Helices and β-pleated sheets are patterns of regular structure with a repeating element, the turn of a helix or a pleat. In contrast, bends, loops, and turns are nonregular secondary structures that do not have a repeating element. They are characterized by an abrupt change of direction and are often found on the protein surface. For example, β-turns are short regions usually involving four successive amino acid residues. They often connect strands of antiparallel β-sheets (Fig. 7.7.). The surface of large globular proteins usually has at least one omega loop, a structure with a neck like the capital Greek letter omega, Ω.

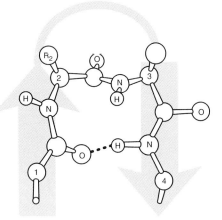

Fig. 7.7. β-turn. The four amino acid residues that form the β-turn (also called a hairpin loop) are held together by hydrogen bonds, which make this an extremely stable structure.

D. Patterns of Secondary Structure

Figure 7.8 is a three-dimensional drawing of a globular domain in the soluble enzyme lactate dehydrogenase (LDH). It illustrates the combination of secondary structural elements to form patterns. This LDH domain is typical of globular proteins, which average approximately 31% α-helical structure and approximately 28% β-pleated sheets (with a wide range of variation.) The helices of globular domains have an average span of approximately 12 residues, corresponding to approximately three to four helical turns, although many are much longer. The β-sheets, represented in diagrams by an arrow for each strand, are an average of six residues long and six strands wide (2–15 strands). Like the β-sheet in the lactate dehydrogenase domain, they generally twist to the right, rather than lie flat (see Fig. 7.8). Most globular domains, such as this LDH domain, also contain motifs. Motifs are relatively small arrangements of secondary structure recognized in many different proteins. For example, certain of the β-strands are connected with α-helices to form the βα βα β structural motif.

The remaining polypeptide segments connecting the helices and β-sheets are said to have a coil or loop conformation (see Fig. 7.8). Although some of the connecting segments recognized in many proteins have been given names (like the Ω-loops), other segments such as those in this LDH domain appear disordered or irregular. These nonregular regions, generally called coils, should never be referred to as "random coils." They are neither truly disordered nor random; they are stabilized through specific hydrogen bonds dictated by the primary sequence of the protein and do not vary from one molecule of the protein to another of the same protein.

The nonregular coils, loops, and other segments are usually more flexible than the relatively rigid helices and β-pleated sheets. They often form hinge regions that allow segments of the polypeptide chain to move as a compound binds or to move as the protein folds around another molecule.

Although it is usually assumed that proteins can have truly disordered regions, the more that is learned about protein structure, the less disordered these regions seem. Even regions that look truly disordered may form a specific binding site for another molecule (e.g., the intracellular C-terminal of transmembrane proteins). Eventually all regions of all proteins may be classified as a particular named pattern.

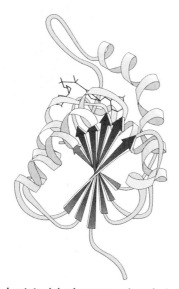

Lactate dehydrogenase domain 1

Fig. 7.8. Ribbon drawing showing the arrangement of secondary structures into a three-dimensional pattern in domain 1 of lactate dehydrogenase. The individual polypeptide strands in the six-stranded β-sheet are shown with arrows. Different strands are connected by helices and by nonrepetitive structures (turns, coils and loops), shown in blue. This domain is the nucleotide binding fold. NAD⁺ is bound to a site created by the helices (upper left of figure.) (Modified from Richardson JS. Adv Protein Chem. The anatomy and taxonomy of protein structure 1981;34:167).

Flexibility is one of the most important features of protein structure. Although every portion of every amino acid in a protein is engaged in bonding to the rest of the protein, to water, or to a ligand, proteins do not have rigid structures. The three-dimensional structure is flexible and dynamic, with rapidly fluctuating movement in the exact position of amino acid side chains and domains. These fluctuations are like wiggling or shaking that can occur without unfolding. They allow ions and water to diffuse through the structure and provide alternate conformations for ligand binding.

IV. TERTIARY STRUCTURE

The tertiary structure of a protein is the folding pattern of the secondary structural elements into a three-dimensional conformation, as shown for the LDH domain in Figure 7.8. As illustrated with examples below, this three-dimensional structure is designed to serve all aspects of the protein's function. It creates specific and flexible binding sites for ligands (the compound that binds), illustrated with actin and myoglobin. The tertiary structure also maintains residues on the surface appropriate for the protein's cellular location, polar residues for cytosolic proteins, and hydrophobic residues for transmembrane proteins (illustrated with the β_2-adrenergic receptor).

A. Domains in the Tertiary Structure

The tertiary structure of large complex proteins is often described in terms of physically independent regions called structural domains. You can usually identify domains from visual examination of a three-dimensional figure of a protein, such as the three-dimensional figure of G-actin shown in Fig. 7.9. Each domain is formed from a continuous sequence of amino acids in the polypeptide chain that are folded into a three-dimensional structure independently of the rest of the protein, and two domains are connected through a simpler structure like a loop (e.g., the hinge region of Fig. 7.9). The structural features of each domain can be discussed independently of another domain in the same protein, and the structural features of one domain may not match that of other domains in the same protein.

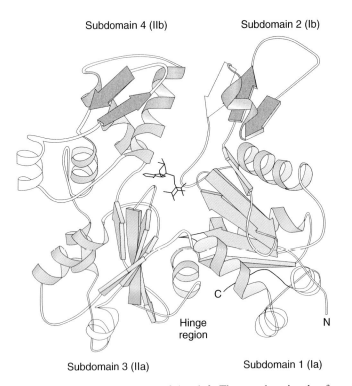

Fig. 7.9. G-Actin. ATP binds in the center of the cleft. The two domains that form the cleft are further subdivided into subdomains 1–4. The overall structure is found in many ATP-binding proteins and is called the actin fold. The conformations of the regions shown in blue are nearly superimposable among the proteins that contain the actin fold. (From Kabsch W, Holmes KC. The actin fold. FASEB J 1995:9:167–174.)

B. Folds in Globular Proteins

Folds are relatively large patterns of three-dimensional structure that have been recognized in many proteins, including proteins from different branches of the phylogenetic tree. A characteristic activity is associated with each fold, such as ATP binding and hydrolysis (the actin fold) or NAD^+ binding (the nucleotide-binding fold). These three examples of fold patterns are discussed below.

1. THE ACTIN FOLD

In the three-dimensional drawing of G-actin shown in Figure 7.9, all four subdomains contribute to a folding pattern called the actin fold, named for the first protein in which it was described. ATP is bound into the middle of the cleft of the actin fold by amino acid residues contributed by domains on both sides; thus, ATP binding promotes a conformational change that closes the cleft. Once bound, ATP is cleaved to ADP and phosphate.

The actin fold is found in proteins as diverse as actin, which polymerizes to form the cytoskeleton, heat shock protein 70 (hsp70), which uses ATP energy in changing the conformation of other proteins and hexokinase, which catalyzes phosphorylation of glucose (see Chapter 8 for further discussion of hexokinase.) Although these proteins have very little sequence identity, three-dimensional drawings of their actin folds are almost superimposable. The amount of sequence identity they do have is consistent with their membership in the same fold family and establishes that they are all homologs of the same ancestral protein. In all of these proteins, ATP binding results in large conformational changes that contribute to the function of the protein.

2. THE NUCLEOTIDE BINDING FOLD

A fold also can be formed by one domain. In the example of secondary structures provided by lactate dehydrogenase (see Fig. 7.8), domain 1 alone forms the nucleotide binding fold. This fold is a binding site for NAD^+ or, in other proteins, molecules with a generally similar structure (e.g., riboflavin). However, many proteins that bind NAD^+ or $NADP^+$ contain a very different fold from a separate fold family. These two different NAD^+ binding folds arise from different ancestral lines and have different structures, but have similar properties and function. They are believed to be the product of convergent evolution.

C. The Solubility of Globular Proteins in an Aqueous Environment

Most globular proteins are soluble in the cell. In general, the core of a globular domain has a high content of amino acids with nonpolar side chains (val, leu, ile, met, and phe), out of contact with the aqueous medium. This hydrophobic core is densely packed to maximize attractive van der Waals forces, which exert themselves over short distances. The charged polar amino acid side chains (arg, his, lys, asp, and glu) are generally located on the surface of the protein, where they form ion pairs (salt bridges) or are in contact with aqueous solvent. Charged side chains often bind inorganic ions (e.g., K^+, PO_4^{3-} or Cl^-) to decrease repulsion between like charges. When charged amino acids are located on the interior, they are generally involved in forming specific binding sites. The polar uncharged amino acid side chains of ser, thr, asn, gln, tyr, and trp are also usually found on the surface of the protein, but may occur in the interior, hydrogen bonded to other side chains. Although cystine disulfide bonds (the bond formed by two cysteine sulfhydryl groups) are sometimes involved in the formation of tertiary structure, they are generally not needed.

More than 1000 folds have now been recognized, and it is predicted that there are only a few thousand different folds for all the proteins that have ever existed. One of the values of classifying proteins into fold patterns is that a specific function, such as ATP binding and hydrolysis, is associated with each fold. Currently, we know the primary structure of many proteins involved in inherited diseases without knowing the function of the protein. However, the function of a domain in a protein can be predicted if its amino acid sequence can be matched to that of other proteins in a fold family with a known function. Classifying proteins into fold families also may be useful for drug design. The structure of a bacterial protein targeted by a drug can be compared with that of human proteins in the same fold family so that an antibacterial drug can be designed that more specifically targets the bacterial protein.

G-actin subunits polymerize to form F-actin, which forms the cytoskeleton (see Chapter 10). The conformational change caused by ATP binding to the G-actin subunits promotes their addition to the growing ends of the F-actin polymers. Hydrolysis of bound ATP to ADP by the G-actin subunit promotes dissociation.

Many features of the adrenaline (β2-adrenergic) receptor are typical of hormone receptors. Each extracellular loop is actually a structural domain, but several loops together form the binding site for the hormone. The binding site is sometimes referred to as a binding domain (a functional domain), even though it is not formed from a continuous segment of the polypeptide chain. The amino terminus (residues 1–34) extends out of the membrane and has branched high mannose oligosaccharides linked through N-glycosidic bonds to the amide of asparagine. It is anchored in the lipid plasma membrane by a palmitoyl group (shown as a squiggle in Fig. 7.10) that forms a thioester with the SH residue of a cysteine. The COOH terminus, which extends into the cytoplasm, has a number of serine and threonine phosphorylation sites (shown as blue circles in Fig. 7.10).

D. Tertiary Structure of Transmembrane Proteins

Transmembrane proteins, such as the β$_2$-adrenergic receptor, contain membrane-spanning domains and intracellular and extracellular domains on either side of the membrane (Fig. 7.10). Many ion channel proteins, transport proteins, neurotransmitter receptors, and hormone receptors contain similar membrane-spanning segments that are α-helices with hydrophobic residues exposed to the lipid bilayer. These rigid helices are connected by loops containing hydrophilic amino acid side chains that extend into the aqueous medium on both sides of the membrane. In the β$_2$-adrenergic receptor, the helices clump together so that the extracellular loops form a surface that acts as a binding site for the hormone adrenaline (epinephrine), our fight or flight hormone. The binding site is sometimes referred to as a binding domain (a functional domain), even though it is not formed from a continuous segment of the polypeptide chain. Once adrenaline binds to the receptor, a conformational change in the arrangement of rigid helical structures is transmitted to the intracellular domains that form a binding site for another signaling protein, a heterotrimeric G protein (a guanosine triphosphate [GTP]-binding protein composed of three different subunits). Thus, receptors require both rigidity and flexibility to transmit signals across the cell membrane.

As discussed in Chapter 6, transmembrane proteins usually have a number of posttranslational modifications that provide additional chemical groups to fulfill requirements of the three-dimensional structure. The amino terminus (residues 1–34) extends out of the membrane and has branched high mannose oligosaccharides linked through N-glycosidic bonds to the amide of asparagine (see Fig. 7.10). It is anchored in the lipid plasma membrane by a palmitoyl group that forms a thioester with the SH residue of a cysteine. The COOH terminus, which extends

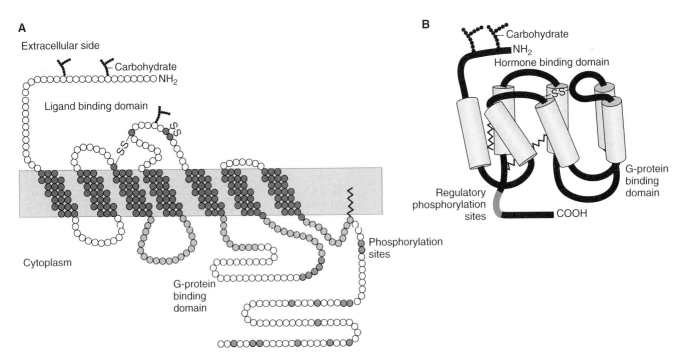

Fig. 7.10. β$_2$-Adrenergic receptor. The receptor has seven α-helix domains that span the membrane and is therefore a member of the heptahelical class of receptors. **A.** The transmembrane domains are drawn in an extended form. **B.** The seven transmembrane helices (shown as tubes) form a cylindrical structure. Loops connecting helices form the hormone binding site on the external side of the plasma membrane, and a binding site for a G-protein is on the intracellular side. The protein also contains oligosaccharide chains, palmityl groups, and phosphorylation sites (shown in blue; see Chapter 6).

into the cytoplasm, has a number of serine and threonine phosphorylation sites (shown as blue circles) that regulate receptor activity.

V. QUATERNARY STRUCTURE

The quaternary structure of a protein refers to the association of individual polypeptide chain subunits in a geometrically and stoichiometrically specific manner. Many proteins function in the cell as dimers, tetramers, or oligomers, proteins in which two, four, or more subunits, respectively, have combined to make one functional protein. The subunits of a particular protein always combine in the same number and in the same way, because the binding between the subunits is dictated by the tertiary structure, which is dictated by the primary structure, which is determined by the genetic code.

A number of different terms are used to describe subunit structure. The prefixes "homo" or "hetero" are used to describe identical or different subunits, respectively, of 2, 3, or 4 subunit proteins (e.g., heterotrimeric G proteins have three different subunits). A protomer is a unit structure composed of nonidentical subunits. In contrast, F-actin is an oligomer, a multisubunit protein composed of identical G-actin subunits. "Multimer" is sometimes used as a more generic term to designate a complex with many subunits of more than one type.

The contact regions between the subunits of globular proteins resemble the interior of a single subunit protein; they contain closely packed nonpolar side chains, hydrogen bonds involving the polypeptide backbones and their side chains, and occasional ionic bonds or salt bridges. The subunits of globular proteins are very rarely held together by interchain disulfide bonds, and never by other covalent bonds. In contrast, fibrous and other structural proteins may be extensively linked to other proteins through covalent bonds.

Assembly into a multisubunit structure increases the stability of a protein. The increase in size increases the number of possible interactions between amino acid residues and therefore makes it more difficult for a protein to unfold and refold. As a result, many soluble proteins are composed of two or four identical or nearly identical subunits with an average size of approximately 200 amino acids.

A multisubunit structure has many advantages besides increased stability. It may enable the protein to exhibit cooperativity between subunits in binding ligands (illustrated later with hemoglobin) or to form binding sites with a high affinity for large molecules (illustrated with antigen binding to the immunoglobulin molecule. IgG). An additional advantage of a multisubunit structure is that the different subunits can have different activities and cooperate in a common function. Examples of enzymes that have regulatory subunits or exist as multiprotein complexes are provided in Chapter 9.

 Creatine phosphokinase (CK), one of the proteins measured to follow **Ann Jeina**'s myocardial infarction (see Chapter 6) is present in cells as dimers (two subunits). The dimers may be homodimers (two identical subunits of either the M [muscle] isozyme or the B [brain] isozyme), or heterodimers (MB) The MB isozyme is produced only by the heart and readily released from injured cardiomyocytes into the blood (see Chapter 6).

Serum levels of lactate dehydrogenase (LDH) were formerly used to diagnose an acute MI. LDH is present in cells as a tetramer of four identical, or nearly identical, subunits. Each subunit is a separate polypeptide chain with a molecular weight of 35 kD (approximately 35,000 g/mole). These subunits are present as two isoforms, the H isoform (for heart) and the M isoform (for skeletal muscle). Although the heart produces principally the H_4 form (four H subunits combined into a tetramer) and skeletal muscles produce principally the M_4 isoform, the heart, skeletal muscle, and other tissues produce several intermediate combinations (e.g., H_3M, H_2M_2). These tetrameric isoforms all have similar activities, but the individual monomeric subunits are inactive. Measurements of LDH isozymes in the serum are no longer used for diagnosis of a recent MI because the enzyme is large, released slowly, and the isozyme pattern is not as specific for the heart as is CK.

Insulin is composed of two nonidentical polypeptide chains attached to each other through disulfide bonds between the chains (see Chapter 6, Fig. 6.13). The subunits of globular proteins are generally not held together by disulfide bonds, but regions of the same chain may be connected by disulfide bonds that form as the chain folds. Insulin actually fits this generalization because it is synthesized as a single polypeptide chain, which forms the disulfide bonds. Subsequently, a proteolytic enzyme in secretory vesicles clips the polypeptide chain into two nonidentical subunits. Generally, each subunit of most protomers and oligomers is synthesized as a separate polypeptide chain. In fibrous proteins, which have a regular, sometimes repeating sequence of amino acids, interchain binding serves different functions. In collagen, for example, extensive interchain binding provides great tensile strength. The structure of collagen is discussed in Chapter 49 on connective tissue.

Equation 7.1. The association constant, K_a for a binding site on a protein.

Consider a reaction in which a ligand (L) binds to a protein (P) to form a ligand–protein complex (LP) with a rate constant of k_1. LP dissociates with a rate constant of k_2.:

$$L + P \underset{k_2}{\overset{k_1}{\rightleftharpoons}} LP$$

then,

$$K_{eq} = \frac{k_1}{k_2} = \frac{[LP]}{[L][P]} = \frac{K_a}{K_d} = 1$$

The equilibrium constant, K_{eq}, is equal to the association constant (K_a) or $1/K_d$, the dissociation constant. Unless otherwise given, the concentrations of L, P, and LP are expressed as mol/L, and K_a has the units of $(mol/L)^{-1}$.

VI. QUANTITATION OF LIGAND BINDING

In the examples of tertiary structure discussed above, the folding of a protein created a three-dimensional binding site for a ligand (NAD^+ for the lactate dehydrogenase domain 1, ATP for hexokinase, or adrenaline for the β_2 adrenergic receptor). The binding affinity of a protein for a ligand is quantitatively described by its association constant, K_a, which is the equilibrium constant for the binding reaction of a ligand (L) with a protein (P) (Eq. 7.1).

K_a is equal to the rate constant (k_1) for association of the ligand with its binding site divided by the rate constant (k_2) for dissociation of the ligand–protein complex (LP). K_d, the dissociation constant for ligand–protein binding, is the reciprocal of K_a. The tighter the binding of the ligand to the protein, the higher is the K_a and the lower is the K_d. The K_a is useful for comparing proteins produced by different alleles, or for describing the affinity of a receptor for different drugs.

VII. STUCTURE–FUNCTION RELATIONSHIPS IN MYOGLOBIN AND HEMOGLOBIN

Myoglobin and hemoglobin are two oxygen-binding proteins with a very similar primary structure (Fig. 7.11). However, myoglobin is a globular protein composed of a single polypeptide chain that has one O_2 binding site. Hemoglobin is a tetramer composed of two different types of subunits (2α and 2β polypeptide chains, referred to as two $\alpha\beta$ protomers). Each subunit has a strong sequence homology to myoglobin and contains an O_2 binding site. A comparison between myoglobin and hemoglobin illustrates some of the advantages of a multisubunit quaternary structure.

The tetrameric structure of hemoglobin facilitates saturation with O_2 in the lungs and release of O_2 as it travels through the capillary beds (Fig. 7.12). When the amount of oxygen bound to myoglobin or hemoglobin is plotted against the partial pressure of oxygen (pO_2), a hyperbolic curve is obtained for myoglobin, whereas that for hemoglobin is sigmoidal. These curves show that when the pO_2 is high, as in the lungs, both myoglobin and hemoglobin are saturated with oxygen. However,

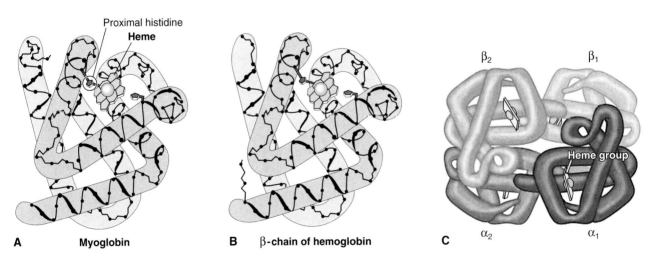

Fig. 7.11. Myoglobin and hemoglobin. Myoglobin consists of a single polypeptide chain, which is similar in structure to the α and β subunits of hemoglobin. In all of the subunits, heme is tightly bound in a hydrophobic binding pocket. The proximal histidine extends down from a helix to bind to the Fe atom. The oxygen binds between the distal histidine and the heme. Panel C displays the quaternary structure of hemoglobin (From Frescht A. Structure and Mechanism in Protein Science. New York: WH Freeman and Company, 1999. Used with permission.)

at the lower levels of pO_2 in oxygen-using tissues, hemoglobin cannot bind oxygen as well as myoglobin (i.e., its percent saturation is much lower). Myoglobin, which is present in heart and skeletal muscle, can bind the O_2 released by hemoglobin, which it stores to meet the demands of contraction. As O_2 is used in the muscle cell for generation of ATP during contraction, it is released from myoglobin and picked up by cytochrome oxidase, a heme-containing enzyme in the electron transport chain that has an even higher affinity for oxygen than myoglobin.

A. Oxygen Binding and Heme

The tertiary structure of myoglobin consists of eight α-helices connected by short coils, a structure that is known as the globin fold (see Fig. 7.11). This structure is unusual for a globular protein in that it has no β-sheets. The helices create a hydrophobic O_2 binding pocket containing tightly bound heme with an iron atom (Fe^{2+}) in its center.

Heme consists of a planar porphyrin ring composed of four pyrrole rings that lie with their nitrogen atoms in the center, binding an Fe^{2+} atom (Fig. 7.13).

Sickle cell anemia is really a disease caused by the wrong quarternary structure. The painful vasoocclusive crises experienced by **Will Sichel** are caused by the polymerization of HbS molecules into long fibers that distort the shape of the red blood cells into sickle cells. The substitution of a hydrophobic valine for a glutamate in the β2 chain creates a knob on the surface of deoxygenated hemoglobin that fits into a hydrophobic binding pocket on the β1 subunit of a different hemoglobin molecule. A third hemoglobin molecule, which binds to the first and second hemoglobin molecules through aligned polar interactions, binds a fourth hemoglobin molecule through its valine knob. Thus the polymerization continues until long fibers are formed.

Myoglobin is readily released from skeletal muscle or cardiac tissue when the cell is damaged. It has a small molecular weight, 17,000 kDa, and is not complexed to other proteins in the cell. (Da is the abbreviation for Dalton, which is a unit of mass approximately equal to one H atom. Thus, a molecular weight of 17,000 kDa is equal to approximately 17,000 g/mole.) Large injuries to skeletal muscle that result from physical crushing or lack of ATP production result in cellular swelling and the release of myoglobin and other proteins into the blood. Myoglobin passes into the urine and turns the urine red because the heme (which is red) remains covalently attached to the protein. During an acute MI, myoglobin is one of the first proteins released into the blood from damaged cardiac tissue. (However, the amount released is not high enough to cause myoglobinuria.) Laboratory measurements of serum myoglobin are used for early diagnosis in patients such as **Ann Jeina**. Because myoglobin is not present in skeletal muscle and the heart as tissue-specific isozymes, and the amount released from the heart is much smaller than the amount that can be released from a large skeletal muscle injury, myoglobin measurements are not specific for an MI.

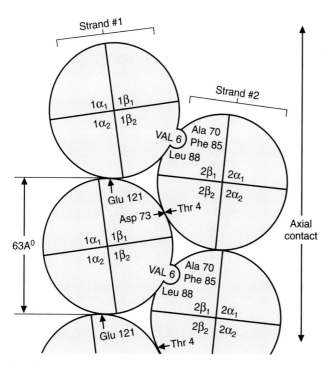

Polymerization of the hemoglobin molecules is highly dependent on the concentration of HbS and is promoted by the conformation of the deoxygenated molecules. At 100% oxygen saturation, even high concentrations of HbS will not polymerize. A red blood cell spends the longest amount of time at the lower oxygen concentrations of the venous capillary bed, where polymerization is most likely initiated.

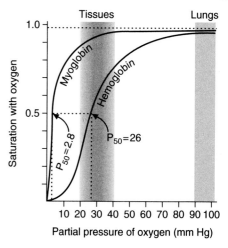

Fig. 7.12. Oxygen saturation curves for myoglobin and hemoglobin. Note that the curve for myoglobin is hyperbolic, whereas that for hemoglobin is sigmoidal. The effect of the tetrameric structure is to inhibit O_2 binding at low O_2 concentrations. P_{50} is the partial pressure of O_2 (pO_2) at which the protein is half-saturated with O_2. P_{50} for myoglobin is 2.8, and that for hemoglobin is 26.

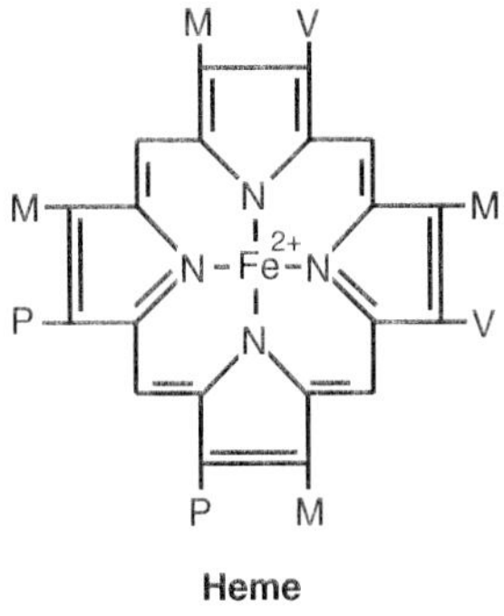

Heme

Fig. 7.13. Heme. The Fe is bound to four nitrogen atoms in the center of the heme porphyrin ring. Methyl (M, CH_3), vinyl (V, -CH = CH_2), and propionate (P, $CH_2CH_3COO^-$) side chains extend out from the four pyrrole rings that constitute the porphyrin ring.

Negatively charged propionate groups on the porphyrin ring interact with arginine and histidine side chains from the hemoglobin, and the hydrophobic methyl and vinyl groups that extend out from the porphyrin ring interact with hydrophobic amino acid side chains from hemoglobin. All together, there are approximately 16 different interactions between myoglobin amino acids and different groups in the porphyrin ring.

Organic ligands that are tightly bound, such as the heme of myoglobin, are called prosthetic groups. A protein with its attached prosthetic group is called a holoprotein; without the prosthetic group, it is called an apoprotein. The tightly bound prosthetic group is an intrinsic part of the protein and does not dissociate until the protein is degraded.

Within the binding pocket of myoglobin, O_2 binds directly to the Fe^{2+} atom on one side of the planar porphyrin ring (Fig. 7.14). The Fe^{2+} atom is able to chelate six different ligands; four of the ligand positions are in a plane and taken by the central nitrogens in the planar porphyrin ring. Two ligand positions are perpendicular to this plane. One of these positions is taken by the nitrogen atom on a histidine, called the proximal histidine, which extends down from a myoglobin helix. The other position is taken by O_2.

The proximal histidine of myoglobin and hemoglobin is sterically repelled by the heme porphyrin ring. Thus, when the histidine binds to the Fe^{2+} in the middle of the

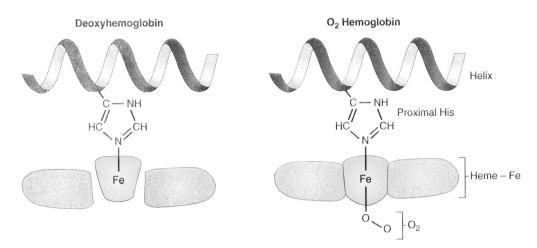

Fig. 7.14. Oxygen binding to the Fe^{2+} of heme in myoglobin. A histidine residue called the proximal histidine binds to the Fe^{2+} on one side of the porphyrin ring; O_2 binds to Fe^{2+} on the other side. O_2 binding causes a conformational change that pulls the Fe^{2+} back into the plane of the ring. As the proximal histidine moves, it moves the helix that contains it.

ring, it pulls the Fe^{2+} above the plane of the ring. When oxygen binds on the other side of the ring, it pulls the Fe^{2+} back into the plane of the ring. The pull of O_2 binding moves the proximal histidine toward the porphyrin ring, which moves the helix containing the proximal histidine. This conformational change has no effect on the function of myoglobin. However, in hemoglobin, the movement of one helix leads to the movement of other helices in that subunit, including one in a corner of the subunit that is in contact with a different subunit through salt bridges. The loss of these salt bridges then induces conformational changes in all other subunits, and all four subunits may change in a concerted manner from their original conformation to a new conformation.

B. Cooperativity of O_2 Binding in Hemoglobin

The cooperativity in oxygen binding in hemoglobin comes from conformational changes in tertiary structure that takes place when O_2 binds (Fig. 7.15). The conformational change of hemoglobin is usually described as changing from a T (tense) state with low affinity for O_2 to an R (relaxed) state with a high affinity for O_2. Breaking the salt bridges in the contacts between subunits is an energy-requiring

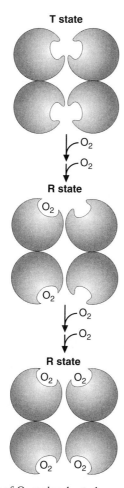

Fig. 7.15. Equilibria for binding of O_2 molecules to hemoglobin according to the concerted model of Monod, Wyman, and Changeux. Hemoglobin exists in two alternate conformations, the T (tense) state with a low affinity for O_2 and the R (relaxed) state with a higher affinity. In the T subunits, the binding sites are hindered, and in the R state the binding sites are open. Each successive addition of O_2 shifts the equilibrium further toward the R state. Because the conformation of all the subunits can change when O_2 binds to one subunit, oxygen binding is said to follow the concerted model. Most of the molecules change to the R state when 2 O_2 molecules have bound.

Amy Lloyd's serum protein electrophoresis indicated the presence of a sharp narrow peak or homogeneous "spike" in the characteristic γ-globulin zone known as an M protein (monoclonal protein) component. A narrow peak of spike in electrophoresis, which separates proteins according to charge distribution of the side chains, suggests an elevation of proteins with a similar or identical structure. Subsequently, it was shown that Amy Lloyd's immunoglobulin M-component was composed of a single homogeneous type of immunoglobulin (just one amino acid sequence in the N-terminal variable region). Thus, the M protein was produced by a single clone of antibody-secreting cells (cells that all arose from proliferation of one cell) in the bone marrow (called plasma cell dyscrasia). In amyloidosis, substitutions of particular amino acids in the light chain variable region are thought to destabilize its native conformation, resulting in fibrillogenesis.

In AL amyloidosis, amyloid is formed from degradation products of the λ or κ light chains that deposit most frequently in the extracellular matrix of the kidney and the heart but also may deposit in the tongue. In other types of amyloidosis, the amyloid arises from other proteins and deposits in a characteristic organ. For example, the amyloid associated with chronic inflammatory conditions, such as tuberculosis or rheumatoid arthritis, is derived from an acute phase serum protein called serum amyloid A that is produced by the liver in response to inflammation. It deposits most frequently in the kidney, and cardiac involvement is rare.

process and, consequently, the binding rate for the first oxygen is very low. When the next oxygen binds, many of the hemoglobin molecules containing one O_2 will already have all four subunits in the R state, and therefore the rate of binding is much higher. With two O_2 molecules bound, an even higher percentage of the hemoglobin molecules will have all four subunits in the R state. This phenomenon, known as positive cooperativity, is responsible for the sigmoidal oxygen saturation curve of hemoglobin (see Fig. 7.12).

VIII. STRUCTURE–FUNCTION RELATIONSHIPS IN IMMUNOGLOBULINS

The immunoglobulins (or antibodies) are one line of defense against invasion of the body by foreign organisms. In this capacity, they function by binding to ligands called antigens on the invading organisms, thereby initiating the process by which these organisms are inactivated or destroyed.

Immunoglobulins all have a similar structure; each antibody molecule contains two identical small polypeptide chains (the light or L chains) and two identical large polypeptide chains (the heavy or H chains) (Fig. 7.16). The chains are joined to each other by disulfide bonds.

The body has five major classes of immunoglobulins. The most abundant immunoglobulins in human blood are the γ-globulins, which belong to the IgG class. The γ-globulins have approximately 220 amino acids in their light chains and 440 in their heavy chains. Like most serum proteins, they have attached oligosaccharides that participate in targeting the protein for clearance from the blood. Both the light and heavy chains consist of domains known as the immunoglobulin fold, which is a collapsed β-barrel made from a number of β-sheets (Fig. 7.17).

Both the light and heavy chains contain regions termed variable (V) and constant (C) regions. The variable regions of the L and H chains (V_L and V_H, respectively) interact to produce a single antigen binding site at each branch of the Y-shaped molecule. Each population (clone) of B cells produces an antibody with a different amino acid composition in the variable region that is complementary to the structure of the antigen eliciting the response. The K_d of antibodies for their specific antigens is extremely small and varies from approximately 10^{-7} to 10^{-11} M. The antigen thus binds very tightly with almost no tendency to dissociate and can be removed from circulation as the antigen–antibody complex is ingested by macrophages. The constant domains that form the Fc part of the antibody are important for binding of the antigen–antibody complex to phagocytic cells for clearance and for other aspects of the immune response.

IX. PROTEIN FOLDING

Although the peptide bonds in a protein are rigid, flexibility around the other bonds in the peptide backbone allow an enormous number of possible conformations for each protein. However, every molecule of the same protein folds into the same stable three-dimensional structure. This shape is known as the native conformation.

The tight binding affinity of immunoglobulins for their specific antigen makes them useful for the measurement of small amounts of other compounds in various radioimmunoassays. The principle of the radioimmunoassay is that the immunoglobulin will specifically bind the compound being measured, and an additional component of the system that is labeled with a radioactive chemical will bind the immunoglobulin. The complex is then separated from the solution and the bound radioactivity measured. The different isozymes of CK and Tn-T used to track **Ann Jeina's** MI are measured with a type of radioimmunassay by using antibodies specific for each isozyme. This method is much faster than the laborious separation of isozymes by electrophoresis. Radioimmunoassays are also useful for measuring the small amounts of hormones present in the blood for diagnosis of endocrine diseases.

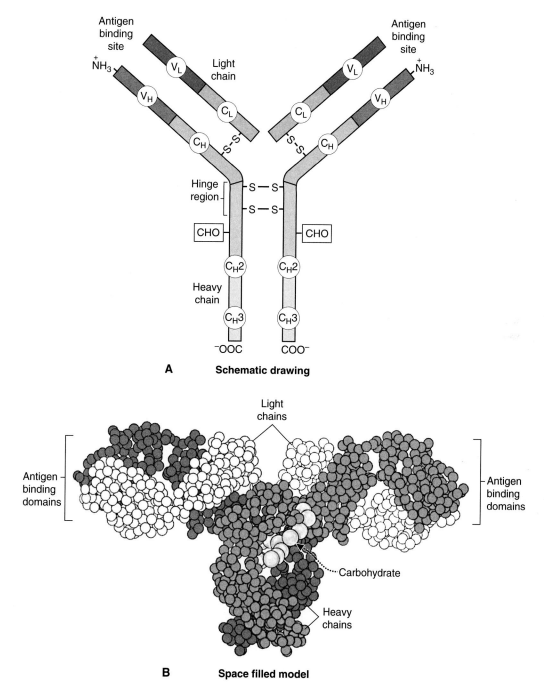

Fig. 7.16. Structure of immunoglobulins. **A.** Each IgG molecule contains two light (L) and two heavy (H) chains joined by disulfide bonds. Each light chain contains two domains, a variable domain (V_L) and a region of constant amino acid sequence (C_L). Each heavy chain has four domains: one variable domain (V_H) and three constant domains (C_H). The conformation of the constant domain contains the β-sheets that are called the immunoglobulin fold. The variable domains are specific for the antigen that is bound, whereas the constant regions are the same for all antibody molecules of a given class. Carbohydrate (CHO) is bound as indicated within the constant region of the heavy chains (CH). The hinge region allows flexibility when the molecule binds antigen. **B.** In the space-filled model, the light chains are light in color and the heavy chains are two different shades of gray. (Modified from Silverton EW, Navia MA, Davies DR, et al. Proc Natl Acad Sci. Three-dimensional structure of an intact human immunoglobulin USA 1977;11:5142)

Very little difference is seen in the energy state of the native conformation and a number of other stable conformations that a protein might assume. It appears that the prion protein, the cause of mad cow disease, is a normal cellular protein that has refolded into a different stable conformation with a lower energy state than its normal functional conformation (discussed under Biochemical Comments, later). If misfolded proteins do not precipitate into aggregates, they can be degraded in the cell by proteolytic reactions, or even refolded.

A. Primary Structure Determines Folding

The primary structure of a protein determines its three-dimensional conformation. More specifically, the sequence of amino acid side chains dictates the fold pattern of the three-dimensional structure and the assembly of subunits into quaternary structure. Under certain conditions, denatured proteins can refold into their native conformation, regaining their original function. Proteins can be denatured with organic solvents such as urea that disrupt hydrophobic interactions and convert the protein to a soluble random coil. Many simple single-subunit proteins like ribonuclease that are denatured in this way spontaneously refold into their native conformation if carefully brought back to physiologic conditions. Even complex multi-subunit proteins containing bound cofactors can sometimes spontaneously renature under the right conditions. Thus, the primary structure essentially specifies the folding pattern.

In the cell, not all proteins fold into their native conformation on their own. As the protein folds and refolds while it is searching for its native low energy state, it passes through many high-energy conformations that slow the process (called kinetic barriers). These kinetic barriers can be overcome by heat shock proteins, which use energy provided by ATP hydrolysis to assist in the folding process (Fig. 7.18). Heat shock proteins were named for the fact that their synthesis in bacteria increased when the temperature was suddenly raised. They are

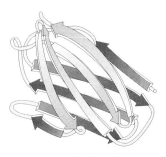

V_L domain

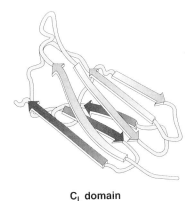

C_L domain

Fig. 7.17. Structure of the V_L and C_L domains of IgG. Layers of antiparallel β-sheets are stacked in these domains, which have been referred to as collapsed β-barrels. The antigen binds between the V_H and V_L immunoglobulin folds, and NOT in the barrel. The C_L domain is also called the immunoglobulin fold. (Top modified from Richardson JS. Adv Protein Chem. The anatomy and taxonomy of protein structure 1981;34:167; bottom reprinted in part with permission from Edmundson AB, Ely KR, Abola EE, et al. Rational allomerism and divergent evolution of domains in immunoglobin light chains. Biochemistry 1975;14:3954. © 1975 American Chemical Society.)

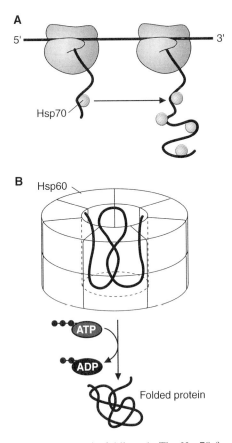

Fig. 7.18. Role of heat shock proteins in folding. **A.** The Hsp70 family of proteins prevent folding of the nascent chain and promote unfolding. The ATPase domain of the protein has the actin fold. **B.** The Hsp60 class of protein has a barrel shape into which the protein fits. It acts as a template, binding and rebinding portions of the unfolded protein until folding is completed. It hydrolyzes many ATP bonds to provide energy for the process.

present in human cells as different families of proteins with different activities. For example, the hsp70 proteins bind to nascent polypeptide chains as their synthesis is being completed to keep the uncompleted chains from folding prematurely. They also unfold proteins prior to their insertion through the membrane of mitochondria and other organelles. The multi-subunit barrel-shaped hsp60 family of proteins is called chaperonins. The unfolded protein fits into the barrel cavity that excludes water and serves as a template for the folding process. The hydrolysis of several ATP molecules is used to overcome the energy barriers to reaching the native conformation.

A *cis-trans* isomerase and a disulfide isomerase also participate in folding. The *cis-trans* isomerase converts a trans peptide bond preceding a proline into the *cis* conformation, which is well suited for making hairpin turns. The disulfide isomerase breaks and reforms disulfide bonds between the -SH groups of two cysteine residues in transient structures formed during the folding process. After the protein has folded, cysteine-SH groups in close contact in the tertiary structure can react to form the final disulfide bonds.

B. Protein Denaturation

1. DENATURATION THROUGH NONENZYMATIC MODIFICATION OF PROTEINS

Amino acids on proteins can undergo a wide range of chemical modifications that are not catalyzed by enzymes, such as nonenzymatic glycosylation or oxidation. Such modifications usually lead to a loss of function and denaturation of the protein, sometimes to a form that cannot be degraded in the cell. In nonenzymatic glycosylation, glucose that is present in blood, or in interstitial or intracellular fluid, binds to an exposed amino group on a protein (Fig. 7.19). The two-step process forms an irreversibly glycosylated protein. Proteins that turn over very slowly in the body, such as collagen or hemoglobin, exist with a significant fraction present in the glycosylated form. Because the reaction is nonenzymatic, the rate of glycosylation is proportionate to the concentration of glucose present, and individuals with hyperglycemia have much higher levels of glycosylated proteins than individuals with normal blood glucose levels. Collagen and other glycosylated proteins in tissues are further modified by nonenzymatic oxidation and form additional cross-links. The net result is the formation of large protein aggregates referred to as AGEs (advanced glycosylation end-products). AGE is a meaningful acronym because AGEs accumulate with age, even in individuals with normal blood glucose levels.

2. PROTEIN DENATURATION BY TEMPERATURE, pH, AND SOLVENT

Proteins can be denatured by changes of pH, temperature, or solvent that disrupt ionic, hydrogen, and hydrophobic bonds. At a low pH, ionic bonds and hydrogen bonds formed by carboxylate groups would be disrupted; at a very alkaline pH, hydrogen and ionic bonds formed by the basic amino acids would be disrupted. Thus, the pH of the body must be maintained within a range compatible with three-dimensional structure. Temperature increases vibrational and rotational energies in the bonds, thereby affecting the energy balance that goes into making a stable three-dimensional conformation.

Hydrophobic molecules can also denature proteins by disturbing hydrophobic interactions in the protein. For example, long-chain fatty acids can inhibit many enzyme-catalyzed reactions by binding nonspecifically to hydrophobic pockets in proteins and disrupting hydrophobic interactions. Thus, long-chain fatty acids and other highly hydrophobic molecules have their own binding proteins in the cell.

Di Abietes' physician used her glycosylated hemoglobin levels, specifically the HbA$_{1c}$ fraction, to determine whether she had sustained hyperglycemia over a long period. The rate of irreversible nonenzymatic glycosylation of hemoglobin and other proteins is directly proportional to the glucose concentration to which they are exposed over the last 4 months. The danger of sustained hyperglycemia is that, over time, many proteins become glycosylated and subsequently oxidized, affecting their solubility and ability to function. The glycosylation of collagen in the heart, for example, is believed to result in a cardiomyopathy in patients with chronic uncontrolled diabetes mellitus. In contrast, glycosylation of hemoglobin has little effect on its function.

Proteins are denatured in the gastric juice of the stomach, which has a pH of 1 to 2. Although this pH cannot break peptide bonds, disruption of the native conformation makes the protein a better substrate for digestive enzymes.

Thermal denaturation is often illustrated by the process of cooking an egg. In the presence of heat, the protein albumin converts from its native translucent state to a denatured white precipitate. Protein precipitates can sometimes be dissolved by amphipathic agents such as urea, guanidine HCl, or SDS (sodium dodecylsulfate) that form extensive hydrogen bonds and hydrophobic interactions with the protein.

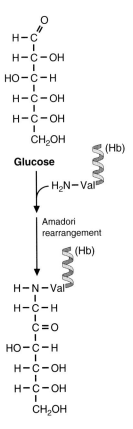

Fig. 7.19. Nonenzymatic glycosylation of hemoglobin. Glucose forms a Schiff base with the N-terminal amino group of the protein, which rearranges to form a stable glycosylated product. Similar nonenzymatc glycosylation reactions occur on other proteins.

CLINICAL COMMENTS

Will Sichel. Will Sichel continues to experience severe low back and lower extremity pain for many hours after admission. The diffuse pains of sickle cell crises are believed to result from occlusion of small vessels in a variety of tissues, thereby depriving cells of oxygen and causing ischemic or anoxic damage to the tissues. In a sickle cell crisis, long hemoglobin polymers form, causing the red blood cells to become distorted and change from a biconcave disc to an irregular shape, such as a sickle (for which the disease was named) or a stellate structure (Fig.7.20). The aggregating Hb polymers damage the cellular membrane and promote aggregation of membrane proteins, increased permeability of the cell, and dehydration. Surface charge and antigens of red blood cells are carried on the transmembrane proteins glycophorin and Band 3 (the erythrocyte anion exchange channel, see Chapter 10). Hemoglobin S binds tightly to the cytoplasmic portion of band 3, contributing to further polymer aggregation and uneven distribution of negative charge on the sickle cell surface. As a result, the affected cells adhere to endothelial cells in capillaries, occluding the vessel and decreasing blood flow to the distal tissues. The subsequent hypoxia in these tissues causes cellular damage and even death.

The sickled cells are sequestered and destroyed mainly by phagocytic cells, particularly those in the spleen. An anemia results as the number of circulating red blood cells decreases and bilirubin levels rise in the blood as hemoglobin is degraded.

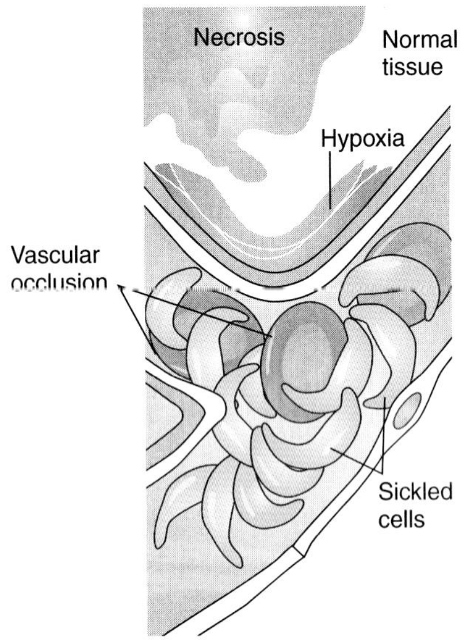

Fig. 7.20 Sickled red blood cells occlude a blood vessel, causing hypoxia (low O_2 in cells) and necrosis (cell death).

After a few days of treatment, **Will Sichel's** crisis was resolved. In the future, should Will suffer a cerebrovascular accident as a consequence of vascular occlusion or have recurrent life-threatening episodes, a course of long-term maintenance blood transfusions to prevent repeated sickle crises may be indicated. Iron chelation would have to accompany such a program to prevent or delay the development of iron overload. Although a few individuals with this disease have survived into the sixth decade, mean survival is probably into the fourth decade. Death usually results from renal failure or cardiopulmonary disease.

Anne Jeina. Mrs. Jeina's diagnosis of an acute myocardial infarction (MI) was based partly on measurements of CK-MB, myoglobin, and cTN-T (the cardiac isozyme of troponin-T, a subunit of the regulatory protein troponin). Early diagnosis is critical for a decision on the type of therapeutic intervention to be used. Of these proteins, myoglobin appears in the blood most rapidly. However, its levels are relatively nonspecific for cardiac injury because the amino acid sequences of cardiac and skeletal muscle myoglobins are identical. Myoglobin measurements do have a very high negative predictive value within the 2- to 6-hour period after the onset of symptoms (i.e., if myoglobin is not elevated, a myocardial infarction did not occur). In contrast, serum cardiac troponin-T is a relatively late, but highly specific, marker of myocardial injury. It is typically detected in an acute MI within 3 to 5 hours after onset of symptoms, is positive in most cases within 8 hours, and approaches 100% sensitivity at 10 to 12 hours. It remains elevated for 5 to 10 days.

Mrs. Jeina stayed in the hospital until she had been free of chest pain for 5 days. She was discharged on a low-fat diet and was asked to participate in the hospital patient exercise program for patients recovering from a recent heart attack. She was scheduled for regular examinations by her physician.

Amy Lloyd. Amy Lloyd has AL amyloidosis, which is characterized by deposition of amyloid fibers derived principally from the variable region of λ or κ immunoglobulin light chains. Increased amounts of the fragments of the light chains called Bence-Jones proteins appeared in her urine. Fibril deposition in the extracellular matrix of her kidney glomeruli has resulted in mild renal failure. Deposition of amyloid in the extracellular matrix of her heart muscle resulted in the cardiac arrhythmia seen on an electrocardiogram. In addition to other signs of right-sided heart failure, she had peripheral edema. The loss of weight may have been caused by infiltrations of amyloid in the gastrointestinal tract or by constipation and diarrhea resulting from involvement of the autonomic nervous system. Treatment may be directed against the plasma cell proliferation, or against the symptomatic results of organ dysfunction.

During Amy Lloyd's evaluation, she developed a cardiac arrhythmia that was refractory to treatment. The extensive amyloid deposits in her heart had disrupted conduction of electrical impulses in the heart muscle, ultimately resulting in cardiac arrest. On autopsy, amyloid deposits were found within the heart, tongue, liver, adipose tissue, and every organ examined except the central nervous system, which had been protected by the blood-brain barrier.

Dianne Abietes. Di Abietes' HbA_{1c} of 8.5% was just above the normal range (5.8–7.2% of total hemoglobin), and her physician decided not to alter her insulin treatment plan. Glycosylation is a nonenzymatic reaction that occurs with a rate directly proportionate to the concentration of glucose in the blood. In the normal range of blood glucose concentrations (approximately 80–140 mg/dL, depending on time after a meal), 6 to 7% of the hemoglobin is glycosylated to form HbA_{1c}. Hemoglobin turns over in the blood as red blood cells are phagocytosed and their hemoglobin degraded and new red blood cells are derived from retic-

Troponin is a heterotrimeric protein involved in the regulation of striated and cardiac muscle contraction. Most troponin in the cell is bound to the actin–tropomyosin complex in the muscle fibril. The three subunits of troponin consist of troponin-C, troponin-T, and troponin-I, each with a specific function in the regulatory process. Troponin-T and troponin-I exist as different isoforms in cardiac and skeletal muscle (sequences with a different amino acid composition), thus allowing the development of specific antibodies against each form. As a consequence, either cardiac troponin-T or cardiac troponin-I may be rapidly measured in blood samples by immunoassay with a good degree of specificity.

Four minor components of adult hemoglobin (HbA) result from posttranslational, nonenzymatic glycosylation of different amino acid residues (HbA_{1a1}, HbA_{1a2}, HbA_{1b1}, and HbA_{1c}). In HbA_{1c}, the fraction that is usually measured, the glycosylation occurs on an N-terminal valine.

Prion diseases are categorized as transmissable spongiform encephalopathies, which are neurodegenerative diseases characterized by spongiform degeneration and astrocytic gliosis in the central nervous system. Frequently, protein aggregates and amyloid plaques are seen. These aggregates are resistant to proteolytic degradation.

Familial prion diseases are caused by point mutations in the gene encoding the Pr protein (point mutations are changes in one base in the DNA nucleotide sequence). The diseases have a variety of names related to the different mutations and the clinical syndrome (e.g., Gertsmann-Straussler-Scheinker disease and familial Creutzfeld-Jakob disease). Familial Creutzfeld-Jakob disease (fCJD) arises from an inherited mutation and has an autosomal dominant pedigree. It typically presents in the fourth decade of life. The mutation lowers the activation energy for refolding and the prion proteins fold into the PrP^{Sc} conformation more readily. It is estimated that the rate of generating prion disease by refolding of PrP^{c} in the normal cell is approximately 3,000 to 4,000 years. Lowering of the activation energy for refolding by mutation presumably decreases this time to the observed 30- to 40-year prodromal period. Sporadic Creutzfeld-Jakob disease may arise from somatic cell mutation or rare spontaneous refoldings that initiate a cascade of refolding into the PrP^{Sc} conformation. The sporadic form of the disease accounts for 85% of all cases of CJD.

ulocytes. The average lifespan of a red blood cell is 120 days. Thus, the extent of hemoglobin glycosylation is a direct reflection of the average serum glucose concentration to which the cell has been exposed over its 120-day lifespan. **Di Abietes'** elevated Hb$_{A1c}$ indicates that her blood glucose levels have been elevated on an average over the preceding 6 weeks to 4 months. An increase of Di's insulin dosage would decrease her hyperglycemia but increase her risk of hypoglycemic events.

BIOCHEMICAL COMMENTS

Protein Misfolding and Prions. Prion proteins are believed to cause a neurodegenerative disease by acting as a template to misfold other cellular prion proteins into a form that cannot be degraded. The word *prion* stands for proteinaceous infectious agent. The prion diseases can be acquired either through infection (mad-cow disease), or from sporadic or inherited mutations (e.g., Creutzfeldt-Jakob disease). Although the infectious prion diseases represent a small proportion of human cases, their link to mad cow disease in the United Kingdom (new variant CJD), to growth hormone inoculations in the United States and France (iatrogenic or "doctor-induced" CJD), and to ritualistic cannibalism in the Fore tribespeople (Kuru) have received the most publicity.

The prion protein is normally found in the brain and is encoded by a gene that is a normal component of the human genome. The disease-causing form of the prion protein has the same amino acid composition but is folded into a different conformation that aggregates into multimeric protein complexes resistant to proteolytic degradation (Fig. 7.21). The normal conformation of the prion protein has been designated PrP^{c} and the disease-causing form PrP^{Sc} (sc for the prion disease scrapies in sheep). Although PrP^{Sc} and PrP^{c} have the same amino acid composition, the PrP^{Sc} conformer is substantially enriched in β-sheet structure compared with the normal PrP^{c} conformer, which has little or no β-sheet structure and is approximately 40% α-helix. This difference favors the aggregation of PrP^{Sc} into multimeric complexes. These two conformations presumably have similar energy levels. Fortunately, spontaneous refolding of PrP proteins into the PrP^{Sc} conformation is prevented by a large activation energy barrier that makes this conversion extremely slow. Thus, very few molecules of PrP^{Sc} are normally formed during a lifetime.

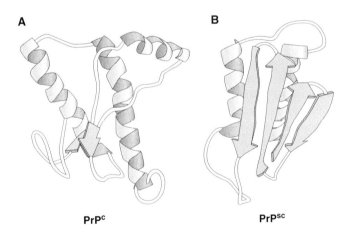

A

B

PrP^{c}

PrP^{sc}

Fig. 7.21. The conformation of PrP^{c} and PrP^{sc}. The prion proteins have two domains, an N-terminal region that binds four Cu^{2+} per chain, and a C-terminal region. In PrP^{c}, the C-terminal regions contain three substantial helices and two 3-residue β strands joined by two to three hydrogen bonds (approximately 40% a-helix and almost no β-sheet structure). It exists as a monomer. In PrP^{sc}, the C-terminal region is folded into an extensive β-sheet. The overall structure is approximately 40 to 50% β-sheet, 20 to 30% α-helices. This conformation promotes aggregation.

The infectious disease occurs with the ingestion of PrP^{Sc} dimers in which the prion protein is already folded into the high β structure. These PrP^{Sc} proteins are thought to act as a template to lower the activation energy barrier for the conformational change, causing native proteins to refold into the PrP^{Sc} conformation much more rapidly (much like the role of chaperonins). The refolding initiates a cascade as each new PrP^{Sc} formed acts as a template for the refolding of other molecules. As the number of PrP^{Sc} molecules increase in the cell, they aggregate into a multimeric assembly that is resistant to proteolytic digestion.

Suggested References

Khan MF, Falk RH. Amyloidosis. Postgrad Med J 2001;77:686–693.

Horwich AL, Weissman JS. Deadly conformations-protein misfolding in prion diseases. Cell 1997;89:499–510.

Raj DSC, Choudhury D, Welbourne TC, Levi M. Advanced glycation end products: a nephrologist's perspective. Am J Kidney Dis 2000;35:365–380.

 REVIEW QUESTIONS—CHAPTER 7

1. Which of the following characterize α-helix regions of proteins?

   (A) They all have the same primary structure.
   (B) They are formed principally by hydrogen bonds between a carbonyl oxygen atom in one peptide bond and the amide hydrogen from a different peptide bond.
   (C) They are formed principally by hydrogen bonds between a carbonyl atom in one peptide bond and the hydrogen atoms on the side chain of another amino acid.
   (D) They are formed by hydrogen bonding between two adjacent amino acids in the primary sequence.
   (E) They require a high content of proline and glycine.

2. Which of the following is a characteristic of globular proteins?

   (A) Hydrophilic amino acids tend to be on the inside.
   (B) Hydrophobic amino acids tend to be on the outside.
   (C) Tertiary structure is formed by hydrophobic and electrostatic interactions between amino acids, and by hydrogen bonds between amino acids and between amino acids and water.
   (D) Secondary structures are formed principally by hydrophobic interactions between amino acids.
   (E) Covalent disulfide bonds are necessary to hold the protein in a rigid conformation.

3. A protein has one transmembrane domain composed entirely of α-helical secondary structure. Which of the following amino acids would you expect to find in the transmembrane domain?

   (A) Proline
   (B) Glutamate
   (C) Lysine
   (D) Leucine
   (E) Arginine

4. Autopsies of patients with Alzheimer's disease show protein aggregates called neurofibrillary tangles and neuritic plaques in various regions of the brain. These plaques exhibit the characteristic staining of amyloid. Which of the following structural features is the most likely characteristic of at least one protein in these plaques?

   (A) A high content of β-pleated sheet structure
   (B) A high content of α-helical structure
   (C) A high content of random coils
   (D) Disulfide bond crosslinks between polypeptide chains
   (E) A low-energy native conformation

5. While studying a novel pathway in a remote species of bacteria, you discover a new globular protein that phosphorylates a substrate, using ATP as the phosphate donor. This protein most likely contains which of the following structures?

    (A) An actin fold
    (B) An immunoglobulin fold
    (C) A nucleotide binding fold
    (D) A globin fold
    (E) A β-barrel

8 Enzymes as Catalysts

*Enzymes are proteins that act as **catalysts,** compounds that increase the rate of chemical reactions (Fig. 8.1). Enzyme catalysts bind reactants (substrates), convert them to products, and release the products. Although enzymes may be modified during their participation in this reaction sequence, they return to their original form at the end. In addition to increasing the speed of reactions, enzymes provide a means for regulating the rate of metabolic pathways in the body. This chapter describes the properties of enzymes that allow them to function as catalysts. The next chapter explains the mechanisms of enzyme regulation.*

*   **Enzyme binding sites.** An enzyme binds the **substrates** of the reaction and converts them to **products.** The substrates are bound to specific **substrate binding sites** on the enzyme through interactions with the amino acid residues of the enzyme. The spatial geometry required for all the interactions between the substrate and the enzyme makes each enzyme **selective for** its **substrates** and ensures that only **specific products** are formed.*

*   **Active catalytic site.** The substrate binding sites overlap in the **active catalytic site** of the enzyme, the region of the enzyme where the reaction occurs. Within the catalytic site, **functional groups** provided by **coenzymes, tightly bound metals,** and, of course, **amino acid residues** of the enzyme, participate in catalysis.*

*   **Activation energy and the transition state.** The functional groups in the catalytic site of the enzyme activate the substrates and decrease the energy needed to form the high-energy intermediate stage of the reaction known as the **transition state complex.** Some of the catalytic strategies employed by enzymes, such as **general acid-base catalysis,** formation of **covalent intermediates,** and **stabilization of the transition state,** are illustrated by **chymotrypsin.***

*   **pH and temperature profiles.** Enzymes have a functional pH range determined by the **pK_as** of functional groups in the active site and the interactions required for three-dimensional structure. Non-denaturing increases of temperature increase the reaction rate.*

*   **Mechanism-based inhibitors.** The effectiveness of many **drugs** and **toxins** depends on their ability to inhibit an enzyme. The strongest inhibitors are **covalent inhibitors,** compounds that form covalent bonds with a reactive group in the enzyme active site, or **transition state analogues** that mimic the transition state complex.*

*   **Enzyme names.** Most enzyme names end in "ase." Enzymes usually have both a common name and a systematic classification that includes a name and an Enzyme Commission (EC) number.*

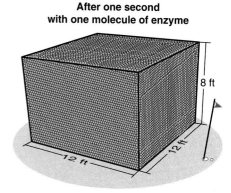

Fig. 8.1. Catalytic power of enzymes. Many enzymes increase the rate of a chemical reaction by a factor of 10^{11} or higher. To appreciate an increase in reaction rate by this order of magnitude, consider a room-sized box of golf balls that "react" by releasing energy and turning blue. The 12 ft × 12 ft × 8 ft box contains 380,000 golf balls. If the rate of the reaction in the absence of enzyme were 100 golf balls per year, the presence of 1 molecule of enzyme would turn the entire box of golf balls blue in 1 second (assuming a 10^{11} increase in reaction rate).

Most, if not all, of the tissues and organs in the body are adversely affected by chronic ingestion of excessive amounts of alcohol, including the liver, pancreas, heart, reproductive organs, central nervous system, and the fetus. Some of the effects of alcohol ingestion, such as the psychotropic effects on the brain or inhibition of vitamin transport, are direct effects caused by ethanol itself. However, many of the acute and chronic pathophysiologic effects of alcohol relate to the pathways of ethanol metabolism (see Chapter 25).

THE WAITING ROOM

A year after recovering from salicylate poisoning (see Chapter 4), **Dennis "the Menace" Veere** was playing in his grandfather's basement. Dennis drank an unknown amount of the insecticide malathion, which is sometimes used for killing fruit flies and other insects (Fig. 8.2). Sometime later when he was not feeling well, Dennis told his grandfather what he had done. Mr. Veere retrieved the bottle and rushed Dennis to the emergency room of the local hospital. On the way, Dennis vomited repeatedly and complained of abdominal cramps. At the hospital, he began salivating and had an uncontrollable defecation.

In the emergency room, physicians passed a nasogastric tube for stomach lavage, started intravenous fluids, and recorded vital signs. Dennis's pulse rate was 48 beats per minute (slow), and his blood pressure was 78/48 mm Hg (low). The physicians noted involuntary twitching of the muscles in his extremities.

Lotta Topaigne was diagnosed with acute gouty arthritis involving her right great toe (see Chapter 5). The presence of insoluble urate crystals within the joint space confirmed the diagnosis. Several weeks after her acute gout attack subsided, Ms. Topaigne was started on allopurinol therapy in an oral dose of 150 mg twice per day.

Al Martini, a 44-year-old man who has been an alcoholic for the past 5 years, had a markedly diminished appetite for food. One weekend he became unusually irritable and confused after drinking two fifths of scotch and eating very little. His landlady convinced him to visit his doctor. Physical examination indicated a heart rate of 104 beats/min. His blood pressure was slightly low, and he was in early congestive heart failure. He was poorly oriented to time, place, and person.

I. THE ENZYME-CATALYZED REACTION

Enzymes, in general, provide speed, specificity, and regulatory control to reactions in the body. Enzymes are usually proteins that act as catalysts, compounds that increase the rate of chemical reactions. Enzyme-catalyzed reactions have three basic steps:

(1) binding of substrate: $\mathbf{E + S \leftrightarrow ES}$
(2) conversion of bound substrate to bound product: $\mathbf{ES \leftrightarrow EP}$
(3) release of product : $\mathbf{EP \leftrightarrow E + P}$

An enzyme binds the substrates of the reaction it catalyzes and brings them together at the right orientation to react. The enzyme then participates in the making and breaking of bonds required for product formation, releases the products, and returns to its original state once the reaction is completed.

Enzymes do not invent new reactions; they simply make reactions occur faster. The catalytic power of an enzyme (the rate of the catalyzed reaction divided by the rate of the uncatalyzed reaction) is usually in the range of 10^6 to 10^{14}. Without the catalytic power of enzymes, reactions such as those involved in nerve conduction, heart contraction, and digestion of food would occur too slowly for life to exist.

Each enzyme usually catalyzes a specific biochemical reaction. The ability of an enzyme to select just one substrate and distinguish this substrate from a group of very similar compounds is referred to as specificity (Fig. 8.3). The enzyme converts

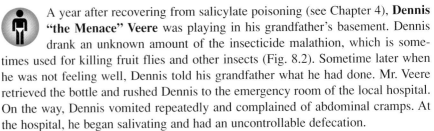

Malathion

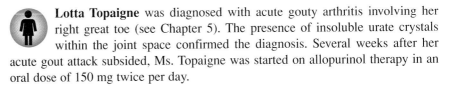

Sarin

Fig. 8.2. Organophosphorous compounds. Malathion and parathion are organophosphorous insecticides. Nausea, coma, convulsions, respiratory failure, and death have resulted from the use of parathion by farmers who have gotten it on their skin. Malathion is similar in structure to parathion, but not nearly as toxic. The nerve gas Sarin, another organophosphorous compound, was used in a terrorist attack in a Japanese subway.

this substrate to just one product. The specificity, as well as the speed, of enzyme-catalyzed reactions result from the unique sequence of specific amino acids that form the three-dimensional structure of the enzyme.

A. The Active Site

To catalyze a chemical reaction, the enzyme forms an enzyme–substrate complex in its active catalytic site (Fig. 8.4). The active site is usually a cleft or crevice in the enzyme formed by one or more regions of the polypeptide chain. Within the active site, cofactors and functional groups from the polypeptide chain participate in transforming the bound substrate molecules into products.

Initially, the substrate molecules bind to their substrate binding sites, also called the substrate recognition sites (see Fig. 8.4B). The three-dimensional arrangement of binding sites in a crevice of the enzyme allows the reacting portions of the substrates to approach each other from the appropriate angles. The proximity of the bound substrate molecules and their precise orientation toward each other contribute to the catalytic power of the enzyme.

The active site also contains functional groups that directly participate in the reaction (see Fig. 8.4C). The functional groups are donated by the polypeptide chain, or by bound cofactors (metals or complex organic molecules called coenzymes). As the substrate binds, it induces conformational changes in the enzyme that promote further interactions between the substrate molecules and the enzyme functional groups. (For example, a coenzyme might form a covalent intermediate with the substrate, or an amino acid side chain might abstract a proton from the reacting substrate.) The activated substrates and the enzyme form a transition state complex, an unstable high-energy complex with a strained electronic configuration that is intermediate between substrate and product. Additional bonds with the enzyme stabilize the transition state complex and decrease the energy required for its formation.

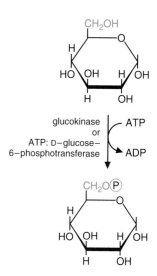

Fig. 8.3. Reaction catalyzed by glucokinase, an example of enzyme reaction specificity. Glucokinase catalyzes the transfer of a phosphate from ATP to carbon 6 of glucose. It cannot rapidly transfer a phosphate from other nucleotides to glucose, or from ATP to closely related sugars such as galactose, or from ATP to any other carbon on glucose. The only products formed are glucose 6-phosphate and ADP.

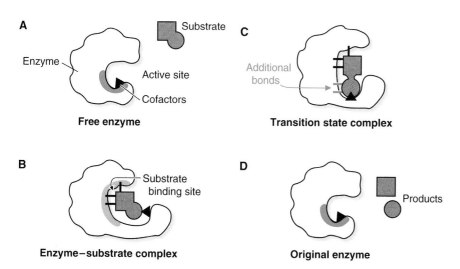

Fig. 8.4. Reaction in the enzyme active catalytic site. **A.** The enzyme contains an active catalytic site, shown in dark blue, with a region or domain where the substrate binds. The active site also may contain cofactors, nonprotein components that assist in catalysis. **B.** The substrate forms bonds with amino acid residues in the substrate binding site, shown in light blue. Substrate binding induces a conformational change in the active site. **C.** Functional groups of amino acid residues and cofactors in the active site participate in forming the transition state complex, which is stabilized by additional noncovalent bonds with the enzyme, shown in blue. **D.** As the products of the reaction dissociate, the enzyme returns to its original conformation.

The transition state complex decomposes to products, which dissociate from the enzyme (see Fig. 8.4D). The enzyme generally returns to its original form. The free enzyme then binds another set of substrates, and repeats the process.

B. Substrate Binding Sites

Enzyme specificity (the enzyme's ability to react with just one substrate) results from the three-dimensional arrangement of specific amino acid residues in the enzyme that form binding sites for the substrates and activate the substrates during the course of the reaction. The "lock-and-key" and the "induced-fit" models for substrate binding describe two aspects of the binding interaction between the enzyme and substrate.

1. LOCK-AND-KEY MODEL FOR SUBSTRATE BINDING

The substrate binding site contains amino acid residues arranged in a complementary three-dimensional surface that "recognizes" the substrate and binds it through multiple hydrophobic interactions, electrostatic interactions, or hydrogen bonds (Fig. 8.5). The amino acid residues that bind the substrate can come from very different parts of the linear amino acid sequence of the enzyme, as seen in glucokinase. The binding of compounds with a structure that differs from the substrate even to a small degree may be prevented by steric hindrance and charge-repulsion. In the lock-and-key model, the complementarity between the substrate and its binding site is compared to that of a key fitting into a rigid lock.

2. "INDUCED FIT" MODEL FOR SUBSTRATE BINDING

Complementarity between the substrate and the binding site is only part of the picture. As the substrate binds, enzymes undergo a conformational change ("induced fit") that repositions the side chains of the amino acids in the active site and increases the number of binding interactions (see Fig. 8.4). The induced fit model for substrate bind-

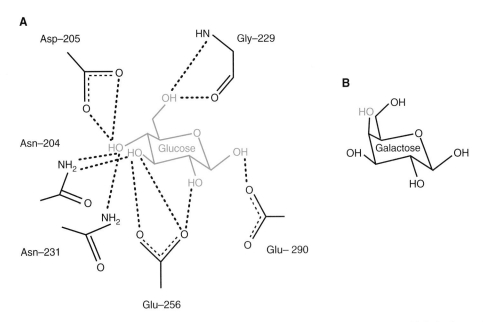

Fig. 8.5. Glucose binding site in glucokinase. A. Glucose, shown in blue, is held in its binding site by multiple hydrogen bonds between each hydroxyl group and polar amino acids from different regions of the enzyme amino acid sequence in the actin fold (see Chapter 7). The position of the amino acid residue in the linear sequence is given by its number. The multiple interactions enable glucose to induce large conformational changes in the enzyme. (Modified from Pilkis SJ, Weber IT, Harisson RW, Bell GI. J Biol Chem. Glucokinase : structaral analysis of a protein involved in susceptibility to diabetes 1994;21925–21928.) B. Enzyme specificity is illustrated by the comparison of galactose and glucose. Galactose differs from glucose only in the position of the -OH group shown in blue. However, it is not phosphorylated at a significant rate by the enzyme. Cells therefore require a separate galactokinase for the metabolism of galactose.

ing recognizes that the substrate binding site is not a rigid "lock" but rather a dynamic surface created by the flexible overall three-dimensional structure of the enzyme.

The function of the conformational change induced by substrate binding, the induced fit, is usually to reposition functional groups in the active site in a way that promotes the reaction, improves the binding site of a cosubstrate, or activates an adjacent subunit through cooperativity. For example, consider the large conformational changes that occur in the actin fold of glucokinase when glucose binds. The induced fit involves changes in the conformation of the whole enzyme that close the cleft of the fold, thereby improving the binding site for ATP, and excluding water (which might interfere with the reaction) from the active site (Fig. 8.6). Thus, the multiple interactions between the substrate and the enzyme in the catalytic site serve both for substrate recognition and for initiating the next stage of the reaction, formation of the transition state complex.

C. The Transition State Complex

For a reaction to occur, the substrates undergoing the reaction need to be activated. If the energy levels of a substrate are plotted as the substrate is progressively converted to product, the curve will show a maximum energy level that is higher than that of either the substrate or the product (Fig. 8.7). This high energy level occurs at the

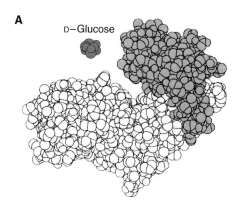

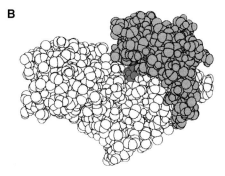

Fig. 8.6. Conformational change resulting from the binding of glucose to hexokinase. (The figure is actually yeast hexokinase, which is more similar to human glucokinase than it is to the other human hexokinase isozymes). The shaded and unshaded areas show the two domains (four subdomains) that form the actin fold with its ATP-binding cleft. **A.** Free enzyme. **B.** With glucose bound, the cleft closes, forming the ATP binding site. The closure of the cleft when glucose binds to hexokinase (or human glucokinase) is one of the largest "induced fits" known. The combination of secondary structures in the actin fold that give hexokinase the flexibility required for this shift are discussed in Chapter 7, section IV.B.1., "The Actin Fold." (From Bennett WS, Steitz TA. J Mol Biol. Structure of a complex between yeast hexokinase A and glucose II. Detailed comparisons of conformation and active site configuration with the native hexokinase B. 1980;211–230.)

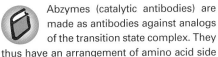

Fig. 8.7. Energy diagram showing the energy levels of the substrates as they progress toward products in the absence of enzyme. The substrates must pass through the high-energy transition state during the reaction. Although a favorable loss of energy occurs during the reaction, the rate of the reaction is slowed by the energy barrier to forming the transition state. The energy barrier is referred to as the activation energy.

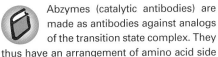

Because the transition state complex binds more tightly to the enzyme than does the substrate, compounds that resemble its electronic and three-dimensional surface (transition state analogs) are more potent inhibitors of an enzyme than are substrate analogs. Consequently, a drug developed as a transition state analog would be highly specific for the enzyme it is designed to inhibit. However, transition state analogs are highly unstable when not bound to the enzyme, and would have great difficulty making it from the digestive tract or injection site to the site of action. Some of the approaches in drug design that are being used to deal with the instability problem include: designing drugs that are almost transition state analogs but have a stable modification; designing a pro-drug that is converted to a transition state analog at the site of action; using the transition state analog to design a complementary antibody.

Abzymes (catalytic antibodies) are made as antibodies against analogs of the transition state complex. They thus have an arrangement of amino acid side chains in their variable regions that is similar to the active site of the enzyme in the transition state. Consequently, they can act as artificial enzymes. For example, abzymes have been developed against analogs of the transition state complex of cocaine esterase, the enzyme that degrades cocaine in the body. These abzymes have esterase activity, and monthly injections of the abzyme drug can be used to rapidly destroy cocaine in the blood, thereby decreasing the dependence of addicted individuals. (See Chapter 7 for antibody structure.)

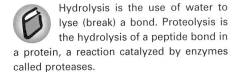

Hydrolysis is the use of water to lyse (break) a bond. Proteolysis is the hydrolysis of a peptide bond in a protein, a reaction catalyzed by enzymes called proteases.

transition state. For some enzyme-catalyzed reactions, the transition state is a condition in which bonds in the substrate are maximally strained. For other enzyme-catalyzed reactions, the electronic configuration of the substrate becomes very strained and unstable as it enters the transition state. The highest energy level corresponds to the most unstable substrate configuration, and the condition in which the changing substrate molecule is most tightly bound to participating functional groups in the enzyme. The difference in energy between the substrate and the transition state complex is called the activation energy.

According to transition state theory, the overall rate of the reaction is determined by the number of molecules acquiring the activation energy necessary to form the transition state complex. Enzymes increase the rate of the reaction by decreasing this activation energy. They use various catalytic strategies, such as electronic stabilization of the transition state complex or acid-base catalysis, to obtain this decrease.

Once the transition state complex is formed, it can collapse back to substrates or decompose to form products. The enzyme does not change the initial energy level of the substrates or the final energy level of the products.

II. CATALYTIC MECHANISM OF CHYMOTRYPSIN

The enzyme chymotrypsin provides a good example of the strategies and amino acid side chains used by enzymes to lower the amount of activation energy required. Chymotrypsin is a digestive enzyme released into the intestine that catalyzes the hydrolysis of specific peptide bonds in denatured proteins. It is a member of the serine protease superfamily, enzymes that use a serine in the active site to form a covalent intermediate during proteolysis. In the overall hydrolysis reaction, an OH^- from water is added to the carbonyl carbon of the peptide bond, and an H^+ to the N, thereby cleaving the bond (Fig. 8.8). The bond that is cleaved is called the scissile bond.

A. The Reaction in the Absence of Enzyme

In the reaction carried out in the absence of enzyme, the negatively charged hydroxyl group of water attacks the carbonyl carbon, which carries a partial positive charge. An unstable oxyanion tetrahedral transition state complex is formed in which the oxygen atom carries a full negative charge. The rate of the chemical reaction in the absence of chymotrypsin is slow because there are too few OH^-

molecules in H_2O with enough energy to form the transition state complex and too few OH^- molecules colliding with the substrate at the right orientation.

B. Catalytic Strategies in the Reaction Catalyzed by Chymotrypsin

In the reaction catalyzed by chymotrypsin, the same oxyanion intermediate is formed by using the hydoxyl group of a serine residue for the attack instead of a free hydroxyl anion. The rate of the chymotrypsin-catalyzed reaction is faster because functional groups in the enzyme active site activate the attacking hydroxyl group, stabilize the oxyanion transition state complexes, form a covalent intermediate, and destabilize the leaving group. The reaction takes place in two stages: (a) cleavage of the peptide bond in the denatured substrate protein and formation of a covalent acyl-enzyme intermediate (Fig. 8.9, steps 1–5), and (b) hydrolysis of the acyl-enzyme intermediate to release the remaining portion of the substrate protein (Fig. 8.9, steps 6–9). The names of the catalytic strategies employed in the various steps are in italics in the following paragraphs.

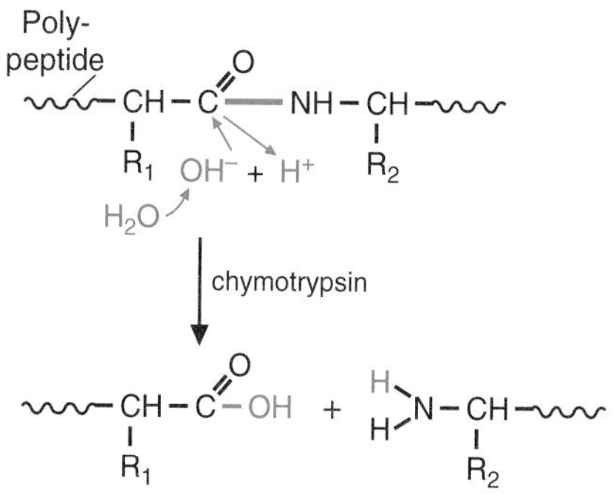

1. SPECIFICITY OF BINDING TO CHYMOTRYPSIN

Chymotrypsin hydrolyzes the peptide bond on the carbonyl side of a phenylalanine, tyrosine, or tryptophan in a denatured protein. The substrate recognition site consists of a hydrophobic binding pocket that holds the hydrophobic amino acid contributing the carbonyl group of the scissile bond (see Fig. 8.9, Step 1). The substrate protein must be denatured to fit into the pocket and be held rigidly in place by glycines in the enzyme peptide backbone. Scissile bond specificity is also provided by the subsequent steps of the reaction, such as moving serine 195 into attacking position (*proximity and orientation*).

2. FORMATION OF THE ACYL-ENZYME INTERMEDIATE IN CHYMOTRYPSIN

In the first stage of the reaction, the peptide bond of the denatured protein substrate is cleaved as an active site serine hydroxyl group attacks the carbonyl carbon of the scissile bond (*nucleophilic catalysis-a nucleophile is a chemical group that is attracted to the positively charged nucleus*) (Fig. 8.9, Step 2). Aspartate and histidine cooperate in converting this hydroxyl group (with a partial negative charge on the oxygen) into a better nucleophilic attacking group by giving it a more negative charge. An active site histidine acts as a base and abstracts a proton from the serine hydroxyl (*acid-base catalysis*). The protonated histidine is stabilized by the negative charge of a nearby aspartate.

The aspartate-histidine-serine combination, referred to as the catalytic triad, is an example of cooperative interactions between amino acid residues in the active site. The strong nucleophilic attacking group created by this charge-relay system has the same general effect on reaction rate as increasing the concentration of hydroxyl ions available for collision in the uncatalyzed reaction.

In the next step of the reaction sequence, an oxyanion tetrahedral transition state complex is formed that is stabilized by hydrogen bonds with –NH groups in the peptide backbone (Fig. 8.9, Step 3). The original view of the way enzymes form transition state complexes was that they stretched the bonds or distorted the bond angles of the reacting substrates. However, most transition state complexes, such as the oxyanion tetrahedral complex, are better described as showing "electronic strain," an electrostatic surface that would be highly improbable if it were not stabilized by bonds with functional groups on the enzyme. *Stabilization of the transition state complex* lowers its energy level and increases the number of molecules that reach this energy level.

Fig. 8.8. Chymotrypsin hydrolyzes certain peptide bonds in proteins. The scissile bond is shown in blue. The carbonyl carbon, which carries a partial positive charge, is attacked by a hydroxyl group from water. An unstable tetrahedral oxyanion intermediate is formed, which is the transition state complex. As the electrons return to the carbonyl carbon, it becomes a carboxylic acid, and the remaining proton from water adds to the leaving group to form an amine.

Q: In the stomach, gastric acid decreases the pH to 1 to 2 to denature proteins through disruption of hydrogen bonding. The protease in the stomach, pepsin, is a member of the aspartate protease superfamily, enzymes that use two aspartate residues in the active site for acid-base catalysis of the peptide bond. Why can they not use histidine like chymotrypsin?

Serine proteases in blood coagulation. The use of an active site serine to cleave a peptide bond is common in the proteolytic enzymes of blood coagulation as well as those of digestion. Blood clots are formed from fibrin, a protein present in the blood as the inactive precursor, fibrinogen. The serine protease thrombin cleaves a peptide bond in fibrinogen to form active fibrin. Thrombin has the same aspartate-histidine-serine catalytic triad found in chymotrypsin and works in essentially the same way. Thrombin is also present as an inactive precursor, prothrombin, which is itself activated through proteolytic cleavage by another blood coagulation serine protease.

1. Substrate binding

2. Histidine activates serine for nucleophilic attack

3. The oxyanion tetrahedral intermediate is stabilized by hydrogen bonds

4. Cleavage of the peptide bond

5. The covalent acyl–enzyme intermediate

6. Water attacks the carbonyl carbon

7. Second oxyanion tetrahedral intermediate

8. Acid catalysis breaks the acyl–enzyme covalent bond

9. The product is free to dissociate

Subsequently, the serine in the active site forms a full covalent bond with the carbon of the carbonyl group as the peptide bond is cleaved (*covalent catalysis*). The formation of a stable covalent intermediate is a catalytic strategy employed by many enzymes and often involves serine or cysteine residues. The covalent intermediate is subsequently hydrolyzed (*acid-base catalysis*). The dissociating products of an enzyme-catalyzed reaction are often "destabilized" by some degree of charge repulsion in the active site. In the case of chymotrypsin, the amino group formed after peptide bond cleavage is destabilized or "uncomfortable" in the presence of the active site histidine (*destabilization of developing product*).

3. HYDROLYSIS OF THE ACYL-CHYMOTRYPSIN INTERMEDIATE

The next sequence of events hydrolyzes the acyl-enzyme intermediate to release the bound carbonyl-side peptide (Fig. 8.9, Steps 6-9). The active site histidine activates water to form an OH^- for a nucleophilic attack, resulting in a second oxyanion transition state complex. When the histidine adds the proton back to serine, the reaction is complete, and the product dissociates.

C. Energy Diagram in the Presence of Chymotrypsin

The number of steps in real enzymatic reactions results in a multi-bump energy diagram (Fig. 8.10). At the initial stage of the reaction, a dip occurs because energy is provided by formation of the initial multiple weak bonds between the substrate and enzyme. As the reaction progresses, the curve rises because additional energy is required for formation of the transition state complex. This energy is provided by the subsequent steps in the reaction replacing the initial weak bonds with progressively tighter bonds. Semi-stable covalent intermediates of the reaction have lower energy levels than do the transition state complexes, and are present in the reaction diagram as dips in the energy curve. The final transition state complex has the highest energy level in the reaction and is therefore the most unstable state. It can collapse back to substrates or decompose to form products.

III. FUNCTIONAL GROUPS IN CATALYSIS

The catalytic strategies employed by chymotrypsin to increase the reaction rate are common to many enzymes. One of these catalytic strategies, proximity and orientation, is an intrinsic feature of substrate binding and part of the catalytic mechanism of all enzymes. All enzymes also stabilize the transition state by electrostatic interactions, but not all enzymes form covalent intermediates.

Great variety occurs in the functional groups employed by different enzymes to carry out these catalytic strategies. Some enzymes, such as chymotrypsin, rely on

 To participate in general acid-base catalysis, the amino acid side chain must be able to abstract a proton at one stage of the reaction, and donate it back at another. Histidine (pK$_a$ 6.3) would be protonated at this low pH, and could not abstract a proton from a potential nucleophile. However, aspartic acid, with a (pK$_a$ of about 2) can release protons at a pH of 2. The two aspartates work together to activate water through the removal of a proton to form the hydroxyl nucleophile.

Fig. 8.9. Catalytic mechanism of chymotrypsin. The substrate (a denatured protein) is in the shaded area. **1.** As the substrate protein binds to the active site, serine-195 and a histidine (his57) are moved closer together and at the right orientation for the nitrogen electrons on histidine to attract the hydrogen of serine. Without this change of conformation on substrate binding, the catalytic triad cannot form. **2.** Histidine serves as a general base catalyst as it abstracts a proton from the serine, increasing the nucleophilicity of the serine-oxygen, which attacks the carbonyl carbon. **3.** The electrons of the carbonyl group form the oxyanion tetrahedral intermediate. The oxyanion is stabilized by the N-H groups of serine-195 and glycine in the chymotrypsin peptide backbone. **4.** The amide nitrogen in the peptide bond is stabilized by interaction with the histidine proton. Here the histidine acts as a general acid catalyst. As the electrons of the carbon-nitrogen peptide bond withdraw into the nitrogen, the electrons of the carboxyanion return to the substrate carbonyl carbon, resulting in cleavage of the peptide bond. **5.** The cleavage of the peptide bond results in formation of the covalent acyl-enzyme intermediate, and the amide half of the cleaved protein dissociates. **6.** The nucleophilic attack by H$_2$O on the carbonyl carbon is activated by histidine, whose nitrogen electrons attract a proton from water. **7.** The second tetrahedral oxyanion intermediate (the transition state complex) is formed. It is again stabilized by hydrogen bonds with the peptide backbone bonds of glycine and serine. **8.** As the histidine proton is donated to the electrons of the bond between the serine oxygen and the substrate carbonyl group, the electrons from the oxyanion return to the substrate carbon to form the carboxylic acid, and the acyl-enzyme bond is broken. **9.** The enzyme, as it releases substrate, returns to its original state.

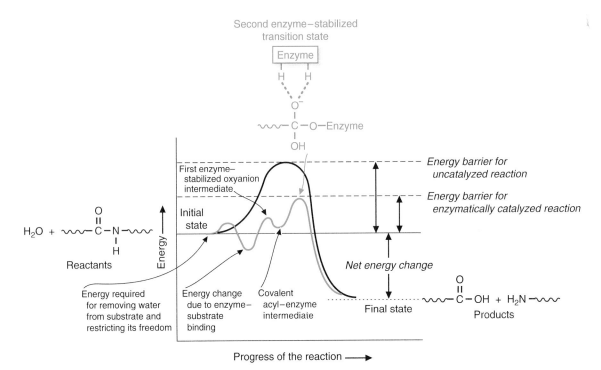

Fig. 8.10. A postulated energy diagram for the reaction catalyzed by chymotrypsin. In the presence of enzyme (blue); in the absence of enzyme (black). The energy barrier to the transition state is lowered in the enzyme-catalyzed reaction by the formation of additional bonds between the substrate and enzyme in the transition state complex. The energy is provided by substrate binding to the enzyme. The enzyme does not, however, change the energy levels of the substrate or product.

Because most vitamins function as coenzymes, the symptoms of vitamin deficiencies reflect the loss of specific enzyme activities dependent on the coenzyme form of the vitamin. Thus, drugs and toxins that inhibit proteins required for coenzyme synthesis (e.g., vitamin transport proteins or biosynthetic enzymes) can cause the symptoms of a vitamin deficiency. This type of deficiency is called a functional deficiency, whereas an inadequate intake is called a dietary deficiency.

Most coenzymes are tightly bound to their enzymes and do not dissociate during the course of the reaction. However, a functional or dietary vitamin deficiency that decreases the level of a coenzyme will result in the presence of the apoenzyme in cells (an enzyme devoid of cofactor).

Ethanol is an "antivitamin" that decreases the cellular content of almost every coenzyme. For example, ethanol inhibits the absorption of thiamine, and acetaldehyde produced from ethanol oxidation displaces pyridoxal phosphate from its protein binding sites, thereby accelerating its degradation.

amino acid residues within the active site. Other enzymes increase their repertoire by employing cofactors to provide a functional group with the right size, shape, and properties. Cofactors are nonprotein compounds that participate in the catalytic process. They are generally divided into three categories: coenzymes, metal ions (e.g., Fe^{2+}, Mg^{2+}, or Zn^{2+}), and metallocoenzymes (similar to the Fe^{2+}-heme in hemoglobin, see Chapter 7).

A. Functional Groups on Amino Acid Side Chains

Almost all of the polar amino acids participate directly in catalysis in one or more enzymes (Table 8.1). Serine, cysteine, lysine, and histidine can participate in covalent

Table 8.1. Some Functional Groups in the Active Site

Function of Amino Acid	Enzyme Example
Covalent intermediates	
Cysteine–SH	Glyceraldehyde 3–phosphate dehydrogenase
Serine–OH	Acetylcholinesterase
Lysine–NH₂	Aldolase
Histidine–NH	Phosphoglucomutase
Acid–base catalysis	
Histidine–NH	Chymotrypsin
Aspartate–COOH	Pepsin
Stabilization of anion formed during the reaction	
Peptide backbone–NH	Chymotrypsin
Arginine–NH	Carboxypeptidase A
Serine–OH	Alcohol dehydrogenase
Stabilization of cation formed during the reaction	
Aspartate–COO⁻	Lysozyme

catalysis. Histidine, because it has a pK_a that can donate and accept a proton at neutral pH, often participates in acid-base catalysis. Most of the polar amino acid side chains are nucleophilic and participate in nucleophilic catalysis by stabilizing more positively charged groups that develop during the reaction.

B. Coenzymes in Catalysis

Coenzymes are complex nonprotein organic molecules that participate in catalysis by providing functional groups, much like the amino acid side chains. In the human, they are usually (but not always) synthesized from vitamins. Each coenzyme is involved in catalyzing a specific type of reaction for a class of substrates with certain structural features. Coenzymes can be divided into two general classes: activation-transfer coenzymes and oxidation-reduction coenzymes.

1. ACTIVATION-TRANSFER COENZYMES

The activation-transfer coenzymes usually participate directly in catalysis by forming a covalent bond with a portion of the substrate; the tightly held substrate moiety is then activated for transfer, addition of water, or some other reaction. The portion of the coenzyme that forms a covalent bond with the substrate is its functional group. A separate portion of the coenzyme binds tightly to the enzyme.

Thiamine pyrophosphate provides a good illustration of the manner in which coenzymes participate in catalysis (Fig. 8.11). It is synthesized in human cells from the vitamin thiamine by the addition of a pyrophosphate. This pyrophosphate provides negatively charged oxygen atoms that chelate Mg^{2+}, which then binds tightly to the enzyme. The functional group that extends into the active site is the reactive carbon atom with a dissociable proton (see Fig. 8.11). In all of the enzymes that use thiamine pyrophosphate, this reactive thiamine carbon forms a covalent bond with a substrate keto group while cleaving the adjacent carbon–carbon bond. However, each thiamine-containing enzyme catalyzes the cleavage of a different substrate (or group of substrates with very closely related structures).

Coenzymes have very little activity in the absence of the enzyme and very little specificity. The enzyme provides specificity, proximity, and orientation in the substrate recognition site, as well as other functional groups for stabilization of the transition state, acid-base catalysis, etc. For example, thiamine is made into a better nucleophilic attacking group by a basic amino acid residue in the enzyme that removes the dissociable proton (EnzB: in Fig. 8.11), thereby generating a negatively charged thiamine carbon anion. Later in the reaction, the enzyme returns the proton.

Coenzyme A (CoA), biotin, and pyridoxal phosphate are also activation-transfer coenzymes synthesized from vitamins. CoA (CoASH), which is synthesized from the vitamin pantothenate, contains an adenosine 3′, 5′-bisphosphate which binds reversibly, but tightly, to a site on an enzyme (Fig. 8.12A). Its functional group, a sulfhydryl group at the other end of the molecule, is a nucleophile that always

 Nucleophiles carry full or partial negative charges (like the oxygen atom in the serine -OH) or have a nitrogen that can act as an electron-donating group by virtue of its two unpaired electrons. Covalent catalysis and acid-base catalysis are carried out by nucleophilic groups. Electrophiles carry full or partial positive charges (e.g., the peptide backbone-NH was used as an electrophilic group in chymotrypsin). In general, nucleophilic and electrophilic catalysis occur when the respective nucleophilic or electrophilic groups on the enzyme stabilize substrate groups of the opposite polarity that develop during the reaction.

 Although coenzymes look as though they should be able to catalyze reactions autonomously (on their own), they have almost no catalytic power when not bound to the enzyme. Why?

 Many alcoholics such as **Al Martini** develop thiamine deficiency because alcohol inhibits the transport of thiamine through the intestinal mucosal cells. In the body, thiamine is converted to thiamine pyrophosphate (TPP). TPP acts as a coenzyme in the decarboxylation of α-keto acids such as pyruvate and α-ketoglutarate (see Fig. 8.11) and in the utilization of pentose phosphates in the pentose phosphate pathway. As a result of thiamine deficiency, the oxidation of α-keto acids is impaired. Dysfunction occurs in the central and peripheral nervous system, the cardiovascular system, and other organs.

Most coenzymes, such as functional groups on the enzyme amino acids, are regenerated during the course of the reaction. However, CoASH and a few of the oxidation-reduction coenzymes are transformed during the reaction into products that dissociate from the enzyme at the end of the reaction (e.g., CoASH is converted to an acyl CoA derivative, and NAD^+ is reduced to NADH). These dissociating coenzymes are nonetheless classified as coenzymes rather than substrates because they are common to so many reactions, the original form is regenerated by subsequent reactions in a metabolic pathway, they are synthesized from vitamins, and the amount of coenzyme in the cell is nearly constant.

For a substrate to react with a coenzyme, it must collide with a coenzyme at exactly the right angle. The probability of the substrate and coenzyme in free solution colliding in exactly the right place at the exactly right angle is very small. In addition to providing this proximity and orientation, enzymes contribute in other ways, such as activating the coenzyme by abstracting a proton (e.g., thiamine-pyrophosphate and coenzyme A) or polarizing the substrate to make it more susceptible to nucleophilic attack.

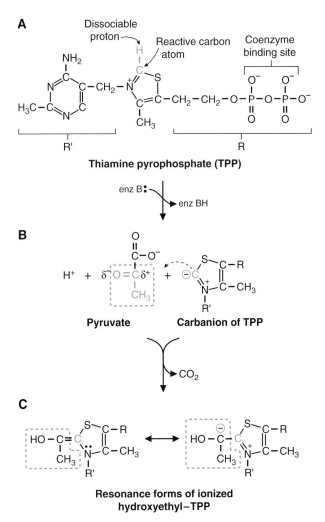

Fig. 8.11. The role of the functional group of thiamine pyrophosphate (the reactive carbon shown in blue) in formation of a covalent intermediate. A. A base on the enzyme (B) abstracts a proton from thiamine, creating a carbanion (general acid-base catalysis). B. The carbanion is a strong nucleophile and attacks the partially positively charged keto group on the substrate. C. A covalent intermediate is formed, which is stabilized by resonance forms. The uncharged intermediate is the stabilized transition state complex.

attacks carbonyl groups and forms acyl thioesters (in fact, the "A" in Co**A** stands for the **a**cyl group that becomes attached).

Biotin, which does not contain a phosphate group, is covalently bound to a lysine in enzymes called carboxylases (see Fig. 8.12B). Its functional group is a nitrogen atom that covalently binds a CO_2 group in an energy-requiring reaction. This bound CO_2 group is activated for addition to another molecule. In the human, biotin functions only in carboxylation reactions.

Pyridoxal phosphate is synthesized from the vitamin pyridoxine, which is also called vitamin B_6 (Fig. 8.13). The reactive aldehyde group usually functions in enzyme-catalyzed reactions by forming a covalent bond with the amino groups on amino acids. The positively charged ring nitrogen withdraws electrons from a bond in the bound amino acid, resulting in cleavage of that bond. The enzyme participates by removing protons from the substrate and by keeping the amino acid and the pyridoxal group in a single plane to facilitate shuttling of electrons.

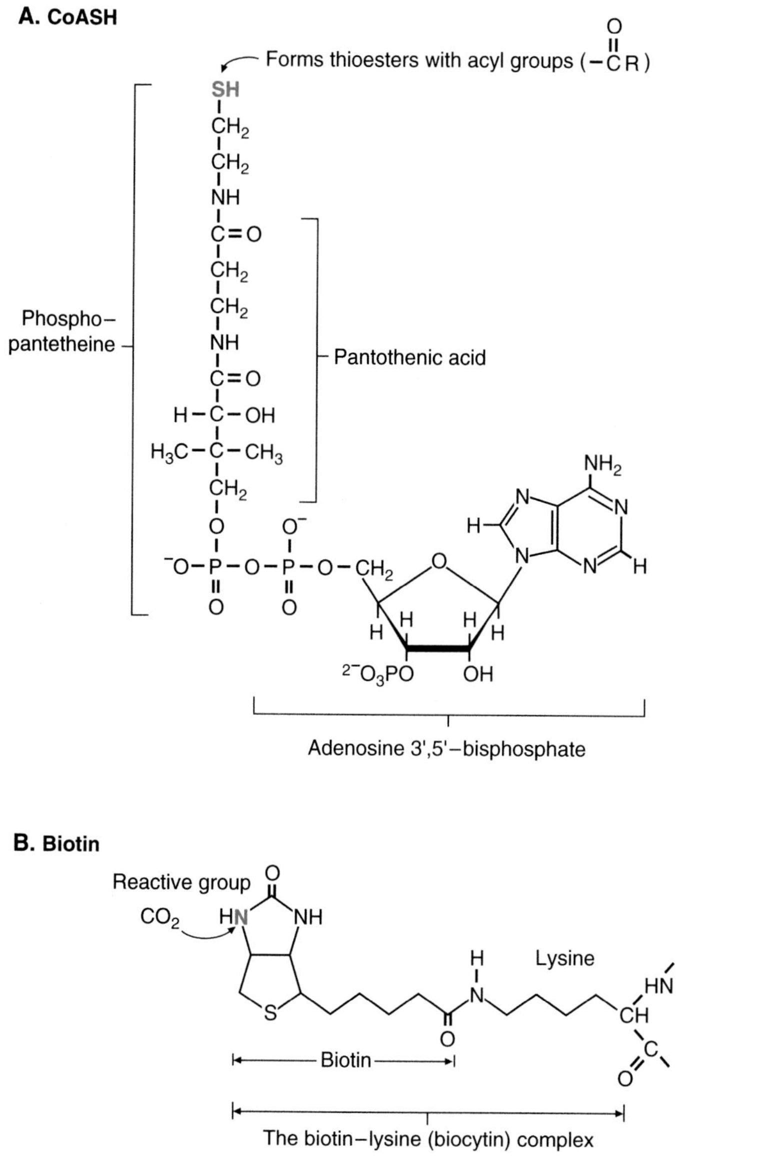

A. CoASH

B. Biotin

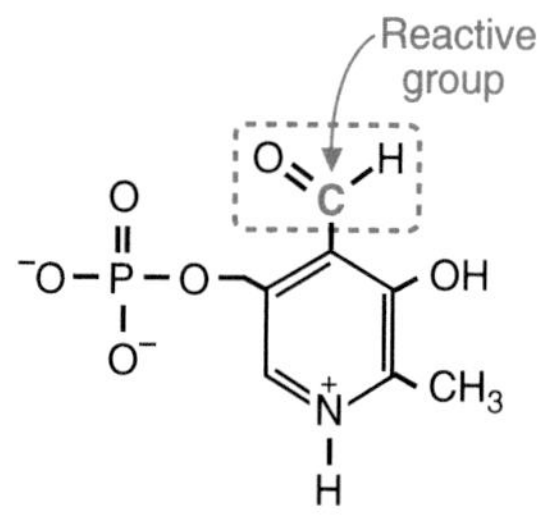

Pyridoxal phosphate (PLP)

Fig. 8.13 Reactive sites of pyridoxal phosphate. The functional group of pyridoxal phosphate is a reactive aldehyde (shown in blue) that forms a covalent intermediate with amino groups of amino acids (a Schiff base). The positively charged pyridine ring is a strong electron-withdrawing group that can pull electrons into it (electrophilic catalysis).

Fig. 8.12. CoA and biotin, activation-transfer coenzymes. A. Coenzyme A (CoA or CoASH) and phosphopantetheine are synthesized from the vitamin pantothenate (pantothenic acid). The active sulfhydryl group, shown in blue, binds to acyl groups (e.g., acetyl, succinyl, or fatty acyl) to form thioesters. B. Biotin activates and transfers CO_2 to compounds in carboxylation reactions. The reactive N is shown in blue. Biotin is covalently attached to a lysine residue in the carboxylase enzyme.

These coenzymes illustrate three features all activation-transfer coenzymes have in common: (1) a specific chemical group involved in binding to the enzyme, (2) a separate and different functional or reactive group that participates directly in the catalysis of one type of reaction by forming a covalent bond with the substrate, and (3) dependence on the enzyme for additional specificity of substrate and additional catalytic power.

2. OXIDATION-REDUCTION CCOENZYMES

A large number of coenzymes are involved in oxidation-reduction reactions catalyzed by enzymes categorized as oxidoreductases. Some coenzymes, such as

In general, coenzymes are nonprotein organic cofactors that participate in reactions. They may be covalently bound to enzymes (like biotin), dissociate during deficiency (thiaminepyrophosphate), or freely dissociate at the end of the reaction (CoASH). Cofactors that are covalently or very tightly bound to nonenzyme proteins are usually called prosthetic groups. A prosthetic group, such as the heme in hemoglobin, usually does not dissociate from a protein until the protein is degraded.

When a compound is oxidized, it loses electrons. As a result, the oxidized carbon has fewer H atoms or gains an O atom. The reduction of a compound is the gain of electrons, which shows in its structure as the gain of H, or loss of O. In the oxidation of lactate to pyruvate (see Fig. 8.14), lactate loses two electrons as a hydride ion, and a proton (H^+) is released; NAD^+, which accepts the hydride ion, is reduced to NADH. The carbon atom with the keto group is now at a higher oxidation state because both of the electrons in bonds between carbon and oxygen are counted as belonging to oxygen, whereas the two electrons in the C-H bond are shared equally between carbon and hydrogen.

The catalysis of oxidation-reduction reactions is carried out by a class of enzymes called oxidoreductases. A subclass of oxidoreductases is given the common name dehydrogenases (such as lactate dehydrogenase), because they transfer hydrogen (hydrogen atoms or hydride atoms) from the substrate to an electron-accepting coenzyme, such as NAD^+.

nicotinamide adenine dinucleotide (NAD^+) and flavin adenine dinucleotide (FAD), can transfer electrons together with hydrogen and have unique roles in the generation of ATP from the oxidation of fuels. Other oxidation-reduction coenzymes work with metals to transfer single electrons to oxygen. Vitamin E and vitamin C (ascorbic acid) are oxidation-reduction coenzymes that can act as antioxidants and protect against oxygen free radical injury. The different functions of oxidation-reduction coenzymes in metabolic pathways are explained in Chapters 19 through 22.

Oxidation-reduction coenzymes follow the same principles as activation-transfer coenzymes, except that they do not form covalent bonds with the substrate. Each coenzyme has a unique functional group that accepts and donates electrons and is specific for the form of electrons it transfers (e.g., hydride ions, hydrogen atoms, oxygen). A different portion of the coenzyme binds the enzyme. Like activation-transfer coenzymes, oxidation-reduction coenzymes are not good catalysts without participation from amino acid side chains on the enzyme.

The enzyme lactate dehydrogenase, which catalyzes the transfer of electrons from lactate to NAD^+, illustrates these principles (Fig. 8.14). The coenzyme nicotinamide adenine dinucleotide (NAD^+) is synthesized from the vitamin niacin (which forms the nicotinamide ring), and from ATP (which contributes an AMP). The ADP portion of the molecule binds tightly to the enzyme and causes conformational

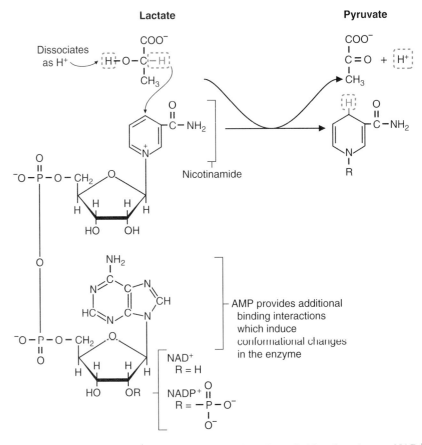

Fig. 8.14 The coenzyme NAD^+ accepting a hydride ion, shown in blue, from lactate. NAD^+-dependent dehydrogenases catalyze the transfer of a hydride ion (H:) from a carbon to NAD^+ in oxidation reactions such as the oxidation of alcohols to ketones or aldehydes to acids. The positively charged pyridine ring nitrogen of NAD^+ increases the electrophilicity of the carbon opposite it in the ring. This carbon then accepts the negatively charged hydride ion. The proton from the alcohol group is released into water. NADP functions by the same mechanism, but it is usually involved in pathways of reductive synthesis.

changes in the enzyme. The functional group of NAD^+ is the carbon on the nicotinamide ring opposite the positively charged nitrogen. This carbon atom accepts the hydride ion (a hydrogen atom that has two electrons) transferred from a specific carbon atom on the substrate. The H^+ from the substrate alcohol (OH) group then dissociates, and a keto group (C = O) is formed. One of the roles of the enzyme is to contribute a histidine nitrogen that can bind the dissociable proton on lactate, thereby making it easier for NAD^+ to pull off the other hydrogen with both electrons. Finally, NADH dissociates.

C. Metal Ions in Catalysis

Metal ions, which have a positive charge, contribute to the catalytic process by acting as electrophiles (electron-attracting groups). They assist in binding of the substrate, or they stabilize developing anions in the reaction. They can also accept and donate electrons in oxidation-reduction reactions.

The ability of certain metals to bind multiple ligands in their coordination sphere enables them to participate in binding substrates or coenzymes to enzymes. For example, Mg^{2+} plays a role in the binding of the negatively charged phosphate groups of thiamine pyrophosphate to anionic or basic amino acids in the enzyme (see Fig. 8.11). The phosphate groups of ATP are usually bound to enzymes through Mg^{2+} chelation.

The metals of some enzymes bind anionic substrates or intermediates of the reaction to alter their charge distribution, thereby contributing to catalytic power. The enzyme alcohol dehydrogenase, which transfers electrons from ethanol to NAD^+ to generate acetaldehyde and NADH, illustrates this role (Fig. 8.15). In the active site of alcohol dehydrogenase, an activated serine pulls a proton off the ethanol –OH group, leaving a negative charge on the oxygen that is stabilized by zinc. This electronic configuration allows the transfer of a hydride ion to NAD^+. Zinc is essentially fulfilling the same function in alcohol dehydrogenase that histidine fulfills in lactate dehydrogenase.

D. Noncatalytic Roles of Cofactors

Cofactors sometimes play a noncatalytic structural role in certain enzymes, binding different regions of the enzyme together to form the tertiary structure. They also can serve as substrates that are cleaved during the reaction.

IV. OPTIMAL pH AND TEMPERATURE

If the activity of most enzymes is plotted as a function of the pH of the reaction, an increase of reaction rate is usually observed as the pH goes from a very acidic level to the physiologic range; a decrease of reaction rate occurs as the pH goes from the physiologic range to a very basic range (Fig. 8.16). The shape of this curve in the acid region usually reflects the ionization of specific functional groups in the active site (or in the substrate) by the increase of pH, and the more general formation of hydrogen bonds important for the overall conformation of the enzyme. The loss of activity on the basic side usually reflects the inappropriate ionization of amino acid residues in the enzyme.

In humans, most of ingested ethanol is oxidized to acetaldehyde in the liver by alcohol dehydrogenase (ADH):

Ethanol + NAD$^+$ ↔ Acetaldehyde + NADH + H$^+$

ADH is active as a dimer, with an active site containing zinc present in each subunit. The human has at least seven genes that encode isozymes of ADH, each with a slightly different range of specificities for the alcohols it oxidizes.

The acetaldehyde produced from ethanol is highly reactive, toxic, and immunogenic. In **Al Martini** and other patients with chronic alcoholism, acetaldehyde is responsible for much of the liver injury associated with chronic alcoholism

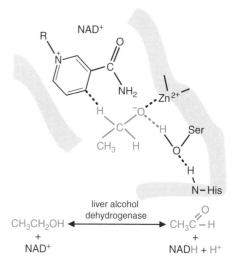

Fig. 8.15. Liver alcohol dehydrogenase catalyzes the oxidation of ethanol (shown in blue) to acetaldehyde. The active site of liver alcohol dehydrogenase contains a bound zinc atom, and a serine side chain –OH and a histidine nitrogen that participate in the reaction. The histidine pulls an H^+ off the active site serine, which pulls the H^+ off of the substrate –OH group, leaving the oxygen with a negative charge that is stabilized by zinc.

The parietal cells of the stomach secrete HCl into the lumen of the stomach, resulting in a pH between 1 and 2. This strongly acidic environment is capable of irreversibly denaturing most proteins by protonating amino acids, thereby preventing the hydrogen bond formation necessary for tertiary structure. Many of the peptide bonds in proteins would not be accessible to digestive proteases unless the protein was denatured. Pepsin, a digestive protease present in the stomach, is an exceptional enzyme because its pH optimum is approximately 1.6 and it is active in the acidic environment of the stomach. As denatured dietary proteins pass into the intestinal lumen, the pH of the gastric juice is raised above 6 by secretion of bicarbonate from the exocrine pancreas. At this higher pH, chymotrypsin and other proteases from the pancreas can act on the denatured proteins.

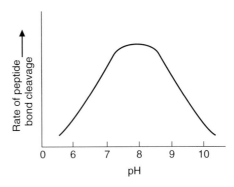

Fig. 8.16. pH profile of an enzyme. The rate of the reaction increases as the pH increases from 6 to 7.4. The exact shape of the curve depends on the protonation state of active site amino acid residues or on the hydrogen bonding required for maintenance of three-dimensional structure in the enzyme. For the enzyme shown in the figure, the increase of reaction rate corresponds to deprotonation of the active site histidine. At a pH above 8.5, deprotonation of an amino-terminal $-NH_3^+$ alters the conformation at the active site and the activity decreases. Other enzymes might have a lower pH maximum, a broader peak, or retain their activity in the basic side of the curve.

Most human enzymes function optimally at a temperature of approximately 37°C. An increase of temperature from 0°C to 37°C increases the rate of the reaction by increasing the vibrational energy of the substrates. The maximum activity for most human enzymes occurs near 37°C because denaturation (loss of secondary and tertiary structure) occurs at higher temperatures.

V. MECHANISM-BASED INHIBITORS

Inhibitors are compounds that decrease the rate of an enzymatic reaction. Mechanism-based inhibitors mimic or participate in an intermediate step of the catalytic reaction. The term includes transition state analogs and compounds that can react irreversibly with functional groups in the active site.

A. Covalent Inhibitors

Covalent inhibitors form covalent or extremely tight bonds with functional groups in the active catalytic site. These functional groups are activated by their interactions with other amino acid residues, and are therefore far more likely to be targeted by drugs and toxins than amino acid residues outside the active site.

The lethal compound diisopropyl phosphofluoridate (DFP, or diisopropylfluorophosphate) is an organophosphorus compound that served as a prototype for the development of the nerve gas Sarin and other organophosphorus toxins, such as the insecticides malathion and parathion (Fig. 8.17). DFP exerts its toxic effect by forming a covalent intermediate in the active site of acetylcholinesterase, thereby preventing the enzyme from degrading the neurotransmitter acetylcholine. Once the covalent bond is formed, the inhibition by DFP is essentially irreversible, and activity can only be recovered as new enzyme is synthesized. DFP also inhibits many other enzymes that use serine for hydrolytic cleavage, but the inhibition is not as lethal.

Aspirin (acetylsalicylic acid) provides an example of a pharmacologic drug that exerts its effect through the covalent acetylation of an active site serine in the enzyme prostaglandin endoperoxide synthase (cycloxygenase). Aspirin resembles a portion of the prostaglandin precursor that is a physiologic substrate for the enzyme.

 The symptoms experienced by **Dennis Veere** resulted from inhibition of acetylcholinesterase. Acetylcholinesterase cleaves the neurotransmitter acetylcholine to acetate and choline in the postsynaptic terminal, thereby terminating the transmission of the neural signal (see Fig. 8.17). Malathion is metabolized in the liver to a toxic derivative (malaoxon) that binds to the active site serine in acetylcholinesterase and other enzymes, an action similar to that of diisopropylfluorophosphate. As a result, acetylcholine accumulates and overstimulates the autonomic nervous system (the involuntary nervous system, including heart, blood vessels, glands), thereby accounting for Dennis's vomiting, abdominal cramps, salivation, and sweating. Acetylcholine is also a neurotransmitter for the somatic motor nervous system, where its accumulation resulted in Dennis's involuntary muscle twitching (muscle fasciculations).

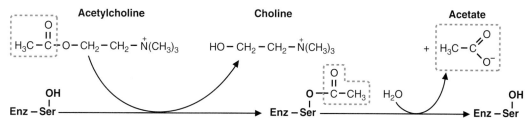

A. Normal reaction of acetylcholinesterase

Fig. 8.17 A. Acetylcholinesterase normally catalyzes inactivation of the neurotransmitter acetylcholine in a hydrolysis reaction. The active site serine forms a covalent intermediate with a portion of the substrate during the course of the reaction. **B.** Diisopropyl phosphofluoridate (DFP), the ancestor of current organophosphorus nerve gases and pesticides, inactivates acetylcholinesterase by forming a covalent complex with the active site serine that cannot be hydrolysed by water. The result is that the enzyme cannot carry out its normal reaction, and acetylcholine accumulates.

B. Transition State Analogs and Compounds that Resemble Intermediate Stages of the Reaction

Transition state analogs are extremely potent and specific inhibitors of enzymes because they bind so much more tightly to the enzyme than do substrates or products. Drugs cannot be designed that precisely mimic the transition state because of its highly unstable structure. However, substrates undergo progressive changes in their overall electrostatic structure during the formation of a transition state complex, and effective drugs often resemble an intermediate stage of the reaction more closely than they resemble the substrate. Medical literature often refers to such compounds as substrate analogs, even though they bind more tightly than substrates.

1. PENICILLIN

The antibiotic penicillin is a transition state analog that binds very tightly to glycopeptidyl transferase, an enzyme required by bacteria for synthesis of the cell wall (Fig. 8.18). Glycopeptidyl transferase catalyzes a partial reaction with penicillin that covalently attaches penicillin to its own active site serine. The reaction is favored by the strong resemblance between the peptide bond in the β-lactam ring of penicillin and the transition state complex of the natural transpeptidation reaction. Active site inhibitors such as penicillin that undergo partial reaction to form irreversible inhibitors in the active site are sometimes termed "suicide inhibitors."

2. ALLOPURINOL

Allopurinol, a drug used to treat gout, decreases urate production by inhibiting xanthine oxidase. This inhibition provides an example of an enzyme that commits suicide by converting a drug to a transition state analog. The normal physiologic

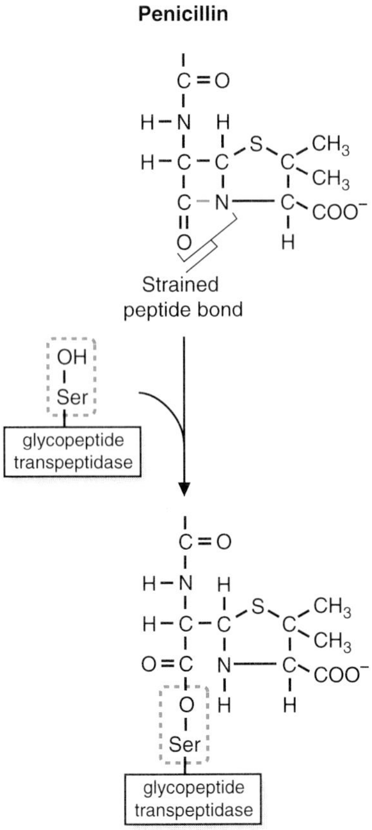

Penicillin

Fig. 8.18 The antibiotic penicillin inhibits the bacterial enzyme glycopeptide transpeptidase. The transpeptidase is a serine protease involved in cross-linking components of bacterial cell walls and is essential for bacterial growth and survival. It normally cleaves the peptide bond between two D-alanine residues in a polypeptide. Penicillin contains a strained peptide bond within the β-lactam ring that resembles the transition state of the normal cleavage reaction, and thus penicillin binds very readily in the enzyme active site. As the bacterial enzyme attempts to cleave this penicillin peptide bond, penicillin becomes irreversibly covalently attached to the enzyme's active site serine, thereby inactivating the enzyme.

Lotta Topaigne is being treated with allopurinol for gout, which is caused by an accumulation of sodium urate crystals in joints and joint fluid, particularly in the ankle and great toe. Allopurinol is a suicide inhibitor of the enzyme xanthine oxidase, which is involved in the degradation of purine nucleotides AMP and GMP to uric acid (urate). Although hypoxanthine levels increase in the presence of allopurinol, hypoxanthine does not participate in urate crystal formation and precipitation at this concentration. It is excreted in the urine.

function of xanthine oxidase is the oxidation of hypoxanthine to xanthine and xanthine to uric acid (urate) in the pathway for degradation of purines (Fig. 8.19). The enzyme contains a molybdenum–sulfide (Mo-S) complex that binds the substrates and transfers the electrons required for the oxidation reactions. Xanthine oxidase oxidizes the drug allopurinol to oxypurinol, a compound that binds very tightly to a molybdenum–sulfide complex in the active site. As a result, the enzyme has committed suicide and is unable to carry out its normal function, the generation of uric acid (urate).

D. Heavy Metals

Heavy metal toxicity is caused by tight binding of a metal such as mercury (Hg), lead (Pb), aluminum (Al), or iron (Fe), to a functional group in an enzyme. Heavy metals are relatively nonspecific for the enzymes they inhibit, particularly if the metal is associated with high dose toxicity. Mercury, for example, binds to so many enzymes, often at reactive sulfhydryl groups in the active site, that it has been difficult to determine which of the inhibited enzymes is responsible for mercury toxicity. Lead provides an example of a metal that inhibits through replacing the normal functional metal in an enzyme. Its developmental and neurologic toxicity may be caused by its

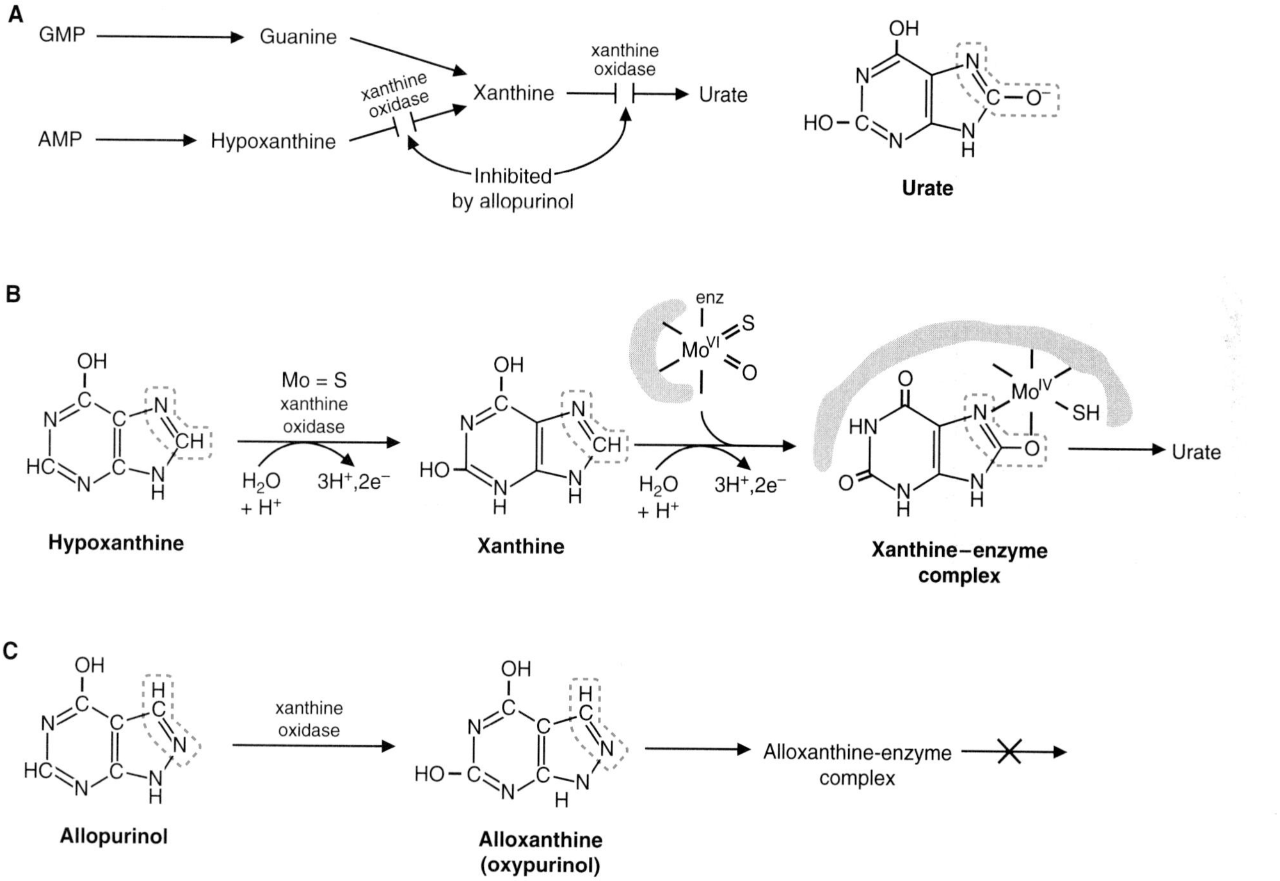

A

B

C

Fig. 8.19. Allopurinol is a suicide inhibitor of xanthine oxidase. A. Xanthine oxidase catalyzes the oxidation of hypoxanthine to xanthine, and xanthine to uric acid (urate) in the pathway for degradation of purine nucleotides. B. The oxidations are performed by a molybdenum-oxo-sulfide coordination complex in the active site that complexes with the group being oxidized. Oxygen is donated from water. The enzyme can work either as an oxidase (O_2 accepts the $2e^-$ and is reduced to H_2O_2) or as a dehydrogenase (NAD^+ accepts the $2e^-$ and is reduced to NADH.) C. Xanthine oxidase is able to perform the first oxidation step and convert allopurinol to alloxanthine (oxypurinol). As a result, the enzyme has committed suicide; the oxypurinol remains bound in the molybdenum coordination sphere, where it prevents the next step of the reaction.

ability to replace Ca^{2+} in two regulatory proteins important in the central nervous system and other tissues, Ca^{2+}-calmodulin and protein kinase C.

CLINICAL COMMENTS

Dennis Veere. Dennis Veere survived his malathion intoxication because he had ingested only a small amount of the chemical, vomited shortly after the agent was ingested, and was rapidly treated in the emergency room. Lethal doses of oral malathion are estimated at 1 g/kg of body weight for humans. Emergency room physicians used a drug (oxime) to reactivate the acetylcholinesterase in Dennis before the aged complex formed. They also used intravenous atropine, an anticholinergic (antimuscarinic) agent, to antagonize the action of the excessive amounts of acetylcholine accumulating in cholinergic receptors throughout his body.

After several days of intravenous therapy, the signs and symptoms of acetylcholine excess abated, and therapy was slowly withdrawn. Dennis made an uneventful recovery.

 Once ingested, the liver converts malathion to the toxic reactive compound, malaoxon, by replacing the sulfur with an oxygen. Malaoxon then binds to the active site of acetylcholinesterase and reacts to form the covalent intermediate. Unlike the complex formed between diisopropylfluorophosphate and acetylcholinesterase, this initial acylenzyme intermediate is reversible. However, with time, the enzyme-inhibitor complex "ages" (dealkylation of the inhibitor and enzyme modification) to form an irreversible complex.

Lotta Topaigne. Within several days of starting allopurinol therapy, Ms. Topaigne's serum uric acid level began to decrease. Several weeks later, the level in her blood was normal. However, while Lotta was adapting to allopurinol therapy, she experienced a mild gout attack, which was treated with a low dose of colchicine (see Chapter 10).

Al Martini. Al Martini was admitted to the hospital after intravenous thiamine was initiated at a dose of 100 mg/day (compared with an RDA of 1.4 mg/day). His congestive heart failure was believed to be the result, in part, of the cardiomyopathy (heart muscle dysfunction) of acute thiamine deficiency known as beriberi heart disease. This nutritional cardiac disorder and the peripheral nerve dysfunction usually respond to thiamine replacement. However, an alcoholic cardiomyopathy can also occur in well-nourished patients with adequate thiamine levels. Exactly how ethanol, or its toxic metabolite acetaldehyde, causes alcoholic cardiomyopathy in the absence of thiamine deficiency is unknown.

BIOCHEMICAL COMMENTS

Basic Reactions and Classes of Enzymes. In the following chapters of the text, students will be introduced to a wide variety of reaction pathways and enzyme names. Although it may seem that the number of reactions is infinite, many of these reactions are similar and occur frequently in different pathways. Recognition of the type of reaction can aid in remembering the pathways and enzyme names, thereby reducing the amount of memorization required. You may wish to use this section for reference as you go through your first biochemical pathways.

The Enzyme Commission has divided the basic reaction types and the enzymes catalyzing them into six broad numbered classes: (1) oxidoreductases, (2) transferases, (3) hydrolases, (4) lyases, (5) isomerases, and (6) ligases. Each broad class of enzymes includes subsets of enzymes with a systematic name and a common name (e.g., dehydrogenases and kinases).

Oxidoreductases. Oxidation-reduction reactions are very common in biochemical pathways and are catalyzed by a broad class of enzymes called oxidoreductases. Whenever an oxidation-reduction reaction occurs, at least one substrate gains electrons and becomes reduced, and another substrate loses electrons and becomes oxidized. One subset of reactions is catalyzed by *dehydrogenases*, which accept and donate electrons in the form of hydride ions ($H:^-$) or hydrogen atoms. Usually an electron-transferring coenzyme, such as $NAD^+/NADH$, acts as an electron donor or acceptor (e.g., see Fig. 8.14 and Fig. 8.15).

In another subset of reactions, O_2 donates either one or both of its oxygen atoms to an acceptor (for example, see xanthine oxidase, Fig. 8.19). When this occurs, O_2 becomes reduced, and an electron donor is oxidized. Enzymes participating in reactions with O_2 are called *hydroxylases* and *oxidases* when one oxygen atom is incorporated into a substrate and the other oxygen atom into water, or both atoms are incorporated into water. They are called *oxygenases* when both atoms of oxygen are incorporated into the acceptor. Most hydroxylases and oxidases require metal ions, such as Fe^{2+}, for electron transfer.

Transferases. Transferases catalyze group transfer reactions—the transfer of a functional group from one molecule to another. If the transferred group is a high-energy phosphate (as shown in Fig. 8.3), the enzyme is a *kinase*; if the transferred group is a carbohydrate residue, the enzyme is a

At low concentrations of ethanol, liver alcohol dehydrogenase is the major route of ethanol oxidation to acetaldehyde, a highly toxic chemical. Acetaldehyde not only damages the liver, it can enter the blood and potentially damage the heart and other tissues. At low ethanol intakes, much of the acetaldehyde produced is safely oxidized to acetate in the liver by acetaldehyde dehydrogenases.

Enzymes have been systematically classified by the Enzyme Commission of the International Union of Biochemists and Molecular Biologists into six major groups according to the type of reaction catalysed. The major groups are further subdivided so that each enzyme has an individual Enzyme Commission number. Most enzymes have systematic names, reflecting their activities. In addition, most enzymes have common or trivial names, which are shorter, reflect the activity of the enzyme in a less standardized way, and may not end in "ase". For example, glucokinase (common name) has the systematic name of ATP:D-hexose 6-phosphotransferase, and its enzyme commission number is EC 2.7.1.2. The "2" is the Enzyme Commission (EC) number of the general class (transferase), followed by a period and "7", the number of the subclass for transfer of phosphorus-containing groups. The "1" denotes transfer to an alcohol acceptor, and the final "2" is the specific number of the enzyme.

Xanthine oxidase uses molybdenum for electron transfer to O_2. This enzyme accounts for the human dietary requirement for molybdenum, which is classified as a trace mineral.

glycosyltransferase; if it is a fatty acyl group, the enzyme is an *acyltransferase.* A common feature of these reactions is that the group being transferred exists as a good leaving group on the donor molecule.

Another subset of group transfer reactions consists of transaminations (Fig. 8.20). In this type of reaction, the nitrogen group from an amino acid is donated to an α-keto acid, forming a new amino acid and the α-keto acid corresponding to the donor amino acid. Enzymes catalyzing this last type of reaction are called *transaminases* or *aminotransferases.* The coenzyme pyridoxal phosphate is required for all transaminases (see Fig. 8.13).

When the physiologically important aspect of the reaction is the compound synthesized, the transferase may be called a *synthase.* For example, the enzyme commonly called glycogen synthase transfers a glucosyl residue from UDP-glucose to the end of a glycogen molecule. Its systematic name is UDP-glucose-glycogen glycosyltransferase.

Hydrolases. In hydrolysis reactions, C-O, C-N, or C-S bonds are cleaved by the addition of H_2O in the form of OH^- and H^+ to the atoms forming the bond (see, for example, Fig. 8.8). The enzyme class names specify the group being cleaved (e.g., the enzyme commonly named chymotrypsin is a protease, a hydrolase that cleaves peptide bonds in proteins).

Lyases. The lyase class of enzymes consists of a diverse group of enzymes cleaving C-C, C-O, and C-N bonds by means other than hydrolysis or oxidation. Some of the enzymes catalyzing C-C bond cleavage are called *aldolases, decarboxylases* (when carbon dioxide is released from a substrate), and *thiolases* (when the sulfur-containing nucleophile of cysteine or CoASH is used to break a carbon-carbon bond) (Fig. 8.21). The structures amenable to carbon–carbon bond cleavage usually require a carbonyl carbon that can act as an electron sink to stabilize the carbanion transiently formed when the carbon–carbon bond breaks.

This broad class of enzymes also includes dehydratases and many synthases. *Dehydratases* remove the elements of water from two adjacent carbon–carbon bonds to form a double bond. Certain enzymes in this group, such as certain group transferases, are commonly called synthases when the physiologically important direction of the reaction favors the formation of a carbon–carbon bond (e.g., citrate synthase).

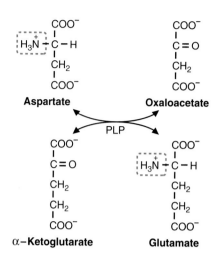

Fig. 8.20. Transamination reactions. Pyridoxal phosphate (PLP) on aspartate aminotransferase transfers an amino group from aspartate to the α-keto acid (α-ketoglutarate) to form a new amino acid (glutamate). The enzyme used to be called glutamate-oxaloacetate transaminase.

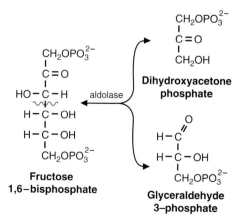

Fig. 8.21. Aldolases catalyze carbon–carbon cleavage in reactions that are usually reversible. In glycolysis, the enzyme fructose 1,6-bisphosphate aldolase cleaves a carbon–carbon bond in fructose 1,6-bisphosphate. Aldolases have a lysine epsilon amino group in the active site that participates in the reaction.

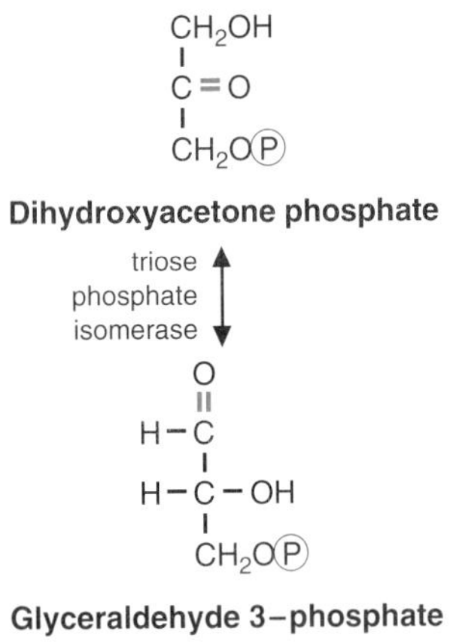

CH₂OH
|
C = O
|
CH₂O(P)

Dihydroxyacetone phosphate

triose
phosphate
isomerase

O
‖
H – C
|
H – C – OH
|
CH₂O(P)

Glyceraldehyde 3–phosphate

Fig. 8.22. Isomerases rearrange atoms within a molecule. In the pathway of glycolysis, triose phosphate isomerase converts dihydroxyacetone phosphate to glyceraldehydes 3-phosphate by rearranging hydrogen atoms. No other substrates or products of the reaction exist.

Isomerases. Many biochemical reactions simply rearrange the existing atoms of a molecule, that is, create isomers of the starting material (Fig. 8.22). Enzymes rearranging the bond structure of a compound are called *isomerases*, whereas enzymes catalyzing movement of a phosphate from one atom to another are called *mutases*.

Ligases. Ligases synthesize C-C, C-S, C-O, and C-N bonds in reactions coupled to the cleavage of a high-energy phosphate bond in ATP or another nucleotide. *Carboxylases*, for example, add CO_2 to another compound in a reaction requiring ATP cleavage to provide energy (see Fig. 8.12B). Most carboxylases require the coenzyme biotin. Other ligases are named *synthetases* (e.g., fatty acyl CoA synthetase). Synthetases differ from the synthases mentioned under "lyases" and "group transferases" in that synthetases derive the energy for new bond formation from cleavage of high-energy phosphate bonds, and synthases use a different source of energy.

Suggested References

Dressler D, Potter H. Discovering enzymes. Scientific American Library. New York: W.H. Freeman, 1991.
Fersht A. Structure and Mechanism in Protein Science. New York: W.H. Freeman, 1999.
EPA has a good website for information on organophosphate compounds at www.epa.gov/pesticides.
The ENZYME database (http://www.expasy.ch/enzyme/) provides basic information about specific enzymes. It is based on the recommendations of the Nomenclature Committee of the International Union of Biochemistry and Molecular Biology. In this database, you can obtain the EC number of any enzyme, its recommended name, alternative names, cofactors, and human diseases associated with the enzyme. You can trace the enzyme from its name to the reaction it catalyses—to the metabolic pathway(s) in which it participates—to the large and intricate Boehringer Mannheim Biochemical Pathways Wallchart. You also can search the database by metabolites or pathways.

REVIEW QUESTIONS—CHAPTER 8

Questions below cover material from Chapters 6 and 7, as well as Chapter 8 (including Biochemical Comments).

1. A patient was born with a congenital mutation in an enzyme, severely affecting its ability to bind an activation-transfer coenzyme. As a consequence,

   (A) the enzyme would be unable to bind the substrate of the reaction.
   (B) the enzyme would be unable to form the transition state complex.
   (C) the enzyme would normally use a different activation-transfer coenzyme.
   (D) the enzyme would normally substitute the functional group of an active site amino acid residue for the coenzyme.
   (E) the reaction could be carried out by the free coenzyme, provided the diet carried an adequate amount of its vitamin precursor.

2. An individual had a congenital mutation in glucokinase in which a proline was substituted for a leucine on a surface helix far from the active site, but within the hinge region of the actin fold. This mutation would be expected to

   (A) have no effect on the rate of the reaction because it is not in the active site.
   (B) have no effect on the rate of the reaction because proline and leucine are both nonpolar amino acids.
   (C) have no effect on the number of substrate molecules reaching the transition state.
   (D) probably affect the binding of ATP or a subsequent step in the reaction sequence.
   (E) probably cause the reaction to proceed through an alternate mechanism.

3. A patient developed a bacterial overgrowth in his intestine that decreased the pH of the luminal contents from their normal pH of approximately 6.5 down to 5.5. This decrease of pH is likely to

   (A) denature proteins reaching the intestine with their native structure intact.
   (B) disrupt hydrogen bonding essential for maintenance of tertiary structure.
   (C) inhibit intestinal enzymes dependent on histidine for acid-base catalysis.
   (D) inhibit intestinal enzymes dependent on an active site lysine for binding substrate.
   (E) have little effect on hydrolases.

   Questions 4 and 5 refer to the reaction shown below:

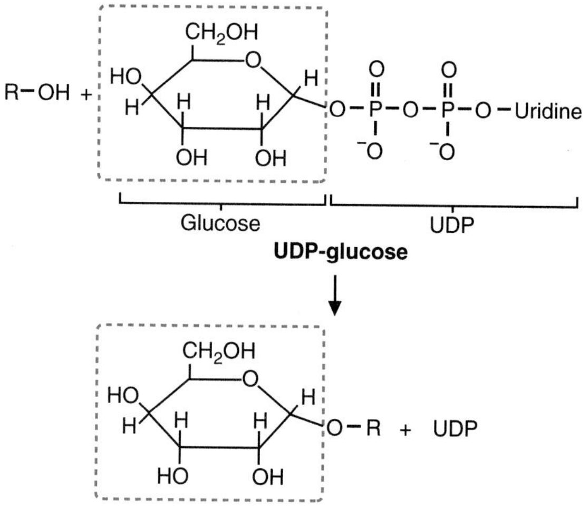

4. The type of reaction shown above fits into which of the following classifications?

   (A) Group transfer
   (B) Isomerization
   (C) Carbon–carbon bond breaking
   (D) Carbon–carbon bond formation
   (E) Oxidation-reduction

5. The type of enzyme catalyzing this reaction is a

   (A) kinase
   (B) dehydrogenase
   (C) glycosyltransferase
   (D) transaminase
   (E) isomerase

9 Regulation of Enzymes

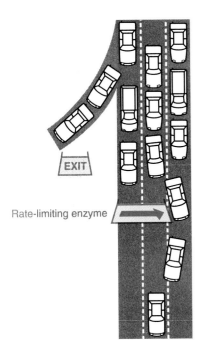

Fig. 9.1. The flux of substrates down a metabolic pathway is analogous to cars traveling down a highway. The rate-limiting enzyme is the portion of the highway that is narrowed to one lane by a highway barrier. This single portion of the highway limits the rate at which cars can arrive at their final destination miles later. Cars will back up before the barrier (similar to the increase in concentration of a precursor when a rate-limiting enzyme is inhibited). Some cars may exit and take an alternate route (similar to precursors entering another metabolic pathway.) Moving the barrier just a little to open an additional lane is like activating a rate-limiting enzyme; it increases flow through the entire length of the pathway.

In the body, thousands of diverse enzymes are regulated to fulfil their individual functions without waste of dietary components. Thus, with changes in our physiologic state, time of eating, environment, diet, or age, the rates of some enzymes must increase and others decrease. In this chapter, we describe the mechanisms for regulation of enzyme activity and the strategies employed to regulate the metabolic pathways in which they reside.

Regulation matches function. *Changes in the rate of a metabolic pathway occur because at least one enzyme in that pathway, the **regulatory enzyme**, has been **activated** or **inhibited,** or the amount of enzyme has increased or decreased. Regulatory enzymes usually catalyze the **rate-limiting**, or slowest, step in the pathway, so that increasing or decreasing their rate changes the rate of the entire pathway (Fig. 9.1). The mechanisms used to regulate the rate-limiting enzyme in a pathway reflect the function of the pathway.*

Substrate concentration. *The rate of all enzymes is dependent on substrate concentration. Enzymes exhibit **saturation kinetics**; their rate increases with increasing substrate concentration [S], but reaches a maximum velocity (V_{max}) when the enzyme is saturated with substrate. For many enzymes, the **Michaelis-Menten equation** describes the relationship between v_i (the initial velocity of a reaction), [S], V_{max}, and the K_m (the substrate concentration at which $v_i = \frac{1}{2} V_{max}$).*

Reversible inhibition. *Enzymes are reversibly inhibited by **structural analogs** and **products**. These inhibitors are classified as **competitive, noncompetitive**, or **uncompetitive,** depending on their effect on formation of the **enzyme–substrate complex.***

Allosteric enzymes. *Allosteric **activators** or **inhibitors** are compounds that bind at sites other than the active catalytic site and regulate the enzyme through **conformational changes** affecting the catalytic site.*

Covalent modification. *Enzyme activity also may be regulated by a covalent modification, such as **phosphorylation** of a serine, threonine, or tyrosine residue by a **protein kinase**.*

Protein–protein interactions. *Enzyme activity can be modulated through the reversible binding of a **modulator protein**, such as Ca^{2+} **calmodulin**. **Monomeric G proteins** (GTP-binding proteins) activate target proteins through reversible binding.*

Zymogen cleavage. *Some enzymes are synthesized as inactive precursors, called zymogens, that are activated by **proteolysis** (e.g., the digestive enzyme chymotrypsin).*

Changes in enzyme concentration. *The concentration of an enzyme can be regulated by changes in the rate of enzyme synthesis (e.g., induction of gene transcription) or the rate of degradation.*

Regulation of metabolic pathways. *The regulatory mechanisms for the rate-limiting enzyme of a pathway always reflects the **function of the pathway in a particular tissue**. In **feedback regulation,** the end product of a pathway directly or indirectly controls its own rate of synthesis; in **feedforword regulation,** the* *substrate controls the rate of the pathway.* **Biosynthetic** *and* **degradative** *pathways are controlled through different but* **complementary regulation**. *Pathways are also regulated through* **compartmentation** *of enzymes.*

THE WAITING ROOM

Al Martini is a 44-year-old man who has been an alcoholic for the past 5 years. He was recently admitted to the hospital for congestive heart failure (see Chapter 8). After being released from the hospital, he continued to drink. One night he arrived at a friend's house at 7:00 P.M. Between his arrival and 11:00 P.M., he drank four beers and five martinis (for a total ethanol consumption of 9.5 oz). His friends encouraged him to stay an additional hour and drink coffee to sober up. Nevertheless, he ran his car off the road on his way home. He was taken to the emergency room of the local hospital and arrested for driving under the influence of alcohol. His blood alcohol concentration at the time of his arrest was 240 mg/dL, compared with the legal limit of ethanol for driving of 80 mg/dL.

Ann O'Rexia, a 23-year old woman, 5 feet 7 inches tall, is being treated for anorexia nervosa (see Chapters 1–3). She has been gaining weight, and is now back to 99 lb from a low of 85 lb. Her blood glucose is still below normal (fasting blood glucose of 72 mg/dL, compared with a normal range of 80-100 mg/dL). She complains to her physician that she feels tired when she jogs, and she is concerned that the "extra weight" she has gained is slowing her down.

We will generally be using the pathways of fuel oxidation to illustrate the role of various mechanisms of enzyme regulation in metabolic pathways. Chapters 1 through 3 provide an overview of the names and functions of these pathways, including the TCA cycle, glycolysis, glycogen synthesis, glycogenolysis, and fatty acid oxidation.

Al Martini was not able to clear his blood ethanol rapidly enough to stay within the legal limit for driving. Ethanol is cleared from the blood at about $\frac{1}{2}$ ounce/hr (15 mg/dL per hour). Liver metabolism accounts for more than 90% of ethanol clearance from the blood. The major route of ethanol metabolism in the liver is the enzyme liver alcohol dehydrogenase (ADH), which oxidizes ethanol to acetaldehyde with generation of NADH.

$$\text{Ethanol} + \text{NAD}^+ \rightarrow \text{Acetaldehyde} + \text{NADH} + \text{H}^+$$

The multienzyme complex MEOS (**m**icrosomal **e**thanol **o**xidizing **s**ystem), which is also called cytochrome P450-2E1, provides an additional route for ethanol oxidation to acetaldehyde in the liver.

Although the regulation of metabolic pathways is an exceedingly complex subject, dealt with in most of the subsequent chapters of this text, a number of common themes are involved. Physiologic regulation of a metabolic pathway depends on the ability to alter flux through the pathway by activating the enzyme catalyzing the rate-limiting step in the pathway (see Fig. 9.1). The type of regulation employed always reflects the function of the pathway and the need for that pathway in a particular tissue or cell type. Pathways producing a necessary product are usually feedback-regulated through a mechanism directly or indirectly involving the concentration of product (e.g., allosteric inhibition or induction/repression of enzyme synthesis). The concentration of product signals when enough of the product has been synthesized. Storage and toxic disposal pathways are usually regulated directly or indirectly through a feedforward mechanism reflecting the availability of precursor. Regulatory enzymes are often tissue-specific isozymes whose properties reflect the different functions of a pathway in particular tissues. Pathways are also regulated through compartmentation, collection of enzymes with a common function within a particular organelle or at a specific site in the cell.

The mechanisms employed to regulate enzymes have been organized into three general categories: regulation by compounds that bind reversibly in the active site (including dependence of velocity on substrate concentration and product levels); regulation by changing the conformation of the active site (including allosteric regulators, covalent modification, protein–protein interactions, and zymogen cleavage); and regulation by changing the concentration of enzyme (enzyme synthesis and degradation).

One of the fuels used by **Ann O' Rexia**'s skeletal muscles for jogging is glucose, which is converted to glucose 6-phosphate (glucose 6-P) by the enzymes hexokinase (HK) and glucokinase (GK). Glucose 6-P is metabolized in the pathway of glycolysis to generate ATP. This pathway is feedback regulated, so that as her muscles use ATP, the rate of glycolysis will increase to generate more ATP.

Glycogen

Glycogen synthesis Glycogenolysis

Glucose ⟶ Glucose-6-P
hexokinase
glucokinase

Glycolysis

Energy, ATP

When she is resting, her muscles and liver will convert glucose 6-phosphate to glycogen (a fuel storage pathway, shown in blue). Glycogen synthesis is feed-forward regulated by the supply of glucose and by insulin and other hormones that signal glucose availability.

Glycogenolysis (glycogen degradation) is activated during exercise to supply additional glucose 6-P for glycolysis. Unless Ann consumes sufficient calories, her glycogen stores will not be replenished after exercise, and she will tire easily.

I. REGULATION BY SUBSTRATE AND PRODUCT CONCENTRATION

A. Velocity and Substrate Concentration

The velocity of all enzymes is dependent on the concentration of substrate. This dependence is reflected in conditions such as starvation, in which a number of pathways are deprived of substrate. In contrast, storage pathways (e.g., glucose conversion to glycogen in the liver) and toxic waste disposal pathways (e.g., the urea cycle, which prevents NH_4^+ toxicity by converting NH_4^+ to urea) are normally regulated to speed up when more substrate is available. In the following sections, we use the Michaelis-Menten equation to describe the response of an enzyme to changes in substrate concentration and use glucokinase to illustrate the role of substrate supply in regulation of enzyme activity.

1. MICHAELIS-MENTEN EQUATION

The equations of enzyme kinetics provide a quantitative way of describing the dependence of enzyme rate on substrate concentration. The simplest of these equations, the Michaelis-Menten equation, relates the initial velocity (v_i) to the concentration of substrate [S] and the two parameters K_m and V_{max} (Equation 9.1) The V_{max} of the enzyme is the maximal velocity that can be achieved at an infinite concentration of substrate, and the K_m of the enzyme for a substrate is the concentration of substrate required to reach ½ V_{max}. The Michaelis-Menten model of enzyme kinetics applies to a simple reaction in which the enzyme and substrate form an enzyme–substrate complex (ES) that can dissociate back to the free enzyme and substrate. The initial velocity of product formation, v_i, is proportionate to the concentration of enzyme–substrate complexes [ES]. As substrate concentration is increased, the concentration of enzyme–substrate complexes increases, and the reaction rate increases proportionately.

The Michaelis-Menten equation relates the initial velocity of the reaction (v_i) to the concentration of enzyme substrate complexes (ES). This equation is derived for a reaction in which a single substrate, S, is converted to a single product, P. The enzyme (E) and S associate to form ES with the rate constant of k_1. The complex dissociates with the rate constant of k_2, or is converted to P with the rate constant k_3. Under conditions in which [S] >> [E], [P] is negligible, and the rate of conversion of ES to an enzyme-product complex is very fast, $v_i = k_3$ [ES]. The concentration of ES is a fraction of E_T, the total amount of enzyme present as ES and E.

Therefore,

$$v_i = k_3[ES] = \frac{k_3[E_T][S]}{K_m + [S]}$$

Where $K_m = (k_2 + k_3)/k_1$. Substitution of V_{max} for k_3 [ET] gives the Michaelis-Menten equation (see Equation 9.1)

The graph of the Michaelis-Menten equation (v_i as a function of substrate concentration) is a rectangular hyperbola that approaches a finite limit, V_{max}, as the fraction of total enzyme present as enzyme–substrate complex increases (Fig. 9.2).

Equation 9.1. The Michaelis-Menten equation:

For the reaction

$$E + S \underset{k_2}{\overset{k_1}{\rightleftharpoons}} ES \overset{k_3}{\rightarrow} P$$

the Michaelis-Menten equation is given by

$$v_i = \frac{V_{max}[S]}{K_m + [S]}$$

where $K_m = (k_2 + k_3)/k_1$
and $V_{max} = k_3 [E_T]$

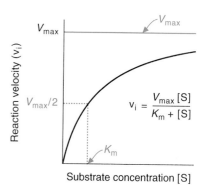

$$v_i = \frac{V_{max}[S]}{K_m + [S]}$$

Fig. 9.2. A graph of the Michaelis-Menten equation. V_{max} (solid blue line) is the initial velocity extrapolated to infinite [S]. K_m (dashed blue line) is the concentration of S at which $v_i = V_{max}/2$.

At a hypothetical infinitely high substrate concentration, all of the enzyme molecules contain bound substrate, and the reaction rate is at V_{max}. The approach to the finite limit of V_{max} is called saturation kinetics because velocity cannot increase any further once the enzyme is saturated with substrate. Saturation kinetics is a characteristic property of all rate processes dependent on the binding of a compound to a protein.

The K_m of the enzyme for a substrate is defined as the concentration of substrate at which v_i equals ½ V_{max}. The velocity of an enzyme is most sensitive to changes in substrate concentration over a concentration range below its K_m (see Fig. 9.2). At substrate concentrations less than ¹⁄₁₀th of the K_m, a doubling of substrate concentration nearly doubles the velocity of the reaction; at substrate concentrations 10 times the K_m, doubling the substrate concentration has little effect on the velocity.

The K_m of an enzyme for a substrate is related to the dissociation constant, K_d, which is the rate of substrate release divided by the rate of substrate binding. For example, a genetic mutation that decreases the rate of substrate binding to the enzyme decreases the affinity of the enzyme for the substrate and increases the K_d and K_m of the enzyme for that substrate. The higher the K_m, the higher is the substrate concentration required to reach ½ V_{max}.

MODY. Patients with maturity onset diabetes of the young (MODY) have a rare genetic form of diabetes mellitus in which the amount of insulin being secreted from the pancreas is too low, resulting in hyperglycemia. The disease is caused by mutations in the gene for pancreatic glucokinase (a closely related isozyme of liver glucokinase) that affect its kinetic properties (K_m or V_{max}). Glucokinase is part of the mechanism controlling release of insulin from the pancreas. A decreased activity of glucokinase results in lower insulin secretion for a given blood glucose level.

2. HEXOKINASE ISOZYMES HAVE DIFFERENT K_m VALUES FOR GLUCOSE

A comparison between the isozymes of hexokinase found in red blood cells and in the liver illustrates the significance of the K_m of an enzyme for its substrate. Hexokinase catalyses the first step in glucose metabolism in most cells, the transfer of a phosphate from ATP to glucose to form glucose 6-phosphate. Glucose 6-phosphate may then be metabolized in glycolysis, which generates energy in the form of ATP, or converted to glycogen, a storage polymer of glucose. Hexokinase I, the isozyme in red blood cells (erythrocytes), has a K_m for glucose of approximately 0.05 mM (Fig. 9.3). The isozyme of hexokinase, called glucokinase, which is found in the liver and pancreas, has a much higher K_m of approximately 5 to 6 mM. The red blood cell is totally dependent on glucose metabolism to meet its needs for ATP. At the low K_m of the erythrocyte hexokinase, blood glucose could fall drastically below its normal fasting level of approximately 5 mM, and the red blood cell could still phosphorylate glucose at rates near V_{max}. The liver, however, stores large amounts of "excess" glucose as glycogen or converts it to fat. Because glucokinase has a K_m of approximately 5 mM, the rate of glucose phosphorylation in the liver will tend to increase as blood glucose increases after a high-carbohydrate meal, and decrease as blood glucose levels fall. The high K_m of hepatic glucokinase thus promotes the storage of glucose as liver glycogen or as fat, but only when glucose is in excess supply.

As **Ann O'Rexia** eats a high carbohydrate meal, her blood glucose will rise to approximately 20 mM in the portal vein, and much of the glucose from her carbohydrate meal will enter the liver. How will the activity of glucokinase in the liver change as glucose is increased from 4 mM to 20 mM? (Hint: Calculate v_i as a fraction of V_{max} for both conditions, using a K_m for glucose of 5 mM and the Michaelis-Menten equation).

Glucokinase, which has a high K_m for glucose, phosphorylates glucose to glucose 6-phosphate about twice as fast after a carbohydrate meal than during fasting. Substitute the values for S and K_m into the Michaelis-Menten equation. The initial velocity will be 0.44 times V_{max} when blood glucose is at 4 mM and about 0.80 times V_{max} when blood glucose is at 20 mM. In the liver, glucose 6-phosphate is a precursor for both glycogen and fat synthesis. Thus, these storage pathways are partially regulated through a direct effect of substrate supply. They are also partially regulated through an increase of insulin and a decrease of glucagon, two hormones that signal the supply of dietary fuel.

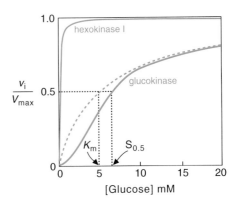

Fig. 9.3. A comparison between hexokinase I and glucokinase. The initial velocity (v_i) as a fraction of V_{max} is graphed as a function of glucose concentration. The plot for glucokinase (heavy blue line) is slightly sigmoidal (S-shaped), possibly because the rate of an intermediate step in the reaction is so slow that the enzyme does not follow Michaelis-Menten kinetics. The dashed blue line has been derived from the Michaelis-Menten equation fitted to the data for concentrations of glucose above 5 mM. For S-shaped curves, the concentration of substrate required to reach half V_{max}, or half-saturation, is sometimes called the $S_{0.5}$ or $K_{0.5}$, rather than K_m. At $v_i/V_{max} = 0.5$, the K_m is 5 mM, and the $S_{0.5}$ is 6.7 mM.

3.   VELOCITY AND ENZYME CONCENTRATION

The rate of a reaction is directly proportional to the concentration of enzyme; if you double the amount of enzyme, you will double the amount of product produced per minute, whether you are at low or at saturating concentrations of substrate. This important relationship between velocity and enzyme concentration is not immediately apparent in the Michaelis-Menten equation because the concentration of total enzyme present (E_t) has been incorporated into the term V_{max} (that is, V_{max} is equal to the rate constant k_3 times E_t.) However, V_{max} is most often expressed as product produced per minute per milligram of enzyme and is meant to reflect a property of the enzyme that is not dependent on its concentration.

4.   MULTISUBSTRATE REACTIONS

Most enzymes have more than one substrate, and the substrate binding sites overlap in the catalytic (active) site. When an enzyme has more than one substrate, the sequence of substrate binding and product release affect the rate equation. As a

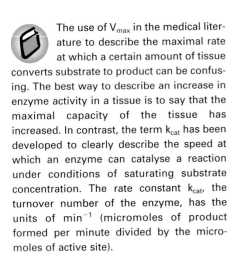

The use of V_{max} in the medical literature to describe the maximal rate at which a certain amount of tissue converts substrate to product can be confusing. The best way to describe an increase in enzyme activity in a tissue is to say that the maximal capacity of the tissue has increased. In contrast, the term k_{cat} has been developed to clearly describe the speed at which an enzyme can catalyse a reaction under conditions of saturating substrate concentration. The rate constant k_{cat}, the turnover number of the enzyme, has the units of min^{-1} (micromoles of product formed per minute divided by the micromoles of active site).

The liver alcohol dehydrogenase most active in oxidizing ethanol has a very low K_m for ethanol of approximately 0.04 mM, and is at over 99% of its V_{max} at the legal limit of blood alcohol concentration for driving (80 mg/dL or about 17 mM). In contrast, the MEOS isozyme most active toward ethanol has a K_m of approximately 11 mM. Thus, MEOS makes a greater contribution to ethanol oxidation and clearance from the blood at higher ethanol levels than lower ones. Liver damage, such as cirrhosis, results partly from toxic byproducts of ethanol oxidation generated by MEOS. **Al Martini**, who has blood alcohol levels of 240 mg/dL (approximately 52 mM), is drinking enough to potentially cause liver damage, as well as his car accident and arrest for driving under the influence of alcohol. The various isozymes and polymorphisms of alcohol dehydrogenase and MEOS are discussed in more detail in Chapter 25.

consequence, an apparent value of K_m ($K_{m,app}$) depends on the concentration of cosubstrate or product present.

5. RATES OF ENZYME-CATALYZED REACTIONS IN THE CELL

Equations for the initial velocity of an enzyme-catalyzed reaction, such as the Michaelis-Menten equation, can provide useful parameters for describing or comparing enzymes. However, many multisubstrate enzymes, such as glucokinase, have kinetic patterns that do not fit the Michaelis-Menten model (or do so under nonphysiologic conditions). The Michaelis-Menten model is also inapplicable to enzymes present in a higher concentration than their substrates. Nonetheless, the term "K_m" is still used for these enzymes to describe the approximate concentration of substrate at which velocity equals $\frac{1}{2}\,V_{max}$.

B. Reversible Inhibition within the Active Site

One of the ways of altering enzyme activity is through compounds binding in the active site. If these compounds are not part of the normal reaction, they inhibit the enzyme. An inhibitor of an enzyme is defined as a compound that decreases the velocity of the reaction by binding to the enzyme. It is a reversible inhibitor if it is not covalently bound to the enzyme and can dissociate at a significant rate. Reversible inhibitors are generally classified as competitive, noncompetitive, or uncompetitive with respect to their relationship to a substrate of the enzyme. In most reactions, the products of the reaction are reversible inhibitors of the enzyme producing them.

1. COMPETITIVE INHIBITION

A competitive inhibitor "competes" with a substrate for binding at the enzyme's substrate recognition site and therefore is usually a close structural analog of the substrate (Fig. 9.4). An increase of substrate concentration can overcome competitive inhibition; when the substrate concentration is increased to a sufficiently high level, the substrate binding sites are occupied by substrate, and inhibitor molecules cannot bind. Competitive inhibitors, therefore, increase the apparent K_m

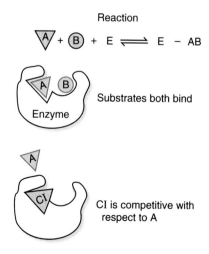

Fig. 9.4. Competitive inhibition with respect to substrate A. A and B are substrates for the reaction forming the enzyme substrate complex (E-AB). The enzyme has separate binding sites for each substrate, which overlap in the active site. The competitive inhibitor (CI) competes for the binding site of A, the substrate it most closely resembles.

Some of **Al Martini**'s problems have arisen from product inhibition of liver alcohol dehydrogenase by NADH. As ethanol is oxidized in liver cells, NAD^+ is reduced to NADH and the $NADH/NAD^+$ ratio rises. NADH is an inhibitor of alcohol dehydrogenase, competitive with respect to NAD^+, so the increased $NADH/NAD^+$ ratio slows the rate of ethanol oxidation and ethanol clearance from the blood.

NADH is also a product inhibitor of enzymes in the pathway that oxidizes fatty acids. Consequently, these fatty acids accumulate in the liver, eventually contributing to the alcoholic fatty liver.

of the enzyme ($K_{m,app}$) because they raise the concentration of substrate necessary to saturate the enzyme. They have no effect on V_{max}.

2. NONCOMPETITIVE AND UNCOMPETITIVE INHIBITION

If an inhibitor does not compete with a substrate for its binding site, the inhibitor is either a noncompetitive or uncompetitive inhibitor with respect to that particular substrate (Fig. 9.5). To illustrate noncompetitive inhibition, consider a multisubstrate reaction in which substrates A and B react to form a product. An inhibitor (NI) that is a structural analog of substrate B would fit into substrate B's binding site, but the inhibitor would be a noncompetitive inhibitor with regard to the other substrate, substrate A. An increase of A will not prevent the inhibitor from binding to substrate B's binding site. The inhibitor, in effect, lowers the concentration of the active enzyme and therefore changes the V_{max} of the enzyme. If the inhibitor has absolutely no effect on the binding of substrate A, it will not change the K_m for A (a pure noncompetitive inhibitor).

Some inhibitors, such as metals, might not bind at either substrate recognition site. In this case, the inhibitor would be noncompetitive with respect to both substrates.

An inhibitor that is uncompetitive with respect to a substrate will bind only to enzyme containing that substrate. Suppose, for example, that in Figure 9.5 an inhibitor that is a structural analog of B and binds to the B site could only bind to an enzyme that contains A. That inhibitor would be called uncompetitive with respect to A. It would decrease both the V_{max} of the enzyme and its apparent K_m for A.

3. SIMPLE PRODUCT INHIBITION IN METABOLIC PATHWAYS

All products are reversible inhibitors of the enzymes that produce them and may be competitive, noncompetitive, or uncompetitive relative to a particular substrate. Simple product inhibition, a decrease in the rate of an enzyme caused by the accumulation of its own product, plays an important role in metabolic pathways; it prevents one enzyme in a sequence of reactions from generating a product faster than it can be used by the next enzyme in that sequence.

Product inhibition of hexokinase by glucose 6-phosphate conserves blood glucose for tissues needing it. Tissues take up glucose from the blood and phosphorylate it to glucose 6-phosphate, which can then enter a number of different pathways (including glycolysis and glycogen synthesis). As these pathways become more active, glucose 6-phosphate concentration decreases, and the rate of hexokinase increases. When these pathways are less active, glucose 6-phosphate concentration increases, hexokinase is inhibited, and glucose remains in the blood for other tissues.

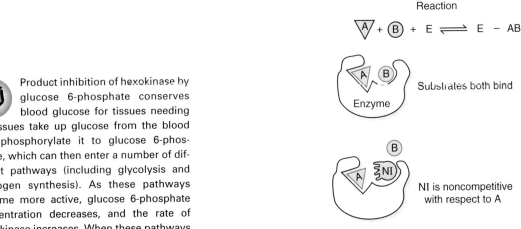

Fig. 9.5. NI is a noncompetitive inhibitor with respect to substrate A. A can still bind to its binding site in the presence of NI. However, NI is competitive with respect to B because it binds to the B binding site. In contrast, an inhibitor that is uncompetitive with respect to A might also resemble B, but it could only bind to the B site after A is bound.

III. REGULATION THROUGH CONFORMATIONAL CHANGES

In substrate response and product inhibition, the rate of the enzyme is affected principally by the binding of a substrate or a product within the catalytic site. Most rate-limiting enzymes are also controlled through regulatory mechanisms that change the conformation of the enzyme in a way that affects the catalytic site. These regulatory mechanisms include: (1) allosteric activation and inhibition; (2) phosphorylation or other covalent modification; (3) protein–protein interactions between regulatory and catalytic subunits, or between two proteins; and (4) proteolytic cleavage. These types of regulation can rapidly change an enzyme from an inactive form to a fully active conformation.

In the sections below, we describe the general characteristics of these regulatory mechanisms and illustrate the first three with glycogen phosphorylase, glycogen phosphorylase kinase, and protein kinase A.

A. Conformational Changes in Allosteric Enzymes

Allosteric activators and inhibitors (allosteric effectors) are compounds that bind to the allosteric site (a site separate from the catalytic site) and cause a conformational change that affects the affinity of the enzyme for the substrate. Usually an allosteric enzyme has multiple interacting subunits that can exist in active and inactive conformations, and the allosteric effector promotes or hinders conversion from one conformation to another.

1. COOPERATIVITY IN SUBSTRATE BINDING TO ALLOSTERIC ENZYMES

Allosteric enzymes usually contain two or more subunits and exhibit positive cooperativity; the binding of substrate to one subunit facilitates the binding of substrate to another subunit (Fig. 9.6). The first substrate molecule has difficulty in binding to the enzyme because all of the subunits are in the conformation with a low affinity for substrate (the taut "T" conformation) (see Chapter 7, section VII.B.). The first substrate molecule to bind changes its own subunit and at least one adjacent subunit to the high-affinity conformation (the relaxed "R" state.) In the example of the tetramer hemoglobin, discussed in Chapter 7, the change in one subunit facilitated changes in all four subunits, and the molecule generally changed to the new conformation in a concerted fashion. However, most allosteric enzymes follow a more stepwise (sequential) progression through intermediate stages (see Fig. 9.6)

2. ALLOSTERIC ACTIVATORS AND INHIBITORS

Allosteric enzymes bind activators at the allosteric site, a site physically separate from the catalytic site. The binding of an allosteric activator changes the conformation of the catalytic site in a way that increases the affinity of the enzyme for the substrate.

In general, activators of allosteric enzymes bind more tightly to the high-affinity R state of the enzyme than the T state (i.e., the allosteric site is open only in the R enzyme) (Fig. 9.7). Thus, the activators increase the amount of enzyme in the active state, thereby facilitating substrate binding in their own and other subunits. In contrast, allosteric inhibitors bind more tightly to the T state, so either substrate concentration or activator concentration must be increased to overcome the effects of the allosteric inhibitor. Allosteric inhibitors might have their own binding site on the enzyme, or they might compete with the substrate at the active site and prevent cooperativity. Thus, the term "allosteric inhibitor" is more generally applied to any inhibitor of an allosteric enzyme.

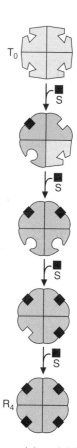

Fig. 9.6. A sequential model for an allosteric enzyme. The sequential model is actually the preferred path from the T_0 (taut, with 0 substrate bound) low-affinity conformation to the R_4 (relaxed, with four substrate molecules bound) conformation, taken from an array of all possible equilibrium conformations that differ by the conformation of only one subunit. The final result is a stepwise path in which intermediate conformations exist, and subunits may change conformations independently, depending on their geometric relationship to the subunits already containing bound substrate.

A model of an allosteric enzyme

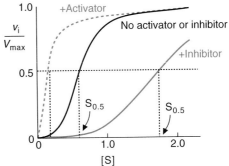

Fig. 9.7. Activators and inhibitors of an allosteric enzyme (simplified model). This enzyme has two identical subunits, each containing three binding sites: one for the substrate (s), one for the allosteric activator (blue triangle), and one for the allosteric inhibitor (two-pronged shape). The enzyme has two conformations, a relaxed active conformation (R) and an inactive conformation (T). The activator binds only to its activator site when the enzyme is in the R configuration. The inhibitor binding site is open only when the enzyme is in the T state.

A plot of velocity (v_i/V_{max}) versus substrate concentration reveals that binding of the substrate at its binding site stabilizes the active conformation so that the second substrate binds more readily, resulting in an S (sigmoidal)-shaped curve. The graph of v_i/V_{max} becomes hyperbolic in the presence of activator (which stabilizes the high-affinity R form), and more sigmoidal with a higher $S_{0.5}$ in the presence of inhibitor (which stabilizes the low-affinity form).

Some of the rate-limiting enzymes in the pathways of fuel oxidation (e.g., muscle glycogen phosphorylase in glycogenolysis, phosphofructokinase-1 in glycolysis and isocitrate dehydrogenase in the TCA cycle) are allosteric enzymes regulated by changes in the concentration of ADP or AMP, which are allosteric activators. The function of fuel oxidation pathways is the generation of ATP. When the concentration of ATP in a muscle cell begins to decrease, ADP and AMP increase; ADP activates isocitrate dehydrogenase, and AMP activates glycogen phosphorylase and phosphofructokinase-1. The response is very fast, and small changes in the concentration of activator can cause large changes in the rate of the reaction.

In the absence of activator, a plot of velocity versus substrate concentration for an allosteric enzyme usually results in a sigmoid or S-shaped curve (rather than the rectangular hyperbola of Michaelis-Menten enzymes) as the successive binding of substrate molecules activates additional subunits (see Fig. 9.7). In plots of velocity versus substrate concentration, the effect of an allosteric activator generally makes the sigmoidal S-shaped curve more like the rectangular hyperbola, with a substantial decrease in the $S_{0.5}$ (K_m) of the enzyme, because the activator changes all of the subunits to the high-affinity state. Such allosteric effectors are "K effectors"; they change the K_m but not the V_{max} of the enzyme. An allosteric inhibitor makes it more difficult for substrate or activators to convert the subunits to the most active conformation, and therefore inhibitors generally shift the curve to the right, either increasing the $S_{0.5}$ alone, or increasing it together with a decrease in the V_{max}.

3. ALLOSTERIC ENZYMES IN METABOLIC PATHWAYS

Regulation of enzymes by allosteric effectors provides several advantages over other methods of regulation. Allosteric inhibitors usually have a much stronger effect on enzyme velocity than competitive, noncompetitive, and uncompetitive inhibitors in the active catalytic site. Because allosteric effectors do not occupy the catalytic site, they may function as activators. Thus, allosteric enzymes are not limited to regulation through inhibition. Furthermore, the allosteric effector need not bear any resemblance to substrate or product of the enzyme. Finally, the effect of an allosteric effector is rapid, occurring as soon as its concentration changes in the cell. These features of allosteric enzymes are often essential for feedback regulation of metabolic pathways by endproducts of the pathway or by signal molecules that coordinate multiple pathways.

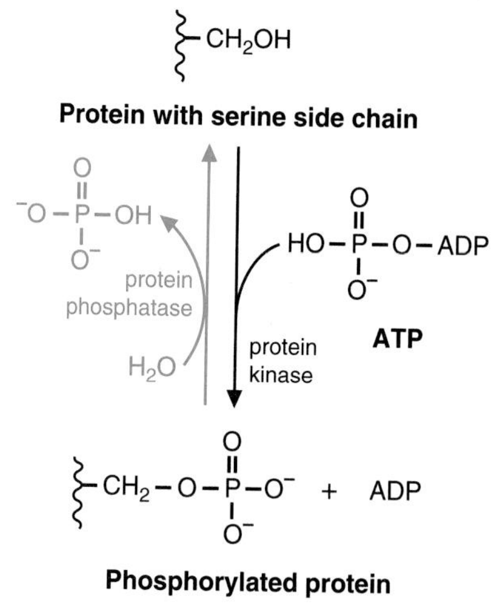

B. Conformational Changes from Covalent Modification

1. PHOSPHORYLATION

The activity of many enzymes is regulated through phosphorylation by a protein kinase or dephosphorylation by a protein phosphatase (Fig. 9.8). Serine/threonine protein kinases transfer a phosphate from ATP to the hydroxyl group of a specific serine (and sometimes threonine) on the target enzyme; tyrosine kinases transfer a phosphate to the hydroxyl group of a specific tyrosine residue. Phosphate is a bulky, negatively charged residue that interacts with other nearby amino acid residues of the protein to create a conformational change at the catalytic site. The conformational change makes certain enzymes more active and other enzymes less active. The effect is reversed by a specific protein phosphatase that removes the phosphate by hydrolysis.

2. MUSCLE GLYCOGEN PHOSPHORYLASE

Muscle glycogen phosphorylase, the rate-limiting enzyme in the pathway of glycogen degradation, degrades glycogen to glucose 1-phosphate. It is regulated by the allosteric activator AMP, which increases in the cell as ATP is used for muscular contraction (Fig. 9.9). Thus, a rapid increase in the rate of glycogen degradation to glucose 1-phosphate is achieved when an increase of AMP signals that more fuel is needed for ATP generation in the glycolytic pathway.

Glycogen phosphorylase also can be activated through phosphorylation by glycogen phosphorylase kinase. Either phosphorylation or AMP binding can change the enzyme to the same fully active conformation. The phosphate is removed by protein

Fig. 9.8. Protein kinases and protein phosphatases.

When **Ann O'Rexia** begins to jog, AMP activates her muscle glycogen phosphorylase, which degrades glycogen to glucose 1-phosphate. This compound is converted to glucose 6-phosphate, which feeds into the glycolytic pathway to generate ATP for muscle contraction. As she continues to jog, her adrenaline (epinephrine) levels rise, producing the signal that activates glycogen phosphorylase kinase. This enzyme phosphorylates glycogen phosphorylase, causing it to become even more active than with AMP alone (see Fig. 9.9).

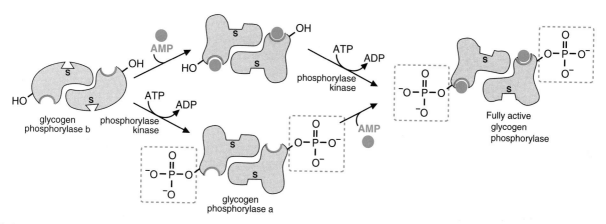

Fig. 9.9. Activation of muscle glycogen phosphorylase by AMP and by phosphorylation. Muscle glycogen phosphorylase is composed of two identical subunits. The substrate binding sites in the active catalytic site are denoted by S. AMP binds to the allosteric site, a site separate from the active catalytic site. Glycogen phosphorylase kinase can transfer a phosphate from ATP to one serine residue in each subunit. Either phosphorylation or binding of AMP causes a change in the active site that increases the activity of the enzyme. The first event at one subunit facilitates the subsequent events that convert the enzyme to the fully active form.

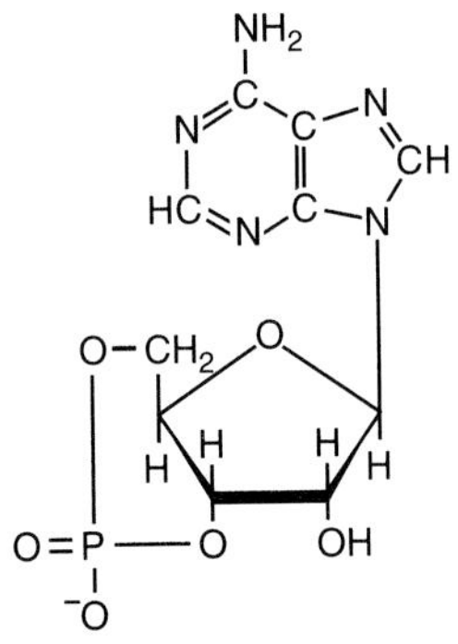

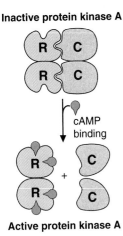

Fig. 9.10. Structure of cAMP ($3',5'$ -cyclic AMP.) The phosphate group is attached to hydroxyl groups on both the 3rd ($3'$) and 5th ($5'$) carbons of ribose, forming a cycle.

Inactive protein kinase A

cAMP binding

+

Active protein kinase A

Fig. 9.11. Protein kinase A. When the regulatory subunits (R) of protein kinase A bind the allosteric activator, cAMP, they dissociate from the enzyme, thereby releasing active catalytic subunits (C).

phosphatase-1. Glycogen phosphorylase kinase links the activation of muscle glycogen phosphorylase to changes in the level of the hormone adrenaline in the blood. It is regulated through phosphorylation by protein kinase A and by activation of Ca^{2+}-calmodulin (a modulator protein) during contraction.

3. PROTEIN KINASE A

Some protein kinases, called dedicated protein kinases, are tightly bound to a single protein and regulate only the protein to which they are tightly bound. However, other protein kinases and protein phosphatases will simultaneously regulate a number of rate-limiting enzymes in a cell to achieve a coordinated response. For example, protein kinase A, a serine/threonine protein kinase, phosphorylates a number of enzymes that regulate different metabolic pathways. One of these enzymes is glycogen phosphorylase kinase (see Fig. 9.9).

Protein kinase A provides a means for hormones to control metabolic pathways. Adrenaline and many other hormones increase the intracellular concentration of the allosteric regulator $3', 5'$-cyclic AMP (cAMP), which is referred to as a hormonal second messenger (Fig. 9.10). cAMP binds to regulatory subunits of protein kinase A, which dissociate and release the activated catalytic subunits (Fig. 9.11). Dissociation of inhibitory regulatory subunits is a common theme in enzyme regulation. The active catalytic subunits phosphorylate glycogen phosphorylase and other enzymes at serine residues.

In the example shown in Figure 9.9, adrenaline indirectly increases cAMP, which activates protein kinase A, which phosphorylates phosphorylase kinase, which phosphorylates glycogen phosphorylase. The sequence of events in which one kinase phosphorylates another kinase is called a phosphorylation cascade. Because each stage of the phosphorylation cascade is associated with one enzyme molecule activating many enzyme molecules, the initial activating event is greatly amplified.

4. OTHER COVALENT MODIFICATIONS

A number of proteins are covalently modified by the addition of groups such as acetyl, ADP-ribose, or lipid moieties (see Chapter 6). These modifications may directly activate or inhibit the enzyme. However, they also may modify the ability of the enzyme to interact with other proteins or to reach its correct location in the cell.

C. Conformational Changes from Protein–Protein Interactions

Changes in the conformation of the active site also can be regulated by direct protein–protein interaction. This type of regulation is illustrated by Ca^{2+}-calmodulin and small (monomeric) G proteins.

1. THE CALCIUM-CALMODULIN FAMILY OF MODULATOR PROTEINS

Modulator proteins bind to other proteins and regulate their activity by causing a conformational change at the catalytic site or by blocking the catalytic site (steric hindrance). They are protein allosteric effectors that can either activate or inhibit the enzyme or protein to which they bind.

Ca^{2+}-calmodulin is an example of a dissociable modulator protein that binds to a number of different proteins and regulates their function. It also exists in the cytosol and functions as a Ca^{2+} binding protein (Fig. 9.12). The center of the symmetric molecule is a hinge region that bends as Ca^{2+}-calmodulin folds over the protein it is regulating.

One of the enzymes activated by Ca^{2+}-calmodulin is muscle glycogen phosphorylase kinase, which is also activated by protein kinase A (see Fig. 9.9). When a

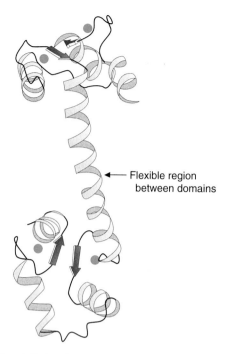

Fig. 9.12. Calcium-calmodulin has four binding sites for calcium (shown in blue). Each calcium forms a multiligand coordination sphere by simultaneously binding several amino acid residues on calmodulin. Thus, it can create large conformational changes in proteins when it binds. Calmodulin has a flexible region in the middle connecting the two domains.

neural impulse triggers Ca^{2+} release from the sarcoplasmic reticulum, Ca^{2+} binds to the calmodulin subunit of muscle glycogen phosphorylase kinase, which undergoes a conformational change. This activated kinase then phosphorylates glycogen phosphorylase, ultimately increasing the generation of ATP to supply energy for muscle contraction. Simultaneously, Ca^{2+} binds to troponin-C, a member of the Ca^{2+}-calmodulin superfamily that serves as a nondissociable regulatory subunit of troponin, a regulator of muscle contraction. Calcium binding to troponin prepares the muscle for contraction. Thus, the supply of energy for contraction is activated simultaneously with the contraction machinery.

2. SMALL (MONOMERIC) G PROTEINS REGULATE THROUGH CONFORMATIONAL CHANGES

The masters of regulation through reversible protein association in the cell are the monomeric G proteins, small single-subunit proteins that bind and hydrolyze GTP. GTP (guanosine triphosphate) is a purine nucleotide that, like ATP, contains high-energy phosphoanhydride bonds that release energy when hydrolyzed. When G proteins bind GTP, their conformation changes so that they can bind to a target protein, which is then either activated or inhibited in carrying out its function (Fig. 9.13, step 1).

G proteins are said to possess an internal clock because they are GTPases that slowly hydrolyze their own bound GTP to GDP and phosphate. As they hydrolyze GTP, their conformation changes and the complex they have formed with the target protein disassembles (see Fig. 9.13, step 2). The bound GDP on the inactive G protein is eventually replaced by GTP, and the process can begin again (see Fig. 9.13, step 3).

The activity of many G proteins is regulated by accessory proteins (GAPs, GEFs, and GDIs), which may, in turn, be regulated by allosteric effectors. GAPs (**G**TPase **a**ctivating **p**roteins) increase the rate of GTP hydrolysis by the G protein, and therefore the rate of dissociation of the G protein-target protein complex (see Fig. 9.13,

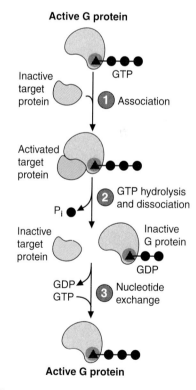

Fig. 9.13. Monomeric G proteins. (1) When GTP is bound, the conformation of the G protein allows it to bind target proteins, which are then activated. (2) The G protein hydrolyzes a phosphate from GTP to form GDP, which changes the G-protein conformation and causes it to dissociate from the target protein. (3) GDP is exchanged for GTP, which reactivates the G protein.

step 2). When a GEF protein (**g**uanine nucleotide **e**xchange **f**actor) binds to a G-protein, it increases the rate of GTP exchange for a bound GDP, and therefore activates the G-protein (see Fig. 9.13, step 3). GDI proteins (**G**DP **d**issociation **i**nhibitor) bind to the GDP-G protein complex and inhibit dissociation of GDP, thereby keeping the G protein inactive.

The Ras superfamily of small G proteins is divided into five families: Ras, Rho, Arf, Rab, and Ran. These monomeric G proteins play major roles in the regulation of growth, morphogenesis, cell motility, axonal guidance, cytokinesis, and trafficking through the Golgi, nucleus, and endosomes. They are generally bound to a lipid membrane through a lipid anchor, such as a myristoyl group or farnesyl group, and regulate the assembly and activity of protein complexes at these sites. The small G protein Ras, for example, is involved in regulation of cellular proliferation by a number of hormones called growth factors (Fig. 9.14). It is attached to the plasma membrane by a farnesyl group (see Chapter 6, section IV.B.). The activity of Ras is regulated by a guanine nucleotide exchange protein called SOS (**s**on **o**f **s**evenless). When SOS is in its active conformation, it binds to Ras, thereby activating dissociation of GDP and binding of GTP. When Ras binds GTP, it is activated, allowing it to bind and activate a protein kinase called Raf. The net effect will be the activation of transcription of certain genes. (Rho, Arf, Rab, and Ran are illustrated in Chapter 10, and the function of Ras is discussed in greater detail in Chapter 11).

D. Proteolytic Cleavage

Although many enzymes undergo some cleavage during synthesis, others enter lysosomes, secretory vesicles or are secreted as proenzymes, which are precursor proteins that must undergo proteolytic cleavage to become fully functional. Unlike most other forms of regulation, proteolytic cleavage is irreversible.

The precursor proteins of proteases (enzymes that cleave specific peptide bonds) are called zymogens. To denote the inactive zymogen form of an enzyme, the name is modified by addition of the suffix "ogen" or the prefix "pro." The synthesis of zymogens as inactive precursors prevents them from cleaving proteins prematurely at their sites of synthesis or secretion. Chymotrypsinogen, for example, is stored in vesicles within pancreatic cells until secreted into ducts leading to the intestinal lumen. In the digestive tract, chymotrypsinogen is converted to chymotrypsin by the proteolytic enzyme trypsin, which cleaves off a small peptide from the N-terminal region (and two internal peptides). This cleavage activates chymotrypsin by causing

Most of the proteases involved in blood clotting are zymogens, such as fibrinogen and prothrombin, which circulate in blood in the inactive form. They are cleaved to the active form (fibrin and thrombin, respectively) by other proteases, which have been activated by their attachment to the site of injury in a blood vessel wall. Thus, clots form at the site of injury and not randomly in circulation.

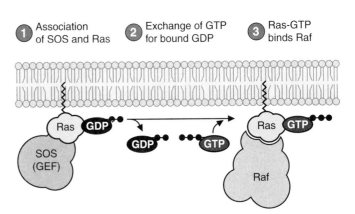

Fig. 9.14. The monomeric G protein Ras. When SOS is activated, it binds to Ras, a monomeric G protein anchored to the plasma membrane. SOS is a guanine nucleotide exchange protein that activates the exchange of GTP for bound GDP on Ras. Activated Ras containing GTP binds the target enzyme Raf, thereby activating it.

a conformational change in the spacing of amino acid residues around the binding site for the denatured protein substrate and around the catalytic site.

IV. REGULATION THROUGH CHANGES IN AMOUNT OF ENZYME

Tissues continuously adjust the rate at which different proteins are synthesized to vary the amount of different enzymes present. The expression for V_{max} in the Michaelis-Menten equation incorporates the concept that the rate of a reaction is proportional to the amount of enzyme present. Thus, the maximal capacity of a tissue can change with increased protein synthesis, or with increased protein degradation.

A. Regulated Enzyme Synthesis

Protein synthesis begins with the process of gene transcription, transcribing the genetic code for that protein from DNA into messenger RNA. The code in messenger RNA is then translated into the primary amino acid sequence of the protein. Generally the rate of enzyme synthesis is regulated by increasing or decreasing the rate of gene transcription, processes generally referred to as induction (increase) and repression (decrease). However, the rate of enzyme synthesis is sometimes regulated through stabilization of the messenger RNA. (These processes are covered in Section Three). Compared with the more immediate types of regulation discussed above, regulation by means of induction/repression of enzyme synthesis is usually slow in the human, occurring over hours to days.

B. Regulated Protein Degradation

The content of an enzyme in the cell can be altered through selective regulated degradation as well as through regulated synthesis. Although all proteins in the cell can be degraded with a characteristic half-life within lysosomes, protein degradation via two specialized systems, proteosomes and caspases, is highly selective and regulated. Protein degradation is dealt with in more detail in Chapter 37.

V. REGULATION OF METABOLIC PATHWAYS

The different means of regulating enzyme activity described above are used to control metabolic pathways, cellular events, and physiologic processes to match the body's requirements. Although many metabolic pathways are present in the body, a few common themes or principles are involved in their regulation. Of course, the overriding principle is: ***Regulation of a pathway matches its function.***

A. Principles of Pathway Regulation

Metabolic pathways are a series of sequential reactions in which the product of one reaction is the substrate of the next reaction (Fig. 9.15). Each step or reaction is usually catalyzed by a separate enzyme. The enzymes of a pathway have a common function—conversion of substrate to the final endproducts of the pathway. A pathway also may have a branchpoint at which an intermediate becomes the precursor for another pathway.

1. REGULATION OCCURS AT THE RATE-LIMITING STEP

Pathways are principally regulated at one key enzyme, the regulatory enzyme, which catalyzes the rate-limiting step in the pathway. This is the slowest step and is usually not readily reversible. Thus, changes in the rate-limiting step can influence flux through the rest of the pathway (see Fig. 9.1). The rate-limiting step is usually the first committed step in a pathway, or a reaction that is related to, or influenced

The maximal capacity of MEOS (cytochrome P450-2E1) is increased in the liver with continued ingestion of ethanol through a mechanism involving induction of gene transcription. Thus, **Al Martini** has a higher capacity to oxidize ethanol to acetaldehyde than a naive drinker (a person not previously subjected to alcohol). Nevertheless, the persistence of his elevated blood alcohol level shows he has saturated his capacity for ethanol oxidation (V-maxed out). Once his enzymes are operating near V_{max}, any additional ethanol he drinks will not appreciably increase the rate of ethanol clearance from his blood.

During fasting or infective stress, protein degradation in skeletal muscle is activated to increase the supply of amino acids in the blood for gluconeogenesis, or for the synthesis of antibodies and other component of the immune response. Under these conditions, synthesis of ubiquitin, a protein that targets proteins for degradation in proteosomes, is increased by the steroid hormone cortisol.

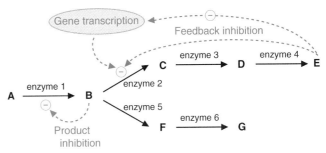

Fig. 9.15. A common pattern for feedback inhibition of metabolic pathways. The letters represent compounds formed from different enzymes in the reaction pathway. Compound B is at a metabolic branchpoint: it can go down one pathway to E or down an alternate pathway to G. The endproduct of the pathway, E, might control its own synthesis by allosterically inhibiting enzyme 2, the first committed step of the pathway, or inhibiting transcription of the gene for enzyme 2. As a result of the feedback inhibition, B accumulates and more B enters the pathway for conversion to G, which could be a storage, or disposal pathway. In this hypothetical pathway, B is a product inhibitor of enzyme 1, competitive with respect to A. Precursor A might induce the synthesis of enzyme 1, which would allow more A to go to G.

The pathways of energy production must be regulated by a mechanism that can respond rapidly to requirements for more ATP, such as the allosteric regulation of glycogen phosphorylase by AMP. However, storage pathways or biosynthetic pathways can be regulated by a mechanism that responds more slowly to changing conditions. For example, cholesterol partially feedback regulates its own rate of synthesis by decreasing transcription of the gene for the rate-limiting enzyme (HMG-CoA reductase). The enzyme concentration of a tissue may change even more slowly in response to developmental changes.

When **Ann O'Rexia** jogs, the increased use of ATP for muscle contraction results in an increase of AMP, which allosterically activates both the allosteric enzyme phosphofructokinase-1, the rate-limiting enzyme of glycolysis, and glycogen phosphorylase, the rate-limiting enzyme of glycogenolysis. This is an example of *feedback regulation* by the ATP/AMP ratio. Unfortunately, her low caloric consumption has not allowed *feed-forward activation* of the rate-limiting enzymes in her fuel storage pathways, and she has very low glycogen stores. Consequently, she has inadequate fuel stores to supply the increased energy demands of exercise.

by, the first committed step. Additional regulated enzymes occur after each metabolic branchpoint to direct flow into the branch. (e.g., in Fig. 9.15, feedback inhibition of enzyme 2 results in accumulation of B, which enzyme 5 then uses for synthesis of compound G). Inhibition of the rate-limiting enzyme in a pathway usually leads to accumulation of the pathway precursor.

2. FEEDBACK REGULATION

Feedback regulation refers to a situation in which the endproduct of a pathway controls its own rate of synthesis (see Fig. 9.15). Feedback regulation usually involves allosteric regulation of the rate-limiting enzyme by the endproduct of a pathway (or a compound that reflects changes in the concentration of the endproduct). The endproduct of a pathway may also control its own synthesis by inducing or repressing the gene for transcription of the rate-limiting enzyme in the pathway. This type of regulation is much slower to respond to changing conditions than allosteric regulation.

3. FEED-FORWARD REGULATION

Certain pathways, such as those involved in the disposal of toxic compounds, are feed-forward regulated. Feed-forward regulation may occur through an increased supply of substrate to an enzyme with a high K_m, allosteric activation of a rate-limiting enzyme through a compound related to substrate supply, substrate-related induction of gene transcription (e.g., induction of cytochrome P450-2E1 by ethanol), or increased concentration of a hormone that stimulates a storage pathway by controlling enzyme phosphorylation state.

4. TISSUE ISOZYMES OF REGULATORY PROTEINS

The human body is composed of a number of different cell types that perform specific functions unique to that cell type and synthesize only the proteins consistent with their functions. Because regulation matches function, regulatory enzymes of pathways usually exist as tissue-specific isozymes with somewhat different regulatory properties unique to their function in different cell types. For example, hexokinase and glucokinase are tissue-specific isozymes with different kinetic properties.

5. COUNTER-REGULATION OF OPPOSING PATHWAYS

A pathway for the synthesis of a compound usually has one or more enzymatic steps that differ from the pathway for degradation of that compound. A biosynthetic pathway can therefore have a different regulatory enzyme than the opposing degradative pathway, and one pathway can be activated while the other is inhibited (e.g., glycogen synthesis is activated while glycogen degradation is inhibited).

6. SUBSTRATE CHANNELING THROUGH COMPARTMENTATION

In the cell, compartmentation of enzymes into multienzyme complexes or organelles provides a means of regulation, either because the compartment provides unique conditions or because it limits or channels access of the enzymes to substrates. Enzymes or pathways with a common function are often assembled into organelles. For example, enzymes of the TCA cycle are all located within the mitochondrion. The enzymes catalyze sequential reactions, and the product of one reaction is the substrate for the next reaction. The concentration of the pathway intermediates remains much higher within the mitochondrion than in the surrounding cellular cytoplasm.

Another type of compartmentation involves the assembly of enzymes catalyzing sequential reactions into multi-enzyme complexes so that intermediates of the pathway can be directly transferred from the active site on one enzyme to the active site on another enzyme, thereby preventing loss of energy and information.

7. LEVELS OF COMPLEXITY

You may have noticed by now that regulation of metabolic pathways in the human is exceedingly complex; this might be called the second principle of metabolic regulation. As you study different pathways in the subsequent chapters of the text, it may help to develop diagrams such as Fig. 9.15 to keep track of the function and rationale behind different regulatory interactions.

The different isozymes of hexokinase (e.g., hexokinase I and glucokinase) are tissue-specific isozymes that arose through gene duplication. Glucokinase, the low-affinity enzyme found in liver, is a single polypeptide chain with a molecular weight of 55 kDa that contains one active catalytic site. The hexokinases found in erythrocytes, skeletal muscles, and most other tissues are 110 kDa and are essentially two mutated glucokinase molecules synthesized as one polypeptide chain. However, only one catalytic site is functional. All of the tissue-specific hexokinases but glucokinase have K_ms for glucose that are less than 0.2 mM.

An example of a multi-enzyme complex is provided by MEOS (microsomal ethanol oxidizing system), which is composed of two different subunits with different enzyme activities. One subunit transfers electrons from NADPH to a cytochrome Fe-heme group on the 2nd subunit, which then transfers the electrons to O_2.

CLINICAL COMMENTS

Al Martini. In the Emergency Room, **Al Martini** was evaluated for head injuries. From the physical examination and blood alcohol levels, it was determined that his mental state resulted from his alcohol consumption. Although his chronic ethanol consumption had increased his level of MEOS (and, therefore, rate of ethanol oxidation in his liver), his excessive drinking resulted in a blood alcohol level greater than the legal limit of 80 mg/dL. He suffered bruises and contusions but was otherwise uninjured. He left in the custody of the police officer.

Ann O'Rexia. Ann O'Rexia's physician explained that she had inadequate fuel stores for her exercise program. To jog, her muscles require an increased rate of fuel oxidation to generate the ATP for muscle contraction. The fuels used by muscles for exercise include glucose from muscle glycogen, fatty acids from adipose tissue triacylglycerols, and blood glucose supplied by liver glycogen. These fuel stores were depleted during her prolonged bout of starvation. In addition, starvation resulted in the loss of muscle mass as muscle protein was being degraded to supply amino acids for other processes, including gluconeogenesis (the synthesis of glucose from amino acids and other noncarbohydrate precursors). Therefore, Ann will need to increase her caloric consumption to rebuild her fuel stores. Her physician helped her calculate the

The hormone epinephrine (released during stress and exercise) and glucagon (released during fasting) activate the synthesis of cAMP in a number of tissues. cAMP activates protein kinase A. Because protein kinase A is able to phosphorylate key regulatory enzymes in many pathways, these pathways can be coordinately regulated. In muscle, for example, glycogen degradation is activated while glycogen synthesis is inhibited. At the same time, fatty acid release from adipose tissue is activated to provide more fuel for muscle. The regulation of glycolysis, glycogen metabolism, and other pathways of metabolism is much more complex than we have illustrated here and is discussed in many subsequent chapters of this text.

additional amount of calories her jogging program will need, and they discussed which foods she would eat to meet these increased caloric requirements. He also helped her visualize the increase of weight as an increase in strength.

BIOCHEMICAL COMMENTS

The Lineweaver-Burk transformation. The K_m and V_{max} for an enzyme can be visually determined from a plot of $1/v_i$ versus $1/S$, called a Lineweaver-Burk or a double reciprocal plot. The reciprocal of both sides of the Michaelis-Menten equation generates an equation that has the form of a straight line, $y = mx + b$ (Fig. 9.16). K_m and V_{max} are equal to the reciprocals of the intercepts on the abscissa and ordinate, respectively. Although double reciprocal plots are often used to illustrate certain features of enzyme reactions, they are not directly used for the determination of K_m and V_{max} values by researchers.

For the reaction in which an enzyme forms a complex with both substrates, the K_m for one substrate can vary with the concentration of cosubstrate (Fig. 9.17). At each constant concentration of cosubstrate, the plot of $1/v_i$ vs $1/[S]$ is a straight line. To obtain V_{max}, the graph must be extrapolated to saturating concentrations of both substrates, which is equivalent to the intersection point of these lines for different cosubstrate concentrations.

Lineweaver-Burk plots provide a good illustration of competitive inhibition and pure noncompetitive inhibition (Fig. 9.18). In competitive inhibition, plots of $1/v$ vs $1/[S]$ at a series of inhibitor concentrations intersect on the ordinate. Thus, at infinite substrate concentration, or $1/[S] = 0$, there is no effect of the inhibitor. In pure noncompetitive inhibition, the inhibitor decreases the velocity even when [S] has been extrapolated to an infinite concentration. However, if the inhibitor has no effect on the binding of the substrate, the K_m is the same for every concentration of inhibitor, and the lines intersect on the abcissa.

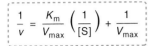

$$\frac{1}{v} = \frac{K_m}{V_{max}} \left(\frac{1}{[S]} \right) + \frac{1}{V_{max}}$$

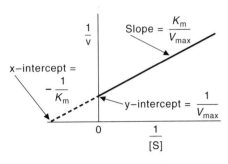

Fig. 9.16. The Lineweaver-Burk transformation (shown in blue) for the Michaelis-Menten equation converts it to a straight line of the form $y = mx + b$. When [S] is infinite, $1/[S] = 0$, and the line crosses the ordinate (y-axis) at $1/v = 1/V_{max}$. The slope of the line is K_m/V_{max}. Where the line intersects the abscissa (x-axis), $1/[S] = -1/K_m$.

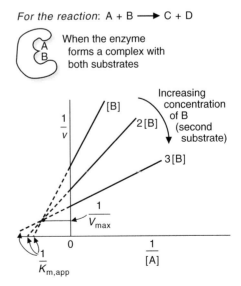

Fig. 9.17. A Lineweaver-Burk plot for a two-substrate reaction in which A and B are converted to products. In the graph, $1/[A]$ is plotted against $1/v$ for three different concentrations of the cosubstrate, [B], 2[B], and 3[B]. As the concentration of B is increased, the intersection on the abscissa, equal to $1/K_{m,app}$ is increased. The "app" represents "apparent", as the $K_{m,app}$ is the K_m at whatever concentration of cosubstrate, inhibitor, or other factor is present during the experiment.

A. Competitive inhibition

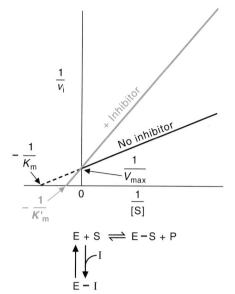

B. Pure noncompetitive inhibition

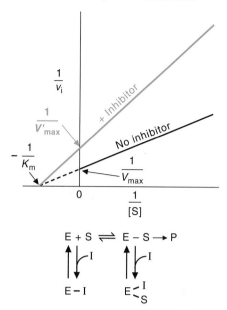

Fig. 9.18. Lineweaver-Burk plots of competitive and pure noncompetitive inhibition. A. $1/v_i$ versus $1/[S]$ in the presence of a competitive inhibitor. The competitive inhibitor alters the intersection on the abscissa. The new intersection is $1/K_{m,app}$ (also called $1/K'_m$). A competitive inhibitor does not affect V_{max}. B. $1/v_i$ versus $1/[S]$ in the presence of a pure noncompetitive inhibitor. The noncompetitive inhibitor alters the intersection on the ordinate, $1/V_{max,app}$ or $1/V'_{max}$, but does not affect $1/K_m$. A pure noncompetitive inhibitor binds to E and ES with the same affinity. If the inhibitor has different affinities for E and ES, the lines will intersect above or below the abscissa, and the noncompetitive inhibitor will change both the K'_m and the V'_m.

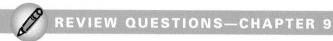

REVIEW QUESTIONS—CHAPTER 9

1. Which of the following describes a characteristic feature of an enzyme obeying Michaelis-Menten kinetics?

    (A) The enzyme velocity is at ½ the maximal rate when 100% of the enzyme molecules contain bound substrate.
    (B) The enzyme velocity is at ½ the maximal rate when 50% of the enzyme molecules contain bound substrate.
    (C) The enzyme velocity is at its maximal rate when 50% of the enzyme molecules contain bound substrate.
    (D) The enzyme velocity is at its maximal rate when all of the substrate molecules in solution are bound by the enzyme.
    (E) The velocity of the reaction is independent of the concentration of enzyme.

2. The pancreatic glucokinase of a patient with MODY had a mutation replacing a leucine with a proline. The result was that the K_m for glucose was decreased from a normal value of 6 mM to a value of 2.2 mM, and the V_{max} was changed from 93 units/mg protein to 0.2 units/mg protein. Which of the following best describes the patient's glucokinase compared with the normal enzyme?

    (A) The patient's enzyme requires a lower concentration of glucose to reach ½ V_{max}.
    (B) The patient's enzyme is faster than the normal enzyme at concentrations of glucose below 2.2 mM.
    (C) The patient's enzyme is faster than the normal enzyme at concentrations of glucose above 2.2 mM.
    (D) At near saturating glucose concentration, the patient would need 90 to 100 times more enzyme than normal to achieve normal rates of glucose phosphorylation.
    (E) As blood glucose levels increase after a meal from a fasting value of 5 mM to 10 mM, the rate of the patient's enzyme will increase more than the rate of the normal enzyme.

3. Methanol (CH_3OH) is converted by alcohol dehydrogenases to formaldehyde (CHO), a compound that is highly toxic in the human. Patients who have ingested toxic levels of methanol are sometimes treated with ethanol (CH_3CH_2OH) to inhibit methanol oxidation by alcohol dehydrogenase. Which of the following statements provides the best rationale for this treatment?

   (A) Ethanol is a structural analog of methanol, and might therefore be an effective noncompetitive inhibitor.
   (B) Ethanol is a structural analog of methanol that would be expected to compete with methanol for its binding site on the enzyme.
   (C) Ethanol would be expected to alter the V_{max} of alcohol dehydrogenase for the oxidation of methanol to formaldehyde.
   (D) Ethanol would be an effective inhibitor of methanol oxidation regardless of the concentration of methanol.
   (E) Ethanol would be expected to inhibit the enzyme by binding to the formaldehyde binding site on the enzyme, even though it cannot bind at the substrate binding site for methanol.

4. Which of the following describes a characteristic of most allosteric enzymes?

   (A) They are composed of single subunits.
   (B) In the absence of effectors, they generally follow Michaelis-Menten kinetics.
   (C) They show cooperativity in substrate binding.
   (D) They have allosteric activators that bind in the catalytic site.
   (E) They have irreversible allosteric inhibitors that bind at allosteric sites.

5. A rate-limiting enzyme catalyzes the first step in the conversion of a toxic metabolite to a urinary excretion product. Which of the following mechanisms for regulating this enzyme would provide the most protection to the body?

   (A) The product of the pathway should be an allosteric inhibitor of the rate-limiting enzyme.
   (B) The product of the pathway should act through gene transcription to decrease synthesis of the enzyme.
   (C) The toxin should act through gene transcription to increase synthesis of the enzyme.
   (D) The enzyme should have a high K_m for the toxin.
   (E) The product of the first enzyme should allosterically activate the subsequent enzyme in the pathway.

10 Relationship between Cell Biology and Biochemistry

The basic unit of a living organism is the cell. In the human, each tissue is composed of similar cell types, which differ from those in other tissues. The diversity of cell types serves the function of the tissue and organs in which they reside, and each cell type has unique structural features that reflect its role. In spite of their diversity in structure, human cell types have certain architectural features in common, such as the plasma membrane, membranes around the nucleus and organelles, and a cytoskeleton (Fig. 10.1). In this chapter, we review some of the chemical characteristics of these common features, the functions of organelles, and the transport systems for compounds into cells and between organelles.

Plasma membrane. *The cell membrane is a **lipid bilayer** that serves as a selective barrier; it restricts the entry and exit of compounds. Within the plasma membrane, different **integral proteins** facilitate the **transport** of specific compounds by*

The cells of humans and other animals are eukaryotes (eu, good; karyon, nucleus) because the genetic material is organized into a membrane-enclosed nucleus. In contrast, bacteria are prokaryotes (pro, before; karyon, nucleus); they do not contain nuclei or other organelles found in eukaryotic cells.

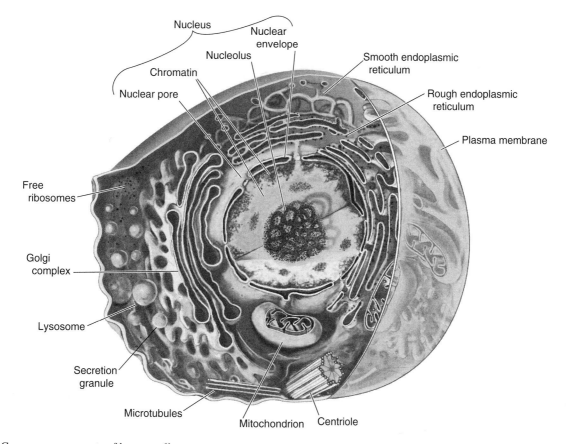

Fig. 10.1. Common components of human cells.

The cytoplasm of the cell is the portion of the cell between the cell membrane and the nucleus. Mitochondria, lysososmes and peroxisomes are referred to as cytoplasmic organelles. The Golgi and the endoplasmic reticulum are referred to as cytoplasmic membrane systems. The plasma membrane can be gently disrupted by detergents or shear stress without damage to the other membrane systems. When a suspension that has been treated this way is centrifuged for a long period of time (100,000g for 1 hour), the organelles and membrane systems will collect at the bottom of the tube. The remaining clear liquid of soluble enzymes, cofactors, and metabolites is the cytosol.

energy-requiring active transport, *facilitated diffusion*, or by forming **pores** or **gated-channels**. *The plasma membrane is supported by a **membrane skeleton** composed of proteins.*

Organelles *and* **cytoplasmic membrane systems**. *Most organelles within the cell are compartments surrounded by a membrane system that restricts exchange of compounds and information with other compartments (see Fig. 10.1). In general, each organelle has unique functions that are served by the enzymes and other compounds it contains, or the environment it maintains.* **Lysosomes** *contain* **hydrolytic enzymes** *that degrade proteins and other large molecules. The* **nucleus** *contains the genetic material and carries out* **gene replication** *and* **transcription** *of* **DNA***, the first step of protein synthesis. The last phase of protein synthesis occurs on* **ribosomes***. For certain proteins, the ribosomes become attached to the complex membrane system called the* **endoplasmic reticulum***; for other proteins, synthesis is completed on ribosomes that remain in the cytoplasm. The* **endoplasmic reticulum** *is also involved in lipid synthesis and transport of molecules to the Golgi. The* **Golgi** *forms vesicles for transport of molecules to the plasma membrane and other membrane systems, and for secretion.* **Mitochondria** *are organelles of* **fuel oxidation** *and* **ATP generation***.* **Peroxisomes** *contain many enzymes that use or produce* **hydrogen peroxide***. The* **cytosol** *is the intracellular compartment free of organelles and membrane systems.*

Cytoskeleton*. The* **cytoskeleton** *is a flexible fibrous protein support system that maintains the geometry of the cell, fixes the position of organelles, and moves compounds within the cell or the cell itself. It is composed principally of* **actin microfilaments***,* **intermediate filaments***,* **tubulin microtubules***, and their attached proteins.*

THE WAITING ROOM

Al Martini had been drinking heavily when he drove his car off the road and was taken to the hospital emergency room (see Chapters 8 and 9). Although he suffered only minor injuries, his driving license was suspended.

Two years after **Dennis "the Menace" Veere** successfully recovered from his malathion poisoning, he visited his grandfather, **Percy Veere**. Mr. Veere took Dennis with him to a picnic at the shore, where they ate steamed crabs. Later that night, Dennis experienced episodes of vomiting and watery diarrhea, and Mr. Veere rushed him to the hospital emergency room. Dennis's hands and feet were cold, he appeared severely dehydrated, and he was approaching hypovolemic shock (a severe drop in blood pressure). He was diagnosed with cholera, caused by the bacteria *Vibrio cholerae*.

V. cholerae epidemics are associated with unsanitary conditions affecting the drinking water supply and are rare in the United States. However, these bacteria grow well under the alkaline conditions found in seawater and attach to chitin in shellfish. Thus, sporadic cases occur in the southeast United States associated with the ingestion of contaminated shellfish.

Before **Lotta Topaigne** was treated with allopurinol (see Chapter 8), her physician administered colchicine (acetyltrimethylcolchicinic acid) for the acute attack of gout affecting her great toe. After taking a high dose of colchicine divided over several-hour intervals, the throbbing pain in her toe had abated significantly. The redness and swelling also seemed to have lessened slightly.

Cell lysis, the breaking of the cell membrane and release of cell contents, occurs when the continuity of the cell membrane is disrupted.

I.   COMPARTMENTATION IN CELLS

Membranes are lipid structures that separate the contents of the compartment they surround from its environment. An outer plasma membrane separates the cell from the external aqueous environment. Organelles (such as the nucleus, mitochondria, lysosomes, and peroxisomes) are also surrounded by a membrane system that separates the internal compartment of the organelle from the cytosol. The function of these membranes is to collect or concentrate enzymes and other molecules serving a common function into a compartment with a localized environment. The transporters and receptors in each membrane system control this localized environment and communication of the cell or organelle with the surrounding milieu.

The following sections describe various organelles and membrane systems found in most human cells and outline the relationship between their properties and function. Each organelle has different enzymes and carries out different general functions. For example, the nucleus contains the enzymes for DNA and RNA synthesis.

Not all cells in the human are alike. Different cell types differ quantitatively in their organelle content, or their organelles may contain vastly different amounts of a particular enzyme, *consistent with the function of the cell.* For example, liver mitochondria contain a key enzyme for synthesizing ketone bodies, but they lack a key enzyme for their use. The reverse is true in muscle mitochondria. Thus, the enzymic content of the organelles varies somewhat from cell type to cell type.

II. PLASMA MEMBRANE

A. Structure of the Plasma Membrane

All mammalian cells are enclosed by a plasma membrane composed of a lipid bilayer (two layers) containing embedded proteins (Fig. 10.2). The membranes are continuous and sealed so that the hydrophobic lipid bilayer selectively restricts the exchange of polar compounds between the external fluid and the intracellular compartment. The membrane is referred to as a fluid mosaic because it consists of a mosaic of proteins and lipid molecules that can, for the most part, move laterally in the plane of the membrane. The proteins are classified as integral proteins, which span the cell membrane, or peripheral proteins, which are attached to the membrane surface through electrostatic bonds to lipids or integral proteins. Many of the proteins and lipids on the external leaflet contain covalently bound carbohydrate chains and therefore are glycoproteins and glycolipids. This layer of carbohydrate on the outer surface of the cell is called the glycocalyx.

1. LIPIDS IN THE PLASMA MEMBRANE

Each layer of the plasma membrane lipid bilayer is formed primarily by phospholipids, which are arranged with their hydrophilic head groups facing the aqueous medium and their fatty acyl tails forming a hydrophobic membrane core (see Fig. 10.2). The principle phospholipids in the membrane are the glycerol lipids phosphatidylcholine, phosphatidylethanolamine, and phosphatidylserine and the sphingolipid sphingomyelin (Fig. 10.3). The lipid composition varies among different cell types, with phosphatidylcholine being the major plasma membrane lipid in most cell types and sphingolipids the most variable.

The lipid composition of the bilayer is asymmetric, with a higher content of phosphatidylcholine and sphingomyelin in the outer leaflet and a higher content of phosphatidylserine and phosphatidylethanolamine in the inner leaflet. Phosphatidylserine contains a net negative charge that contributes to the membrane potential and might be important for binding positively charged molecules within the cell. Phosphatidylinositol, which is found only in the inner membrane, functions in the transfer of information from hormones and neurotransmitters across the cell membrane into the cell (Fig. 10.4).

Bacteria are single cells surrounded by a cell membrane and a cell wall exterior to the membrane. They are prokaryotes, which do not contain nuclei or other organelles (i.e. membrane-surrounded subcellular structures) found in eukaryotic cells. Nonetheless, bacteria carry out many similar metabolic pathways, with the enzymes located in either the intracellular compartment or the cell membrane.

The *Vibrio cholerae* responsible for **Dennis Veere's** cholera are gram-negative bacteria. Their plasma membrane is surrounded by a thin cell wall composed of a protein–polysaccharide structure called peptidoglycan and an outer membrane. In contrast, gram-positive bacteria have a plasma membrane and a thick peptidoglycan cell wall that retains the Gram stain. *Vibrio* grow best under aerobic conditions, but also can grow under low oxygen conditions. They possess enzymes similar to those in human cells for glycolysis, the TCA cycle, and oxidative phosphorylation. They have a low tolerance for acid, which partially accounts for their presence in slightly basic seawater and shellfish.

The variable carbohydrate components of the glycolipids on the cell surface function as cell recognition markers. For example, the A, B, or O blood groups are determined by the carbohydrate composition of the glycolipids. Cell surface glycolipids may also serve as binding sites for viruses and bacterial toxins before penetrating the cell. For example, the cholera AB toxin binds to GM_1-gangliosides on the surface of the intestinal epithelial cells. The toxin is then endocytosed in caveolae (invaginations or "caves" that can form in specific regions of the membrane).

One of the bacterial toxins secreted by *Clostridium perefringens,* the bacteria that cause gas gangrene, is a lipase that hydrolyzes phosphocholine from phosphatidylcholine and from sphingomyelin. The resulting lysis of the cell membrane releases intracellular contents that provide the bacteria with nutrients for rapid growth. These bacteria are strict anaerobes and grow only in the absence of oxygen. As their toxins lyse membranes in the endothelial cells of blood vessels, the capillaries are destroyed, and the bacteria are protected from oxygen transported by the red blood cells. They are also protected from antibiotics and components of the immune system carried in the blood.

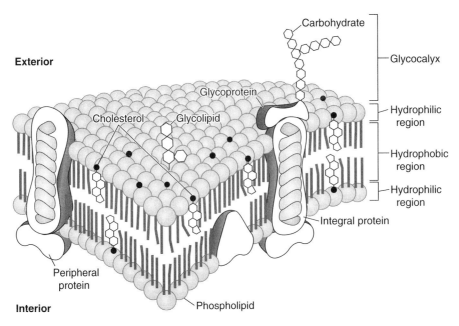

Fig. 10.2. Basic structure of an animal cell membrane.

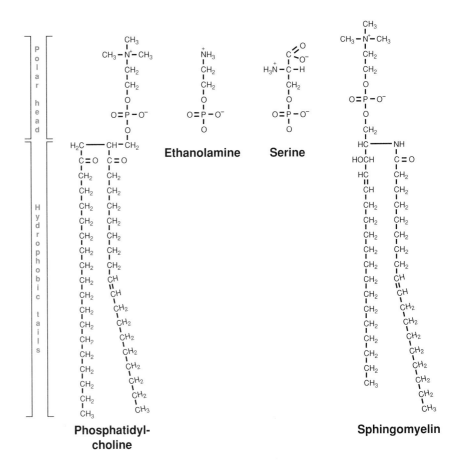

Fig. 10.3. Common phospholipids in the mammalian cell membrane. The polar head groups shown for ethanolamine and serine replace the choline in phosphatidylcholine to form phosphatidylethanolamine and phosphatidylserine, respectively. Phosphatidylcholine, phosphatidylethanolamine, and phosphatidylserine are phosphoacylglycerols. In contrast, sphingomyelin does not contain the glycerol backbone but has a sphingosine backbone and is a sphingolipid.

**Phosphatidylinositol
4,5–bisphosphate
(PIP$_2$)**

Fig. 10.4. Phosphatidylinositol bisphosphate (PIP$_2$). R1 and R2 are fatty acyl chains. The portion of PIP$_2$ that becomes inositol triphosphate, the polar head group extending into the cytosol, is shown in blue.

Cholesterol, which is interspersed between the phospholipids, maintains membrane fluidity. In the phosphoacylglycerols, unsaturated fatty acid chains bent into the *cis* conformation form a pocket for cholesterol, which binds with its hydroxyl group in the external hydrophilic region of the membrane and its hydrophobic steroid nucleus in the hydrophobic membrane core (Fig. 10.5). The presence of cholesterol and the *cis* unsaturated fatty acids in the membrane prevent the hydrophobic chains from packing too closely together. As a consequence, lipid and protein molecules that are not bound to external or internal structural proteins can rotate and move laterally in the plane of the leaflet. This movement enables the plasma membrane to partition between daughter cells during cell division, to

Al Martini is suffering from both short-term and long-term effects of ethanol on his central nervous system. Data support the theory that the short-term effects of ethanol on the brain partially arise from an increase in membrane fluidity caused when ethanol intercalates between the membrane lipids. The changes in membrane fluidity may affect proteins that span the membrane (integral proteins), such as ion channels and receptors for neurotransmitters involved in conducting the nerve impulse.

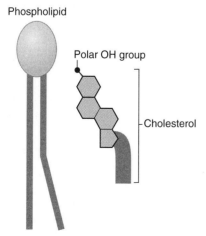

Fig. 10.5. Cholesterol in the plasma membrane. The polar hydroxyl group of cholesterol is oriented toward the surface. The hydrocarbon tail and the steroid nucleus (blue) lie in the hydrophobic core. A *cis* double bond in the fatty acyl chain of a phospholipid bends the chain to create a hydrophobic binding site for cholesterol.

deform as cells pass through capillaries, and to form and fuse with vesicle membranes. The fluidity of the membrane is partially determined by the unsaturated fatty acid content of the diet.

The composition of the membrane is dynamic. Sections of membrane form buds that pinch off into vesicles and membrane vesicles formed in the Golgi and elsewhere bring new and recycled components back to the membrane. Individual fatty acyl chains turn over as they are hydrolyzed from the lipids and replaced, and enzymes called flipases transfer lipids between leaflets.

2.   PROTEINS IN THE PLASMA MEMBRANE

The integral proteins contain transmembrane domains with hydrophobic amino acid side chains that interact with the hydrophobic portions of the lipids to seal the membrane (see Fig. 10.2). Hydrophilic regions of the proteins protrude into the aqueous medium on both sides of the membrane. Many of these proteins function as either channels or transporters for the movement of compounds across the membrane, as receptors for the binding of hormones and neurotransmitters, or as structural proteins (Fig. 10.6).

Peripheral membrane proteins, which were originally defined as those proteins that can be released from the membrane by ionic solvents, are bound through weak electrostatic interactions with the polar head groups of lipids or with integral proteins. One of the best-characterized classes of peripheral proteins is the spectrin family of proteins, which are bound to the intracellular membrane surface and provide mechanical support for the membrane. Spectrin is bound to actin, which together form a structure that is called the inner membrane skeleton or the cortical skeleton (see Fig. 10.6).

A third classification of membrane proteins consists of lipid-anchored proteins bound to the inner or outer surface of the membrane. The glycophosphatidylinositolglycan (GPI) anchor is a covalently attached lipid that anchors proteins to the

Two of the prominent integral proteins in the red blood cell membrane are glycophorin, which provides an external negative charge that repels other cells, and band 3, which is a channel for bicarbonate and chloride exchange. The transport of bicarbonate into the red blood cell in exchange for chloride helps to carry the bicarbonate to the lungs, where it is expired as CO_2.

All cells contain an inner membrane skeleton of spectrin-like proteins. Red blood cell spectrin was the first member of the spectrin family described. The protein dystrophin present in skeletal muscle cells is a member of the spectrin family. Genetic defects in the dystrophin gene are responsible for Duchenne's and Becker's muscular dystrophies.

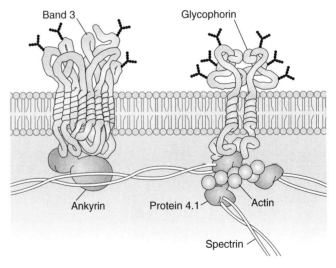

Fig. 10.6. Proteins in the red blood cell membrane. The proteins named Band 3 (the bicarbonate-chloride exchange transporter) and glycophorin contain nonpolar α-helical segments spanning the lipid bilayer. These proteins contain a large number of polar and charged hydrophilic amino acids in the intracellular and extracellular domains. On the inside of the cell, they are attached to peripheral proteins constituting the inner membrane skeleton. Band 3 is connected to spectrin filaments via the protein ankyrin. Glycophorin is connected to short actin filaments and spectrin via protein 4.1.

external surface of the membrane (Fig.10.7). A number of proteins involved in hormonal regulation are anchored to the internal surface of the membrane through palmityl (C16) or myristyl (C14) fatty acyl groups or through geranylgeranyl (C20) or farnesyl (C15) isoprenyl groups (see Ras, Chapter 9, Fig. 9.14, or Chapter 6, Fig. 6.14). However, many integral proteins also contain attached lipid groups to increase their stability in the membrane.

3.   THE GLYCOCALYX OF THE PLASMA MEMBRANE

Some of the proteins and lipids on the external surface of the membrane contain short chains of carbohydrates (oligosaccharides) that extend into the aqueous medium. Carbohydrates therefore constitute 2 to10% of the weight of plasma membranes. This hydrophilic carbohydrate layer, called the glycocalyx, protects the cell against digestion and restricts the uptake of hydrophobic compounds.

The glycoproteins generally contain branched oligosaccharide chains of approximately 15 sugar residues that are attached through N-glycosidic bonds to the amide nitrogen of an asparagine side chain (N-glycosidic linkage), or through a glycosidic bond to the oxygen of serine (O-glycoproteins). The membrane glycolipids are usually galactosides or cerebrosides. Specific carbohydrate chains on the glycolipids serve as cell recognition molecules (see Chapter 5 for structures of classes of compounds).

B. Transport of Molecules across the Plasma Membrane

Membranes form hydrophobic barriers around cells to control the internal environment by restricting the entry and exit of molecules. As a consequence, cells require transport systems to permit entry of small polar compounds that they need (e.g., glucose) to concentrate compounds inside the cell (e.g., K^+) and to expel other

 The prion protein, present in neuronal membranes, provides an example of a protein attached to the membrane through a GPI anchor. This is the protein that develops an altered pathogenic conformation in both mad cow disease and Creutzfeldt-Jakob disease (see Chapter 7, Biochemical Comments).

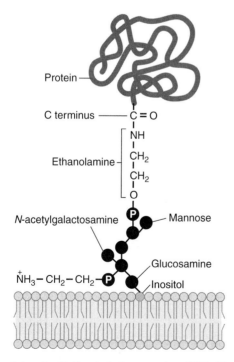

Fig. 10.7. The glycosylphosphatidylinositol glycan anchor (GPI). The carboxy terminus of the protein is attached to phosphoethanolamine, which is bound to a branched oligosaccharide that is attached to the inositol portion of phosphatidylinositol. The hydrophobic fatty acyl chains of the phosphatidylinositol portion are bound in the hydrophobic core of the membrane.

compounds (e.g., Ca^{2+} and Na^+). The transport systems for small organic molecules and inorganic ions fall into four categories: simple diffusion through the lipid bilayer or through a large pore; facilitative diffusion; gated channels; and active transport pumps (Fig. 10.8). These transport mechanisms are classified as passive if energy is not required, or active if energy is required. The energy is often provided by the hydrolysis of ATP.

In addition to these mechanisms for the transport of small individual molecules, cells engage in endocytosis. The plasma membrane extends or invaginates to surround a particle, a foreign cell, or extracellular fluid, which then closes into a vesicle that is released into the cytoplasm (see Fig. 10.8).

1. SIMPLE DIFFUSION

Gases such as O_2 and CO_2 and lipid-soluble substances (such as steroid hormones) can cross membranes by simple diffusion (see Fig. 10.8). In simple diffusion (free diffusion), molecules move by engaging in random collisions with other like molecules. There is a net movement from a region of high concentration to a region of low concentration because molecules keep bumping into each other where their concentration is highest. Energy is not required for diffusion, and compounds that are uncharged eventually reach the same concentrations on both sides of the membrane.

Water is considered to diffuse through membranes by unspecific movement through ion channels, pores, or around proteins embedded in the lipids. Certain cells (e.g., renal tubule cells) also contain large protein pores, called aquaporins, which permit a high rate of water flow from a region of a high water concentration (low solute concentration) to one of low water concentration (high solute concentration).

2. FACILITATIVE DIFFUSION THROUGH BINDING
TO TRANSPORTER PROTEINS

Facilitative diffusion requires that the transported molecule bind to a specific carrier or transport protein in the membrane (Fig. 10.9). The transporter protein

Dennis Veere has become dehydrated because he has lost so much water through vomiting and diarrhea (see Chapter 4). Cholera toxin increases the efflux of sodium and chloride ions from his intestinal mucosal cells into the intestinal lumen. The increase of water in his stools results from the passive transfer of water from inside the cell and body fluids, where it is in high concentration (i.e., intracellular Na^+ and Cl^- concentrations are low), to the intestinal lumen and bowel, where water is in lower concentration (relative to high Na^+ and Cl^-). The watery diarrhea is also high in K^+ ions and bicarbonate. All of the signs and symptoms of cholera generally derive from this fluid loss.

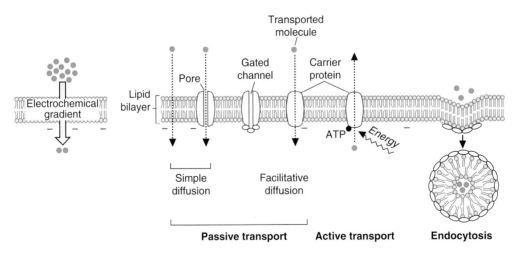

Fig. 10.8. Common types of transport mechanisms for human cells. The electrochemical gradient consists of the concentration gradient of the compound and the distribution of charge on the membrane, which affects the transport of charged ions such as Cl^-. Both protein amino acid residues and lipid polar head groups contribute to the net negative charge on the inside of the membrane. Generally, the diffusion of uncharged molecules (passive transport) is net movement from a region of high concentration to a low concentration, and active transport (energy-requiring) is net movement from a region of low concentration to one of high concentration.

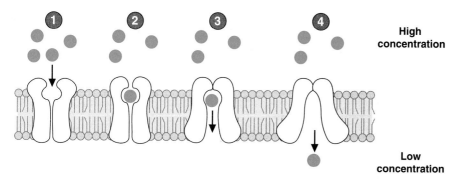

High concentration

Low concentration

Fig. 10.9. Facilitative transport. Although the molecule being transported must bind to the protein transporter, the mechanism is passive diffusion, and the molecule moves from a region of high concentration to one of low concentration. "Passive" refers to the lack of an energy requirement for the transport.

 All of the cells in the body have facilitative glucose transporters that transport glucose across the plasma membrane down an electrochemical (concentration) gradient as it is rapidly metabolized in the cell. In muscle and adipose tissue, insulin increases the content of facilitative glucose transporters in the cell membrane, thus increasing the ability of these tissues to take up glucose. Patients with type 1 diabetes mellitus, who do not produce insulin (e.g., **Di Abietes**, see Chapter 7), have a decreased ability to transport glucose into these tissues, thereby contributing to hyperglycemia (high blood glucose).

then undergoes a conformational change that allows the transported molecule to be released on the other side of the membrane. Although the transported molecules are bound to proteins, the transport process is still classified as diffusion because energy is not required, and the compound equilibrates (achieves a balance of concentration and charge) on both sides of the membrane.

Transporter proteins, like enzymes, exhibit saturation kinetics; when all the binding sites on all of the transporter proteins in the membrane are occupied, the system is saturated and the rate of transport reaches a plateau (the maximum velocity). By analogy to enzymes, the concentration of a transported compound required to reach ½ the maximum velocity is often called the K_m (Fig. 10.10). Facilitative transporters are similar to enzymes with respect to two additional features: they are relatively specific for the compounds they bind and they can be inhibited by compounds that block their binding sites or change their conformation.

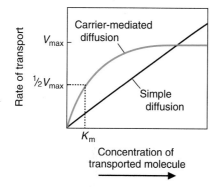

Fig. 10.10. Saturation kinetics of transporter proteins. When a compound must bind to a protein to be transported across a membrane, the velocity of transport depends on the amount of compound bound. It reaches a maximum rate when the compound's concentration is raised so high that all of the transporter binding sites are occupied. The curve is a rectangular hyperbola that approaches V_{max} at infinite substrate concentration, identical to that of Michaelis-Menten enzymes. The K_m of transport is the concentration of compound required for ½ V_{max}. In contrast, simple diffusion of a compound does not require its binding to a protein, and the rate of transport increases linearly with increasing concentration of the compound.

3. GATED CHANNELS IN PLASMA MEMBRANES

In gated channels, transmembrane proteins form a pore for ions that is either opened or closed in response to a stimulus: voltage changes across the membrane (voltage-gated channels), the binding of a compound (ligand-gated channels), or a regulatory change in the intracellular domain (phosphorylation-gated and pressure-gated channels). For example, the conduction of a nerve impulse along the axon depends on the passive flux of Na^+ ions through a voltage-gated channel that is opened by depolarization of the membrane. CFTR (**c**ystic **f**ibrosis **t**ransmembrane conductance **r**egulator) is a Cl^- channel that provides an example of a ligand-gated channel regulated through phosphorylation (phosphorylation-gated) (Fig. 10.11). CFTR is a member of the ABC (adenine nucleotide binding cassette, or ATP binding cassette) superfamily of transport proteins. It has two transmembrane domains that form a closed channel, each connected to an ATP binding site, and a regulatory domain that sits in front of the channel. When the regulatory domain is phosphorylated by a kinase, its conformation changes and it moves away from the ATP binding domains. As ATP binds and is hydrolyzed, the transmembrane domains change conformation and open the channel, and chloride ions diffuse through. As the conformation reverts back to its original form, the channel closes.

Transport through a ligand-gated channel is considered diffusion, although ATP is involved, because only a few ATP molecules are being used to open and close the channel through which many, many chloride ions diffuse. However, the distinction between ligand-gated channels and facilitative transporters is not always as clear. Many gated channels show saturation kinetics at very high concentrations of the compounds being transported.

4. ACTIVE TRANSPORT REQUIRES ENERGY AND TRANSPORTER PROTEINS

Both active transport and facilitative transport are mediated by protein transporters (carriers) in the membrane. However, in facilitative transport, the compound is transported down an electrochemical gradient (the balance of concentration and charge across a membrane), usually from a high concentration to a low concentration, to equilibrate between the two sides of the membrane. In active transport, energy is used to concentrate the compound on one side of the membrane. If energy is directly applied to the transporter (e.g., ATP hydrolysis by Na^+,K^+-ATPase), the transport is called primary active transport; if energy is used to establish an ion gradient (e.g., the Na^+ gradient), and the gradient is used to concentrate another compound, the transport is called secondary active transport.

The Na^+,K^+-ATPase spans the plasma membrane, much like a gated pore, with a binding site for 3 Na^+ ions open to the intracellular side (Fig. 10.12). Energy from

The cystic fibrosis transmembrane conductance regulator (CFTR) was named for its role in cystic fibrosis. A mutation in the gene encoding its transmembrane subunits results in dried mucus accumulation in the airways and pancreatic ducts.

The CFTR is also involved in the dehydration experienced by cholera patients such as **Dennis Veere**. In intestinal mucosal cells, cholera A toxin indirectly activates phosphorylation of the regulatory domain of CFTR by protein kinase A. Thus, the channel stays open and Cl^- and H_2O flow from the cell into the intestinal lumen, resulting in dehydration.

Protein-mediated transport systems, whether facilitative or active, are classified as antiports if they specifically exchange compounds of similar charge across a membrane; they are called symports or cotransporters if they simultaneously transport two molecules across the membrane in the same direction. Band 3 in the red blood cell membrane, which exchanges chloride ion for bicarbonate, provides an example of an antiport.

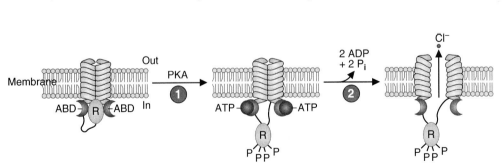

Fig. 10.11. CFTR, a ligand-gated channel controlled by phosphorylation. Two intracellular binding domains control opening of the channel, an adenine nucleotide binding domain (ABD) and a regulatory domain (R). **1.** Phosphorylation of the regulatory subunit by protein kinase A causes a conformational change that allows ATP to bind to the adenine nucleotide binding domain (ABD). **2.** Hydrolysis of bound ATP opens the channel so that chloride ions can diffuse through.

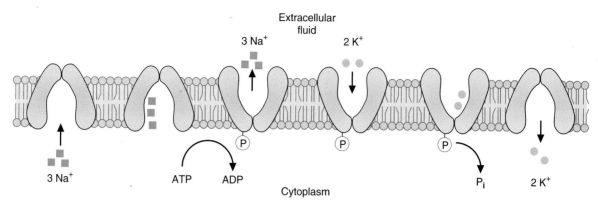

Fig. 10.12. Active transport by Na^+,K^+-ATPase. Three sodium ions bind to the transporter protein on the cytoplasmic side of the membrane. When ATP is hydrolyzed to ADP, the carrier protein is phosphorylated and undergoes a change in conformation that causes the sodium ions to be released into the extracellular fluid. Two potassium ions then bind on the extracellular side. Dephosphorylation of the carrier protein produces another conformational change, and the potassium ions are released on the inside of the cell membrane. The transporter protein then resumes its original conformation, ready to bind more sodium ions.

ATP hydrolysis is used to phosphorylate an internal domain and change the transporters' conformation so that bound Na^+ ions are released to the outside, and two external K^+ ions bind. K^+ binding triggers hydrolysis of the bound phosphate group and a return to the original conformation, accompanied by release of K^+ ions inside the cell. As a consequence, cells are able to maintain a much lower intracellular Na^+ concentration and much higher intracellular K^+ ion concentration than present in the external fluid.

The Na^+ gradient, which is maintained by primary active transport, is used to power the transport of glucose, amino acids, and many other compounds into the cell through secondary active transport. An example is provided by the transport of glucose into cells of the intestinal epithelium in conjunction with Na^+ ions (Fig. 10.13).

 The Ca^{2+}-ATPase, a calcium pump, uses a mechanism similar to that of Na^+,K^+-ATPase to maintain intracellular Ca^{2+} concentration below 10^{-7} M in spite of the high extracellular concentration of 10^{-3} M. This transporter is inhibited by binding of the regulatory protein calmodulin. When the intracellular Ca^{2+} concentration increases, Ca^{2+} binds to calmodulin, which dissociates from the transporter, thereby activating it to pump Ca^{2+} out of the cell (see Chapter 9 for the structure of calmodulin). High levels of intracellular Ca^{2+} are associated with irreversible progression from cell injury to cell death.

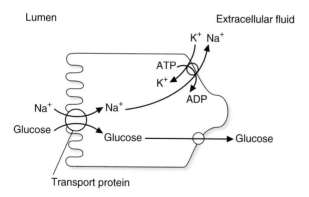

Fig. 10.13. Secondary active transport of glucose by the Na^+-glucose cotransporter. One sodium ion binds to the carrier protein in the luminal membrane, stimulating the binding of glucose. After a conformational change, the protein releases Na^+ and glucose into the cell and returns to its original conformation. Na^+,K^+-ATPase in the basolateral membrane pumps Na^+ against its concentration gradient into the extracellular fluid. Thus, the Na^+ concentration in the cell is low, and Na^+ moves from the lumen down its concentration gradient into the cell and is pumped against its gradient into the extracellular fluid. Glucose, consequently, moves against its concentration gradient from the lumen into the cell by traveling on the same carrier as Na^+. Glucose then passes down its concentration gradient into the extracellular fluid on a passive transporter protein.

The dehydration of cholera is often treated with an oral rehydration solution containing Na^+, K^+, and glucose or a diet of rice (which contains glucose and amino acids). Glucose is absorbed from the intestinal lumen via the Na^+-dependent glucose cotransporters, which cotransport Na^+ into the cells together with glucose. Many amino acids are also absorbed by Na^+-dependent cotransport. With the return of Na^+ to the cytoplasm, water efflux from the cell into the intestinal lumen decreases.

The vitamin folate provides an example of a compound transported into cells by caveolae, which form around the occupied folate receptor. In contrast, endocytosis of many compounds such as membrane hormone receptors occurs through clathrin-coated pits. The receptors are targeted for these pits by adaptor proteins that bind to a specific amino acid sequence in the receptor.

These cells create a gradient in Na^+ and then use this gradient to drive the transport of glucose from the intestinal lumen into the cell against its concentration gradient.

D. Vesicular Transport across the Plasma Membrane

Vesicular transport occurs when a membrane completely surrounds a compound, particle, or cell and encloses it into a vesicle. When the vesicle fuses with another membrane system, the entrapped compounds are released. Endocytosis refers to vesicular transport into the cell, and exocytosis to transport out of the cell. Endocytosis is further classified as phagocytosis if the vesicle forms around particulate matter (such as whole bacterial cells or metals and dyes from a tattoo), and pinocytosis if the vesicle forms around fluid containing dispersed molecules. Receptor-mediated endocytosis is the name given to the formation of clathrin-coated vesicles that mediate the internalization of membrane-bound receptors in vesicles coated on the intracellular side with subunits of the protein clathrin (Fig. 10.14). Potocytosis is the name given to endocytosis that occurs via caveolae (small invaginations or "caves"), which are regions of the cell membrane with a unique lipid and protein composition (including the protein caveolin-1).

III. LYSOSOMES

Lysosomes are the intracellular organelles of digestion enclosed by a single membrane that prevents the release of its digestive enzymes into the cytosol. They are central to a wide variety of body functions that involve elimination of unwanted material and recycling their components, including destruction of

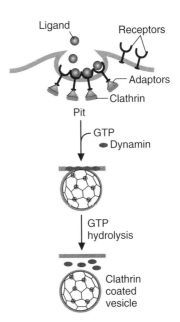

Fig. 10.14. Formation of a clathrin-coated vesicle. Ligands entering the cell through receptor-mediated endocytosis bind to receptors that cluster in an area of the membrane. Adaptor proteins bind to the receptor tails and to the clathrin molecules to enclose the budding membrane in a cage-like clathrin coat.

Molecules of a monomeric G protein called dynamin (from the Rab family) constrict the neck of the vesicle and pinch it off from the membrane as GTP is hydrolyzed.

infectious bacteria and yeast, recovery from injury, tissue remodeling, involution of tissues during development, and normal turnover of cells and organelles.

A. Lysosomal Hydrolases

The lysosomal digestive enzymes include nucleases, phosphatases, glycosidases, esterases, and proteases called cathepsins (Fig. 10.15). These enzymes are all hydrolases, enzymes that cleave amide, ester, and other bonds through the addition of water. Many of the products of lysosomal digestion, such as the amino acids, return to the cytosol. Lysosomes are therefore involved in recycling compounds.

Most of these lysosomal hydrolases have their highest activity near a pH of approximately 5.5 (the pH optimum). The intralysosmal pH is maintained near 5.5 principally by *v*-ATPases (vesicular ATPases), which actively pump protons into the lysosome. The cytosol and other cellular compartments have a pH nearer 7.2 and are therefore protected from escaped lysosomal hydrolases.

B. Endocytosis, Phagocytosis, and Autophagy

Lysosomes are formed from digestive vesicles called endosomes, which are involved in receptor-mediated endocytosis. They also participate in digestion of foreign cells acquired through phagocytosis and the digestion of internal contents in the process of autophagocytosis.

1. RECEPTOR-MEDIATED ENDOCYTOSIS

Lysosomes are involved in the digestion of compounds brought into the cells in endocytotic clathrin-coated vesicles formed by the plasma membrane (Fig. 10.16). These vesicles fuse to form multivesicular bodies called early endosomes. The early endosomes mature into late endosomes as they recycle clathrin, lipids, and other

Lysosomal storage diseases. Genetic defects in lysosomal enzymes, or in proteins such as the mannose 6-phosphate receptors required for targeting the enzymes to the lysosome, lead to an abnormal accumulation of undigested material in lysosomes that may be converted to residual bodies. The accumulation may be so extensive that normal cellular function is compromised, particularly in neuronal cells. Genetic diseases such as the Tay-Sachs disease (an accumulation of partially digested gangliosides in lysosomes), and Pompe's disease (an accumulation of glycogen particles in lysosomes) are caused by the absence or deficiency of specific lysosomal enzymes.

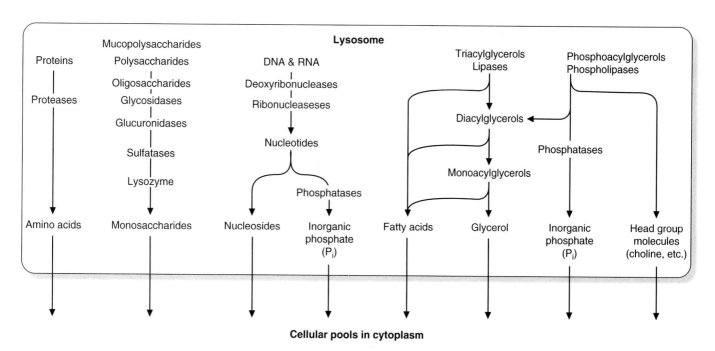

Fig. 10.15. Lysosomal reactions. Most lysosomal enzymes are hydrolases, which cleave peptide, ester, and glycosidic bonds by adding the components of water across the bond. These enzymes are active at the acidic pH of the lysosome and inactive if accidentally released into the cytosol.

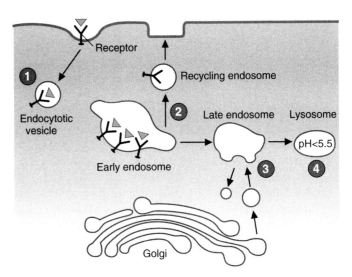

Fig. 10.16. Lysosomes in receptor-mediated endocytosis via clathrin-coated pits. **1.** Endocytotic vesicles fuse to form early endosomes. **2.** Vesicle contents are sorted, and receptors, clathrin, and lipids are sent back to the plasma membrane. **3.** Transport vesicles from the trans-Golgi carry lysosomal hydrolases to the late endosome. **4.** Lysosomes containing concentrated hydrolases digest proteins and other components acquired from endocytotic vesicles.

The elevated level of uric acid in **Lotta Topaigne**'s blood led to the deposition of monosodium urate crystals in the joint space (synovial fluid) of her right great toe, resulting in podagra (painful great toe). Neutrophils, the mediators of the acute inflammation that followed, attempted to phagocytose the urate crystals. The engulfed urate crystals were deposited in the late endosomes and lysosomes of the neutrophil. Because urate crystals are particles that cannot be degraded by any of the lysosomal acid hydolases, their accumulation caused lysis of the lysosomal membranes, followed by cell lysis and release of lysosomal enzymes into the joint space. The urate crystals also resulted in release of chemical mediators of inflammation that recruited other cells into the area. This further amplified the acute inflammatory reaction in the tissues of the joint caspsule (synovitis), leading to the extremely painful swelling of acute gouty arthritis.

Phagocytosis and autophagy are part of the normal turnover of body components, such as degradation of cells that have a shorter lifespan than the whole organism and remodeling of tissues during pregnancy. For example, phagocytes, located mainly in the spleen and liver, remove approximately 3×10^{11} red blood cells from the circulation each day. During pregnancy, breast tissue is remodeled to develop the capacity for lactation; after weaning of an infant, the lactating breast returns to its original state (involution).

membrane components back to the plasma membrane in vesicles called recycling endosomes. The late endosomes mature into lysosomes as they progressively accumulate newly synthesized acid hydrolases and vesicular proton pumps brought to them in clathrin-coated vesicles from the Golgi. Thus, lysosomes do not acquire their full digestive power until after sorting of membrane lipids and proteins for recycling.

Within the Golgi, enzymes are targeted for endosomes (and eventually lysosomes) by addition of mannose 6-phosphate residues that bind to mannose 6-phosphate receptor proteins in the Golgi membrane. The mannose 6-phosphate receptors together with their bound acid hydrolases are incorporated into the clathrin-coated Golgi transport vesicles and released. The transport vesicles lose their clathrin coat and then fuse with the late endosomal membrane. The acidity of the endosome releases the acid hydrolases from the receptors into the vesicle lumen. The receptors are eventually recycled back to the Golgi.

2. PHAGOCYTOSIS AND AUTOPHAGY

One of the major roles of lysosomes is phagocytosis (Fig. 10.17). Neutrophils and macrophages, the major phagocytic cells, devour pathogenic microorganisms and clean up wound debris and dead cells, thus aiding in repair. As bacteria or other particles are enclosed into clathrin-coated pits in the plasma membrane, these vesicles bud off to form intracellular phagosomes. The phagosomes fuse with lysosomes, where the acidity and digestive enzymes destroy the contents. Pinocytotic vescicles also may fuse with lysosomes.

In autophagy (self-eating), intracellular components such as organelles or glycogen particles are surrounded by a membrane derived from ER vesicles, forming an autophagosome. The autophagosome fuses with a lysosome, and the contents of the phagolysosome are digested by lysosomal enzymes. Organelles usually turn over much more rapidly than the cells in which they reside (e.g., approximately four mitochondria in each liver cell are degraded per hour). Cells that are damaged but still viable recover, in part, by using autophagy to eliminate damaged components.

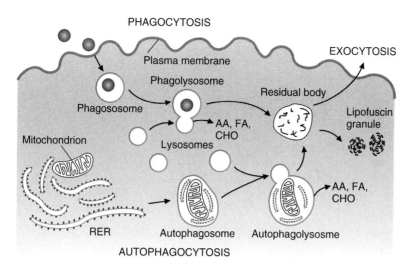

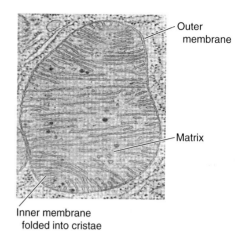

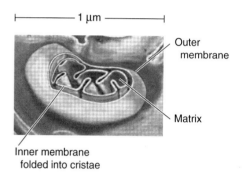

Fig. 10.17. Phagocytosis and autophagy. Cells and large particles are phagocytosed. The phagosomes fuse with lysosomes to form phagolysosomes. Recyclable amino acids (AA), fatty acids (FA), and carbohydrates (CHO) are released into the cytosol. Autophagosomes are formed in the ER as the cell digests mitochondria and its own large particles. These also merge with lysosomes. Undigested material may remain in the lysosomes to form residual bodies, which are either extruded or remain in the cell as lipofuscin granules.

Fig. 10.18. Mitochondrion. Electron micrograph (top); three-dimensional drawing (bottom).

If a significant amount of undigestible material remains within the lysosome after the digestion process is completed, the lysosome is called a residual body. Depending on the cell type, residual bodies may be expelled (exocytosis) or remain indefinitely in the cell as lipofuscin granules that accumulate with age.

IV. MITOCHONDRIA

Mitochondria contain most of the enzymes for the pathways of fuel oxidation and oxidative phosphorylation and thus generate most of the ATP required by mammalian cells. Each mitochondrion is surrounded by two membranes, an outer membrane and an inner membrane, separating the mitochondrial matrix from the cytosol (Fig. 10.18). The inner membrane forms invaginations known as cristae containing the electron transport chain and ATP synthase. Most of the enzymes for the TCA cycle and other pathways for oxidation are located in the mitochondrial matrix, the compartment enclosed by the inner mitochondrial membrane. (The TCA cycle and electron transport chain are described in more detail in Chapters 20 and 21.)

The inner mitochondrial membrane is highly impermeable, and the proton gradient that is built up across this membrane during oxidative phosphorylation is essential for ATP generation from ADP and phosphate. The transport of ions occurs principally through facilitative transporters in a type of secondary active transport powered by the proton gradient established by the electron transport chain. The outer membrane contains pores made from proteins called porins and is permeable to molecules with a molecular weight up to about 1000 g/mole.

Mitochondria can replicate by division; however, most of their proteins must be imported from the cytosol. Mitochondria contain a small amount of DNA, which encodes for only 13 different subunits of proteins involved in oxidative phosphorylation. Most of the enzymes and proteins in mitochondria are encoded by nuclear DNA and synthesized on cytoplasmic ribosomes. They are imported

Mitochondial diseases. Mitochondria contain DNA and can reproduce by replicating their DNA and then dividing in half. Although nuclear DNA encodes most of the enzymes found in mitochondria, mitochondrial DNA encodes some of the subunits of the electron transport chain proteins and ATP synthase. Mutations in mitochondrial DNA result in a number of genetic diseases that affect skeletal muscle, neuronal, and renal tissues. They are implicated in aging.

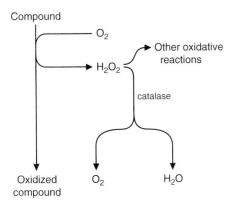

Fig. 10.19. Types of reactions in peroxisomes.

Peroxisomal Diseases. Peroxisomal diseases are caused by mutations affecting either the synthesis of functional peroxisomal enzymes or their incorporation into peroxisomes. For example, adrenoleukodystrophy probably involves a mutation that decreases the content of a transporter in the peroxisomal membrane. Zellweger's syndrome is caused by the failure to complete the synthesis of peroxisomes.

through membrane pores by a receptor-mediated process involving members of the heat shock family of proteins.

V. PEROXISOMES

Peroxisomes are cytoplasmic organelles, similar in size to lysosomes, that are involved in oxidative reactions using molecular oxygen (Fig. 10.19). These reactions produce the toxic chemical hydrogen peroxide (H_2O_2), which is subsequently used or degraded within the peroxisome by catalase and other enzymes. Peroxisomes function in the oxidation of very long chain fatty acids (containing 20 or more carbons) to shorter chain fatty acids, the conversion of cholesterol to bile acids, and the synthesis of ether lipids called plasmalogens. They are bounded by a single membrane.

Like mitochondria, peroxisomes can replicate by division. However, they are dependent on the import of proteins to function. They contain no DNA.

VI. NUCLEUS

The largest of the subcellular organelles of animal cells is the nucleus (Fig. 10.20). Most of the genetic material of the cell is located in the chromosomes of the nucleus, which are composed of DNA, an equal weight of small, positively charged proteins called histones, and a variable amount of other proteins. This nucleoprotein

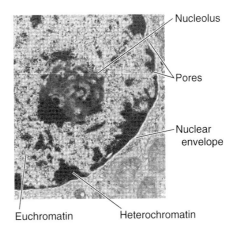

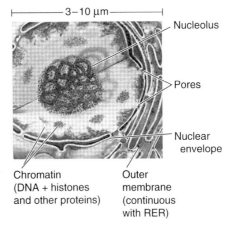

Fig. 10.20. Nucleus. Electron micrograph (top); three-dimensional drawing (bottom).

complex is called chromatin. The nucleolus, a substructure of the nucleus, is the site of rRNA transcription and processing, and of ribosome assembly. Replication, transcription, translation, and the regulation of these processes are the major focus of the molecular biology section of this text (see Section Three).

The nucleus is separated from the rest of the cell (the cytoplasm) by the nuclear envelope, which consists of two membranes joined at nuclear pores. The outer nuclear membrane is continuous with the rough endoplasmic reticulum. To convert the genetic code of the DNA into the primary sequence of a protein, DNA is transcribed into RNA, which is modified and edited into mRNA. The mRNA travels through the nuclear pores into the cytoplasm, where it is translated into the primary sequence of a protein on ribosomes (Fig. 10.21). Ribosomes, which are generated in the nucleolus, also must travel through nuclear pores to the cytoplasm. Conversely, proteins required for replication, transcription, and other processes pass into the nucleus through these pores. Thus, transport through the pore is specific for the molecule and the direction of transport.

Specificity and direction of travel through the nuclear pore (import vs. export) is dictated by binding proteins (importins vs. exportins), by a small GTP protein called Ran, and by the location of the regulatory protein, RanGAP (GTPase activating protein) only on the cytoplasmic side (Fig. 10.22). Proteins transported into the nucleus have a nuclear localization signal that causes them to bind to one of the subunits of cytosolic proteins called importins. The other subunit of the importin molecule binds to cytoplasmic filaments attached to the outer ring of the nuclear pore. As the importin-protein complex enters the nucleus, the small GTP-binding protein Ran binds to an importin subunit, causing release of the transported protein into the nucleus. The Ran-importin complex is returned to the cytosol, where RanGAP (GTPase activating protein) activates hydrolysis of bound GTP to GDP and phosphate. The energy released by GTP hydrolysis changes the conformation of Ran and the complex dissociates. The free importin can then bind another protein.

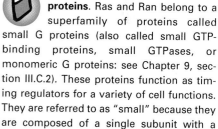

The Ras family of monomeric G proteins. Ras and Ran belong to a superfamily of proteins called small G proteins (also called small GTP-binding proteins, small GTPases, or monomeric G proteins: see Chapter 9, section III.C.2). These proteins function as timing regulators for a variety of cell functions. They are referred to as "small" because they are composed of a single subunit with a weight of 20 to 40 kDa, and they are called GTPases because they slowly hydrolyze bound GTP. When small G proteins contain bound GTP, they bind to and activate their target proteins. As their bound GTP is hydrolyzed to GDP and Pi, their conformation changes dramatically, and they dissociate from the target protein. They thus serve as "automatic clocks" that shut themselves off. Many of the monomeric GTP binding proteins are regulated by GAPs (GTPase activating proteins), GEFs (GTP exchange proteins which stimulate GDP dissociation and GTP binding), or GDIs (GDP-dissociation inhibitory proteins). (See Chapter 9 for a more complete discussion of these regulators). The function of each of the five major classes of Ras monomeric G proteins in cell biology is summarized in Table 10.1.

Table 10.1 Monomeric G Proteins in the Ras Superfamily

G-Protein Family	Function	Some Family Members	Location and Membrane Attachment Site
Ras	Regulator of gene expression and cell growth, found in mutated oncogenic forms in many human tumors	H-Ras, K-Ras, N-Ras, Ral A, Rad, Rap, Rit,	Anchored to plasma membrane by farnesyl, palmitoyl, or other lipid groups
Rho	Controls organization of actin cytoskeleton and gene expression (F-actin bundling, myosin filament assembly)	Rho (A-E), Cdc42, Rac (1-3)	Anchored to plasma membrane by lipids, and translocates to cytosol
Arf/Sar	Assembly of coatomer-coated vesicles (COPI and COPII) for vesicular trafficking pathways originating in the Golgi	Arf (1-6), Sar 1a,1b; Arl (1-7)	Arf is anchored to vesicular membranes by myristyl groups, but Sar is anchored by the protein itself.
Rab	Targeting of vesicles involved in secretory and endocytotic pathways and formation of v-SNARE–t-SNARE complexes	Dynamin, Rab (11-33)	Anchored to lipid membranes with geranylgeranyl (C20 isoprenoid) groups and other lipids
Ran	Transport through nuclear pore complexes.	Ran	Not anchored to lipid membrane. Found in cytosol and nucleus

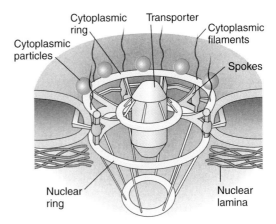

Fig. 10.21. The nuclear pore complex. The approximately 100 different polypeptide chains of the nuclear pore complex form an assembly of 8 spokes attached to two ring structures (a cytoplasmic ring in the outer nuclear membrane and a nuclear ring through the inner membrane) with a transporter "plug" in the center. Small molecules, ions, and proteins with less than a 50-kDa mass passively diffuse through the pore in either direction. However, RNAs and most proteins are too large to diffuse through, and are actively transported in a process that requires energy, is selective for the molecule transported, is unidirectional, and can be regulated.

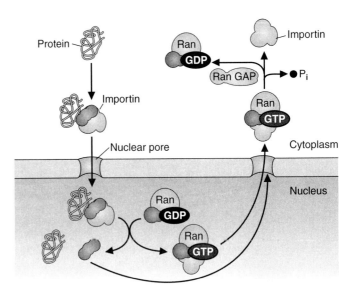

Fig. 10.22. Nuclear import. Proteins with the nuclear localization signal bind to importins, which carry them through the nuclear pore into the nucleus. The monomeric G protein Ran containing bound GTP binds to one of the subunits of importin. This causes dissociation of the importin subunits and release of the imported protein in the nucleus. The Ran-importin complex exits a nuclear pore. On the cytoplasmic side, a RanGAP (GTPase activating protein) activates the hydrolysis of GTP to GDP, which causes dissociation of the complex. RanGDP is subsequently returned to the nucleus, where an accessory protein activates dissociation of GDP and association of GTP.

RNAs are transported from the nucleus to the cytoplasm as ribonucleoproteins, which are targeted for export by a specific amino acid sequence called the nuclear export signal. The nucleoprotein forms a complex with additional proteins called exportins and with Ran. This complex is transported through the pore to the cytoplasm, where RanGAP activates hydrolysis of the bound GTP. In the absence of GTP, the complex dissociates with the release of RNA into the cytoplasm, and the exportins and Ran are transported back to the nucleus.

VII. ENDOPLASMIC RETICULUM

The endoplasmic reticulum (ER) is a network of membranous tubules within the cell consisting of smooth endoplasmic reticulum (SER), which lacks ribosomes, and rough endoplasmic reticulum (RER), which is studded with ribosomes (Fig. 10.23). The SER has a number of functions. It contains enzymes for the synthesis of many lipids, such as triacylglycerols and phospholipids. It also contains the cytochrome P450 oxidative enzymes involved in metabolism of drugs and toxic chemicals such as ethanol and the synthesis of hydrophobic molecules such as steroid hormones. Glycogen is stored in regions of liver cells that are rich in SER.

The RER is involved in the synthesis of certain proteins. Ribosomes attached to the membranes of the RER give them their "rough" appearance. Proteins produced on these ribosomes enter the lumen of the RER, travel to the Golgi complex in vesicles, and are subsequently either secreted from the cell, sequestered within membrane-enclosed organelles such as lysosomes, or embedded in the plasma membrane. Posttranslational modifications of these proteins, such as the initiation of N-linked glycosylation and the addition of GPI anchors, occur in the RER. In contrast, proteins encoded by the nucleus and found in the cytosol, peroxisomes, or mitochondria are synthesized on free ribosomes in the cytosol and are seldom modified by the attachment of oligosaccharides.

Chronic ingestion of ethanol has increased the content of MEOS, the microsomal ethanol oxidizing system, in **Al Martini's** liver. MEOS is a cytochrome P450 enzyme that catalyzes the conversion of ethanol, NADPH and O_2 to acetaldehyde, $NADP^+$, and 2 H_2O (see Chapter 9). The adjective *microsomal* is a term derived from experimental cell biology that is sometimes used for processes occurring in the ER. When cells are lysed in the laboratory, the ER is fragmented into vesicles called *microsomes,* which can be isolated by centrifugation. Microsomes, as such, are not actually present in cells.

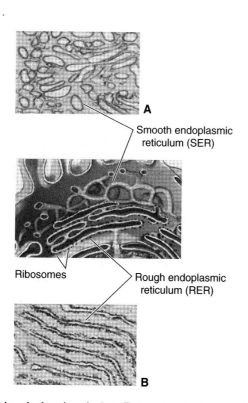

Smooth endoplasmic reticulum (SER)

Ribosomes

Rough endoplasmic reticulum (RER)

Fig. 10.23 A. Smooth endoplasmic reticulum. **B.** Rough endoplasmic reticulum. A and B are electron micrographs. A three-dimensional drawing is in the middle.

VIII.   GOLGI COMPLEX

The Golgi complex is involved in modifying proteins produced in the RER and in sorting and distributing these proteins to the lysosomes, secretory vesicles, or the plasma membrane. It consists of a curved stack of flattened vesicles in the cytoplasm that is generally divided into three compartments: the *cis*-Golgi network, which is often convex and faces the nucleus; the *medial* Golgi stacks; and the *trans* Golgi network, which often faces the plasma membrane (Fig. 10.24).

Proteins are transported to and from the Golgi in at least three kinds of vesicles: coatomer-coated COP I vesicles, coatomer-coated COP II vesicles, and clathrin-coated vesicles (see Fig. 10.24). Proteins produced on the RER travel in COP II vesicles to an endoplasmic reticulum-Golgi intermediate compartment (ERGIC), and then to the *cis*-Golgi network, where they enter the lumen. Here N-linked oligosaccharide chains that were added to proteins in the RER are modified, and O-linked oligosaccharides are added. COP I vesicles recycle material from the Golgi back to the ER and possibly transfer material from the Golgi to other sites.

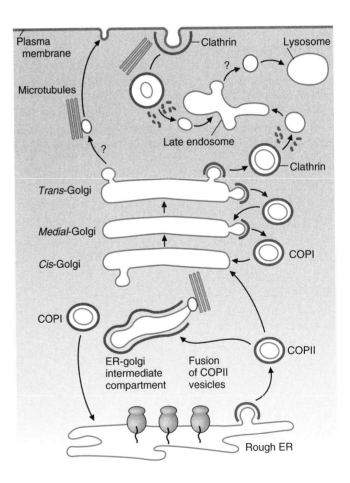

Fig. 10.24. Vesicular transport to and from the Golgi complex. COP II vesicles (coatomer-coated) form in the rough ER and move to the Golgi. COP I vesicles generally go from the trans to the cis Golgi to the ER. Vesicles that go to late endosomes (eventually lysosomes) from the Golgi or the plasma membrane are clathrin-coated. Less is known about exocytotic vesicles. Vesicle transport, as well as transport of organelles and secretory proteins, occurs along microtubules (structures formed from the protein tubulin).

Vesicles released from the *trans* face of the Golgi complex travel to endosomes as clathrin-coated vesicles.

COP vesicles are coated with a complex composed of coatomer proteins (COP), an Arf family monomeric G protein that mediates vesicle assembly, and other proteins (Fig. 10.25). COP I vesicles contain the monomeric G protein Arf (**ADP-ribosylating factor**), and COP II vesicles contain the monomeric G protein Sar (another member of the Arf family). In both types of vesicles, hydrolysis of GTP causes dissociation of the G-protein and disassembly of the vesicle coat. The vesicle components are then recycled. Glycoproteins or glycolipids once anchored in the membrane of the vesicle remain in the plasma membrane when the vesicular and plasma membranes fuse.

Vesicles that have lost their coats are ready to fuse with the target membrane. The vesicle membranes contain proteins called v-SNARES (vesicle-SNARES) (see Fig. 10.25). Each type of v-SNARE is able to recognize and bind to its complementary t-SNARE (target SNARE) on the target membrane, thus ensuring that

The monomeric G protein Arf was named for its contribution to the pathogenesis of cholera and not for its normal function in the assembly of COP I vesicles. However, it is also required for the transport of *V. cholerae* A-toxin. The cholera toxin is endocytosed in caveolae vesicles that subsequently merge with lysosomes (or are transformed into lysosomes), where the acidic pH contributes to activation of the toxin. As the toxin is transported through the Golgi and ER, it is further processed and activated. Arf forms a complex with the A-toxin that promotes its travel between compartments. The A-toxin is actually an ADP-ribosylase (an enzyme that cleaves NAD and attaches the ADP portion to a protein) (see Chapter 6, Fig. 6.14), and hence, Arf became known as the ADP-ribosylating factor. The ADP-ribosylation of proteins regulating the CFTR chloride channel leads to **Dennis Veere's** dehydration and diarrhea.

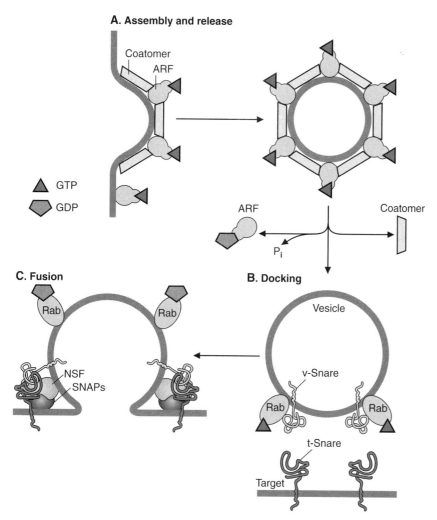

Fig. 10.25. Transport in COP-coated vesicles. **A.** Assembly and release. Arf with bound GTP assembles a region of the trans-Golgi membrane containing receptors for the protein cargo and coatomers. As GTP is hydrolyzed to GDP, the coat is released. **B.** Docking. The small G protein Rab assists in docking. v-Snares in the vesicle membrane recognize complementary t-Snares in the target membrane. **C.** Fusion. NSF and SNAP are fusion proteins.

Secretory vesicles. The hormone insulin is synthesized as a prohormone, proinsulin, which is incorporated into secretory vesicles. These vesicles contain a protease that is activated by the acidic pH of the secretory vesicle. It cleaves proinsulin into the A, B, and C chains (see Fig. 6.13).

the vesicle contents are delivered to the right location. Several additional proteins are required for fusion of the vesicle with the target membrane, including Rab (another monomeric G protein) and two additional proteins called SNAP (**s**oluble **N**SF **a**ttachment **p**roteins) and NSF (**N**-ethylmaleimide **s**ensitive **f**actor).

Exocytotic vesicles release proteins into the extracellular space after fusion of the vesicular and plasma cell membranes. Exocytotic vesicles containing hormones also may contain proteases that cleave the prohormone at a specific site and *v*-ATPases that acidify the vesicle and activate the protease (similar to lysosomes).

IX. CYTOSKELETON

The structure of the cell, the shape of the cell surface, and the arrangement of subcellular organelles is organized by three major protein components: microtubules composed of tubulin, which move and position organelles and vesicles; thin filaments composed of actin, which form a cytoskeleton, and intermediate filaments composed of different fibrous proteins. Actin and tubulin, which are involved in cell movement, are dynamic structures composed of continuously associating and dissociating globular subunits. Intermediate filaments, which play a structural role, are composed of stable fibrous proteins that turn over more slowly.

A. Microtubules

Microtubules, cylindrical tubes composed of tubulin subunits, are present in all nucleated cells and the platelets in blood (Fig. 10.26). They are responsible for the positioning of organelles in the cell cytoplasm and the movement of vesicles, including phagocytic vesicles, exocytotic vesicles, and the transport vesicles between the ER, Golgi, and endosomes (see Fig. 10.24). They also form the spindle apparatus for cell division. The microtubule network (the minus end) begins in the nucleus at the centriole and extends outward to the plasma membrane (usually the plus end). Microtubule-associated proteins (MAPs) attach microtubules to other cellular components, and can determine cell shape and polarity.

Lotta Topaigne was given colchicine, a drug that is frequently used to treat gout. One of its actions is to prevent phagocytic activity by binding to dimers of the α and β subunits of tubulin. When the tubulin dimer–colchicine complexes bind to microtubules, further polymerization of the microtubules is inhibited, depolymerization predominates, and the microtubules disassemble. Microtubules are necessary for vesicular movement of urate crystals during phagocytosis and release of mediators that activate the inflammatory response. Thus, colchicine diminishes the inflammatory response, swelling and pain caused by formation of urate crystals.

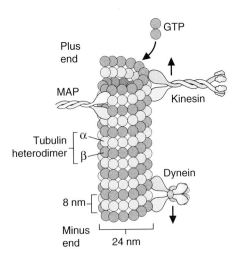

Fig. 10.26. Microtubules composed of αβ tubulin heterodimers. MAP, microtubule-associated protein. These proteins project outward to attach the microtubules to other cellular components. The microtubule grows by the addition of αβ dimers containing bound GTP to the plus end of the polymer. Kinesin and dyneins are motor proteins that transport cargo (e.g., vesicles) along the microtubule.

Motor proteins called kinesins and cytoplasmic dyneins use ATP energy to move cargo along the microtubules. Kinesins moves molecules, vesicles, and organelles toward the plus end of microtubules, usually toward the plasma membrane. Cytoplasmic dyneins are huge proteins that move vesicles and organelles to the minus end, generally toward the nucleus. They are also involved in the positioning of the Golgi complex and the movement of chromosomes during mitosis.

Microtubules consist of polymerized arrays of α and β tubulin dimers that form 13 protofilaments organized around a hollow core (see Fig. 10.26). Three different tubulin polypeptides (α, β, and γ) of similar amino acid composition are encoded by related genes; α and β dimers polymerize to form most microtubules, and γ-tubuluin is found only in the centrosome. Tubulin dimers composed of one α and one β subunit bind GTP, which creates a conformational change in the dimer that favors addition of dimers to the tubulin polymer. The dimers can add to and dissociate from both ends of the tubulin, but the end to which they add more rapidly (the plus end) has a net rate of growth, and the end to which they add more slowly (the minus end) has a net rate of loss. As GTP is hydrolyzed to GDP, the binding of tubulin subunits is weakened, resulting in their dissociation (dynamic instability). Thus, the net rate and direction of growth is dictated by the fastest growing end of the microtubule.

B. Actin Filaments

Actin filaments form a network controlling the shape of the cell and movement of the cell surface, thereby allowing cells to move, divide, engulf particles, and contract. Actin is present in all living cells. The actin polymer, called F-actin, is composed of a helical arrangement of globular G-actin subunits (Fig. 10.27). Within the polymer, each G-actin subunit contains a bound ATP or ADP that

A variety of human cells have cilia and flagella, hairlike projections from the surface that have a stroke-like motion. These projections contain a flexible organized array of microtubules. Fluid or mucus is propelled over the surface of ciliated epithelial cells by the coordinated beating of cilia. A sperm cell swims by means of a flagellum.

Colchicine has a narrow therapeutic index (i.e., the amount of drug that produces the desirable therapeutic effect is not much lower than the amount that produces an adverse effect). Its therapeutic effect depends on inhibiting tubulin synthesis in neutrophils, but it can also prevent tubulin synthesis (and, thus, cell division and other cellular processes) in other cells. Fortunately, neutrophils concentrate colchicine, so they are affected at lower intakes than other cell types. Neutrophils lack the transport protein P-glycoprotein, a member of the ABC cassette family (which includes the CFTR channel). In most other cell types, P-glycoprotein exports chemicals such as colchicine, thus preventing their accumulation.

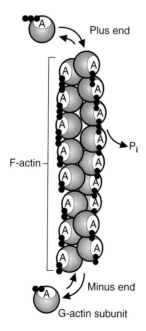

Fig. 10.27. Actin filaments. The polymer F-actin is assembled from G-actin subunits containing bound ATP. While bound, the ATP is slowly hydrolyzed to ADP. The conformational change shifts the equilibrium so that dissociation of the G-actin subunits is favorable at the minus end of the polymer. Once dissociated, the actin subunits exchange ADP for ATP, which may again associate with the actin polymer. At the plus end of the molecule, association is favored over dissociation.

holds the actin fold into a closed conformation (see Chapter 7). The actin polymer is dynamic. New subunits of G-actin containing ATP continuously combine with the assembled F-actin polymer at the plus end. As F-actin elongates, bound ATP is hydrolyzed to ADP, so that most of the polymer contains G-actin-ADP subunits. The conformation of ADP-actin favors dissociation from the minus end of the polymer; thus, the polymer is capable of lengthening from the plus end. This directional growth can account for certain types of cell movement and shape changes: the formation of pseudopodia that surround other cells during phagocytosis, the migration of cells in the developing embryo, or the movement of white blood cells through tissues.

Actin polymers form the thin filaments (also called microfilaments) in the cell that are organized into compact ordered bundles or loose network arrays by cross-linking proteins. Short actin filaments bind to the cross-linking protein spectrin to form the cortical actin skeleton network (see Fig. 10.6). In muscle cells, long actin filaments combine with thick filaments, composed of the protein myosin, to produce muscle contraction. The assembly of G-actin subunits into polymers, bundling of fibers, and attachments of actin to spectrin and to the plasma membrane proteins and organelles, are mediated by a number of actin-binding proteins and G-proteins from the Rho family.

C. Intermediate Filaments

Intermediate filaments (IF) are composed of fibrous protein polymers that provide structural support to membranes of the cells and scaffolding for attachment of other cellular components. Each IF subunit is composed of a long rod-like α-helical core containing globular spacing domains, and globular N- and C-terminal domains. The α-helical segments of two subunits coil around each other to form a coiled coil, and then combine with another dimer coil to form a tetramer. Depending on the type of filament, the dimers may be either hetero- or homo-dimers. The tetramers join end-to end to form protofilaments and approximately eight proto filaments combine to form filaments (Fig. 10.28). Filament assembly is partially controlled through phosphorylation.

In contrast to actin thin filaments, the 50 or so different types of intermediate filaments are each composed of a different protein having the same general structure described above (Table 10.2). Some of the intermediate filaments, such as the nuclear lamins, are common to all cell types. These filaments provide a lattice-like support network attached to the inner nuclear membrane. Other intermediate filaments are specific for types of cells (e.g., epithelial cells have cytokeratins, and neurons have neurofilaments). These provide an internal network that helps to support the shape and resilience of the cell.

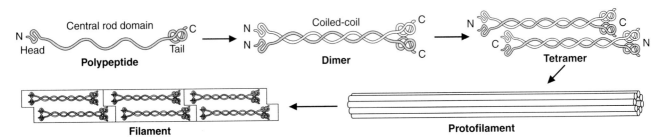

Fig. 10.28. Formation of a cytokeratin filament. The central rod of the keratin monomer is principally α-helical structure. A specific acidic keratin monomer combines with a specific basic keratin monomer to form a heterodimer coil (a coiled coil structure). Two dimers combine in antiparallel fashion to form a tetramer, and the tetramers combine head-to-tail to form protofilaments. Approximately eight protofilaments combine to form a filament. The filament is thicker than actin filaments (called thin filaments or microfilaments) and is thinner than microtubules (thick tubes) and is therefore called an intermediate filament.

Table 10.2 Intermediate Filaments

Type	Protein	Location
Type I	Acidic keratins	Different epithelial cells express different keratins.
Type II	Basic keratins	Epithelial cells. Each cell type has a specific acidic and a specific basic keratin.
Type III	Vimentin-like	Cells of mesenchymal origin
	Vimentin Desmin	Muscle
	Glial fibrillary acid protein	Glial cells in the central nervous system
Type IV	Neurofilaments (NF-L, NF-M, NF-H)	Neurons, particularly long thin motor axons
Type V	Nuclear lamins A, B, and C	Forms a mesh-like network in the inner lining of cellular nuclear envelopes.
Type VI	Nestin	Stem cells of central nervous system

CLINICAL COMMENTS

 Al Martini. Al Martini has been drinking for 5 years and has begun to exhibit mental and systemic effects of chronic alcohol consumption. In his brain, ethanol has altered the fluidity of neuronal lipids, causing changes in their response to neurotransmitters released from exocytotic vesicles. In his liver, increased levels of MEOS (CYP2E1) located in the smooth ER increased his rate of ethanol oxidation to acetaldehyde, a compound that is toxic to the cell. His liver also continues to oxidize ethanol to acetaldehyde through a cytosolic enzyme, liver alcohol dehydrogenase.

One of the toxic effects of acetaldehyde is inhibition of tubulin polymerization. Tubulin is used in the liver for secretion of very low-density lipoprotein (VLDL) particles containing newly synthesized triacylglycerols. As a result, these triacylglycerols accumulate in the liver, and he has begun to develop a fatty liver. Acetaldehyde may also damage protein components of the inner mitochondrial membrane and affect its ability to pump protons to the cytosol.

 Lotta Topaigne had a rapid and gratifying clinical response to the hourly administration of colchicine. This drug diminishes phagocytosis and the subsequent release of the lysosomal enzymes that initiate the inflammatory response in synovial tissue.

The inflammatory response that causes the symptoms of an acute gout attack begins when neutrophils and macrophages ingest urate crystals. In neutrophils, urate activates the conversion of the polyunsaturated fatty acid arachidonic acid (present in membrane phospholipids) to leukotriene B_4. The release of this prostaglandin contributes to the pain. Colchicine, through its effect on tubulin, inhibits phagocytosis, leukotriene B_4 release, and recruitment and cell division of additional cells involved in inflammation. Colchicine also inhibits the tubulin-dependent release of histamine from mast cells. As a result, there was a rapid improvement in the pain and swelling in Lotta's great toe.

After the gout attack subsided, Ms. Topaigne was placed on allopurinol, a drug that inhibits urate production (see Chapter 8). During the next 6 months of allopurinol therapy, Ms. Topaigne's blood urate levels decreased. She did not have another gout attack during this time.

Dennis Veere. Dennis Veere was diagnosed with cholera. He was placed on intravenous rehydration therapy, followed by oral rehydration therapy with high glucose and Na^+-containing fluids (to be continued in Chapter 11).

Vibrio cholerae secrete an A toxin that is processed and transported in the cell in conjunction with the monomeric G protein Arf (ADP-ribosylation factor). The A

 In epidermolysis bullosa simplex, the skin blisters in response to a very slight mechanical stress. The familial form of the disease is generally caused by mutations in either of the two forms of keratin that constitute the keratin heterodimers of the basal layer of the epidermis. The weakened keratin cytoskeleton results in cytolysis when stress is applied. The disease also can be caused by mutations in plektin, the protein that attaches keratin to the membrane protein integrin in hemidesmosomes (a structure involved in attaching cells to the extracellular matrix).

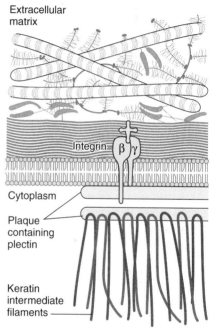

toxin ADP-ribosylates the G_α subunit of a heterotrimeric G protein (a process discussed in Chapter 11.) The net result is activation of protein kinase A, which then phosphorylates the CFTR (cystic fibrosis transmembrane conductance regulator) chloride channel so that it remains permanently open. The subsequent efflux of chloride, sodium, and water into the bowel lumen is responsible for Dennis Veere's diarrhea and subsequent dehydration.

BIOCHEMICAL COMMENTS

Differences between bacteria and human cells. Different species of bacteria have some common structural features that distinguish them from animal cells. They are single-cell organisms that are prokaryotes ("before nucleus"). Their genetic material (DNA) is concentrated in the central region of the cell called a nucleoid, rather than a nucleus, because it is not separated from the rest of the cellular contents by a membrane. Likewise, bacteria contain no cytoplasmic organelles defined by membranes. They do have a plasma membrane that encloses the cytoplasm. External to this membrane is a peptidoglycan cell wall composed of extensively cross-linked polysaccharides that form a protective shield on the surface of the cell.

The mitochondria of eukaryotic cells have many features in common with prokaryotic cells and, in fact, may have originated when primordial anaerobic eukaryotes engulfed ancient aerobic prokaryotes, establishing a symbiotic relationship. These prokaryotes provided eukaryotes with a more efficient mechanism for oxidizing fuels to obtain energy.

Bacterial cells obtain nutrients from the medium on which they grow. Many of their metabolic pathways for fuel oxidation are similar to those in eukaryotes and generate NADH and ATP; however, individual steps in these pathways may use different coenzymes or very different enzymes for catalysis than do human cells. Like human cells, bacteria use intermediates of glycolysis and other basic degradative pathways to serve as precurors for biosynthetic pathways, and energy acquired from catabolic pathways is used in anabolic pathways. Aerobic bacteria, such as *Escherichia coli*, contain enzymes of the tricarboxylic acid (TCA) cycle and the components of the electron transport chain, which are located in the cell membrane. However, many bacteria are anaerobes and can function in the absence of oxygen.

Many of the metabolic differences between human cells and bacteria are related to their interactions with their environment. Some bacteria, such as *E. coli*, can adapt to adverse or changing conditions (high versus low O_2 tension or a single supply of nutrients from which to synthesize everything) by dramatic shifts in the genes that are transcribed. Other bacteria find a unique environmental niche where they do not have to compete with other bacteria for nutrients (e.g., *Lactobaccili* in yogurt are adapted to an acidic pH). In contrast, the human cells are adapted to interacting with blood and interstitial fluid, which provides a well-controlled pH, a constant nutrient supply, and a medium for communication between very distant cells. As a consequence of their constant environment, adult human cells seldom need to adapt (or can adapt) to widely fluctuating conditions through large variations in the genes transcribed. As a consequence of being organized into a multicellular organism, human cell types have been able to specialize in function, structure, and enzyme content.

Suggested References

Emmerson BT. The management of gout. N Engl J Med. 1996;334:445–451.

Takai Y, Sasaki T, Matozaki T. Small GTP-binding proteins. Physiol Rev 2001;81:153–208. Although this is a lengthy review for medical students, it is very useful in identifying the roles of different G proteins.

A number of extremely good cell and molecular biology textbooks have recently been published. Some of the most recent textbooks that we found helpful include:

Karp G. Cell and Molecular Biology: Concepts and Experiments. 3rd Ed. New York: John Wiley and Sons, 2002.

Cooper GM. The Cell: A Molecular Approach. 2nd Ed. Washington, DC: ASM Press, Sinauer Assoc., 2000.
Lodish H, Berk A, Zipursky SL, Matsudaira P, Baltimore D, Darnell J. Molecular Cell Biology. 4th
Ed. New York: W.H. Freeman, 2000. The section on cell structure is particularly good.
Alberts B, Johnson A, Lewis J, Raff M, Roberts K, Walter P. Molecular Biology of the Cell. 4th Ed.
New York: Garland Science, 2002.

 REVIEW QUESTIONS—CHAPTER 10

1. Which of the following is a characteristic of the plasma membrane?

    (A) It is composed principally of triacylglycerols and cholesterol.
    (B) It contains principally nonpolar lipids.
    (C) It contains phospholipids with their acyl groups extending into the cytosol.
    (D) It contains more phosphatidylserine in the inner than the outer leaflet.
    (E) It contains oligosaccharides sandwiched between the inner and outer leaflets.

2. Transmembrane proteins

    (A) can usually be dissociated from membranes without disrupting the lipid bilayer.
    (B) are classified as peripheral membrane proteins.
    (C) contain hydrophobic amino acid residues at their carboxy terminus.
    (D) contain hydrophilic amino acid residues extending into the lipid bilayer.
    (E) contain membrane-spanning regions that are α-helices.

Use the following case history for questions 3 and 4.
   A patient had a sudden heart attack caused by inadequate blood flow through the vessels of the heart. As a consequence, there was an inadequate supply of oxygen to generate ATP in his cardiomyocytes.

3. The compartment of the cardiomyocyte most directly involved in ATP generation is the

    (A) mitochondrion.
    (B) peroxisome.
    (C) lyosome.
    (D) nucleus.
    (E) Golgi.

4. The transport process most directly affected by his decreased rate of ATP generation is

    (A) active transport of Na^+ out of the cell.
    (B) facilitative transport of glucose into the cell.
    (C) passive diffusion of H_2O into the cell.
    (D) ion flux through ligand-gated channels.
    (E) receptor-mediated endocytosis.

Use the following case history for question 5.
   A patient in a nursing home who developed severe diarrhea was diagnosed with a *Clostridium difficile* infection. The severe diarrhea associated with *C. difficile* is caused principally by two toxins that are UDP-glucosyltransferases. These toxins modify a monomeric G protein, thereby disrupting cellular attachments associated with the actin skeleton.

5. On the basis of its effect, which of the following G protein families is the most likely target of this modification?

    (A) Ras
    (B) Ran
    (C) Rho
    (D) Rab
    (E) Arf

11 Cell Signaling by Chemical Messengers

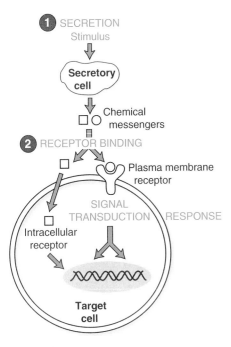

1 SECRETION
Stimulus

Secretory cell

Chemical messengers

2 RECEPTOR BINDING

Plasma membrane receptor

SIGNAL TRANSDUCTION   RESPONSE

Intracellular receptor

Target cell

Fig. 11.1. General features of chemical messengers.

Within a complex organism such as the human, different organs, tissues, and individual cell types have developed specialized functions. Yet each cell must contribute in an integrated way as the body grows, differentiates, and adapts to changing conditions. Such integration requires communication that is carried out by chemical messengers traveling from one cell to another or by direct contact of cells with the extracellular matrix or with each other. The eventual goal of such signals is to change actions carried out in target cells by intracellular proteins (metabolic enzymes, gene regulatory proteins, ion channels, or cytoskeletal proteins). In this chapter, we present an overview of signaling by chemical messengers.

Chemical messengers. Chemical messengers (also called signaling molecules) transmit messages between cells. They are **secreted** from one cell in **response to a specific stimulus** and **travel to a target cell**, where they **bind to a specific receptor** and **elicit a response** (Fig. 11.1). In the nervous system, these chemical messengers are called **neurotransmitters**; in the **endocrine system**, they are **hormones**, and in **the immune system**, they are called **cytokines**. Additional chemical messengers include **retinoids**, **eicosanoids**, and **growth factors**. Depending on the distance between the secreting and target cells, chemical messengers can be classified as **endocrine** (travel in the blood), **paracrine** (travel between nearby cells), or **autocrine** (act on the same cell or on nearby cells of the same type).

Receptors and Signal Transduction. Receptors are proteins containing a binding site specific for a single chemical messenger and another binding site involved in transmitting the message (see Fig. 11.1). The second binding site may interact with another protein or with DNA. They may be either **plasma membrane receptors** (which span the plasma membrane and contain an extracellular binding domain for the messenger) or **intracellular binding proteins** (for messengers able to diffuse into the cell) (see Fig. 11.1). Most plasma membrane receptors fall into the categories of **ion channel receptors**, **tyrosine kinase receptors**, **tyrosine-kinase associated receptors (JAK-STAT receptors)**, **serine-threonine kinase receptors**, or **heptahelical receptors** (proteins with seven α-helices spanning the membrane). When a chemical messenger binds to a receptor, the signal it is carrying must be converted into an intracellular response. This conversion is called **signal transduction**.

Signal Transduction for Intracellular Receptors. Most intracellular receptors are **gene-specific transcription factors**, proteins that bind to DNA and regulate the transcription of certain genes (Gene transcription is the process of copying the genetic code from DNA to RNA.).

Signal Transduction for Plasma Membrane Receptors. Mechanisms of signal transduction that follow the binding of signaling molecules to plasma membrane receptors include phosphorylation of receptors at tyrosine residues (**receptor tyrosine kinase** activity), conformational changes in **signal transducer proteins** (e.g., proteins with **SH2** domains, the **monomeric G protein Ras, heterotrimeric G proteins**) or increases in the levels of **intracellular second messengers**. Second messengers are nonprotein molecules generated inside the cell in response to *hormone binding that continue transmission of the message. Examples include 3′,5′-cyclic AMP (**cAMP**), inositol trisphosphate (**IP₃**), and diacylglycerol (**DAG**).*

Signaling often requires a rapid response and rapid termination of the message, which may be achieved by degradation of the messenger or second messenger, the automatic G protein clock, deactivation of signal transduction kinases by phosphatases, or other means.

THE WAITING ROOM

Mya Sthenia is a 37-year-old woman who complains of increasing muscle fatigue in her lower extremities with walking. If she rests for 5 to 10 minutes, her leg strength returns to normal. She also notes that if she talks on the phone, her ability to form words gradually decreases. By evening, her upper eyelids droop to the point that she has to pull her upper lids back in order to see normally. These symptoms are becoming increasingly severe. When Mya is asked to sustain an upward gaze, her upper eyelids eventually drift downward involuntarily. When she is asked to hold both arms straight out in front of her for as long as she is able, both arms begin to drift downward within minutes. Her physician suspects that **Mya Sthenia** has myasthenia gravis and orders a test to determine whether she has antibodies in her blood directed against the acetylcholine receptor.

Ann O'Rexia, who suffers from anorexia nervosa, has increased her weight to 102 lb from a low of 85 lb (see Chapter 9). On the advice of her physician, she has been eating more to prevent fatigue during her daily jogging regimen. She runs about 10 miles before breakfast every second day and forces herself to drink a high-energy supplement immediately afterward.

Dennis Veere was hospitalized for dehydration resulting from cholera toxin (see Chapter 10). In his intestinal mucosal cells, cholera A toxin indirectly activated the CFTR channel, resulting in secretion of chloride ion and Na^+ ion into the intestinal lumen. Ion secretion was followed by loss of water, resulting in vomiting and watery diarrhea. Dennis is being treated for hypovolemic shock.

I. GENERAL FEATURES OF CHEMICAL MESSENGERS

Certain universal characteristics to chemical messenger systems are illustrated in Figure 11.1. Signaling generally follows the sequence: (1) the chemical messenger is secreted from a specific cell in response to a stimulus; (2) the messenger diffuses or is transported through blood or other extracellular fluid to the target cell; (3) a receptor in the target cell (a plasma membrane receptor or intracellular receptor) specifically binds the messenger; (4) binding of the messenger to the receptor elicits a response; (5) the signal ceases and is terminated. Chemical messengers elicit their response in the target cell without being metabolized by the cell.

Another general feature of chemical messenger systems is that the specificity of the response is dictated by the type of receptor and its location. Generally, each receptor binds only one specific chemical messenger, and each receptor initiates a characteristic signal transduction pathway that will ultimately activate or inhibit certain processes in the cell. Only certain cells, the target cells, carry receptors for that messenger and are capable of responding to its message.

The means of signal termination is an exceedingly important aspect of cell signaling, and failure to terminate a message contributes to a number of diseases, such as cancer.

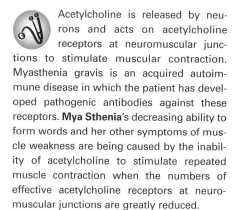

Acetylcholine is released by neurons and acts on acetylcholine receptors at neuromuscular junctions to stimulate muscular contraction. Myasthenia gravis is an acquired autoimmune disease in which the patient has developed pathogenic antibodies against these receptors. **Mya Sthenia**'s decreasing ability to form words and her other symptoms of muscle weakness are being caused by the inability of acetylcholine to stimulate repeated muscle contraction when the numbers of effective acetylcholine receptors at neuromuscular junctions are greatly reduced.

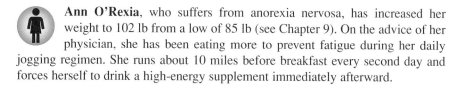

Endocrine hormones enable **Ann O'Rexia** to mobilize fuels from her adipose tissue during her periods of fasting and during jogging. While she fasts overnight, α-cells of her pancreas increase secretion of the polypeptide hormone glucagon. The stress of prolonged fasting and chronic exercise stimulates release of cortisol, a steroid hormone, from her adrenal cortex. The exercise of jogging also increases secretion of the hormones epinephrine and norepinephrine from the adrenal medulla. Each of these hormones is being released in response to a specific signal and causes a characteristic response in a target tissue, enabling her to exercise. However, each of these hormones binds to a different type of receptor and works in a different way.

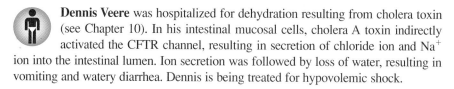

Ann O'Rexia's fasting is accompanied by high levels of the endocrine hormone glucagon, which is secreted in response to low blood glucose levels. It enters the blood and acts on the liver to stimulate a number of pathways, including the release of glucose from glycogen stores (glycogenolysis) (see Chapter 3). The specificity of its action is determined by the location of receptors. Although liver parenchymal cells have glucagon receptors, skeletal muscle and many other tissues do not. Therefore, glucagon cannot stimulate glycogenolysis in these tissues.

Most chemical messengers (including neurotransmitters, cytokines, and endocrine hormones) are contained in vesicles that fuse with a region of the cell membrane when the cell receives a stimulus to release the messenger. Most secretory cells use a similar set of proteins to enable vesicle fusion, and fusion is usually triggered by Ca^{2+} influx, as seen with the release of acetylcholine.

Myasthenia gravis is a disease of autoimmunity caused by the production of an antibody directed against the acetylcholine receptor in skeletal muscle. In this disease, B and T lymphocytes cooperate in producing a variety of antibodies against the nicotinic acetylcholine receptor. The antibodies then bind to various locations in the receptor and cross-link the receptors, forming a multireceptor antibody complex. The complex is endocytosed and incorporated into lysosomes, where it is degraded. **Mya Sthenia**, therefore, has fewer functional receptors for acetylcholine to activate.

A. General Features of Chemical Messenger Systems Applied to the Nicotinic Acetylcholine Receptor

The individual steps involved in cell signaling by chemical messengers are illustrated with acetylcholine, a neurotransmitter that acts on nicotinic acetylcholine receptors on the plasma membrane of certain muscle cells. This system exhibits the classic features of chemical messenger release and specificity of response.

Neurotransmitters are secreted from neurons in response to an electrical stimulus called the action potential (a voltage difference across the plasma membrane, caused by changes in Na^+ and K^+ gradients, that is propagated along a nerve). The neurotransmitters diffuse across a synapse to another excitable cell, where they elicit a response (Fig. 11.2). Acetylcholine is the neurotransmitter at neuromuscular junctions, where it transmits a signal from a motor nerve to a muscle fiber that elicits contraction of the fiber. Before release, acetylcholine is sequestered in vesicles clustered near an active zone in the presynaptic membrane. This membrane also has voltage-gated Ca^{2+} channels that open when the action potential reaches them, resulting in an influx of Ca^{2+}. Ca^{2+} triggers fusion of the vesicles with the plasma membrane, and acetylcholine is released into the synaptic cleft. Thus, the chemical messenger is released from a specific cell in response to a specific stimulus.

Acetylcholine diffuses across the synaptic cleft to bind to plasma membrane receptors on the muscle cells called nicotinic acetylcholine receptors (Fig. 11.3). The subunits are assembled around a channel, which has a funnel-shaped opening in the center. As acetylcholine binds to the receptor, a conformational change opens the narrow portion of the channel (the gate), allowing Na^+ to diffuse in and K^+ to diffuse out (A uniform property of all receptors is that signal transduction begins with conformational changes in the receptor.). The change in ion concentration

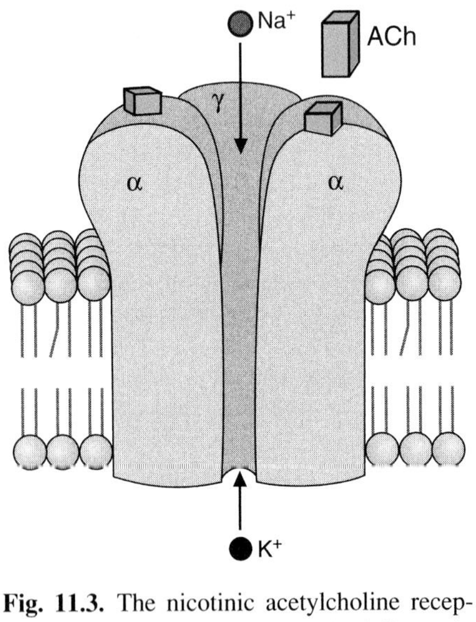

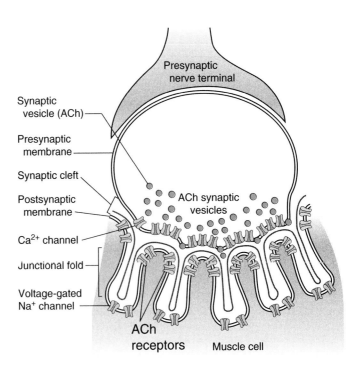

Fig. 11.3. The nicotinic acetylcholine receptor. Each receptor is composed of five subunits, and each subunit has four membrane-spanning helical regions. The two α subunits are identical and contain binding sites for acetylcholine. When two acetylcholine molecules are bound, the subunits change their conformation so that the channel in the center of the receptor is open, allowing K^+ ions to diffuse out and Na^+ ions to diffuse in.

Fig. 11.2. Acetylcholine receptors at the neuromuscular junction. A motor nerve terminates in several branches; each branch terminates in a bulb-shaped structure called the presynaptic bouton. Each bouton synapses with a region of the muscle fiber containing junctional folds. At the crest of each fold, there is a high concentration of acetylcholine receptors, which are gated ion channels.

activates a sequence of events that eventually triggers the cellular response—
contraction of the fiber.

Once acetylcholine secretion stops, the message is rapidly terminated by acetylcholinesterase, an enzyme located on the postsynaptic membrane that cleaves
acetylcholine. It is also terminated by diffusion of acetylcholine away from the
synapse. Rapid termination of message is a characteristic of systems requiring a
rapid response from the target cell.

B. Endocrine, Paracrine, and Autocrine

The actions of chemical messengers are often classified as endocrine, paracrine, or
autocrine (Fig. 11.4). Each endocrine hormone is secreted by a specific cell type

 Mya Sthenia was tested with an
inhibitor of acetylcholinesterase,
edrophonium chloride, administered intravenously (see Chapter 8, Fig.
8.18). After this drug inactivates acetylcholinesterase, acetylcholine that is released
from the nerve terminal accumulates in the
synaptic cleft. Even though Mya expresses
fewer acetylcholine receptors on her muscle
cells (due to the auto-antibody–induced
degradation of receptors), by increasing the
local concentration of acetylcholine, these
receptors have a higher probability of being
occupied and activated. Therefore, acute
intravenous administration of this short-
acting drug briefly improves muscular weakness in patients with myasthenia gravis.

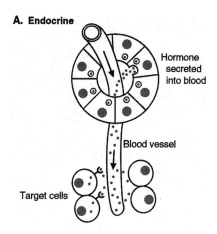
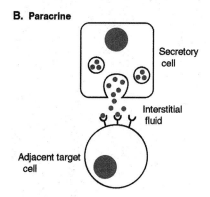
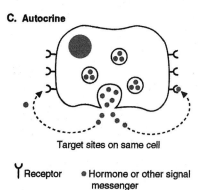

Fig. 11.4. Endocrine, autocrine, and paracrine actions of hormones and other chemical messengers.

(generally in an endocrine gland), enters the blood, and exerts its actions on specific target cells, which may be some distance away. In contrast to endocrine hormones, paracrine actions are those performed on nearby cells, and the location of the cells plays a role in specificity of the response. Synaptic transmission by acetylcholine and other neurotransmitters (sometimes called neurocrine signaling) is an example of paracrine signaling. Acetylcholine activates only those acetylcholine receptors located across the synaptic cleft from the signaling nerve and not all muscles with acetylcholine receptors. Paracrine actions are also very important in limiting the immune response to a specific location in the body, a feature that helps prevent the development of autoimmune disease. Autocrine actions involve a messenger acting on the cell from which it is secreted, or on nearby cells that are the same type as the secreting cells.

C. Types of Chemical Messengers

Three major signaling systems in the body employ chemical messengers: the nervous system, the endocrine system, and the immune system. Some messengers are difficult to place in just one such category.

1. THE NERVOUS SYSTEM

The nervous system secretes two types of messengers: small molecule neurotransmitters, often called biogenic amines, and neuropeptides. Small molecule neurotransmitters are nitrogen-containing molecules, which can be amino acids or are derivatives of amino acids (e.g., acetylcholine and γ-aminobutyrate, Fig. 11.5). Neuropeptides are usually small peptides (between 4 and 35 amino acids), secreted by neurons, that act as neurotransmitters at synaptic junctions or are secreted into the blood to act as neurohormones.

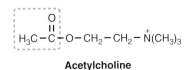

Acetylcholine

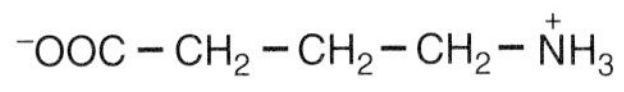

$$^-OOC - CH_2 - CH_2 - CH_2 - \overset{+}{N}H_3$$

γ-aminobutyrate (GABA)

Fig. 11.5. Small molecule neurotransmitters.

The catecholamine hormone epinephrine (also called adrenaline) is the fight, fright, and flight hormone. Epinephrine and the structurally similar hormone norepinephrine are released from the adrenal medulla in response to a variety of immediate stresses, including pain, hemorrhage, exercise, hypoglycemia, and hypoxia. Thus, as **Ann O'Rexia** begins to jog, there is a rapid release of epinephrine and norepinephrine into the blood.

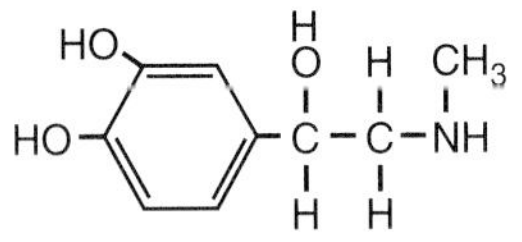

Epinephrine

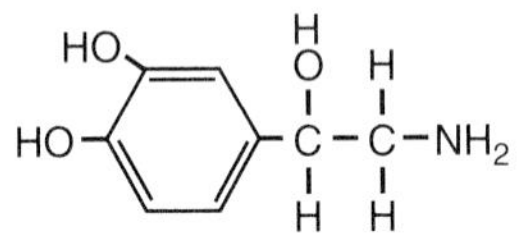

Norepinephrine

2. THE ENDOCRINE SYSTEM

Endocrine hormones are defined as compounds, secreted from specific endocrine cells in endocrine glands, that reach their target cells by transport through the blood. Insulin, for example, is an endocrine hormone secreted from the β cells of the pancreas. Classic hormones are generally divided into the structural categories of polypeptide hormones (e.g., insulin –see Chapter 6, Fig. 6.15 for the structure of insulin), catecholamines such as epinephrine (which is also a neurotransmitter), steroid hormones (which are derived from cholesterol), and thyroid hormone (which is derived from tyrosine). Many of these endocrine hormones also exert paracrine or autocrine actions. The hormones that regulate metabolism are discussed throughout this chapter and in subsequent chapters of this text.

Some compounds normally considered hormones are more difficult to categorize. For example, retinoids, which are derivatives of vitamin A (also called retinol) and vitamin D (which is also derived from cholesterol) are usually classified as hormones, although they are not synthesized in endocrine cells.

3. THE IMMUNE SYSTEM

The messengers of the immune system, called cytokines, are small proteins with a molecular weight of approximately 20,000 daltons. Cytokines regulate a network of responses designed to kill invading microorganisms. The different classes of cytokines (interleukins, tumor necrosis factors, interferons, and colony-stimulating factors) are secreted by cells of the immune system and usually alter the behavior of other cells in the immune system by activating the transcription of genes for proteins involved in the immune response.

Selection and Proliferation of B Cells Producing the Desired Antibody. Interleukins, a class of cytokine, illustrate some of the signaling involved in the immune response. Interleukins are polypeptide factors with molecular weights ranging from 15,000 to 25,000 Daltons. They participate in a part of the immune response called humoral immunity, which is carried out by a population of lymphoid B cells producing just one antibody against one particular antigen. The proliferation of cells producing that particular antibody is mediated by receptors and by certain interleukins.

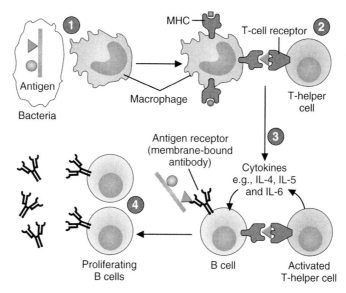

Bacteria phagocytized by macrophages are digested by lysosomes. (1) A partially digested fragment of the bacterial protein (the blue antigen) is presented on the extracellular surface of the macrophage by a membrane protein called an MHC (**m**ajor **h**istocompatibility **c**omplex). (2) Certain lymphoid cells called T-helper cells contain receptors that can bind to the displayed antigen–MHC complex, a process that activates the T-cell (direct cell-to-cell signaling, requiring recognition molecules). (3) The activated T-helper cell then finds and binds to a B cell whose antigen receptor binds a soluble fragment of that same bacterially derived antigen molecule (again, direct cell-to-cell signaling). The bound T cell secretes interleukins, which act on the B cell (a paracrine signal). The interleukins thus stimulate proliferation of only those B cells capable of synthesizing and secreting the desirable antibody. Furthermore, the interleukins determine which class of antibody is produced.

4. THE EICOSANOIDS

The eicosanoids (including prostaglandins [PG], thromboxanes, and leukotrienes) control cellular function in response to injury (Fig. 11.6) These compounds are all derived from arachidonic acid, a 20-carbon polyunsaturated fatty acid that is usually present in cells as part of the membrane lipid phosphatidylcholine (see Chapter 5, Fig. 5.21). Although almost every cell in the body produces an eicosanoid in response to tissue injury, different cells produce different eicosanoids. The eicosanoids act principally in paracrine and autocrine functions, affecting the cells that produce them or their neighboring cells. For example, vascular endothelial cells (cells lining the vessel wall) secrete the prostaglandin PGI_2 (prostacyclin), which acts on nearby smooth muscle cells to cause vasodilation (expansion of the blood vessel).

5. GROWTH FACTORS

Growth factors are polypeptides that function through stimulation of cellular proliferation. For example, platelets aggregating at the site of injury to a blood vessel secrete

Lotta Topaigne suffered enormously painful gout attacks affecting her great toe (see Clinical Comments, Chapter 8). The extreme pain was caused by the release of a leukotriene that stimulated pain receptors. The precipitated urate crystals in her big toe stimulated recruited inflammatory cells to release the leukotriene.

Arachidonic acid
($C_{20:4}, \Delta^{5,8,11,14}$)

Prostacyclin
PGI_2

Fig. 11.6. Eicosanoids are derived from arachidonic acid and retain its original 20 carbons (thus the name *eicosanoids*). All prostaglandins, such as prostacyclin, also have an internal ring.

PDGF (**p**latelet-**d**erived **g**rowth **f**actor). PDGF stimulates the proliferation of nearby smooth muscle cells, which eventually form a plaque covering the injured site. Some growth factors are considered hormones, and some have been called cytokines.

Each of the hundreds of chemical messengers has its own specific receptor, which will usually bind no other messenger.

II. INTRACELLULAR TRANSCRIPTION FACTOR RECEPTORS

A. Intracellular Versus Plasma Membrane Receptors

The structural properties of a messenger determine, to some extent, the type of receptor it binds. Most receptors fall into two broad categories: intracellular receptors or plasma membrane receptors (Fig. 11.7) Messengers using intracellular receptors must be hydrophobic molecules able to diffuse through the plasma membrane into cells. In contrast, polar molecules such as peptide hormones, cytokines, and catecholamines cannot rapidly cross the plasma membrane and must bind to a plasma membrane receptor.

Most of the intracellular receptors for lipophilic messengers are gene-specific transcription factors. A transcription factor is a protein that binds to a specific site on DNA and regulates the rate of transcription of a gene (i.e., synthesis of the mRNA). External signaling molecules bind to transcription factors that bind to a specific sequence on DNA and regulate the expression of only certain genes; they are called gene-specific or site-specific transcription factors.

B. The Steroid Hormone/Thyroid Hormone Superfamily of Receptors

Lipophilic hormones that use intracellular gene-specific transcription factors include the steroid hormones, thyroid hormone, retinoic acid (active form of vitamin A), and vitamin D (Fig. 11.8). Because these compounds are water-insoluble, they are transported in the blood bound to serum albumin, which has a hydrophobic binding pocket, or to a more specific transport protein, such as steroid hormone-binding globulin (SHBG) and thyroid hormone-binding globulin (TBG). The intracellular receptors for these hormones are structurally similar and are referred to as the steroid hormone/thyroid hormone superfamily of receptors.

The steroid hormone/thyroid hormone superfamily of receptors reside primarily in the nucleus, although some are found in the cytoplasm. The glucocorticoid receptor, for example, exists as cytoplasmic multimeric complexes associated with heat shock proteins. When the hormone cortisol (a glucocorticoid) binds, the receptor undergoes a conformational change and dissociates from the heat shock proteins, exposing a nuclear translocation signal (see Chapter 10, Section VI.) The receptors dimerize, and the complex (including bound hormone) translocates to the nucleus, where it binds to a portion of the DNA called the hormone response element (e.g.,

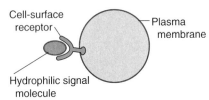

Cell-surface receptors

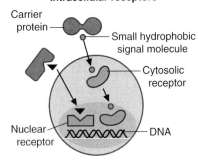

Intracellular receptors

Fig. 11.7. Intracellular vs. plasma membrane receptors. Plasma membrane receptors have extracellular binding domains. Intracellular receptors bind steroid hormones or other messengers able to diffuse through the plasma membrane. Their receptors may reside in the cytoplasm and translocate to the nucleus, reside in the nucleus bound to DNA, or reside in the nucleus bound to other proteins.

 The steroid hormone cortisol is synthesized and released from the adrenal cortex in response to the polypeptide hormone ACTH (adrenal corticotrophic hormone). Chronic stress (pain, hypoglycemia, hemorrhage, and exercise) signals are passed from the brain cortex to the hypothalamus to the anterior pituitary, which releases ACTH. Cortisol acts on tissues to change enzyme levels and redistribute nutrients in preparation for acute stress. For example, it increases transcription of the genes for regulatory enzymes in the pathway of gluconeogenesis, thereby increasing the content of these enzymes (called gene-specific activation of transcription, or induction of protein synthesis). Induction of gluconeogenic enzymes prepares the liver to respond rapidly to hypoglycemia with increased synthesis of glucose. **Ann O'Rexia**, who has been frequently fasting and exercising, has an increased capacity for gluconeogenesis in her liver.

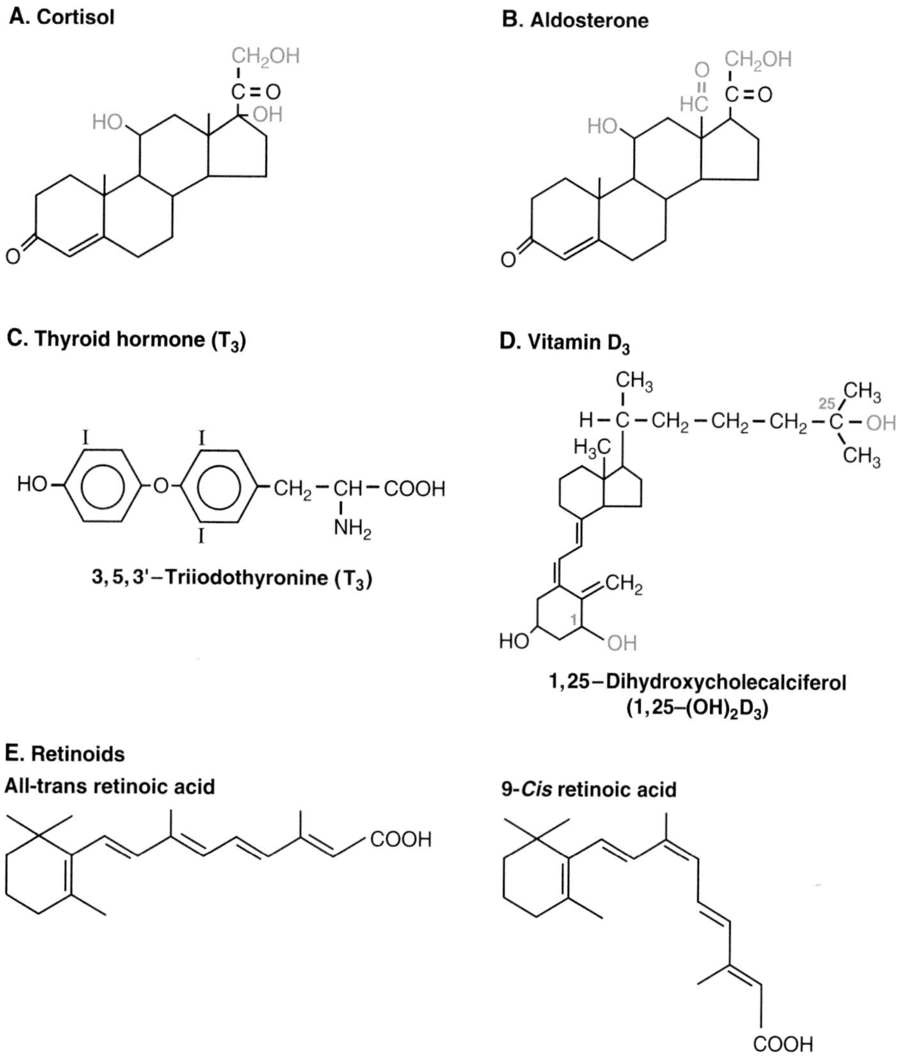

A. Cortisol

B. Aldosterone

C. Thyroid hormone (T$_3$)

3,5,3'-Triiodothyronine (T$_3$)

D. Vitamin D$_3$

1,25-Dihydroxycholecalciferol
(1,25-(OH)$_2$D$_3$)

E. Retinoids
All-trans retinoic acid

9-*Cis* retinoic acid

Fig. 11.8. Steroid hormone/thyroid hormone superfamily. A. Cortisol (a glucocorticoid). B. Aldosterone (an androgen). C. Thyroid hormone D. Vitamin D$_3$. E. Retinoids.

the glucocorticoid receptor binds to the glucocorticoid response element, GRE). Most of the intracellular receptors reside principally in the nucleus, and some of these are constitutively bound, as dimers, to their response element in DNA (e.g., the thyroid hormone receptor). Binding of the hormone changes its activity and its ability to associate with, or disassociate from, DNA. Regulation of gene transcription by these receptors is described in Chapter 16.

Recently several nuclear receptors have been identified that play important roles in intermediary metabolism, and they have become the target of lipid-lowering drugs. These include the peroxisome proliferator activated receptors (PPAR α, β and γ), the liver X-activated receptor (LXR), the farnesoid X-activated receptors (FXR), and the pregnane X receptor (PXR). These receptors form heterodimers with the 9-*cis* retinoic acid receptor (RXR) and bind to their appropriate response elements in DNA in an inactive state. When the activating ligand binds to the receptor (oxysterols for LXR, bile salts for FXR, secondary bile salts for PXR, and fatty acids and their derivatives for the PPARs), the complex is activated, and gene expression is altered. Unlike the cortisol receptor, these receptors reside in the nucleus and are activated once their ligands enter the nucleus and bind to them.

III. PLASMA MEMBRANE RECEPTORS AND SIGNAL TRANSDUCTION

All plasma membrane receptors are proteins with certain features in common: an extracellular domain that binds the chemical messenger, one or more membrane-spanning domains that are α-helices, and an intracellular domain that initiates signal transduction. As the ligand binds to the extracellular domain of its receptor, it causes a conformational change that is communicated to the intracellular domain through the rigid α-helix of the transmembrane domain. The activated intracellular domain initiates a characteristic signal transduction pathway that usually involves the binding of a specific intracellular signal transduction protein.

The pathways of signal transduction for plasma membrane receptors have two major types of effects on the cell: (1) rapid and immediate effects on cellular ion levels or activation/inhibition of enzymes and/or (2) slower changes in the rate of gene expression for a specific set of proteins. Often, a signal transduction pathway will diverge to produce both kinds of effects.

A. Major Classes of Plasma Membrane Receptors

Individual plasma membrane receptors are grouped into the categories of ion channel receptors, receptors that are kinases or bind kinases, and receptors that work through second messengers. This classification is based on the receptor's general structure and means of signal transduction.

1. ION CHANNEL RECEPTORS

The ion channel receptors are similar in structure to the nicotinic acetylcholine receptor (see Fig. 11.3). Signal transduction consists of the conformational change when ligand binds. Most small molecule neurotransmitters and some neuropeptides use ion channel receptors.

2. RECEPTORS THAT ARE KINASES OR BIND KINASES

Several types of receptors that are kinases or bind kinases are illustrated in Figure 11.9. Their common feature is that the intracellular domain of the receptor (or an associated protein) is a kinase that is activated when the messenger binds to the extracellular domain. The receptor kinase phosphorylates an amino acid residue on the receptor (autophosphorylation) or an associated protein. The message is propagated through signal transducer proteins that bind to the activated messenger-receptor complex (e.g., Grb2, STAT, or Smad).

Signal transduction pathways, like a river, run in one direction. From a given point in a signal transduction pathway, events closer to the receptor are referred to as "upstream," and events closer to the response are referred to as "downstream."

Protein kinases transfer a phosphate group from ATP to the hydroxyl group of a specific amino acid residue in the protein. Tyrosine kinases transfer the phosphate group to the hydroxyl group of a specific tyrosine residue and serine/threonine protein kinases to the hydroxyl of a specific serine or threonine residue (serine is more often phosphorylated than threonine in target proteins). Different protein kinases have specificity for distinct amino acid sequences (containing a tyrosine, serine, or threonine). Thus, two different protein kinases target distinct sequences (and usually different proteins) for phosphorylation. A protein containing both target sequences could be a substrate for both protein kinases.

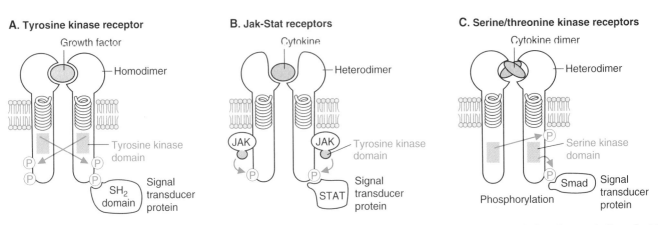

Fig. 11.9. Receptors that are kinases or bind kinases. The kinase domains are shown in blue, and the phosphorylation sites are indicated with blue arrows. A. Tyrosine kinase receptors. B. JAK-STAT receptors. C. Serine/threonine kinase receptors.

3. HEPTAHELICAL RECEPTORS

Heptahelical receptors (which contain 7-membrane spanning α-helices) are the most common type of plasma membrane receptor. They work through second messengers, which are small nonprotein compounds, such as cAMP, generated inside the cell in response to messenger binding to the receptor (Fig. 11.10). They continue intracellular transmission of the message from the hormone/cytokine/neurotransmitter, which is the "first" messenger. Second messengers are present in low concentrations so that their concentration, and hence the message, can be rapidly initiated and terminated.

B. Signal Transduction through Tyrosine Kinase Receptors

The tyrosine kinase receptors are summarized in Figure 11.9A. They generally exist in the membrane as monomers with a single membrane-spanning helix. One molecule of the growth factor generally binds two molecules of the receptor and promotes their dimerization (Fig. 11.11). Once the receptor dimer has formed, the intracellular tyrosine kinase domains of the receptor phosphorylate each other on certain tyrosine residues (autophosphorylation). The phosphotyrosine residues form specific binding sites for signal transducer proteins.

1. RAS AND THE MAP KINASE PATHWAY

One of the domains of the receptor containing a phosphotyrosine residue forms a binding site for intracellular proteins with a specific three-dimensional structure known as the SH2 domain (the Src homology 2 domain, named for the first protein in which it was found, the src protein of the Rous sarcoma virus). The adaptor

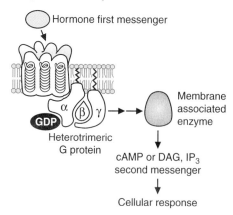

Heptahelical receptors

Fig. 11.10. Heptahelical Receptors and Second Messengers. The secreted chemical messenger (hormone, cytokine, or neurotransmitter) is the first messenger, which binds to a plasma membrane receptor such as the heptahelical receptors. The activated hormone–receptor complex activates a heterotrimeric G protein and via stimulation of membrane-bound enzymes, different G-proteins lead to generation of one or more intracellular second messengers, such as cAMP, diacylglycerol (DAG), or inositol trisphosphate (IP_3).

 Although many different signal transducer proteins have SH2 domains, and many receptors have phosphotyrosine residues, each signal transducer protein is specific for one type of receptor. This specificity of binding results from the fact that each phosphotyrosine residue has a different amino acid sequence around it that forms the binding domain. Likewise, the SH2 domain of the transducer protein is only part of its binding domain.

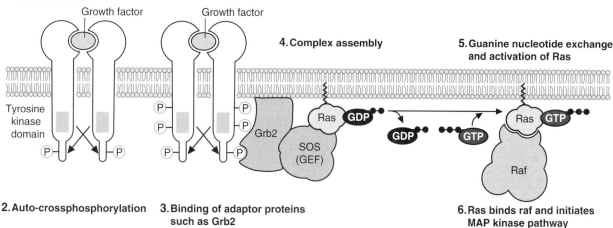

Fig. 11.11. Signal transduction by tyrosine kinase receptors. (1) Binding and dimerizaion. (2) Autophosphorylation. (3) Binding of Grb2 and SOS. (4) SOS is a GEF (guanine nucleotide exchange protein) that binds Ras, a monomeric G protein anchored to the plasma membrane. (5) GEF activates the exchange of GTP for bound GDP on Ras. (6) Activated Ras containing GTP binds the target enzyme Raf, thereby activating it.

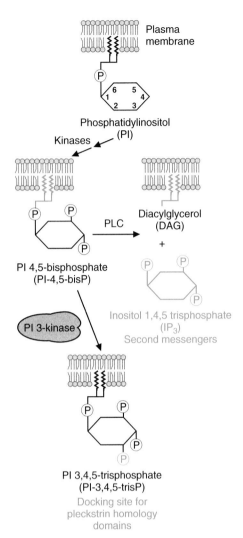

Fig. 11.12. Major route for generation of the phosphatidyl inositide signal molecules, inositol 1,4,5-trisphosphate (IP$_3$) and phosphatidylinositol 3,4,5 trisphosphate (PI-3,4,5-trisP). PI 3-kinase phosphorylates PI-4,5-bisP and PI-4P at the 3 position. Prime symbols are sometimes used in these names to denote the inositol ring. DAG is also a second messenger.

protein Grb2, which is bound to a membrane phosphoinositide, is one of the proteins with an SH2 domain that binds to phosphotyrosine residues on growth factor receptors. Binding to the receptor causes a conformational change in Grb2 that activates another binding site called an SH3 domain. These activated SH3 domains bind the protein SOS (SOS is an acronym for "son of sevenless," a name unrelated to the function or structure of the compound). SOS is a guanine nucleotide exchange factor (GEF) for Ras, a monomeric G protein located in the plasma membrane (see Chapter 9, Section III.C.2.) SOS activates exchange of guanosine triphosphate (GTP) for guanosine diphosphate (GDP) on Ras, causing a conformational change in Ras that promotes binding of the protein Raf. Raf is a serine protein kinase that is also called MAPKKK (**m**itogen **a**ctivated **p**rotein **k**inase **k**inase **k**inase.) Raf begins a sequence of successive phosphorylation steps called a phosphorylation cascade (When a kinase in a cascade is phosphorylated, it binds and phosphorylates the next enzyme in the cascade.). The MAP kinase cascade terminates at a gene transcription factor, thereby regulating transcription of certain genes involved in cell survival and proliferation.

Many tyrosine kinase receptors (as well as heptahelical receptors) also have additional signaling pathways involving phosphatidylinositol phosphates.

2.   PHOSPHATIDYLINOSITOL PHOSPHATES IN SIGNAL TRANSDUCTION

Phosphatidylinositol phosphates serve two different functions in signal transduction: (1) Phosphatidylinositol 4′,5′ bisphosphate (PI-4,5-bisP) can be cleaved to generate the two intracellular second messengers, diacylglycerol (DAG) and inositol trisphosphate (IP$_3$); and (2) Phosphatidylinositol 3′,4′,5′ trisphosphate (PI-3,4,5-trisP) can serve as a plasma membrane docking site for signal transduction proteins.

Phosphatidyl inositol, which is present in the inner leaflet of the plasma membrane, is converted to PI-4,5-bisP by kinases that phosphorylate the inositol ring at the 4′ and 5′ positions (Fig. 11.12). PI-4,5-bisP, which has three phosphate groups, is cleaved by a phospholipase C-isozyme to generate IP$_3$ and DAG. The phospholipase isozyme C$_\gamma$ (PLC$_\gamma$) is activated by tyrosine kinase growth factor receptors, and phospholipase Cβ is activated by a heptahelical receptor–G protein signal transduction pathway.

PI-4,5-bisP can also be phosphorylated at the 3′ position of inositol by the enzyme phosphatidylinositol 3′ kinase (PI 3-kinase) to form PI -3,4,5- trisP (see Fig. 11.12). PI-3,4,5- tris P (and PI -3,4 bis P) form membrane docking sites for proteins containing a certain sequence of amino acids called the pleckstrin homology (PH) domain. PI 3- kinase contains an SH2 domain and is activated by binding to a specific phosphotyrosine site on a tyrosine kinase receptor or receptor-associated protein.

3.   THE INSULIN RECEPTOR

The insulin receptor, a member of the tyrosine kinase family of receptors, provides a good example of divergence in the pathway of signal transduction. Unlike other growth factor receptors, the insulin receptor exists in the membrane as a preformed dimer, with each half containing an α and a β subunit (Fig. 11.13). The β subunits

   Insulin is a growth factor that is essential for cell viability and growth. It increases general protein synthesis, which strongly affects muscle mass. However, it also regulates immediate nutrient availability and storage, including glucose transport into skeletal muscle and glycogen synthesis. Thus, **Di Abietes** and other patients with type I diabetes mellitus who lack insulin rapidly develop hyperglycemia once insulin levels drop too low. They also exhibit muscle "wasting." To mediate the diverse regulatory roles of insulin, the signal transduction pathway diverges after activation of the receptor and phosphorylation of IRS, which has multiple binding sites for different signal mediator proteins.

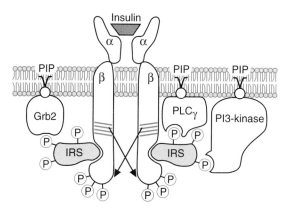

Fig. 11.13. Insulin receptor signaling. The insulin receptor is a dimer of two membrane-spanning α–β pairs. The tyrosine kinase domains are shown in blue, and arrows indicate auto-crossphosphorylation. The activated receptor binds IRS molecules (insulin receptor substrates) and phosphorylates IRS at multiple sites, thereby forming binding sites for proteins with SH2 domains: Grb2, phospholipase Cγ(PLCγ), and PI 3-kinase. These proteins are associated with various phosphatidylinositol phosphates (all designated with PIP) in the plasma membrane.

autophosphorylate each other when insulin binds, thereby activating the receptor. The activated phosphorylated receptor binds a protein called IRS (insulin receptor substrate). The activated receptor kinase phosphorylates IRS at multiple sites, creating multiple binding sites for different proteins with SH2 domains. One of the sites binds Grb2, leading to activation of Ras and the MAP kinase pathway. Grb2 is anchored to PI-3,4,5-trisP in the plasma membrane through its PH (pleckstrin homology) domain. At another phosphotyrosine site, PI 3-kinase binds and is activated. At a third site, phospholipase C_γ(PLC$_\gamma$) binds and is activated. The insulin receptor can also transmit signals through a direct docking with other signal transduction intermediates.

The signal pathway initiated by the insulin receptor complex involving PI 3-kinase leads to activation of protein kinase B, a serine-threonine kinase that mediates many of the downstream effects of insulin (Fig. 11.14). PI 3- kinase binds and phosphorylates PI-4,5- bis P in the membrane to form PI-3,4,5- trisP. Protein kinase

Protein kinase B is a serine-threonine kinase, also known as Akt. One of the signal transduction pathways from protein kinase B (Akt) leads to the effects of insulin on glucose metabolism. Other pathways, long associated with Akt, result in the phosphorylation of a host of other proteins that affect cell growth, cell cycle entry, and cell survival. In general, phosphorylation of these proteins by Akt inhibits their action and promotes cell survival.

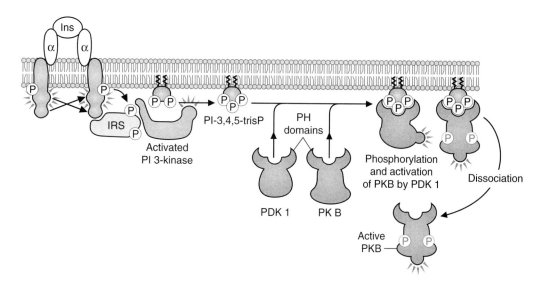

Fig. 11.14. The insulin receptor–protein kinase B signaling pathway. Abbreviations: Ins, insulin; IRS, insulin receptor substrate; PH domains, pleckstrin homology domains; PDK1, phosphoinositide-dependent protein kinase 1; PKB, protein kinase B. The final phosphorylation step that activates PKB is shown in blue.

B and PDK1 (phosphoinositide-dependent kinase-1) are recruited to the membrane by their PH domains, where PDK1 phosphorylates and activates protein kinase B. Many other signal transducer proteins have PH domains and are docked at the membrane, where they can find and bind each other. Thus, the insulin signal diverges again and again. Insulin is covered in more detail in Chapters 26, 36 and 43.

C. Signal Transduction by JAK-STAT Receptors

Tyrosine kinase-associated receptors called Jak-STAT receptors are often used by cytokines to regulate the proliferation of certain cells involved in the immune response (see Fig. 11.9B). The receptor itself has no intrinsic kinase activity but binds (associates with) the tyrosine kinase Jak (**ja**nus **k**inase). Their signal transducer proteins, called STATs (**s**ignal **t**ransducer and **a**ctivator of **t**ranscription), are themselves gene-specific transcription factors. Thus, Jak-STAT receptors have a more direct route for propagation of the signal to the nucleus than tyrosine kinase receptors.

Each receptor monomer has an extracellular domain, a membrane-spanning region, and an intracellular domain. As the cytokine binds to these receptors, they form dimers (either homodimers or heterodimers, between two distinct receptor molecules) and may cluster (Fig. 11.15). The activated Jaks phosphorylate each other and intracellular tyrosine residues on the receptor, forming phosphotyrosine-binding sites for the SH2 domain of a STAT. STATs are inactive in the cytoplasm until they bind to the receptor complex, where they are also phosphorylated by the bound JAK. Phosphorylation changes the conformation of the STAT, causing it to dissociate from the receptor and dimerize with another phosphorylated STAT, thereby forming an activated transcription factor. The STAT dimer translocates to the nucleus and binds to a response element on DNA, thereby regulating gene transcription.

There are many different STAT proteins, each with a slightly different amino acid sequence. Receptors for different cytokines bind different STATs, which then form heterodimers in various combinations. This microheterogeneity allows different cytokines to target different genes.

D. Receptor Serine/Threonine Kinases

Proteins in the transforming growth factor superfamily use receptors that have serine/threonine kinase activity and associate with proteins from the Smad family, which are gene-specific transcription factors (see Fig. 11.9C). This superfamily includes transforming growth factor β (TGF-β), a cytokine/hormone involved in tissue repair, immune regulation, and cell proliferation, and bone morphogenetic proteins (BMPs), which control proliferation, differentiation, and cell death during development.

Although Jak is an acronym for **ja**nus **k**inase, it has been suggested that it stands for "just another kinase". It was named for Janus, a two-headed god of the Romans.

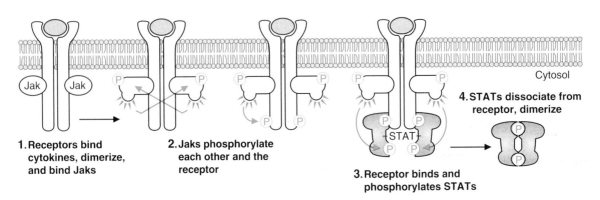

Fig. 11.15. Steps in Jak-STAT receptor signaling.

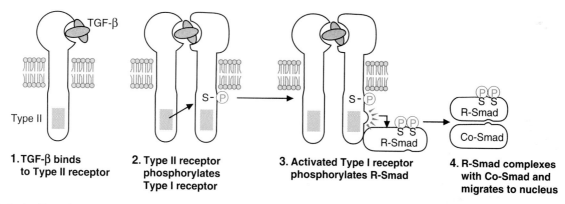

1. TGF-β binds
   to Type II receptor

2. Type II receptor
   phosphorylates
   Type I receptor

3. Activated Type I receptor
   phosphorylates R-Smad

4. R-Smad complexes
   with Co-Smad and
   migrates to nucleus

Fig. 11.16. Serine/threonine receptors and Smad proteins. TGF-β (transforming growth factor β), which is composed of two identical subunits, communicates through a receptor dimer of type I and type II subunits that have serine kinase domains. The type I receptor phosphorylates an R-Smad (receptor-specific Smad), which binds a Co-Smad (common Smad, also called Smad 4).

A simplified version of TGF-β1 binding to its receptor complex and activating Smads is illustrated in Fig. 11.16 The TGF-β receptor complex is composed of two different single membrane-spanning receptor subunits (type I and type II), which have different functions even though they both have serine kinase domains. TGF-β binds to a type II receptor. The activated type II receptor recruits a type I receptor, which it phosphorylates at a serine residue, forming an activated receptor complex. The type I receptor then binds a receptor-specific Smad protein (called R-Smads), which it phosphorylates at serine residues. The phosphorylated R-Smad undergoes a conformational change and dissociates from the receptor. It then forms a complex with another member of the Smad family, Smad 4 (Smad 4 is known as the common Smad, Co-Smad, and is not phosphorylated). The Smad complex, which may contain several Smads, translocates to the nucleus, where it activates or inhibits the transcription of target genes. Receptors for different ligands bind different Smads, which bind to different sites on DNA and regulate the transcription of different genes.

E. Signal Transduction through Heptahelical Receptors

The heptahelical receptors are named for their 7-membrane spanning domains, which are α-helices (see Fig. 11.10; see also Chapter 7, Fig. 7.10). Although hundreds of hormones and neurotransmitters work through heptahelical receptors, the extracellular binding domain of each receptor is specific for just one polypeptide hormone, catecholamine, or neurotransmitter (or its close structural analog). Heptahelical receptors have no intrinsic kinase activity but initiate signal transduction through heterotrimeric G proteins composed of α, β and γ subunits. However, different types of heptahelical receptors bind different G proteins, and different G proteins exert different effects on their target proteins.

1. HETEROTRIMERIC G PROTEINS

The function of heterotrimeric G proteins is illustrated in Figure 11.17 using a hormone that activates adenylyl cyclase (e.g., glucagon or epinephrine). While the α subunit contains bound GDP, it remains associated with the β and γ subunits, either free in the membrane or bound to an unoccupied receptor (see Fig. 11.17, part 1). When the hormone binds, it causes a conformational change in the receptor that activates GDP dissociation and GTP binding. The exchange of GTP for bound GDP causes dissociation of the α subunit from the receptor and from the βγ subunits (see Fig. 11.17, part 2). The α and β subunits are tethered to the intracellular side of the

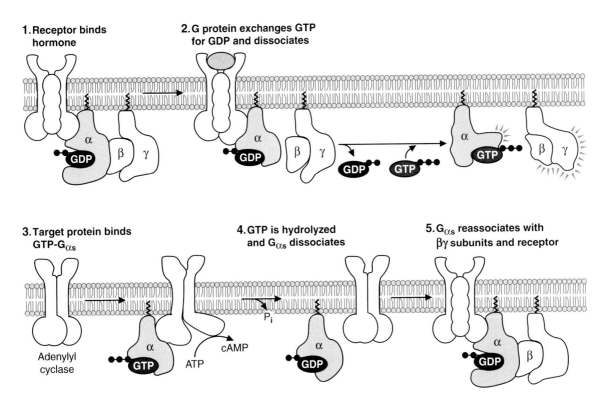

Fig. 11.17. Heptahelical receptors and heterotrimeric G proteins. (1) The intracellular domains of the receptor form a binding site for a G protein containing GDP bound to the α-subunit. (2) Hormone binding to the receptor promotes the exchange of GTP for GDP. As a result, the complex disassembles, releasing the G protein α-subunit from the βγ complex. (3) The Gs α-subunit binds to a target enzyme, thereby changing its activity. The βγ complex may simultaneously target another protein and change its activity. (4) Over time, bound GTP is hydrolysed to GDP, causing dissociation of the α-subunit from adenylyl cyclase. The GDP-α-subunit reassociates with the βγ subunit and the receptor.

The importance of signal termination is illustrated by the "internal clock" of G proteins, which is the rate of spontaneous hydrolysis of GTP to GDP. Mutations in *ras* (the gene encoding Ras) that decrease the rate of GTP hydrolysis are found in about 20 to 30% of all human cancers, including approximately 25% of lung cancers, 50% of colon cancers, and more than 90% of pancreatic cancers. In these mutations of Ras, GTP hydrolysis is decreased and Ras remains locked in the active GTP-bound form, rather than alternating normally between inactive and active state in response to extracellular signals. Consequently, MAP kinase pathways are continuously stimulated and drive cell proliferation, even in the absence of growth factors that would be required for *ras* activation in normal cells.

plasma membrane through lipid anchors, but can still move around on the membrane surface. The GTP-α subunit binds its target enzyme in the membrane, thereby changing its activity. In this example, the α-subunit binds and activates adenylyl cyclase, thereby increasing synthesis of cAMP (see Fig. 11.17, part 3).

With time, the Gα subunit inactivates itself by hydrolyzing its own bound GTP to GDP and P$_i$. This action is unrelated to the number of cAMP molecules formed. Like the monomeric G proteins, the GDP-α subunit then dissociates from its target protein, adenylyl cyclase (see Fig. 11.16, part 4). It reforms the trimeric G protein complex, which may return to bind the empty hormone receptor. As a result of this GTPase "internal clock," sustained elevations of hormone levels are necessary for continued signal transduction and elevation of cAMP.

A large number of different heterotrimeric G protein complexes are generally categorized according to the activity of the α subunit (Table 11.1). The 20 or more different isoforms of Gα fall into four broad categories: Gα$_s$, Gα$_{i/0}$, Gα$_{q/11}$, and Gα12/13$_{13}$. Gα$_s$ refers to α subunits, which, like the one in Figure 11.17, stimulate adenylyl cyclase (hence the *s*). Gα subunits that inhibit adenylyl cyclase are called Gα$_i$. The βγ subunits likewise exist as different isoforms, which also transmit messages.

Acetylcholine has two types of receptors: nicotinic ion channel receptors, the receptors inhibited by antibodies in myasthenia gravis, and muscarinic receptors, which exist as a variety of subtypes. The M2 muscarinic receptors activate a Gα$_{i/o}$ heterotrimeric G protein in which release of the βγ subunit controls K$^+$ channels and pacemaker activity in the heart. Epinephrine has several types and subtypes of heptahelical receptors: β receptors work through a Gα$_s$ and stimulate adenylyl cyclase; α$_2$ receptors in other cells work through a Gα$_i$ protein and inhibit adenylyl cyclase; α$_1$ receptors work through Gα$_q$ subunits and activate phospholipase Cβ. This variety in receptor types allows a messenger to have different actions in different cells.

Table 11.1 Subunits of Heterotrimeric G Proteins

Gα subunit	Action	Some Physiologic Uses
α_s; Gα (s) *	**s**timulates adenyl cyclase	Glucagon and epinephrine to regulate metabolic enzymes, regulatory polypeptide hormones to control steroid hormone and thyroid hormone synthesis, and by some neurotransmitters (e.g., dopamine) to control ion channels
$\alpha_{i/o}$; Gα (i/o) (signal also flows through βγ subunits)	**i**nhibits adenylyl cyclase	Epinephrine, many neurotransmitters including acetylcholine, dopamine, serotonin. Has a role in the transducin pathway, which mediates detection of light in the eye.
$\alpha_{q/11}$; Gα (q/11)	activates phospholipase C_β	Epinephrine, acetylcholine, histamine, thyroid-stimulating hormone (TSH), interleukin 8 , somatostatin, angiotensin
$\alpha_{12/13}$; Gα (12/13)	Physiologic connections are not yet well established	Thromboxane A2, lysophosphatidic acid

*There is a growing tendency to designate the heterotrimeric G protein subunits without using subscripts so that they are actually visible to the naked eye.

2. ADENYLYL CYCLASE AND CAMP PHOSPHODIESTERASE

cAMP is referred to as a second messenger because changes in its concentration reflect changes in the concentration of the hormone (the first messenger). When a hormone binds and adenylyl cyclase is activated, it synthesizes cAMP from adenosine triphosphate (ATP). cAMP is hydrolyzed to AMP by cAMP phosphodiesterase, which also resides in the plasma membrane (Fig. 11.18). The concentration of cAMP and other second messengers is kept at very low levels in cells by balancing the activity of these two enzymes so that cAMP levels can change rapidly when hormone levels change. Some hormones change the concentration of cAMP by targeting the phosphodiesterase enzyme rather than adenylyl cyclase. For example, insulin lowers cAMP levels by causing phosphodiesterase activation.

cAMP exerts diverse effects in cells. It is an allosteric activator of protein kinase A (see Chapter 9, section III.B.3), which is a serine/threonine protein kinase that phosphorylates a large number of metabolic enzymes, thereby providing a rapid response to hormones such as glucagon and epinephrine. The catalytic subunits of protein kinase A also enter the nucleus and phosphorylate a gene-specific transcription factor called CREB (cyclic AMP response element-binding protein). Thus, cAMP also activates a slower response pathway, gene transcription. In other cell types, cAMP directly activates ligand-gated channels.

3. PHOSPHATIDYLINOSITOL SIGNALING BY HEPTAHELICAL RECEPTORS

Certain heptahelical receptors bind the q isoform of the Gα subunit ($Gα_q$), which activates the target enzyme phospholipase C_β (see Fig.11.12). When activated, phospholipase C_β hydrolyzes the membrane lipid phosphatidyl inositol bis phosphate (PI-4,5-bisP) into two second messengers, diacylglycerol (DAG) and 1,4,5-inositol trisphosphate (IP_3). IP_3 has a binding site in the sarcoplasmic reticulum and the endoplasmic reticulum that stimulates the release of Ca^{2+} (Fig. 11.19). Ca^{2+} activates enzymes containing the calcium–calmodulin subunit, including a protein kinase. Diacylglycerol, which remains in the membrane, activates protein kinase C, which then propagates the response by phosphorylating target proteins.

F. Changes in Response to Signals

Tissues vary in their ability to respond to a message through changes in receptor activity or number. Many receptors contain intracellular phosphorylation sites that alter their ability to transmit signals. Receptor number is also varied through

Dennis Veere was hospitalized for dehydration resulting from cholera toxin (see Chapter 10). Cholera A toxin was absorbed into the intestinal mucosal cells, where it was processed and complexed with Arf (ADP-ribosylation factor), a small G protein normally involved in vesicular transport. Cholera A toxin is an NAD-glycohydrolase, which cleaves NAD and transfers the ADP ribose portion to other proteins. It ADP-ribosylates the $Gα_s$ subunit of heterotrimeric G proteins, thereby inhibiting their GTPase activity. As a consequence, they remain actively bound to adenylyl cyclase, resulting in increased production of cAMP. The CFTR channel is activated, resulting in secretion of chloride ion and Na^+ ion into the intestinal lumen. The ion secretion is followed by loss of water, resulting in vomiting and watery diarrhea.

Some signaling pathways cross from the MAP kinase pathway to phosphorylate CREB, and all heterotrimeric G protein pathways diverge to include a route to the MAP kinase pathway. These types of complex interconnections in signaling pathways are sometimes called hormone cross-talk.

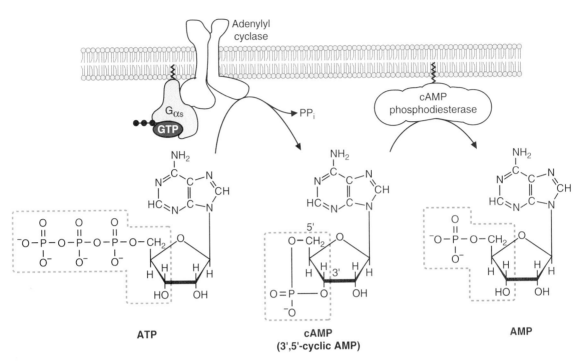

Fig. 11.18. Formation and cleavage of the cyclic phosphodiester bond in cAMP. When activated by Gαs, adenyl cyclase converts ATP to 3′,5′-cyclic AMP + PPi . cAMP phosphodiesterase hydrolyzes cAMP to AMP.

In myasthenia gravis, increased endocytosis and degradation of acetylcholine receptors lead to a signal transduction pathway that decreases synthesis of new receptors. Thus, downregulation of acetylcholine receptors is part of this disease.

down-regulation. After a hormone binds to the receptor, the hormone–receptor complex may be taken into the cell by the process of endocytosis in clathrin-coated pits (see Chapter 10, Section III.B.1.) The receptors may be degraded or recycled back to the cell surface. This internalization of receptors decreases the number available on the surface under conditions of constant high hormone levels when more of the receptors are occupied by hormones and results in decreased synthesis of new receptors. Hence, it is called down-regulation.

IV. SIGNAL TERMINATION

Some signals, such as those that modify the metabolic responses of cells or transmit neural impulses, need to turn off rapidly when the hormone is no longer being produced. Other signals, such as those that stimulate proliferation, turn off more slowly. In contrast, signals regulating differentiation may persist throughout our lifetime. Many chronic diseases are caused by failure to terminate a response at the appropriate time.

The first level of termination is the chemical messenger itself (Fig.11.20). When the stimulus is no longer applied to the secreting cell, the messenger is no longer secreted, and existing messenger is catabolized. For example, many polypeptide hormones such as insulin are taken up into the liver and degraded. Termination of the acetylcholine signal by acetylcholinesterase has already been mentioned.

Within each pathway of signal transduction, the signal may be turned off at specific steps. The receptor might be desensitized to the messenger by phosphorylation. G proteins, both monomeric and heterotrimeric, automatically terminate messages as they hydrolyze GTP. Termination also can be achieved through degradation of the second messenger (e.g., phosphodiesterase cleavage of cAMP). Each of these terminating processes is also highly regulated.

Another important pathway for reversing the message is through protein phosphatases, enzymes that reverse the action of kinases by removing phosphate groups

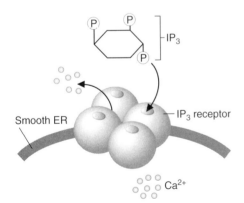

Fig. 11.19. IP_3 signaling calcium release from the endoplasmic reticulum.

from proteins. Specific tyrosine or serine/threonine phosphatases (enzymes that remove the phosphate group from specific proteins) exist for all of the sites phosphorylated by signal transduction kinases. Some receptors are even protein phosphatases.

CLINICAL COMMENTS

Mya Sthenia. Mya Sthenia has myasthenia gravis, an autoimmune disease caused by the production of antibodies directed against the nicotinic acetylcholine receptor in skeletal muscles. The diagnosis is made by history (presence of typical muscular symptoms), physical examination (presence of inability to do specific repetitive muscular activity over time), and tests such as the inhibition of acetylcholinesterase activity. The diagnosis can be further confirmed with an electromyogram (EMG) showing a partial blockade of ion flux across muscular membranes and a diagnostic procedure involving repetitive electrical nerve stimulation.

Ann O'Rexia. Anorexia nervosa presents as a distorted visual self-image often associated with compulsive exercise. Although Ann has been gaining weight, she is still relatively low on stored fuels needed to sustain the metabolic requirements of exercise. Her prolonged starvation has resulted in release of the steroid hormone cortisol and the polypeptide hormone glucagon, whereas levels of the polypeptide hormone insulin have decreased. Cortisol activates transcription of genes for some of the enzymes of gluconeogenesis (the synthesis of glucose from amino acids and other precursors; see Chapter 3.) Glucagon binds to heptahelical receptors in liver and adipose tissue and, working through cAMP and protein kinase A, activates many enzymes involved in fasting fuel metabolism. Insulin, which is released when she drinks her high-energy supplement, works through a specialized tyrosine kinase receptor to promote fuel storage. Epinephrine, a catecholamine released when she exercises, promotes fuel mobilization.

Dennis Veere. In the emergency room, Dennis received intravenous rehydration therapy (normal saline [0.9% NaCl]) and oral hydration therapy with a glucose-electrolyte solution to increase his glucose-dependent Na^+ uptake from the intestinal lumen (see Chapter 10). Dennis quickly recovered from his bout of cholera. Cholera is self-limiting, possibly because the bacteria remain in the intestine, where they are washed out of the system by the diffuse watery diarrhea. Over the past three years, **Percy Veere** has persevered through the death of his wife and the subsequent calamities of his grandson Dennis "the Menace" Veere, including salicylate poisoning, suspected malathion poisoning, and now cholera. Mr. Veere decided to send his grandson home for the remainder of the summer.

BIOCHEMICAL COMMENTS

Death domain receptors. The cytokine TNF (**t**umor **n**ecrosis **f**actor) uses a type of receptor called the death domain receptor (Fig. 11.21). These receptors function as a trimer when they bind TNF (which is also a trimer). On TNF binding, an inhibitory protein called the "silencer of death" is released from the receptor. The receptor then binds and activates several adaptor proteins. One adaptor protein, FADD (**f**as-**a**ssociated **d**eath **d**omain), recruits and activates the zymogen form of a proteolytic enzyme called caspase. Caspases

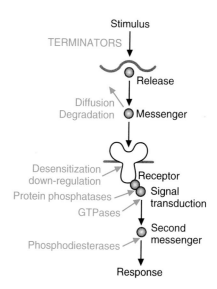

Fig. 11.20. Sites of signal termination. Processes that terminate signals are shown in blue.

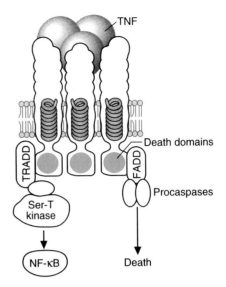

Fig. 11.21. Death domain receptors. The portion of the receptor shown in blue is called the death domain because it binds adaptor proteins that initiate different signaling pathways leading to cell death. The adaptor protein FADD forms a scaffold on which proteolytic procaspases cleave each other, thereby initiating a death pathway. The adaptor protein TRADD binds a protein that binds a serine-threonine kinase (Ser-T kinase) that initiates another signaling pathway leading to activation of the transcription factor NF-κB.

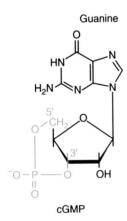

Caspases are proteolytic enzymes that have a critical role in programmed cell death (also called apoptosis) (see Chapter 16). Caspases are present as latent zymogens until their autoproteolysis (self-cleavage) is activated by "death signals" to the receptor complex. Once activated, they work systematically to dismantle a cell through degrading a wide variety of proteins, such as DNA repair enzymes and cellular structural proteins.

initiate a signal transduction pathway leading to apoptosis (programmed cell death) (see Chapter 18). Another adaptor protein, TRADD (**T**NF **r**eceptor-**a**ssociated **d**eath **d**omain), initiates signaling pathways that lead to activation of the gene-specific transcription factors Jun and NF-κB (nuclear factor-κB). Through these pathways, TNF mediates cell-specific responses, such as cell growth and death, the inflammatory response, and immune function.

Guanylyl cyclase receptors. Guanylyl cyclase receptors convert GTP to the second messenger $3',5'$ cyclic GMP (cGMP), which is analogous to cAMP (Fig. 11.22). Like cAMP, cGMP is degraded by a membrane-bound phosphodiesterase. Elevated cGMP activates protein kinase G, which then phosphorylates target proteins to propagate the response.

One type of guanylyl cyclase exists in the cytoplasm and is a receptor for nitric oxide (NO), a neurotransmitter/neurohormone. NO is a lipophilic gas that is able to diffuse into the cell. This receptor thus is an exception to the rule that intracellular receptors are gene transcription factors. The other type of guanyl cyclase receptor is a membrane-spanning receptor in the plasma membrane with an external binding domain for a signal molecule (e.g., natriuretic peptide).

Fig. 11.22. Structure of $3',5'$-cyclic GMP (cGMP).

Suggested References

Signaling Pathways. The May 31, 2002 issue of Science, Vol 296, provides a 2–3-page synopsis of many signaling pathways. The articles most relevant to the pathways discussed in this chapter are:

Aaronson DA, Horvath CM. A road map for those who don't know JAK-STAT. Science 2002;296:1653–1655.
Cantley LC. The phosphoinositide 3-kinase pathway. Science 2002;296:1655–1657.
Attisano L, Wrana, JL. Signal transduction by the TGF-β superfamily. Science 2002;296:1646–1647.
Neves SR, Ram PT, Iyengar R. G protein pathways. Science 2002;296:1636–1639.
Chen Q, Goeddel DV. TNF-R1 signaling: A beautiful pathway. Science 2002;296:1634–1635.

REVIEW QUESTIONS—CHAPTER 11

1. Which of the following is a general characteristic of all chemical messengers?

    (A) They are secreted by one cell, enter the blood, and act on a distant target cell.
    (B) To achieve a coordinated response, each messenger is secreted by several types of cells.
    (C) Each messenger binds to a specific protein receptor in a target cell.
    (D) Chemical messengers must enter cells to transmit their message.
    (E) Chemical messengers are metabolized to intracellular second messengers to transmit their message.

2. Which of the following is a characteristic of chemical messengers that bind to intracellular transcription factor receptors?

    (A) They are usually cytokines or polypeptide hormones.
    (B) They are usually small molecule neurotransmitters.
    (C) They exert rapid actions in cells.
    (D) They are transported through the blood bound to proteins.
    (E) They are always present in high concentrations in the blood.

    Use the following case history for questions 3 and 4. To answer this question, you do not need to know more about parathyroid hormone or pseudophypoparathyroidism than the information given.

    Pseudohypoparathyroidism is a heritable disorder caused by target organ unresponsiveness to parathyroid hormone (a polypeptide hormone secreted by the parathyroid gland). One of the mutations causing this disease occurs in the gene encoding $G_s\alpha$ in certain cells.

3. The receptor for parathyroid hormone is most likely

    (A) an intracellular transcription factor.
    (B) a cytoplasmic guanylyl cyclase.
    (C) a receptor that must be endocytosed in clathrin-coated pits to transmit its signal.
    (D) a heptahelical receptor.
    (E) a tyrosine kinase receptor.

4. This mutation most likely

    (A) is a gain-of-function mutation.
    (B) decreases the GTPase activity of the $G_{\alpha s}$ subunit.
    (C) decreases synthesis of cAMP in response to parathyroid hormone.
    (D) decreases generation of IP_3 in response to parathyroid hormone.
    (E) decreases synthesis of phosphatidylinositol 3,4,5-trisphosphate in response to parathyroid hormone.

5. SH2 domains on proteins are specific for which of the following sites?

    (A) Certain sequences of amino acids containing a phosphotyrosine residue
    (B) PI-3,4,5 trisphosphate in the membrane
    (C) GTP-activated Ras
    (D) Ca^{2+}-calmodulin
    (E) Receptor domains containing phosphoserine residues

Gene Expression and the Synthesis of Proteins

In the middle of the 20th century, DNA was identified as the genetic material, and its structure was determined. Using this knowledge, researchers then discovered the mechanisms by which genetic information is inherited and expressed. During the last quarter of the 20th century, our understanding of this critical area of science, known as molecular biology, grew at an increasingly rapid pace. We now have techniques to probe the human genome that will completely revolutionize the way medicine is practiced in the 21st century.

The genome of a cell consists of all its genetic information, encoded in DNA (deoxyribonucleic acid). In eukaryotes, DNA is located mainly in nuclei, but small amounts are also found in mitochondria. Nuclear genes are packaged in chromosomes that contain DNA and protein in tightly coiled structures (Chapter 12).

The molecular mechanism of inheritance involves a process known as replication, in which the strands of parental DNA serve as templates for the synthesis of DNA copies (Fig. 1) (Chapter 13). After DNA replication, cells divide, and these DNA copies are passed to daughter cells. Alterations in genetic material occur by recombination (the exchange of genetic material between chromosomes) and by mutation (the result of chemical changes that alter DNA). DNA repair mechanisms correct much of this damage, but, nevertheless, many gene alterations are passed to daughter cells.

The expression of genes within cells requires two processes: transcription and translation (see Fig. 1) (Chapters 14 and 15). DNA is transcribed to produce ribonucleic acid (RNA). Three major types of RNA are transcribed from DNA and subsequently participate in the process of translation (The synthesis of proteins). Messenger RNA (mRNA) carries the genetic information from the nucleus to the cytoplasm, where translation occurs on ribosomes, structures containing proteins complexed with ribosomal RNA (rRNA). Transfer RNA (tRNA) carries individual amino acids to the ribosomes, where they are joined in peptide linkage to form proteins. During translation, the sequence of nucleic acid bases in mRNA is read in sets of three (each set of three bases constitutes a codon). The sequence of codons in the mRNA dictates the sequence of amino acids in the protein. Proteins function in cell structure, signaling, and catalysis and, therefore, determine the appearance and behavior of cells and the organism as a whole. The regulation of gene expression (Chapter 16) determines which proteins are synthesized and the amount synthesized at any time, thus allowing cells to undergo development and differentiation and to respond to changing environmental conditions.

Research in molecular biology has produced a host of techniques, known collectively as recombinant DNA technology, biotechnology, or genetic engineering, that can be used for the diagnosis and treatment of disease (Chapter 17). These techniques can detect a number of genetic diseases that previously could only be diagnosed after symptoms appeared. Diagnosis of these diseases can now be made with considerable accuracy even before birth, and carriers of these diseases also can be identified.

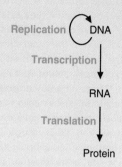

Fig. 1. Replication, transcription, and translation. Replication: DNA serves as a template for producing DNA copies. Transcription: DNA serves as a template for the synthesis of RNA. Translation: RNA provides the information for the synthesis of proteins.

Many drugs used in medicine to treat bacterial infections are targeted to interfere with their ability to synthesize RNA and proteins. Thus, medical students need to know the basics of bacterial DNA replication, RNA synthesis, and protein synthesis.

Ethical dilemmas have come along with technological advances in moleuclar biology. Consider the case of a patient with a mild case of ornithine transcarbamoylase deficiency, a urea cycle defect that, if untreated, leads to elevated ammonia levels and nervous system dysfunction. The patient was being effectively treated by dietary restriction of protein. However, in 1999, he was treated with a common virus carrying the normal gene for ornithine transcarbamoylase. The patient developed a severe immune response to the virus and died as a result of the treatment. This case history raises the issues of appropriate patient consent, appropriate criteria to be included in this type of study, and the types of diseases for which gene therapy is appropriate. These are issues that you, the student, will be facing as you enter your practice of medicine.

Tumors may be benign or malignant. A tumor is malignant if it invades locally or if cells break away from the tumor and travel to other parts of the body, where they establish new growths (a process called metastasis), resulting in destruction of the tissues they invade. Many of the drugs used to treat malignant tumors are directed toward inhibition of DNA replication. These chemotherapeutic drugs are more toxic to cancer cells than normal cells, because the cancer cells divide more rapidly. However, such drugs also may inhibit normal rapidly dividing cells, such as the cells of the bone marrow (causing a decrease in white blood cell count) or cells in the hair follicles (resulting in hair loss during chemotherapy).

With recent developments in the field of gene therapy, diseases that for centuries have been considered hopeless are now potentially curable. Much of the therapy for these diseases is currently experimental. However, during the 21st century, physicians may be using genetic engineering techniques routinely for both the diagnosis and treatment of their patients.

Replication and cell division are highly regulated processes in the human. Cancer is a group of diseases in which a cell in the body has been transformed and begins to grow and divide out of control (Chapter 18). It results from multiple mutations or changes in DNA structure in the genes that activate cell growth, called proto-oncogenes, and those that ensure that DNA replication and repair are normal, called growth suppressor or tumor suppressor genes. Mutations that activate proto-oncogenes to oncogenes disturb the regulation of the cell cycle and the rate of cell proliferation. Mutations disrupting tumor suppressor genes lead to an increased incidence of these proto-oncogene–activating mutations. Such mutations may be inherited, causing a predisposition to a type of cancer. They also may arise from DNA replication or copying errors that remain uncorrected, from chemicals or radiation that damages DNA, from translocation of pieces of chromosomes from one chromosome to another during replication, or from incorporation of viral encoded DNA into the genome.

12 Structure of the Nucleic Acids

Nucleotides in DNA and RNA. Nucleotides *are the monomeric units of the nucleic acids, DNA (deoxyribonucleic acid) and RNA (ribonucleic acid). Each nucleotide consists of a heterocyclic **nitrogenous base**, a **sugar**, and **phosphate**. **DNA** contains the purine bases **adenine** (A) and **guanine** (G) and the pyrimidine bases **cytosine** (C) and **thymine** (T). **RNA** contains A, G, and C, but it has **uracil** (U) instead of thymine. In DNA, the sugar is **deoxyribose**, whereas in RNA it is **ribose**.*

*Polynucleotides such as DNA and RNA are linear sequences of nucleotides linked by **3'- to 5'-phosphodiester bonds** between the sugars (Fig. 12.1). The bases of the nucleotides can interact with other bases or with proteins.*

DNA Structure. *Genetic information is encoded by the sequence of different nucleotide bases in DNA. **DNA** is **double-stranded**; it contains **two antiparallel polynucleotide strands**. The two strands are joined by hydrogen bonding between their bases to form **base-pairs**. **Adenine** pairs with **thymine**, and **guanine** pairs with **cytosine**. The two DNA strands run in **opposite directions**. One strand runs 5' to 3', and the other strand runs 3' to 5'. The two DNA strands wind around each other, forming a **double helix**.*

*Transcription of a gene generates a **single-stranded RNA** that is identical in nucleotide sequence to one of the strands of the duplex DNA. The three major types of RNA are **messenger RNA** (mRNA), **ribosomal RNA** (rRNA), and **transfer RNA** (tRNA).*

RNA Structures. mRNAs *contain the nucleotide sequence that is converted into the amino acid sequence of a protein in the process of translation. Eukaryotic mRNA has a structure known as a **cap** at the 5'-end, a sequence of adenine nucleotides (a **poly(A) tail**) at the 3'-end, and a **coding region** in the center containing **codons** that dictate the sequence of amino acids in a protein or relay a signal. Each codon in the genetic code is a different sequence of three nucleotides.*

*rRNAs and tRNAs are part of the apparatus for protein synthesis, but do not encode proteins. **rRNA** has **extensive internal base pairing** and complexes with proteins to form **ribonucleoprotein particles** called **ribosomes**. The ribosomes bind mRNA and tRNAs during translation. Each **tRNA** binds and **activates a specific amino acid** for insertion into the polypeptide chain and therefore has a somewhat different nucleotide sequence than other tRNAs. A unique trinucleotide sequence on each tRNA called an **anticodon** binds to a complementary codon on the mRNA, thereby ensuring insertion of the correct amino acid. In spite of their differences, all tRNAs contain a number of unusual nucleotides and assume a similar **cloverleaf** structure.*

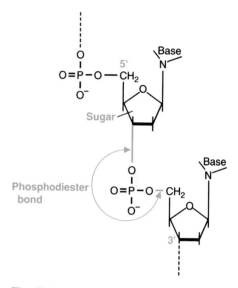

Fig. 12.1. Structure of a polynucleotide. The 5'-carbon of the top sugar and the 3'-carbon of the bottom sugar are indicated.

THE WAITING ROOM

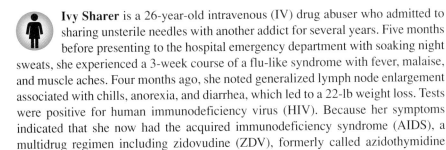

Ivy Sharer is a 26-year-old intravenous (IV) drug abuser who admitted to sharing unsterile needles with another addict for several years. Five months before presenting to the hospital emergency department with soaking night sweats, she experienced a 3-week course of a flu-like syndrome with fever, malaise, and muscle aches. Four months ago, she noted generalized lymph node enlargement associated with chills, anorexia, and diarrhea, which led to a 22-lb weight loss. Tests were positive for human immunodeficiency virus (HIV). Because her symptoms indicated that she now had the acquired immunodeficiency syndrome (AIDS), a multidrug regimen including zidovudine (ZDV), formerly called azidothymidine (AZT), was initiated.

Colin Tuma had intestinal polyps at age 45, which were removed via a colonoscope. However, he did not return for annual colonoscopic examinations as instructed. At age 56, he reappeared, complaining of tar-colored stools (melena), which are caused by intestinal bleeding. The source of the blood loss was an adenocarcinoma growing from a colonic polyp of the large intestine. At surgery, it was found that the tumor had invaded the gut wall and perforated the visceral peritoneum. Several pericolic lymph nodes contained cancer cells, and several small nodules of metastatic cancer were found in the liver. After resection of the tumor, the oncologist began treatment with 5-fluorouracil (5-FU) combined with other chemotherapeutic agents.

Agneu ("neu") Moania complains to his physician of a fever and cough. His cough produces thick yellow-brown sputum. A stain of his sputum shows many Gram-positive, bullet-shaped diplococci. A sputum culture confirms that he has pneumonia, a respiratory infection caused by *Streptococcus pneumoniae*, which is sensitive to penicillin, erythromycin, tetracycline, and other antibiotics. Because of a history of penicillin allergy, he is started on oral erythromycin therapy.

An adenoma is a mass of rapidly proliferating cells, called a neoplasm (neo = new; plasm = growth), that is formed from epithelial cells growing into a glandlike structure. The cells lining all the external and internal organs are epithelial cells, and most human tumors are adenocarcinomas. Adenematous polyps are adenomas that grow into the lumen of the colon or rectum. The term *malignant* applied to a neoplasm refers to invasive unregulated growth. **Colin Tuma** has an adenocarcinoma, which is a malignant adenoma that has started to grow through the wall of the colon into surrounding tissues. Cells from adenocarcinomas can break away and spread through the blood or lymph to other parts of the body, where they form "colony" tumors. This process is called metastasis.

I.   DNA STRUCTURE

A.   Location of DNA

DNA and RNA serve as the genetic material for prokaryotic and eukaryotic cells, for viruses, and for plasmids, each of which stores it in a different arrangement or location. In prokaryotes, DNA is not separated from the rest of the cellular contents. In eukaryotes, however, DNA is located in the nucleus, where it is separated from the rest of the cell by the nuclear envelope (see Fig. 10.20). Eukaryotic DNA is bound to proteins, forming a complex called chromatin. During interphase (when cells are not dividing), some of the chromatin is diffuse (euchromatin) and some is dense (heterochromatin), but no distinct structures can be observed. However, before mitosis (when cells divide), the DNA is replicated, resulting in two identical chromosomes called sister chromatids. During metaphase (a period in mitosis), these condense into discrete, visible chromosomes.

Less than 0.1% of the total DNA in a cell is present in mitochondria. The genetic information in a mitochondrion is encoded in less than 20,000 base pairs of DNA; the information in a human haploid nucleus (i.e., an egg or a sperm cell) is encoded in approximately 3×10^9 (3 billion) base pairs. The DNA and protein synthesizing systems in mitochondria more closely resemble the systems in bacteria, which do

DNA is a double-stranded molecule that forms base pairs (bp) between strands. The bp designation is often used to indicate the size of a DNA molecule. For example, in a stretch of DNA 200 bp long, both strands are included with 200 bases in each strand, for a total of 400 bases.

not have membrane-enclosed organelles, than those in the eukaryotic nucleus and cytoplasm. It has been suggested that mitochondria were derived from ancient bacterial invaders of primordial eukaryotic cells.

Viruses are small infectious particles consisting of a DNA or RNA genome (but not both), proteins required for pathogenesis or replication, and a protein coat. They lack, however, complete systems for replication, transcription, and translation and, consequently, viruses must invade other cells and commandeer their DNA, RNA, and protein-synthesizing machinery to reproduce. Both eukaryotes and prokaryotes can be infected by viruses. Viruses that infect bacteria are known as bacteriophage (or more simply as phage).

Plasmids are small, circular DNA molecules that can enter bacteria and replicate autonomously, that is, outside the host genome. In contrast to viruses, plasmids are not infectious; they do not convert their host cells into factories devoted to plasmid production. Genetic engineers use plasmids as tools for transfer of foreign genes into bacteria because segments of DNA can readily be incorporated into plasmids.

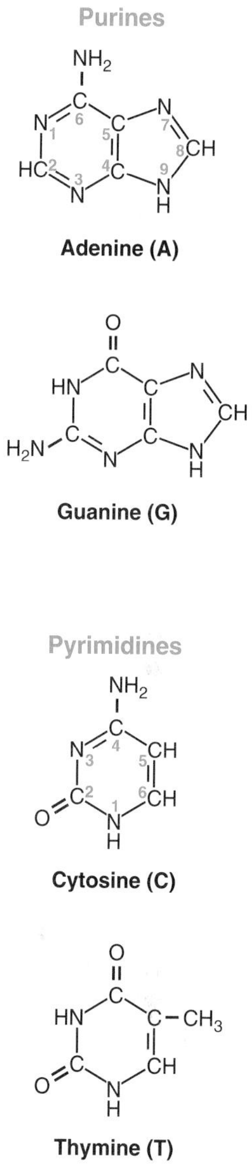

B. Determination of the Structure of DNA

In 1865, Frederick Meischer first isolated DNA, obtaining it from pus scraped from surgical bandages. Initially, scientists speculated that DNA was a cellular storage form for inorganic phosphate, an important but unexciting function that did not spark widespread interest in determining its structure. In fact, the details of DNA structure were not fully determined until 1953, almost 90 years after it had first been isolated, but only 9 years after it had been identified as the genetic material.

Early in the 20th century, the bases of DNA were identified as the purines adenine (A) and guanine (G), and the pyrimidines cytosine (C) and thymine (T) (Fig. 12.2). The sugar was found to be deoxyribose, a derivative of ribose, lacking a hydroxyl group on carbon 2 (Fig. 12.3).

Nucleotides, composed of a base, a sugar, and phosphate, were found to be the monomeric units of the nucleic acids (Table 12.1). In nucleosides, the nitrogenous base is linked by an *N*-glycosidic bond to the anomeric carbon of the sugar, either ribose or deoxyribose. A nucleotide is a nucleoside with an inorganic phosphate attached to a 5′-hydroxyl group of the sugar in ester linkage (Fig. 12.4). The names and abbreviations of nucleotides specify the base, the sugar, and the number of phosphates attached (MP, **m**ono**p**hosphate; DP, **d**i**p**hosphate; TP, **t**ri**p**hosphate). In deoxynucleotides, the prefix "d" precedes the abbreviation. For example, GDP is guanosine diphosphate (the base guanine attached to a ribose that has two phosphate groups) and dATP is deoxyadenosine triphosphate (the base adenine attached to a deoxyribose with three phosphate groups).

Purines

Adenine (A)

Guanine (G)

Pyrimidines

Cytosine (C)

Thymine (T)

Fig. 12.2. Purine and pyrimidine bases in DNA.

Table 12.1. Names of Bases and Their Corresponding Nucleosides[a]

Base	Nucleoside
Adenine (A)	Adenosine
Guanine (G)	Guanosine
Cytosine (C)	Cytidine
Thymine (T)	Thymidine
Uracil (U)	Uridine
Hypoxanthine (I)	Inosine[b]

[a] If the sugar is deoxyribose rather than ribose, the nucleoside has "deoxy" as a prefix (e.g., deoxyadenosine). Nucleotides are given the name of the nucleoside plus mono, di, or triphosphate (e.g., adenosine triphosphate or deoxyadenosine triphosphate).
[b] The base hypoxanthine is not found in DNA but is produced during degradation of the purine bases. It is found in certain tRNA molecules. Its nucleoside, inosine, is produced during synthesis of the purine nucleotides (see Chapter 41).

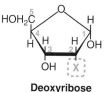

Deoxyribose

Fig. 12.3. Deoxyribose and ribose, the sugars of DNA and RNA. The carbon atoms are numbered from 1 to 5. When the sugar is attached to a base, the carbon atoms are numbered from 1′ to 5′ to distinguish it from the base. In deoxyribose the X = H; in ribose the X = OH.

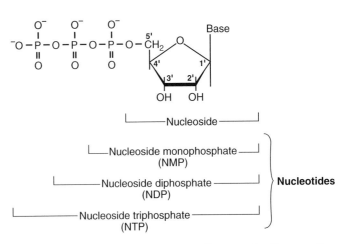

Fig. 12.4. Nucleoside and nucleotide structures. Shown with ribose as the sugar. The corresponding deoxyribonucleotides are abbreviated dNMP, dNDP, and dNTP. N = any base (A, G, C, U, or T).

After **Ivy Sharer** was diagnosed with AIDS, she was treated with a mixture of drugs including zidovudine (ZDV), formerly called AZT. This drug is an analog of the thymine nucleotide found in DNA (the modified group is shown in the dashed box). ZDV is phosphorylated in the body by the kinases that normally phosphorylate nucleosides and nucleotides. As the viral DNA chain is being synthesized in a human cell, ZDV is then added to the growing 3'-end by viral reverse transcriptase. However, ZDV lacks a 3' OH group and, therefore, no additional nucleotides can be attached through a 5'→3' bond. Thus, chain elongation of the DNA is terminated. Reverse transcriptase has a higher affinity for ZDV than does normal human cellular DNA polymerases, enabling the drug to target viral replication more specifically than cellular replication.

ZDV,
an analogue of deoxythymidine

In 1944, after Oswald Avery's experiments establishing DNA as the genetic material were published, interest in determining the structure of DNA intensified. Digestion with enzymes of known specificity proved that inorganic phosphate joined the nucleotide monomers, forming a phosphodiester bond between the 3'-carbon of one sugar and the 5'-carbon of the next sugar along the polynucleotide chain (Fig. 12.5). Another key to DNA structure was provided by Erwin Chargaff. He analyzed the base composition of DNA from various sources and concluded that, on a molar basis, the amount of adenine was always equal to the amount of thymine, and the amount of guanine was equal to the amount of cytosine.

During this era, James Watson and Francis Crick joined forces and, using the x-ray diffraction data of Maurice Wilkins and Rosalind Franklin, incorporated the available information into a model for DNA structure. In 1953, they published a brief paper, describing DNA as a double helix consisting of two polynucleotide strands joined by pairing between the bases (adenine with thymine and guanine with cytosine). The model of base-pairing they proposed is the basis of modern molecular biology.

C. Concept of Base-Pairing

As proposed by Watson and Crick, each DNA molecule consists of two polynucleotide chains joined by hydrogen bonds between the bases. In each base pair, a purine on one strand forms hydrogen bonds with a pyrimidine on the other strand. In one type of base pair, adenine on one strand pairs with thymine on the other strand (Fig. 12.6). This base pair is stabilized by two hydrogen bonds. The other base pair, formed between guanine and cytosine, is stabilized by three hydrogen bonds. As a consequence of base-pairing, the two strands of DNA are complementary, that is, adenine on one strand corresponds to thymine on the other strand, and guanine corresponds to cytosine.

The concept of base-pairing proved to be essential for determining the mechanism of DNA replication (in which the copies of DNA are produced that are distributed to daughter cells) and the mechanisms of transcription and translation (in

Watson and Crick's one-page paper, published in 1953, contained little more than 900 words. However it triggered a major revolution in the biologic sciences and produced the conceptual foundation for the discipline of molecular biology.

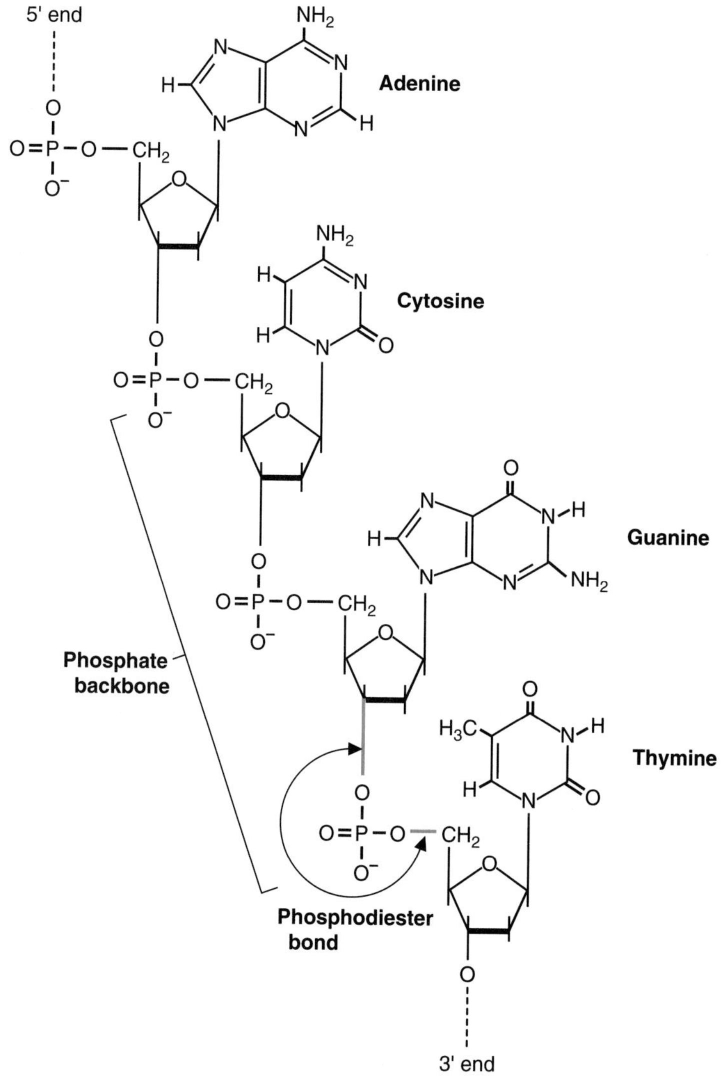

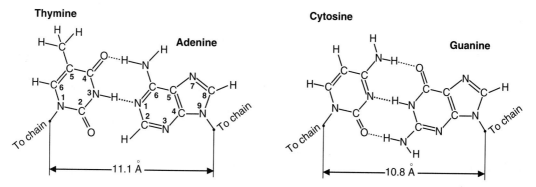

Fig. 12.5. A segment of a polynucleotide chain of DNA. The dashes at the 5'- and 3'-ends indicate that the molecule contains more nucleotides than are shown.

Fig. 12.6. Base pairs of DNA. Note that the pyrimidine bases are "flipped over" from the positions in which they are usually shown (see Fig. 12.5). The bases must be in this orientation to form base pairs. The dotted lines indicate hydrogen bonds between the bases. Although the hydrogen bonds hold the bases and thus the two DNA strands together, they are weaker than covalent bonds and allow the DNA strands to separate during replication and transcription.

"It has not escaped our notice that the specific pairing we have postulated immediately suggests a possible copying mechanism for the genetic material." J.D. Watson and F.H.C. Crick, *Nature,* April 25, 1953.

which mRNA is produced from genes and used to direct the process of protein synthesis). Obviously, as Watson and Crick suggested, base-pairing allows one strand of DNA to serve as a template for the synthesis of the other strand (Fig. 12.7). Base-pairing also allows a strand of DNA to serve as a template for the synthesis of a complementary strand of RNA.

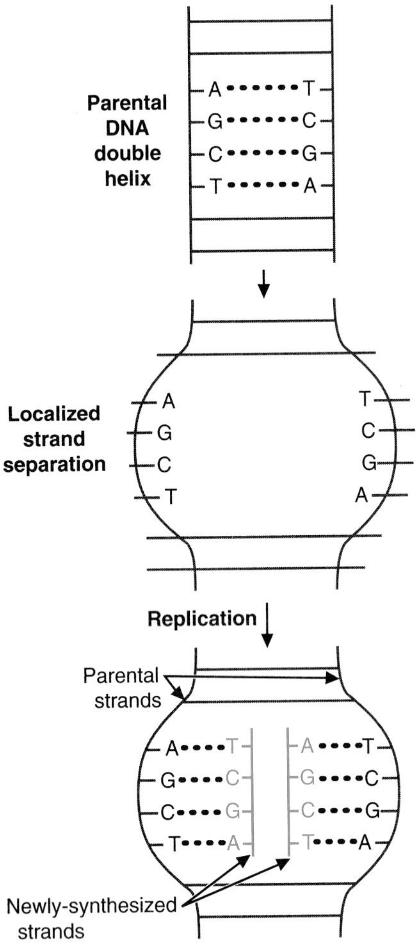

D. DNA Strands Are Antiparallel

As concluded by Watson and Crick, the two complementary strands of DNA run in opposite directions. On one strand, the 5′-carbon of the sugar is above the 3′-carbon (Fig. 12.8). This strand is said to run in a 5′ to 3′ direction. On the other strand, the 3′-carbon is above the 5′-carbon. This strand is said to run in a 3′ to 5′ direction. Thus, the strands are antiparallel (that is, they run in opposite directions.) This concept of directionality of nucleic acid strands is essential for understanding the mechanisms of replication and transcription.

E. The Double Helix

Because each base pair contains a purine bonded to a pyrimidine, the strands are equidistant from each other throughout. If two strands that are equidistant from each other are twisted at the top and the bottom, they form a double helix (Fig. 12.9). In the double helix of DNA, the base pairs that join the two strands are stacked like a spiral staircase along the central axis of the molecule. The electrons of the adjacent base pairs interact, generating stacking forces that, in addition to the hydrogen bonding of the base pairs, help to stabilize the helix.

The phosphate groups of the sugar-phosphate backbones are on the outside of the helix (see Fig. 12.9). Each phosphate has two oxygen atoms forming the phosphodiester bonds that link adjacent sugars. However, the third -OH group on the phosphate is free and dissociates a hydrogen ion at physiologic pH. Therefore, each DNA helix has negative charges coating its surface that facilitate the binding of specific proteins.

The helix contains grooves of alternating size, known as the major and minor grooves (see Fig. 12.9). The bases in these grooves are exposed and therefore can interact with proteins or other molecules.

Fig. 12.7. DNA strands serve as templates. During replication, the strands of the helix separate in a localized region. Each parental strand serves as a template for the synthesis of a new DNA strand.

Multi-drug regimens used to treat cancers (e.g., lymphomas) sometimes include the drug doxorubicin (adriamycin). It is a natural product with a complex multi-ring structure that intercalates or slips in between the stacked base pairs of DNA and inhibits replication and transcription.

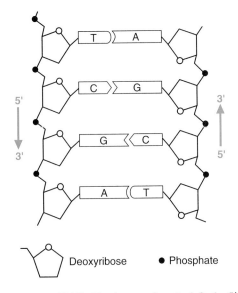

Fig. 12.8. Antiparallel strands of DNA. For the strand on the left, the 5′-carbon of each sugar is above the 3′-carbon, so it runs 5′ to 3′. For the strand on the right, the 3′-carbon of each sugar is above the 5′-carbon, so it runs 3′ to 5′.

Watson and Crick described the B form of DNA, a right-handed helix, containing 3.4 Å between base pairs and 10.4 base pairs per turn. Although this form predominates in vivo, other forms also occur (Fig. 12.10). The A form, which predominates in DNA-RNA hybrids, is similar to the B form, but is more compact (2.3 Å between base pairs and 11 base pairs per turn). In the Z form, the bases of the two DNA strands are positioned toward the periphery of a left-handed helix . There are 3.8 Å between base pairs and 12 base pairs per turn in Z DNA. This form of the helix was designated "Z" because, in each strand, a line connecting the phosphates "zigs" and "zags."

F. Characteristics of DNA

Both alkali and heat cause the two strands of the DNA helix to separate (denature). Many techniques employed to study DNA or to produce recombinant DNA molecules make use of this property. Although alkali causes the two strands of DNA to

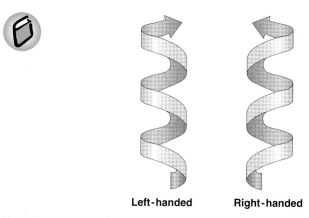

Left-handed   **Right-handed**

If you look up through the bottom of a helix along the central axis and the helix spirals away from you in a clockwise direction (toward the arrowhead in the drawing), it is a right-handed helix. If it spirals away from you in a counterclockwise direction, it is a left-handed helix.

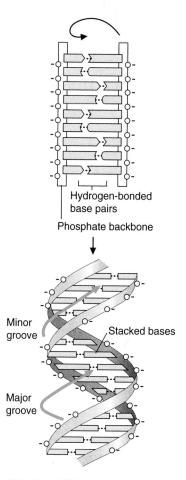

Fig. 12.9. Two DNA strands twist to form a double helix. The distance between the two phosphodiester backbones, shown with a ribbon, is about 11 Å. The hydrogen-bonded base pairs, shown in blue, create stacking forces with adjacent base pairs. Each phosphate group contains one negatively charged oxygen atom that provides the phosphodiester backbone with a negative charge. Because of the twisting of the helix, grooves are formed along the surface, the larger one being the major groove, and the smaller one the minor groove.

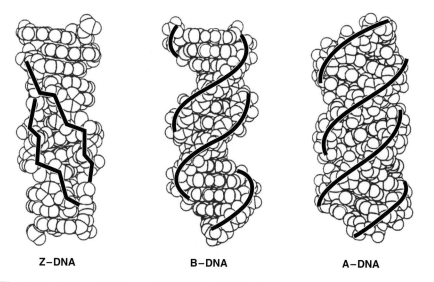

Z–DNA   **B–DNA**   **A–DNA**

Fig. 12.10. Z, B, and A forms of DNA. The solid black lines connect one phosphate group to the next. Modified from Saenger W. Principles of nucleic acid structure. New York: Springer Verlag, 1984:257–286.

Heating and cooling cycles are used to separate and reanneal DNA strands in the polymerase chain reaction (PCR), a technique for obtaining large quantities of DNA from very small samples for research or for clinical and forensic testing (see Chapter 17).

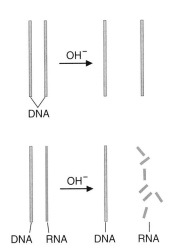

Fig. 12.11. Effect of alkali on DNA and RNA. DNA strands stay intact, but they separate. RNA strands are degraded to nucleotides.

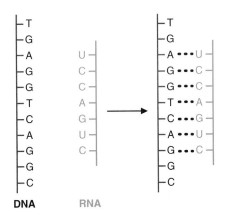

Fig. 12.12. Hybridization of DNA and complementary RNA.

 If histones contain large amounts of arginine and lysine, will their net charge be positive or negative?

separate, it does not break the phosphodiester bonds (Fig. 12.11). In contrast, the phosphodiester bonds of RNA are cleaved by alkali. Therefore, alkali is used to remove RNA from DNA and to separate DNA strands before, or after, electrophoresis on polyacrylamide or agarose gels.

Heat alone converts double-stranded DNA to single-stranded DNA. The separation of strands is called melting, and the temperature at which 50% of the DNA is separated is called the T_m. If the temperature is slowly decreased, complementary single strands can realign and base-pair, re-forming a double helix essentially identical to the original DNA. This process is known as renaturation, reannealing, or hybridization. The process by which a single-stranded DNA anneals with complementary strands of RNA is also called hybridization (Fig. 12.12). Hybridization is used extensively in research and clinical testing.

II. STRUCTURE OF CHROMOSOMES

A. Size of DNA Molecules

A prokaryotic cell generally contains a single chromosome composed of double-stranded DNA that forms a circle. These circular DNA molecules are extremely large. The entire chromosome of the bacterium *Escherichia coli*, composed of a single, circular double-stranded DNA molecule, contains over 4×10^6 base pairs. Its molecular weight is over $2,500 \times 10^6$ g/mol (compared to the molecular weight for a glucose molecule of 180 g/mol). If this molecule were linear, its length would measure almost 2 mm.

DNA from eukaryotic cells is approximately 1,000 times larger than that from bacterial cells. In eukaryotes, each chromosome contains one continuous, linear DNA helix. The DNA of the longest human chromosome is over 7 cm in length. In fact, if the DNA from all 46 chromosomes in a diploid human cell were placed end to end, our total DNA would span a distance of about 2 m (over 6 feet). Our total DNA contains about 6×10^9 base pairs.

B. Packing of DNA

DNA molecules require special packaging to enable them to reside within cells because the molecules are so large. In *E. coli*, the circular DNA is supercoiled and attached to an RNA-protein core. Packaging of eukaryotic DNA is much more complex because it is larger and must be contained within the nucleus of the eukaryotic cell. Eukaryotic DNA binds to an equal weight of histones, which are small basic proteins containing large amounts of arginine and lysine. The complex of DNA and proteins is called chromatin. The organization of eukaryotic DNA into chromatin is essential for controlling transcription, as well as for packaging. When chromatin is extracted from cells, it has the appearance of beads on a string (Fig. 12.13). The beads with DNA protruding from each end are known as nucleosomes, and the beads themselves are known as nucleosome cores (Fig. 12.14). Two molecules of each of four histone classes (histones H2A, H2B, H3, and H4) form the center of the core around which approximately 140 base pairs of double-stranded DNA are wound. The DNA wrapped around the nucleosome core is continuous and joins one

DNA consists of a double helix, with the two strands of DNA wrapping around each other to form a helical structure. To compact, the DNA molecule coils about itself to form a structure called a supercoil. A telephone cord, which connects the handpiece to the phone, displays supercoiling when the coiled cord wraps about itself. When the strands of a DNA molecule separate and unwind over a small local region (which occurs during DNA replication), supercoils are introduced into the remaining portion of the molecule, thereby increasing stress on this portion. Enzymes known as topoisomerases relieve this stress so that unwinding of the DNA strands can occur.

nucleosome core to the next. The DNA joining the cores is complexed with the fifth type of histone, H1. Further compaction of chromatin occurs as the strings of nucleosomes wind into helical, tubular coils called solenoid structures.

Although complexes of DNA and histones form the nucleosomal substructures of chromatin, other types of proteins are also associated with DNA in the nucleus. These proteins were given the unimaginative name of "non-histone chromosomal proteins." The cells of different tissues contain different amounts and types of these proteins, which include enzymes that act on DNA and factors that regulate transcription.

C. The Human Genome

The genome, or total genetic content, of a human haploid cell (a sperm or an egg) is distributed in 23 chromosomes. Haploid cells contain one copy of each chromosome. The haploid egg and haploid sperm cells combine to form the diploid zygote, which continues to divide to form our other cells (mitosis), which are diploid. Diploid cells thus contain 22 pairs of autosomal chromosomes, with each pair composed of two homologous chromosomes containing a similar series of genes (Fig. 12.15). In addition to the autosomal chromosomes, each diploid cell has two sex chromosomes, designated X and Y. A female has two X chromosomes, and a male has one X and one Y chromosome. The total number of chromosomes per diploid cell is 46.

Genes are arranged linearly along each chromosome. A gene, in genetic terms, is the fundamental unit of heredity. In structural terms, a gene encompasses the DNA sequence encoding the structural components of the gene product (whether it be a polypeptide chain or RNA molecule) along with the DNA sequences adjacent to the 5′ end of the gene which regulates its expression. A genetic locus is a specific position or location on a chromosome. Each gene on a chromosome in a diploid cell is matched by an alternate version of the gene at the same genetic locus on the homologous chromosome (Fig. 12.16). These alternate versions of a gene are called alleles. We thus have two alleles of each

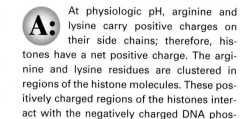

At physiologic pH, arginine and lysine carry positive charges on their side chains; therefore, histones have a net positive charge. The arginine and lysine residues are clustered in regions of the histone molecules. These positively charged regions of the histones interact with the negatively charged DNA phosphate groups.

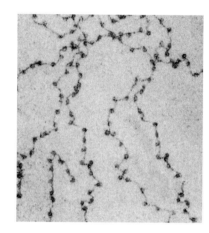

Fig. 12.13. Chromatin showing "beads on a string" structure.

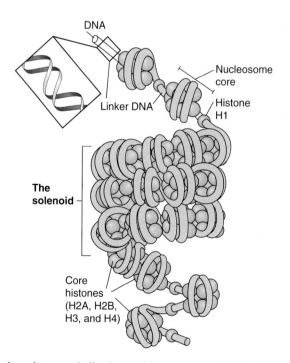

Fig. 12.14. A polynucleosome, indicating the histone cores and linker DNA.

Labels in figure: DNA; Nucleosome core; Linker DNA; Histone H1; The solenoid; Core histones (H2A, H2B, H3, and H4)

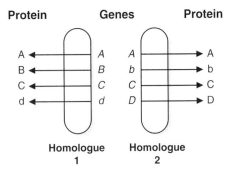

Fig. 12.16. Homologous chromosomes and their protein products. A set of homologous chromosomes is shown diagrammatically. (Of course, during interphase when they are producing their protein products, they cannot be visualized as discrete entities.) Four genes are shown as examples on each homologue. The genes of the homologues are alleles (e.g., *AA, Bb, CC, dD*). They may be identical (e.g., *AA, CC*), or they may differ (e.g., *Bb, dD*) in DNA sequence. Thus the corresponding protein products may be identical or they may differ in amino acid sequence.

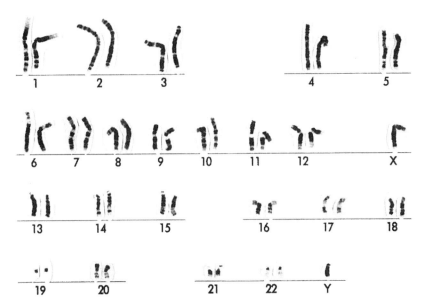

Fig. 12.15. Human chromosomes from a male dipolid cell. Each diploid cell contains 22 pairs of autosomes (the numbered chromosomes 1–22) plus one X and one Y. Each female diploid cell contains two X chromosomes. Each haploid cell contains chromosomes 1 through 22 plus either an X or a Y. From Gelehrter TD, Collins FS, Ginsburg D. Principles of Human Genetics, 2nd Ed. Baltimore: Williams & Wilkins, 1998.

Will Sichel has sickle cell anemia (see Chapters 6 and 7). He has two alleles for the β-globin gene that both generate the mutated form of hemoglobin, HbS. His younger sister Amanda, a carrier for sickle cell trait, has one normal allele (that produces HbA) and one that produces HbS. A carrier would theoretically be expected to produce HbA:HbS in a 50:50 ratio. However, what is generally seen in electrophoresis is 60:40 ratio of HbA:HbS. Dramatic deviations from this ratio imply the occurrence of an additional hemoglobin mutation (e.g., thalassemia).

gene, one from our mother and one from our father. If the alleles are identical in base sequence, we are homozygous for this gene. If the alleles differ, we are heterozygous for this gene and may produce two versions of the encoded protein that differ somewhat in primary structure.

The genomes of prokaryotic and eukaryotic cells differ in size. The genome of the bacterium *E. coli* contains approximately 3,000 genes. All of this bacterial DNA has a function; it either codes for proteins, rRNA, and tRNA, or it serves to regulate the synthesis of these gene products. In contrast, the genome of the human haploid cell contains between 30,000 and 50,000 genes, 10 to 15 times the number in *E. coli*. The function of most of this extra DNA has not been determined (an issue considered in more detail in Chapter 15).

III. STRUCTURE OF RNA

A. General Features of RNA

RNA is similar to DNA. Like DNA, it is composed of nucleotides joined by 3'- to 5'-phosphodiester bonds, the purine bases adenine and guanine, and the pyrimidine base cytosine. However, its other pyrimidine base is uracil rather than thymine. Uracil and thymine are identical bases except that thymine has a methyl group at position 5 of the ring (Fig. 12.17). In RNA, the sugar is ribose, which contains a hydroxyl group on the 2'-carbon (see Fig 12.3. The prime refers to the position on the ribose ring). (The presence of this hydroxyl group allows RNA to be cleaved to its constituent nucleotides in alkaline solutions.)

RNA chains are usually single-stranded and lack the continuous helical structure of double-stranded DNA. However, RNA still has considerable secondary and tertiary structure because base pairs can form in regions where the strand loops back on itself. As in DNA, pairing between the bases is complementary and antiparallel. But in RNA, adenine pairs with uracil rather than thymine (Fig. 12.18). Base-pairing in RNA can be extensive, and the irregular looped structures generated are

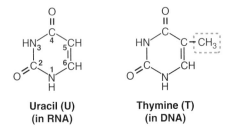

Fig. 12.17. Comparison of the structures of uracil and thymine. They differ in structure only by a methyl group, outlined in blue.

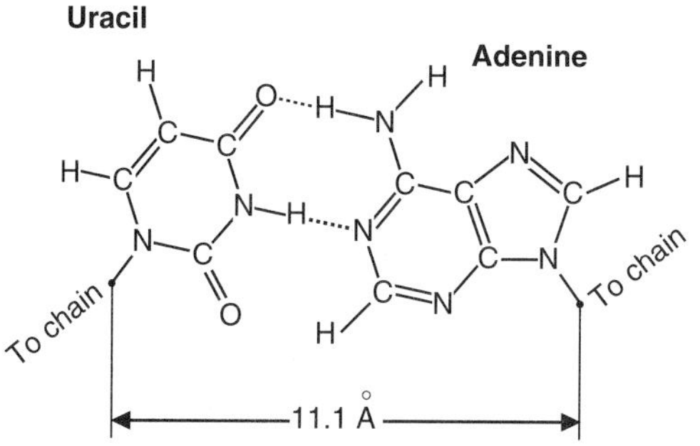

Uracil

Adenine

Fig. 12.18. A uracil–adenine base pair in RNA.

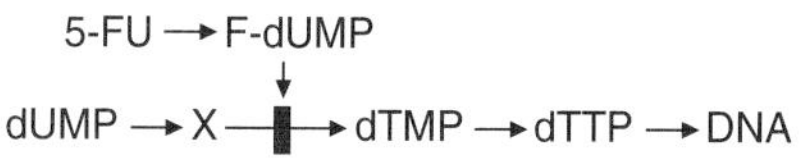

important for the binding of molecules, such as enzymes, that interact with specific regions of the RNA.

The three major types of RNA (mRNA, rRNA, and tRNA) participate directly in the process of protein synthesis. Other less abundant RNAs are involved in replication or in the processing of RNA, that is, in the conversion of RNA precursors to their mature forms.

Some RNA molecules are capable of catalyzing reactions. Thus, RNA, as well as protein, can have enzymatic activity. Certain rRNA precursors can remove internal segments of themselves, splicing the remaining fragments together. Because this RNA is changed by the reaction that it catalyzes, it is not truly an enzyme and therefore has been termed a "ribozyme." Other RNAs act as true catalysts, serving as ribonucleases that cleave other RNA molecules or as a peptidyl transferase, the enzyme in protein synthesis that catalyzes the formation of peptide bonds.

B. Structure of mRNA

Each **mRNA** molecule contains a nucleotide sequence that is converted into the amino acid sequence of a polypeptide chain in the process of translation. In eukaryotes, messenger RNA (mRNA) is transcribed from protein-coding genes as a long primary transcript that is processed in the nucleus to form mRNA. The various processing intermediates, which are mRNA precursors, are called pre-mRNA or hnRNA (**h**eterogenous **n**uclear RNA). mRNA travels through nuclear pores to the cytoplasm, where it binds to ribosomes and tRNAs and directs the sequential insertion of the appropriate amino acids into a polypeptide chain.

Eukaryotic mRNA consists of a leader sequence at the 5′ end, a coding region, and a trailer sequence at the 3′ end (Fig 12.19). The leader sequence begins with a guanosine cap structure at its 5′ end. The coding region begins with a trinucleotide start codon that signals the beginning of translation, followed by the trinucleotide codons for amino acids, and ends at a termination signal. The trailer terminates at its 5′ end with a poly(A) tail that may be up to 200 nucleotides long. Most of the leader sequence, all of the coding region, and most of the trailer are formed by transcription of the complementary nucleotide sequence in DNA. However, the terminal guanosine in the cap structure and the poly(A) tail do not have complementary sequences; they are added posttranscriptionally.

C. Structure of rRNA

Ribosomes are subcellular ribonucleoprotein complexes on which protein synthesis occurs. Different types of ribosomes are found in prokaryotes and in the cytoplasm and mitochondria of eukaryotic cells (Fig. 12.20). Prokaryotic ribosomes contain three types of rRNA molecules with sedimentation coefficients of 16, 23, and 5S. The 30S ribosomal subunit contains the 16S rRNA complexed with proteins, and

 Colin Tuma is being treated with 5-fluorouracil (5-FU), a pyrimidine base similar to uracil and thymine. 5-FU inhibits the synthesis of the thymine nucleotides required for DNA replication. Thymine is normally produced by a reaction catalyzed by thymidylate synthase, an enzyme that converts deoxyuridine monophosphate (dUMP) to deoxythymidine monophosphate (dTMP). 5-FU is converted in the body to F-dUMP, which binds tightly to thymidylate synthase in a transition state complex and inhibits the reaction (recall that thymine is 5-methyl uracil). Thus, thymine nucleotides cannot be generated for DNA synthesis, and the rate of cell proliferation decreases.

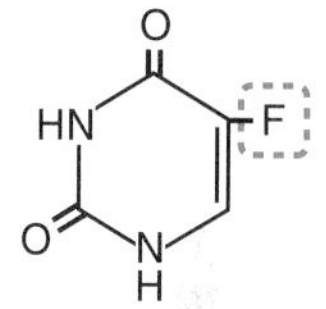

5–Fluorouracil, an analogue of uracil or thymine

5-FU → F-dUMP

dUMP → X ─┃→ dTMP → dTTP → DNA

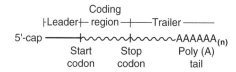

Fig. 12.19. The regions of eukaryotic mRNA. The wavy line indicates the polynucleotide chain of the mRNA and the As constituting the poly(A) tail. The 5′-cap consists of a guanosine residue linked at its 5′ hydroxyl group to three phosphates, which are linked to the 5′-hydroxyl group of the next nucleotide in the RNA chain. The start and stop codons represent where protein synthesis is initiated and terminated from this mRNA.

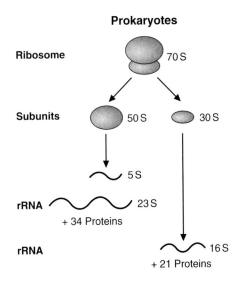

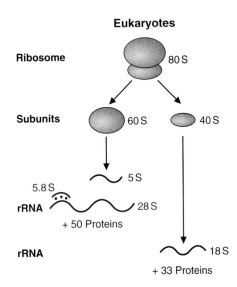

Fig. 12.20. Comparison of prokaryotic and eukaryotic ribosomes. The cytoplasmic ribosomes of eukaryotes are shown. Mitochondrial ribosomes are similar to prokaryotic ribosomes, but they are smaller (55S rather than 70S).

Erythromycin, the antibiotic used to treat **Neu Moania,** inhibits protein synthesis on prokaryotic ribosomes, but not on eukaryotic ribosomes. It binds to the 50S ribosomal subunit, which is absent in eukaryotes. Therefore, it will selectively inhibit bacterial growth. However, because mitochondrial ribosomes are similar to those of bacteria, mitochondrial protein synthesis can also be inhibited. This fact is important in understanding some of the side effects of antibiotics that work by inhibiting bacterial protein synthesis.

A sedimentation coefficient is a measure of the rate of sedimentation of a macromolecule in a high-speed centrifuge (an ultracentrifuge). It is expressed in Svedberg units (S). Although larger macromolecules generally have higher sedimentation coefficients than do smaller macromolecules, sedimentation coefficients are not additive. Because frictional forces acting on the surface of a macromolecule slow its migration through the solvent, the rate of sedimentation depends not only on the density of the macromolecule, but also on its shape.

the 50S ribosomal subunit contains the 23S and 5S rRNAs complexed with proteins. The 30S and 50S ribosomal subunits join to form the 70S ribosome, which participates in protein synthesis.

Cytoplasmic ribosomes in eukaryotes contain four types of rRNA molecules of 18, 28, 5, and 5.8S. The 40S ribosomal subunit contains the 18S rRNA complexed with proteins, and the 60S ribosomal subunit contains the 28, 5, and 5.8S rRNAs complexed with proteins. In the cytoplasm, the 40S and 60S ribosomal subunits combine to form the 80S ribosomes that participate in protein synthesis.

Mitochondrial ribosomes, with a sedimentation coefficient of 55S, are smaller than cytoplasmic ribosomes. Their properties are similar to those of the 70S ribosomes of bacteria.

rRNAs contain many loops and exhibit extensive base-pairing in the regions between the loops (Fig. 12.21). The sequences of the rRNAs of the smaller ribosomal subunits exhibit secondary structures that are common to many different genera.

D. Structure of tRNA

During protein synthesis, tRNA molecules carry amino acids to ribosomes and ensure that they are incorporated into the appropriate positions in the growing polypeptide chain (Fig. 12.22). This is done through base-pairing of three bases of the tRNA (the anticodon) with the three base codons within the coding region of the mRNA. Therefore, cells contain at least 20 different tRNA molecules that differ somewhat in nucleotide sequence, one for each of the amino acids found in proteins. Many amino acids have more than one tRNA.

tRNA molecules contain not only the usual nucleotides, but also derivatives of these nucleotides that are produced by posttranscriptional modifications. In eukaryotic cells, 10 to 20% of the nucleotides of tRNA are modified. Most tRNA molecules contain ribothymidine (T), in which a methyl group is added to uridine to form ribothymidine. They also contain dihydrouridine (D), in which one of the double bonds of the base is reduced; and pseudouridine (Ψ), in which uracil is attached to ribose by a carbon–carbon bond rather than a nitrogen–carbon bond (see Chapter 14). The base at the 5'-end of the anticodon of tRNA is frequently modified.

tRNA molecules are rather small compared with both mRNA and the large rRNA molecules. On average, tRNA molecules contain approximately 80 nucleotides and have a sedimentation coefficient of 4S. Because of their small size and high content of modified nucleotides, tRNAs were the first nucleic acids to be sequenced. Since 1965 when Robert Holley deduced the structure of the first tRNA, the nucleotide sequences of many different tRNAs have been determined. Although their primary sequences differ, all tRNA molecules can form a structure resembling a cloverleaf (discussed in more detail in Chapter 14).

E. Other Types of RNA

In addition to the three major types of RNA described above, other RNAs are present in cells. These RNAs include the oligonucleotides that serve as primers for DNA replication and the RNAs in the small nuclear ribonucleoproteins (snRNPs or snurps) that are involved in the splicing and modification reactions that occur during the maturation of RNA precursors (see Chapter 14).

CLINICAL COMMENTS

 Ivy Sharer. Ivy Sharer's clinical course was typical for the development of full-blown AIDS, in this case caused by the use of needles contaminated with HIV. The progressive immunologic deterioration that accompanies this disease ultimately results in life-threatening opportunistic infections with fungi (e.g., *Candida,* cryptococcus), other viruses (e.g., cytomegalovirus, herpes simplex), and bacteria (e.g., *Mycobacterium, Pneumocystis carinii, Salmonella*). The immunologic incompetence also frequently results in the development of certain neoplasms (e.g., Kaposi's sarcoma, non-Hodgkin's lymphoma) as well as meningitis, neuropathies, and neuropsychiatric disorders causing cognitive dysfunction. Although recent advances in drug therapy can slow the course of the disease, no cure is yet available.

Colin Tuma. Colin Tuma's original benign adenomatous polyp was located in the ascending colon, where 10% of large bowel cancers eventually arise. Because Mr. Tuma's father died of a cancer of the colon, his physician had warned him that his risk for developing colon cancer was three times higher than for the general population. Unfortunately, Mr. Tuma neglected to have his annual colonoscopic examinations as prescribed, and he developed an adenocarcinoma that metastasized.

The most malignant characteristic of neoplasms is their ability to metastasize, that is, form a new neoplasm at a noncontiguous site. The initial site of metastases for a tumor is usually at the first capillary bed encountered by the malignant cells once they are released. Thus, cells from tumors of the gastrointestinal tract often pass through the portal vein to the liver, which is Colin Tuma's site of metastasis. Because his adenocarcinoma has metastasized, there is little hope of eradicating it, and his therapy with 5-FU is palliative (directed toward reducing the severity of the disease and alleviation of the symptoms without actually curing the disease.)

Agneu Moania. Neu Moania's infection was treated with erythromycin, a macrolide antibiotic. Because this agent can inhibit mitochondrial protein synthesis in eukaryotic cells, it has the potential to alter host cell function, leading to such side effects as epigastric distress, diarrhea, and, infrequently, cholestatic jaundice.

BIOCHEMICAL COMMENTS

Retroviruses. RNA also serves as the genome for certain types of viruses, including retroviruses (e.g., the human immunodeficiency virus [HIV] that causes AIDS). Viruses must invade host cells to reproduce. They are not capable of reproducing independently. Some viruses that are pathogenic to

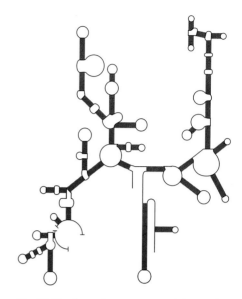

Fig. 12.21. Secondary structure of the portion of 16S-type ribosomal RNA that is common to many species. Darkened areas are base-paired. Circles are unpaired loops. Reproduced with permission, from Annu Rev Biochem. 1984;53:137. © 1984, by Annual Reviews, Inc.

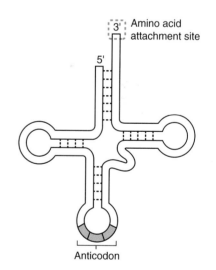

Fig 12.22. The typical cloverleaf structure of tRNA.

 Colin Tuma completed his first course of intravenous 5-fluorouracil (5-FU) in the hospital. He tolerated the therapy with only mild anorexia and diarrhea and with only a mild leukopenia (a decreased white blood cell count; leuko = white). Thirty days after the completion of the initial course, these symptoms abated and he started his second course of chemotherapy with 5-FU as an outpatient.

Because 5-FU inhibits synthesis of thymine, DNA synthesis is affected in all cells in the human body that are rapidly dividing, such as the cells in the bone marrow that produce leukocytes and the mucosal cells lining the intestines. Inhibition of DNA synthesis in rapidly dividing cells contributes to the side effects of 5-FU and many other chemotherapeutic drugs.

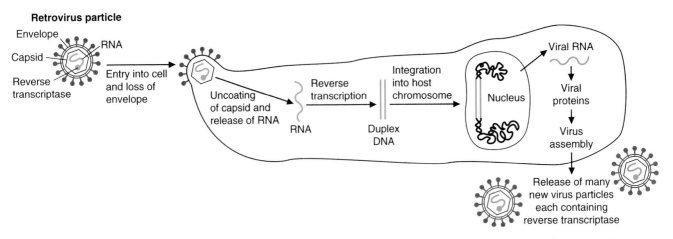

Fig. 12.23. The life cycle of a retrovirus. The virus contains two identical RNA strands, only one of which is shown for clarity. After penetrating the plasma membrane, the single-stranded viral RNA genome is reverse-transcribed to a double-stranded DNA form. The viral DNA migrates to the nucleus and integrates into the chromosomal DNA, where it is transcribed to form a viral RNA transcript. The viral transcript can form the viral RNA genome for progeny viruses, or can be translated to generate viral structural proteins.

humans contain DNA as their genetic material. Others contain RNA as their genetic material.

Some viruses that contain an RNA genome are known as retroviruses. HIV, the human immunodeficiency virus, is the retrovirus that causes AIDS (Fig 12.23). It invades cells of the immune system and prevents the affected individual from mounting an adequate immune response to combat infections.

According to the "central dogma" proposed by Francis Crick, information flows from DNA to RNA to proteins. For the most part, this concept holds true. However, retroviruses provide one violation of this rule. When retroviruses invade cells, their RNA genome is transcribed to produce a DNA copy. The enzyme that catalyzes this process is encoded in the viral RNA and is known as reverse transcriptase. This DNA copy integrates into the genome of the infected cell, and enzymes of the host cell are used to produce many copies of the viral RNA, as well as viral proteins, which can be packaged into new viral particles.

Suggested Readings

Watson JD. The Double Helix. New York: Atheneum, 1968.

Watson JD, Crick FHC. Molecular structure of nucleic acids: a structure for deoxyribose nucleic acid. Nature 1953;171:737–738.

American Cancer Society Web site (http://www.cancer.org): Colorectal cancer. This web site provides information on the cause, treatment and prevention of a number of different cancers, and links to additional resources.

The Human Genome Project Web site (http://www.nhgri.nih.gov/About_NHGRI/Der/Elsi/): This site discusses the ethical issues involved in gene therapy protocols.

REVIEW QUESTIONS—CHAPTER 12

1. For the following DNA sequence, determine the sequence and direction of the complementary strand.
   5′ – ATCGATCGATCGATCG – 3′

   (A) 5′ – ATCTATCGATCGATCG – 3′
   (B) 3′ – ATCGATCGATCGATCG – 5′
   (C) 5′ – CGAUCGAUCAUCGAU – 3′
   (D) 5′ – CGATCGATCGATCGAT – 3′
   (E) 3′ – CGATCGATCGATCGAT – 5′

2. If the DNA strand shown below serves as a template for the synthesis of RNA, which of the following choices gives the sequence and direction of the RNA?
   5′ – GCTATGCATCGTGATCGAATTGCGT – 3′

   (A) 5′ – ACGCAATTCGATCACGATGCATAGC – 3′
   (B) 5′ – UGCGUUAAGCUAGUGCUACGUAUCG – 3′
   (C) 5′ – ACGCAAUUCGAUCACGAUGCAUAGC – 3′
   (D) 5′ – CGAUACGUAGCACUAGCUUAACGCA – 3′
   (E) 5′ – GCTATGCATCGTGATCGAATTGCGT – 3′

3. In DNA, the bond between the deoxyribose sugar and the phosphate is which of the following?

   (A) A polar bond
   (B) An ionic bond
   (C) A hydrogen bond
   (D) A covalent bond
   (E) A van der Waals bond

4. How many double-stranded DNA molecules 8 base pairs long are theoretically possible?

   (A) 12
   (B) 32
   (C) 64
   (D) 256
   (E) 65,536

5. The backbone of a DNA strand is composed of which of the following?

   (A) Sugars and bases
   (B) Phosphates and sugars
   (C) Bases and phosphates
   (D) Nucleotides and sugars
   (E) Phosphates and nucleosides

13 Synthesis of DNA

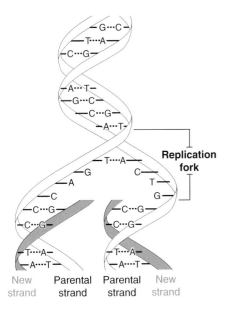

Fig. 13.1. A replicating DNA helix. The parental strands separate at the replication fork. Each parental strand serves as a template for the synthesis of a new strand.

*DNA synthesis occurs by the process of **replication**. During replication, each of the two parental strands of DNA serves as a **template** for the synthesis of a complementary strand. Thus, each DNA molecule generated by the replication process contains one intact parental strand and one newly synthesized strand (Fig. 13.1). In eukaryotes, **DNA replication** occurs during the **S phase** of the **cell cycle,** which is followed by the G_2 phase. The cell **divides** during the next phase (**M**), and each daughter cell receives an exact copy of the DNA of the parent cell.*

*The Replication Fork. In both prokaryotes and eukaryotes, the site at which replication is occurring at any given moment is called the **replication fork**. As replication proceeds, the two parental strands separate in front of the fork. Behind the fork, each newly synthesized strand of DNA base-pairs with its complementary parental template strand. A complex of proteins is involved in replication. **Helicases** and **topoisomerases** unwind the parental strands, and **single-strand binding proteins** prevent them from reannealing.*

*The major enzyme involved in replication is a **DNA polymerase** that copies each parental template strand in the 3' to 5' direction, producing new strands in a 5' to 3' direction. **Deoxyribonucleoside triphosphates** serve as the precursors. One strand of newly synthesized DNA grows continuously, whereas the other strand is synthesized discontinuously in short segments known as **Okazaki fragments**. These fragments are subsequently joined by **DNA ligase**.*

*Initiation. **DNA polymerase cannot initiate** the synthesis of new strands. Therefore, a short **primer** is produced, which contains ribonucleotides (RNA). DNA polymerase can add deoxyribonucleotides to the 3' end of this primer. This RNA primer is subsequently removed and replaced by deoxyribonucleotides.*

*Telomeres. The ends of linear chromosomes are called telomeres. The enzyme **telomerase,** an RNA-dependant DNA polymerase that carries its own RNA template, is required for their replication.*

*Errors and Repair. Errors occurring **during replication** could lead to deleterious **mutations**. However, many errors are corrected by enzyme activities associated with the complex at the replication fork. The **error rate** is thus kept at a very **low** level.*

*Damage to DNA molecules also causes mutations. **Repair mechanisms** correct DNA damage, usually by removing and replacing the damaged region. The intact, undamaged strand serves as a template for the DNA polymerase involved in the repair process.*

*Recombination. Although cells have mechanisms to correct replication errors and to repair DNA damage, some genetic change is desirable. It produces new proteins or variations of proteins that may increase the survival rate of the species. Genetic change is produced by unrepaired mutations and by a mechanism known as **recombination** in which portions of chromosomes are exchanged.*

THE WAITING ROOM

Ivy Sharer is having difficulty complying with her multidrug regimen. She often forgets to take her pills. When she returns for a checkup, she asks whether such a large number of pills are really necessary for treatment of acquired immunodeficiency syndrome (AIDS).

Di Abietes responded to treatment for her diabetes mellitus but subsequently developed a low-grade fever, an increase in urinary urgency and frequency, and burning at the urethral opening with urination (dysuria). A urinalysis showed a large number of white blood cells and many Gram-negative bacilli. A urine culture indicated many colonies of *Escherichia coli*, which is sensitive to several antibiotics, including the quinolone norfloxacin.

Melvin (Mel) Anoma is a 46-year-old man who noted a superficial, brownish-black, 5-mm nodule with irregular borders in the skin on his chest. He was scheduled for outpatient surgery, at which time a wide excision biopsy was performed. (In an excision biopsy, the complete mole is removed and biopsy performed). Examination of the nodule indicated histologic changes characteristic of a malignant melanoma reaching a thickness of only 0.7 mm from the skin surface (Stage I).

Nick O'Tyne is a 62-year-old electrician who has smoked two packs of cigarettes a day for 40 years. He recently noted that his chronic cough had gotten worse. His physician ordered a chest radiograph, which showed a 2-cm nodule in the upper lobe of the right lung. Cytologic study of the sputum by Papanicolaou technique showed cells consistent with the presence of a well-differentiated adenocarcinoma of the lung.

I.   DNA SYNTHESIS IN PROKARYOTES

The basic features of the mechanism of DNA replication are illustrated by the processes occurring in the bacterium *E. coli*. This bacillus grows symbiotically in the human colon. It has been extensively studied and serves as a model for the more complex and, consequently, less well-understood processes that occur in eukaryotic cells.

A.   Replication Is Bidirectional

Replication of the circular, double-stranded DNA of the chromosome of *E. coli* begins with the binding of approximately 30 molecules of the protein DnaA at a single point of origin, designated *oriC*, where the DNA coils around the DnaA core (Fig. 13.2). With the assistance of other proteins (e.g., a helicase, gyrase, and single-stranded binding protein), the two parental strands separate within this region, and both strands are copied simultaneously. Synthesis begins at the origin and occurs at two replication forks that move away from the origin bidirectionally (in both directions at the same time). Replication ends on the other side of the chromosome at a termination point. One round of synthesis, involving the incorporation of over 4 million nucleotides in each new strand of DNA, is completed in approximately 40 minutes. However, a second round of synthesis can begin at the origin before the first round is finished. These multiple initiations of replication allow bacterial multiplication to occur much more quickly than the time it takes to complete a single round of replication.

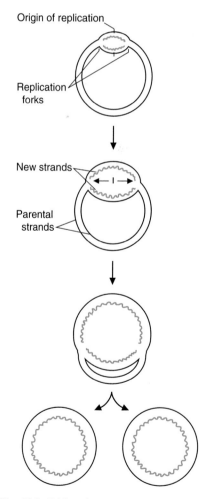

Fig. 13.2. Bidirectional replication of a circular chromosome. Replication begins at the point of origin (*oriC*) and proceeds in both directions at the same time.

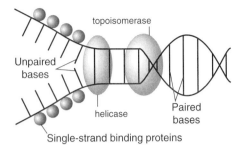

Fig. 13.3. Proteins involved in separating and unwinding parental DNA strands at the replication fork in prokaryotes.

Di Abietes' urinary tract infection was treated with norfloxacin, a fluorinated member of the quinolone family. This group of drugs inhibits bacterial DNA gyrase, a topoisomerase that unwinds the closed circular bacterial DNA helix ahead of the replication fork, and thus inhibits bacterial DNA synthesis. Because eukaryotic cells have linear DNA and do not contain DNA gyrase, they are not affected by quinolones.

One of the drugs used to treat **Ivy Sharer** was didanosine (ddI). It is a dideoxynucleoside, an example of which is shown below.

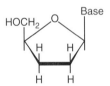

A dideoxynucleoside

The dideoxynucleosides do not have a hydroxyl group on either the 2'- or 3'-carbon. They can be converted to dideoxynucleoside triphosphates in cells and, like ZDV, terminate chain growth when incorporated into DNA. In the case of the dideoxynucleosides, chain termination results from the absence of a hydroxyl group on the 3' carbon. The HIV virus mutates very rapidly (mostly because reverse transcriptase lacks 3' to 5' exonuclease activity, the proofreading activity) and frequently develops resistance to one or more of these drugs. Therefore, it is recommended that AIDS patients take a number of drugs, including more than one reverse transcriptase inhibitor.

B. Replication Is Semiconservative

Each daughter chromosome contains one of the parental DNA strands and one newly synthesized, complementary strand. Therefore, replication is said to be semiconservative; i.e., the parental strands are conserved but are no longer together. Each one is paired with a newly synthesized strand (see Figs. 13.1 and 13.2).

C. Unwinding of Parental Strands

Replication requires separation of the parental DNA strands and unwinding of the helix ahead of the replication fork. Helicases (DnaB) separate the DNA strands and unwind the parental duplex. Single-strand binding proteins prevent the strands from reassociating and protect them from enzymes that cleave single-stranded DNA (Fig. 13.3). Topoisomerases, enzymes that can break phosphodiester bonds and rejoin them, relieve the supercoiling of the parental duplex caused by unwinding. DNA gyrase is a major topoisomerase in bacterial cells.

D. Action of DNA Polymerase

Enzymes that catalyze the synthesis of DNA are known as DNA polymerases. *E. coli* has three DNA polymerases, Pol I, Pol II, and Pol III. Pol III is the major replicative enzyme (Table 13.1). All DNA polymerases that have been studied copy a DNA template strand in its 3' to 5' direction, producing a new strand in the 5' to 3' direction (Fig. 13.4). Deoxyribonucleoside triphosphates (dATP, dGTP, dCTP, and dTTP) serve as substrates for the addition of nucleotides to the growing chain.

The incoming nucleotide forms a base pair with its complementary nucleotide on the template strand. Then an ester bond is formed between the first 5'-phosphate of the incoming nucleotide and the free 3'-hydroxyl group at the end of the growing chain. Pyrophosphate is released. The release of pyrophosphate and its subsequent cleavage by a pyrophosphatase provide the energy that drives the polymerization process.

DNA polymerases that catalyze the synthesis of new strands during replication exhibit a feature called processivity. They remain bound to the parental template strand while continuing to "process" down the chain, rather than dissociating and reassociating as each nucleotide is added. Consequently, synthesis is much more rapid than it would be with an enzyme that was not processive.

E. Elimination of Base-Pairing Errors

In *E. coli*, the replicative enzyme Pol III also performs a proofreading or editing function. This enzyme has 3'–5'-exonuclease activity in addition to its polymerase activity (see Table 13.1). If the nucleotide at the end of the growing chain is incorrectly base-paired with the template strand, Pol III removes this nucleotide before continuing to lengthen the growing chain. This proofreading activity eliminates

Table 13.1. Functions of Bacterial DNA Polymerases

Polymerases	Functions[a]	Exonuclease Activity[b]
Pol I	Filling of gap after removal of RNA primer DNA repair Removal of RNA primer in conjunction with RNAse H	5' to 3' and 3' to 5'
Pol II	DNA repair	3' to 5'
Pol III	Replication – synthesis of DNA	3' to 5'

[a] Synthesis of new DNA strands always occurs 5' to 3'
[b] Exonucleases remove nucleotides from DNA strands and act at the 5' end (cleaving 5' to 3') or at the 3' end (cleaving 3' to 5').

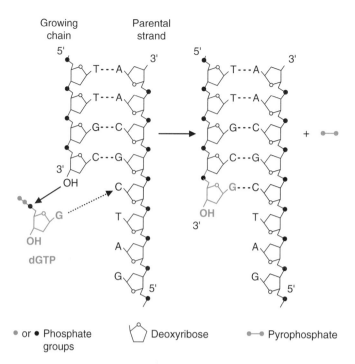

Fig. 13.4. Action of DNA polymerase. Deoxyribonucleoside triphosphates serve as precursors (substrates) used by DNA polymerase to lengthen the DNA chain. DNA polymerase copies the DNA template strand in the 3′ to 5′ direction. The new strand grows 5′ to 3′.

most base-pairing errors as they occur. Only about one base pair in a million is mismatched in the final DNA product; the error rate is about 10^{-6}. If this proofreading activity is experimentally removed from the enzyme, the error rate increases to about 10^{-3}.

After replication, other mechanisms replace mismatched bases that escaped proofreading so that the fidelity of DNA replication is very high. The two processes of proofreading and postreplication mismatch repair result in an overall error rate of about 10^{-10}, that is, less than one mismatched base pair in 10 billion.

F. Function of RNA Primers

DNA polymerase cannot initiate the synthesis of new strands; it requires the presence of a free 3′-OH group to function. Therefore, a primer is required to supply the free 3′-OH group. This primer is an RNA oligonucleotide. It is synthesized in a 5′ to 3′ direction by an RNA polymerase (primase) that copies the DNA template strand. DNA polymerase initially adds a deoxyribonucleotide to the 3′-hydroxyl group of the primer and then continues adding deoxyribonucleotides to the 3′-end of the growing strand (Fig. 13.5).

G. DNA Synthesis at the Replication Fork

Both parental strands are copied at the same time in the direction of the replication fork, an observation difficult to reconcile with the known activity of DNA polymerase, which can produce chains only in a 5′ to 3′ direction. Because the parental strands run in opposite directions relative to each other, synthesis should occur in a 5′ to 3′ direction **toward** the fork on one template strand and in a 5′ to 3′ direction **away** from the fork on the other template strand.

Okazaki resolved this dilemma by showing that synthesis on one strand, called the leading strand, is continuous in the 5′ to 3′ direction toward the fork. The other

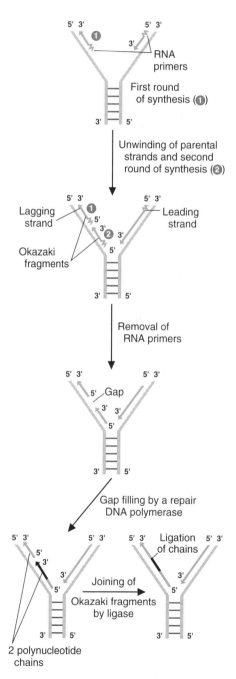

Fig. 13.5. Synthesis of DNA at the replication fork. (See Fig. 13.6 for the ligation reaction.)

RNase H is a ribonuclease that specifically degrades RNA from an RNA-DNA hybrid. The HIV virus (see Chapter 12) converts an RNA genome to a double-stranded DNA copy using the enzyme reverse transcriptase. An intermediate in the conversion of the single-stranded RNA genome to double-stranded DNA is an RNA-DNA hybrid. To remove the RNA so a double-stranded DNA molecule can be made, reverse transcriptase contains RNase H activity. Scientists are currently attempting to target the RNase H activity of reverse transcriptase with inhibitors as a means of controlling spread of the virus.

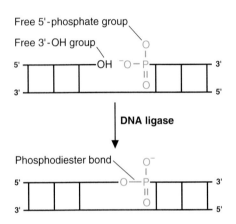

Fig. 13.6. Action of DNA ligase. Two polynucleotide chains, one with a free 3′-OH group and one with a free 5′-phosphate group, are joined by DNA ligase, which forms a phosphodiester bond.

strand, called the lagging strand, is synthesized discontinuously in short fragments (see Fig. 13.5). These fragments, named for Okazaki, are produced in a 5′ to 3′ direction (away from the fork), but then joined together so that, overall, synthesis proceeds toward the replication fork.

H. Function of DNA Ligase

As replication progresses, the RNA primers are removed from Okazaki fragments, probably by the combined action of DNA polymerase I (Pol I, using its $5' \rightarrow 3'$ exonuclease activity) and RNase H. Pol I fills in the gaps produced by removal of the primers. Because DNA polymerases cannot join two polynucleotide chains together, an additional enzyme, DNA ligase, is required to perform this function. The 3′-hydroxyl group at the end of one fragment is ligated to the phosphate group at the 5′-end of the next fragment (Fig. 13.6).

II. DNA SYNTHESIS IN EUKARYOTES

The process of replication in eukaryotes is similar to that in prokaryotes. Differences in the processes are related mainly to the vastly larger amount of DNA in eukaryotic cells (over 1,000 times the amount in *E. coli*) and the association of eukaryotic DNA with histones in nucleosomes. Enzymes with DNA polymerase, primase, ligase, helicase, and topoisomerase activity are all present in eukaryotes, although these enzymes differ in some respects from those of prokaryotes.

A. Eukaryotic Cell Cycle

The cell cycle of eukaryotes consists of four phases (Fig. 13.7). The first three phases (G_1, S, and G_2) constitute interphase. Cells spend most of their time in these three phases, carrying out their normal metabolic activities. The fourth phase is mitosis, the process of cell division. This phase is very brief.

The first phase of the cell cycle, G_1 (the first "gap" phase), is the most variable in length. Late in G_1, the cells prepare to duplicate their chromosomes (e.g., by producing nucleotide precursors). In the second or S phase, DNA replicates. Nucleosomes disassemble as the replication forks advance. Throughout S phase, the synthesis of histones and other proteins associated with DNA is markedly increased.

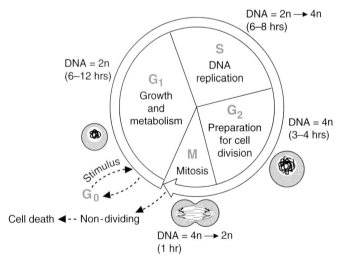

Fig. 13.7. Eukaryotic cell cycle. The times given for the length of each phase are for cells growing in culture.

The amount of DNA and histones both double, and chromosomes are duplicated. Histones complex with DNA, and nucleosomes are formed very rapidly behind the advancing replication forks.

During the third phase of the cell cycle, G_2 (the second "gap" phase), the cells prepare to divide and synthesize tubulin for construction of the microtubules of the spindle apparatus. Finally, division occurs in the brief mitotic or M phase.

After mitosis, some cells reenter G_1, repeatedly going through the phases of the cell cycle and dividing. Other cells leave the cycle after mitosis, never to divide again, or they enter an extended G_1 phase (sometimes called G_0), in which they remain for long periods. On the appropriate signal, cells in G_0 are stimulated to reenter the cycle and divide.

B. Points of Origin for Replication

In contrast to bacterial chromosomes (see section I.A. of this chapter), eukaryotic chromosomes have multiple points of origin at which replication begins. "Bubbles" appear at these points on the chromosomes. At each end of a bubble, a replication fork forms; thus, each bubble has two forks. DNA synthesis occurs at each of these forks, as illustrated in Figure 13.8. As the bubbles enlarge, they eventually merge, and replication is completed. Because eukaryotic chromosomes contain multiple points of origin of replication (and, thus, multiple replicons-units of replication), duplication of such large chromosomes can occur within a few hours.

C. Eukaryotic DNA polymerases

At least nine DNA polymerases exist in eukaryotic cells (α, β, γ, δ, ϵ, ζ, κ, η, and ι) (Table 13.2). Polymerase δ (pol δ) is the major replicative enzyme. Pol α and pol ϵ are also involved in relication. Polymerases β and ϵ, as well as pol α, appear to be involved in DNA repair. Pol γ is located in mitochondria and replicates the DNA of this organelle. Polymerases ζ, κ, η and ι, which lack $3' \rightarrow 5'$ exonuclease activity, are used when DNA is damaged.

D. The Eukaryotic Replication Complex

Many proteins bind at or near the replication fork and participate in the process of duplicating DNA (Fig. 13.9)(Table 13.3). Polymerase δ (pol δ) is the major replica-

 HeLa cells, derived from a human cervical carcinoma, are rapidly dividing cells that can be grown in culture flasks. Their cell cycle is approximately 20 hours. Only 1 hour of this time is spent in mitosis.

Cells within the body that divide less frequently, such as liver cells, spend days, weeks, or months in interphase before going through a brief mitotic phase.

 Although Prometheus was chained to a rock as punishment for his theft of fire from the gods, and a vulture pecked at his liver each day, he survived. Can you guess why?

In the human body, many cells cycle frequently, e.g., hair follicles, skin cells, and cells of the duodenal crypts. Other cells, such as the precursors of red blood cells, divide a number of times, then lose their nuclei and leave the cell cycle to form mature red blood cells. These cells transport oxygen and carbon dioxide between the lungs and other tissues for about 120 days, then die. Other cells are normally quiescent (in G_0). However, they can be stimulated to divide. In many instances, the stimuli are growth factors or hormones (e.g., mammary aveolar cells and uterine cells). In the case of liver cells, the stimulus is produced by death of some of the cells.

Table 13.2. Functions of Eukaryotic DNA Polymerases

Polymerase	Functions[a]	Exonuclease Activity
Pol α	Replication (in a complex with primase and aids in starting the primer) DNA repair	None
Pol β	DNA repair exclusively	None
Pol γ	DNA replication in mitochondria	3' to 5'
Pol δ	Replication (processive DNA synthesis on leading and lagging strands) DNA repair	3' to 5'
Pol ϵ	Replication (in some tissues takes the place of Pol d) DNA repair	3' to 5'
Pol κ	DNA repair (bypass polymerase)[b]	None
Pol η	DNA repair (bypass polymerase)	None
Pol ζ	DNA repair (bypass polymerase)	None
Pol ι	DNA repair (bypass polymerase)	None

[a] Synthesis of new DNA strands always occurs 5' to 3'.
[b] Bypass polymerase are able to "bypass" areas of DNA damage and continue DNA replication. Some enzymes are error-free and insert the correct bases; other enzymes are error prone and insert random bases.

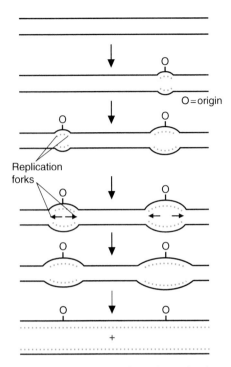

Fig. 13.8. Replication of a eukaryotic chromosome. Synthesis is bidirectional from each point of origin (O) and semiconservative, each daughter DNA helix contains one intact parental strand (solid line) and one newly synthesized strand (dashed line).

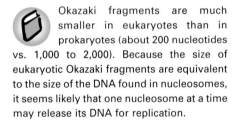

Okazaki fragments are much smaller in eukaryotes than in prokaryotes (about 200 nucleotides vs. 1,000 to 2,000). Because the size of eukaryotic Okazaki fragments are equivalent to the size of the DNA found in nucleosomes, it seems likely that one nucleosome at a time may release its DNA for replication.

A: Liver cells are in G_0. Up to 90% of the human liver can be removed. The remaining liver cells are stimulated to re-enter the cell cycle and divide, regenerating a mass equivalent to the original mass of the liver within a few weeks. The myth of Prometheus indicates that the capacity of the liver to regenerate was recognized even in ancient times.

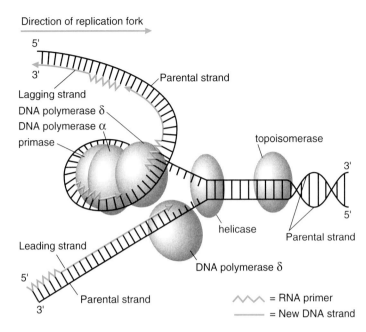

Fig. 13.9. Replication complex in eukaryotes. The lagging strand is shown looped around the replication complex. Single-strand binding proteins (not shown) are bound to the unpaired, single-stranded DNA. Other proteins also participate in this complex (see text).

tive enzyme. However, before it acts, a primase associated with polymerase α (pol δ) produces an RNA primer (approximately 10 nucleotides in length). Then pol α adds about 20 deoxyribonucleotides to this RNA and dissociates from the template, because of the low processivity of pol α. On the leading strand, pol δ adds deoxyribonucleotides to this RNA-DNA primer, continuously producing this strand. Pol δ is a highly processive enzyme.

The lagging strand is produced from a series of Okazaki fragments (see Fig. 13.5). Synthesis of each Okazaki fragment is initiated by pol α and its associated primase, as described above. After pol α dissociates, pol δ adds deoxyribonucleotides to the primer, producing an Okazaki fragment. Pol δ stops synthesizing one fragment when it reaches the start of the previously synthesized Okazaki fragment (see Fig. 13.5). The primer of the previously synthesized Okazaki fragment is

Table 13.3 Major proteins involved in replication

DNA polymerases	- add nucleotides to a strand growing $5' \to 3'$, copying a DNA template $3' \to 5'$
Primase	- synthesizes RNA primers
Helicases	- Separate parental DNA strands, i.e., unwind the double helix
Single-strand binding proteins	- Prevent single strands of DNA from reassociating
Topoisomerases	- Relieve torsional strain on parental duplex caused by unwinding
Enzymes that remove primers	- RNase H – hydrolyzes RNA of DNA-RNA hybrids
	- Flap endonucleases 1 (FEN1) – recognizes "flap" (Unannealed portion of RNA) near 5'-end of primer and cleaves downstream in DNA region of primer
DNA ligase	- Joins, by forming a phosphodiester bond, two adjacent DNA strands that are bound to the same template

removed by flap endonuclease 1 (FEN1) and Rnase H. The gap left by the primer is filled by a DNA polymerase that uses the parental DNA strand as its template and the newly synthesized Okazaki fragment as its primer. DNA ligase subsequently joins the Okazaki fragments together (see Fig. 13.6).

Obviously, eukaryotic replication requires many proteins. The complexity of the fork and the fact that it is not completely understood limits the detail shown in Figure 13.9. One protein not shown is proliferating cell nuclear antigen (PCNA), which is involved in organizing and orchestrating the replication process.

Additional activities that occur during replication include proofreading and DNA repair. Pol δ, which is part of the replication complex, has the $3' \rightarrow 5'$-exonuclease activity required for proofreading. Enzymes that catalyze repair of mismatched bases are also present (see section III.B.3 of this chapter). Consequently, eukaryotic replication occurs with high fidelity; approximately one mispairing occurs for every 10^9 to 10^{12} nucleotides incorporated into growing DNA chains.

Proliferating cell nuclear antigen (PCNA) is used clinically as a diagnostic marker for proliferating cells.

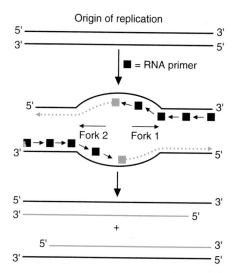

Fig. 13.10. The "end-replication" problem in linear chromosomes. After replication, the telomeres have 3'-overhangs. When these molecules are replicated, chromosome shortening will result. The figure depicts a linear chromosome with one origin of replication. At the origin, two replication forks are generated, each moving in the opposite direction, labeled as Fork I and Fork II. As Fork I moves to the right, the bottom strand is read in the 3' to 5' direction, which means it is the template for the leading strand. The newly synthesized DNA complementary to the upper strand at Fork 1 will be the lagging strand. Now consider Fork 2. As this replication fork moves to the left, the upper strand is read in the 3' to 5' direction, so the newly synthesized DNA complementary to this strand will be the leading strand. For this fork, the newly synthesized DNA complementary to the bottom strand will be the lagging strand.

E. Replication of the Ends of Chromosomes

Eukaryotic chromosomes are linear, and the ends of the chromosomes are called telomeres. As DNA replication approaches the end of the chromosome, a problem develops in the lagging strand (Fig. 13.10). Either primase cannot lay down a primer at the very end of the chromosome, or, after DNA replication is complete, the RNA at the end of the chromosome is degraded. Consequently, the newly synthesized strand is shorter at the 5' end, and there is a 3'-overhang in the DNA strand being replicated. If the chromosome became shorter with each successive replication, genes would be lost. How is this problem solved?

The 3' overhang is lengthened by the addition of telomeres so that primase can bind and synthesize the complementary strand. Telomeres consist of a repeating sequence of bases (TTAGGG for humans), which may be repeated thousands of times. The enzyme telomerase contains both proteins and RNA and acts as an RNA-dependent DNA polymerase (just like reverse transcriptase). The RNA within telomerase contains the complementary copy of the repeating sequence in the telomeres and can base pair with the existing 3'-overhang (Fig. 13.11). The polymerase activity of telomerase then uses the existing 3'-hydroxyl group of the overhang as a primer, and its own RNA as a template, and synthesizes new DNA that lengthens the 3'-end of the DNA strand. The telomerase moves down the DNA toward the new 3'-end and repeats the process a number of times. When the 3'-overhang is sufficiently long, primase binds, and synthesis of the complementary strand is completed. The 3' overhang can also form a complicated structure with telomere binding proteins to protect the ends of the chromosomes from damage and nuclease attack once they have been lengthened

An inability to replicate telomeres has been linked to cell aging and death. Many somatic cells do not express telomerase; when placed in culture they survive a fixed number of population doublings, enter senescence, and then die. Analysis has shown significant telomere shortening in those cells. In contrast, stem cells do express telomerase and appear to have an infinite lifetime in culture. Research is underway to understand the role of telomeres in cell aging, growth, and cancer.

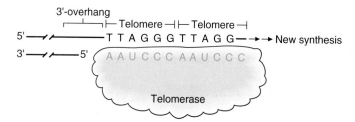

Fig. 13.11. Telomerase action. The RNA present in telomerase base-pairs with the overhanging 3'-end of telomeres and extends it by acting both as a template and a reverse transcriptase. After copying a small number of repeats, the complex moves down to the 3'-end of the overhang and repeats the process.

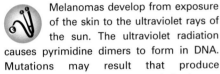 **Nick O'Tyne** has been smoking for 40 years in spite of the warnings on cigarette packs that this habit can be dangerous and even deadly. The burning of tobacco, and, for that matter, the burning of any organic material, produces many different carcinogens, such as benzo[a]pyrene. These carcinogens coat the airways and lungs. They can cross cell membranes and interact with DNA, causing damage to bases that interferes with normal base pairing. If these DNA lesions cannot be repaired or if they are not repaired rapidly enough, a permanent mutation can be produced when the cells replicate. Some mutations are silent, whereas other mutations can lead to abnormal cell growth, and cancer results.

Melanomas develop from exposure of the skin to the ultraviolet rays of the sun. The ultraviolet radiation causes pyrimidine dimers to form in DNA. Mutations may result that produce melanomas, appearing as dark brown growths on the skin.

Fortunately, **Mel Anoma**'s malignant skin lesion was discovered at an early stage. Because there was no evidence of cancer in the margins of the resected mass, full recovery was expected. However, lifelong surveillance for return of the melanoma was planned.

Pyrimidine dimers, most commonly thymine dimers, can be repaired by photoreactivating enzymes that cleave the bonds between the bases by using energy from visible light. In this process, nucleotides are not removed from the damaged DNA. This repair process is used by bacteria and might serve as a very minor repair mechanism in human cells.

III. DNA REPAIR

A. Actions of Mutagens

Despite proofreading and mismatch repair during replication, some mismatched bases do persist. Additional problems may arise from DNA damaged by mutagens, chemicals produced in cells, inhaled, or absorbed from the environment that cause mutations. Mutagens that cause normal cells to become cancer cells are known as carcinogens. Unfortunately, mismatching of bases and DNA damage produce thousands of potentially mutagenic lesions in each cell every day. Without repair mechanisms, we could not survive these assaults on our genes.

DNA damage can be caused by radiation and by chemicals (Fig. 13.12). These agents can directly affect the DNA or they can act indirectly. For example, x-rays, a type of ionizing radiation, act indirectly to damage DNA by exciting water in the cell and generating the hydroxyl radical, which reacts with DNA, thereby altering the structure of the bases or cleaving the DNA strands.

While exposure to x-rays is infrequent, it is more difficult to avoid exposure to cigarette smoke and virtually impossible to avoid exposure to sunlight. Cigarette smoke contains carcinogens such as the aromatic polycyclic hydrocarbon benzo[a]pyrene (see Fig. 13.12). When this compound is oxidized by cellular enzymes, which normally act to make foreign compounds more water soluble and easy to excrete, it becomes capable of forming bulky adducts with guanine residues in DNA. Ultraviolet rays from the sun, which also produce distortions in the DNA helix, excite adjacent pyrimidine bases on DNA strands, causing them to form covalent dimers (Fig. 13.13).

B. Repair Mechanisms

The mechanisms used for the repair of DNA have many similarities (Fig. 13.14). First, a distortion in the DNA helix is recognized, and the region containing the distortion is removed. The gap in the damaged strand is replaced by the action of a DNA polymerase that uses the intact, undamaged strand as a template. Finally, a ligase seals the nick in the strand that has undergone repair.

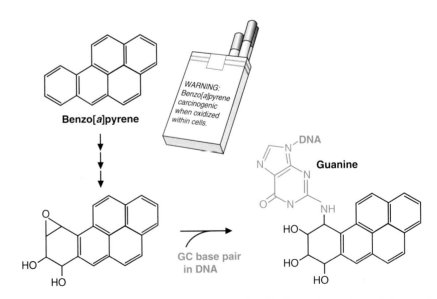

Fig. 13.12. Oxidation of benzo[a]pyrene and covalent binding to DNA. Benzo[a]pyrene is not carcinogenic until it is oxidized within cells. Then it can covalently bind to guanine residues in DNA, interrupting hydrogen bonding in G-C base pairs and producing distortions of the helix.

1. NUCLEOTIDE EXCISION REPAIR

Nucleotide excision repair involves local distortions of the DNA helix, such as mismatched bases or bulky adducts (e.g., oxidized benzo[*a*]pyrene) (Fig. 13.15, see also Fig. 13.14). Endonucleases cleave the abnormal chain and remove the distorted region. The gap is then filled by a DNA polymerase that adds deoxyribonucleotides, one at a time, to the 3′-end of the cleaved DNA, using the intact, complementary DNA strand as a template. The newly synthesized segment is joined to the 5′-end of the remainder of the original DNA strand by a DNA ligase.

2. BASE EXCISION REPAIR

DNA glycosylases recognize small distortions in DNA involving lesions caused by damage to a single base (e.g., the conversion of cytosine to uracil). A glycosylase cleaves the *N*-glycosidic bond that joins the damaged base to deoxyribose (see Fig. 13.15). The sugar–phosphate backbone of the DNA now lacks a base at this site (known as an apurinic or apyrimidinic site, or an AP site). Then an AP endonuclease cleaves the sugar–phosphate strand at this site. Subsequently, the same types of enzymes involved in other types of repair mechanisms restore this region to normal.

3. MISMATCH REPAIR

Mismatched bases (bases that do not form normal Watson-Crick base pairs) are recognized by enzymes of the mismatch repair system. Because neither of the bases in a mismatch is damaged, these repair enzymes must be able to determine which base of the mispair to correct.

The mismatch repair enzyme complex acts during replication when an incorrect, but normal base (i.e., A, G, C, or T) is incorporated into the growing chain (Fig. 13.16). In bacteria, parental DNA strands contain methyl groups on adenine bases in specific sequences. During replication, the newly synthesized strands are not immediately methylated. Before methylation occurs, the proteins involved in mismatch repair can distinguish parental from newly synthesized strands. A region of the new, unmethylated strand, containing the mismatched base, is removed and replaced.

Human enzymes also can distinguish parental from newly synthesized strands and repair mismatches. However, the mechanisms have not yet been as clearly defined as those in bacteria.

Pyrimidine dimers occur frequently in the skin. Usually repair mechanisms correct this damage, and cancer rarely occurs. However, in individuals with xeroderma pigmentosum, cancers are extremely common. These individuals have defects in their DNA repair systems. The first defect to be identified was a deficiency of the endonuclease involved in removal of pyrimidine dimers from DNA. Because of the inability to repair DNA, the frequency of mutation increases. A cancer develops once proto-oncogenes or tumor suppressor genes mutate. By scrupulously avoiding light, these individuals can reduce the number of skin cancers that develop.

Spontaneous deamination occurs frequently in human DNA and converts cytosine bases to uracil. This base is not normally found in DNA and is potentially harmful because U pairs with A, forming U-A base pairs instead of the normal C-G pairs. To prevent this change from occurring, a uracil *N*-glycosylase removes uracil, and it is replaced by a cytosine via base excision repair.

Hereditary nonpolyposis colorectal cancer (a human cancer that does not arise from intestinal polyps) is caused by mutations in genes for proteins involved in mismatch repair (hMSH1, hMSH2, hPMS1, or hPMS2). The inability to repair mismatches increases the mutation frequency, resulting in cancers from mutations in growth regulatory genes.

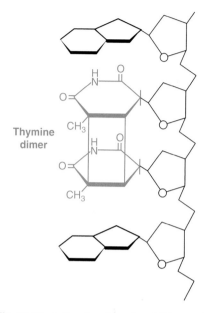

Fig. 13.13. A thymine dimer in a DNA strand. Ultraviolet light can cause two adjacent pyrimidines to form a covalent dimer.

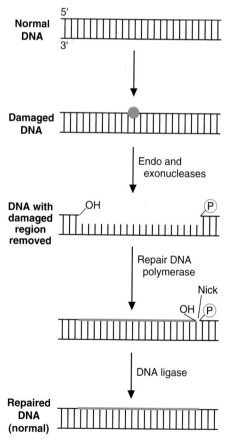

Fig. 13.14. Common steps in DNA repair mechanisms.

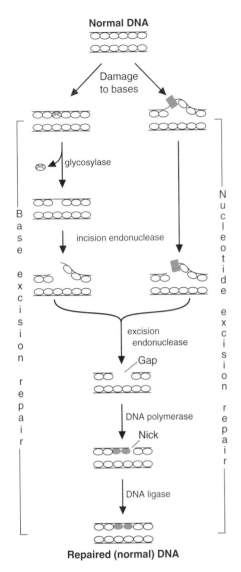

Fig. 13.15. Types of damage and various repair mechanisms. In base excision repair, the glycosylase cleaves the glycosidic bond between the altered base (shown with an X) and ribose. In nucleotide excision repair, the entire nucleotide is removed at once. The gap formed by the incision (cut) and excision (removal) endonucleases is usually several nucleotides wider than the one shown.

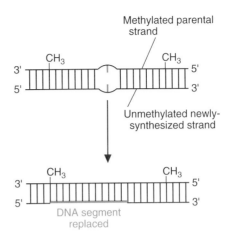

Fig. 13.16. Mismatch repair. Normal, undamaged but mismatched bases bind proteins of the mismatch repair system. In bacteria, these proteins recognize the older, parental strand because it is methylated and replace a segment of newly synthesized (and unmethylated) DNA containing the mismatched base. The mechanism for distinguishing between parental and newly synthesized strands in humans is not as well understood.

4. TRANSCRIPTION-COUPLED REPAIR

Genes that are actively transcribed to produce mRNA are preferentially repaired. The RNA polymerase that is transcribing a gene (see Chapter 14 for a description of the process) stalls when it encounters a damaged region of the DNA template. Excision repair proteins are attracted to this site and repair the damaged region. Subsequently, RNA polymerase can resume transcription.

IV. GENETIC REARRANGEMENTS

The exchange of segments between DNA molecules occurs quite frequently and is responsible for genetic alterations that can have beneficial or devastating consequences for the affected individuals and, in some instances, for their offspring. The DNA segments that are exchanged may be homologous (that is, of very similar sequence) or they may be totally unrelated. The size of these segments can range from a few nucleotides to tens of thousands and can include many different genes or portions of genes. Many of the enzymes involved in these exchanges are the same as or similar to those used for replication and repair and include endonucleases, exonucleases, unwinding enzymes, topoisomerases, DNA polymerases, and ligases.

One type of genetic rearrangement that has been observed for many years is "crossing-over" between homologous chromosomes during meiosis. Another type occurs in stem cells as they differentiate into lymphocytes. Segments of the genes of stem cells are rearranged so that the mature cell is capable of producing only a single type of antibody (see Chapter 16). Other types of genetic exchanges involve transposable elements (transposons) that can move from one site in the genome to another or produce copies that can be inserted into new sites. Translocations occur when chromosomes break and portions randomly become joined to other chromosomes, producing gross changes that can be observed under the light microscope. Genetic exchanges can even occur between species, for example, when foreign DNA is inserted into the human genome as a result of viral infection.

A. General or Homologous Recombination

Various models, supported by experimental evidence, have been proposed for the mechanism of recombination between homologous DNA sequences. Although these mechanisms are complex, a simplified scheme for one type of recombination is presented in Figure 13.17.

Initially, two homologous chromosomes or segments of double-helical (duplex) DNA that have very similar, but not necessarily identical, sequences become aligned (see Fig. 13.17). One strand of one duplex is nicked by an enzyme and invades the other DNA duplex, base-pairing with a region of complementary sequence. The match between the sequences does not have to be perfect, but a significant number of bases must pair so that the strand displaced from its partner can form a displacement (D) loop. This D loop is nicked, and the displaced strand now base-pairs with the former partner of the invading strand. Ligation occurs, and a Holliday structure is generated (see Fig. 13.17). The branch point of the Holliday structure can migrate and may move many thousands of nucleotides from its original position. The Holliday structure, named for the scientist who discovered it, is finally cleaved and then religated, forming two chromosomes that have exchanged segments. In addition to enzymes similar to those used in DNA replication, enzymes for strand invasion, branch migration, and cleavage of the Holliday structure are required.

B. Translocations

Breaks in chromosomes, caused by agents such as x-rays or chemical carcinogens, can result in gross chromosomal rearrangements (Fig. 13.18). If the free ends of the DNA at the break point reseal with the free ends of a different broken chromosome, a translocation is produced. These exchanges of large portions of chromosomes can have deleterious effects and are frequently observed in cancer cells.

C. Transposable Elements

Movable (or transposable) genetic elements, "jumping genes," were first observed by Barbara McClintock in the 1940s. Her work, initially greeted with skepticism, was ultimately accepted, and she was awarded the Nobel Prize in 1983.

Transposons are segments of DNA that can move from their original position in the genome to a new location (Fig. 13.19). They are found in all organisms. Transposons contain the gene for an enzyme called a transposase, which is involved in cleaving the transposon from the genome and moving it from one location to another.

Retroposons are similar to transposons except that they involve an RNA intermediate. Reverse transcriptase (see below) makes a single-stranded DNA copy of the RNA. A double-stranded DNA is then produced that is inserted into the genome at a new location.

V. REVERSE TRANSCRIPTASE

Reverse transcriptase is an enzyme that uses a single-stranded RNA template and makes a DNA copy (Fig. 13.20). The RNA template can be transcribed from DNA by RNA polymerase or obtained from another source, such as an RNA virus. The DNA copy of the RNA produced by reverse transcriptase is known as complementary DNA (because it is complementary to the RNA template), or cDNA. Retroviruses (RNA viruses) contain a reverse transcriptase, which copies the viral RNA genome. A double-stranded cDNA is produced, which can become integrated into the human genome (see Fig. 12.23). After integration, the viral genes may be inactive, or they may be transcribed, sometimes causing diseases such as AIDS or cancer (see Chapter 18).

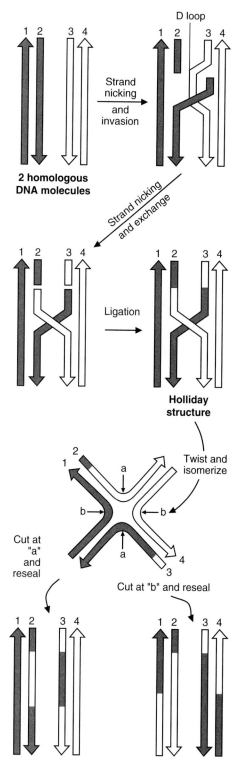

Fig. 13.17. Key steps in recombination.

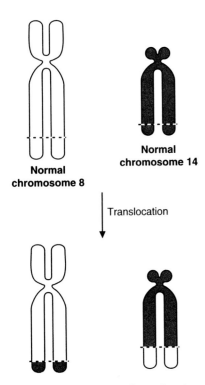

Fig. 13.18. A chromosomal translocation. A portion of the long arm of chromosome 8 is exchanged for a portion of the long arm of chromosome 14. This chromosomal translocation occurs in Burkitt's lymphoma.

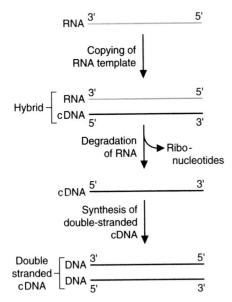

Fig. 13.20. Action of reverse transcriptase. This enzyme catalyzes the production of a DNA copy from an RNA template. The RNA of a DNA-RNA hybrid is degraded, and the single DNA strand is used as a template to make double-stranded DNA. This figure is a simplified version of a more complex process.

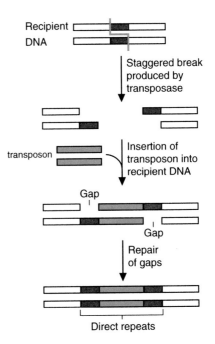

Fig. 13.19. Transposons. The steps involved in transposition are shown. Direct repeats are regions of DNA that have the same base sequence in the 5′ → 3′ direction.

CLINICAL COMMENTS

Ivy Sharer. Ivy Sharer contracted AIDS when she used needles contaminated with HIV to inject drugs intravenously. Intravenous drug abusers account for 15 to 20% of new AIDS cases in the United States. HIV mutates rapidly, and, therefore, current treatment involves a combination of drugs that affect different aspects of its life cycle. This multidrug therapy lowers the viral titer (the number of viral particles found in a given volume of blood), sometimes to undetectable levels. However, if treatment is not followed carefully (i.e., if the patient is not "compliant"), the titer increases rapidly. Therefore, Ivy's physician emphasized that she must carefully follow her drug regimen.

Di Abietes. Di Abietes' poorly controlled diabetes mellitus predisposed her to a urinary tract infection because glucose in the urine serves as a "culture medium" for bacterial growth. The kidney glomerulotubular unit reabsorbs filtered glucose so that normally, the urine is glucose-free. However, when serum blood glucose levels exceed 175 to 185 mg/dL (the tubular threshold for glucose), the capacity for reabsorption is exceeded. In Ms. Abietes' case, blood glucose levels frequently exceed this threshold.

Mel Anoma. The average person has 20 moles on the body surface; however, only seven people of every 100,000 develop a malignant melanoma. The incidence of malignant melanoma, however, is rising rapidly. Because 35 to 40% of patients with malignant melanoma die as a result of this cancer, the physician's decision to perform a biopsy on a pigmented mole with an irregular border and variation of color probably saved **Mel Anoma's** life.

Nick O'Tyne. Lung cancer currently accounts for one fifth of all cancers in men and one tenth in women. The overall 5-year survival rate is still less than 15%. For those who smoke two or more packs of cigarettes daily, as does

Nick O'Tyne, the death rate is 265 per 100,000 population. Thankfully, cigarette smoking has declined in the United States. Whereas 50% of men and 32% of women smoked in 1965, these figures have currently fallen to 26% and 24%, respectively.

BIOCHEMICAL COMMENTS

Chemical carcinogens and tumor promoters. Once it was realized that a number of chemicals react with DNA, leading to mutations, and that mutations may lead to tumor formation, toxicologists searched for chemicals with the ability to cause skin tumors in rats. To test a chemical, it was applied to an area of shaved skin on the back of a rat to see whether a tumor would develop. The chemicals fell into two groups: Group I, the initiators, caused mutations in DNA and group II, the promoters, greatly enhanced the probability that cells that had been previously initiated would develop a tumor. Compounds falling into group II activate a protein kinase (protein kinase C), which is usually only transiently activated when normal cells are stimulated to grow. Tumor promoters, however, are long-lived, and lead to an enhanced activation of protein kinase C.

Is there an easy way to determine whether a compound is an initiator? Bruce Ames developed a rapid and simple test to determine whether chemicals are mutagens. The basic test uses bacteria that have a mutation in a gene necessary for histidine biosynthesis and require histidine for growth. The bacteria are treated with the test chemicals and the number that can grow in the absence of histidine measured. Bacteria that no longer require histidine for growth must have acquired a second, chemically induced mutation that opposed the inactivating, original mutation. In this fashion, the ability of chemicals to alter DNA can be determined. Because many chemicals (such as benz[o]pyrene) do not become carcinogenic in humans until they are metabolized by the liver, the Ames test also involves incubating the chemical with a liver extract, and then testing the metabolized extract for DNA-modifying activity.

Suggested References

Hanawalt P. Transcription-coupled repair and human disease. Science 1994;266:1957–1958.
Kunkel T. DNA replication fidelity. J Biol Chem 1992;267:18251–18254.
Modrich P. Mismatch repair, genetic stability, and cancer. Science 1994;266:1959–1960.
Sancar A. Mechanisms of DNA excision repair. Science 1994;266:1954–1956.
Waga S, Stillman B. The DNA replication fork in eukaryotic cells. Annu Rev Biochem 1998;67:721-751.

REVIEW QUESTIONS—CHAPTER 13

1. Reverse transcriptase, an RNA-dependant DNA polymerase, differs from DNA polymerase δ by which of the following?

    (A) Synthesizes DNA in the 5′ to 3′ direction
    (B) Contains 3′ to 5′ exonuclease activity
    (C) Follows Watson-Crick base pair rules
    (D) Synthesizes DNA in the 3′ to 5′ direction
    (E) Can insert inosine into a growing DNA chain

2. If a 1,000-kilobase fragment of DNA has 10 evenly spaced and symmetric replication origins and DNA polymerase moves at 1 kilobase per second, how many seconds will it take to produce two daughter molecules (ignore potential problems at the ends of this linear piece of DNA)? Assume that the 10 origins are evenly spaced from each other, but not from the ends of the chromosome.

   (A) 20
   (B) 30
   (C) 40
   (D) 50
   (E) 100

3. Primase is not required during DNA repair processes because of which of the following?

   (A) All of the primase is associated with replication origins.
   (B) RNA would be highly mutagenic at a repair site.
   (C) DNA polymerase I does not require a primer.
   (D) DNA polymerase III does not require a primer.
   (E) DNA polyemerase I or III can use any 3' -OH for elongation.

4. Which of the following enzymes is required to actively enhance the separation of DNA strands during replication?

   (A) Helicase
   (B) 3' to 5' exonuclease
   (C) DNA ligase
   (D) Primase
   (E) AP endonuclease

5. The key mechanistic failure in patients with xeroderma pigmentosum involves which of the following?

   (A) Mutation in the primase gene
   (B) Inability to excise a section of the UV-damaged DNA
   (C) Mutation of one of the mismatch repair components
   (D) Inability to synthesize DNA across the damaged region
   (E) Loss of proofreading capacity

14 Transcription: Synthesis of RNA

*Synthesis of RNA from a **DNA template** is called **transcription**. Genes are transcribed by enzymes called **RNA polymerases** that generate a **single-stranded RNA** identical in sequence (with the exception of U in place of T) to one of the strands of the double-stranded DNA. The DNA strand that directs the sequence of nucleotides in the RNA by **complementary base-pairing** is the template strand. The RNA strand that is initially generated is **the primary transcript**. The DNA **template is copied** in the **3′ to 5′** direction, and the **RNA transcript is synthesized** in the **5′ to 3′** direction. RNA polymerases differ from DNA polymerases in that they can **initiate** the **synthesis** of new strands in the absence of a primer.*

*In addition to catalyzing the polymerization of **ribonucleotides**, RNA polymerases must be able to recognize the appropriate gene to transcribe, the appropriate strand of the double-stranded DNA to copy, and the **startpoint** of transcription (Fig. 14.1). Specific sequences on DNA, called **promoters**, determine where the RNA polymerase binds and how frequently it initiates transcription. Other regulatory sequences, such as **promoter-proximal elements** and **enhancers**, also affect the frequency of transcription.*

*In **bacteria**, a **single RNA polymerase** produces the primary transcript precursors for all three major classes of RNA: messenger RNA (mRNA), ribosomal RNA (rRNA), and transfer RNA (tRNA). Because bacteria do not contain nuclei, ribosomes bind to mRNA as it is being transcribed, and protein synthesis occurs simultaneously with transcription.*

Eukaryotic genes are transcribed in the nucleus by **three different RNA polymerases**, each principally responsible for one of the major classes of RNA. The primary transcripts are **modified** and **trimmed** to produce the mature RNAs. The precursors of **mRNA** (called **pre-mRNA**) have a **guanosine** "cap" added at the 5′-end and a **poly(A)** "tail" at the 3′-end. **Exons**, which contain the coding sequences for the proteins, are separated in **pre-mRNA** by **introns**, regions that have no coding function. During **splicing reactions**, introns are removed and the exons connected to form the mature mRNA. In eukaryotes, tRNA and rRNA precursors are also modified and trimmed, although not as extensively as pre-mRNA.*

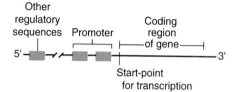

Fig. 14.1. Regions of a gene. A gene is a segment of DNA that functions as a unit to generate an RNA product or, through the processes of transcription and translation, a polypeptide chain. The transcribed region of a gene contains the template for synthesis of an RNA, which begins at the startpoint. A gene also includes regions of DNA that regulate production of the encoded product, such as a promoter region. In a structural gene, the transcribed region contains the coding sequences that dictate the amino acid sequence of a polypeptide chain.

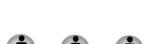

THE WAITING ROOM

Anne Niemick is a 4-year-old girl of Mediterranean ancestry whose height and body weight are below the 20th percentile for girls of her age. She is listless, tires easily, and complains of loss of appetite and shortness of breath on exertion. A dull pain has been present in her right upper quadrant for

237

The thalassemias are a heterogeneous group of hereditary anemias that constitute the most common gene disorder in the world, with a carrier rate of almost 7%. The disease was first discovered in countries around the Mediterranean Sea and was named for the Greek word "thalassa" meaning "sea". However, it is also present in areas extending into India and China that are near the equator.

The thalassemia syndromes are caused by mutations that decrease or abolish the synthesis of the α or β chains in the adult hemoglobin A tetramer. Individual syndromes are named according to the chain whose synthesis is affected and the severity of the deficiency. Thus, in β^0 thalassemia, the superscript 0 denotes none of the β chain is present; in β^+ thalassemia, the + denotes a partial reduction in the synthesis of the β chain. More than 170 different mutations have been identified that cause β thalassemia; most of these interfere with the transcription of β-globin mRNA or its processing or translation.

the last 3 months. Her complexion is slate-gray and she appears pale. Initial laboratory studies indicate a severe anemia (decreased red blood cell count) with a hemoglobin of 6.2 g/dL (reference range, 12–16). A battery of additional hematologic tests shows that Anne has β^+-thalassemia, intermediate type.

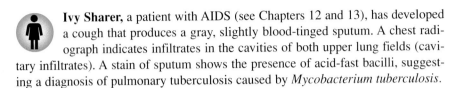

Ivy Sharer, a patient with AIDS (see Chapters 12 and 13), has developed a cough that produces a gray, slightly blood-tinged sputum. A chest radiograph indicates infiltrates in the cavities of both upper lung fields (cavitary infiltrates). A stain of sputum shows the presence of acid-fast bacilli, suggesting a diagnosis of pulmonary tuberculosis caused by *Mycobacterium tuberculosis.*

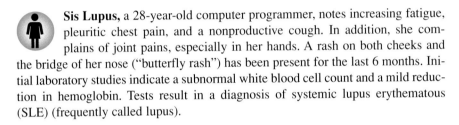

Amanda Tin picked mushrooms in a wooded area near her home. A few hours after eating one small mushroom, she experienced mild nausea and diarrhea. She brought a mushroom with her to the hospital emergency room. A poison expert identified it as *Amanita phalloides* (the "death cap"). These mushrooms contain the toxin α-amanitin.

Sis Lupus, a 28-year-old computer programmer, notes increasing fatigue, pleuritic chest pain, and a nonproductive cough. In addition, she complains of joint pains, especially in her hands. A rash on both cheeks and the bridge of her nose ("butterfly rash") has been present for the last 6 months. Initial laboratory studies indicate a subnormal white blood cell count and a mild reduction in hemoglobin. Tests result in a diagnosis of systemic lupus erythematous (SLE) (frequently called lupus).

I. ACTION OF RNA POLYMERASE

Transcription, the synthesis of RNA from a DNA template, is carried out by RNA polymerases (Fig. 14.2). Like DNA polymerases, RNA polymerases catalyze the formation of ester bonds between nucleotides that base-pair with the complementary nucleotides on the DNA template. Unlike DNA polymerases, RNA polymerases can initiate the synthesis of new chains in the absence of primers. They also lack the 3′ to 5′ exonuclease activity found in DNA polymerases. A strand of DNA serves as the template for RNA synthesis and is copied in the 3′ to 5′ direction. Synthesis of the new RNA molecule occurs in the 5′ to 3′ direction. The ribonucleoside triphosphates ATP, GTP, CTP, and UTP serve as the precursors. Each nucleotide base sequentially pairs with the complementary deoxyribonucleotide base on the DNA template (A, G, C, and U pair with T, C, G and A, respectively). The polymerase forms an ester bond between the α-phosphate on the ribose 5′-hydroxyl of the nucleotide precursor and the ribose 3′-hydroxyl at the end of the growing RNA chain. The cleavage of a high-energy phosphate bond in the nucleotide triphosphate and release of pyrophosphate (from the β and γ phosphates) provides the energy for this polymerization reaction. Subsequent cleavage of the pyrophosphate by a pyrophosphatase also helps to drive the polymerization reaction forward by removing a product.

RNA polymerases must be able to recognize the startpoint for transcription of each gene and the appropriate strand of DNA to use as a template. They also must be sensitive to signals that reflect the need for the gene product and control the frequency of transcription. A region of regulatory sequences called the promoter, usually contiguous with the transcribed region, controls the binding of RNA polymerase to DNA and identifies the startpoint (see Fig. 14.1). The frequency of transcription is controlled by regulatory sequences within the promoter, nearby the promoter (promoter-proximal elements), and by other regulatory sequences, such as enhancers, that may be located at considerable distances, sometimes thousands of nucleotides, from the startpoint. Both the promoter-proximal elements, and the enhancers interact with proteins that stabilize RNA polymerase binding to the promoter.

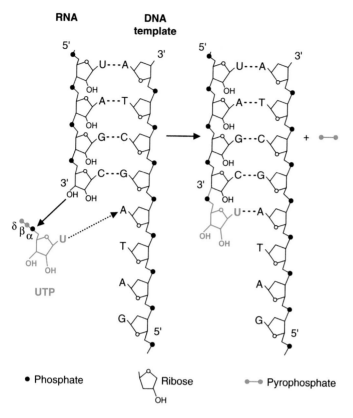

Fig. 14.2. RNA synthesis. The α-phosphate from the added nucleotide (shown in black) connects the ribosyl groups.

II. TYPES OF RNA POLYMERASES

Bacterial cells have a single RNA polymerase that transcribes DNA to generate all of the different types of RNA (mRNA, rRNA, and tRNA). The RNA polymerase of *Escherichia coli* contains four subunits ($\alpha_2\beta\beta'$), which form the core enzyme. Another protein called a σ (sigma) factor binds the core enzyme and directs binding of RNA polymerase to specific promoter regions of the DNA template. The σ factor dissociates shortly after transcription begins. *E. coli* has a number of different σ factors that recognize the promoter regions of different groups of genes. The major σ factor is σ^{70}, a designation related to its molecular weight of 70,000 Daltons.

In contrast to prokaryotes, eukaryotic cells have three RNA polymerases (Table 14.1). Polymerase I produces most of the rRNAs, polymerase II produces mRNA, and polymerase III produces small RNAs, such as tRNA and 5S rRNA. All of these RNA polymerases have the same mechanism of action. However, they recognize different types of promoters.

A. Sequences of Genes

Double-stranded DNA consists of a coding strand and a template strand (Fig. 14.3) The DNA template strand is the strand that is actually used by RNA polymerase during the process of transcription. It is complementary and antiparallel both to the coding (nontemplate) strand of the DNA and to the RNA transcript produced from the template. Thus, the coding strand of the DNA is identical in base sequence and direction to the RNA transcript, except, of course, that wherever this DNA strand contains a T, the RNA transcript contains a U. By convention, the

 Patients with acquired immune deficiency syndrome (AIDS) frequently develop tuberculosis. After **Ivy Sharer's** sputum stain suggested that she had tuberculosis, a multidrug antituberculous regimen, which includes an antibiotic of the rifamycin family (rifampin), was begun. A culture of her sputum was taken to confirm the diagnosis.

Rifampin inhibits bacterial RNA polymerase, selectively killing the bacteria that cause the infection. The nuclear RNA polymerase from eukaryotic cells is not affected. Although rifampin can inhibit the synthesis of mitochondrial RNA, the concentration required is considerably higher than that used for treatment of tuberculosis.

Table 14.1 Products of Eukaryotic RNA Polymerases

RNA polymerase I:	RNA
RNA polymerase II:	mRNA
RNA polymerase III:	tRNA + other small RNAs

The mushrooms picked by **Amanda Tin** contained α-amanitin, an inhibitor of eukaryotic RNA polymerases. It is particularly effective at blocking the action of RNA polymerase II. This toxin initially causes gastrointestinal disturbances, then electrolyte imbalance and fever, followed by liver and kidney dysfunction. Between 40 and 90% of the individuals who ingest α-amanitin die within a few days.

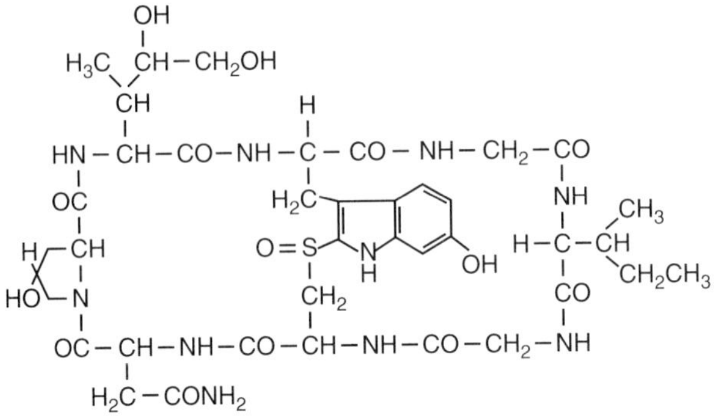

α–Amanitin

nucleotide sequence of a gene is represented by the letters of the nitrogenous bases of the coding strand of the DNA duplex. It is written from left to right in the 5′ to 3′ direction.

During translation, mRNA is read 5′ to 3′ in sets of three bases, called codons, that determine the amino acid sequence of the protein (see Fig. 14.3) Thus, the base sequence of the coding strand of the DNA can be used to determine the amino acid sequence of the protein. For this reason, when gene sequences are given, they refer to the coding strand.

A gene consists of the transcribed region and the regions that regulate transcription of the gene (e.g., promoter and enhancer regions)(Fig. 14.4). The base in the coding strand of the gene serving as the startpoint for transcription is numbered +1. This nucleotide corresponds to the first nucleotide incorporated into the RNA at the 5′-end of the transcript. Subsequent nucleotides within the transcribed region of the gene are numbered +2, +3, etc., toward the 3′-end of the gene. Untranscribed sequences to the left of the startpoint, known as the 5′-flanking region of the gene, are numbered −1, −2, −3, etc., starting with the nucleotide (−1) immediately to the left of the startpoint (+1) and moving from right to left. By analogy to a river, the sequences to the left of the startpoint are said to be upstream from the startpoint and those to the right are said to be downstream.

B. Recognition of Genes by RNA Polymerase

For genes to be expressed, RNA polymerase must recognize the appropriate point to start transcription and the strand of the DNA to transcribe (the template strand).

The two strands of DNA are antiparallel, with complementary nucleotides at each position. Thus, each strand would produce a different mRNA, resulting in different codons for amino acids and a different protein product. Therefore, it is critical that RNA polymerase transcribe the correct strand.

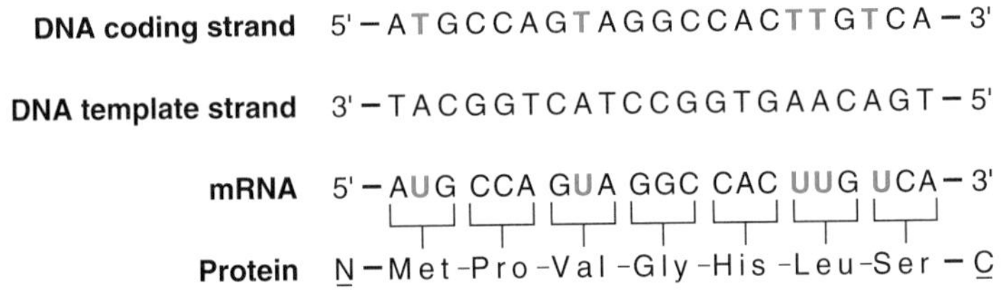

DNA coding strand   5′ − A T G C C A G T A G G C C A C T T G T C A − 3′

DNA template strand   3′ − T A C G G T C A T C C G G T G A A C A G T − 5′

mRNA   5′ − AUG CCA GUA GGC CAC UUG UCA − 3′

Protein   N − Met − Pro − Val − Gly − His − Leu − Ser − C

Fig. 14.3. Relationship between the coding strand of DNA, the DNA template strand, the mRNA transcript, and the protein produced from the gene. The bases in mRNA are used in sets of three (called codons) to specify the order of the amino acids inserted into the growing polypeptide chain during the process of translation (see Chapter 15).

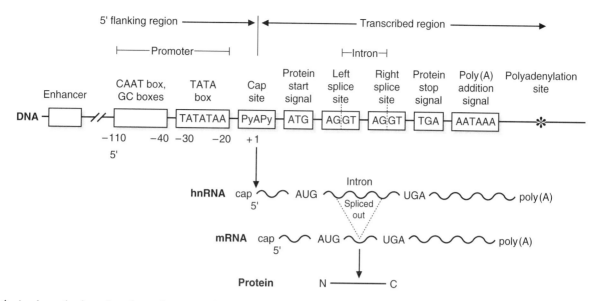

Fig. 14.4. A schematic view of a eukaryotic gene, and steps required to produce a protein product. The gene consists of promoter and transcribed regions. The transcribed region contains introns, which do not contain coding sequence for proteins, and exons, which do carry the coding sequences for proteins. The first RNA form produced is heterogenous nuclear RNA (hn RNA), which contains both intronic and exonic sequences. The hnRNA is modified such that a cap is added at the 5′ end (cap site), and a poly-A tail added to the 3′ end. The introns are removed (a process called splicing) to produce the mature mRNA, which leaves the nucleus to direct protein synthesis in the cytoplasm. Py is pyrimidine (C or T).

RNA polymerase also must recognize which genes to transcribe because transcribed genes are only a small fraction of the total DNA. The genes that are transcribed differ from one type of cell to another and change with changes in physiologic conditions. The signals in DNA that RNA polymerase recognizes are called promoters. Promoters are sequences in DNA (often composed of smaller sequences called boxes or elements) that determine the startpoint and the frequency of transcription. Because they are located on the same molecule of DNA and near the gene they regulate, they are said to be *cis* acting (i.e., "cis" refers to acting on the same side). Proteins that bind to these DNA sequences and facilitate or prevent the binding of RNA polymerase are said to be *trans* acting.

C. Promoter Regions of Genes for mRNA

The binding of RNA polymerase and the subsequent initiation of gene transcription involves a number of consensus sequences in the promoter regions of the gene (Fig. 14.5). A consensus sequence is the sequence most commonly found in a given region when many genes are examined. In both prokaryotes and eukaryotes, an adenine- and thymine-rich consensus sequence in the promoter determines the startpoint of transcription by binding proteins that facilitate the binding of RNA polymerase. In the prokaryote *E. coli*, this consensus sequence is TATAAT, which is known as the TATA or Pribnow box. It is centered about −10 and is recognized by the sigma factor σ^{70}. A similar sequence in the −25 region of eukaryotic genes has a consensus sequence of TATA(A/T)A. (The (A/T) in the fifth position indicates that either A or T occurs with equal frequency.) This eukaryotic sequence is also known as a TATA box, but is sometimes named the Hogness or Hogness-Goldberg box after its discoverers. Other consensus sequences involved in binding of RNA polymerase are found further upstream in the promoter region (see Fig. 14.5). Bacterial promoters contain a sequence TTGACA in the −35 region. Eukaryotes frequently have CAAT boxes and GC-rich sequences in the region between −40 and −110. Eukaryotic genes also contain promoter-proximal elements (in the region of −100

 Anne Niemick has a β⁺ thalassemia classified clinically as β-thalassemia intermedia. She produces an intermediate amount of functional β globin chains (her hemoglobin is 6.2 g/dL; normal is 12–16). β-thalassemia intermedia is usually the result of two different mutations (one that mildly affects the rate of synthesis of β-globin and one severely affecting its rate of synthesis), or, less frequently, homozygosity for a mild mutation in the rate of synthesis, or a complex combination of mutations. For example, mutations within the promoter region of the β-globin gene could result in a significantly decreased rate of β-globin synthesis in an individual who is homozygous for the allele, without completely abolishing synthesis of the protein.

Two of the point mutations that result in a β⁺ phenotype are within the TATA box (A→ G or A→ C in the −28 to −31 region). These mutations reduce the accuracy of the startpoint of transcription so that only 20 to 25% of the normal amount of β-globin is synthesized. Other mutations that also reduce the frequency of β-globin transcription have been observed further upstream in the promoter region (−87 C→ G and −88 C→T).

Prokaryotic promoters

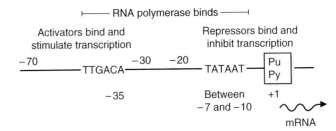

Eukaryotic promoters

Fig. 14.5. Prokaryotic and eukaryotic promoters. The promoter-proximal region contains binding sites for transcription factors which that can accelerate the rate at which RNA polymerase binds to the promoter. Pu = purine; Py = pyrimidine.

Q: What property of an AT-rich region of a DNA double helix makes it suitable to serve as a recognition site for the startpoint of transcription?

to –200), which are sites that bind other gene regulatory proteins. Genes vary in the number of such sequences present.

In bacteria, a number of protein-producing genes may be linked together and controlled by a single promoter. This genetic unit is called an operon (Fig. 14.6). Proteins bind to the promoter and either inhibit or facilitate transcription of the operon. Repressors are proteins that bind to a region in the promoter known as the operator and inhibit transcription by preventing the binding of RNA polymerase to DNA. Activators are proteins that stimulate transcription by binding within the –35 region or upstream from it, facilitating the binding of RNA polymerase. (Operons are described in more detail in Chapter 16.)

In eukaryotes, proteins known as general transcription factors (or basal factors) bind to the TATA box and facilitate the binding of RNA polymerase II, the polymerase that transcribes mRNA (Fig. 14.7). This binding process involves at least six basal transcription factors (labeled as TFIIs, transcription factors for RNA polymerase II). The TATA-binding protein (TBP), which is a component of TFIID, initially binds to the TATA box. TFIID consists of both the TBP and a number of transcriptional coactivators. TFIIA and TFIIB interact with TBP. RNA polymerase II binds to the complex of transcription factors and to DNA, and is aligned at the startpoint for transcription. TFIIE, TFIIF, and TFIIH subsequently bind, cleaving adenosine triphosphate (ATP), and transcription of the gene is initiated.

With only these transcription (or basal) factors and RNA polymerase II attached (the basal transcription complex), the gene is transcribed at a low or basal rate.

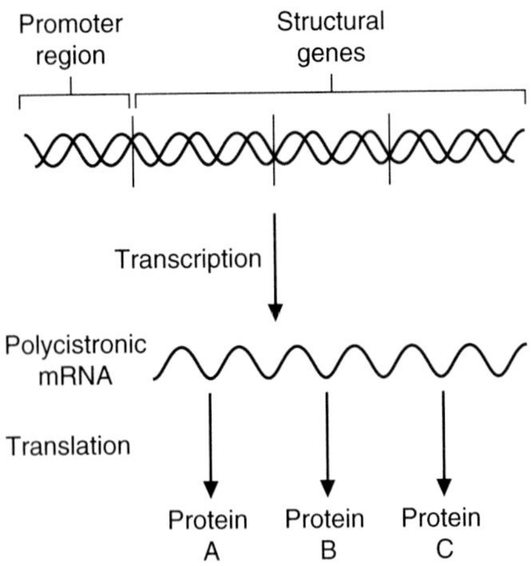

Fig. 14.6. Bacterial operon. A cistron encodes a single polypeptide chain. In bacteria, a single promoter may control transcription of an operon containing many cistrons. A single polycistronic mRNA is transcribed. Its translation produces a number of polypeptide chains.

TFIIH plays a number of roles in both transcription and DNA repair. In both processes, it acts as an ATP-dependent DNA helicase, unwinding DNA for either transcription or repair to occur. Two of the forms of xeroderma pigmentosum (XPB and XPD; see Chapter 13) arise from mutations within two different helicase subunits of TFIIH. TFIIH also contains a kinase activity, and RNA polymerase II is phosphorylated by this factor during certain phases of transcription.

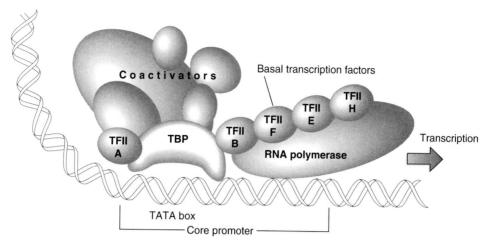

Fig. 14.7. Transcription apparatus. The TATA-binding protein (TBP), a component of TFIID, binds to the TATA box. Transcription factors TFII A and B bind to TBP. RNA polymerase binds, then TFII E, F, and H bind. This complex can transcribe at a basal level. Some coactivator proteins are present as a component of TFIID, and these can bind to other regulatory DNA binding proteins (called specific transcription factors or transcriptional activators).

The rate of transcription can be further increased by binding of other regulatory DNA binding proteins to additional gene regulatory sequences (such as the promoter proximal or enhancer regions). These regulatory DNA binding proteins are called gene-specific transcription factors (or transactivators) because they are specific to the gene involved (see Chapter 16). They interact with coactivators in the basal transcription complex.

III. TRANSCRIPTION OF BACTERIAL GENES

In bacteria, binding of RNA polymerase with a σ factor to the promoter region of DNA causes the two DNA strands to unwind and separate within a region approximately 10 to 20 nucleotides in length. As the polymerase transcribes the DNA, the untranscribed region of the helix continues to separate, whereas the transcribed region of the DNA template rejoins its DNA partner (Fig. 14.8). The sigma factor is released when the growing RNA chain is approximately 10 nucleotides long. The elongation reactions continue until the RNA polymerase encounters a transcription termination signal. One type of termination signal involves the formation of a hairpin loop in the transcript, preceding a number of U residues. The second type of

A: In regions in which DNA is being transcribed, the two strands of the DNA must be separated. AT base pairs in DNA are joined by only two hydrogen bonds, whereas GC pairs have three hydrogen bonds. Therefore, in AT-rich regions of DNA, the two strands can be separated more readily than in regions that contain GC base pairs.

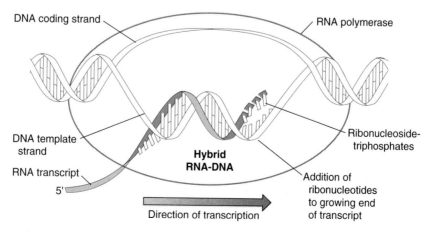

Fig. 14.8. Mechanism of transcription.

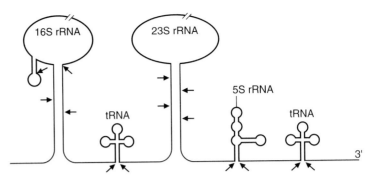

Fig. 14.9. Bacterial rRNA and tRNA transcripts. One large precursor is cleaved (at arrows) to produce 16S, 23S, and 5S rRNA and some tRNAs.

mechanism for termination involves the binding of a protein, the rho factor, which causes release of the RNA transcript from the template. The signal for both termination processes is the sequence of bases in the newly synthesized RNA.

A cistron is a region of DNA that encodes a single polypeptide chain. In bacteria, mRNA is usually generated from an operon as a polycistronic transcript (one that contains the information to produce a number of different proteins). The polycistronic transcript is translated as it is being transcribed. This transcript is not modified and trimmed, and it does not contain introns (regions within the coding sequence of a transcript that are removed before translation occurs). Several different proteins are produced during translation of the polycistronic transcript, one from each cistron (see Fig. 14.6).

In prokaryotes, rRNA is produced as a single, long transcript that is cleaved to produce the 16S, 23S, and 5S ribosomal RNAs. tRNA is also cleaved from larger transcripts (Fig. 14.9). One of the cleavage enzymes, RNase P, is a protein containing an RNA molecule. This RNA actually catalyzes the cleavage reaction.

IV. TRANSCRIPTION OF EUKARYOTIC GENES

The process of transcription in eukaryotes is similar to that in prokaryotes. RNA polymerase binds to the transcription factor complex in the promoter region and to the DNA, the helix unwinds within a region near the startpoint of transcription, DNA strand separation occurs, synthesis of the RNA transcript is initiated, and the RNA transcript is elongated, copying the DNA template. The DNA strands separate as the polymerase approaches and rejoin as the polymerase passes.

One of the major differences between eukaryotes and prokaryotes is that eukaryotes have more elaborate mechanisms for processing the transcripts, particularly the precursors of mRNA (pre-mRNA). Eukaryotes also have three polymerases, rather than just the one present in prokaryotes. Other differences include the facts that eukaryotic mRNA usually contains the coding information for only one polypeptide chain and that eukaryotic RNA is transcribed in the nucleus and migrates to the cytoplasm where translation occurs.

A. Synthesis of Eukaryotic mRNA

In eukaryotes, extensive processing of the primary transcript occurs before the mature mRNA is formed and can migrate to the cytosol, where it is translated into a protein product. RNA polymerase II synthesizes a large primary transcript from the template strand that is capped at the 5′ end as it is transcribed (Fig. 14.10). The transcript also rapidly acquires a poly(A) tail at the 3′ end. Pre-mRNAs thus contain untranslated regions at both the 5′ and 3′ ends (the leader and trailing sequences, respectively). These untranslated regions are retained in the mature

Although each eukaryotic mRNA only codes for one polypeptide chain, a number of proteins can contain different polypeptide chains or have multiple active sites, allowing the protein to catalyze more than one reaction.

The terms hnRNA (heterogeneous nuclear RNA) and pre-mRNA are both used to denote mRNA precursors. The term hnRNA was originally applied to a pool of RNA molecules in the nucleus that were rapidly synthesized and varied greatly in size. These RNA molecules are now known to be the mRNA precursors that vary greatly in size because they contain exons that encode different sizes of polypeptide chains and introns that vary in amount and size.

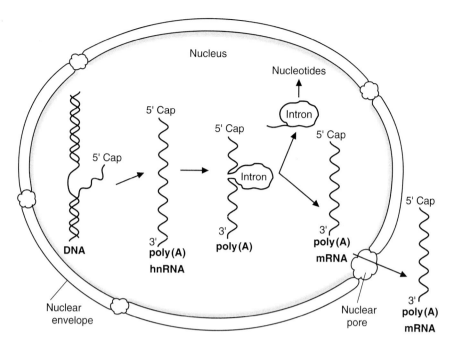

Fig. 14.10. Overview of mRNA synthesis. Transcription produces hnRNA from the DNA template. hnRNA processing involves addition of a 5′-cap and a poly(A) tail and splicing to join exons and remove introns. The product, mRNA, migrates to the cytoplasm, where it will direct protein synthesis.

mRNA. The coding region of the pre-mRNA, which begins with the start codon for protein synthesis and ends with the stop codon, contains both exons and introns. Exons consist of the nucleotide codons that dictate the amino acid sequence of the eventual protein product. Between the exons, interspersing regions called introns contain nucleotide sequences that are removed by splicing reactions to form the mature RNA. The mature RNA thus contains a leader sequence (that includes the cap), a coding region comprising exons, and a tailing sequence that includes the poly(A) tail.

This mature mRNA complexes with the poly(A) binding protein and other proteins. It travels through pores in the nuclear envelope into the cytoplasm. There it combines with ribosomes and directs the incorporation of amino acids into proteins.

1. TRANSCRIPTION AND CAPPING OF mRNA

"Capping" of the primary transcript synthesized by RNA polymerase II occurs at its 5′-end as it is being transcribed (Fig.14.11). The 5′- terminal, the initial nucleotide of the transcript, is a pyrimidine with three phosphate groups attached to the 5′- hydroxyl of the ribose. To form the cap, the terminal triphosphate loses one phosphate, forming a 5′-diphosphate. The β-phosphate of the diphosphate then attacks the α-phosphate of GTP, liberating pyrophosphate, and forming an unusual 5′ to 5′ triphosphate linkage. A methyl group is transferred from S-adenosylmethionine (SAM), a universal methyl donor, to position 7 of the added guanine ring. Methylation also occurs on the ribose 2′-hydroxyl group in the terminal nucleotide to which the cap is attached, and sometimes the 2′-hydroxyl group of the adjacent nucleotide ribose. This cap "seals" the 5′ end of the primary transcript and decreases the rate of degradation. It also serves as a recognition site for the binding of the mature mRNA to a ribosome at the initiation of protein synthesis.

Once SAM (S-adenosylmethionine) donates its methyl group, it must be regenerated by reactions that require the vitamins folate and B_{12}. Thus formation of mRNA is also one of the processes affected by a deficiency of these vitamins.

There are three different types of methyl caps, shown in blue: CAP0 refers to the methylated guanosine (on the nitrogen at the seven position, N^7) added in the 5′ to 5′ linkage to the mRNA; CAP1 refers to CAP0 with the addition of a methyl to the 22′ carbon of ribose on the nucleotide (N_1) at the 5′ end of the chain; and CAP2 refers to CAP1 with the addition of another 2′ methyl group to the next nucleotide (N_2). The methyl groups are donated by S-adenosylmethionine (SAM).

$$CH_3 (n^7) \quad \boxed{CAP\ 0}$$
$$G - 5' - P\ P\ P - 5' - N_1\ N_2\ N_3 - - - - CAP\ 0$$
$$\downarrow (CH_3)\text{-SAM}$$
$$\boxed{CAP\ 1}$$
$$CH_3 (n^7) \downarrow \qquad CH_3$$
$$G - 5' - P\ P\ P - 5' - N_1 - N_2\ N_3 - - - - CAP\ 1$$
$$\downarrow (CH_3)\text{-SAM}$$
$$\boxed{CAP\ 2}$$
$$CH_3 (n^7) \qquad CH_3\ CH_3$$
$$G - 5' - P\ P\ P - 5' - N_1 - N_2 - N_3 - - - - CAP\ 2$$

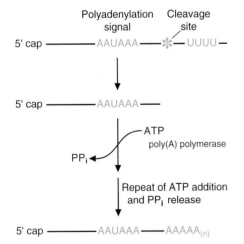

Fig. 14.11. The cap structure in eukaryotic mRNA. The phosphates in blue originated from the original RNA transcript; the phosphate in black comes from GTP.

2. ADDITION OF A POLY(A) TAIL

After the RNA polymerase transcribes the stop codon for protein translation, it passes a sequence called the polyadenylation signal (AAUAAA) (Fig. 14.12). It continues past the polyadenylation signal until it reaches an unknown, and possibly unspecific, termination signal many nucleotides later. However, as the primary transcript is released from the RNA polymerase elongation complex, an enzyme complex binds to the polyadenylation signal and cleaves the primary transcript approximately 10 to 20 nucleotides downstream, thereby forming the 3′ end. After this cleavage, a poly(A) tail that can be over 200 nucleotides in length is added to the 3′-end. Thus, there is no poly(dT) sequence in the DNA template that corresponds to this tail; it is added posttranscriptionally. ATP serves as the precursor for the sequential addition of the adenine nucleotides. They are added one at a time, with poly(A) polymerase catalyzing each addition. The poly(A) tail is a protein binding site that protects the mRNA from degradation.

Fig. 14.12. Synthesis of the poly(A) tail. As RNA polymerase continues to transcribe the DNA, enzymes cleave the transcript (hnRNA) at a point 10–20 nucleotides beyond an AAUAAA sequence, just before a run of Us (or Gs). Approximately 250 adenine nucleotides are then added to the 3′-end of the hnRNA, one at a time, by poly(A) polymerase.

Within a few days of initiation of treatment for tuberculosis, laboratory staining results of **Ivy Sharer's** sputum confirmed the diagnosis of pulmonary tuberculosis caused by *M. tuberculosis*. Therefore, the multidrug therapy, which included the antibiotic rifampin, was continued. Rifampin binds to the RNA polymerases of several bacteria. *M. tuberculosis* rapidly develops resistance to rifampin through mutations that result in an RNA polymerase that cannot bind the complex structure. Simultaneous treatment with a drug that works through a different mechanism decreases the selective advantage of the mutation and the rate at which resistance develops.

The presence of a poly (A) tail on eukaryotic mRNA allows this form of RNA to be easily separated from the more abundant rRNA. After extracting all of the RNA from a cell, the total RNA is applied to a column of beads to which oligo-dT has been covalently attached. As the mRNA flows through the column, its poly (A) tail will base pair with the oligo-dT, and the mRNA will become bound to the column. All other types of RNA will flow through the column and not bind to the beads. The bound mRNA can then be eluted from the column by changing the ionic strength of the buffer.

3. REMOVAL OF INTRONS

Eukaryotic pre-mRNA transcripts contain regions known as exons and introns. Exons appear in the mature mRNA; introns are removed from the transcript and are not found in the mature mRNA (see Fig. 14.10). Introns, therefore, do not contribute to the amino acid sequence of the protein. Some genes contain 50 or more introns. These introns are carefully removed from the pre-mRNA transcript and the exons spliced together, so that the appropriate protein is produced from the gene.

The consensus sequences at the intron/exon boundaries of the pre-mRNA are AGGU (AGGT in the DNA). The sequences vary to some extent on the exon side of the boundaries, but almost all introns begin with a 5' GU and end with a 3' AG (Fig. 14.13). These intron sequences at the left splice site and the right splice site are, therefore, invariant. Because every 5' GU and 3' AG combination does not result in a functional splice site, clearly other features within the exon or intron help to define the appropriate splice sites. These features, which are currently being identified, involve the presence of positive- and negative-acting *cis*-regulatory sequences within the intron.

A complex structure known as a spliceosome ensures that exons are spliced together with great accuracy (Fig. 14.14). Small nuclear ribonucleoproteins

⊢Exon─┼──Intron──┼─Exon⊣

hnRNA 5' cap ──── AG⸬GU⸬──── ⸬AG⸬G(U) ── 3'

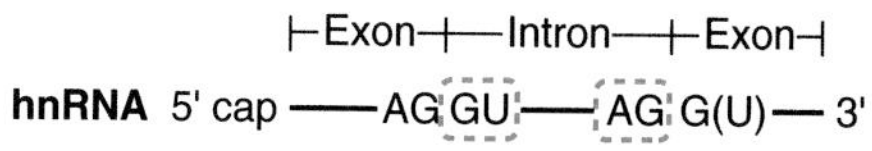

Fig. 14.13. Splice junctions in hnRNA. The intron sequences shown in blue dashed boxes are invariant. They always appear at this position in introns. The sequences on the exon side of the splice sites are more variable.

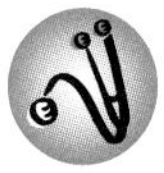

Anne Niemick has β⁺-thalassemia (enough of the β-chain is produced to maintain blood hemoglobin levels above 6.0 g/dL). One mutation resulting in β⁺-thalassemia is a point mutation (AATAAA → AACAAA) that changes the sequence in hnRNA at the polyadenylation signal site from AAUAAA to AACAAA. Homozygous individuals with this mutation produce only one-tenth the amount of normal β-globin mRNA.

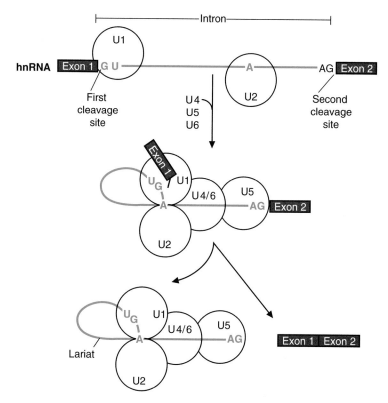

Fig. 14.14. Splicing process. Nuclear ribonucleoproteins (snurps U_1 to U_6) bind to the intron, causing it to form a loop. The complex is called a splicesosome. The U1 snurp binds near the first exon/intron junction, and U2 binds within the intron in a region containing an adenine nucleotide residue. Another group of snurps, U4, U5, and U6, binds to the complex, and the loop is formed. The phosphate attached to the G residue at the 5'-end of the intron forms a 2'–5' linkage with the 2'-hydroxyl group of the adenine nucleotide residue. Cleavage occurs at the end of the first exon, between the AG residues at the 3' end of the exon and the GU residues at the 5' end of the intron. The complex continues to be held in place by the spliceosome. A second cleavage occurs at the 3'-end of the intron after the AG sequence. The exons are joined together. The intron, shaped like a lariat, is released and degraded to nucleotides.

Some types of β^0-thalassemia (little or none of the hemoglobin β chain produced) are caused by homozygous mutations in the splice junction sequences at intron/exon boundaries. In some individuals, an AT replaces a GT in the gene at the 5' end of the first or second intron. Mutations also occur within the splice junction sequences at the 3'-end of introns (GT at the donor site 5'-end and AG at the acceptor site 3'-end). Mutations at either site totally abolish normal splicing and result in β^0 thalassemia.

(snRNPs), called "snurps," are involved in formation of the spliceosome. Because snurps are rich in uracil, they are identified by numbers preceded by a U.

Exons frequently code for separate functional or structural domains of proteins. Proteins with similar functional regions (e.g., ATP or NAD binding regions) frequently have similar domains, although their overall structure and amino acid sequence is quite different. A process known as exon shuffling has probably occurred throughout evolution, allowing new proteins to develop with functions similar to those of other proteins.

B. Synthesis of Eukaryotic rRNA

Ribosomal RNAs (rRNAs) form the ribonucleoprotein complexes on which protein synthesis occurs. In eukaryotes, the rRNA gene exists as many copies in the nucleolar organizer region of the nucleus (Fig. 14.15, circle 1). Each gene produces a large, 45S transcript that is cleaved to produce the 18S, 28S, and 5.8S rRNAs. Approximately 1,000 copies of this gene are present in the human genome. The genes are linked in tan-

Systemic lupus erythematous is an autoimmune disease characterized by a particular spectrum of autoantibodies against many cellular components, including chromatin, ribonucleoprotein, and cell membrane phospholipids. In this disorder, the body makes these antibodies against its own components. snRNPs are one of the targets of these antibodies. In fact, snRNPs were discovered as a result of studies using antibodies obtained from patients with SLE.

Tests were performed on **Sis Lupus's** blood to detect elevated levels of antinuclear antibodies (including antibodies to DNA, antibodies to histone, antibodies to ribonucleoproteins, and antibodies to nuclear antigens). The tests were strongly positive and, in conjunction with her symptoms, led to a diagnosis of systemic lupus erythematosus (SLE).

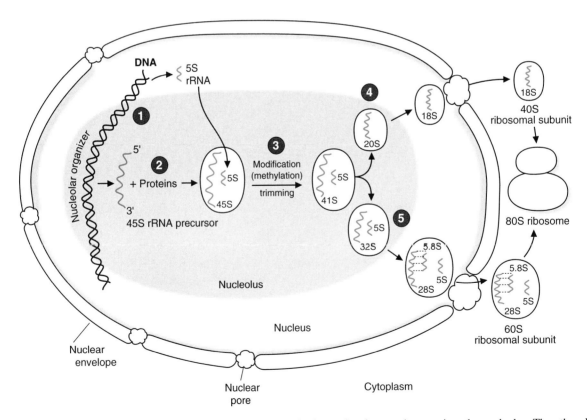

Fig. 14.15. rRNA and ribosome synthesis. The 5S rRNA is transcribed in the nucleoplasm and moves into the nucleolus. The other rRNAs are transcribed from DNA and mature in the nucleolus, forming the 40S and 60S ribosomal subunits, which migrate to the cytoplasm.

dem, separated by spacer regions that contain the termination signal for one gene and the promoter for the next. Promoters for rRNA genes are located in the 5′-flanking region of the genes and extend into the region surrounding the startpoint. rRNA genes caught in the act of transcription by electron micrographs show that many RNA polymerase I molecules can be attached to a gene at any given time, all moving toward the 3′ end as the 45S rRNA precursors are synthesized.

As the 45S rRNA precursors are released from the DNA, they complex with proteins, forming ribonucleoprotein particles that generate the granular regions of the nucleolus (see Fig. 14.15, circle 2). Processing of the transcript occurs in the granular regions. 5S rRNA, produced by RNA polymerase III from genes located outside the nucleolus in the nucleoplasm, migrates into the nucleolus and joins the ribonucleoprotein particles.

One to two percent of the nucleotides of the 45S precursor become methylated, primarily on the 2′-hydroxyl groups of ribose moieties (see Fig. 14.15, circle 3). These methyl groups may serve as markers for cleavage of the 45S precursors and are conserved in the mature rRNA. A series of cleavages in the 45S transcripts occur to produce the mature rRNAs (Fig. 14.16).

In the production of cytoplasmic ribosomes in human cells, one portion of the 45S rRNA precursor becomes the 18S rRNA that, complexed with proteins, forms the small 40S ribosomal subunit (Fig. 14.15, circle 4). Another segment of the precursor folds back on itself and is cleaved, forming 28S rRNA, hydrogen-bonded to the 5.8S rRNA. The 5S rRNA, transcribed from nonnucleolar genes, and a number of proteins complex with the 28S and 5.8S rRNAs to form the 60S ribosomal subunit (Fig. 14.15, circle 5). The ribosomal subunits migrate through the nuclear pores. In the cytoplasm, the 40S and 60S ribosomal subunits interact with mRNA, forming the 80S ribosomes on which protein synthesis occurs.

C. Synthesis of Eukaryotic tRNA

A transfer RNA has one binding site for a specific sequence of three nucleotides in mRNA (the anticodon site) and another binding site for the encoded amino acid. tRNAs thus ensure that the genetic code is translated into the correct sequence of

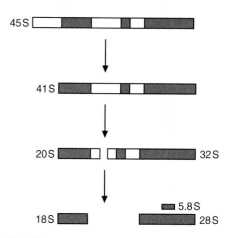

Fig. 14.16 Maturation of the 45S rRNA precursor. The clear regions are removed, and the shaded regions become the mature rRNAs. (The 5S rRNA is not produced from this precursor.)

 Some rRNA precursors contain introns within the regions that become the mature rRNAs. These introns are removed by the rRNA precursors themselves, which undergo self-splicing reactions. The rRNA precursors that catalyze their own splicing are known as ribozymes (see Chapter 12, III.A).

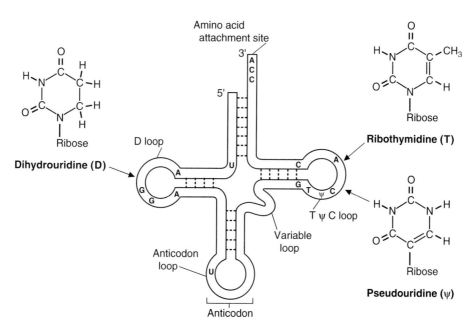

Fig. 14.17. The tRNA cloverleaf. Bases that commonly occur in a particular position are indicated by letters. Base-pairing in stem regions is indicated by lines between the strands. The locations of the modified bases dihydrouridine (D), ribothymidine (T), and pseudouridine (Ψ) are indicated.

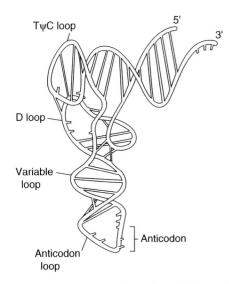

Fig. 14.18. The three-dimensional folding of tRNA. (Reprinted with permission from Kim SH, et al. Science 1974;185:436. Copyright 1974 American Association for the Advancement of Science.)

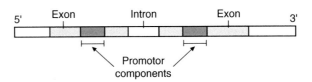

Fig. 14.19. Promoter for tRNA transcription. The segments of the genes from which the mature tRNA is produced are indicated by the light blue color. The two regions of the promoter lie within these segments, and are indicated by the dark blue color.

amino acids. At least 20 types of tRNAs occur in cells, one for every amino acid that is incorporated into growing polypeptide chains during the synthesis of proteins. tRNAs have a cloverleaf structure that folds into a three-dimensional L shape, and contains a number of bases that are modified posttranscriptionally (Fig. 14.17). The loop closest to the 5'-end is known as the D-loop because it contains dihydrouridine (D). The second, or anticodon, loop contains the trinucleotide anticodon that base-pairs with the codon on mRNA. The third loop (the TΨC loop) contains both ribothymidine (T) and pseudouridine (Ψ). A fourth loop, known as the variable loop because it varies in size, is frequently found between the anticodon and TΨC loops. Base-pairing occurs in the stem regions of tRNA, and a three-nucleotide sequence (e.g., CCA) at the 3'-end is the attachment site for the specific amino acid carried by each tRNA. Different tRNAs bind different amino acids. The three-dimensional structure of tRNA has been determined and is shown in Figure 14.18. tRNA is produced by RNA polymerase III, which recognizes a split promoter within the transcribed region of the gene (Fig. 14.19). One segment of the promoter is located between +8 and +19. A second segment is 30 to 60 base pairs downstream from the first.

tRNA precursors of approximately 100 nucleotides in length are generated. (Fig. 14.20, circle 1). The pre-tRNA assumes a cloverleaf shape and is subsequently cleaved at the 5'- and 3'-ends (see Fig. 14.20, circle 2). The enzyme that acts at the

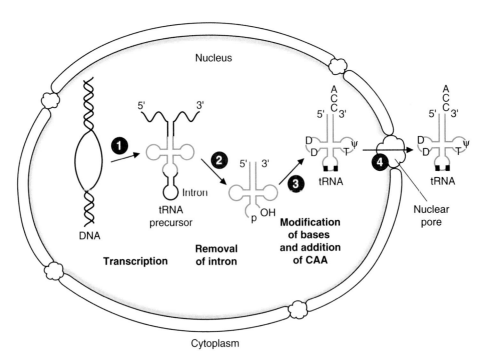

Fig. 14.20. Overview of tRNA synthesis. D, T, Ψ, and ■ indicate modified bases. D = dihydrouracil, T = ribothymine, ψ = pseudouridine, ■ = other modified bases

5'-end is RNase P, similar to the RNase P of bacteria. Both enzymes contain a small RNA (M1) that has catalytic activity and serves as an endonuclease. Some tRNA precursors contain introns that are removed by endonucleases. To close the opening, a 2'- or 3'-phosphate group from one end is ligated to a 5'-hydroxyl on the other end by an RNA ligase.

The bases are modified at the same time the endonucleolytic cleavage reactions are occurring (see Fig. 14.20, circle 3). Three modifications occur in most tRNAs: (1) Uracil is methylated by *S*-adenosylmethionine (SAM) to form thymine; (2) one of the double bonds of uracil is reduced to form dihydrouracil;, and (3) a uracil residue (attached to ribose by an *N*-glycosidic bond) is rotated to form pseudouridine, which contains uracil linked to ribose by a carbon–carbon bond. (see Fig. 14.17). Other, less common but more complex, modifications also occur and involve bases other than uracil. Of particular note is the deamination of adenosine to form the base inosine.

The final step in forming the mature tRNA is the addition of a CCA sequence at its 3'-end (see Fig 14.20, circle 4). These nucleotides are added one at a time by nucleotidyltransferase. The tRNA then migrates to the cytoplasm. The terminal adenosine at the 3'-end is the site at which the specific amino acid for each tRNA is bound and activated for incorporation into a protein.

V. DIFFERENCES IN SIZE BETWEEN EUKARYOTIC AND PROKARYOTIC DNA

A. Human Cells Are Diploid

Except for the germ cells, most normal human cells are diploid. Therefore, they contain two copies of each chromosome, and each chromosome contains genes that are alleles of the genes on the homologous chromosome. Because one chromosome in each set of homologous chromosomes is obtained from each parent, the alleles can be identical, containing the same DNA sequence, or they can differ. A diploid human cell contains 2,000 times more DNA than the genome of the bacterium in the haploid *E. coli* cell (approximately 4×10^6 base pairs).

B. Human Genes Contain Introns

Eukaryotic introns contribute to the DNA size difference between bacteria and human cells. In eukaryotic genes, introns (noncoding regions) occur within sequences that code for proteins. Consequently, the primary transcript (heterogeneous nuclear RNA or hnRNA) averages roughly 10 times longer than the mature mRNA produced by removal of the introns. In contrast, bacterial genes do not contain introns.

C. Repetitive Sequences in Eukaryotic DNA

Although diploidy and introns account for some of the difference between the DNA content of humans and bacteria, a large difference remains that is related to the greater complexity of the human organism. Bacterial cells have a single copy of each gene, called unique DNA, and they contain very little DNA that does not produce functional products. Eukaryotic cells contain substantial amounts of DNA that does not code for functional products (i.e., proteins or rRNA and tRNA). In addition, some genes that encode functional products are present in multiple copies,

The removal of introns in pre-tRNA has been most extensively studied in yeast. The intron, less than 20 nucleotides long, is located within the anticodon loop at the 3'-end. Removal of the intron by endonucleases leaves the two halves of the tRNA, which remain held together by hydrogen bonds between base pairs in the stem regions. The opening is closed by an RNA ligase.

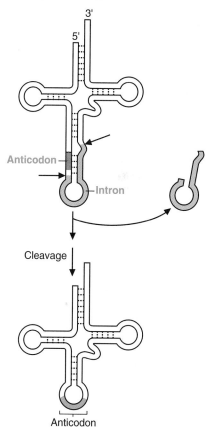

Calculate the number of different proteins, 300 amino acids in length, which could be produced from the *E. coli* genome (4×10^6 base pairs of DNA).

A number of differences between eukaryotes and prokaryotes affect the processes of replication, transcription, and translation, in addition to the content of their DNA. Eukaryotic DNA is complexed with histones, and prokaryotic DNA is not. In eukaryotic cells, the process of transcription, which occurs in the nucleus, is separated by the nuclear envelope from the process of translation (protein synthesis from the mRNA template), which occurs in the cytoplasm. Because prokaryotes lack nuclei, the processes of transcription and translation occur simultaneously. Transcription of bacterial DNA requires only one promoter per operon. In contrast, human DNA requires one promoter for each gene.

Complexity may explain some of the differences between the DNA content of bacteria and humans. But an extension of this line of reasoning would lead to the conclusion that frogs are more complex than humans, because frogs have 8 feet of DNA per diploid nucleus compared to the 6 feet in a human cell. Logic, or perhaps vanity, suggests that the amount of DNA per cell does not necessarily reflect the complexity of the organism. One of the features of frog DNA that may explain its length is that frogs have more repetitive DNA than humans. More than 75% of the frog genome is in the moderately and highly repetitive category, whereas only about 35% of the human genome is repetitive.

 Four million base pairs contain $4 \times 10^6/3$ or 1.33 million codons. If each protein contained approximately 300 amino acids, *E. coli* could produce about 4,000 different proteins ($1.33 \times 10^6/300$).

called highly repetitive or moderately repetitive DNA. Approximately 64% of the DNA in the human genome is unique, consisting of DNA sequences present in one or a very few copies in the genome (Fig. 14.21). Unique DNA sequences are transcribed to generate mRNA, which is translated to produce proteins.

Highly repetitive DNA consists of sequences approximately 6 to- 100 base pairs in length that are present in hundreds of thousands to millions of copies, clustered within a few locations in the genome (see Fig. 14.21). It occurs in centromeres (which join sister chromatids during mitosis) and in telomeres (the ends of chromosomes). This DNA represents approximately 10% of the human genome. It is not transcribed.

Moderately repetitive DNA is present in a few to tens of thousands of copies in the genome (see Fig. 14.21). This fraction constitutes approximately 25% of the human genome. It contains DNA that is functional and transcribed to produce rRNA, tRNA, and also some mRNA. The histone genes, present in a few hundred copies in the genome, belong to this class. Moderately repetitive DNA also includes some gene sequences that are functional but not transcribed. Promoters and enhancers (which are involved in regulating gene expression) are examples of gene sequences in this category. Other groups of moderately repetitive gene sequences that have been found in the human are called the Alu sequences (approximately 300 base pairs in length). Alu

 Alu sequences in DNA were named for the enzyme Alu (obtained from **A**rthrobacter **lu**teus), that which is able to cleave them. Alu sequences make up 6 to 8% of the human genome. In some cases of familial hypercholesterolemia, homologous recombination is believed to have occurred between two Alu repeats, resulting in a large deletion in the low- density lipoprotein (LDL) receptor gene. The LDL receptor mediates uptake of the cholesterol-containing LDL particle into many cell types and, in the absence of functional LDL receptors, blood cholesterol levels are elevated. Patients who are homozygous for this mutation may die from of cardiac disease as early as in their second or third decade of life.

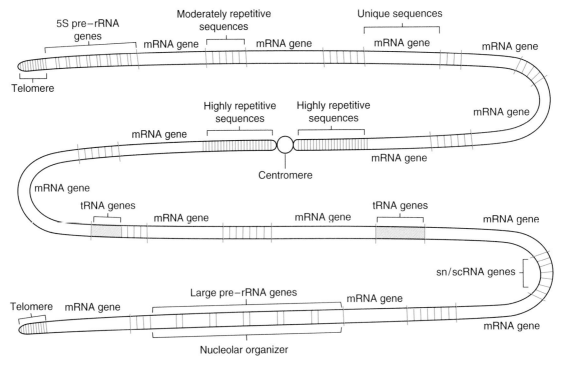

Fig. 14.21. Distribution of unique, moderately repetitive, and highly repetitive sequences in a hypothetical human chromosome. Unique genes encode mRNA. These genes occur in single copies. The genes for the large rRNA and the tRNA precursors occur in multiple copies that are clustered in the genome. The large rRNA genes form the nucleolar organizer. Moderately repetitive sequences are dispersed throughout the genome, and highly repetitive sequences are clustered around the centromere and at the ends of the chromosome (the telomeres). From Wolfe SL. Mol Cell Biol 1993:761.

Table 14.2. Differences between Eukaryotes and Prokaryotes

	Eukaryotes (human)	Prokaryotes (E. coli)
Nucleus	Yes	No
Chromosomes		
Number	23 per haploid cell	1 per haploid cell
DNA	Linear	Circular
Histones	Yes	No
Genome		
Diploid	Somatic cells	No
Haploid	Germ cells	All cells
Size	3×10^9 base pairs per haploid cell	4×10^6 base pairs
Genes		
Unique	64%	100%
Repetitive		
Moderately	25%	None
Highly	10%	None
Operons	No	Yes
mRNA		
Polycistronic	No	Yes
Introns (hnRNA)	Yes	No
Translation	Separate from transcription	Coupled with transcription

sequences are also examples of SINEs (**S**hort **IN**terspersed **E**lements). The LINE sequences (**L**ong **IN**terspersed **E**lements) are 6,000 to 7,000 base pairs in length. The function of the Alu and LINE sequences has not been determined.

Major differences between prokaryotic and eukaryotic DNA and RNA are summarized in Table 14.2.

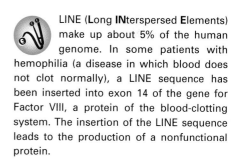

LINE (**L**ong **IN**terspersed **E**lements) make up about 5% of the human genome. In some patients with hemophilia (a disease in which blood does not clot normally), a LINE sequence has been inserted into exon 14 of the gene for Factor VIII, a protein of the blood-clotting system. The insertion of the LINE sequence leads to the production of a nonfunctional protein.

CLINICAL COMMENTS

Anne Niemick. Patients with β^+-thalassemia who maintain their hemoglobin levels above 6.0 to 7.0 g/dL are usually classified as having thalassemia intermedia. In the β-thalassemias, the α chains of adult hemoglobin A ($\alpha_2\beta_2$) continue to be synthesized at a normal rate. These chains accumulate in the bone marrow, where the red blood cells are synthesized in erythropoiesis (generation of red blood cells). The accumulation of α chains diminishes erythopoiesis, resulting in an anemia. Individuals who are homozygous for a severe mutation require constant transfusions.

Individuals with thalassemia intermedia, such as **Anne Niemick,** could have inherited two different defective alleles, one from each parent. One parent may be a "silent" carrier, with one normal allele and one mildly affected allele. This parent produces enough functional β-globin, so no clinical symptoms of thalassemia appear. (However, they generally have a somewhat decreased amount of hemoglobin, resulting in microcytic hypochromic red blood cells.) When this parent contributes the mildly defective allele and the other heterozygous parent contributes a more severely defective allele,

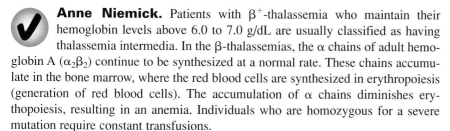

The mutations that cause the thalassemias affect the synthesis of either the α- or the β-chains of adult hemoglobin, causing an anemia. They are classified by the chain affected (α- or β-) and by the amount of chain synthesized (0 for no synthesis and + for synthesis of some functional chains). They are also classified as major, intermediate, or minor, according to the severity of the clinical disorder. β-thalassemia major (also called homozygous β-thalassemia) is a clinically severe disorder requiring frequent blood transfusions. It is caused by the inheritance of two alleles for a severe mutation. In β-thalassemia intermedia, the patient exhibits a less severe clinical phenotype and is able to maintain hemoglobin levels above 6 g/dL. It is usually the result of two different mild mutations or homozygosity for a mild mutation. β-thalassemia minor (also known as β-thalassemia trait) is a heterozygous disorder involving a single mutation that is often clinically asymptomatic.

During embryonic and fetal life, the β-chain is replaced by the ε and γ chains. As a result, patients with severe mutations in the α-chain tend to die in utero, whereas those with mutations in the β chains exhibit symptoms postnatally, as hemoglobin F is normally replaced with adult hemoglobin A.

thalassemia intermedia occurs in the child. The child is thus heterozygous for two different defective alleles.

Ivy Sharer. Ivy Sharer was treated with a multidrug regimen for tuberculosis because the microbes that cause the disease frequently become resistant to the individual drugs. Rifampin in combination with the drug isoniazid (which affects metabolism of vitamin B_6 in the pathogenic bacteria) is usually effective, but months of treatment are required.

Just as bacteria can become resistant to drugs, so can HIV. A great concern to physicians treating patients with AIDS is the appearance of resistant strains of HIV-1 in patients taking a single drug, such as ZDV (zidovudine), for 6 months or more. Therefore, multidrug regimens are used that include other nucleoside reverse transcriptase inhibitors, such as dideoxyinosine (didanosine, formerly called ddI) and dideoxycytidine (zalcitabine, formerly called ddC). The multidrug therapy often includes nonnucleoside inhibitors (e.g., efavirenz), which acts allosterically on reverse transcriptase, and protease inhibitors (e.g., indinavir), which prevent the HIV polyprotein from being cleaved into its mature products (see Biochemical Comments).

Recent studies have indicated that a failure to properly dispose of cellular debris, a normal byproduct of cell death, may lead to the induction of auto-antibodies directed against chromatin in patients with SLE. Normal cells have a finite lifetime, and are programmed to die (apoptosis) through a distinct biochemical mechanism. One of the steps in this mechanism is the stepwise degradation of cellular DNA (and other cellular components). If the normal intracellular components are exposed to the immune system, auto-antibodies against them may be generated. The enzyme in cells that degrades DNA is deoxyribonuclease I (DNase I), and individuals with SLE have reduced serum activity levels of DNase I compared with individuals who do not have the disease. Through an understanding of the molecular mechanism whereby auto-antibodies are generated, it may be possible to develop therapies to combat this disorder.

Amanda Tin. The toxin α-amanitin is capable of causing irreversible hepatocellular and renal dysfunction through inhibition of mammalian RNA polymerases. Fortunately, **Amanda Tin's** toxicity proved mild. She developed only gastrointestinal symptoms and slight changes in her hepatic and renal function, which returned to normal within a few weeks. Treatment was primarily supportive, with fluid and electrolyte replacement for that lost through the gastrointestinal tract. No effective antidote is available for the *A. phalloides* toxin.

Sis Lupus. SLE is a multisystem disease of unknown origin characterized by inflammation related to the presence of autoantibodies in the blood. These autoantibodies react with antigens normally found in the nucleus, cytoplasm, and plasma membrane of the cell. Such "self" antigen–antibody (autoimmune) interactions initiate an inflammatory cascade that produces the broad symptom profile of multiorgan dysfunction found in **Sis Lupus.**

Pharmacological therapy for SLE, directed at immunosuppression, includes high doses of corticosteroids, which suppress the immune response. In refractory cases that do not respond to corticosteroids, cytotoxic drugs inhibiting the synthesis of antibody-producing cells by the bone marrow are also used to cause immunosuppression.

BIOCHEMICAL COMMENTS

Production of the Virus That Causes AIDS. AIDS is caused by the human immuno-deficiency virus (HIV). Two forms of the virus have been discovered, HIV-1, which is prevalent in industrialized countries, and HIV-2, which is prevalent in certain regions of Africa. Eight to ten years or more can elapse between the initial infection and development of the full-blown syndrome.

The reverse transcriptase that copies the viral genome has a high error rate because it does not have proofreading capability. Because incorporation of mismatched bases leads to evolution of the virus, new populations develop rapidly in response to changes in the environment. Mutations in the viral reverse transcriptase gene cause the enzyme to become resistant to drugs such as ZDV. Current vaccines developed experimentally against the gp120 surface protein may not be effective because this protein also mutates. As a consequence of the rapid mutation rate of HIV, current treatments for AIDS have limited effectiveness, and a cure has proved elusive.

Proteins in the viral coat bind to membrane receptors (named CD4) of helper T lymphocytes, a class of cells involved in the immune response. Subsequently, conformational changes occur that allow the viral coat proteins to bind to a chemokine coreceptor in the cell membrane. The lipid in the viral coat then fuses with the cell membrane, and the viral core enters the cell, releasing its RNA and enzymes (including the reverse transcriptase) by a process called "uncoating." Reverse transcriptase uses the viral RNA as a template to produce a single-stranded DNA copy, which then serves as a template for synthesis of a double-stranded DNA. An integrase enzyme, also carried by the virus, enables this DNA to integrate into the host cell genome as a provirus (Fig. 14.22).

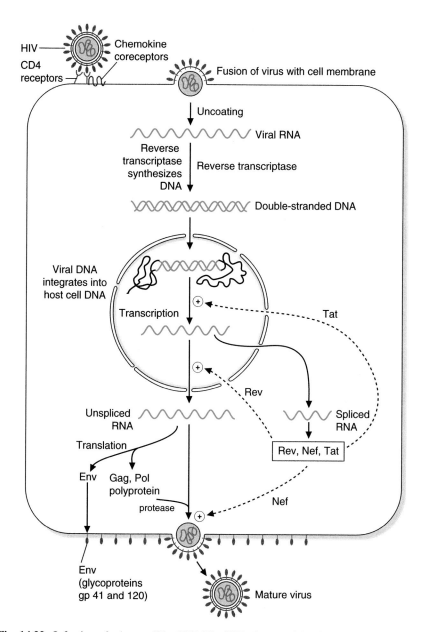

Fig. 14.22. Infection of a host cell by HIV. The HIV virus particle binds to the CD4 receptor and a chemokine coreceptor in the host cell membrane. The virus enters the cell and uncoats, releasing its RNA and proteins. The viral enzyme reverse transcriptase produces a double-stranded DNA copy that is integrated into the host cell genome. HIV is now a provirus. Transcripts of the viral DNA are spliced and translated to produce the proteins Tat, Rev, and Nef. Tat stimulates transcription of the viral DNA, and Rev causes the viral RNA transcripts to leave the nucleus unspliced. The unspliced RNA serves as the viral genome and also codes for the proteins of the viral core and envelope. The envelope proteins (gp41 and gp120, which are derived from the env protein) enter the cell membrane. The viral core proteins are synthesized as a polyprotein, which is cleaved by a protease as the viral particles form and bud from the cell membrane. The particles carry membrane lipid as a coat that contains gp41 and gp120. Nef indirectly aids in the assembly of viral particles. Pol is the reverse transcriptase produced from the viral RNA. ⊕ = stimulates.

In the initial stage of transcription of the provirus, the transcript is spliced, and three proteins, Nef, Tat, and Rev, are produced. Tat stimulates transcription of the viral genes. As Rev accumulates, it allows unspliced viral RNA to leave the nucleus and to produce proteins of the viral envelope and viral core, including reverse transcriptase. Two of the envelope glycoproteins (gp41 and gp120, which are derived from the env gene product) form a complex that embeds in the cell membrane. The other proteins, which are translated as a polyprotein and cleaved by the viral protease, combine with the full-length viral RNA to form core viral particles, which bud from the cell membrane. Thus, the virus obtains its lipid coat from the host cell membrane, and the coat contains the viral proteins gp41 and gp120. These surface proteins of the virus bind to CD4 receptors on other human helper T lymphocytes, and the infection spreads.

In an uninfected person, helper T lymphocytes usually number approximately 1,000/mL. Infection with HIV causes the number of these cells to decrease, which results in a deficiency of the immune system. When the number of T lymphocytes drops below 200/mL, the disease is in an advanced stage, and opportunistic infections, such as tuberculosis, occur. Although macrophages and dendritic cells lack CD4 receptors, they can also become infected with HIV and can carry the virus to the central nervous system.

The most effective means of combating HIV infection involves the use of drugs that inhibit the viral reverse transcriptase or the viral protease. However, these drugs only hold the infection at bay; they do not effect a cure.

Drugs currently used to treat AIDS act on the viral reverse transcriptase or the protease (see Fig. 14.22). The nonnucleoside drugs (e.g., efavirenz) bind to reverse transcriptase and inhibit its action. The nucleoside analogs (e.g., ZDV) add to the 3′ end of the growing DNA transcript produced by reverse transcriptase and prevent further elongation. The protease inhibitors (e.g., indinavir) bind to the protease and prevent it from cleaving the polyprotein.

Suggested References

A more complete coverage of transcription can be found in:

Lewin B. Chapter 5: mRNA. In: Genes VII. Oxford: Oxford University Press, 2000:119–138.

Lewin B. Chapter 9: mRNA and Transcription. In: Genes VII. Oxford: Oxford University Press, 2000:232–272.

Lewin, B. Chapter 20: Initiation of transcription. In: Genes VII. Oxford: Oxford University Press, 2000:649–684.

Tjian R. Molecular machines that control genes. Sci Am 1995;272:54–61.

References covering diseases discussed in this chapter:

Clumeck N. Choosing the best initial therapy for HIV-1 infection. N Engl J Med 1999;341:1925–1926. [See also the accompanying articles.]

Frankel AD, Young JAT. HIV-1: Fifteen proteins and an RNA. Annu Rev Biochem 1998;67:1–25.

Weatherall DJ, Clegg JB, Higgs DR, Wood WG. The hemoglobinopathies. Vol. III. In: Scriver CR, Beaudet AL, Sly WS, Valle B., eds. The Metabolic and Molecular Bases of Inherited Disease. 8th Ed. New York: McGraw Hill, 2001: 4571–4636.

Walport MJ. Lupus, DNase and defective disposal of cellular debris. Nature Ggenetics 2000;25:135–136.

 REVIEW QUESTIONS—CHAPTER 14

1. The short transcript AUCCGUACG would be derived from which of the following template DNA sequences? (Note all sequences are written from 5′ to 3′)

    (A) ATCCGTACG
    (B) CGTACGGAT
    (C) AUCCGUACG
    (D) TAGGCATGC
    (E) GCATGCCTA

2. Given that the LD_{50} (the dose at which 50% of the recipients die) of amanitin is 0.1 mg per kg body weight, and that the average mushroom contains 7 mg amanitin, how many mushrooms must be consumed by Amanda Tin (50 kg body weight) to be above the LD_{50}?

    (A) 1
    (B) 2
    (C) 3
    (D) 4
    (E) 5

3. Which of the following eukaryotic DNA control sequences does not need to be in a fixed location, and is most responsible for high rates of transcription of particular genes?

    (A) Promoter
    (B) Promoter-proximal element
    (C) Enhancer
    (D) Operator
    (E) Splice donor site

4. Which of the following is true of both eukaryotic and prokaryotic gene expression?

    (A) After transcription, a 3′ poly A tail and a 5′ cap are added to mRNA.
    (B) Translation of mRNA can begin before transcription is complete.
    (C) mRNA is synthesized in the 3′ to 5′ direction.
    (D) RNA polymerase binds at a promoter region upstream of the gene.
    (E) Mature mRNA is always precisely co-linear to the gene from which it was transcribed.

5. In a segment of a transcribed gene, the nontemplate strand of DNA has the following sequence:
    5′...AGCTCACTG...3′
    What will be the corresponding sequence in the RNA produced from this segment of the gene?

    (A) CAGUGAGCU
    (B) AGCUCACUG
    (C) CAGTGAGCT
    (D) UCGAGUGAC
    (E) GTCACTCGA

15 Translation: Synthesis of Proteins

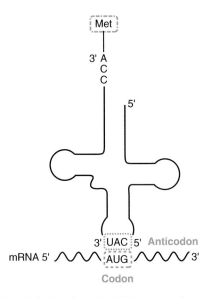

Fig. 15.1. Binding of tRNA to a codon on mRNA. The tRNA contains an amino acid at its 3'-end that corresponds to the codon on mRNA with which the anticodon of the tRNA can base-pair. Note that the codon–anticodon pairing is complementary and antiparallel.

*Proteins are produced by the process of **translation**, which occurs on **ribosomes** and is directed by **mRNA**. The genetic message encoded in DNA is first transcribed into mRNA, and the **nucleotide sequence** in the coding region of the mRNA is then translated into the **amino acid sequence** of the protein.*

*   **Translation of the code**. The portion of mRNA that specifies the amino acid sequence of the protein is read in **codons**, which are **sets of three nucleotides** that specify individual amino acids (Fig 15.1). The codons on mRNA are read sequentially in the 5' to 3' direction, starting with the 5'-**AUG** (or "**start**" codon) that specifies **methionine** and sets the **reading frame** and ending with a 3'-**termination** (or "**stop**") codon (**UAG**, **UGA**, or **UAA**). The protein is synthesized from its **N-terminus** to its **C-terminus**.*

*   Each amino acid is carried to the ribosome by an **aminoacyl-tRNA** (i.e., a tRNA with an amino acid covalently attached). **Base-pairing** between the **anticodon** of the tRNA and the **codon** on the mRNA ensures that each amino acid is inserted into the growing polypeptide at the appropriate position.*

*   **Synthesis of the protein. Initiation** involves formation of a complex containing the initial **methionyl-tRNA** bound to the AUG "**start**" codon of the **mRNA** and to the "**P**" site of the **ribosome**. It requires **GTP** and proteins known as **eukaryotic initiation factors (eIFs)**.*

*   **Elongation** of the polypeptide involves **three steps**: (a) **binding** of an **aminoacyl-tRNA** to the "**A**" site on the ribosome where it base-pairs with the second codon on the mRNA; (b) **formation** of a **peptide bond** between the first and second amino acids; and (c) **translocation**, movement of the mRNA relative to the ribosome, so that the third mRNA codon moves into the "**A**" site. These three **elongation steps** are **repeated** until a **termination** codon aligns with the site on the ribosome where the next aminoacyl-tRNA would normally bind. **Release factors** bind instead, causing the completed protein to be released from the ribosome.*

*   After one ribosome binds and moves along the mRNA, translating the polypeptide, another ribosome can bind and begin translation. The complex of a single mRNA with multiple ribosomes is known as a **polysome**.*

*   **Folding and modification and targeting of the protein. Folding** of the polypeptide into its three-dimensional configuration occurs as the polypeptide is being translated. This process involves proteins called **chaperones. Modification** of amino acid residues in a protein occurs during or after translation. Proteins synthesized on **cytosolic ribosomes** are released into the cytosol or transported into mitochondria, peroxisomes, and nucleus. Proteins synthesized on ribosomes attached to the **rough endoplasmic reticulum (RER)** are destined for lysosomes, cell membranes, or secretion from the cell. These proteins are transferred to the **Golgi complex**, where they are modified and **targeted** to their ultimate locations.*

THE WAITING ROOM

Anne Niemick, a 4-year old patient with β^+-thalassemia intermedia (see Chapter 14), showed no improvement in her symptoms at her second visit. Her hemoglobin level was 7.0 g/dL (reference range for females = 12–16 g/dL).

Jay Sakz is a 9-month-old male infant of Ashkenazi Jewish parentage. His growth and development were normal until age 5 months, when he began to exhibit mild, generalized muscle weakness. By 7 months, he had poor head control, slowed development of motor skills, and was increasingly inattentive to his surroundings. His parents also noted unusual eye movements and staring episodes. On careful examination of his retinae, his pediatrician observed a "cherry-red" spot within a pale macula. The physician suspected Tay-Sachs disease and sent whole blood samples to the molecular biology-genetics laboratory.

Neu Moania returned to his physician's office after 1 week of erythromycin therapy (see Chapter 12). The sputum sample from his previous visit had been cultured. The results confirmed that his respiratory infection was caused by *Streptococcus pneumoniae* and that the organism was sensitive to penicillin, macrolides (e.g., erythromycin, clarithromycin), tetracycline, and other antibiotics.

Erna Nemdy, a 25-year-old junior medical student ("earn an M.D."), brings her healthy 4-month-old daughter, **Beverly**, to the pediatrician for her second diphtheria, pertussis, tetanus (DPT-2) immunization. Erna tells the doctor that her great, great aunt had died of diphtheria during an epidemic many years ago.

The results of tests performed in the molecular biology laboratory show that **Jay Sakz** has an insertion in exon 11 of the β-chain of the hexosaminidase A gene, the most common mutation found in patients of Ashkenazi Jewish background who have Tay-Sachs disease.

I. THE GENETIC CODE

Transcription, the transfer of the genetic message from DNA to RNA, and translation, the transfer of the genetic message from the nucleotide language of nucleic acids to the amino acid language of proteins, both depend on base-pairing. In the late 1950s and early 1960s, molecular biologists attempting to decipher the process of translation recognized two problems. The first involved decoding the relationship between the "language" of the nucleic acids and the "language" of the proteins, and the second involved determining the molecular mechanism by which translation between these two languages occurs.

Twenty different amino acids are commonly incorporated into proteins, and, therefore, the protein "alphabet" has 20 characters. The nucleic acid alphabet, however, has only four characters, corresponding to the four nucleotides of mRNA (A, G, C, and U). If two nucleotides constituted the code for an amino acid, then only 4^2 or 16 amino acids could be specified. Therefore, the number of nucleotides that code for an amino acid has to be three, providing 4^3 or 64 possible combinations or "codons," more than required, but not overly excessive.

Scientists set out to determine the specific codons for each amino acid. In 1961, Marshall Nirenberg produced the first crack in the genetic code (the collection of codons that specify all the amino acids found in proteins). He showed that poly(U), a polynucleotide in which all the bases are uracil, produced polyphenylalanine in a cell-free protein-synthesizing system. Thus, UUU must be

A. Codons for alanine

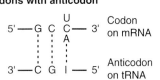

B. Base pairing of alanine codons with anticodon

Fig. 15.2. Base-pairing of codons for alanine with 5′-IGC-3′. A. Note that the variation is in the third base. B. The first three of these codons can pair with a tRNA that contains the anticodon 5′-IGC-3′. Hypoxanthine (I) is an unusual base found in tRNA that can form base pairs with U, C, or A. It is formed by the deamination of adenine.

Hypoxanthine is the base attached to ribose in the nucleoside inosine. The single-letter abbreviation for hypoxanthine is "I," in reference to the nucleoside inosine. (In other cases, the first letter of the base is also the first letter of the nucleoside and the single letter abbreviation. For example, A is the base adenine and the nucleoside adenosine.)

the codon for phenylalanine. As a result of experiments using synthetic polynucleotides in place of mRNA, other codons were identified.

The pioneering molecular biologists recognized that, because amino acids cannot bind directly to the sets of three nucleotides that form their codons, "adapters" are required. The "adapters" were found to be tRNA molecules. Each tRNA molecule contains an anticodon and covalently binds a specific amino acid at its 3′-end (see Chapters 12 and 14). The anticodon of a tRNA molecule is a set of three nucleotides that can interact with a codon on mRNA (Fig. 15.2). To interact, the codon and anticodon must be complementary (i.e., they must be able to form base pairs in an antiparallel orientation). Thus, the anticodon of a tRNA serves as the link between an mRNA codon and the amino acid that the codon specifies.

Obviously, each codon present within mRNA must correspond to a specific amino acid. Nirenberg found that trinucleotides of known base sequence could bind to ribosomes and induce the binding of specific aminoacyl-tRNAs (i.e., tRNAs with amino acids covalently attached). As a result of these and the earlier experiments, the relationship between all 64 codons and the amino acids they specify (the entire genetic code) was determined by the mid-1960s (Table 15.1).

Three of the 64 possible codons (UGA, UAG, and UAA) terminate protein synthesis and are known as "stop" or nonsense codons. The remaining 61 codons specify amino acids. Two amino acids each have only one codon (AUG = methionine; UGG = tryptophan). The remaining amino acids have multiple codons.

A. The Code Is Degenerate, But Unambiguous

Because many amino acids are specified by more than one codon, the genetic code is described as "degenerate," which means that an amino acid may have more than one codon. However, each codon specifies only one amino acid, and the genetic code is, thus, unambiguous.

Inspection of a codon table shows that in most instances of multiple codons for a single amino acid, the variation occurs in the third base of the codon (see Table 15.1). Crick noted that the pairing between the 3′-base of the codon and the 5′-base of the anticodon does not always follow the strict base-pairing rules that he and Watson had previously discovered (i.e., A pairs with U, and G with C). This observation resulted in the "wobble" hypothesis.

At the third base of the codon (the 3′-position of the codon and the 5′-position of the anticodon), the base pairs can "wobble", e.g., G can pair with U; and A, G, or U can pair with the unusual base hypoxanthine (I) found in tRNA. Thus, three of

Table 15.1. The Genetic Code

First Base	Second Base				Third Base
(5′)	**U**	**C**	**A**	**G**	**(3′)**
U	Phe	Ser	Tyr	Cys	U
	Phe	Sor	Tyr	Cys	C
	Leu	Ser	Stop	Stop	A
	Leu	Ser	Stop	Trp	G
C	Leu	Pro	His	Arg	U
	Leu	Pro	His	Arg	C
	Leu	Pro	Gln	Arg	A
	Leu	Pro	Gln	Arg	G
A	Ile	Thr	Asn	Ser	U
	Ile	Thr	Asn	Ser	C
	Ile	Thr	Lys	Arg	A
	Met	Thr	Lys	Arg	G
G	Val	Ala	Asp	Gly	U
	Val	Ala	Asp	Gly	C
	Val	Ala	Glu	Gly	A
	Val	Ala	Glu	Gly	G

the four codons for alanine (GCU, GCC, and GCA) can pair with a single tRNA that contains the anticodon 5′-IGC-3′ (see Fig. 15.2). If each of the 61 codons for amino acids required a distinct tRNA, cells would contain 61 tRNAs. However, because of "wobble" between the codon and anticodon, fewer than 61 tRNAs are required to translate the genetic code.

B. The Code Is Almost Universal

All organisms studied so far use the same genetic code, with some rare exceptions. One exception occurs in human mitochondrial mRNA, where UGA codes for tryptophan instead of serving as a stop codon, AUA codes for methionine instead of isoleucine, and CUA codes for threonine instead of leucine.

C. The Code Is Nonoverlapping and without Punctuation

mRNA does not contain punctuation to separate one codon from the next and the codons do not overlap. Each nucleotide is read only once. Beginning with a start codon (AUG) near the 5′-end of the mRNA, the codons are read sequentially, ending with a stop codon (UGA, UAG, or UAA) near the 3′-end of the mRNA.

II. RELATIONSHIP BETWEEN mRNA AND THE PROTEIN PRODUCT

The start codon (AUG) sets the reading frame, the order in which the sequence of bases in the mRNA is sorted into codons (Fig. 15.3). The order of the codons in the mRNA determines the sequence in which amino acids are added to the growing polypeptide chain. Thus, the order of the codons in the mRNA determines the linear sequence of amino acids in the protein.

III. EFFECTS OF MUTATIONS

Mutations that result from damage to the nucleotides of DNA molecules or from unrepaired errors during replication (see Chapter 13) can be transcribed into mRNA, and, therefore, can result in the translation of a protein with an abnormal amino acid sequence. Various types of mutations can occur that have different effects on the encoded protein (Table 15.2).

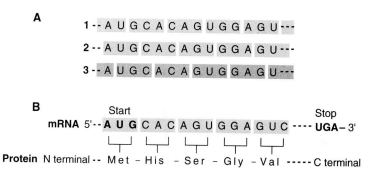

Fig. 15.3. Reading frame of mRNA. A. For any given mRNA sequence, there are three possible reading frames (1, 2, and 3). B. An AUG near the 5′-end of the mRNA (the start codon) sets the reading frame for translation of a protein from the mRNA. The codons are read in linear order, starting with this AUG. (The other potential reading frames are not used. They would give proteins with different amino acid sequences.)

Table 15.2. Types of Mutations

Type	Description	Example
Point	A single base change	
Silent	A change that specifies the same amino acid	CGA → CGG Arg → Arg
Missense	A change that specifies a different amino acid	CGA → CCA Arg → Pro
Nonsense	A change that produces a stop codon	CGA → UGA Arg → Stop
Insertion	An addition of one or more bases	
Deletion	A loss of one or more bases	

A. Point Mutations

Point mutations occur when only one base in DNA is altered, producing a change in a single base of an mRNA codon. There are three basic types of point mutations: silent mutations, missense mutations, and nonsense mutations. Point mutations are said to be "silent" when they do not affect the amino acid sequence of the protein. For example, a codon change from CGA to CGG does not affect the protein because both of these codons specify arginine (see Table 15.1). In missense mutations, one amino acid in the protein is replaced by a different amino acid. For example, a change from CGA to CCA causes arginine to be replaced by proline. A "nonsense" mutation causes the premature termination of a polypeptide chain. For example, a codon change from CGA to UGA causes a codon for arginine to be replaced by a stop codon and synthesis of the mutant protein terminates at this point.

Sickle cell anemia is caused by a missense mutation. In each of the alleles for β-globin, **Will Sichel's** DNA has a single base change (see Chapter 6). In the sickle cell gene, GTG replaces the normal GAG. Thus, in the mRNA, the codon GUG replaces GAG and a valine residue replaces a glutamate residue in the protein.

B. Insertions, Deletions, and Frameshift Mutations

An insertion occurs when one or more nucleotides are added to DNA. If the insertion does not generate a stop codon, a protein with more amino acids than normal could be produced.

When one or more nucleotides are removed from DNA, the mutation is known as a deletion. If the deletion does not affect the normal start and stop codons, a protein with fewer than the normal number of amino acids could be produced.

A frameshift mutation occurs when the number of inserted or deleted nucleotides is not a multiple of three (Fig. 15.4). The reading frame shifts at the point where the insertion or deletion begins. Beyond that point, the amino acid sequence of the protein translated from the mRNA differs from the normal protein.

One type of thalassemia is caused by a nonsense mutation. Codon 17 of the β-globin chain is changed from UGG to UGA. This change results in the conversion of a codon for a tryptophan residue to a stop codon.

Is it likely that **Anne Niemick** has this mutation in codon 17?

Some types of thalassemia are caused by deletions in the globin genes. Patients have been studied who have large deletions in either the 5′ or the 3′ coding region of the β-globin gene, removing almost one third of the DNA sequence.

Is it likely that **Anne Niemick** has a large deletion in the β-globln gene?

IV. FORMATION OF AMINOACYL-tRNA

A tRNA that contains an amino acid covalently attached to its 3′-end is called an aminoacyl-tRNA and is said to be "charged." Aminoacyl-tRNAs are named both for the amino acid and the tRNA that carries the amino acid. For example, the tRNA

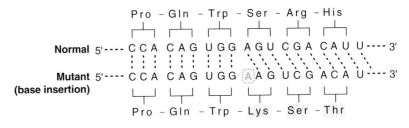

Fig. 15.4. A frameshift mutation. The insertion of a single nucleotide (the A in the dotted box) causes the reading frame to shift, so that the amino acid sequence of the protein translated from the mRNA is different after the point of insertion. A similar effect can result from the insertion or deletion of nucleotides if the number inserted or deleted is not a multiple of 3.

for alanine (tRNA^Ala) acquires alanine to become alanyl-tRNA^ala. A particular tRNA recognizes only the AUG start codon that initiates protein synthesis and not other AUG codons that specify insertion of methionine within the polypeptide chain. This initiator methionyl-tRNA^Met is denoted by the subscript "i" in methionyl-tRNA_i^Met.

Amino acids are attached to their tRNAs by highly specific enzymes known as aminoacyl-tRNA synthetases. Twenty different synthetases exist, one for each amino acid. Each synthetase recognizes a particular amino acid and all of the tRNAs that carry that amino acid.

The formation of the ester bond that links the amino acid to the tRNA by an aminoacyl-tRNA synthetase is an energy-requiring process that occurs in two steps. The amino acid is activated in the first step when its carboxyl group reacts with adenosine triphosphate (ATP) to form an enzyme/aminoacyl–AMP complex and pyrophosphate (Fig. 15.5). The cleavage of a high-energy bond of ATP in this reaction provides energy, and the subsequent cleavage of pyrophosphate by a pyrophosphatase helps to drive the reaction by removing one of the products. In the second step, the activated amino acid is transferred to the 2'- or 3'-hydroxyl group (depending on the type of aminoacyl-tRNA synthetase catalyzing the reaction) of the 3' terminal A residue of the tRNA, and AMP is released (recall that all tRNAs have a CCA added to their 3' end posttranscriptionally). The energy in the aminoacyl-tRNA ester bond is subsequently used in the formation of a peptide bond during the process of protein synthesis.

Some aminoacyl-tRNA synthetases use the anticodon of the tRNA as a recognition site as they attach the amino acid to the hydroxyl group at the 3'-end of the tRNA (Fig. 15.6). However, other synthetases do not use the anticodon but recognize only bases located at other positions in the tRNA. Nevertheless, insertion of the amino acid into a growing polypeptide chain depends solely on the bases of the anticodon, through complementary base-pairing with the mRNA codon.

V. PROCESS OF TRANSLATION

Translation of a protein involves three steps: initiation, elongation, and termination. It begins with the formation of the initiation complex. Subsequently, synthesis of the polypeptide occurs by a series of elongation steps that are repeated as each

 A nonsense mutation at codon 17 would cause premature termination of translation. A nonfunctional peptide containing only 16 amino acids would result, producing a β⁰-thalassemia if the mutation occurred in both alleles. A large deletion in the coding region of the gene could also produce a truncated protein. If **Anne Niemick** has a nonsense mutation or a large deletion, it could only be in one allele. The mutation in the other allele must be milder, since she produces some normal β-globin. Her hemoglobin is 7 g/dL, typical of thalassemia intermedia (a β⁺-thalassemia).

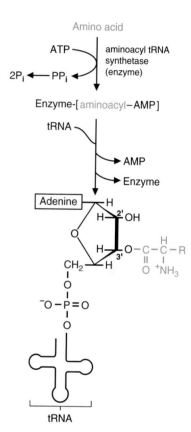

Fig. 15.5. Formation of aminoacyl-tRNA. The amino acid is first activated by reacting with ATP. The amino acid is then transferred from the aminoacyl-AMP to tRNA.

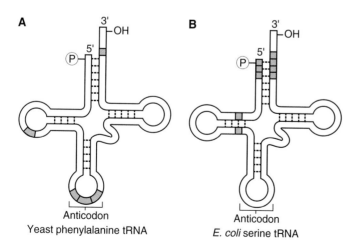

Fig. 15.6. Some aminoacyl-tRNA synthetase recognition sites on tRNA. Each aminoacyl-tRNA synthetase is specific for one tRNA, which it "recognizes" by binding the sequences of nucleotides called the recognition sites, shown in blue. In some cases, the anticodon is a recognition site; in others, it is not. This is true for human tRNAs as well as those shown here.

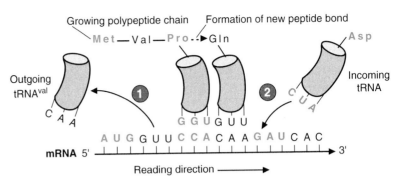

Fig. 15.7. Overview of the process of translation. 1. Once a tRNA has donated its amino acid to the growing polypeptide chain, it is released from the mRNA. 2. A new aminoacyl-tRNA binds to the correct codon in the mRNA to donate its amino acid to the growing polypeptide chain.

amino acid is added to the growing chain (Fig. 15.7). Termination occurs where the mRNA contains an in-frame stop codon, and the completed polypeptide chain is released.

A. Initiation of Translation

Eukaryotic initiation factor 2 (eIF2) and also elongation factor 1 (EF1) are types of heterotrimeric G proteins (see Chapter 11). They dramatically change their conformation and actively form complexes when they bind GTP but become inactive and dissociate when they hydrolyze this GTP to GDP. GTP can then displace the bound GDP to reactivate the initiation factor eIF2 or the elongation factor EF1.

In eukaryotes, initiation of translation involves formation of a complex composed of methionyl-tRNA$_i^{Met}$, mRNA, and a ribosome (Fig. 15.8). Methionyl-tRNA$_i^{Met}$ (also known as Met-tRNA$_i^{Met}$) initially forms a complex with the protein eukaryotic initiation factor 2 (eIF2), which binds GTP. This complex then binds to the small (40S) ribosomal subunit. The cap at the 5'-end of the mRNA binds an initiation factor known as the cap binding protein (CBP). CBP contains a number of subunits, including eIF4E. Several other eIFs join, and the mRNA then binds to the eIFs-Met-tRNA$_i^{Met}$ – 40S ribosome complex. In a reaction requiring hydrolysis of ATP (due to the helicase activity of an eIF subunit), this complex unwinds a hairpin loop in the mRNA and scans the mRNA until it locates the AUG start codon (usually the

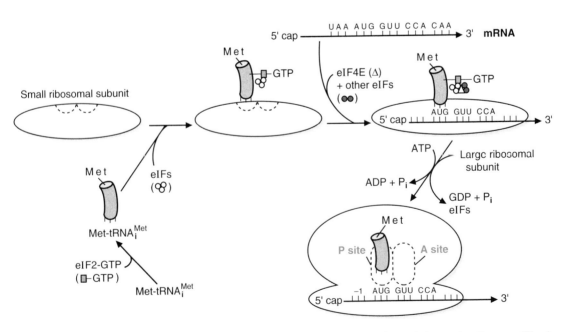

Fig. 15.8. Initiation of protein synthesis. P site = peptidyl site on the ribosome; A site = aminoacyl site on the ribosome (The A and P sites or portions of them are indicated by dashed lines); eIF = eukaryotic initiation factor.

Table 15.3. Differences between Eukaryotes and Prokaryotes in the Initiation of Protein Synthesis

	Eukaryotes	Prokaryotes
Binding of mRNA to small ribosomal subunit	Cap at 5' end of mRNA binds eIFs and 40S ribosomal subunit containing tRNA$_i^{met}$. mRNA is scanned for AUG start codon	Shine-Dalgarno sequence upstream of initiating AUG binds to complementary sequence in 16S rRNA
First amino acid	Methionine	Formyl-methionine
Initiation factors	eIFs (12 or more)	IFs (3)
Ribosomes	80S (40S and 60S subunits)	70S (30S and 50S subunits)

first AUG). GTP is hydrolyzed, the initiation factors are released, and the large ribosomal (60S) subunit binds. The ribosome is now complete. It contains one small and one large subunit, and has two binding sites for tRNA, known as the P (peptidyl) and A (aminoacyl) sites. During initiation, Met-tRNA$_i^{Met}$ binds to the ribosome at the P site.

The initiation process differs for prokaryotes and eukaryotes (Table 15.3). In bacteria, the initiating methionyl-tRNA is formylated, producing a formyl-methionyl-tRNA$_f^{Met}$ that participates in formation of the initiation complex (Fig. 15.9). Only three initiation factors (IFs) are required to generate this complex in prokaryotes, compared with the dozen or more required by eukaryotes. The ribosomes also differ in size. Prokaryotes have 70S ribosomes, composed of 30S and 50S subunits, and eukaryotes have 80S ribosomes, composed of 40S and 60S subunits. Unlike eukaryotic mRNA, bacterial mRNA is not capped. Identification of the initiating AUG triplet in prokaryotes occurs when a sequence in the mRNA (known as the Shine–Dalgarno sequence) binds to a complementary sequence near the 3'-end of the 16S rRNA of the small ribosomal subunit.

B. Elongation of Polypeptide Chains

After the initiation complex is formed, addition of each amino acid to the growing polypeptide chain involves binding of an aminoacyl-tRNA to the A site on the ribosome, formation of a peptide bond, and translocation of the peptidyl-tRNA to the P site (Fig. 15.10). The peptidyl-tRNA contains the growing polypeptide chain.

1. BINDING OF AMINOACYL-tRNA TO THE A SITE

When Met-tRNA$_i$ (or a peptidyl-tRNA) is bound to the P site, the mRNA codon in the A site determines which aminoacyl-tRNA will bind to that site. An aminoacyl-tRNA binds when its anticodon is antiparallel and complementary to the mRNA codon. In eukaryotes, the incoming aminoacyl-tRNA first combines with elongation

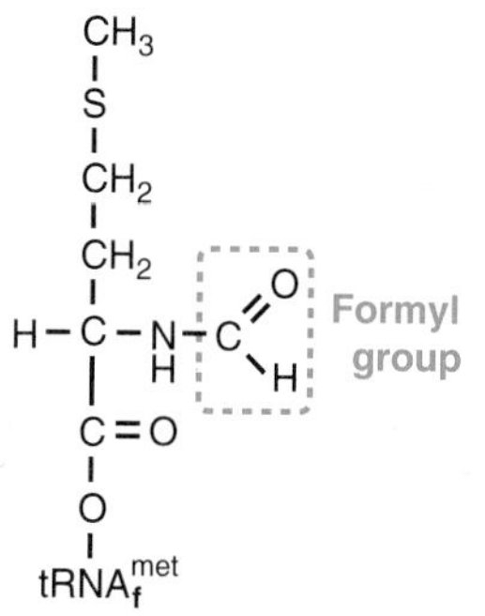

Insulin, an anabolic hormone, stimulates general protein synthesis by activating the initiation factor eIF4E. Normally, eIF4E is bound to an inhibitor protein, 4E binding protein (4E-BP). When insulin binds to its cell surface receptor, it initiates an intracellular sequence of events resulting in phosphorylation of 4E-BP. Phosphorylated 4E-BP no longer binds to eIF4E, and eIF4E is now free to participate in the initiation of protein synthesis.

eIF2 is a regulator of the initiation step in protein synthesis. When it is phosphorylated, it is inactive, and protein synthesis cannot begin. Conditions such as starvation, heat shock, and viral infection result in phosphorylation of eIF2 by a specific kinase.

The regulation of globin synthesis by heme in reticulocytes illustrates the role of eIF2 in regulation of translation. Reticulocytes, which are the precursors of red blood cells, synthesize the oxygen-carrying hemoglobin molecules from the globin polypeptide chains and the Fe-binding pigment, heme. In the absence of heme, the rate of initiation of globin synthesis decreases. Heme acts by inhibiting the phosphorylation of the initiation factor eIF2. Thus, eIF2 is active in the presence of heme and globin synthesis is initiated.

Many antibiotics that are used to combat bacterial infections in humans take advantage of the differences between the mechanisms for protein synthesis in prokaryotes and eukaryotes. For example, streptomycin binds to the 30S ribosomal subunit of prokaryotes. It interferes with initiation of protein synthesis and causes misreading of mRNA.

Although the bacterium causing his infection was sensitive to streptomycin, this drug was not used to treat **Neu Moania** because it can cause permanent hearing loss. Its use is, therefore, confined mainly to the treatment of tuberculosis or other infections that do not respond adequately to other antibiotics.

The antibiotic tetracycline binds to the 30S ribosomal subunit of prokaryotes and inhibits binding of aminoacyl-tRNA to the A site of the ribosome. The bacterium causing **Neu Moania's** infection was found to be sensitive to tetracycline.

CH$_3$
|
S
|
CH$_2$
|
CH$_2$
|
H—C—N—C⟨O,H⟩ Formyl group
| |
H
|
C=O
|
O
|
tRNA$_f^{met}$

Fig. 15.9. Bacterial tRNA containing formyl-methionine. The initial methionine is not formylated in eukaryotic protein synthesis.

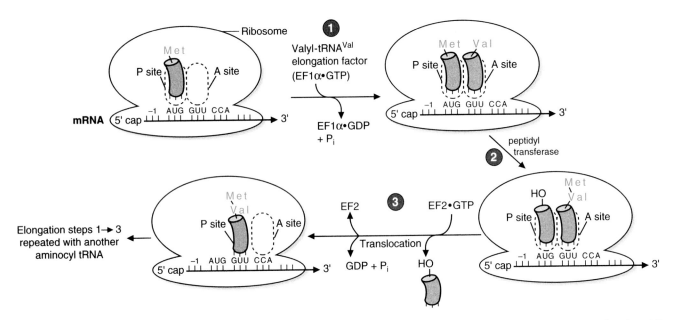

Fig. 15.10. Elongation of a polypeptide chain. 1. Binding of valyl-tRNA^{Val} to the A site. 2. Formation of a peptide bond. 3. Translocation. After step 3, step 1 is repeated using the aminoacyl-tRNA for the new codon in the A site. Steps 2 and 3 follow. These three steps keep repeating until termination occurs. (In prokaryotes, an exit site called the E site binds the t-RNA after it is displaced from the P site). EF = elongation factor.

factor EF1α containing bound GTP before binding to the mRNA–ribosome complex (EF1α is the GTP-binding α subunit of a heterotrimeric G protein, which is activated for association with other proteins when it contains GTP; see Chapter 11). When the aminoacyl-tRNA-EF1α-GTP complex binds to the A site, GTP is hydrolyzed to GDP. This prompts dissociation of EF1α-GDP from the aminoacyl-tRNA ribosomal complex, thereby allowing protein synthesis to continue (Fig. 15.11).

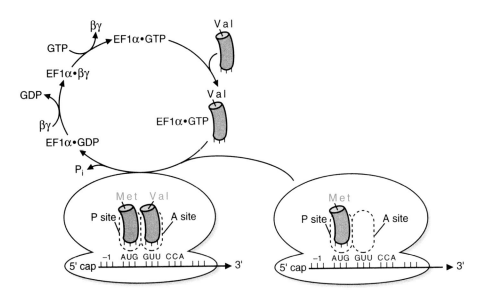

Fig. 15.11. Recycling of EF1 in eukaryotes. Note that EF1 is a heterotrimeric G protein. Its α-subunit binds GTP and activates the process whereby an aminoacyl-tRNA binds to the A site of the ribosome. GTP is hydrolyzed, and EF1α binds to the EF1βγ subunits, releasing GDP. GTP binds to the α subunit, the βγ subunits are released, and EF1α GTP is ready for another round. In prokaryotes, EF1α is EF-Tu and the protein corresponding to βγ is EF-Ts.

The free EF1α-GDP reassociates with the EF1βγ subunits, and GDP is released. Subsequently, GTP binds and the βγ subunits dissociate. Thus, EF1α-GTP is ready to bind another aminoacyl-tRNA molecule.

The process of elongation is very similar in prokaryotes, except that the corresponding factor for EF1α is named EF-Tu and the associating elongation factors are called EF-Ts instead of EF1βγ.

2. FORMATION OF A PEPTIDE BOND

In the first round of elongation, the amino acid on the tRNA in the A site forms a peptide bond with the methionine on the tRNA in the P site. In subsequent rounds of elongation, the amino acid on the tRNA in the A site forms a peptide bond with the peptide on the tRNA in the P site (see Fig. 15.10). Peptidyltransferase, which is not a protein but the rRNA of the large ribosomal subunit, catalyzes the formation of the peptide bond. The tRNA in the A site now contains the growing polypeptide chain, and the tRNA in the P site is uncharged (i.e., it no longer contains an amino acid or peptide).

3. TRANSLOCATION

Translocation in eukaryotes involves another G protein, elongation factor EF2 (EF-G in prokaryotes) that complexes with GTP and binds to the ribosome, causing a conformational change that moves the mRNA and its base-paired tRNAs with respect to the ribosome. The uncharged tRNA moves from the P site and is released from the ribosome. The peptidyl-tRNA moves into the P site, and the next codon of the mRNA occupies the A site. During translocation, GTP is hydrolyzed to GDP, which is released from the ribosome along with the elongation factor (see Fig. 15.10).

C. Termination of Translation

The three elongation steps are repeated until a termination (stop) codon moves into the A site on the ribosome. Because no tRNAs with anticodons that can pair with stop codons normally exist in cells, release factors bind to the ribosome instead, causing peptidyltransferase to hydrolyze the bond between the peptide chain and tRNA. The newly synthesized polypeptide is released from the ribosome, which dissociates into its individual subunits, releasing the mRNA.

Currently, some parents are not having their children immunized. The decrease in the incidence of infectious disease in the United States has led to complacency. Other parents who lack health insurance cannot afford to have their children vaccinated. Anyone who remembers the summertime fear of poliomyelitis in the 1940s and 1950s realizes that immunizations are a blessing that should be available to all children.

Protein synthesis requires a considerable amount of energy. Formation of each aminoacyl-tRNA requires the equivalent of two high-energy phosphate bonds because ATP is converted to AMP and pyrophosphate, which is cleaved to form two inorganic phosphates. As each amino acid is added to the growing peptide chain, two GTPs are hydrolyzed, one at the step involving EF1 and the second at the translocation step. Thus, four high-energy bonds are cleaved for each amino acid of the polypeptide. In addition, energy is required for initiation of synthesis of a polypeptide chain and for synthesis from nucleotide triphosphate precursors of the mRNA, tRNA, and rRNA involved in translation.

The macrolide antibiotics (e.g., erythromycin, clarithromycin) bind to the 50S ribosomal subunit of bacteria and inhibit translocation. Clarithromycin was used to treat **Neu Moania** because he had taken it previously without difficulty. It has less serious side effects than many other antibiotics and is used as an alternative drug in patients, such as **Mr. Moania,** who are allergic to penicillin. After 1 week of therapy, **Mr. Moania** recovered from his infection.

Chloramphenicol is an antibiotic that interferes with the peptidyltransferase activity of the 50S ribosomal subunit of bacteria. It was not used to treat **Neu Moania** because it is very toxic to humans, partly because of its effect on mitochondrial protein synthesis.

Diphtheria is a highly contagious disease caused by a toxin secreted by the bacterium *Corynebacterium diphtheriae*. Although the toxin is a protein, it is not produced by a bacterial gene, but by a gene brought into the bacterial cell by an infecting bacteriophage.

Diphtheria toxin is composed of two protein subunits. The B subunit binds to a cell surface receptor, facilitating the entry of the A subunit into the cell. In the cell, the A subunit catalyzes a reaction in which the ADP-ribose (ADPR) portion of NAD is transferred to EF2 (ADP-ribosylation). In this reaction, the ADPR is covalently attached to a post-translationally modified histidine residue, known as diphthamide. ADP-ribosylation of EF2 inhibits protein synthesis, leading to cell death. Children, including **Erna Nemdy's** daughter, are usually immunized against this often fatal disease at an early age.

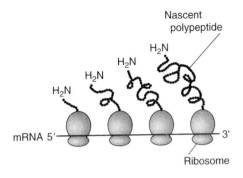

Fig. 15.12. A polysome. The complex of mRNA and multiple ribosomes, each of which is producing a polypeptide chain, is called a polysome.

VI. POLYSOMES

As one ribosome moves along the mRNA, producing a polypeptide chain, a second ribosome can bind to the vacant 5'-end of the mRNA. Many ribosomes can simultaneously translate a single mRNA, forming a complex known as a polysome (Fig. 15.12). A single ribosome covers approximately 80 nucleotides of mRNA. Therefore, ribosomes are positioned on mRNA at intervals of approximately 100 nucleotides. The growing polypeptide chains attached to the ribosomes become longer as each ribosome moves from the 5'-end toward the 3'-end of the mRNA.

VII. PROCESSING OF PROTEINS

Nascent polypeptide chains (i.e., polypeptides that are in the process of being synthesized) are processed. As they are being produced, they travel through a tunnel in the ribosome, which can hold roughly 30 amino acid residues. As polymerization of the chain progresses, the amino acid residues at the N-terminal end begin to emerge from this protected region within the ribosome and to fold and refold into the three-dimensional conformation of the polypeptide. Proteins bind to the nascent polypeptide and mediate the folding process. These mediators are called chaperones (see Chapter 7) because they prevent improper interactions from occurring. Disulfide bond formation between cysteine residues is catalyzed by disulfide isomerases and may also be involved in producing the three-dimensional structure of the polypeptide.

VIII. POSTTRANSLATIONAL MODIFICATIONS

After proteins emerge from the ribosome, they may undergo posttranslational modifications. The initial methionine is removed by specific proteases; methionine is not the N-terminal amino acid of all proteins. Subsequently, other specific cleavages also may occur that convert proteins to more active forms (e.g., the conversion of proinsulin to insulin). In addition, amino acid residues within the peptide chain can be enzymatically modified to alter the activity or stability of the proteins, direct it to a subcellular compartment, or prepare it for secretion from the cell.

Amino acid residues are enzymatically modified by the addition of various types of functional groups. (Box 15.1) For example, the N-terminal amino acid is sometimes acetylated, and methyl groups can be added to lysine residues. These changes alter the charge on the protein. Proline and lysine residues can be modified by hydroxylation. In collagen, hydroxylations lead to stabilization of the protein. Carboxylations are important, especially for the function of proteins involved in blood coagulation. Formation of γ-carboxylglutamate allows these proteins to chelate Ca^{2+}, a step in clot formation. Fatty acids or other hydrophobic groups (e.g., prenyl groups) anchor the protein in membranes. An ADP–ribose group can be transferred from NAD^+ to certain proteins. The addition and removal of phosphate groups (which bind covalently to serine, threonine, or tyrosine residues) serve to regulate the activity of many proteins (e.g., the enzymes of glycogen degradation and regulators of gene transcription.) Glycosylation, the addition of carbohydrate groups, is a common modification that occurs mainly on proteins that are destined to be secreted or incorporated into lysosomes or cellular membranes.

Box 15.1 Posttranslational Modifications of Proteins

Acetylation
ADP-ribosylation
Carboxylation
Fatty acylation
Glycosylation
Hydroxylation
Methylation
Phosphorylation
Prenylation

IX. TARGETING OF PROTEINS TO SUBCELLULAR AND EXTRACELLULAR LOCATIONS

Many proteins are synthesized on polysomes in the cytosol. After they are released from ribosomes, they remain in the cytosol, where they carry out their functions. Other proteins synthesized on cytosolic ribosomes enter organelles,

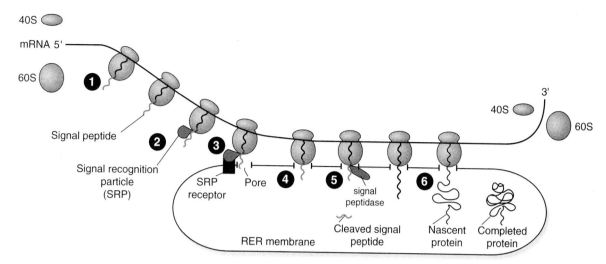

Fig. 15.13. Synthesis of proteins on the RER. **1.** Translation of the protein begins in the cytosol. **2.** As the signal peptide emerges from the ribosome, a signal recognition particle (SRP) binds to it and to the ribosome and inhibits further synthesis of the protein. **3.** The SRP binds to the SRP receptor in the RER membrane, docking the ribosome on the RER. **4.** The SRP is released and protein synthesis resumes. **5.** As the signal peptide moves through a pore into the RER, a signal peptidase removes the signal peptide. **6.** Synthesis of the nascent protein continues, and the completed protein is released into the lumen of the RER.

such as mitochondria or nuclei. These proteins contain amino acid sequences called targeting sequences or signal sequences that facilitate their transport into a certain organelle. Another group of proteins are synthesized on ribosomes bound to the RER. These proteins are destined for secretion or for incorporation into various subcellular organelles (e.g., lysosomes, endoplasmic reticulum [ER], Golgi complex) or cellular membranes, including the plasma membrane. Proteins that enter the RER as they are being synthesized have signal peptides near their N-termini that do not have a common amino acid sequence. However, they do contain a number of hydrophobic residues and are 15 to 30 amino acids in length (Fig. 15.13). A signal recognition particle (SRP) binds to the ribosome and to the signal peptide as the nascent polypeptide emerges from the tunnel in the ribosome, and translation ceases. When the SRP subsequently binds to an SRP receptor (docking protein) on the RER, translation resumes, and the polypeptide begins to enter the lumen of the RER. The signal peptide is removed by the signal peptidase, and the remainder of the newly synthesized protein enters the lumen of the RER. These proteins are transferred in small vesicles to the Golgi complex.

The Golgi complex serves to process the proteins it receives from the RER and to sort them so that they are delivered to their appropriate destinations (Fig. 15.14). Processing, which can be initiated in the endoplasmic reticulum, involves glycosylation, the addition of carbohydrate groups, and modification of existing carbohydrate chains. Sorting signals permit delivery of proteins to their target locations. For example, glycosylation of enzymes destined to become lysosomal enzymes results in the presence of a mannose 6-phosphate residue on an oligosaccharide attached to the enzyme. This residue is recognized by the mannose 6-phosphate receptor protein, which incorporates the enzyme into a clathrin-coated vesicle. The vesicle travels to endosomes, and is eventually incorporated into lysosomes. Other proteins containing a KDEL (lys-asp-glu-leu) sequence at their carboxyl terminal are returned to the ER from the Golgi. Proteins with hydrophobic regions can embed in various membranes. Some proteins, whose sorting signals have not yet been determined, enter secretory vesicles and travel to the cell membrane, where they are secreted by the process of exocytosis.

 I-cell disease (Mucolipidosis II) is a disorder of protein targeting. Lysosomal proteins are not sorted properly from the Golgi to the lysosomes, and lysosomal enzymes end up secreted from the cell. This is because of a mutation in the enzyme N-acetylglucosamine phosphotransferase, which is a required first step for attaching the lysosomal targeting signal, mannose-6-phosphate, to lysosomal proteins. Thus, lysosomal proteins cannot be targeted to the lysosomes, and these organelles become clogged with materials that cannot be digested, destroying overall lysosomal function. This leads to a lysosomal storage disease of severe consequence, with death before the age of 8.

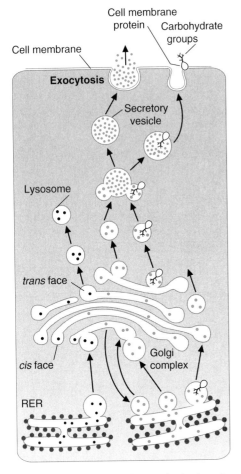

Fig. 15.14. Fate of proteins synthesized on the RER. Proteins synthesized on ribosomes attached to the ER travel in vesicles to the *cis* face of the Golgi complex. After the membranes fuse, the proteins enter the Golgi complex. Structural features of the proteins determine their fate. Some remain in the Golgi complex, and some return to the RER. Others bud from the *trans* face of the Golgi complex in vesicles. These vesicles can become lysosomes or secretory vesicles, depending on their contents. Secretory proteins are released from the cell when secretory vesicles fuse with the cell membrane (exocytosis). Proteins with hydrophobic regions embedded in the membrane of secretory vesicles become cell membrane proteins. See Chapter 10 for descriptions of the endoplasmic reticulum, Golgi complex, lysosomes, and the cell membrane, and also for an explanation of the process of exocytosis.

CLINICAL COMMENTS

✔ **Ann Niemick** has a β^+ thalassemia classified clinically as β-thalassemia intermedia. She produces an intermediate amount of functional β globin chains (her hemoglobin is 7 g/dL; normal is 12–16). In β^0-thalassemia, little or none of the hemoglobin β chain is produced. β-thalassemia intermedia is usually the result of two different mutations (one that mildly affects the rate of synthesis of β-globin and one severely affecting its rate of synthesis), or, less frequently, homozygosity for a mild mutation in the rate of synthesis, or a complex combination of mutations. The mutations that cause the thalassemias have been studied extensively and are summarized in Table 15.4. For each of these mutations, you should now be able to explain whether it is most likely to result in a β^+ or β^0 thalassemia.

✔ **Jay Sakz.** The molecular biology genetics laboratory's report on Jay Sakz's white blood cells indicated that he had a deficiency of hexosaminidase A caused by a defect in the gene encoding the α subunit of this enzyme (variant B, Tay-Sachs disease). Hexosaminidases are lysosomal enzymes necessary for the normal degradation of glycosphingolipids, such as the gangliosides. Gangliosides are found in high concentrations in neural ganglia, although they are produced in many areas of the nervous system. When the activity of these degradative enzymes is absent or subnormal, partially degraded gangliosides accumulate in lysosomes in various cells of the central nervous system, causing a wide array of neurologic disorders known collectively as gangliosidoses.

Table 15.4 Some Examples of Mutations in β-Thalassemia

Type of Mutation	Phenotype	Origin
Nonsense		
Codon 17 (A → T)	β^0	Chinese
Codon 39 (C → T)	β^0	Mediterranean
Codon 121 (A → T)	β^0	Polish
Frameshift		
Codon 6 (-1 bp)	β^0	Mediterranean
Codon 16 (-1 bp)	β^0	Asian Indian
Codon 41/42 (-4 bp)	β^0	Asian Indian, Chinese
Codon 71/72 (+1 bp)	β^0	Chinese
Promoter		
Position -88 (C → T)	β^+	African American
Position -31 (A → G)	β^+	Japanese
Position -28 (A → C)	β^+	Kurdish
Cap Site		
Position +1 (A → C)	β^+	Asian Indian
Splice Junction		
Intron 1, position 1 (G → A)	β^0	Mediterranean
Intron 1, 3'-end (-25 bp)	β^0	Asian Indian
Intron 2, position 1 (G → A)	β^0	Mediterranean
Intron 2, 3'-end (A → G)	β^0	African American
Intron, internal		
Intron 1, position 5 (G → T)	β^+	Mediterranean
Intron 1, position 6 (T → C)	β^+	Mediterranean
Intron 2, position 110 (G → A)	β^+	Mediterranean
Intron 2, position 654 (C → T)	β^0	Chinese
Intron 2, position 745 (C → G)	β^+	Mediterranean
Exon, internal		
Codon 24 (T → A)	β^+	African American
Codon 26 (G → A)	β^E	Southeast Asian
Codon 27 (G → T)	$\beta^{Knossos}$	Mediterranean
RNA cleavage/polyadenylation		
AATAAA ≠ AACAAA	β^+	African American

Data from Scriver CR, et al. The Metabolic and Molecular Basis of Inherited Diseases, Vol III. New York: McGraw-Hill, 1995:3456–3457.

When the enzyme deficiency is severe, symptoms appear within the first 3–5 months of life. Eventually symptoms include upper and lower motor neuron deficits, visual difficulties that can progress to blindness, seizures, and increasing cognitive dysfunction. By the second year of life, the patient may regress into a completely vegetative state, often succumbing to bronchopneumonia caused by aspiration or an inability to cough.

Erna Nemdy. With the availability of diphtheria toxoid as part of the almost universal DPT immunization practices in the United States, fatalities due to infection by the Gram-positive bacillus *C. diphtheriae* are rare. Most children, as is the case with Erna Nemdy's daughter Beverly, are immunized. In unimmunized individuals, however, symptoms are caused by a bacterial exotoxin encoded by a phage that infects the bacterial cells. The toxin enters human cells, inhibiting protein synthesis and, ultimately, causing cell death. Complications related to cardiac and nervous system involvement are the major cause of morbidity and mortality. Patients for whom a definitive diagnosis of diphtheria is established are treated with equine diphtheria antitoxin.

BIOCHEMICAL COMMENTS

Antibiotics That Inhibit Protein Synthesis. The processes of translation on bacterial ribosomes and on the cytoplasmic ribosomes of eukaryotic cells have many similarities, but there are a number of subtle differences. Antibiotics act at steps at which these differences occur, and different antibiotics target each of the major steps of protein synthesis (Table 15.5). Therefore, these compounds can be used selectively to prevent bacterial protein synthesis and inhibit bacterial proliferation, while having little or no effect on human cells. Caution must be exercised in their use, however, because some of the antibiotics affect human mitochondria, which have a protein-synthesizing system similar to that of bacteria. Another problem with these drugs is that bacteria can become resistant to their action. Mutations in genes encoding the proteins or RNA of bacterial ribosomes can cause resistance. Resistance also results when bacteria take up plasmids carrying genes for inactivation of the antibiotic. Because of the widespread and often indiscriminate use of antibiotics, strains of bacteria are rapidly developing that are resistant to all known antibiotics.

Streptomycin. Streptomycin inhibits initiation by binding to three proteins and probably the 16S rRNA of the 30S ribosomal subunit of bacteria. Abnormal initiation complexes, known as streptomycin monosomes, accumulate. Streptomycin can also cause misreading of mRNA, resulting in premature termination of translation or in the incorporation of incorrect amino acids into polypeptide chains that already have been initiated. The use of this antibiotic is limited because it causes ototoxicity that can result in loss of hearing.

Table 15.5 Inhibitors of Protein Synthesis in Prokaryotes

Antibiotic	Mode of Action
Streptomycin	Binds to the 30S ribosomal subunit of prokaryotes, thereby preventing formation of the initiation complex. It also causes misreading of mRNA
Tetracycline	Binds to the 30S ribosomal subunit and inhibits binding of aminoacyl-tRNA to the A site
Chloramphenicol	Binds to the 50S ribosomal subunit and inhibits peptidyltransferase
Erythromycin	Binds to the 50S ribosomal subunit and prevents translocation

Tetracycline. Tetracycline binds to the 30S ribosomal subunit of bacteria and prevents an aminoacyl-tRNA from binding to the A site on the ribosome. This effect of the drug is reversible; thus, when the drug is removed, bacteria resume protein synthesis and growth, resulting in a rekindling of the infection. Furthermore, tetracycline is not absorbed well from the intestine, and its concentration can become elevated in the contents of the gut, leading to changes in the intestinal flora. Because it has been used to treat human infections and added to animal feed to prevent animal infections, humans have had extensive exposure to tetracycline. As a result, resistant strains of bacteria have developed.

Chloramphenicol. Chloramphenicol binds to the 50S ribosomal subunit of bacteria and prevents binding of the amino acid portion of the aminoacyl-tRNA, effectively inhibiting peptidyltransferase action. This antibiotic is used only for certain extremely serious infections, such as meningitis and typhoid fever. Chloramphenicol readily enters human mitochondria, where it inhibits protein synthesis. Cells of the bone marrow often fail to develop in patients treated with chloramphenicol, and use of this antibiotic has been linked to fatal blood dyscrasias, including an aplastic anemia.

Erythromycin. Erythromycin and the other macrolide antibiotics bind to the 50S ribosomal subunit of bacteria near the binding site for chloramphenicol. They prevent the translocation step, the movement of the peptidyl-tRNA from the "A" to the "P" site on the ribosome. Because the side effects are less severe and more readily reversible than those of many other antibiotics, the macrolides are often used to treat infections in persons who are allergic to penicillin, an antibiotic that inhibits bacterial cell wall synthesis. However, bacterial resistance to erythromycin is increasing. Therefore, its close relative, clarithromycin, is often used.

Suggested References

Translation:
Pestova TV, Hellen CUT. Ribosome recruitment and scanning. TIBS 1999;24:85–87.
Lewin B. Genes VII. Protein synthesis. Translation: expressing genes as proteins. Oxford: Oxford University Press, 2000:139–166.
Tay-Sachs:
Gravel R, Clarke J, Kaback M, et al. The Gm2 gangliosidoses. In: Scriver C, Beaudet A, Sly W, Valle D (eds). The Metabolic and Molecular Bases of Inherited Disease. 8th Ed. Vol III. New York: McGraw-Hill, 2001:3827–3876.
Thalassemia:
Weatherall D, Clegg J, Higgs D, Wood W. The hemoglobinopathies. In: Scriver C, Beaudet A, Sly W, Valle D, eds. The Metabolic and Molecular Bases of Inherited Disease. 8th Ed. Vol III. New York: McGraw-Hill, 2001:4571–4636.
Antibiotics that inhibit protein synthesis:
Hardman JG, Limbird LE, et al. Goodman and Gilman's The Pharmacological Basis of Therapeutics. New York: McGraw-Hill, 1996:1103–1153.

 REVIEW QUESTIONS—CHAPTER 15

1.   In the read-out of the genetic code in prokaryotes, which one of the following processes acts before any of the others?

(A) tRNA$_i$ alignment with mRNA
(B) Termination of transcription
(C) Movement of the ribosome from one codon to the next
(D) Recruitment of termination factors to the A site
(E) Export of mRNA from the nucleus

2. tRNA charged with cysteine can be chemically treated so that the amino acid changes its identity to alanine. If some of this charged tRNA is added to a protein-synthesizing extract that contains ALL the normal components required for translation, which of the following statements represents THE MOST LIKELY OUTCOME after adding an mRNA that has both cys and ala codons in the normal reading frame?

    (A) Cysteine would be added each time the alanine codon was translated.
    (B) Alanine would be added each time the cysteine codon was translated.
    (C) The protein would have a deficiency of cysteine residues.
    (D) The protein would have a deficiency of alanine residues.
    (E) The protein would be entirely normal.

3. The genetic code is said to be degenerate because of which of the following?

    (A) Many codons have pairs of identical bases next to each other.
    (B) Some triplets are made up of repeating purines or pyrimidines.
    (C) Many of the amino acids have more than one triplet code.
    (D) There is wobble in the bond between the first base of the anticodon and the third base of the codon.
    (E) All triplets seem to have at least one uracil.

4. Which of the following is responsible for retaining the enzyme protein disulfide isomerase in the ER?

    (A) Glycosylation
    (B) The presence of a KDEL sequence at the C-terminal
    (C) Retention of the signal peptide
    (D) Phosphorylation of Ser 22
    (E) Attachment of a fatty acid

5. The reason there are 64 possible codons is which of the following?

    (A) There are 64 aminoacyl tRNA synthetases.
    (B) Each base is able to participate in wobbling.
    (C) All possible reading frames can be used this way.
    (D) There are four possible bases at each of three codon positions.
    (E) The more codons, the faster protein synthesis can be accomplished.

16 Regulation of Gene Expression

The prokaryotic bacterium *Escherichia coli* can use a wide range of different nutrients to sustain growth. It accomplishes this partially by turning on and off expression of the genes required for synthesis of enzymes in different metabolic pathways. For example, enzymes encoded by the *lac* operon allow *E. coli* to use lactose for energy and the presence of lactose activates transcription of these genes. Thus, the nutrient itself is involved in regulating gene expression.

In contrast, the cells of the adult human are exposed to a nearly constant and safe environment composed of blood and interstitial fluid. Hormones maintain this nearly constant environment, in spite of changes in nutrient demand and availability, partially by regulating gene transcription. The immune system protects cells against foreign organisms, partially by controlling the expression of genes required for the immune response. However, some nutrient regulation of gene expression also occurs. For example, iron controls expression of the genes for its storage and transport proteins at the level of their mRNAs.

Gene expression, the generation of a protein or RNA product from a particular gene, is controlled by complex mechanisms. Normally, only a fraction of the genes in a cell are expressed at any time. Gene expression is regulated differently in prokaryotes and eukaryotes.

Regulation of gene expression in prokaryotes. In prokaryotes, gene expression is regulated mainly by controlling the **initiation of gene transcription.** *Sets of genes encoding proteins with related functions are organized into* **operons,** *and each operon is under the control of* **a single promoter** *(or regulatory region). Regulatory proteins called* **repressors** *bind to the promoter and inhibit the binding of RNA polymerase* **(negative control),** *whereas* **activator proteins** *facilitate RNA polymerase binding* **(positive control).** *Repressors are controlled by nutrients or their metabolites, classified as* **inducers** *or corepressors. Regulation also may occur through* **attenuation of transcription.**

*Eukaryotes: Regulation of gene expression at the level of DNA. In eukaryotes, activation of a gene requires changes in the state of chromatin (**chromatin remodeling**) that are facilitated by* **acetylation of histones and methylation of bases.** *These changes in DNA determine which genes are available for transcription.*

Regulation of eukaryotic gene transcription. Transcription of specific genes is regulated by proteins (called **specific transcription factors or transactivators)** *that bind to* **gene regulatory sequences** *(called* **promoter-proximal elements, response elements, or enhancers)** *that activate or inhibit assembly of the basal transcription complex and RNA polymerase at the TATA box. These specific transcription factors, which may bind to DNA sequences some distance from the promoter, interact with coactivators or corepressors that bind to components of the basal transcription complex. These protein factors are said to work in* **"trans"**; *the DNA sequences to which they bind are said to work in* **"cis."**

Other sites for regulation of eukaryotic gene expression. Regulation also occurs during the **processing** *of RNA, during RNA* **transport** *from the nucleus to the cytoplasm, and at the level of* **translation** *in the cytoplasm. Regulation can occur simultaneously at multiple levels for a specific gene, and many factors act in concert to stimulate or inhibit expression of a gene.*

THE WAITING ROOM

Arlyn Foma, a 68-year old man, complained of fatigue, loss of appetite, and a low-grade fever. An open biopsy of a lymph node indicated the presence of non-Hodgkin's lymphoma, follicular type. Computed tomography and other noninvasive procedures showed a diffuse process with bone marrow involvement. He is receiving multidrug chemotherapy with AV/CM (doxorubicin [adriamycin], vincristine, cyclophosphamide, and methotrexate). His disease is not responding well to this regimen, and the follicular lymphoma appears to be evolving into a more aggressive process. Because recombinant interferon α-2b has been reported to have synergistic or additive effects with these agents, it is added to the protocol. Although resistance to methotrexate is considered, the drug is continued as part of the combined therapeutic approach.

Mannie Weitzels is a 56-year-old male who complains of headaches, weight loss related to a declining appetite for food, and a decreasing tolerance for exercise. He notes discomfort and fullness in the left upper quadrant of his abdomen. On physical examination, he is noted to be pale and to have ecchymoses (bruises) on his arms and legs. His spleen is markedly enlarged.

Initial laboratory studies show a hemoglobin of 10.4 g/dL (normal = 13.5–17.5 g/dL) and a leukocyte (white blood cell) count of 86,000 cells/mm³ (normal = 4,500–11,000 cells/mm³). Most of the leukocytes are granulocytes (white blood cells arising from the myeloid lineage), some of which have an "immature" appearance. The percentage of lymphocytes in the peripheral blood is decreased. A bone marrow aspiration and biopsy show the presence of an abnormal chromosome (the Philadelphia chromosome) in dividing marrow cells.

Ann O'Rexia, who has anorexia nervosa, has continued on an almost meat-free diet (see Chapters 1, 3, 9, and 11). She now appears emaciated and pale. Her hemoglobin is 9.7 g/dL (normal = 12−16 g/dL), her hematocrit (volume of packed red cells) is 31% (reference range for women = 36−46%), and her mean corpuscular hemoglobin (the average amount of hemoglobin per red cell) is 21 pg/cell (reference range = 26−34 pg/cell). These values indicate an anemia that is microcytic (small red cells) and hypochromic (light in color, indicating a reduced amount of hemoglobin per red cell). Her serum ferritin (the cellular storage form of iron) was also subnormal. Her plasma level of transferrin (the iron transport protein in plasma) was greater than normal, but its percent saturation with iron was below normal. This laboratory profile is consistent with changes that occur in an iron deficiency state.

I. GENE EXPRESSION IS REGULATED FOR ADAPTATION AND DIFFERENTIATION

Although most cells of an organism contain identical sets of genes, at any given time only a small number of the total genes in each cell are expressed (that is, generate a protein or RNA product). The remaining genes are inactive. Organisms gain a number of advantages by regulating the activity of their genes. For example, both prokaryotic and eukaryotic cells adapt to changes in their environment by turning the expression of genes on and off. Because the processes of RNA transcription and protein synthesis consume a considerable amount of energy, cells conserve fuel by making proteins only when they are needed.

In addition to regulating gene expression to adapt to environmental changes, eukaryotic organisms alter expression of their genes during development. As a fertilized egg becomes a multicellular organism, different kinds of proteins are synthesized in varying quantities. In the human, as the child progresses through adolescence and then into adulthood, physical and physiologic changes result from variations in gene expression and, therefore, of protein synthesis. Even after an organism has reached the adult stage, regulation of gene expression enables certain cells to undergo differentiation to assume new functions.

 Each of the drugs used by **Arlyn Foma** inhibits the proliferation of cancer cells in a different way. Doxorubicin (adriamycin) is a large nonpolar molecule synthesized by fungi that intercalates between DNA bases, inhibiting replication and transcription and forming DNA with single- and double-stranded breaks. Vincristine binds to tubulin and inhibits formation of the mitotic spindle, thereby preventing cell division. Cyclophosphamide is an alkylating agent that damages DNA by covalently attaching alkyl groups to DNA bases. Methotrexate is an analogue of the vitamin folate. It inhibits folate-requiring enzymes in the pathways for synthesis of thymine and purines, thereby depriving cells of precursors for DNA synthesis.

E. coli is a facultative anaerobe, which means that it can grow in the presence or absence of oxygen. The switch to oxygen-requiring pathways for fuel metabolism is under control of *arc*, the **a**erobic **r**espiration **c**ontrol gene. When *arc* is activated, transcription is increased by 1,000-fold or more for enzymes in the pathways that ultimately transfer electrons to oxygen (e.g., proteins of the respiratory chain, the TCA cycle, and fatty acid oxidation). In the absence of oxygen (i.e., anaerobic, without air), these proteins are not synthesized, an energy-saving feature useful for bacteria growing in the largely anaerobic colon. Most human cells, in contrast, express constant (constitutive) levels of respiratory enzymes and die without oxygen.

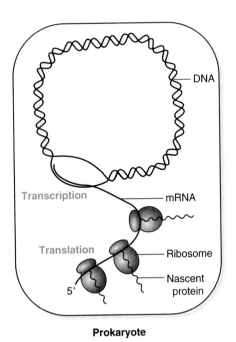

Prokaryote

Fig. 16.1. *E. coli* cell. In prokaryotes, DNA is not separated from the rest of the cellular contents by a nuclear envelope; therefore, simultaneous transcription and translation occur in bacteria. Once a small piece of mRNA is synthesized, ribosomes bind to the mRNA, and translation begins.

II. REGULATION OF GENE EXPRESSION IN PROKARYOTES

Prokaryotes are single-celled organisms and, therefore, require less complex regulatory mechanisms than the multicellular eukaryotes (Fig. 16.1). The most extensively studied prokaryote is the bacterium *Escherichia coli*, an organism that thrives in the human colon, usually enjoying a symbiotic relationship with its host. Based on the size of its genome (4×10^6 base pairs), *E. coli* should be capable of making several thousand proteins. However, under normal growth conditions, they synthesize only about 600 to 800 different proteins. Obviously, many genes are inactive, and only those genes are expressed that generate the proteins required for growth in that particular environment.

All *E. coli* cells of the same strain are morphologically similar and contain an identical circular chromosome (see Fig. 16.1). As in other prokaryotes, DNA is not complexed with histones, no nuclear envelope separates the genes from the contents of the cytoplasm, and gene transcripts do not contain introns. In fact, as mRNA is being synthesized, ribosomes bind and begin to produce proteins, so that transcription and translation occur simultaneously. The mRNAs in *E. coli* have very short half-lives and are degraded within a few minutes so that an mRNA must be constantly generated from transcription to maintain synthesis of its proteins. Thus, regulation of transcription, principally at the level of initiation, is sufficient to regulate the level of proteins within the cell.

A. Operons

The genes encoding proteins are called structural genes. In the bacterial genome, the structural genes for proteins involved in performing a related function (such as the enzymes of a biosynthetic pathway) are often grouped sequentially into units called operons (Fig. 16.2). The genes in an operon are coordinately expressed; that is, they are either all "turned on" or all "turned off." When an operon is expressed, all of its genes are transcribed. A single polycistronic mRNA is produced that codes for all the proteins of the operon. This polycistronic mRNA contains multiple sets of start and stop codons that allow a number of different proteins to be produced from this single transcript at the translational level. Transcription of the genes in an operon is regulated by its promoter, which is located in the operon at the 5′-end, upstream from the structural genes.

B. Regulation of RNA Polymerase Binding by Repressors

In bacteria, the principle means of regulating gene transcription is through repressors, which are regulatory proteins that prevent the binding of RNA polymerase to the promoter and, thus, act on initiation of transcription (Fig. 16.3). In general,

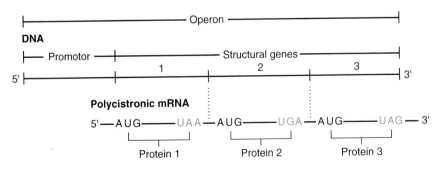

Fig. 16.2. An operon. The structural genes of an operon are transcribed as one long polycistronic mRNA. During translation, different start (AUG) and stop (shown in blue) codons lead to a number of distinct proteins being produced from this single mRNA.

regulatory mechanisms such as repressors that work through inhibition of gene transcription are referred to as negative control, and mechanisms that work through stimulation of gene transcription are called positive control.

The repressor is encoded by a regulatory gene (see Fig. 16.3). Although this gene is considered part of the operon, it is not always located near the remainder of the operon. Its product, the repressor protein, diffuses to the promoter and binds to a region of the operon called the operator. The operator is located within the promoter or near its 3'-end, just upstream from the transcription startpoint. When a repressor is bound to the operator, the operon is not transcribed because the repressor blocks the binding of RNA polymerase to the promoter. Two regulatory mechanisms work through controlling repressors: induction (an inducer inactivates the repressor), and repression (a co-repressor is required to activate the repressor).

1. INDUCERS

Induction involves a small molecule, known as an inducer, which stimulates expression of the operon by binding to the repressor and changing its conformation so that it can no longer bind to the operator (Fig. 16.4). The inducer is either a nutrient or a metabolite of the nutrient. In the presence of the inducer, RNA polymerase can therefore bind to the promoter and transcribe the operon. The key to this mechanism is that *in the absence of the inducer, the repressor is active, transcription is repressed, and the genes of the operon are not expressed.*

Consider, for example, induction of the *lac* operon of *E.* coli by lactose (Fig. 16.5). The enzymes for metabolizing glucose by glycolysis are produced constitutively; that is, they are constantly being made. If the milk sugar lactose is available, the cells adapt and begin to produce the three additional enzymes required for lactose metabolism, which are encoded by the *lac* operon. A metabolite of lactose (allolactose) serves as an inducer, binding to the repressor and inactivating it. Because the inactive repressor no longer binds to the operator, RNA polymerase can bind to the promoter and transcribe the structural genes of the *lac* operon, producing a polycistronic mRNA that encodes for the three additional proteins. However, the presence of glucose can prevent activation of the lac operon (see "Stimulation of RNA polymerase binding," below).

2. COREPRESSORS

In a regulatory model called repression, the repressor is inactive until a small molecule called a corepressor (a nutrient or its metabolite) binds to the repressor, activating it (Fig. 16.6). The repressor–corepressor complex then binds to the operator, preventing binding of RNA polymerase and gene transcription. Consider, for example, the trp operon, which encodes the five enzymes required for the synthesis of the amino acid tryptophan. When tryptophan is available, *E. coli* cells save energy by no longer making these enzymes. Tryptophan is a corepressor that binds to the inactive repressor, causing it to change conformation and bind to the operator, thereby inhibiting transcription of the operon. *Thus, in the repression model, the repressor is inactive without a corepressor; in the induction model, the repressor is active unless an inducer is present.*

If one of the *lac* operon enzymes induced by lactose is lactose permease (which increases lactose entry into the cell), how does lactose initially get into the cell to induce these enzymes? A small amount of the permease exists even in the absence of lactose, and a few molecules of lactose enter the cell and are metabolized to allolactose, which begins the process of inducing the operon. As the amount of the permease increases, more lactose can be transported into the cell.

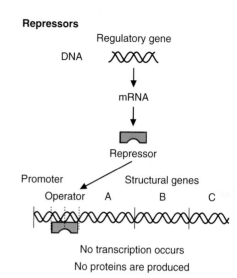

Repressors

No transcription occurs
No proteins are produced

Fig. 16.3. Regulation of operons by repressors. When the repressor protein is bound to the operator, RNA polymerase cannot bind, and transcription therefore does not occur.

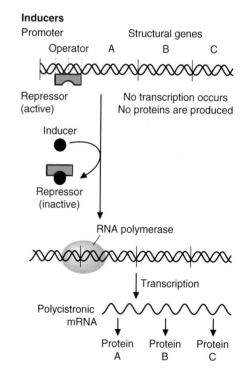

Inducers

No transcription occurs
No proteins are produced

Fig. 16.4. An inducible operon. In the absence of an inducer, the repressor binds to the operator, preventing the binding of RNA polymerase. When the inducer is present, the inducer binds to the repressor, inactivating it. The inactive repressor no longer binds to the operator. Therefore, RNA polymerase can bind to the promoter region and transcribe the structural genes.

The lac operon

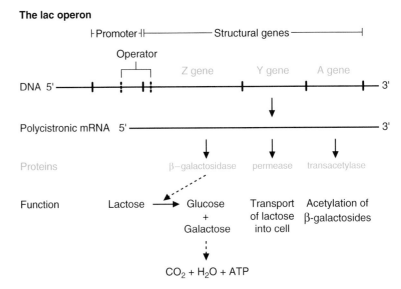

Fig. 16.5. The protein products of the *lac* operon. Lactose is a disaccharide that is hydrolyzed to glucose and galactose by β-galactosidase (the Z gene). Both glucose and galactose can be oxidized by the cell for energy. The permease (Y gene) enables the cell to take up lactose more readily. The A gene produces a transacetylase that acetylates β-galactosides. The function of this acetylation is not clear. The promoter binds RNA polymerase and the operator binds a repressor protein. Lactose is converted to allolactose, an inducer that binds the repressor protein and prevents it from binding to the operator. Transcription of the lac operon also requires activator proteins that are inactive when glucose levels are high.

C. Stimulation of RNA Polymerase Binding

In addition to regulating transcription by means of repressors that inhibit RNA polymerase binding to promoters (negative control), bacteria regulate transcription by means of activating proteins that bind to the promoter and stimulate the binding of RNA polymerase (positive control). Transcription of the *lac* operon, for example, can be induced by allolactose only if glucose is absent. The presence or absence of glucose is communicated to the promoter by a regulatory protein named the cyclic adenosine monophosphate (cAMP) receptor protein (CRP)

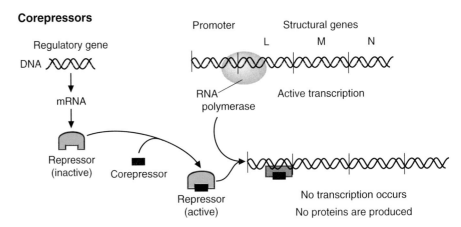

Fig. 16.6. A repressible operon. The repressor is inactive until a small molecule, the corepressor, binds to it. The repressor–corepressor complex binds to the operator and prevents transcription.

A. In the presence of lactose and glucose

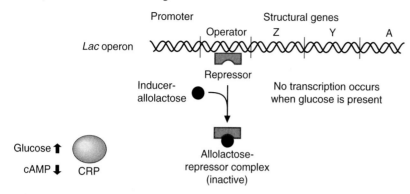

B. In the presence of lactose and absence of glucose

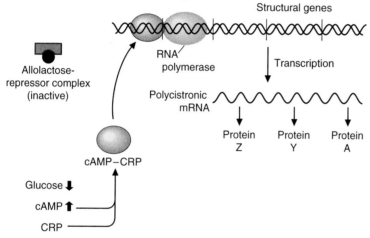

Fig. 16.7. Catabolite repression of stimulatory proteins. The *lac* operon is used as an example. **A.** The inducer allolactose (a metabolite of lactose) inactivates the repressor. However, because of the absence of the required coactivator, cAMP-CRP, no transcription occurs unless glucose is absent. **B.** In the absence of glucose, cAMP levels rise. cAMP forms a complex with the cAMP receptor protein (CRP). The binding of the cAMP–CRP complex to a regulatory region of the operon permits the binding of RNA polymerase to the promoter. Now the operon is transcribed, and the proteins are produced.

(Fig. 16.7). This regulatory protein is also called a catabolite activator protein (CAP). A decrease in glucose levels increases levels of the intracellular second messenger cAMP by a mechanism that is not well understood. cAMP binds to CRP, and the cAMP-CRP complex binds to a regulatory region of the operon, stimulating binding of RNA polymerase to the promoter and transcription. When glucose is present, cAMP levels decrease, CRP assumes an inactive conformation that does not bind to the operon, and transcription is inhibited. Thus, the enzymes encoded by the *lac* operon are not produced if cells have an adequate supply of glucose, even if lactose is present at very high levels.

Nutrient regulation of gene expression may occur through the nutrient itself, or through a metabolite of the nutrient synthesized inside the cell. Sometimes both the nutrient and its metabolite are grouped into the term "catabolite," as in "catabolite repression."

D. Regulation of RNA Polymerase Binding by Sigma Factors

E. coli has only one RNA polymerase. Sigma factors bind to this RNA polymerase, stimulating its binding to certain sets of promoters, thus simultaneously activating transcription of several operons. The standard sigma factor in *E. coli* is

σ^{70}, a protein with a molecular weight of 70,000 daltons (see Chapter 14). Other sigma factors also exist. For example, σ^{32} helps RNA polymerase recognize promoters for the different operons that encode the "heat shock" proteins. Thus, increased transcription of the genes for heat shock proteins, which prevent protein denaturation at high temperatures, occurs in response to elevated temperatures.

E. Attenuation of Transcription

Some operons are regulated by a process that interrupts (attenuates) transcription after it has been initiated (Fig. 16.8). For example, high levels of tryptophan attenuate transcription of the E. coli *trp* operon, as well as repress its transcription. As mRNA is being transcribed from the *trp* operon, ribosomes bind and rapidly begin to translate the transcript. Near the 5′-end of the transcript, there are a number of codons for tryptophan. Initially, high levels of tryptophan in the cell result in high levels of trp-tRNA^{trp} and rapid translation of the transcript. However, rapid translation generates a hairpin loop in the mRNA that serves as a termination signal for RNA polymerase, and transcription terminates. Conversely, when tryptophan levels are low, levels of trp-tRNA^{trp} are low, and ribosomes stall at codons for tryptophan. A different hairpin loop forms in the mRNA that does not terminate transcription, and the complete mRNA is transcribed.

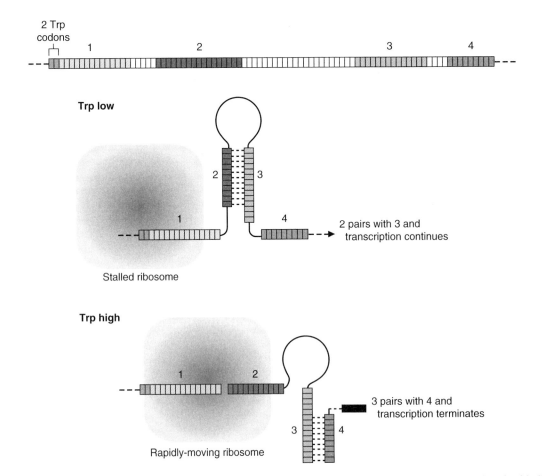

Fig. 16.8. Attenuation of the *trp* operon. Sequences 2, 3, and 4 in the mRNA transcript can form base pairs (2 with 3 or 3 with 4) that generate hairpin loops. When tryptophan levels are low, the ribosome stalls at the adjacent trp codons in sequence 1, the 2–3 loop forms, and transcription continues. When tryptophan levels are high, translation is rapid and the ribosome blocks formation of the 2–3 loop. Under these conditions, the 3–4 loop forms and terminates transcription.

The tryptophan, histidine, leucine, phenylalanine, and threonine operons are regulated by attenuation. Repressors and activators also act on the promoters of some of these operons, allowing the levels of these amino acids to be very carefully and rapidly regulated.

III. REGULATION OF PROTEIN SYNTHESIS IN EUKARYOTES

Multicellular eukaryotes are much more complex than single-celled prokaryotes. As the human embryo develops into a multicellular organism, different sets of genes are turned on, and different groups of proteins are produced, resulting in differentiation into morphologically distinct cell types able to perform different functions. Even beyond the reproductive age, certain cells within the organism continue to differentiate, such as those that produce antibodies in response to an infection, renew the population of red blood cells, and replace digestive cells that have been sloughed into the intestinal lumen. All of these physiologic changes are dictated by complex alterations in gene expression.

A. Regulation of Eukaryotic Gene Expression at Multiple Levels

Differences between eukaryotic and prokaryotic cells result in different mechanisms for regulating gene expression. DNA in eukaryotes is organized into the nucleosomes of chromatin, and genes must be in an active structure to be expressed in a cell. Furthermore, operons are not present in eukaryotes, and the genes encoding proteins that function together are usually located on different chromosomes. Thus, each gene needs its own promoter. In addition, the processes of transcription and translation are separated in eukaryotes by intracellular compartmentation (nucleus and cytosol, or endoplasmic reticulum [ER]) and by time (eukaryotic hnRNA must be processed and translocated out of the nucleus before it is translated). Thus, regulation of eukaryotic gene expression occurs at multiple levels:

- DNA and the chromosome, including chromosome remodeling and gene rearrangement
- Transcription, primarily through transcription factors affecting binding of RNA polymerase
- Processing of transcripts
- Initiation of translation and stability of mRNA

Once a gene is activated through chromatin remodeling, the major mechanism of regulating expression affects initiation of transcription at the promoter.

B. Regulation of Availability of Genes for Transcription

Once a haploid sperm and egg combine to form a diploid cell, the number of genes in human cells remains approximately the same. As cells differentiate, different genes are available for transcription. A typical nucleus contains chromatin that is condensed (heterochromatin) and chromatin that is diffuse (euchromatin)(Fig. 16.9) (see Chapter 12). The genes in heterochromatin are inactive, whereas those in euchromatin produce mRNA. Long-term changes in the activity of genes occur during development as chromatin goes from a diffuse to a condensed state or vice versa.

The cellular genome is packaged together with histones into nucleosomes, and initiation of transcription is prevented if the promoter region is part of a nucleosome. Thus, activation of a gene for transcription requires changes in the state of the chromatin, called chromatin remodeling. The availability of genes for transcription

The globin chains of hemoglobin provide an example of functionally related proteins that are on different chromosomes. The gene for the α-globin chain is on chromosome 16, whereas the gene for the β-globin chain is on chromosome 11. As a consequence of this spatial separation, each gene must have its own promoter. This situation is different from that of bacteria, in which genes encoding proteins that function together are often sequentially arranged in operons controlled by a single promoter.

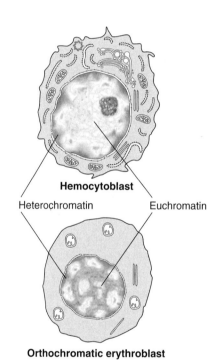

Hemocytoblast

Heterochromatin   Euchromatin

Orthochromatic erythroblast

Reticulocyte

Fig. 16.9. Inactivation of genes during development of red blood cells. Diffuse chromatin (euchromatin) is active in RNA synthesis. Condensed chromatin (heterochromatin) is inactive. As red blood cell precursors mature, their chromatin becomes more condensed. Eventually, the nucleus is extruded.

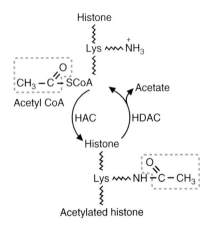

Fig. 16.10. Histone acetylation. Abbreviations: HAC, histone acetylase; HDAC, histone deacetylase.

also can be affected in certain cells, or under certain circumstances, by gene rearrangements, amplification, or deletion. For example, during lymphocyte maturation, genes are rearranged to produce a variety of different antibodies.

1. CHROMATIN REMODELING

The remodeling of chromatin generally refers to displacement of the nucleosome from specific DNA sequences so that transcription of the genes in that sequence can be initiated. This occurs through two different mechanisms. The first mechanism is by an adenosine triphosphate (ATP)-driven chromatin remodeling complex, which uses energy from ATP hydrolysis to unwind certain sections of DNA from the nucleosome core. The second mechanism is by covalent modification of the histone tails through acetylation (Fig. 16.10). Histone acetyltransferases (HAT) transfer an acetyl group from acetyl CoA to lysine residues in the tail (the amino terminal ends of histones H2A, H2B, H3, and H4). This reaction removes a positive charge from the ε-amino group of the lysine, thereby reducing the electrostatic interactions between the histones and the negatively charged DNA, making it easier for DNA to unwind from the histones. The acetyl groups can be removed by histone deacetylases (HDAC). Each histone has a number of lysine residues that may be acetylated and, through a complex mixing of acetylated and nonacetylated sites, different segments of DNA can be freed from the nucleosome. A number of transcription factors and co-activators also contain histone acetylase activity, which facilitates the binding of these factors to the DNA and simultaneous activation of the gene and initiation of its transcription.

2. METHYLATION OF DNA

Cytosine residues in DNA can be methylated to produce 5-methylcytosine. The methylated cytosines are located in GC-rich sequences (called GC-islands), which are often near or in the promoter region of a gene. In certain instances, genes that are methylated are less readily transcribed than those that are not methylated. For example, globin genes are more extensively methylated in nonerythroid cells (cells which are not a part of the erythroid, or red blood cell, lineage) than in the cells in which these genes are expressed (such as the erythroblast and reticulocyte). Methylation is a mechanism for regulating gene expression during differentiation, particularly in fetal development.

Methylation has been implicated in genomic imprinting, a process occurring during the formation of the eggs or sperm that blocks the expression of the gene in the fertilized egg. Males methylate a different set of genes than females. This sex-dependant differential methylation has been most extensively studied in two human disorders, Prader-Willi syndrome and Angelman syndrome. Both syndromes, which have very different symptoms, result from deletions of the same region of chromosome 15 (a microdeletion of less than 5 megabases in size). If the deletion is inherited from the father, Prader-Willi syndrome is seen in the child; if the deletion is inherited from the mother, Angelman's syndrome is observed. A disease occurs when a gene that is in the deleted region of one chromosome is methylated on the other chromosome. The mother methylates different genes than the father, so different genes are expressed depending on which parent transmitted the intact chromosome. For example, if genes 1, 2, and 3 are deleted in the paternal chromosome in the Prader-Willi syndrome, and gene 2 is methylated in the maternal chromosome, only genes 1 and 3 will be expressed. If in the Angelman syndrome, genes 1, 2 and 3 are deleted on the maternal chromosome and gene 1 is methylated on the paternal chromosome, only genes 2 and 3 would be expressed.

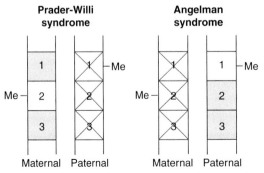

3. GENE REARRANGEMENT

Segments of DNA can move from one location to another in the genome, associating with each other in various ways so that different proteins are produced (Fig. 16.11). The most thoroughly studied example of gene rearrangement occurs in cells that produce antibodies. Antibodies contain two light chains and two heavy chains, each of which contains both a variable and a constant region (see Chapter 7, section V.B, Fig. 7.19). Cells called B cells make antibodies. In the precursors of B cells, hundreds of V_H sequences, approximately 20 D_H sequences, and approximately 6 J_H sequences are located in clusters within a long region of the chromosome. During the production of the immature B cells, a series of recombinational events occur that join one V_H, one D_H, and one J_H sequence into a single exon. This now encodes the variable region of the heavy chain of the antibody. Given the large number of immature B cells that are produced, virtually every recombinational possibility occurs, such that all VDJ combinations are represented within this cell population. Later in development, during differentiation of mature B cells, recombinational events join a VDJ sequence to one of the nine heavy chain elements. When the immune system encounters an antigen, the one immature B cell that can bind to that antigen (because of its unique manner in forming the VDJ exon) is stimulated to proliferate (clonal expansion) and to produce antibodies against the antigen.

4. GENE AMPLIFICATION

Gene amplification is not the usual physiologic means of regulating gene expression in normal cells, but it does occur in response to certain stimuli if the cell can obtain a growth advantage by producing large amounts of a protein. In gene amplification, certain regions of a chromosome undergo repeated cycles of DNA replication. The newly synthesized DNA is excised and forms small, unstable chromosomes called "double minutes." The double minutes integrate into other chromosomes throughout the genome, thereby amplifying the gene in the process. Normally, gene amplification occurs through errors during DNA replication and cell division and, if the environmental conditions are correct, cells containing amplified genes may have a growth advantage over those without the amplification.

Although rearrangements of short DNA sequences are difficult to detect, microscopists have observed major rearrangements for many years. Such major rearrangements, known as translocations, can be observed in metaphase chromosomes under the microscope.

Mannie Weitzels has such a translocation, known as the Philadelphia chromosome because it was first observed in that city. The Philadelphia chromosome is produced by a balanced exchange between chromosomes 9 and 22.

Arlyn Foma has been treated with a combination of drugs that includes methotrexate, a drug that inhibits cell proliferation by inhibiting dihydrofolate reductase. Dihydrofolate reductase reduces dihydrofolate to tetrahydrofolate, a cofactor required for synthesis of thymine and purine nucleotides. Because Arlyn Foma has not been responding well, the possibility that he has become resistant to methotrexate was considered. Sometimes, rapidly dividing cancer cells treated with methotrexate amplify the gene for dihydrofolate reductase, producing hundreds of copies in the genome. These cells generate large amounts of difhydrofolate reductase, and normal doses of methotrexate are no longer adequate. Gene amplification is one of the mechanisms by which patients become resistant to a drug.

In fragile X syndrome, a GCC triplet is amplified on the 5'-side of a gene (FMR-1) associated with the disease. This gene is located on the X chromosome. The disease is named for the finding that in the absence of folic acid (which impairs nucleotide production and hence, the replication of DNA) the X chromosome develops single and double-stranded breaks in its DNA. These were termed fragile sites. It was subsequently determined that the FMR-1 gene was located in one of these fragile sites. A normal person has about 30 copies of the GCC triplet, but in affected individuals, thousands of copies can be present. This syndrome, which is a common form of inherited mental retardation, affects about 1 in 1,250 males and 1 in 2,000 females.

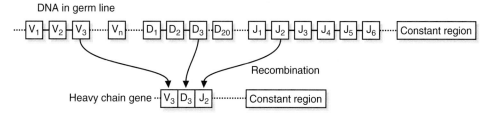

Fig. 16.11. Rearrangement of DNA. The heavy chain gene from which lymphocytes produce immunoglobulins is generated by combining specific segments from among a large number of potential sequences in the DNA of precursor cells. The variable and constant regions of immunoglobulins (antibodies) are described in Chapter 7.

5.   GENE DELETIONS

With a few exceptions, the deletion of genetic material is likewise not a normal means of controlling transcription, although such deletions do result in disease. Gene deletions can occur through errors in DNA replication and cell division and are usually only noticed if a disease results. For example, various types of cancers result from the loss of a good copy of a tumor suppressor gene, leaving the cell with a mutated copy of the gene (see Chapter 18).

C.   Regulation at the Level of Transcription

The transcription of active genes is regulated by controlling assembly of the basal transcription complex containing RNA polymerase and its binding to the TATA box of the promoter (see Chapter 14). The basal transcription complex contains the TATA binding protein (TBP, a component of TFIID) and other proteins called general (basal) transcription factors (such as TFIIA, etc.) that form a complex with RNA polymerase II. Additional transcription factors that are ubiquitous to all promoters bind upstream at various sites in the promoter region. They increase the frequency of transcription and are required for a promoter to function at an adequate level. Genes that are regulated solely by these consensus elements in the promoter region are said to be constitutively expressed.

The control region of a gene also contains DNA regulatory sequences that are specific for that gene and may increase its transcription 1,000-fold or more (Fig. 16.12). Gene-specific transcription factors (also called transactivators or activators) bind to these regulatory sequences and interact with a mediator protein, such as a coactivator. By forming a loop in the DNA, coactivators interact with the basal transcription complex and can activate its assembly at the initiation site on the promoter. These DNA regulatory sequences might be some distance from the promoter and may be either upstream or downstream of the initiation site.

1.   GENE-SPECIFIC REGULATORY PROTEINS

The regulatory proteins that bind directly to DNA sequences are most often called transcription factors or gene-specific transcription factors (if it is necessary to distinguish them from the general transcription factors of the basal transcription complex). They also can be called activators (or transactivators), inducers, repressors, or nuclear receptors. In addition to their DNA-binding domain, these proteins usually have a domain that binds to mediator proteins (coactivators, corepressors, or TATA binding protein associated factors–TAFs). Coactivators, corepressors, and other mediator proteins do not bind directly to DNA but generally bind to components of the basal transcription complex and mediate its assembly at the promoter. They can be specific for a given gene transcription factor or general and bind many different gene-specific transcription factors. Certain coactivators have histone acetylase activity, and certain corepressors have histone deacetylase activity. When the appropriate interactions between the transactivators, coactivators, and the basal transcription complex occur, the rate of transcription of the gene is increased (induction).

Some regulatory DNA binding proteins inhibit (repress) transcription and may be called repressors. Repression can occur in a number of ways. A repressor bound to its specific DNA sequence may inhibit binding of an activator to its regulatory sequence. Alternately, the repressor may bind a corepressor that inhibits binding of a coactivator to the basal transcription complex. The repressor may directly bind a component of the basal transcription complex. Some steroid hormone receptors that are transcription factors bind either coactivators or corepressors, depending on whether the receptor contains bound hormone. Furthermore, a particular transcription factor may induce transcription when bound to the regulatory sequence of one gene and may repress transcription when bound to the regulatory sequence of another gene.

 The terminology used to describe components of gene-specific regulation varies somewhat, depending on the system. For example, in the original terminology, DNA regulatory sequences called enhancers bound transactivators, which bound coactivators. Similarly, silencers bound corepressors. Hormones bound to hormone receptors, which bound to hormone response elements in DNA. Although these terms are still used, they are often replaced with more general terms such as "DNA regulatory sequences" and "specific transcription factors," in recognition of the fact that many transcription factors activate one gene while inhibiting another or that a specific transcription factor may be changed from a repressor to an activator by phosphorylation.

Histone acetylase activity has been associated with a number of transcription factors and co-activators. The proteins ACTR (activator of the thyroid and retinoic acid receptor) and SRC-1 (steroid receptor co-activator) are involved in activation of transcription by several ligand-bound nuclear receptors, and both contain histone acetylase activity. TAF250, a component of TFIID, also contains histone acetylase activity, as does the co-activator p300/CBP (CREB binding protein), which interacts with the transcription factor CREB.

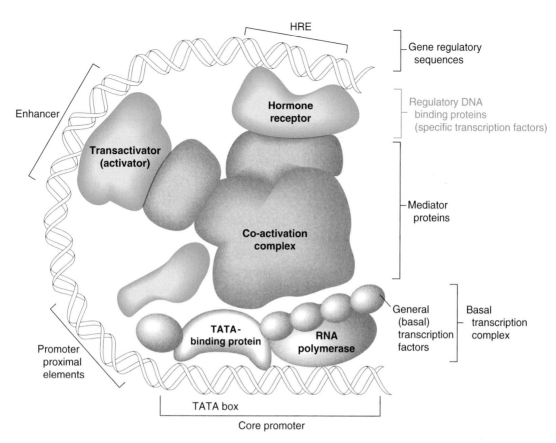

Fig. 16.12. The gene regulatory control region consists of the promoter region and additional gene regulatory sequences, including enhancers and hormone response elements (shown in blue). Gene regulatory proteins that bind directly to DNA (regulatory DNA binding proteins) are usually called specific transcription factors or transactivators; they may be either activators or repressors of the transcription of specific genes. The specific transcription factors bind mediator proteins (co-activators or corepressors) that interact with the general transcription factors of the basal transcription complex. The basal transcription complex contains RNA polymerase and associated general transcription factors (TFII factors) and binds to the TATA box of the promoter, initiating gene transcription.

2. TRANSCRIPTION FACTORS THAT ARE STEROID HORMONE/THYROID HORMONE RECEPTORS

In the human, steroid hormones and other lipophilic hormones activate or inhibit transcription of specific genes through binding to nuclear receptors that are gene-specific transcription factors (Fig. 16.13A). The nuclear receptors bind to DNA regulatory sequences called hormone response elements and induce or repress transcription of target genes. The receptors contain a hormone (ligand) binding domain, a DNA binding domain, and a dimerization domain that permits two receptor molecules to bind to each other, forming characteristic homodimers or heterodimers. A transactivation domain binds the coactivator proteins that interact with the basal transcription complex. The receptors also contain a nuclear localization signal domain that directs them to the nucleus at various times after they are synthesized.

Various members of the steroid hormone/thyroid hormone receptor family work in different ways. The glucocorticoid receptor, which binds the steroid hormone cortisol, resides principally in the cytosol bound to heat shock proteins. As cortisol binds, the receptor dissociates from the heat shock proteins, exposing the nuclear localization signal (see Fig. 16.13B). The receptors form homodimers that are translocated to the nucleus, where they bind to the hormone response elements (glucocorticoid response elements–GRE) in the DNA control region of certain genes. The transactivation domains of the receptor dimers bind mediator proteins, thereby activating transcription of specific genes and inhibiting transcription of others.

In a condition known as testicular feminization, patients produce androgens (the male sex steroids), but target cells fail to respond to these steroid hormones because they lack the appropriate intracellular transcription factor receptors. Therefore, the transcription of the genes responsible for masculinization is not activated. A patient with this condition has an XY (male) karyotype (set of chromosomes) but looks like a female. External male genitalia do not develop, but testes are present, usually in the inguinal region.

A. Domains of the steroid hormone receptor

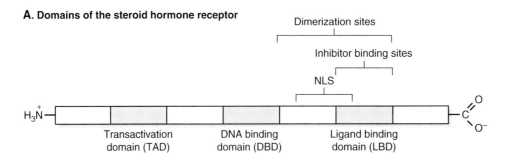

B. Transcriptional regulation by steroid hormone receptors

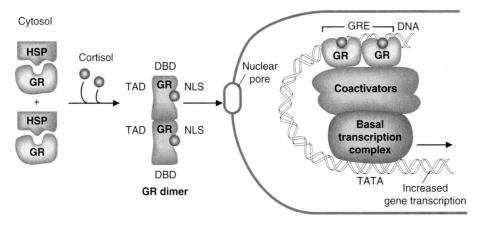

Fig. 16.13. Steroid hormone receptors. A. Domains of the steroid hormone receptor. The transactivation domain (TAD) binds coactivators; DNA-binding domain (DBD) binds to hormone response element in DNA; ligand-binding domain (LBD) binds hormone; NLS is the nuclear localization signal; the dimerization sites are the portions of the protein involved in forming a dimer. The inhibitor binding site binds heat shock proteins and masks the nuclear localization signal. B. Transcriptional regulation by steroid hormone receptors. Additional abbreviations: HSP, heat shock proteins; GRE, glucocorticoid response element; GIZ, glucocorticoid receptor.

Other members of the steroid hormone/thyroid hormone family of receptors are also gene-specific transactivation factors but generally form heterodimers that constitutively bind to a DNA regulatory sequence in the absence of their hormone ligand and repress gene transcription (Fig. 16.14). For example, the thyroid hormone receptor forms a heterodimer with the retinoid X receptor (RXR) that binds to thyroid hormone response elements and to corepressors (including one with deacetylase activity), thereby inhibiting expression of certain genes. When thyroid hormone binds, the receptor dimer changes conformation, and the transactivation domain binds coactivators, thereby initiating transcription of the genes.

The RXR receptor, which binds the retinoid 9-cis retinoic acid, can form heterodimers with at least eight other nuclear receptors. Each heterodimer has a different DNA binding specificity. This allows the RXR to participate in the regulation of a wide variety of genes, and to regulate gene expression differently, depending on the availability of other active receptors.

3. STRUCTURE OF DNA BINDING PROTEINS

Several unique structural motifs have been characterized for specific transcription factors. Each of these proteins has a distinct recognition site (DNA binding domain) that binds to the bases of a specific sequence of nucleotides in DNA. Four of the best-characterized structural motifs are zinc fingers, b-zip proteins (including leucine zippers), helix-turn-helix, and helix-loop-helix.

To regulate gene transcription, two estrogen receptors combine to form a dimer that binds to a palindrome in the promoter region of certain genes (see Figs. 16.12 and 16.13). A palindrome is a sequence of bases that is identical on the antiparallel strand when read in the opposite direction. For example, the sequence ATCGCGAT base-pairs to form the sequence TAGCGCTA, which when read in the opposite direction is ATCGCGAG. Each estrogen receptor is approximately 73 amino acids long and contains two zinc fingers. Each zinc is chelated to two cysteines in an α-helix and two cysteines in a β-sheet region. The position of the nucleotide recognition sequence in an α-helix keeps the sequence in a relatively rigid conformation as it fits into the major groove of DNA. The zinc finger that lies closest to the carboxyl terminal is involved in dimerization with the second estrogen receptor, thus inverting the nucleotide recognition sequence to match the other half of the palindrome. The dimer-palindrome requirement enormously enhances the specificity of binding, and, consequently, only certain genes are affected.

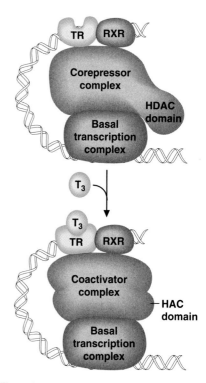

Zinc finger motifs (commonly found in the DNA binding domain of steroid hormone receptors) contain a bound zinc chelated at four positions with either histidine or cysteine in a sequence of approximately 20 amino acids (Fig. 16.15). The result is a relatively small, tight, autonomously-folded domain. The zinc is required to maintain the tertiary structure of this domain. Eukaryotic transcription factors generally have two to six zinc finger motifs that function independently. At least one of the zinc fingers forms an α-helix containing a nucleotide recognition signal, a sequence of amino acids that specifically fits into the major groove of DNA (Fig. 16.16A).

Leucine zippers also function as dimers to regulate gene transcription (see Fig. 16.16B). The leucine zipper motif is an α-helix of 30 to 40 amino acid residues that contains a leucine every seven amino acids, positioned so that they align on the same side of the helix. Two helices dimerize so that the leucines of one helix align with the

Fig. 16.14. Activity of the thyroid hormone receptor–retinoid receptor dimer (TR-RXR) in the presence and absence of thyroid hormone (T_3). Abbrev: HAC, histone acetylase; HDAC, histone deacetylase.

 A wide variety of transcription factors contain the zinc finger motif, including the steroid hormone receptors, such as the estrogen and the glucocorticoid receptor. Other transcription factors that contain zinc finger motifs include Sp1 and polymerase III transcription factor TFIIIA (part of the basal transcription complex), which has nine zinc finger motifs.

 Leucine zipper transcription factors function as homodimers or heterodimers. For example, AP1 is a heterodimer whose subunits are encoded by the genes *fos* and *jun*.

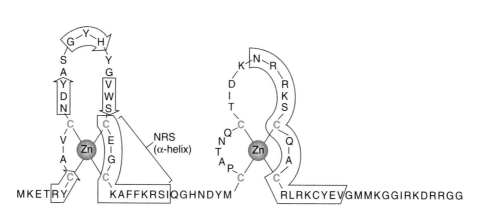

Fig. 16.15. Zinc fingers of the estrogen receptor. In each of the two zinc fingers, one zinc ion is coordinated with four cysteine residues, shown in blue. The region labeled α-helix with NRS forms an α-helix that contains a nucleotide recognition signal (NRS). This signal consists of a sequence of amino acid residues that bind to a specific base sequence in the major groove of DNA. Regions enclosed in boxed arrows participate in rigid helices.

A. Zinc fingers   **B. Leucine zipper**   **C. Helix-turn-helix**   **D. Helix-loop-helix**

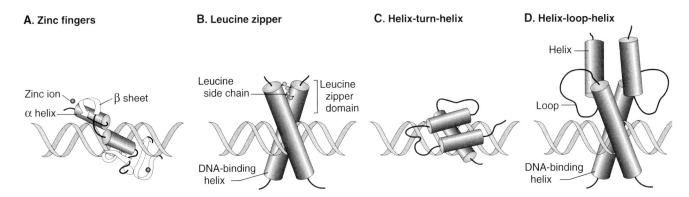

Fig. 16.16. Interaction of DNA binding proteins with DNA. (A) Zinc finger motifs consist of an α-helix and a β sheet in which 4 cysteine and/or histidine residues coordinately bind a zinc ion. The nucleotide recognition signal (contained within the α-helix) of at least one zinc finger binds to a specific sequence of bases in the major groove of DNA. (B) Leucine zipper motifs form from two distinct polypeptide chains. Each polypeptide contains a helical region in which leucine residues are exposed on one side. These leucines form hydrophobic interactions with each other, causing dimerization. The remaining helices interact with DNA. (C) Helix-turn-helix motifs contain three (or sometimes four) helical regions, one of which binds to DNA, whereas the others lie on top and stabilize the interaction. (D) Helix-loop-helix motifs contain helical regions that bind to DNA like leucine zippers. However, their dimerization domains consist of two helices, each of which is connected to its DNA binding helix by a loop.

The helix-turn-helix motif is found in homeodomain proteins (proteins that play critical roles in the regulation of gene expression during development).

Many of the transcription factors containing the helix-loop-helix motif are involved in cellular differentiation (such as myogenin in skeletal muscle, neurogenin in neurogenesis and SCL/tal-1 in hematopoeisis, blood cell development).

other helix through hydrophobic interactions to form a coiled coil. The portions of the dimer adjacent to the zipper "grip" the DNA through basic amino acid residues (arginine and lysine) that bind to the negatively charged phosphate groups. This DNA binding portion of the molecule also contains a nucleotide recognition signal.

In the helix-turn-helix motif, one helix fits into the major groove of DNA, making most of the DNA binding contacts (see Fig. 16.16C). It is joined to a segment containing two additional helices that lie across the DNA binding helix at right angles. Thus, a very stable structure is obtained without dimerization.

Helix-loop-helix transcription factors are a fourth structural type of DNA binding protein (see Fig. 16.16D). They also function as dimers that fit around and grip DNA in a manner geometrically similar to leucine zipper proteins. The dimerization region consists of a portion of the DNA-gripping helix and a loop to another helix. Like leucine zippers, helix-loop-helix factors can function as either hetero or homodimers. These factors also contain regions of basic amino acids near the amino terminus and are also called basic helix-loop-helix (bHLH) proteins.

4. REGULATION OF TRANSCRIPTION FACTORS

The activity of gene-specific transcription factors is regulated in a number of different ways. Because transcription factors need to interact with a variety of coactivators to stimulate transcription, the availability of coactivators or other mediator proteins is critical for transcription factor function. If a cell upregulates or downregulates its synthesis of coactivators, the rate of transcription can also be increased or decreased. Transcription factor activity can be modulated by changes in the amount of transcription factor synthesized (see section 5, "Multiple regulators of promoters"), by binding a stimulatory or inhibitory ligand (such as steroid hormone binding to the steroid hormone receptors), and by stimulation of nuclear entry (illustrated by the glucocorticoid receptor). The ability of a transcription factor to influence the transcription of a gene is also augmented or antagonized by the presence of other transcription factors. For example, the thyroid hormone receptor is critically dependent on the concentration of the retinoid receptor to provide a dimer partner. Another example is provided by the phosphoenol pyruvate (PEP) carboxykinase gene, which is induced or repressed by a variety of hormone-activated transcription factors (see section 5). Frequently, transcription factor activity is regulated through phosphorylation.

Growth factors, cytokines, polypeptide hormones, and a number of other signal molecules regulate gene transcription through phosphorylation of specific transcription factors by receptor kinases.

For example, STAT proteins are transcription factors phosphorylated by JAK-STAT receptors, and SMAD proteins are transcription factors phosphorylated by serine-threonine kinase receptors such as the transforming growth factor-β(TGF-β) receptor (see Chapter 11).

Nonreceptor kinases, such as protein kinase A, also regulate transcription factors through phosphorylation. Many hormones generate the second messenger **cAMP,** which activates protein kinase A. Activated protein kinase A enters the nucleus and phosphorylates the transcription factor CREB (**c**AMP **r**esponse **e**lement **b**inding protein). CREB is constitutively bound to the DNA response element CRE (**c**AMP **r**esponse **e**lement) and is activated by phosphorylation. Other hormone signaling pathways, such as the MAP kinase pathway, also phosphorylate CREB (as well as many other transcription factors).

5.   MULTIPLE REGULATORS OF PROMOTERS

The same transcription factor inducer can activate transcription of many different genes if the genes each contain a common response element. Furthermore, a single inducer can activate sets of genes in an orderly, programmed manner (Fig. 16.17). The inducer initially activates one set of genes. One of the protein products of this set of genes can then act as a specific transcription factor for another set of genes. If this process is repeated, the net result is that one inducer can set off a series of events that result in the activation of many different sets of genes.

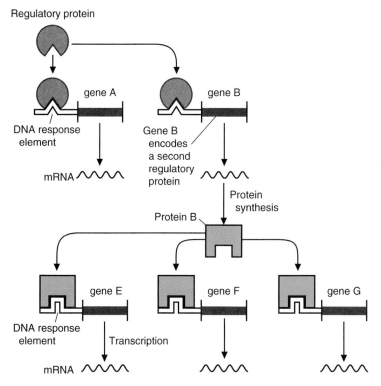

Fig. 16.17. Activation of sets of genes by a single inducer. Each gene in a set has a common DNA regulatory element, so one regulatory protein can activate all the genes in the set. In the example shown, the first regulatory protein stimulates the transcription of genes A and B, which have a common DNA regulatory sequence in their control regions. The protein product of gene B is itself a transcriptional activator, which in turn stimulates the transcription of genes E, F, and G, which likewise contain common response elements.

 Interferons, cytokines produced by cells that have been infected with a virus, bind to the JAK-STAT family of cell surface receptors. When an interferon binds, JAK (a receptor-associated tyrosine kinase) phosphorylates STAT transcription factors bound to the receptors (see Chap. 11). The phosphorylated STAT proteins are released, dimerize, enter the nucleus, and bind to specific gene regulatory sequences. Different combinations of phosphorylated STAT proteins bind to different sequences and activate transcription of a different set of genes. One of the genes activated by interferon produces the oligonucleotide 2′-5′-oligo(A), which is an activator of a ribonuclease. This RNase degrades mRNA, thus inhibiting synthesis of the viral proteins required for its replication.

In addition to antiviral effects, interferons have antitumor effects. The mechanisms of the antitumor effects are not well understood, but are probably likewise related to stimulation of specific gene expression by STAT proteins. Interferon-α, produced by recombinant DNA technology, has been used to treat patients such as **Arlyn Foma** who have certain types of nodular lymphomas and patients, such as **Mannie Weitzels,** who have chronic myelogenous leukemia.

 An example of a transcriptional cascade of gene activation is observed during adipocyte (fat cell) differentiation. Fibroblast-like cells can be induced to form adipocytes by the addition of dexamethasome (a steroid hormone) and insulin to the cells. These factors induce the transient expression of two similar transcription factors named C/EPBβ and C/EPBγ. The names stand for CCAAT enhancer binding protein, and β and γ are two forms of these factors which recognize CCAAT sequences in DNA. The C/EPB transcription factors then induce the synthesis of yet another transcription factor, named the peroxisome proliferator-activated receptor γ (PPARγ), which forms heterodimers with RXR to regulate the expression of two more transcription factors, C/EPB α and STAT5. The combination of PPARγ, STAT5, and C/EPBα then leads to the expression of adipocyte-specific genes.

The enzyme PEP carboxykinase (PEPCK) is required for the liver to produce glucose from amino acids and lactate. **Ann O'Rexia,** who has an eating disorder, needs to maintain a certain blood glucose level to keep her brain functioning normally. When her blood glucose levels drop, cortisol (a glucocorticoid) and glucagon (a polypeptide hormone) are released. In the liver, glucagon increases intracellular cAMP levels, resulting in activation of protein kinase A and subsequent phosphorylation of CREB. Phosphorylated CREB binds to its response element in DNA, as does the cortisol receptor. Both transcription factors enhance transcription of the PEPCK gene (see Figure 16.17). Insulin, which is released when blood glucose levels rise after a meal, can inhibit expression of this gene.

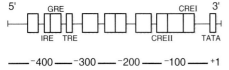

Fig. 16.18. A simplified view of the regulatory region of the PEPCK gene. Boxes represent various response elements in the 5′-flanking region of the gene. Not all elements are labeled. Regulatory proteins bind to these DNA elements and stimulate or inhibit the transcription of the gene. This gene encodes the enzyme phosphoenolpyruvate carboxykinase (PEPCK), which catalyzes a reaction of gluconeogenesis (the pathway for production of glucose) in the liver. Synthesis of the enzyme is stimulated by glucagon (by a cAMP-mediated process), by glucocorticoids, and by thyroid hormone. Synthesis of PEPCK is inhibited by insulin. CRE = cAMP response element; TRE = thyroid hormone response element; GRE = glucocorticoid response element; IRE = insulin response element.

An individual gene contains many different response elements and enhancers, and genes that encode different protein products contain different combinations of response elements and enhancers. Thus, each gene does not have a single, unique protein that regulates its transcription. Rather, as different proteins are stimulated to bind to their specific response elements and enhancers in a given gene, they act cooperatively to regulate expression of that gene (Fig. 16.18). Overall, a relatively small number of response elements and enhancers and a relatively small number of regulatory proteins generate a wide variety of responses from different genes.

D. Posttranscriptional Processing of RNA

After the gene is transcribed (i.e., posttranscription), regulation can occur during processing of the RNA transcript (hnRNA) into the mature mRNA. The use of alternative splice sites or sites for addition of the poly(A) tail (polyadenylation sites) can result in the production of different mRNAs from a single hnRNA and, consequently, in the production of different proteins from a single gene.

1. ALTERNATIVE SPLICING AND POLYADENYLATION SITES

Processing of the primary transcript involves the addition of a cap to the 5′-end, removal of introns, and polyadenylation (the addition of a poly(A) tail to the 3′-end) to produce the mature mRNA (see Chapter 14). In certain instances, the use of alternative splicing and polyadenylation sites causes different proteins to be produced from the same gene (Fig. 16.19). For example, genes that code for antibodies are regulated by alterations in the splicing and polyadenylation sites, in addition to undergoing gene rearrangement (Fig. 16.20). At an early stage of maturation, pre-B lymphocytes produce IgM antibodies that are bound to the cell membrane. Later, a shorter protein (IgD) is produced that no longer binds to the cell membrane, but rather is secreted from the cell.

2. RNA EDITING

In some instances, RNA is "edited" after transcription. Although the sequence of the gene and the primary transcript (hnRNA) are the same, bases are altered or nucleotides are added or deleted after the transcript is synthesized so that the mature mRNA differs in different tissues (Fig. 16.21).

E. Regulation at the Level of Translation and the Stability of mRNA

1. INITIATION OF TRANSLATION

In eukaryotes, regulation of gene transcription at the level of translation usually involves the initiation of protein synthesis by eIFs (eukaryotic initiation factors), which are regulated through mechanisms involving phosphorylation (see Chapter 15, section V.B.). For example, heme regulates translation of globin mRNA in reticulocytes by controlling the phosphorylation of eIF2 (Fig. 16.22). In reticulocytes (red blood cell precursors), globin is produced when heme levels in the cell are high but not when they are low. Because reticulocytes lack nuclei, globin synthesis must be regulated at the level of translation rather than transcription. Heme acts by preventing phosphorylation of eIF2 by a specific kinase (heme kinase) that is inactive when heme is bound. Thus, when heme levels are high, eIF2 is not phosphorylated and is active, resulting in globin synthesis. Similarly, in other cells, conditions such as starvation, heat shock, or viral infections

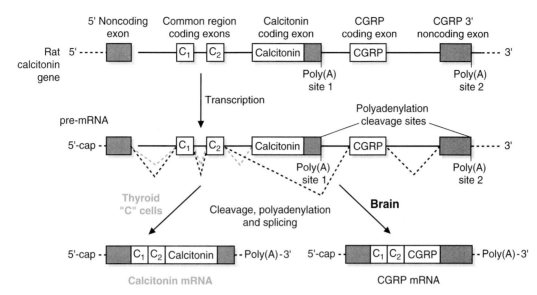

Fig. 16.19. Alternative splicing of the calcitonin gene produces an mRNA for calcitonin in thyroid cells and an mRNA for CGRP in neurons. In thyroid cells, the pre-mRNA from the calcitonin gene is processed to form an mRNA that codes for calcitonin. Cleavage occurs at poly(A) site 1, and splicing occurs along the blue dashed lines. In the brain, the pre-mRNA of this gene undergoes alternative splicing and polyadenylation to produce calcitonin gene-related protein (CGRP). Cleavage occurs at poly(A) site 2, and splicing occurs along the black dashed lines. CGRP is involved in the sensation of taste.

may result in activation of a specific kinase that phosphorylates eIF2 to an inactive form. Another example is provided by insulin, which stimulates general protein synthesis by activating the phosphorylation of an inhibitor of eIF4E, called 4E-BP. When 4E-BP is phosphorylated, it dissociates, leaving eIF4E in the active form.

A different mechanism for regulation of translation is illustrated by iron regulation of ferritin synthesis (Fig. 16.23). Ferritin, the protein involved in the storage of iron within cells, is synthesized when iron levels increase. The mRNA for ferritin has an iron response element (IRE), consisting of a hairpin loop near its 5′-end, which can bind a regulatory protein called the iron response element binding protein (IRE-BP). When IRE-BP does not contain bound iron, it binds to the IRE and prevents initiation of translation. When iron levels increase and IRE-BP binds iron, it changes to a conformation that can no longer bind to the IRE on the ferritin mRNA. Therefore, the mRNA is translated and ferritin is produced.

F. Transport and stability of mRNA

Stability of an mRNA also plays a role in regulating gene expression, because mRNAs with long half-lives can generate a greater amount of protein than can those with shorter half-lives. The mRNA of eukaryotes is relatively stable (with half-lives measured in hours to days), although it can be degraded by nucleases in the nucleus or cytoplasm before it is translated. To prevent degradation during transport from the nucleus to the cytoplasm, mRNA is bound to proteins that help to prevent its degradation. Sequences at the 3′-end of the mRNA appear to be involved in determining its half-life and binding proteins that prevent degradation. One of these is the poly(A) tail, which protects the mRNA from attack by nucleases. As mRNA ages, its poly(A) tail becomes shorter.

An example of the role of mRNA degradation in control of translation is provided by the transferrin receptor mRNA (Fig. 16.24) The transferrin receptor is a

In addition to stimulating degradation of mRNA, interferon also causes eIF2 to become phosphorylated and inactive. This is a second mechanism by which interferon prevents synthesis of viral proteins.

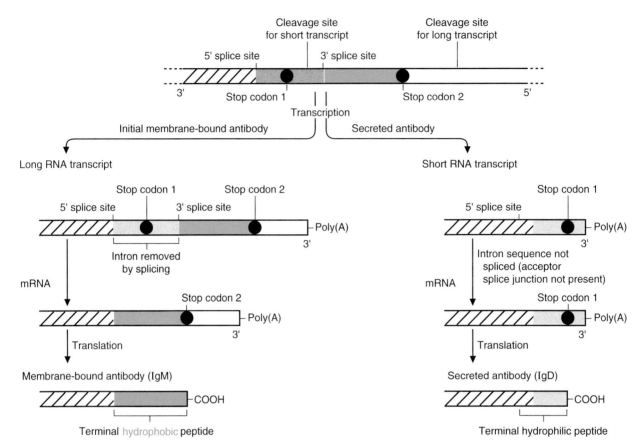

Fig. 16.20. Production of a membrane-bound antibody (IgM) and a smaller secreted antibody (IgD) from the same gene. Initially, the lympho-cytes produce a long transcript that is cleaved and polyadenylated after the second stop codon. The intron that contains the first stop codon is removed by splicing between the 5'- and 3'-splice sites. Therefore, translation ends at the second stop codon, and the protein contains a hydrophobic exon at its C-terminal end that becomes embedded in the cell membrane. After antigen stimulation, the cells produce a shorter tran-script by using a different cleavage and polyadenylation site. This transcript lacks the 3'-splice site for the intron, so the intron is not removed. In this case, translation ends at the first stop codon. The IgD antibody does not contain the hydrophobic region at its C-terminus, so it is secreted from the cell.

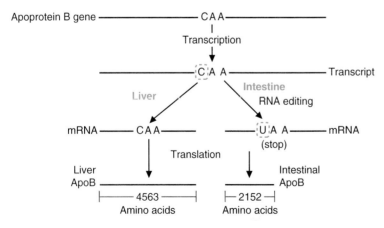

Fig. 16.21. RNA editing. In liver, the apoprotein B (ApoB) gene produces a protein that con-tains 4,563 amino acids. In intestinal cells, the same gene produces a protein that contains only 2,152 amino acids. Conversion of a C to a U (through deamination) in the RNA tran-script generates a stop codon in the intestinal mRNA. Thus, the protein produced in the intes-tine (B-48) is only 48% of the length of the protein produced in the liver (B-100).

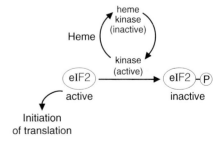

Fig. 16.22. Heme prevents inactivation of eIF2. When eIF2 is phosphorylated by heme kinase, it is inactive, and protein synthesis can-not be initiated. Heme inactivates heme kinase, thereby preventing phosphorylation of eIF2 and activating translation of the globin mRNA.

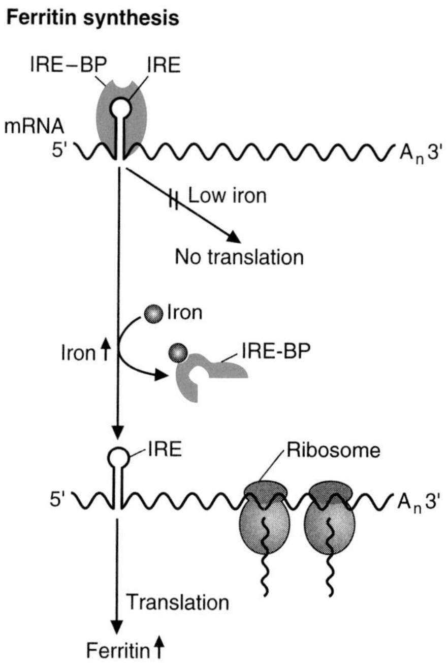

Ferritin synthesis

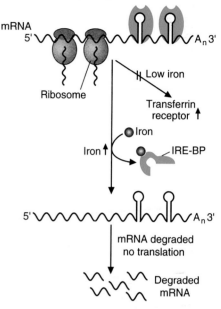

Fig. 16.23. Translational regulation of ferritin synthesis. The mRNA for ferritin has an iron response element (IRE). When the iron response element binding protein, IRE-BP does not contain bound iron, it binds to IRE, preventing translation. When IRE-BP binds iron, it dissociates, and the mRNA is translated.

Transferrin receptor synthesis

Fig. 16.24. Regulation of degradation of the mRNA for the transferrin receptor. Degradation of the mRNA is prevented by binding of the iron response element binding protein (IRE-BP) to iron response elements (IRE), which are hairpin loops located at the 3′-end of the transferrin receptor mRNA. When iron levels are high, IRE-BP binds iron and is not bound to the mRNA. The mRNA is rapidly degraded, preventing synthesis of the transferrin receptor.

protein located in cell membranes that permits cells to take up transferrin, the protein that transports iron in the blood. The rate of synthesis of the transferrin receptor increases when intracellular iron levels are low, enabling cells to take up more iron. Synthesis of the transferrin receptor, like that of the ferritin receptor, is regulated by the binding of the iron response element binding protein (IRE-BP) to the iron response elements (IRE). However, in the case of the transferrin receptor mRNA, the IREs are hairpin loops located at the 3′-end of the mRNA, and not at the 5′end where translation is initiated. When the IRE-BP does not contain bound iron, it has a high affinity for the IRE hairpin loops. Consequently, IRE-BP prevents degradation of the mRNA when iron levels are low, thus permitting synthesis of more transferrin receptor so that the cell can take up more iron. Conversely, when iron levels are elevated, IRE-BP binds iron and has a low affinity for the IRE hairpin loops of the mRNA. Without bound IRE-BP at its 3′end, the mRNA is rapidly degraded and the transferrin receptor is not synthesized. (Note: When IRE-BP is bound to IRE hairpin loops at the 3′-end of the mRNA, the IRE-BP prevents degradation of the mRNA)

CLINICAL COMMENTS

Arlyn Foma. Follicular lymphomas are the most common subset of non-Hodgkin's lymphomas (25–40% of cases). Patients with a more aggressive course, as seen in Arlyn Foma, die within 3 to 5 years after diagnosis if left untreated. In patients pretreated with multidrug chemotherapy (in this case AV/CM), a response rate of 50% has been reported when interferon-α is added to this regimen. In addition, a significantly longer event-free survival has been reported when using this approach.

Ominipotent stem cells in the bone marrow normally differentiate and mature in a highly selective and regulated manner, becoming red blood cells, white blood cells, or platelets. Cytokines stimulate differentiation of the stem cells into the lymphoid and myeloid lineages. The lymphoid lineage gives rise to B and T lymphocytes, which are white blood cells that generate antibodies for the immune response. The myeloid lineage gives rise to three types of progenitor cells: erythroid, granulocytic–monocytic, and megakaryocytic. The erythroid progenitor cells differentiate into red blood cells (erythrocytes), and the other myeloid progenitors give rise to nonlymphoid white blood cells and platelets. Various medical problems can affect this process. In **Mannie Weitzels,** who has chronic myelogenous leukemia (CML), a single line of primitive myeloid cells produces leukemic cells that proliferate abnormally, causing a large increase in the number of white blood cells in the circulation. In **Anne Niemick,** who has a deficiency of red blood cells caused by her β⁺ thalassemia (see Chapter 15), differentiation of precursor cells into mature red blood cells is stimulated to compensate for the anemia.

Ann O'Rexia has a hypochromic anemia, which means that her red blood cells are pale because they contain low levels of hemoglobin. Because of her iron deficiency, she is not producing adequate amounts of heme. Consequently, eIF2 is phosphorylated in her reticulocytes and cannot activate inititation of globin translation.

Mannie Weitzels. Mannie Weitzels has CML (chronic myelogenous leukemia), a hematologic disorder in which the proliferating leukemic cells are believed to originate from a single line of primitive myeloid cells. Although classified as one of the myeloproliferative disorders, CML is distinguished by the presence of a specific cytogenetic abnormality of the dividing marrow cells known as the Philadelphia chromosome, found in more than 90% of cases. In most instances, the cause of CML is unknown, but the disease occurs with an incidence of around 1.5 per 100,000 population in Western societies.

Ann O'Rexia. Ann O'Rexia's iron stores are depleted. Normally, about 16 to 18% of total body iron is contained in ferritin, which contains a spherical protein (apoferritin) that is capable of storing as many as 4,000 atoms of iron in its center. When an iron deficiency exists, serum and tissue ferritin levels fall. Conversely, the levels of transferrin (the blood protein that transports iron) and the levels of the transferrin receptor (the cell surface receptor for transferrin) increase.

BIOCHEMICAL COMMENTS

Regulation of transcription by iron. A cell's ability to acquire and store iron is a carefully controlled process. Iron obtained from the diet is absorbed in the intestine and released into the circulation, where it is bound by transferrin, the iron transport protein in plasma. When a cell requires iron, the plasma iron–transferrin complex binds to the transferrin receptor in the cell membrane and is internalized into the cell. Once the iron is freed from transferrin, it then binds to ferritin, which is the cellular storage protein for iron. Ferritin has the capacity to store up to 4,000 molecules of iron per ferritin molecule. Both transcriptional and translational controls work to maintain intracellular levels of iron (see Figs. 16.23 and 16.24). When iron levels are low, the iron response element binding protein (IRE-BP) binds to specific looped structures on both the ferritin and transferrin receptor mRNAs. This binding event stabilizes the transferrin receptor mRNA so that it can be translated and the number of transferrin receptors in the cell membrane increased. Consequently, cells will take up more iron, even when plasma transferrin/iron levels are low. The binding of IRE-BP to the ferritin mRNA, however, blocks translation of the mRNA. With low levels of intracellular iron, there is little iron to store and less need for intracellular ferritin. Thus, the IRE-BP can stabilize one mRNA, and block translation from a different mRNA.

What happens when iron levels rise? Iron will bind to the IRE-BP, thereby decreasing its affinity for mRNA. When the IRE-BP dissociates from the transferrin receptor mRNA, the mRNA becomes destabilized and is degraded, leading to less receptor being synthesized. Conversely, dissociation of the IRE-BP from the ferritin mRNA allows that mRNA to be translated, thereby increasing intracellular levels of ferritin and increasing the cells capacity for iron storage.

Why does an anemia result from iron deficiency? When an individual is deficient in iron, the reticulocytes do not have sufficient iron to produce heme, the required prosthetic group of hemoglobin. When heme levels are low, the eukaryotic initiation factor eIF2 (see Fig. 16.22) is phosphorylated, and inactive. Thus, globin mRNA cannot be translated because of the lack of heme. This results in red blood cells with inadequate levels of hemoglobin for oxygen delivery, and an anemia.

Suggested Readings

Regulation of gene expression in prokaryotic and eukaryotic cells:
Lewin B. Genes VII. Oxford: Oxford University Press, 2000:273–318, 649–684.
Thalassemias:
Watson J, Gilman M, Witkowski J, Zoller M. Recombinant DNA. Scientific American Books. New York: WH Freeman, 1992:540–544.
Weatherall DJ, Clegg JB, Higgs DR, Wood WG. The hemoglobinopathies. In Scriver CR, Beaudet AL, Slv WS, Valle D. The Metabolic and Molecular Bases of Inherited Disease. 8th Ed. New York: McGraw-Hill, 2001:4571–4636.
Leukemias and Lymphomas:
Goldman L, Bennet JC. Cecil Textbook of Medicine. 21st Ed. Philadelphia: WB Saunders, 2000:945–977.

 REVIEW QUESTIONS—CHAPTER 16

1. Which of the following explains why several different proteins can be synthesized from a typical prokaryotic mRNA?

    (A) Any of the three reading frames can be used.
    (B) There is redundancy in the choice of codon/tRNA interactions.
    (C) The gene contains several operator sequences from which to initiate translation.
    (D) Alternative splicing events are commonly found.
    (E) Many RNAs are organized in a series of consecutive translational cistrons.

2. In *E. Coli,* under high lactose, high glucose conditions, which of the following could lead to maximal transcription activation of the *lac* operon?

    (A) A mutation in the lac I gene (which encodes the repressor)
    (B) A mutation in the CRP binding site leading to enhanced binding
    (C) A mutation in the operator sequence
    (D) A mutation leading to enhanced cAMP levels
    (E) A mutation leading to lower binding of repressor

3. A mutation in the I (repressor) gene of a "non-inducible" strain of *E. coli* resulted in an inability to synthesize any of the proteins of the *lac* operon. Which of the following provides a rational explanation?

    (A) The repressor has lost its affinity for inducer.
    (B) The repressor has lost its affinity for operator.
    (C) A trans acting factor can no longer bind to the promoter.
    (D) The CAP protein is no longer made.
    (E) Lactose feedback inhibition becomes constitutive.

4. Which of the following double-stranded DNA sequences shows perfect dyad symmetry (the same sequence of bases on both strands)?

    (A) GAACTGCTAGTCGC
    (B) GGCATCGCGATGCC
    (C) TAATCGGAACCAAT
    (D) GCAGATTTTAGACG
    (E) TGACCGGTGACCGG

5. Which of the following describes a common theme in the structure of DNA binding proteins?

    (A) The presence of a specific helix that lies across the major groove of DNA
    (B) The ability to recognize RNA molecules with the same sequence
    (C) The ability to form multiple hydrogen bonds between the protein peptide backbone and the DNA phosphodiester backbone
    (D) The presence of zinc
    (E) The ability to form dimers with disulfide linkages

17 Use of Recombinant DNA Techniques in Medicine

The rapid development of techniques in the field of molecular biology is revolutionizing the practice of medicine. The potential uses of these techniques for the diagnosis and treatment of disease are vast.

Clinical applications. Polymorphisms, *inherited differences in DNA base sequences, are abundant in the human population, and many alterations in DNA sequences are associated with diseases. Tests for DNA sequence variations are more sensitive than many other techniques (such as enzyme assays) and permit recognition of diseases at earlier and therefore potentially more treatable stages. These tests can also identify carriers of inherited diseases so they can receive appropriate counseling. Because genetic variations are so distinctive,* **DNA "*fingerprinting*"** *(analysis of DNA sequence differences) can be used to determine family relationships or to help identify the perpetrators of a crime.*

Techniques of molecular biology are used in the ***prevention*** *and* ***treatment*** *of disease. For example, recombinant DNA techniques provide human insulin for the treatment of diabetes, Factor VIII for the treatment of hemophilia, and vaccines for the prevention of hepatitis. Although treatment of disease by gene therapy is in the experimental phase of development, the possibilities are limited only by the human imagination and, of course, by ethical considerations.*

Techniques. *To recognize normal or pathologic genetic variations, DNA must be isolated from the appropriate source, and adequate amounts must be available for study. Techniques for* ***isolating*** *and* ***amplifying*** *genes and studying and* ***manipulating*** *DNA sequences involve the use of* ***restriction enzymes, cloning vectors, polymerase chain reaction (PCR), gel electrophoresis, blotting onto nitrocellulose paper,*** *and the preparation of* ***labeled probes that hybridize*** *to the appropriate target DNA sequences.* ***Gene therapy*** *involves isolating normal genes and inserting them into diseased cells so that the normal genes are expressed, permitting the diseased cells to return to a normal state. Students must have at least a general understanding of recombinant DNA techniques to appreciate their current use and the promise they hold for the future.*

THE WAITING ROOM

Erna Nemdy, a third-year medical student, has started working in the hospital blood bank two nights per week (see Chapter 15 for an introduction to Erna Nemdy and her daughter, Beverly). Because she will be handling human blood products, she must have a series of hepatitis B vaccinations. She has reservations about having these vaccinations and inquires about the efficacy and safety of the vaccines currently in use.

Cystic fibrosis is a disease caused by an inherited deficiency in the CFTR (cystic fibrosis transmembrane conductance regulator) protein, which is a chloride channel (see Chapter 10, Fig. 10.11). In the absence of chloride secretion, dried mucus blocks the pancreatic duct, resulting in decreased secretion of digestive enzymes into the intestinal lumen. The resulting malabsorption of fat and other foodstuffs decreases growth and may lead to varying degrees of small bowel obstruction. Liver and gallbladder secretions may be similarly affected. Eventually, atrophy of the secretory organs or ducts may occur. Dried mucus also blocks the airways, markedly diminishing air exchange and predisposing the patient to stasis of secretions, diminished immune defenses, and increased secondary infections. Defects in the CFTR chloride channel also affect sweat composition, increasing the sodium and chloride contents of the sweat, thereby providing a diagnostic tool.

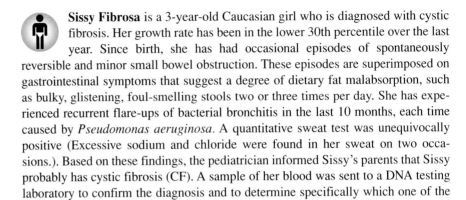

Sissy Fibrosa is a 3-year-old Caucasian girl who is diagnosed with cystic fibrosis. Her growth rate has been in the lower 30th percentile over the last year. Since birth, she has had occasional episodes of spontaneously reversible and minor small bowel obstruction. These episodes are superimposed on gastrointestinal symptoms that suggest a degree of dietary fat malabsorption, such as bulky, glistening, foul-smelling stools two or three times per day. She has experienced recurrent flare-ups of bacterial bronchitis in the last 10 months, each time caused by *Pseudomonas aeruginosa*. A quantitative sweat test was unequivocally positive (Excessive sodium and chloride were found in her sweat on two occasions.). Based on these findings, the pediatrician informed Sissy's parents that Sissy probably has cystic fibrosis (CF). A sample of her blood was sent to a DNA testing laboratory to confirm the diagnosis and to determine specifically which one of the many potential genetic mutations known to cause CF was present in her cells.

Carrie Sichel, Will Sichel's 19-year-old sister, is considering marriage. Her growth and development have been normal, and she is free of symptoms of sickle cell anemia. Because a younger sister, Amanda, was tested and found to have sickle trait, and because of Will's repeated sickle crises, Carrie wants to know whether she also has sickle trait (see Chapters 6 and 7 for Will Sichel's history). A hemoglobin electrophoresis is performed that shows the composition of her hemoglobin to be 58% HbA, 39% HbS, 1% HbF, and 2% HbA_2, a pattern consistent with the presence of sickle cell trait. The hematologist who saw her in the clinic on her first visit is studying the genetic mutations of sickle cell trait and asks Carrie for permission to draw additional blood for more sophisticated analysis of the genetic disturbance that causes her to produce HbS. Carrie informed her fiancé that she has sickle cell trait and that she wants to delay their marriage until he is tested.

Victoria Tim (Vicky Tim) was a 21-year-old woman who was the victim of a rape and murder. She left her home and drove to the local convenience store. When she had not returned home an hour later, her father drove to the store, looking for Vicky. He found her car still parked in front of the store and called the police. They searched the area around the store, and found Vicky Tim's body in a wooded area behind the building. She had been sexually assaulted and strangled. Medical technologists from the police laboratory collected a semen sample from vaginal fluid and took samples of dried blood from under the victim's fingernails. Witnesses identified three men who spoke to Vicky Tim while she was at the convenience store. DNA samples were obtained from these suspects to determine whether any of them was the perpetrator of the crime.

Ivy Sharer's cough is slightly improved on a multidrug regimen for pulmonary tuberculosis, but she continues to have night sweats. She is tolerating her current AIDS therapy well but complains of weakness and fatigue. The man with whom she has shared "dirty" needles to inject drugs accompanies Ivy to the clinic and requests that he be tested for the presence of HIV.

I. RECOMBINANT DNA TECHNIQUES

Techniques for joining DNA sequences into new combinations (recombinant DNA) were originally developed as research tools to explore and manipulate genes but are now also being used to identify defective genes associated with disease and to correct genetic defects. Even a cursory survey of the current literature demonstrates that these techniques will soon replace many of the current clinical testing procedures. At least a basic appreciation of recombinant DNA techniques is required to understand the ways in which genetic variations among individuals are determined and how these differences can be used to diagnose disease. The first steps in determining individual variations in genes involve isolating the genes (or fragments of DNA) that contain variable sequences and obtaining adequate quantities for study.

A. Strategies for Obtaining Fragments of DNA and Copies of Genes

1. RESTRICTION FRAGMENTS

Enzymes called restriction endonucleases enable molecular biologists to cleave segments of DNA from the genome of various types of cells or to fragment DNA obtained from other sources. A restriction enzyme is an endonuclease that specifically recognizes a short sequence of DNA, usually 4 to 6 base pairs (bp) in length, and cleaves a phosphodiester bond in both DNA strands within this sequence (Fig. 17.1). A key feature of restriction enzymes is their specificity. A restriction enzyme always cleaves at the same DNA sequence and only cleaves at that particular sequence. Most of the DNA sequences recognized by restriction enzymes are palindromes, that is, both strands of DNA have the same base sequence when read in a 5′ to 3′ direction. The cuts made by these enzymes are usually "sticky" (that is, the products are single-stranded at the ends, with one strand overhanging the other). However, sometimes they are blunt (the products are double-stranded at the ends, with no overhangs). Hundreds of restriction enzymes with different specificities have been isolated (Table 17.1).

Restriction fragments of DNA can be used to identify variations in base sequence in a gene. However, they also can be used to synthesize a recombinant DNA (also called chimeric DNA), which is composed of molecules of DNA from different

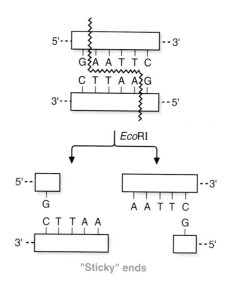

Fig. 17.1. Action of restriction enzymes. Note that the DNA sequence shown is a palindrome; each strand of the DNA, when read in a 5′ to 3′ direction, has the same sequence. Cleavage of this sequence by *Eco*RI produces single-stranded (or "sticky") ends or tails. Not shown is an example of an enzyme that generates blunt ends (see Table 17.1).

🐛 In sickle cell anemia, the point mutation that converts a glutamate residue to a valine residue (**GAG** to **GTG**) occurs in a site that is cleaved by the restriction enzyme *Mst*II (recognition sequence CCTNAGG, where N can be any base) within the normal β-globin gene. The sickle cell mutation causes the β-globin gene to lose this *Mst*II restriction site. Therefore, because **Will Sichel** is homozygous for the sickle cell gene, neither of the two alleles of his β-globin gene will be cleaved at this site.

Q: Which **ONE** of the following sequences is most likely to be a restriction enzyme recognition sequence?

(A)   (5′) G T C C T G (3′)
         C A G G A C
(B)   (5′) T A C G A T (3′)
         A T G C T A
(C)   (5′) C T G A G (3′)
         G A C T C
(D)   (5′) A T C C T A (3′)
         T A G G A T

📖 Restriction endonucleases were discovered in bacteria in the late 1960s and 1970s. These enzymes were named for the fact that bacteria use them to "restrict" the growth of viruses (bacteriophage) that infect the bacterial cells. They cleave the phage DNA into smaller pieces so the phage cannot reproduce in the bacterial cells. However, they do not cleave the bacterial DNA, because its bases are methylated at the restriction sites by DNA methylases. Restriction enzymes also restrict uptake of DNA from the environment, and they restrict mating with nonhomologous species.

Table 17.1. Sequences Cleaved by Selected Restriction Enzymes*

Restriction Enzyme	Source	Cleavage Site
*Alu*I	*Arthrobacter luteus*	5′ - A G↓C T - 3′ 3′ - T C↑G A - 5′
*Bam*HI	*Bacillus amyloliquefaciens* H	5′ - G↓G A T C C - 3′ 3′ - C C T A G↑G - 5′
*Eco*RI	*Escherichia coli* RY13	5′ - G↓A A T T C - 3′ 3′ - C T T A A↑G - 5′
*Hae*III	*Haemophilus aegyptius*	5′ - G G↓C C - 3′ 3′ - C C↑G G - 5′
*Hind*III	*Haemophilus influenzae* R$_d$	5′ - A↓A G C T T - 3′ 3′ - T T C G A↑A - 5′
*Msp*I	*Moraxella* species	5′ - C↓C G G - 3′ 3′ - G G C↑C - 5′
*Mst*II	*Microcoleus*	5′ - C C↓T N A G G - 3′ 3′ - G G A N T↑C C - 5′
*Not*I	*Nocardia otitidis*	5′ - G C↓G G C C G C - 3′ 3′ - C G C C G G↑C G - 5′
*Pst*I	*Providencia stuartii* 164	5′ - C T G C A↓G - 3′ 3′ - G↑A C G T C - 5′
*Sma*I	*Serratia marcescens* S$_b$	5′ - C C C↓G G G - 3′ 3′ - G G G↑C C C - 5′

*Restriction enzymes are named for the bacterium from which they were isolated (e.g., *ECO* is from *Escherichia coli*).

A: The answer is C. C follows a palindromic sequence of CTNAG, where N can be any base. None of the other sequences is this close to a palindrome. Although most restriction enzymes recognize a "perfect" palindrome, where the sequence of bases in each strand are the same, others can have intervening bases between the regions of identity, as in this question. Note also the specificity of the enzyme *Mst*II in Table 1.

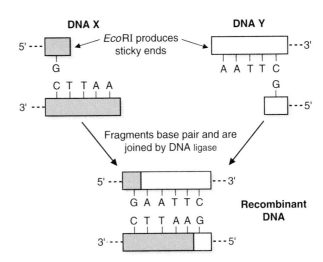

Fig. 17.2. Production of recombinant DNA molecules with restriction enzymes and DNA ligase. The dashes at the 5′ and 3′-ends indicate that this sequence is part of a longer DNA molecule.

sources that have been recombined in vitro (outside the organism, e.g., in a test tube). The sticky ends of two unrelated DNA fragments can be joined to each other if they have sticky ends that are complementary. Complementary ends are obtained by cleaving the unrelated DNAs with the same restriction enzyme (Fig. 17.2). After the sticky ends of the fragments base-pair with each other, the fragments can be covalently attached by the action of DNA ligase.

2. DNA PRODUCED BY REVERSE TRANSCRIPTASE

If mRNA transcribed from a gene is isolated, this mRNA can be used as a template by the enzyme reverse transcriptase, which produces a DNA copy (cDNA) of the RNA. In contrast to DNA fragments cleaved from the genome by restriction enzymes, DNA produced by reverse transcriptase does not contain introns because mRNA, which has no introns, is used as a template.

3. CHEMICAL SYNTHESIS OF DNA

Automated machines can synthesize oligonucleotides (short molecules of single-stranded DNA) up to 100 nucleotides in length. These machines can be programmed to produce oligonucleotides with a specified base sequence. Although entire genes cannot yet be synthesized in one piece, oligonucleotides can be prepared that will base-pair with segments of genes. These oligonucleotides can be used in the process of identifying, isolating, and amplifying genes.

B. Techniques for Identifying DNA Sequences

1. PROBES

A probe is a single-stranded polynucleotide of DNA or RNA that is used to identify a complementary sequence on a larger single-stranded DNA or RNA molecule (Fig. 17.3). Formation of base pairs with a complementary strand is called annealing or hybridization. Probes can be composed of cDNA (produced from mRNA by reverse transcriptase), fragments of genomic DNA (cleaved by restriction enzymes from the genome), chemically synthesized oligonucleotides, or, occasionally, RNA.

To identify the target sequence, the probe must carry a label (see Fig. 17.3). If the probe has a radioactive label such as ^{32}P, it can be detected by autoradiography. An autoradiogram is produced by covering the material containing the probe with a sheet of x-ray film. Electrons (β particles) emitted by disintegration of the

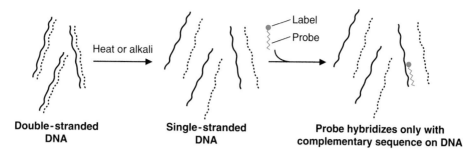

Fig. 17.3. Use of probes to identify DNA sequences. The probe can be either DNA or RNA.

radioactive atoms expose the film in the region directly over the probe. A number of techniques can be used to introduce labels into these probes. Not all probes are radioactive. Some are chemical adducts (compounds that bind covalently to DNA) that can be identified, for example, by fluorescence.

2. GEL ELECTROPHORESIS

Gel electrophoresis is a technique that uses an electrical field to separate molecules on the basis of size. Because DNA contains negatively charged phosphate groups, it will migrate in an electrical field toward the positive electrode (Fig. 17.4). Shorter molecules migrate more rapidly through the pores of a gel than do longer molecules, so separation is based on length. Gels composed of polyacrylamide, which can separate DNA molecules that differ in length by only one nucleotide, are used to determine the base sequence of DNA. Agarose gels are used to separate longer DNA fragments that have larger size differences.

The bands of DNA in the gel can be visualized by various techniques. Staining with dyes such as ethidium bromide allows direct visualization of DNA bands under ultraviolet light. Specific sequences are generally detected by means of a labeled probe.

3. DETECTION OF SPECIFIC DNA SEQUENCES

To detect specific sequences, DNA is usually transferred to a solid support, such as a sheet of nitrocellulose paper. For example, if bacteria are growing on an agar plate, cells from each colony will adhere to a nitrocellulose sheet pressed against the

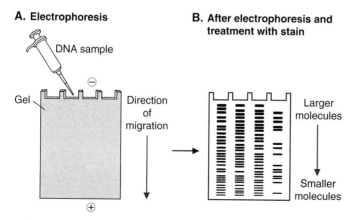

Fig. 17.4. Gel electrophoresis of DNA. **A.** DNA samples are placed into depressions ("wells") at one end of a gel, and an electrical field is applied. The DNA migrates toward the positive electrode at a rate that depends on the size of the DNA molecules. Shorter molecules migrate more rapidly than longer molecules. **B.** The gel is removed from the apparatus. The bands are not visible until techniques are performed to visualize them (see Fig. 17.6).

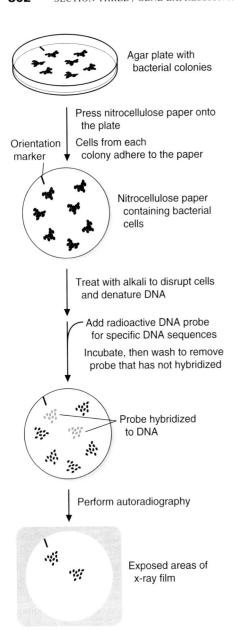

Agar plate with bacterial colonies

Press nitrocellulose paper onto the plate

Cells from each colony adhere to the paper

Orientation marker

Nitrocellulose paper containing bacterial cells

Treat with alkali to disrupt cells and denature DNA

Add radioactive DNA probe for specific DNA sequences

Incubate, then wash to remove probe that has not hybridized

Probe hybridized to DNA

Perform autoradiography

Exposed areas of x-ray film

Fig. 17.5. Identification of bacterial colonies containing specific DNA sequences. The autoradiogram can be used to identify bacterial colonies on the original agar plate that contain the desired DNA sequence. Note that an orientation marker is placed on the nitrocellulose and the agar plate so the results of the autoradiogram can be properly aligned with the original plate of bacteria.

agar, and an exact replica of the bacterial colonies can be transferred to the nitrocellulose paper (Fig. 17.5). A similar technique is used to transfer bands of DNA from electrophoretic gels to nitrocellulose sheets. After bacterial colonies or bands of DNA are transferred to nitrocellulose paper, the paper is treated with an alkaline solution. Alkaline solutions denature DNA (that is, separate the two strands of each double helix). The single-stranded DNA is then hybridized with a probe, and the regions on the nitrocellulose blot containing DNA that base-pairs with the probe are identified.

E. M. Southern developed the technique, which bears his name, for identifying DNA sequences on gels. Southern blots are produced when DNA on a nitrocellulose blot of an electrophoretic gel is hybridized with a DNA probe. Molecular biologists decided to continue with this geographic theme as they named two additional techniques. Northern blots are produced when RNA on a nitrocellulose blot is hybridized with a DNA probe. A slightly different but related technique, known as a Western blot, involves separating proteins by gel electrophoresis and probing with labeled antibodies for specific proteins (Fig. 17.6).

4. DNA SEQUENCING

The most common procedure for determining the sequence of nucleotides in a DNA strand was developed by Frederick Sanger and involves the use of dideoxynucleotides. Dideoxynucleotides lack a 3'-hydroxyl group (in addition to lacking the 2' hydroxyl group normally absent from DNA deoxynucleotides). Thus, once they are incorporated into the growing chain, the next nucleotide cannot add, and polymerization is terminated. In this procedure, only one of the four dideoxynucleotides (ddATP, ddTTP, ddGTP, or ddCTP) is added to a tube containing all four normal deoxynucleotides, DNA polymerase, a primer, and the template strand for the DNA that is being sequenced (Fig. 17.7). As DNA polymerase catalyzes the sequential addition of complementary bases to the 3' end, the dideoxynubleotide competes with its corresponding normal nucleotide for insertion. Whenever the dideoxynucleotide is incorporated, further polymerization of the strand cannot occur, and synthesis is terminated. Some of the chains will terminate at each of the locations in the template strand that is complementary to the dideoxnucleotide. Consider, for example, a growing polynucleotide strand in which adenine (A) should add at positions 10, 15, and 17. Competition between ddATP and dATP for each position results in some chains terminating at position 10, some at 15, and some at 17. Thus, DNA strands of varying lengths are produced from a template. The shortest strands are closest to the 5'-end of the growing DNA strand because the strand grows in a 5' to 3' direction.

Four separate reactions are performed, each with only one of the dideoxynucleotides present (ddATP, ddTTP, ddGTP, ddCTP) plus a complete mixture of normal nucleotides (see Fig. 17.7B.). In each tube, some strands are terminated whenever the complementary base for that dideoxynucleotide is encountered. If these strands are subjected to gel electrophoresis, the sequence 5'→3' of the DNA strand complementary to the template can be determined by "reading" from the bottom to the top of the gel, that is, by noting the lanes (A, G, C, or T) in which bands appear, starting at the bottom of the gel and moving sequentially toward the top.

 Western blots are one of the tests for the AIDS virus. Viral proteins in the blood are detected by antibodies. Tests performed on **Ivy Sharer's** friend showed that he was HIV positive. Unlike Ivy, however, he has not yet developed the symptoms of AIDS.

Ivy Sharer is being treated with didanosine. This drug is a purine nucleoside composed of the base hypoxanthine linked to dideoxyribose. In cells, didanosine is phosphorylated to form a nucleotide that adds to growing DNA strands. Because dideoxynucleotides lack both 2'- and 3'-hydroxyl groups, DNA synthesis is terminated. Reverse transcriptase has a higher affinity for the dideoxynucleotides than does the cellular DNA polymerase, so the use of this drug will affect reverse transcriptase to a greater extent than the cellular enzyme.

Q: In the early studies on cystic fibrosis, DNA sequencing was used to determine the type of defect in patients. Buccal cells were obtained from washes of the mucous membranes of the mouth, DNA isolated from these cells was amplified by PCR, and DNA sequencing of the CF gene was performed. A sequencing gel for the region in which the normal gene differs from the mutant gene is shown below.

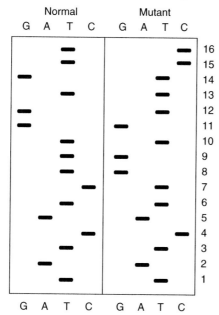

What is the difference between the normal and the mutant CF gene sequence shown on the gel, and what effect would this difference have on the protein produced from this gene?

C. Techniques for Amplifying DNA Sequences

To study genes or other DNA sequences, adequate quantities of material must be obtained. It is often difficult to isolate significant quantities of DNA from the original source. For example, an individual cannot usually afford to part with enough tissue to provide the amount of DNA required for clinical testing. Therefore, the available quantity of DNA has to be amplified.

1. CLONING OF DNA

The first technique developed for amplifying the quantity of DNA is known as cloning (Fig. 17.8). The DNA that you want amplified (the "foreign" DNA) is attached to a vector (a carrier DNA), which is introduced into a host cell that makes multiple copies of the DNA. The foreign DNA and the vector DNA are usually cleaved with the same restriction enzyme, which produces complementary sticky ends in both DNAs. The foreign DNA is then added to the vector. Base pairs form between the complementary single-stranded regions, and DNA ligase joins the molecules to produce a chimera, or recombinant DNA. As the host cells divide, they replicate their own DNA, and they also replicate the DNA of the vector, which includes the foreign DNA.

If the host cells are bacteria, commonly used vectors are bacteriophage (viruses that infect bacteria), plasmids (extrachromosomal pieces of circular DNA that are taken up by bacteria), or cosmids (plasmids that contain DNA sequences from the lambda phage). When eukaryotic cells are used as the host, the vectors are often retroviruses, adenoviruses, free DNA, or DNA coated with a lipid layer (liposomes). The foreign DNA sometimes integrates into the host cell genome or it exists as eipsomes (extrachromosomal fragments of DNA) (See section III.D. of this chapter.)

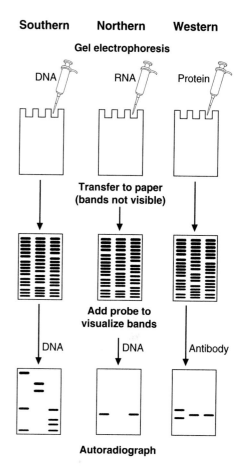

Fig. 17.6. Southern, Northern, and Western blots. For Southern blots, DNA molecules are separated by electrophoresis, denatured, transferred to nitrocellulose paper (by "blotting"), and hybridized with a DNA probe. For Northern blots, RNA is electrophoresed and treated similarly except that alkali is not used. (First, alkali hydrolyzes RNA, and second, RNA is already single stranded.) For Western blots, proteins are electrophoresed, transferred to nitrocellulose, and probed with a specific antibody.

A genomic "library" in molecular biologists' terms is a set of host cells that collectively contain all of the DNA sequences from the genome of another organism. A cDNA library is a set of host cells that collectively contain all the DNA sequences produced by reverse transcriptase from the mRNA obtained from cells of a particular type. Thus, a cDNA library contains all the genes expressed in that cell type, at the stage of differentiation when the mRNA was isolated.

In individuals of northern European descent, 70% of the cases of cystic fibrosis (CF) are caused by a deletion of three bases in the CF gene. In the region of the gene shown on the gels, the base sequence (read from the bottom to the top of the gel) is the same for the normal and mutant gene for the first 6 positions, and the bases in positions 10 through 16 of the normal gene are the same as the bases in positions 7 through 13 of the mutant gene. Therefore, a 3-base deletion in the mutant gene corresponds to bases 7 through 9 of the normal gene.

```
              Ile   Ile   Phe   Gly
Normal sequence:  T A T C A T C T T T G G T
CF sequence:      T A T C A T - - - T G G T
              Ile   Ile         Gly
```

Loss of 3 bp (indicated by the dashes) maintains the reading frame, so only the single amino acid phenylalanine (F) is lost. Phenylalanine would normally appear as residue 508 in the protein. Therefore, the deletion is referred to as ΔF_{508}. The rest of the amino acid sequence of the normal and the mutant proteins is identical.

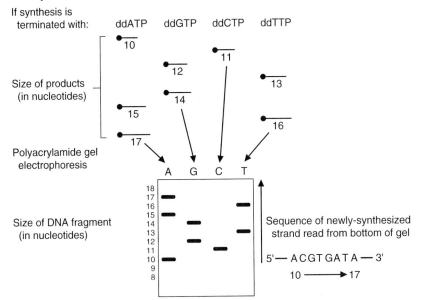

Fig. 17.7. The Sanger method. (A). A reaction mixtures contain one of the dideoxynucleotides, such as ddATP, and some of the normal nucleotide, dATP, which compete for incorporation into the growing polypeptide chain. When a T is encountered on the template strand (position 10), some of the molecules will incorporate a ddATP, and the chain will be terminated. Those that incorporate a normal dATP will continue growing until position 15 is reached, where they will incorporate either a ddATP or the normal dATP. Only those that incorporate a dATP will continue growing to position 17. Thus, strands of different length from the 5' end are produced, corresponding to the position of a T in the template strand. (B). DNA sequencing by the dideoxynucleotide method. Four tubes are used. Each one contains DNA polymerase, a DNA template hybridized to a primer, plus dATP, dGTP, dCTP, and dTTP. Either the primer or the nucleotides must have a radioactive label, so bands can be visualized on the gel by autoradiography. Only one of the four dideoxyribonucleotides (ddNTPs) is added to each tube. Termination of synthesis occurs where the ddNTP is incorporated into the growing chain. The template is complementary to the sequence of the newly synthesized strand.

Host cells that contain recombinant DNA are called transformed cells if they are bacteria, or transfected cells if they are eukaryotes. Markers in the vector DNA are used to identify cells that have been transformed, and probes for the foreign DNA can be used to determine that the host cells actually contain the foreign DNA. If the host cells containing the foreign DNA are incubated under conditions in which they replicate rapidly, large quantities of the foreign DNA can be isolated from the cells. With the appropriate vector and growth conditions that

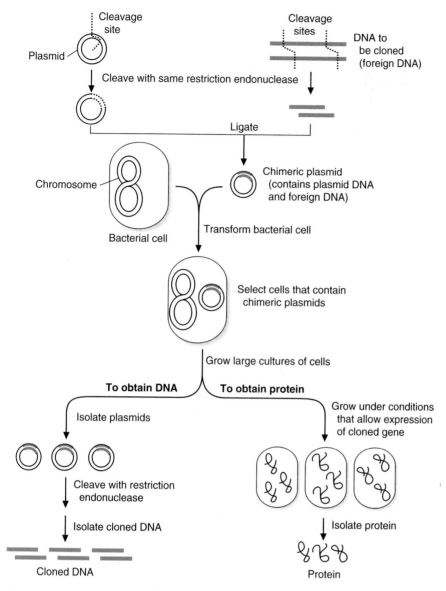

Fig. 17.8. Simplified scheme for cloning of DNA in bacteria. A plasmid is a specific type of vector, or carrier, which can contain inserts of foreign DNA of up to 2.0 kb in size. For clarity, the sizes of the pieces of DNA are not drawn to scale (for example, the bacterial chromosomal DNA should be much larger than the plasmid DNA).

permit expression of the foreign DNA, large quantities of the protein produced from this DNA can be isolated.

2. POLYMERASE CHAIN REACTION (PCR)

PCR is an in vitro method that can be used for rapid production of very large amounts of specific segments of DNA. It is particularly suited for amplifying regions of DNA for clinical or forensic testing procedures because only a very small sample of DNA is required as the starting material. Regions of DNA can be amplified by PCR from a single strand of hair or a single drop of blood or semen.

First, a sample of DNA containing the segment to be amplified must be isolated. Large quantities of primers, the four deoxyribonucleoside triphosphates, and a heat-stable DNA polymerase are added to a solution in which the DNA is heated to separate the strands (Fig. 17.9). The primers are two synthetic oligonu-

Although only small amounts of semen were obtained from **Vicky Tim's** body, the quantity of DNA in these specimens could be amplified by PCR. This technique provided sufficient amounts of DNA for comparison with DNA samples from the three suspects.

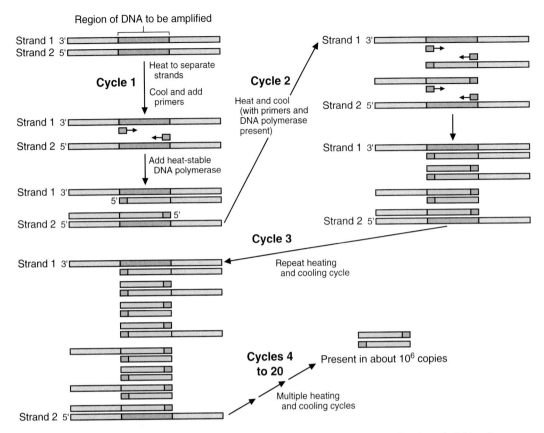

Fig. 17.9. Polymerase chain reaction (PCR). Strand 1 and strand 2 are the original DNA strands. The short dark blue fragments are the primers. After multiple heating and cooling cycles, the original strands remain, but most of the DNA consists of amplified copies of the segment (shown in lighter blue) synthesized by the heat-stable DNA polymerase.

The DNA polymerase used for PCR is isolated from *Thermus aquaticus,* a bacterium that grows in hot springs. This polymerase can withstand the heat required for separation of DNA strands.

cleotides; one oligonucleotide is complementary to a short sequence in one strand of the DNA to be amplified, and the other is complementary to a sequence in the other DNA strand. As the solution is cooled, the oligonucleotides form base pairs with the DNA and serve as primers for the synthesis of DNA strands by the heat-stable DNA polymerase. The process of heating, cooling, and new DNA synthesis is repeated many times until a large number of copies of the DNA are obtained. The process is automated, so that each round of replication takes only a few minutes and in 20 heating and cooling cycles, the DNA is amplified over a million-fold.

II. USE OF RECOMBINANT DNA TECHNIQUES FOR DIAGNOSIS OF DISEASE

A. DNA Polymorphisms

Polymorphisms are variations among individuals of a species in DNA sequences of the genome. They serve as the basis for using recombinant DNA techniques in the diagnosis of disease. The human genome probably contains millions of different polymorphisms. Some polymorphisms involve point mutations, the substitution of one base for another. Deletions and insertions are also responsible for variations in DNA sequences. Some polymorphisms occur within the coding region of genes. Others are found in noncoding regions closely linked to genes involved in the cause of inherited disease, in which case they can be used as a marker for the disease.

B. Detection of Polymorphisms

1. RESTRICTION FRAGMENT LENGTH POLYMORPHISMS

Occasionally, a point mutation occurs in a recognition site for one of the restriction enzymes. The restriction enzyme therefore can cut at this restriction site in DNA from most individuals, but not in DNA from individuals with this mutation. Consequently, the restriction fragment that binds a probe for this region of the genome will be larger for a person with the mutation than for most members of the population. Mutations also can create restriction sites that are not commonly present. In this case, the restriction fragment from this region of the genome will be smaller for a person with the mutation than for most individuals. These variations in the length of restriction fragments are known as restriction fragment length polymorphisms (RFLPs).

In some cases, the mutation that causes a disease affects a restriction site within the coding region of a gene. However, in many cases, the mutation affects a restriction site that is outside the coding region but tightly linked (i.e., physically close on the DNA molecule) to the abnormal gene that causes the disease. This RFLP could still serve as a biologic marker for the disease. Both types of RFLPs can be used for genetic testing to determine whether an individual has the disease.

2. DETECTION OF MUTATIONS BY ALLELE-SPECIFIC OLIGONUCLEOTIDE PROBES

Other techniques have been developed to detect mutations, because many mutations associated with genetic diseases do not occur within restriction enzyme recognition sites or cause detectable restriction fragment length differences when digested with restriction enzymes. For example, oligonucleotide probes (containing 15-20 nucleotides) can be synthesized that are complementary to a DNA sequence that includes a mutation. Different probes are produced for alleles that contain mutations and for those that have a normal DNA sequence. The region of the genome that contains the abnormal gene is amplified by PCR, and the samples of DNA are placed in narrow bands on nitrocellulose paper ("slot blotting"). The paper is then treated with the radioactive probe for either the normal or the mutant sequence. Autoradiograms indicate whether the normal or mutant probe has preferentially base-paired (hybridized) with the DNA, that is, whether the alleles are normal or mutated. Carriers, of course, have two different alleles, one that binds to the normal probe and one that binds to the mutant probe.

So how does one determine the DNA sequence of a gene that contains a mutation to develop specific probes to that mutation? Initially the gene causing the disease must be identified. This is done by a process known as positional cloning, which involves linking polymorphic markers to the disease. Individuals who express the disease should contain a specific variant of these polymorphic markers, whereas individuals who do not express the disease would not contain these markers. Once such polymorphic markers are identified, they are used as probes to screen a human genomic library. This will identify pieces of human DNA containing the polymorphic marker. These pieces of DNA are then used as probes to expand the region of the genome surrounding this marker. Potential genes within this region are identified (using data available from the sequencing of the human genome), and the sequence of bases within each gene compared with the sequence of bases in the genes of individuals with the disease. The one gene that shows an altered sequence in disease-carrying individuals as compared with normal individuals is the tentative disease gene. Through the sequencing of genes from many people afflicted with the disease, the types of mutations that lead to this disease can be characterized and specific tests developed to look for these specific mutations.

The mutation that causes sickle cell anemia abolishes a restriction site for the enzyme *Mst*II in the β-globin gene. The consequence of this mutation is that the restriction fragment produced by *Mst*II that includes the 5′-end of the β-globin gene is larger (1.3 kilobases [kb]) for individuals with sickle cell anemia than for normal individuals (1.1 kb). Analysis of restriction fragments provides a direct test for the mutation. In **Will Sichel's** case, both alleles for β-globin lack the *Mst*II site and produce 1.3-kb restriction fragments; thus, only one band is seen in a Southern blot.

Carriers have both a normal and a mutant allele. Therefore, their DNA will produce both the larger and the smaller *Mst*II restriction fragments. When **Will Sichel's** sister **Carrie Sichel** was tested, she was found to have both the small and the large restriction fragments, and her status as a carrier of sickle cell anemia, initially made on the basis of protein electrophoresis, was confirmed.

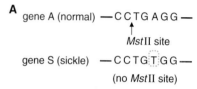

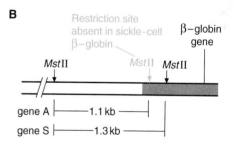

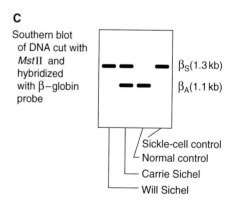

Testing for cystic fibrosis by DNA sequencing is time-consuming and expensive. Therefore, another technique that uses allele-specific oligonucleotide probes has been developed. **Sissy Fibrosa** and her family were tested by this method. Oligonucleotide probes, complementary to the region where the 3-base deletion is located, have been synthesized. One probe binds to the mutant (ΔF_{508}) gene, and the other to the normal gene.

DNA was isolated from Sissy, her parents, and two siblings and amplified by PCR. Samples of the DNA were spotted on nitrocellulose paper, treated with the oligonucleotide probes, and the following results were obtained. (Dark spots indicate binding of the probe.)

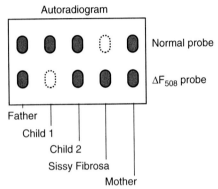

Which members of Sissy's family have CF, which are normal, and which are carriers?

3. TESTING FOR MUTATIONS BY PCR

If an oligonucleotide complementary to a DNA sequence containing a mutation is used as a primer for PCR, a DNA sample used as the template will be amplified only if it contains the mutation. If the DNA is normal, the primer will not hybridize with it, and the DNA will not be amplified. This concept is extremely useful for clinical testing. In fact, a number of oligonucleotides, each specific for a different mutation and each containing a different label, can be used as primers in a single PCR reaction. This procedure results in rapid and relatively inexpensive testing for multiple mutations.

4. DETECTION OF POLYMORPHISMS CAUSED BY REPETITIVE DNA

Human DNA contains many sequences that are repeated in tandem a variable number of times at certain loci in the genome. These regions are called highly variable regions because they contain a variable number of tandem repeats (VNTR). Digestion with restriction enzymes that recognize sites that flank the VNTR region produces fragments containing these loci, which differ in size from one individual to another, depending on the number of repeats that are present. Probes used to identify these restriction fragments bind to or near the sequence that is repeated (Fig. 17.10).

The restriction fragment patterns produced from these loci can be used to identify individuals as accurately as the traditional fingerprint. In fact, this restriction fragment technique has been called "DNA fingerprinting" and is gaining widespread use in forensic analysis. Family relationships can be determined by this method, and it can be used to help acquit or convict suspects in criminal cases.

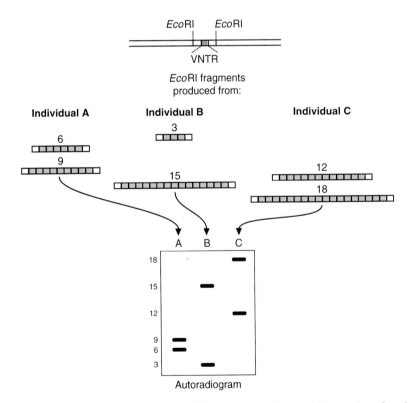

Fig. 17.10. Restriction fragments produced from a gene with a variable number of tandem repeats (VNTR). Each individual has two homologues of every somatic chromosome and thus two genes each containing this region with a VNTR. Cleavage of each individual's genomic DNA with a restriction enzyme produces two fragments containing this region. The length of the fragments depends on the number of repeats they contain. Electrophoresis separates the fragments, and a labeled probe that binds to the fragments allows them to be visualized. Each short blue block represents one repeat.

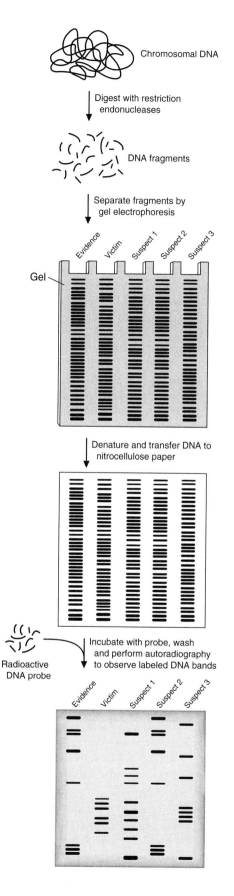

 Obviously, the father and mother are both carriers of the defective allele, as is one of the two siblings (Child 2). Sissy has the disease, and the other sibling (Child 1) is normal.

DNA samples were obtained from each of the three suspects in **Vicky Tim's** rape and murder case, and these samples were compared with the victim's DNA by using DNA fingerprinting. Because **Vicky Tim's** sample size was small, PCR was used to amplify the regions containing the VNTRs. The results, using a probe for one of the repeated sequences in human DNA, are shown below to illustrate the process. For more positive identification, a number of different restriction enzymes and probes were used. The DNA from suspect 2 produced the same restriction pattern as the DNA from the semen obtained from the victim. If the other restriction enzymes and probes corroborate this finding, suspect 2 can be identified by DNA fingerprinting as the rapist/murderer.

The huge amount of information now available from the sequencing of the human genome, and the results available from gene chip experiments, has greatly expanded the field of Bioinformatics. Bioinformatics can be defined as the gathering, processing, data storage, data analysis, information extraction, and visualization of biologic data. Bioinformatics also provides the scientist with the capability of organizing vast amounts of data in a manageable form that allows easy access and retrieval of data. Powerful computers are required to perform these analyses. As an example of an experiment requiring these tools, suppose you want to compare the effects of two different immunosuppressant drugs on gene expression in lymphocytes. Lymphocytes would be treated with either nothing (the control) or with the drugs (experimental samples). RNA would be isolated from the cells during drug treatment, and the RNA converted to fluorescent cDNA using the enzyme reverse transcriptase and a fluorescent nucleotide analog. The cDNA produced from your three samples would be used as probes for a gene chip containing DNA fragments from more than 5,000 human genes. The samples would be allowed to hybridize to the chips, and you would then have 15,000 results to interpret (the extent of hybridization of each cDNA sample with each of the 5,000 genes on the chip). Computers are used to analyze the fluorescent spots on the chips and to compare the levels of fluorescent intensity from one chip to another. In this way, you can group genes showing similar levels of stimulation or inhibition in the presence of the drugs and compare the two drugs with respect to which genes have activated or inhibited expression.

Individuals who are closely related genetically will have restriction fragment patterns (DNA fingerprints) that are more similar than those who are more distantly related. Only monozygotic twins will have identical patterns.

5. DNA CHIPS

A recently introduced technique will permit the screening of many genes to determine which alleles of these genes are present in samples obtained from patients. The surface of a small chip is dotted with thousands of pieces of single-stranded DNA, each representing a different gene or segment of a gene. The chip is then incubated with a sample of a patient's DNA, and the pattern of hybridization is determined by computer analysis. The results of the hybridization analysis could be used, for example, to determine which one of the many known mutations for a particular genetic disease is the specific defect underlying a patient's problem. An individual's gene chip also may be used to determine which alleles of drug-metabolizing enzymes are present and, therefore, the likelihood of that individual having an adverse reaction to a particular drug.

Another use for a DNA chip is to determine which genes are being expressed. If the mRNA from a tissue specimen is used to produce a cDNA by reverse transcriptase, the cDNA will hybridize with only those genes being expressed in that tissue. In the case of a cancer patient, this technique could be used to determine the classification of the cancer much more rapidly and more accurately than the methods traditionally used by pathologists. The treatment then could be more specifically tailored to the individual patient. This technique also can be used to identify the genes required for tissue specificity (e.g., the difference between a muscle cell and a liver cell) and differentiation (the conversion of precursor cells into the different cell types). Experiments using gene chips are helping us to understand differentiation and may open the opportunity to artificially induce differentiation and tissue regeneration in the treatment of disease.

Although development of this DNA or biochip technology is in its infancy, the technique has astonishing potential for the future diagnosis and treatment of disease.

III. USE OF RECOMBINANT DNA TECHNIQUES FOR THE PREVENTION AND TREATMENT OF DISEASE

A. Vaccines

Before the advent of recombinant DNA technology, vaccines were made exclusively from infectious agents that had been either killed or attenuated (altered so that they can no longer multiply in an inoculated individual). Both types of vaccines were potentially dangerous because they could be contaminated with the live, infectious agent. In fact, in a small number of instances, disease has actually been caused by vaccination. The human immune system responds to antigenic proteins on the surface of an infectious agent. By recombinant DNA techniques, these antigenic proteins can be produced, completely free of the infectious agent, and used in a vaccine. Thus, any risk of infection is eliminated. The first successful recombinant DNA vaccine to be produced was for the hepatitis B virus.

When **Erna Nemdy** began working with patients, she received the hepatitis B vaccine. The hepatitis B virus (HBV) infects the liver, causing severe damage. The virus contains a surface antigen (HBsAg) or coat protein for which the gene has been isolated. However, because the protein is glycosylated, it could not be produced in *E. coli*. (Bacteria, because they lack subcellular organelles, cannot produce glycosylated proteins.) Therefore, a yeast (eukaryotic) expression system was used that produced a glycosylated form of the protein. The viral protein, separated from the small amount of contaminating yeast protein, is used as a vaccine for immunization against HBV infection.

B. Production of Therapeutic Proteins

1. INSULIN AND GROWTH HORMONE

Recombinant DNA techniques are used to produce proteins that have therapeutic properties. One of the first such proteins to be produced was human insulin. Recombinant DNA corresponding to the A chain of human insulin was prepared and inserted into plasmids that were used to transform *E. coli* cells. The bacteria then synthesized the insulin chain, which was purified. A similar process was used to obtain B chains. The A and B chains were then mixed and allowed to fold and form disulfide bonds, producing active insulin molecules (Fig. 17.11). Insulin is not glycosylated, so there was no problem with differences in glycosyltransferase activity between *E. coli* and human cell types.

Human growth hormone has also been produced in *E. coli* and is used to treat children with growth hormone deficiencies. Before production of recombinant growth hormone, growth hormone isolated from cadaver pituitary tissue was used, which was in short supply.

2. COMPLEX HUMAN PROTEINS

More complex proteins have been produced in mammalian cell culture using recombinant DNA techniques. The gene for Factor VIII, a protein involved in blood clotting, is defective in individuals with hemophilia. Before genetically engineered Factor VIII became available, a number of hemophiliac patients died of AIDS or hepatitis that they contracted from transfusions of contaminated blood or from Factor VIII isolated from contaminated blood.

Tissue plasminogen activator (TPA) is a protease in blood that converts plasminogen to plasmin. Plasmin is a protease that cleaves fibrin (a major component of blood clots), and, thus, TPA administration dissolves blood clots. Recombinant TPA, produced in mammalian cell cultures, is frequently administered during or immediately after a heart attack to dissolve the thrombi that occlude coronary arteries and prevent oxygen from reaching the heart muscle.

Hematopoietic growth factors also have been produced in mammalian cell cultures by recombinant DNA techniques. Erythropoietin can be used in certain types of anemias to stimulate the production of red blood cells. Colony-stimulating factors (CSFs) and interleukins (ILs) can be used after bone marrow transplants and after chemotherapy to stimulate white blood cell production and decrease the risk of infection.

Recombinant β-interferon is the first drug known to decrease the frequency and severity of episodes resulting from the effects of demyelination in patients with multiple sclerosis.

A method for producing human proteins that is being tested involves transgenic animals. These animals (usually goat or sheep) have been genetically engineered to produce human proteins in the mammary gland and secrete them into milk. The gene of interest is engineered to contain a promoter that is only active in the mammary glands under lactating conditions. The vector containing the gene and promoter is inserted into the nucleus of a freshly fertilized egg, which is then implanted into a foster mother. The female animal progeny are tested for the presence of this transgene, and milk from the positive animals is collected. Large quantities of the protein of interest can then be isolated from the relatively small number of proteins present in milk.

C. Genetic Counseling

One means of preventing disease is to avoid passing defective genes to offspring. If individuals are tested for genetic diseases, particularly in families known to carry a

 Di Abietes is using a recombinant human insulin called lispro (Humalog) (see Chapter 6, Fig. 6.13). Lispro was genetically engineered so that lysine is at position 28 and proline is at position 29 of the B chain (the reverse of their positions in normal human insulin). Di injects a Humalog mixture that contains 75% lispro protamine suspension (intermediate-acting) and 25% lispro solution (rapid-acting). The switch of position of the two amino acids leads to a faster-acting insulin homolog. The lispro is absorbed from the site of injection much more quickly than other forms of insulin, and it acts to lower blood glucose levels much more rapidly than the other insulin forms.

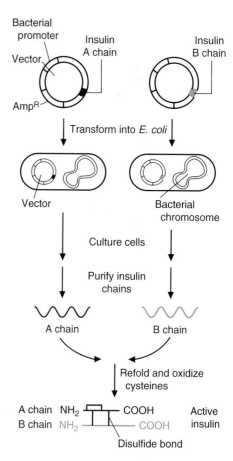

Fig. 17.11. Production of human insulin in *E. coli*. Amp^R = the gene for ampicillin resistance. The presence of Amp^R allows bacterial cells that contain the vector to grow in the presence of ampicillin. Cells lacking the Amp^R gene die in the presence of ampicillin. Because *E. coli* cannot process preproinsulin, a synthetic scheme was developed whereby each individual chain of insulin was expressed, produced, and purified, and then the two chains were linked together in a test tube.

Carrie Sichel's fiancé decided to be tested for the sickle cell gene. He was found to have both the 1.3-kb and the 1.1-kb *Mst*II restriction fragments that include a portion of the β-globin gene. Therefore, like Carrie, he also is a carrier for the sickle cell gene.

Retroviral vector

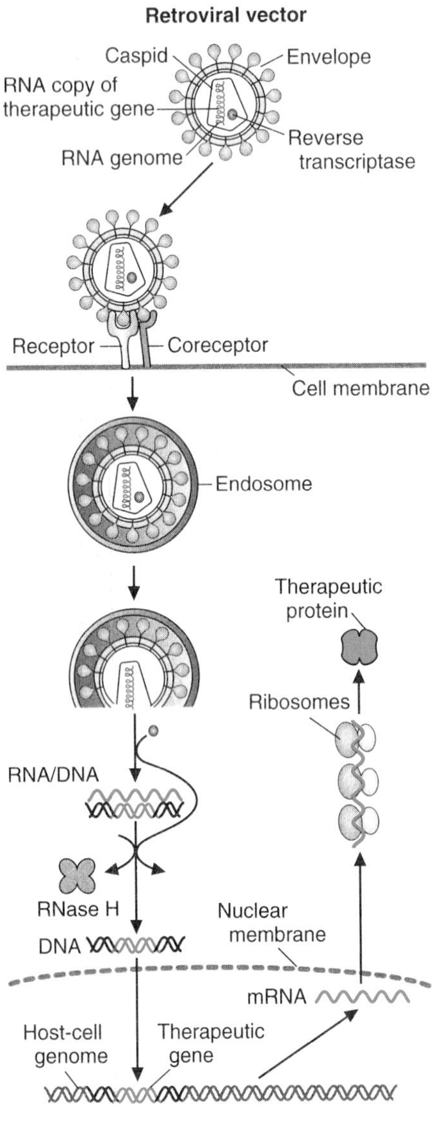

Fig. 17.12. Use of retroviruses for gene therapy. The retrovirus carries an RNA copy of the therapeutic gene into the cell. The endosome that contains the virus dissolves, and the RNA and viral reverse transcriptase are released. This enzyme copies the RNA, making a double-stranded DNA that integrates into the host cell genome. Transcription and translation of this DNA (the therapeutic gene) produces the therapeutic protein. (The virus does not multiply because its genes were removed and replaced by the RNA copy of the therapeutic gene.)

defective gene, genetic counselors can inform them of their risks and options. With this information, individuals can decide in advance whether to have children.

Screening tests, based on the recombinant DNA techniques outlined in this chapter, have been developed for many inherited diseases. Although these tests are currently rather expensive, particularly if entire families have to be screened, the cost may be trivial compared with the burden of raising children with severe disabilities. Obviously, ethical considerations must be taken into account, but recombinant DNA technology has provided individuals with the opportunity to make choices.

Screening can be performed on the prospective parents before conception. If they decide to conceive, the fetus can be tested for the genetic defect. In some cases, if the fetus has the defect, treatment can be instituted at an early stage, even in utero. For certain diseases, early therapy leads to a more positive outcome.

D. Gene Therapy

The ultimate cure for genetic diseases is to introduce normal genes into individuals who have defective genes. Currently, gene therapy is being attempted in animals, cell cultures, and human subjects. It is not possible at present to replace a defective gene with a normal gene at its usual location in the genome of the appropriate cells. However, as long as the gene is expressed at the appropriate time and produces adequate amounts of the protein to return the person to a normal state, the gene does not have to integrate into the precise place in the genome. Sometimes the gene does not even have to be in the cells that normally contain it.

Retroviruses were the first vectors used to introduce genes into human cells. Normally, retroviruses enter target cells, their RNA genome is copied by reverse transcriptase, and the double-stranded DNA copy is integrated into the host cell genome (see Fig. 14.22). If the retroviral genes (e.g., *gag, pol,* and *env*) are first removed and replaced with the therapeutic gene, the retroviral genes integrated into the host cell genome will produce the therapeutic protein rather than the viral proteins (Fig. 17.12). This process works only when the human host cells are undergoing division, so it has limited applicability. Other problems with this technique are that it can only be used with small genes (=8 kb), and it may disrupt other genes because the insertion point is random, thereby possibly resulting in cancer.

A defect in the adenosine deaminase (ADA) gene causes severe combined immunodeficiency syndrome (SCID). When ADA is defective, deoxyadenosine and dATP accumulate in rapidly dividing cells, such as lymphocytes, and prove toxic to these cells. Cells of the immune system cannot proliferate at a normal rate, and children with SCID usually die at an early age because they cannot combat infections. To survive, they must be confined to a sterile, environmental "bubble." When an appropriate donor is available, bone marrow transplantation can be performed with a reasonable degree of success.

In 1990, a 4-year-old girl, for whom no donor was available, was treated with infusions of her own lymphocytes that had been treated with a retrovirus containing a normal ADA gene. Although she had not responded to previous therapy, she improved significantly after this attempt at gene therapy. This disease is still being treated with gene therapy, in combination with replacement enzyme infusion.

In familial hypercholesterolemia, a condition associated with a high incidence of heart attacks, the low-density lipoprotein (LDL) receptor is deficient. Attempts to correct this defect with gene therapy involved removal of a segment of liver and preparation of hepatocytes that had been grown in tissue culture. After these dividing cells were infected with a retrovirus containing the gene for the LDL receptor, they were reinfused into the hepatic portal vein of the patient. The early efforts using this approach met with only limited success.

Adenoviruses, which are natural human pathogens, can also be used as vectors. As in retroviral gene therapy, the normal viral genes required for synthesis of viral particles are replaced with the therapeutic genes. The advantages to using an adenovirus are that the introduced gene can be quite large (~36 kb), and infection does not require division of host cells. The disadvantage is that genes carried by the adenovirus do not stably integrate into the host genome, resulting in only transient expression of the therapeutic proteins (but preventing disruption of host genes). Thus, the treatment must be repeated periodically. Another problem with adenoviral gene therapy is that the host can mount an immune response to the pathogenic adenovirus, causing complications.

To avoid the problems associated with viral vectors, researchers are employing treatment with DNA alone or with DNA coated with a layer of lipid (i.e., in liposomes). Adding a ligand for a receptor located on the target cells could aid delivery of the liposomes to the appropriate host cells. Many problems still plague the field of gene therapy. In many instances, the therapeutic genes must be targeted to the cells where they normally function—a difficult task at present. Deficiencies in dominant genes are more difficult to treat than those in recessive genes, and the expression of the therapeutic genes often needs to be carefully regulated. Although the field is moving forward, progress is slow.

Another approach to gene therapy involves the use of antisense oligonucleotides rather than vectors. These oligonucleotides are designed to hybridize either with the target gene to prevent transcription or with mRNA to prevent translation. Again technical problems have plagued the development of therapy based on this theoretically promising idea.

E. Transgenic Animals

The introduction of normal genes into somatic cells with defective genes corrects the defect only in the treated individuals, not in their offspring. To eliminate the defect for future generations, the normal genes must be introduced into the germ cell line (the cells that produce sperm in males or eggs in females). Experiments with animals indicate that gene therapy in germ cells is feasible. Genes can be introduced into fertilized eggs from which transgenic animals develop, and these transgenic animals can produce apparently normal offspring.

In fact, if the nucleus isolated from the cell of one animal is injected into the enucleated egg from another animal of the same species and the egg is implanted in a foster mother, the resulting offspring is a "clone" of the animal from which the nucleus was derived (Fig. 17.13). Clones of sheep and pigs have been produced, and similar techniques could be used to clone humans. Obviously, these experiments raise many ethical questions that will be difficult to answer.

Adenoviral vectors have been used in a aerosol spray to deliver normal copies of the CFTR (cystic fibrosis transmembrane conductance regulator) gene to cells of the lung. Some cells took up this gene, and the patients experienced moderate improvement. However, stable integration of the gene into the genome did not occur, and cells affected by the disease other than those in the lung (e.g., pancreatic cells) did not benefit. Nevertheless, this approach marked a significant forward step in the development of gene therapy.

In an attempt to treat ornithine transcarbamoylase deficiency (a disorder of nitrogen metabolism) using adenoviral vectors, a volunteer died of a severe immune response to the vector. This unfortunate result has led to a reevaluation of the safety of viral vectors for gene therapy.

One approach to in vivo gene therapy involves the direct injection of DNA for certain HLA antigens into malignant melanomas (skin cancers). The HLA gene chosen for therapy should not be the one expressed by the patient. Thus, if the gene is incorporated into the cells and expressed, the body should recognize the tumor cells as foreign tissue and mount an immune attack. Preliminary results using this strategy were encouraging.

CLINICAL COMMENTS

Erna Nemdy. In reading about development of the hepatitis B vaccine, **Erna Nemdy** learned that the first vaccine available for HBV, marketed in 1982, was a purified and "inactivated" vaccine containing HBV virus that had been chemically killed. The virus was derived from the blood of known HBV carriers. Later, "attenuated" vaccines were used in which the virus remained live but was altered so that it no longer multiplied in the inoculated host. Both the inactivated and the attenuated vaccines are potentially dangerous because they can be contaminated with live infectious HBV.

The modern "subunit" vaccines, first marketed in 1987, were made by recombinant DNA techniques described earlier in this chapter. Because this vaccine consists solely of the viral surface protein or antigen to which the immune system responds, there is no risk for infection with HBV.

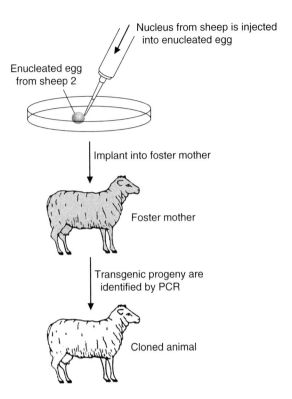

Fig. 17.13. Cloning of a mammalian organism.

The most common CF mutation is a 3-bp deletion that causes the loss of phenylalanine at position 508 (delta 508). This mutation is present in more than 70% of CFTR patients. The defective protein is synthesized in the endoplasmic reticulum, but is misfolded. It is therefore not transported to the Golgi, but is degraded by a proteolytic enzyme complex called the proteosome. Other mutations responsible for CF generate an incomplete mRNA because of premature stop signals, frame shifts, or abnormal splice sites or create a CFTR channel in the membrane that does not function properly.

Sissy Fibrosa. Cystic fibrosis (CF) is a genetically determined autosomal recessive disease that can be caused by a variety of mutations within the CF gene located on chromosome 7. **Sissy Fibrosa** was found to have a 3-bp deletion at residue 508 of the CF gene (the mutation present in approximately 70% of Caucasian patients with CF in the United States). This mutation is generally associated with a more severe clinical course than many other mutations causing the disease. However, other genes and environmental factors may modify the clinical course of the disease, so it is not currently possible to counsel patients accurately about prognosis based on their genotype.

CF is a relatively common genetic disorder in the United States, with a carrier rate of approximately 5% in Caucasians. The disease occurs in 1 per 1,600 to 2,000 Caucasian births in the country (1 per 17,000 in African Americans and 1 per 100,000 in Asians).

Carrie Sichel. After learning the results of their tests for the sickle cell gene, **Carrie Sichel** and her fiancé consulted a genetic counselor. The counselor informed them that, because they were both carriers of the sickle cell gene, their chance of having a child with sickle cell anemia was fairly high (approximately 1 in 4). She told them that prenatal testing was available with fetal DNA obtained from cells by amniocentesis or chorionic villus sampling. If these tests indicated that the fetus had sickle cell disease, abortion was a possibility. Carrie, because of her religious background, was not sure that abortion was an option for her. But having witnessed her brother's sickle cell crises for many years, she also was not sure that she wanted to risk having a child with the disease. Her fiancé also felt that, at 25 years of age, he was not ready to deal with such difficult problems. They mutually agreed to cancel their marriage plans.

Vicky Tim. DNA fingerprinting represents an important advance in forensic medicine. Before development of this technique, identification of criminals was far less scientific. The suspect in the rape and murder of **Vicky Tim** was arrested and convicted mainly on the basis of the results of DNA fingerprint analysis.

This technique has been challenged in some courts on the basis of technical problems in statistical interpretation of the data and sample collection. It is absolutely necessary for all of the appropriate controls to be run, including samples from the victim's DNA as well as the suspect's DNA. Another challenge to the fingerprinting procedure has been raised because PCR is such a powerful technique that it can amplify minute amounts of contaminating DNA from a source unrelated to the case.

BIOCHEMICAL COMMENTS

Mapping of the Human Genome. The Human Genome Project began in 1990, and by the summer of 2000, the entire human genome had been mapped. This feat was accomplished in far less than the expected time as a result of both cooperative and competitive interactions of laboratories in the private as well as the public sector.

The human genome contains over 3×10^9 (3 billion) bp. A large percentage of this genome (<95%) does not code for the amino acid sequences of proteins or for functional RNA (such as rRNA or tRNA) but is composed of repetitive sequences, introns, and other noncoding elements of unknown function. The human genome is estimated to contain only about 30,000 to 50,000 genes.

As the announcement of the identification of a wayward gene appears in the morning newspaper, the average citizen expects the cure for the genetic disease to be described in the evening edition. Although knowledge of the chromosomal location and the sequence of genes will result in the rapid development of tests to determine whether an individual carries a defective gene, the development of a treatment for the genetic disease caused by the defective gene will not be that easy or that rapid. As outlined in the section on gene therapy above, many technical problems need to be solved before gene therapy becomes commonplace. In addition to solving the molecular puzzles involved in gene therapy, we also will have to deal with many difficult questions.

Is it appropriate to replace defective genes in somatic cells to relieve human suffering? Many people may agree with this goal. But there is a related question: is it appropriate to replace defective genes **in the germ cell line** to relieve human suffering? Fewer people may agree with this goal. Genetic manipulation of somatic cells affects only one generation; these cells die with the individual. Germ cells, however, live on, producing each successive generation.

The techniques developed to explore the human genome could be used for many purposes. What are the limits for the application of the knowledge gained by advances in molecular biology? Who should decide what the limits are, and who should serve as the genetic police? If we permit experiments that involve genetic manipulation of the human germ cell line, however nobly conceived, could we, in our efforts to "improve" ourselves, genetically engineer the human race into extinction?

What are the statistical issues relating to DNA fingerprinting? Through the analysis of 1,000 individuals of different ethnicities, one can determine the frequency of a particular DNA polymorphism within that distinct population. By matching four or five polymorphisms from DNA at the crime scene with DNA from a suspect, one can determine the odds of that match happening by chance. For example, let us assume that a suspect's DNA was compared with DNA found at the crime scene for four unique polymorphisms within the suspect's ethnic group. The frequency of polymorphism A in that population is 1 in 20; of polymorphism B, 1 in 30; of polymorphism C, 1 in 50; and of polymorphism D, 1 in 100. The odds of the suspect DNA matching the DNA found at the crime scene for all four polymorphisms would be the product of each individual probability, or $(1/20) \times (1/30) \times (1/50) \times (1/100)$. This comes out to a 1 in 3 million chance that an individual would have the same polymorphisms in their DNA as that found at the crime scene. The question left to the courts is whether the 1 in 3 million match is sufficient to convict the suspect of the crime. Given that there may be 30 million individuals in the United States within the same ethnic group as the suspect, there would then be 30 people within the country who would match the DNA polymorphisms found at the scene of the crime. Can the court be sure that the suspect is the correct individual? Clearly, the use of DNA fingerprinting is much clearer when a match is not made, for that immediately indicates that the suspect was not at the scene of the crime.

Suggested References

- Housman D. DNA on trial—the molecular basis of DNA fingerprinting. N Engl J Med 1995;332:534–535.
- Trent RJ. Molecular Medicine. New York: Churchill Livingstone, 1993.

- Watson JD, Gilman M, Witkowski J, Zoller M. Recombinant DNA. 2nd Ed. New York: Scientific American Books, WH Freeman, 1992.
- Gelehrter TD, Collins FS, Ginsburg D. Principles of Medical Genetics. 2nd Ed. Baltimore: Williams & Wilkins, 1998.
- Welsh MJ. Cystic Fibrosis. Chapter 76. In: Goldman L, Bennett JC, eds. Cecil Textbook of Medicine. 21st Ed, Volume 1, pp 401–405. Philadelphia: WB Saunders, 2000.

REVIEW QUESTIONS—CHAPTER 17

1. Electrophoresis resolves double-stranded DNA fragments based on which of the following?

    (A) Sequence
    (B) Molecular weight
    (C) Isoelectric point
    (D) Frequency of CTG repeats
    (E) Secondary structure

2. If a restriction enzyme recognizes a six-base sequence, how frequently, on average, will this enzyme cut a large piece of DNA?

    (A) Once every 16 bases
    (B) Once every 64 bases
    (C) Once every 256 bases
    (D) Once every 1,024 bases
    (E) Once every 4,096 bases

3. Which of the following sets of reagents are required for dideoxy chain DNA synthesis in the Sanger technique for DNA sequencing? .

    (A) Deoxyribonucleotides, Taq polymerase, DNA primer
    (B) Dideoxyribonucleotides, deoxyribonucleotides, template DNA
    (C) Dideoxyribonucleotides, DNA primer, reverse transcriptase
    (D) Two DNA primers, template DNA, Taq polymerase
    (E) mRNA, dideoxynucleotides, reverse transcriptase

4. Which of the following statements correctly describe a feature of DNA electrophoresis?

    (A) Larger DNA fragments migrate farther in the gel.
    (B) DNA fragments migrate toward the negative charge (anode).
    (C) DNA can be visualized using UV light and the dye ethidium bromide.
    (D) Total human genomic DNA cut by a specific restriction endonuclease will generate three distinctly separable bands.
    (E) DNA must be denatured before it can be run in the gel.

5. The best method to determine whether albumin is transcribed in the liver of a mouse model of hepatocarcinoma is which of the following?

    (A) Genomic library screening
    (B) Genomic Southern blot
    (C) Tissue Northern blot
    (D) Tissue Western blot
    (E) VNTR analysis

18 The Molecular Biology of Cancer

The term **cancer** applies to a group of diseases in which **cells grow abnormally** and form a **malignant tumor**. Malignant cells can invade nearby tissues and **metastasize** (i.e., travel to other sites in the body, where they establish secondary areas of growth). This aberrant growth pattern results from **mutations in genes that regulate proliferation, differentiation, and survival of cells** in a multicellular organism. Because of these genetic changes, cancer cells no longer respond to the signals that govern growth of normal cells (Fig. 18.1.)

Oncogenes and Tumor Suppressor Genes. The genes involved in the development of cancer are classified as **oncogenes** or **tumor suppressor genes.** **Oncogenes** are mutated derivatives of normal genes (**proto-oncogenes**) whose function is to promote proliferation or cell survival. These genes can code for **growth factors, growth factor receptors, signal transduction proteins, intracellular kinases, and transcription factors.** The process of transformation into a malignant cell may begin with a **"gain of function"** mutation in only one copy of a proto-oncogene. As the mutated cell proliferates, additional mutations can occur. **Tumor suppressor genes** (normal growth suppressor genes) encode proteins that **inhibit proliferation, promote cell death, or repair DNA;** both alleles need to be inactivated for transformation (**a loss of function**). Growth suppressor genes have been called the guardians of the cell.

Cell Cycle Suppression and Apoptosis. Normal cell growth depends on a balanced regulation of **cell cycle** progression and **apoptosis** (programmed cell death) by proto-oncogenes and growth suppressor genes. At **checkpoints** in the **cell cycle** products of **tumor suppressor genes** slow growth in response to signals from the cell's environment, including external growth inhibitory factors, or to allow time for repair of damaged DNA, or in response to other adverse circumstances in cells. Alternately, cells with damaged DNA are targeted for apoptosis so that they will not proliferate. Many growth-stimulatory pathways involving proto-oncogenes, and growth-inhibitory controls involving a variety of tumor suppressor genes, converge to regulate the activity of some key protein kinases, the **cyclin-dependent kinases.** These kinases act to control progression at specific points in the cell growth cycle. Apoptosis is initiated by either **death receptor activation** or intracellular signals leading to release of the **mitochondrial protein, cytochrome c.**

Mutations. Mutations in DNA that give rise to cancer may be inherited or caused by **chemical carcinogens, radiation, viruses,** and by **replication errors** that are not repaired. A cell population must accumulate **multiple mutations** for transformation to malignant cells.

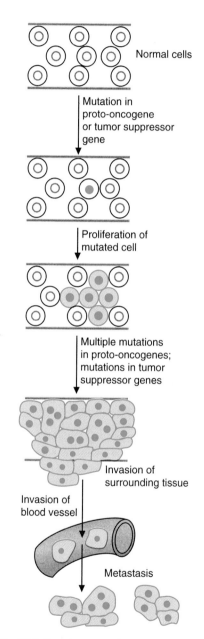

Fig. 18.1. Development of cancer. Accumulation of mutations in a number of genes results in transformation. Cancer cells change morphologically, proliferate, invade other tissues, and metastasize.

THE WAITING ROOM

 Patients with leukemia experience a variety of hemorrhagic (bleeding) manifestations caused by a decreased number of platelets. Platelets are small cells that initiate clot formation at the site of endothelial injury. Because of the uncontrolled proliferation of white cells within the limited space of the marrow, the normal platelet precursor cells (the megakaryocytes) in the marrow are "squeezed" or crowded and fail to develop into mature platelets. Consequently, the number of mature platelets (thrombocytes) in the circulation falls, and a thrombocytopenia develops. Because there are fewer platelets to contribute to clot formation, bleeding problems are common.

 Malignant neoplasms (new growth, a tumor) of epithelial cell origin (including the intestinal lining, cells of the skin, and cells lining the airways of the lungs) are called carcinomas. If the cancer grows in a gland-like pattern, it is an adenocarcinoma. Thus, **Nick O'Tyne** and **Colin Tuma** have adenocarcinomas. **Mel Anoma** had a carcinoma arising from melanocytes, which is technically a melanocarcinoma, but is usually referred to as a melanoma.

 Moles (also called nevi) are tumors of the skin. They are formed by melanocytes that have been transformed from highly dendritic single cells interspersed among other skin cells to round oval cells that grow in aggregates or "nests." (Melanocytes produce the dark pigment melanin that protects against sunlight by absorbing UV light.) Additional mutations may transform the mole into a malignant melanoma.

 Mannie Weitzels has chronic myelogenous leukemia, a disease in which a single line of myeloid cells in the bone marrow proliferate abnormally, causing a large increase in the number of nonlymphoid white blood cells (see Chapter 16). His myeloid cells contain the abnormal Philadelphia chromosome, which increases their proliferation. He has recently complained of pain and tenderness in various areas of his skeleton, possibly stemming from the expanding mass of myeloid cells within his bone marrow. He also reports a variety of hemorrhagic signs, including bruises (ecchymoses), bleeding gums, and the appearance of small red spots (petechiae caused by release of red cells into the skin).

 Nick O'Tyne was diagnosed with a well-differentiated adenocarcinoma of the lungs (see Chapter 13). He underwent anatomic staging procedures to determine the location and severity of the tumor. As a result of these tests, he was considered a candidate for surgical resection of the primary tumor aimed at cure. He survived the surgery and was recovering uneventfully until 6 months later when he complained of an increasingly severe right temporal headache. A CT scan of his brain was performed. Results indicated that the cancer, which had originated in his lungs, had metastasized to his brain.

 Colin Tuma has had an intestinal adenocarcinoma resected, but there were several metastatic nodules in his liver (see Chapters 12 and 13). He completed his second course of chemotherapy with 5-fluorouracil (5-FU) and had no serious side effects. He assured his physician at his most recent checkup that, this time, he intended to comply with any instructions his physicians gave him. He ruefully commented that he wished he had returned for regular examinations after his first round of surgery for benign intestinal polyps.

 Mel Anoma returned to his physician after observing a brownish-black irregular mole on his forearm (see Chapter 13). His physician thought the mole looked suspiciously like a malignant melanoma, and performed an excision biopsy (surgical removal for the purposes of biopsy).

I. CAUSES OF CANCER

Cancer is the term applied to a group of diseases in which cells no longer respond to normal restraints on growth. Normal cells in the body respond to signals, such as contact inhibition, that direct them to stop proliferating. Cancer cells do not require growth stimulatory signals and they are resistant to growth inhibitory signals. They are also resistant to apoptosis, the programmed death process whereby unwanted or

 The study of cells in culture was a great impetus to the study of cancer, because the development of a tumor in animals could take months. Once cells could be removed from an animal and propagated in a tissue culture dish, the onset of transformation (the normal cell becoming a cancer cell) could be seen in days.

What are the criteria that distinguish transformed cells from normal cells in culture? The first is the requirement for serum in the cell culture medium to stimulate growth. Transformed cells have a reduced requirement for serum, approximately 10% that required for normal cells to grow. The second is the ability to grow without attachment to a supporting matrix (anchorage dependence). Normal cells (such as fibroblasts, smooth muscle cells) require adherence to a substratum (in this case, the bottom of the plastic dish) and will not grow if suspended in a soft agar mixture (the consistency of loose jello). Transformed cells, however, have lost this anchorage dependence for growth. An additional criterion used to demonstrate that cells are truly transformed is that they form tumors when injected into mice lacking an immune system.

irreparably damaged cells self-destruct. They have an infinite proliferative capacity and do not become senescent (i.e., they are immortalized). Furthermore, they can grow independently of structural support, such as the extracellular matrix (loss of anchorage dependence).

A single cell that divides abnormally eventually forms a mass called a tumor. A tumor can be benign and harmless; the common wart is a benign tumor formed from a slowly expanding mass of cells. In contrast, a malignant neoplasm (malignant tumor) is a proliferation of rapidly growing cells that progressively infiltrate, invade, and destroy surrounding tissue. Tumors develop angiogenic potential, which is the capacity to form new blood vessels and capillaries. Thus, tumors can generate their own blood supply to bring in oxygen and nutrients. Cancer cells also can metastasize, separating from the growing mass of the tumor and traveling through the blood or lymph to unrelated organs, where they establish new growths of cancer cells.

The transformation of a normal cell to a cancer cell begins with damage to DNA (base changes or strand breaks) caused by chemical carcinogens, UV light, viruses, or replication errors (see Chapter 13). Mutations result from the damaged DNA if it is not repaired properly or if it is not repaired before replication occurs. A mutation that can lead to transformation also may be inherited. When a cell with one mutation proliferates, this clonal expansion (proliferation of cells arising from a single cell) results in a substantial population of cells containing this one mutation, from which one cell may acquire a second mutation relevant to control of cell growth or death. With each clonal expansion, the probability of another transforming mutation increases. As mutations accumulate in genes controlling proliferation, subsequent mutations occur even more rapidly until the cells acquire the multiple mutations (in the range of 4–7) necessary for full transformation.

The transforming mutations occur in genes that regulate cellular proliferation and differentiation (proto-oncogenes), suppress growth (tumor suppressor genes), target irreparably damaged cells for apoptosis, or repair damaged DNA. The genes regulating cellular growth are called proto-oncogenes, and their mutated forms are called oncogenes. The term *oncogene* is derived from the Greek word "onkos" meaning bulk or tumor. A transforming mutation in a proto-oncogene increases the activity or amount of the gene product (a gain-of-function mutation). Tumor suppressor genes (normal growth suppressor genes) and repair enzymes protect against uncontrolled cell proliferation. A transforming mutation in these protective genes results in a loss of activity or a decreased amount of the gene product. In summary, cancer is caused by the accumulation of mutations in the genes involved in normal cellular growth and differentiation. These mutations give rise to cancer cells capable of unregulated, autonomous, and infinite proliferation.

II. DAMAGE TO DNA LEADING TO MUTATIONS

A. Chemical and Physical Alterations in DNA

An alteration in the chemical structure of DNA, or of the sequence of bases in a gene, is an absolute requirement for the development of cancer. The function of DNA depends on the presence of various polar chemical groups in DNA bases, capable of forming hydrogen bonds between DNA strands or other chemical reactions. The oxygen and nitrogen atoms in DNA bases are targets for a variety of electrophiles (electron-seeking chemical groups). A typical sequence of events leading to a mutation is shown for dimethylnitrosamine in Figure 18.2. Chemical carcinogens (compounds that can cause transforming mutations) found in the environment and ingested in foods are generally stable lipophilic compounds that, like dimethylnitrosamine, must be activated by metabolism in the body to react with DNA (see also benz[o]pyrene, Action of Mutagens, Chapter 13, section III.A.). Many

 Drs. Michael Bishop and Harold Varmus demonstrated that cancer is not caused by unusual and novel genes, but rather by mutation within existing cellular genes and that for every gene that causes cancer (an oncogene) there was a corresponding cellular gene, called the proto-oncogene. Although this concept seems straightforward today, it was a significant finding when it was first announced and, in 1989, Drs. Bishop and Varmus were awarded the Nobel Prize in Medicine.

 The first experiments to show that oncogenes were mutant forms of proto-oncogenes in human tumors involved cells cultured from a human bladder carcinoma. The DNA sequence of the *ras* oncogene cloned from these cells differed from the normal *c-ras* proto-oncogene. Similar mutations were subsequently found in the *ras* gene of lung and colon tumors. **Colin Tuma's** malignant polyp had a mutation in the *ras* proto-oncogene.

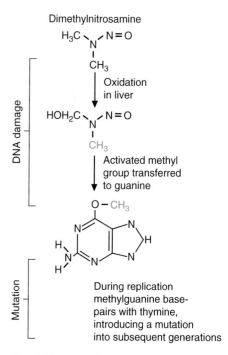

Fig. 18.2. Mutations in DNA caused by nitrosamines. Nitrosamines are consumed in many natural products and are produced in the stomach from nitrites used as preservatives and secondary amines found in foods such as fish. They are believed to be responsible for the high incidence of gastric cancer found in Japan and Iceland, where salt-preserved fish was a major dietary item. Nitrosamine metabolites methylate guanine (the transferred methyl group is shown in blue).

UV rays derived from the skin induce an increased incidence of all skin cancers, including squamous cell carcinoma, basal cell carcinoma, and malignant melanoma of the skin. The wavelength of UV light most associated with skin cancer is UVB (280–320 nm), which forms pyrimidine dimers in DNA. This type of DNA damage is repaired by nucleotide excision repair pathways that require products of at least 20 genes. With excessive exposure to the sun, the nucleotide excision repair pathway is overwhelmed, and some damage remains unrepaired.

 Burkitt's lymphoma, a general name for a number of types of B-cell malignancies, results from a translocation between chromosomes 8 and 14. The translocation of genetic material moves the proto-oncogene transcription factor *c-myc* (normally found on chromosome 8) to chromosome 14. The translocated gene is now under the control of the promoter region for the immunoglobulin heavy chain gene, which leads to inappropriate and over-expression of *c-myc*. The result may be uncontrolled cell proliferation and tumor development. All subtypes of Burkitt's lymphoma contain this translocation. Epstein-Barr virus infection of B cells is also associated with certain types of Burkitt's lymphoma.

 Mannie Weitzels' bone marrow cells contain the Philadelphia chromosome, typical of chronic myelogenous leukemia (CML). The Philadelphia chromosome results from a reciprocal translocation between the long arms of chromosome 9 and 22. As a consequence, a fusion protein is produced containing the N-terminal region of the Bcr protein from chromosome 22 and the C-terminal region of the Abl protein from chromosome 9. *Abl* is a proto-oncogene, and the resulting fusion protein (Bcr-Abl) has lost its regulatory region and is constitutively active. When active, Abl stimulates the Ras pathway of signal transduction, leading to cell proliferation.

The oncogene N-myc (a cell proliferation transcription factor, related to c-myc) is amplified in some neuroblastomas, and amplification of the erb-B2 oncogene (a growth factor receptor) is associated with several breast carcinomas.

chemotherapeutic agents, which are designed to kill proliferating cells by interacting with DNA, may also may act as carcinogens and cause new mutations and tumors while eradicating the old. Structural alterations in DNA also occur through radiation and through UV light, which causes the formation of pyrimidine dimers. More than 90% of skin cancers occur in sunlight-exposed areas. Thus, each chemical carcinogen or reactant creates a characteristic modification in a DNA base. The DNA damage, if not repaired, introduces a mutation into the next generation when the cell proliferates.

B. Gain-of-Function Mutations in Proto-oncogenes

Proto-oncogenes are converted to oncogenes by mutations in the DNA that cause a "gain- in-function," that is, the protein can now function better in the absence of the normal activating events. Several mechanisms that lead to the conversion of proto-oncogenes to oncogenes are known:

- Radiation and chemical carcinogens act (a) by causing a mutation in the regulatory region of a gene, increasing the rate of production of the proto-oncogene protein, or (b) by producing a mutation in the coding portion of the oncogene that results in the synthesis of a protein of slightly different amino acid composition capable of transforming the cell (Fig. 18.3A).
- The entire proto-oncogene or a portion of it may be transposed or translocated, that is, moved from one position in the genome to another (Fig. 18.3B). In its new location, the proto-oncogene may be controlled by a more active promoter and, therefore, overexpressed (increased amounts of the protein product may be produced). If only a portion of the proto-oncogene is translocated, it may be expressed as a truncated protein with altered properties, or it may fuse with another gene and produce a fusion protein containing portions of what normally were two separate proteins. The truncated or fusion protein would be hyperactive and cause inappropriate cell growth.
- The proto-oncogene may be amplified (Fig. 18.3C), so that multiple copies of the gene are produced in a single cell. If more genes are active, more proto-oncogene protein will be produced, increasing the growth rate of the cells.
- If an oncogenic virus infects a cell, its oncogene may integrate into the host cell genome, permitting production of the abnormal oncogene protein. The cell may be transformed and exhibit an abnormal pattern of growth. Rather than inserting an oncogene, a virus may simply insert a strong promoter into the host cell genome. This promoter may cause an increased or untimely expression of a normal proto-oncogene.

The important point to remember is that transformation results from abnormalities in the normal growth regulatory program caused by gain-of-function mutations in proto-oncogenes. However, loss-of-function mutations also must occur in the tumor suppressor genes, repair enzymes, or activators of apoptosis for full transformation to a cancer cell.

C. Mutations in Repair Enzymes

Repair enzymes are the first line of defense preventing conversion of chemical damage in DNA to a mutation (see Chapter 13, section III.B). DNA repair enzymes are tumor suppressor genes in the sense that errors repaired before replication do not become mutagenic. DNA damage is constantly occurring from exposure to sunlight, background radiation, toxins, and replication error. If DNA repair enzymes are absent, mutations accumulate much more rapidly, and once a mutation develops in a growth regulatory gene, a cancer may arise. As an example, inherited mutations in the tumor suppressor genes *brca1* and *brca2* predispose women to the development of breast cancer.

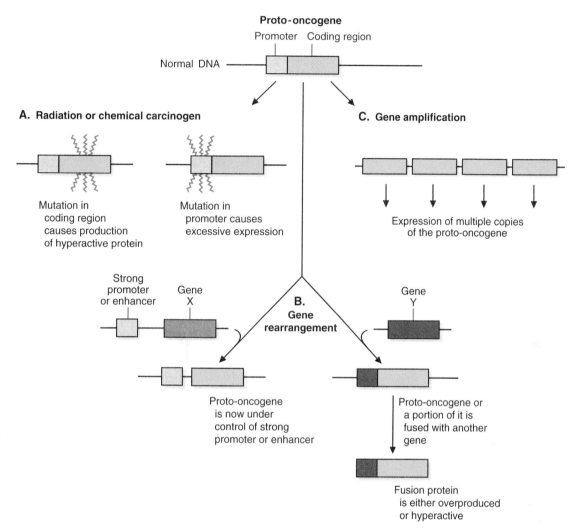

Fig. 18.3. Transforming mutations in proto-oncogenes. (A) Effect of radiation or chemical carcinogens on proto-oncogenes or their promoters. The mutations may be point mutations, deletions, or insertions. (B) Gene rearrangements as caused by transposition or translocation of a proto-oncogene or proto-oncogene fragment. (C) Amplification of a proto-oncogene allows more protein to be produced. The proto-oncogene and the resulting oncogene are shown in blue.

The protein products of these genes play roles in DNA repair, recombination, and regulation of transcription. A second example, HNPCC (hereditary non-polyposis colorectal cancer), was previously introduced in Chapter 13. It results from inherited mutations in enzymes involved in the DNA mismatch repair system.

III. ONCOGENES

Proto-oncogenes control normal cell growth and division. These genes encode proteins that are growth factors, growth factor receptors, signal transduction proteins, transcription factors, cell cycle regulators, and regulators of apoptosis (Table 18.1). (The name representing the gene of an oncogene is referred to in lowercase letters and italics [e.g., *myc*], but the name of the protein product is capitalized and italics are not used [e.g., Myc]). The mutations in oncogenes giving rise to transformation are usually gain-of-function mutations; either a more active protein is produced or an increased amount of the normal protein is synthesized.

 Although mutations in both the brca1 and brca2 genes are linked to breast cancer development in women, there are some fundamental differences in how these genes interact with other proteins at the molecular level. As a result, there are some differences in the diseases expressed by mutations within these genes. For example, *brca1* mutations are also linked to ovarian cancer and *brca2* mutations are not. *Brca2* mutations have been linked to pancreatic cancer, whereas *brca1* mutations have not. Men with inherited *brca2* mutations develop breast cancer; but men who carry *brca1* mutations do not.

Table 18.1 Classes of Oncogenes, Mechanism of Activation, and Associated Human Tumors

Class	Proto-oncogene	Activation Mechanism	Location	Disease
Growth Factors				
Platelet-Derived Growth Factor-β Chain	*sis*	Overexpression	Secreted	Astrocytoma Osteosarcoma
Fibroblast growth factors	*int-2*	Amplification	Secreted	Breast cancer Bladder cancer Melanoma
Growth Factor Receptors				
Epidermal Growth Factor Receptor Family	*erb-B1* *erb-B2*	Overexpression Amplification	Cell membrane Cell membrane	Squamous cell carcinoma of the lung Breast, ovarian, lung, stomach cancer
Platelet- Derived Growth Factor-Receptor	*PDGFR*	Translocation	Cell membrane	Chronic myelomonocytic leukemia
Hedgehog Receptor	*SMO*	Point mutation	Cell membrane	Basal cell carcinoma
Signal Transduction Proteins				
G proteins	*ras*	Point mutation	Cytoplasm	Multiple cancers including lung, colon, thyroid, pancreas, many leukemias
Serine/threonine kinase	*akt2* *raf*	Amplification Overexpression	Cytoplasm Cytoplasm	Ovarian carcinoma Myeloid leukemia
Tyrosine kinase	*abl*	Translocation	Cytoplasm	Chronic myeloid leukemia Acute lymphoblastic leukemia
	src	Overexpression	Cytoplasm	Breast
Hormone Receptors				
Retinoid receptor	*RARα*	Translocation	Nucleus	Acute promyelocytic leukemia
Transcription Factors				
	Hox11 *Myc*	Translocation Translocation Amplification	Nucleus Nucleus nucleus	Acute T cell leukemia Burkitt's lymphoma Neuroblastoma, small cell carcinoma of the lung
	fos, jun	Phosphorylation	Nucleus	Breast cancer
Apoptosis Regulators				
	Bcl-2	Translocation	Mitochondria	Follicular B-cell lymphoma
Cell Cycle Regulators				
Cyclins	Cyclin D	Translocation Amplification	Nucleus Nucleus	Lymphoma Breast, liver, esophageal cancer
Cyclin-dependent kinase	CDK4	Amplification Point mutation	Nucleus Nucleus	Gglioblastoma, sarcoma Melanoma

The gene for the human epidermal growth factor receptor (*HER2, c-erbB-2*) is over-expressed in 10 to 20% of breast cancer cases. When this gene is over-expressed, the prognosis for recovery is poor, as the patients display shorter disease-free intervals, increased risks for metastasis, and a resistance to therapy. Clinical trials are underway using a monoclonal antibody directed against this receptor (herceptin) to inactivate it. Preliminary results are encouraging in that use of this drug, either alone or in combination with others, appears to control the growth of some tumors overexpressing the *HER2* gene. However, not all tumors over-expressing *HER2* are responsive to herceptin. Thus, it appears that a complete genotyping of breast cancer cells may be necessary (using the microarray techniques described in Chapter 17) to specifically develop an effective therapy for each patient with the disease.

A. Oncogenes and Signal Transduction Cascades

All of the proteins in growth factor signal transduction cascades are proto-oncogenes (Fig18.4).

1. GROWTH FACTORS AND GROWTH FACTOR RECEPTORS

The genes for both growth factors and growth factor receptors are oncogenes.

Growth factors generally regulate growth by serving as ligands that bind to cellular receptors located on the plasma membrane (cell-surface receptors) (see Chapter 11). Binding of ligands to these receptors stimulates a signal transduction pathway in the cell activating the transcription of certain genes. If too much of a growth factor or a growth factor receptor is produced, the target cells may respond by proliferating inappropriately. Growth factors receptors may also become oncogenic through translocation or point mutations in domains affecting binding of the growth factor, dimerization, kinase activity, or some other aspect of their signal transmission. In such cases, the receptor transmits a proliferative signal even though the growth factor normally required to activate the receptor is absent. In other words, the receptor is stuck in the "on" position.

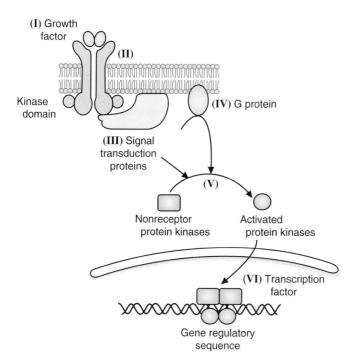

Fig. 18.4. Proto-oncogene sites for transforming mutations in growth factor signaling pathways. I. The amount of growth factor. II. The receptor, which normally must bind the growth factor to dimerize and activate a kinase domain. III. Signal transduction proteins. Some, such as PI 3-kinase, form second messengers. IV. G proteins, and their regulators, which are also signal transduction proteins. V. Nonreceptor protein kinase cascades, which lead to phosphorylation of transcription factors. VI. Nuclear transcription factors normally activated through phosphorylation or binding of a ligand.

2. SIGNAL TRANSDUCTION PROTEINS

The genes encoding proteins involved in growth factor signal transduction cascades may also be proto-oncogenes. Consider, for example, the monomeric G protein Ras. Binding of growth factor leads to the activation of Ras (see Fig 11.11). When Ras binds GTP, it is active, but Ras slowly inactivates itself by hydrolyzing its bound GTP to GDP and Pi. This controls the length of time that Ras is active. Ras is converted to an oncogenic form by point mutations that decrease the activity of the GTPase domain of Ras, thereby increasing the length of time it remains in the active form.

Ras, when active, activates the serine/threonine kinase Raf (a MAP kinase kinase kinase), which activates MEK (a MAP kinase kinase), which activates MAP kinase (Fig. 18.5). Activation of MAP kinase results in the phosphorylation of cytoplasmic and nuclear proteins, followed by increased transcription of the transcription factor proto-oncogenes *myc* and *fos* (see below). Note that mutations in the genes for any of the proteins that regulate MAP kinase activity, as well as those proteins induced by MAP kinase activation, can lead to uncontrolled cell proliferation.

3. TRANSCRIPTION FACTORS

Many transcription factors, such as Myc and Fos, are proto-oncoproteins (the products of proto-oncogenes). MAP kinase, in addition to inducing *myc* and *fos*, also directly activates the AP-1 transcription factor through phosphorylation (see Fig.18.5). AP-1 is a heterodimer formed by the protein products of the *fos* and *jun* families of proto-oncogenes. The targets of AP-1 activation are genes involved in

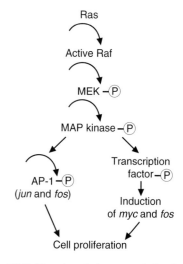

Fig. 18.5. Phosphorylation cascade leading to activation of proto-oncogene transcription factors *myc, fos,* and *jun.*

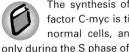

The synthesis of the transcription factor C-myc is tightly regulated in normal cells, and it is expressed only during the S phase of the cell cycle. In a large number of tumor types, this regulated expression is lost, and c-myc becomes inappropriately expressed or overexpressed throughout the cell cycle, driving cells continuously to proliferation.

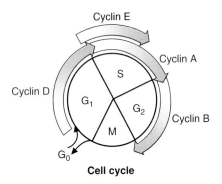

Cell cycle

Fig. 18.6. Cyclin synthesis during different phases of the cell cycle.

The proteins induced by E2F include cyclin E, cyclin A, cdc25A (an activating protein phosphatase), and proteins required to bind at origins of replication to initiate DNA synthesis. The synthesis of cyclin E allows it to complex with cdk2, forming another active cyclin complex that retains activity into S phase (see Fig. 18.6). Cyclin A activates Cdk2. Thus, each phase of the cell cycle activates the next through cyclin synthesis. The cyclins are removed by regulated proteolysis.

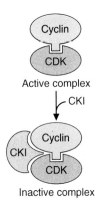

Fig. 18.7. CKI inhibition of cyclin/CDK activity.

cellular proliferation and progression through the cell cycle, as are the targets of the *myc* transcription factor. The net result is increased production of the proteins that carry out the processes required for proliferation.

B. Oncogenes and the Cell Cycle

The growth of human cells, involving DNA replication and cell division in the cell cycle, is activated by growth factors, hormones, and other messengers. These activators work through cyclins and cyclin- dependent kinases (CDKs) that control progression from one phase of the cycle to another (Fig 18.6). For quiescent cells to proliferate, they must leave G_0 and enter the G1 phase of the cell cycle (see Chapter 13, Fig. 13.7). If the proper sequence of events occurs during G1, the cells enter the S phase and are committed to DNA replication and cell division. Similarly, during G2 cells make a commitment to mitotic division. CDKs are made constantly throughout the cell cycle but require binding of a specific cyclin to be active. Different cyclins made at different times in the cell cycle control each of the transitions (G1/S, S/G2, G2/M).

The activity of the cyclin–CDK complex is further regulated through phosphorylation and through inhibitory proteins called cyclin-dependent kinase inhibitors (CKIs) (Fig. 18.7). CKIs slow cell cycle progression by binding and inhibiting the CDK–cyclin complexes. CDKs are also controlled through activating phosphorylation by CAK (cyclin-activating kinases) and inhibitory hyperphosphorylation kinases.

To illustrate the role of these proteins, consider some of the events occurring at the G1/S checkpoint (Fig. 18.8). Because the cell is committed to DNA replication and division once it enters the S phase, multiple regulatory proteins are involved in determining whether the cell is ready to pass this checkpoint. These regulatory proteins include cdk4 and cdk6 (which are constitutively produced throughout the cell cycle), cyclin D (whose synthesis is only induced after growth factor stimulation of a quiescent cell), the retinoblastoma gene product (Rb), and a class of transcription factors known collectively as E2F. In quiescent cells, Rb is complexed with E2F, resulting in inhibition of these transcription factors. On growth factor stimulation, the cyclin Ds are induced (there are three types of cyclin D; D1, D2, and D3). They bind to cdk4 and cdk6, converting them to active protein kinases. One of the targets of cyclin/cdk phosphorylation is the Rb protein. Phosphorylation of Rb releases it from E2F, and E2F is then free to activate the transcription of genes required for entry into S. The Rb protein is a tumor suppressor gene (more below).

Progression through the cell cycle is opposed by the CKIs (see Fig. 18.8). The CKIs regulating cyclin/cdk expression in the G1 phase of the cell cycle fall into two categories: the Cip/Kip family and the INK4 family. The Cip/Kip family members (p21, p27, and p57) have a broad specificity and inhibit all cyclin–CDK complexes. The INK4 family, which consists of p15, p16, p18, and p19, are specific for the cyclin D–cdk4/6 family of complexes (**in**hibitors of cyclin-dependent **k**inase-**4**). The regulation of synthesis of different CKIs is complex, but some are induced by DNA damage to the cell and halt cell cycle progression until the damage can be repaired. For example, the CKI p21 (a protein of 21,000 Daltons) is a key member of this group that responds to specific signals to block cell proliferation. If the damage cannot be repaired, an apoptotic pathway is selected, and the cell dies.

In addition to sunlight and a preexisting nevus, hereditary factors also play a role in the development of malignant melanoma. Ten percent of melanomas tend to run in families. Some of the suspected melanoma-associated genes include the tumor suppressor gene p16 (an inhibitor of cdk 4) and CDK4. **Mel Anoma** was the single child of parents who had died of a car accident in their 50s, and thus, a familial tendency could not be assessed.

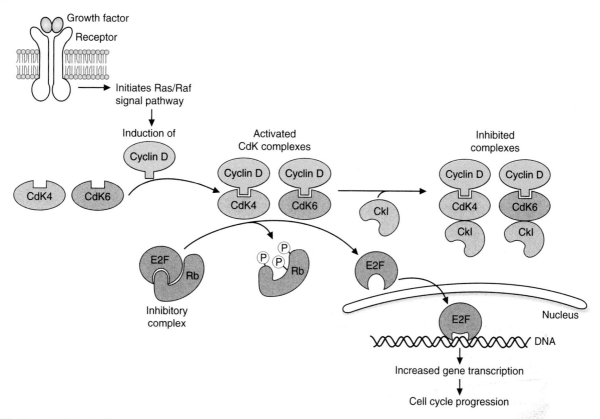

Fig. 18.8. Control of the G1/S transition in the cell cycle. The genes encoding cyclins and CDKs are oncogenes, and the gene encoding the Retinoblastoma protein (Rb) is a tumor suppressor gene. Abbreviations: CDK, cyclin- dependent kinase; CDKI, cyclin-dependent kinase inhibitor.

IV. TUMOR SUPPRESSOR GENES

Like the oncogenes, the tumor suppressor genes encode molecules involved in the regulation of cell proliferation. Table 18.2 provides several examples. The normal function of tumor suppressor proteins is generally to inhibit proliferation in response to certain signals such as DNA damage. The signal is removed when the cell is fully equipped to proliferate; the effect of their elimination of tumor suppressor genes is to remove the brakes on cell growth. They affect cell cycle regulation, signal transduction, transcription, and cell adhesion. The products of tumor suppressor genes frequently modulate pathways that are activated by the products of proto-oncogenes.

Table 18.2 Tumor Suppressors

Class	Protein	Location	Associated Diseases
Adhesion protein	E-cadherin	Cell membrane	Stomach cancer
Receptor	PATCHED	Cell membrane	Basal cell carcinoma
	TGF–β receptor	Cell membrane	Colon cancer
Signal transduction	NF-1	Under cell membrane	Neurofibrosarcoma
	SMAD4/DPC	Cytoplasm/nucleus	Pancreatic and colorectal cancer
Transcription factor	WT-1	Nucleus	Wilms tumor
Cell cycle regulator	p16(INK4)	Nucleus	Melanoma, lung, pancreatic cancer
	Retinoblastoma	Nucleus	Retinblastoma, sarcomas
Cell cycle/apoptosis	p53	Nucleus	Most cancers
DNA repair	BRACA 1	Nucleus	Breast cancer

Tumor suppressor genes contribute to the development of cancer when both copies of the gene are inactivated. This is different from the case of proto-oncogene mutations because only one allele of a proto-oncogene needs to be converted to an oncogene to initiate transformation.

A. Tumor Suppressor Genes That Directly Regulate the Cell Cycle

The two best understood cell cycle regulators that are also tumor suppressors are the retinoblastoma (*rb*) and *p53* genes.

1. THE RETINOBLASTOMA (*rb*) GENE

Inheritance of a mutation in *p53* leads to Li-Fraumeni syndrome, which is characterized by multiple types of tumors. Mutations in *p53* are present in more than 50% of human tumors. These are secondary mutations within the cell, and if *p53* is mutated the overall rate of cellular mutation will increase because there is no p53 to check for DNA damage, to initiate the repair of the damaged DNA, or to initiate apoptosis if the damage is not repaired. Thus, damaged DNA is replicated, and the frequency of additional mutations within the same cell increases remarkably.

As previously discussed, the retinoblastoma gene product, Rb, functions in the transition from G1 to S phase and regulates the activation of members of the E2F family of transcription factors (see Fig. 18.8). If an individual inherits a mutated copy of the *rb* allele, there is a 100% chance of that individual developing retinoblastoma, because of high probability that the second allele of *rb* will gain a mutation (Fig.18.9). This is considered familial retinoblastoma. Individuals who do not inherit mutations in *rb*, but who develop retinoblastoma, are said to have sporadic retinoblastoma, and acquire two specific mutations, one in each *rb* allele of the retinoblast, during their lifetime.

2. p53, THE GUARDIAN OF THE GENOME

The p53 protein is a transcription factor regulating the cell cycle and apoptosis, programmed cell death. Loss of both *p53* alleles is found in over more than 50% of human tumors. p53 acts as the "guardian of the genome" by halting replication in cells that have suffered DNA damage and targeting unrepaired cells to apoptosis.

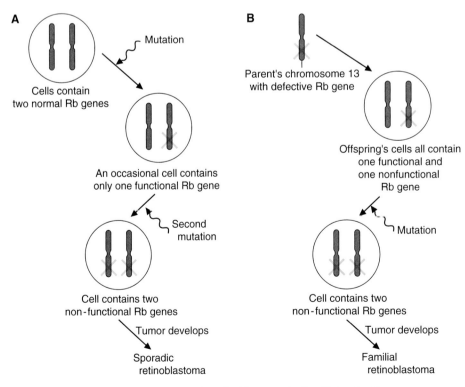

Fig. 18.9. Mutations in the retinoblastoma (Rb) gene. A. Sporadic retinoblastoma. B. Familial retinoblastoma.

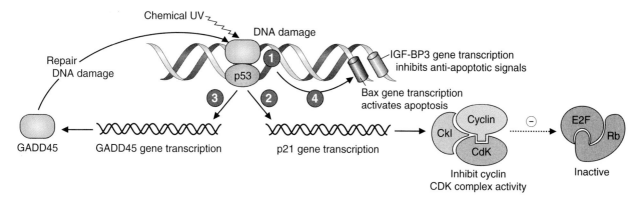

Fig. 18.10. p53 and cell cycle arrest. Mechanisms that recognize DNA damage stop p53 degradation and modify the p53 protein (circle 1). p53 stimulates the transcription of p21 (circle 2) and GADD45 (circle 3). p21 blocks the cyclin/CDK phosphorylation of Rb, which continues to inhibit the E2F family of transcription factors, thereby blocking cell progression through the cell cycle. GADD45 allows the DNA damage to be repaired. If the damage is not repaired, apoptotic genes are activated (circle 4).

In response to DNA-damaging mutagens, ionizing radiation, or ultraviolet light, the level of p53 rises (Fig. 18.10, circle 1). p53, acting as a transcription factor, stimulates transcription of *p21* (a member of the Cip/Kip family of CKIs), as shown in Figure 18.10, circle 2. The p21 gene product inhibits the cyclin/CDK complexes, which prevents the phosphorylation of Rb and release of E2F proteins. The cell is thus prevented from entering S phase. P53 also stimulates the transcription of GADD45 (Growth Arrest and DNA Damage), a DNA repair enzyme (Fig. 18.10, circle 3). If the DNA is successfully repaired, p53 induces its own downregulation. If the DNA repair was not successful, p53 activates two apoptosis genes, *bax* (discussed below) and *IGF-BP3* (Fig. 18.10, circle 4). The IGF-BP3 protein product binds the receptor for insulin-like growth factor, which presumably induces apoptosis by blocking the anti-apoptotic signaling by growth factors, and the cell enters a growth factor deprivation mode.

B. Tumor Suppressor Genes That Affect Receptors and Signal Transduction

Tumor suppressor genes may encode receptors, components of the signaling transduction pathway, or transcription factors.

1. REGULATORS OF RAS

The Ras family of proteins is involved in signal transduction for many hormones and growth factors (see above), and is, therefore, oncogenic. The activity of these pathways is interrupted by GAPs (GTPase-activating proteins; see Chapter 9), which vary among cell types. Neurofibromin, the product of the tumor suppressor gene *NF-1*, is a nervous system-specific GAP that regulates the activity of Ras in neuronal tissues (Fig. 18.11). The growth signal is transmitted so long as the Ras protein binds GTP. Binding of NF-1 to Ras activates the GTPase domain of Ras, which hydrolyzes GTP to GDP, thereby inactivating Ras. Without a functional neurofibromin molecule, Ras is perpetually active.

2. PATCHED AND SMOOTHENED

A good example of tumor suppressors and oncogenes working together is provided by the co-receptor genes *patched* and *smoothened*, which encode the receptor for the hedgehog class of signaling peptides. These co-receptors normally function to control growth during embryogenesis and illustrate the importance of maintaining

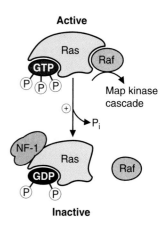

Fig.18.11. NF-1 (neurofibromin) binds to Ras and activates its GTPase activity, thereby decreasing cell proliferation. A mutation in neurofibromin leads to prolonged GTP binding and activation of Ras.

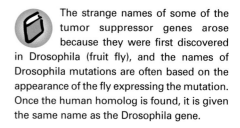
An inherited mutation in *NF-1* can lead to neurofibromatosis, a disease primarily of numerous benign, but painful, tumors of the nervous system. The movie *Elephant Man* was based on an individual who was believed to have this disease. Recent analysis of the patient's remains, however, indicates that he may have suffered from the rare Proteus syndrome, and not neurofibromatosis.

The strange names of some of the tumor suppressor genes arose because they were first discovered in Drosophila (fruit fly), and the names of Drosophila mutations are often based on the appearance of the fly expressing the mutation. Once the human homolog is found, it is given the same name as the Drosophila gene.

A. Catenins and cadherins in cell attachment

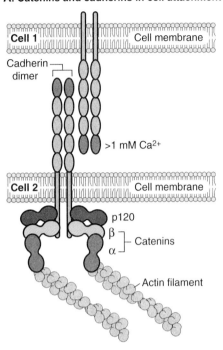

B. β-catenin and APC in gene transcription

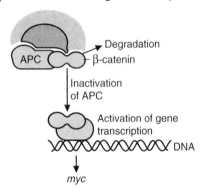

Fig. 18.12. A. Catenins and cadherins. E-cadherin molecules form intercellular, calcium-dependent homodimers with cadherins from another cell, resulting in cell–cell adhesion. The cytoplasmic portion of E-cadherin is complexed to a variety of catenins, which anchor the cadherin to the actin cytoskeleton. B. β-Catenin and APC in transcription. The APC complex activates β-catenin for proteolytic degradation. If APC is inactivated, β-catenin levels increase. It acts as a transcription factor that increases synthesis of *myc* and other genes regulating cell cycle progression.

a balance between oncogenes and tumor suppressor genes. The Patched receptor protein inhibits Smoothened, its co-receptor protein. Binding of a hedgehog ligand to Patched releases the inhibition of Smoothened, which then transmits an activating signal to the nucleus, stimulating new gene transcription. *Smoothened* is a proto-oncogene, and *patched* is a tumor suppressor gene. If *patched* loses its function (definition of a tumor suppressor), then Smoothened can signal the cell to proliferate, even in the absence of a hedgehog signal. Conversely, if *smoothened* undergoes a gain of function mutation (definition of an oncogene), it can signal in the absence of the hedgehog signal, even in the presence of Patched. Inherited mutations in either *smoothened* or *patched* will lead to an increased incidence of basal cell carcinoma.

C. Tumor Suppressor Genes That Affect Cell Adhesion

The cadherin family of glycoproteins mediates calcium- dependent cell–cell adhesion. Cadherins form intercellular complexes binding cells together (Fig. 18.12A). They are anchored intracellularly by catenins, which bind to actin filaments. Loss of E-cadherin expression may contribute to the ability of cancer cells to detach and migrate in metastasis. Individuals who inherit a mutation in E cadherin (this mutation is designated as CDH1) are sharply predisposed to developing diffuse type gastric cancer.

The catenin proteins have two functions; in addition to anchoring cadherins to the cytoskeleton, they act as transcription factors (Fig. 18.12B). β-Catenin also binds to a complex containing the regulatory protein APC (adenomatous polyposis coli), which activates it for degradation. When the appropriate signal activates APC, β-catenin levels increase, and it travels to the nucleus, where it activates *myc* and *cyclin D1* transcription, leading to cell proliferation. APC is a tumor suppressor gene. If it is inactivated, it cannot bind β-catenin and inhibit cell proliferation. Mutations in APC or proteins interacting with it are found in the vast majority of sporadic human colon cancer. Inherited mutations in APC lead to the most common form of hereditary colon cancer, familial adenomatous polyposis.

V. CANCER AND APOPTOSIS

In the body, superfluous or unwanted cells are destroyed by a pathway called apoptosis, or programmed cell death. Apoptosis is a regulated energy-dependent sequence of events by which a cell self-destructs. In this suicidal process, the cell shrinks, the chromatin condenses, and the nucleus fragments. The cell membrane forms blebs (outpouches), and the cell breaks up into membrane-enclosed apoptotic vesicles (apoptotic bodies) containing varying amounts of cytoplasm, organelles, and DNA fragments. Phosphatidylserine, a lipid on the inner leaflet of the cell membrane, is exposed on the external surface of these apoptotic vesicles. It is one of the phagocytic markers recognized by macrophages and other nearby phagocytic cells that engulf the apoptotic bodies.

Apoptosis is a normal part of multiple processes in complex organisms: embryogenesis, the maintenance of proper cell number in tissues, the removal of infected or otherwise injured cells, the maintenance of the immune system, and aging. It can be initiated by injury, radiation, free radicals or other toxins, withdrawal of growth

A form of apoptosis is a normal part of embryonic development. For example, the development of the nervous system uses apoptosis to destroy neurons that have not made the proper connections with target cells. Neurons are produced in excess, and more than 50% of developing neurons are eliminated by programmed cell death. Those neurons that have made the correct connections survive by secreting growth factors that block apoptosis.

factors or hormones, binding of pro-apoptotic cytokines, or interactions with cytotoxic T cells in the immune system. Apoptosis can protect organisms from the negative effect of mutations by destroying cells with irreparably damaged DNA before they proliferate. Just as an excess of a growth signal can produce an excess of unwanted cells, the failure of apoptosis to remove excess or damaged cells can contribute to the development of cancer.

A. Normal Pathways to Apoptosis

Apoptosis can be divided into three general phases: an initiation phase, a signal integration phase, and an execution phase. Apoptosis can be initiated by external signals that work through death receptors, such as tumor necrosis factor (TNF), or deprivation of growth hormones (Fig. 18.13). It can also be initiated by intracellular events that affect mitochondrial integrity (e.g., oxygen deprivation, radiation), and irreparably damaged DNA. In the signal integration phase, these pro-apoptotic signals are balanced against anti-apoptotic cell survival signals by several pathways, including members of the Bcl-2 family of proteins. The execution phase is carried out by proteolytic enzymes called caspases.

1. CASPASES

Caspases are cysteine proteases that cleave peptide bonds next to an aspartate residue. They are present in the cell as procaspases, zymogen-type enzyme precursors activated by proteolytic cleavage of the inhibitory portion of their polypeptide chain. The different caspases are generally divided into two groups according to their function: initiator caspases, which specifically cleave other procaspases, and execution caspases, which cleave other cellular proteins involved in maintaining cellular integrity (see Fig. 18.13). The initiator caspases are activated through two major signaling pathways; the death receptor pathway and the mitochondrial integrity pathway. They activate the execution caspases, which cleave protein kinases involved in cell adhesion, lamins that form the inner lining of the nuclear envelope, actin and other proteins required for cell structure, and DNA repair enzymes. They also cleave an inhibitor protein of the endonuclease CAD (**c**aspase-**a**ctivated **D**Nase). With destruction of the nuclear envelope, additional endonucleases (Ca^{2+}- and Mg^{2+}-dependent) also become activated.

2. THE DEATH RECEPTOR PATHWAY TO APOPTOSIS

The death receptors are a subset of TNF-1 receptors, which includes Fas/CD95, TNF-Receptor 1 (TNF-R1) and Death Receptor 3 (DR3). These receptors form a trimer that binds TNF-1 or another death ligand on its external domain and adaptor proteins to its intracellular domain (Fig.18.14). The activated TNF–receptor complex forms the scaffold for binding two molecules of procaspase 8, which autocatalytically cleave each other to form active caspase 8. Caspase 8 is an initiator caspase that activates execution caspases 3, 6, and 7. Caspase 8 also cleaves a Bcl-2 protein, Bid, to a form that activates the mitochondrial integrity pathway to apoptosis.

3. THE MITOCHONDRIAL INTEGRITY PATHWAY TO APOPTOSIS

Apoptosis is also induced by intracellular signals indicating that cell death should occur. Examples of these signals include growth factor withdrawal, cell injury, the release of certain steroids, and an inability to maintain low levels of intracellular calcium. All of these treatments, or changes, lead to release of cytochrome c from the mitochondria (Fig. 18.15). Cytochrome c is a necessary protein component of the mitochondrial electron transport chain that is a loosely bound to the outside of the inner mitochondrial membrane. Its release initiates apoptosis.

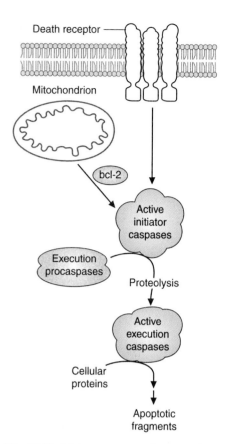

Fig. 18.13. Major components in apoptosis.

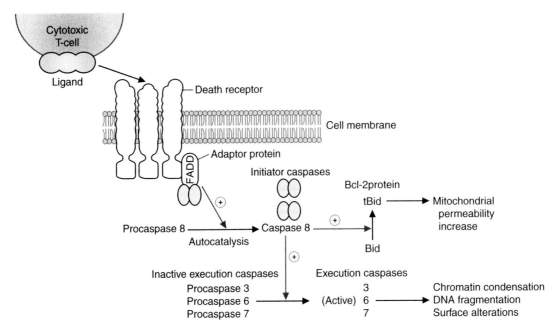

Fig. 18.14. The death receptor pathway to apoptosis. The ligand (usually a cell surface protein on another cell) binds to the death receptor, which makes a scaffold for autocatalytic activation of caspase 8. Active caspase 8 directly cleaves apoptotic execution caspases. However, the pathway also activates Bid, which acts on mitochondrial membrane integrity.

In the cytosol, cytochrome c binds Apaf (pro-**a**poptotic **p**rotease **a**ctivating **f**actor). The Apaf/cytochrome c complex binds caspase 9, an initiator caspase, to form an active complex called the apoptosome. The apoptosome in turn activates execution caspases by zymogen cleavage.

4. INTEGRATION OF PRO- AND ANTI-APOPTOTIC SIGNALS BY THE BCL-2 FAMILY OF PROTEINS

The Bcl-2 family members are decision-makers that integrate prodeath and antideath signals to determine whether the cell should commit suicide. Both pro-apoptotic and anti-apoptotic members of the *Bcl-2* family exist (Table 18.3).

The antiapoptotic *Bcl-2* –type proteins (including Bcl-2, Bcl-xL, Bcl-wL) have at least two ways of antagonizing death signals. They insert into the outer mitochondrial membrane to antagonize channel-forming pro-apoptotic factors, therby decreasing cytochrome c release. They may also bind cytoplasmic Apaf so that it cannot form the apoptosome complex (Fig. 18.16).

These anti-apoptotic Bcl-2 proteins are opposed by pro-apoptotic family members that fall into two categories: ion-channel forming members and the BH3-only members. The pro-death ion channel forming members, such as Bax, are very similar to the anti-apoptotic family members, except that they do not contain the binding domain for Apaf. They have the other structural domains, however, and when they dimerize with

Table 18.3 Bcl-2 Family Members

Anti-apoptotic
  Bcl-2
  Bcl-x
  Bcl-w

Proapoptotic
Channel Forming
  Bax
  Bak
  Bok

Pro-apoptotic
BH3-Only
  Bad
  Bid
  Bod/Bim

Roughly 30 Bcl-2 family members are currently known. These proteins play tissue-specific as well as signal pathway–specific roles in regulating apoptosis. The tissue-specificity is overlapping. For example, Bcl-2 is expressed in hair follicles, kidney, small intestines, neurons, and the lymphoid system, whereas Bcl-x is expressed in the nervous system and hematopoietic cells.

 When *Bcl-2* is mutated, and oncogenic, it is usually overexpressed, for example, in follicular lymphoma and CML (chronic myelogenous leukemia). Overexpression of *Bcl-2* disrupts the normal regulation of pro and anti-apoptotic factors and tips the balance to an anti-apoptotic stand. This leads to an inability to destroy cells with damaged DNA, such that mutations can accumulate within the cell. Bcl-2 is also a multi-drug resistance protein and if over-expressed will block the induction of apoptosis by antitumor agents by rapidly removing them from the cell. Thus, strategies are being developed to reduce Bcl-2 levels in tumors over-expressing it before initiating drug or radiation treatment.

pro-apoptotic BH3-only members in the outer mitochondrial membrane, they form an ion channel that promotes cytochrome c release rather than inhibiting it (see Fig. 18.16). The pro-death BH3-only proteins (e.g., Bim and Bid) contain only the structural domain that allows them to bind to other bcl-2 family members (the BH3 domain), and not the domains for binding to the membrane or forming ion channels. Their binding activates the pro-death family members and inactivates the anti-apoptotic members. When the cell receives a signal from a pro-death agonist, a BH3 protein like Bid is activated (see Fig. 18.16). The BH3 protein activates Bax (an ion-channel forming pro-apoptotic channel member), which stimulates release of cytochrome c. Normally Bcl-2 acts as a death antagonist by binding Apaf and keeping it in an inactive state. However, at the same time that Bid is activating Bax, Bid also binds to Bcl-2, thereby disrupting the Bcl-2/Apaf complex and freeing Apaf to bind to released cytochrome c to form the apoptosome.

B. Cancer Cells Bypass Apoptosis

Apoptosis should be triggered by a number of stimuli, such as withdrawal of growth factors, elevation of p53 in response to DNA damage, monitoring of DNA damage by repair enzymes, or by release of TNF or other immune factors. However, mutations in oncogenes can create apoptosis-resistant cells.

One of the ways this occurs is through activation of growth factor–dependent signaling pathways that inhibit apoptosis, such as the PDGF/Akt/BAD pathway. Nonphosphorylated BAD acts like Bid in promoting apoptosis (see Fig. 18.16). Binding of the platelet-derived growth factor to its receptor activates PI-3 kinase, which phosphorylates and activates the serine/threonine kinase Akt (protein kinase B, see Chapter 11, section III.B.3). Activation of Akt results in the phosphorylation of the pro-apoptotic BH3-only protein BAD, which inactivates it. The PDGF/Akt/BAD pathway illustrates the requirement of normal cells for growth factor stimulation to prevent cell death. One of the features of neoplastic transformation is the loss of growth factor dependence for survival.

The MAP kinase pathway is also involved in regulating apoptosis and sends cell survival signals. MAP kinase kinase phosphorylates and activates another protein kinase known as RSK. Like Akt, RSK phosphorylates BAD and inhibits its activity. Thus, BAD acts as a site of convergence for the PI-3 kinase/Akt and MAP kinase pathways in signaling cell survival. Gain-of-function mutations in the genes controlling these pathways, such as *ras*, creates apoptosis- resistant cells.

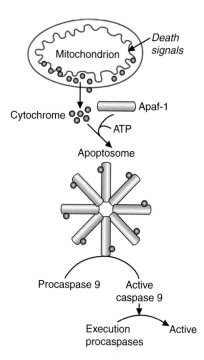

Fig. 18.15. The mitochondrial integrity pathway releases cytochrome c, which binds to Apaf and forms a multimeric complex called the apoptosome. The apoptosome converts procaspase 9 to active caspase, which it releases into the cytosol.

Stimulus

Growth factor deprivation
Steroids
Irradiation
Chemotherapeutic drugs

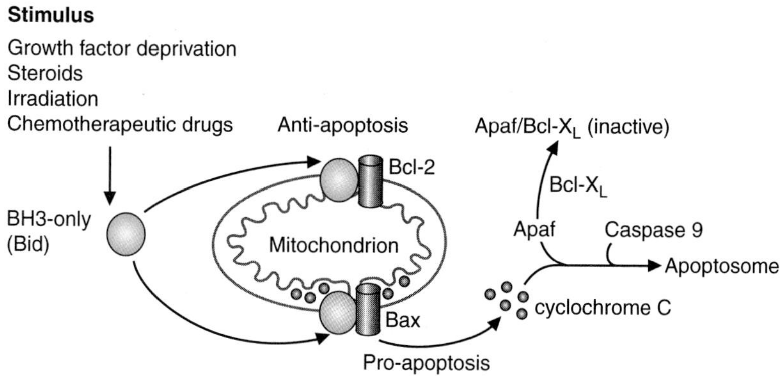

Fig. 18.16. Roles of the Bcl-2 family members in regulating apoptosis. Bcl-2, which is anti-apoptotic, binds Bid (or tBid) and blocks formation of channels that allow cytochrome c release from the mitochondria. Death signals result in activation of a BH3-only protein such as Bid, which can lead to mitochondrial pore formation, swelling, and release of cytochrome c. Bid binds to and activates the membrane ion-channel protein Bax, activating cytochrome c release, which binds to Apaf and leads to formation of the apoptosome.

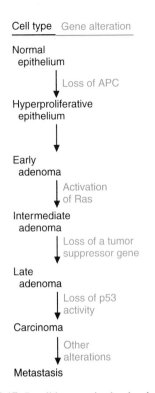

Fig. 18.17. Possible steps in the development of colon cancer. The changes do not always occur in this order, but the most benign tumors have the lowest frequency of mutations, and the most malignant have the highest frequency.

VI. CANCER REQUIRES MULTIPLE MUTATIONS

Cancer takes a long time to develop in humans because multiple genetic alterations are required to transform normal cells into malignant cells (see Fig. 18.1). A single change in one oncogene or tumor suppressor gene in an individual cell is not adequate for transformation. For example, if cells derived from biopsy specimens of normal cells are not already "immortalized," that is, able to grow in culture indefinitely, addition of the *ras* oncogene to the cells is not sufficient for transformation. However, additional mutations in a combination of oncogenes, for example *ras* and *myc*, can result in transformation (Fig. 18.17). Epidemiologists have estimated that four to seven mutations are required for normal cells to be transformed.

Cells accumulate multiple mutations through clonal expansion. When DNA damage occurs in a normally proliferative cell, a population of cells with that mutation is produced. Expansion of the mutated population enormously increases the probability of a second mutation in a cell containing the first mutation. After one or more mutations in proto-oncogenes or tumor suppressor genes, a cell may proliferate more rapidly in the presence of growth stimuli and with further mutations grow autonomously, that is, independent of normal growth controls. Enhanced growth increases the probability of further mutations. Some families have a strong predisposition to cancer. Individuals in these families have inherited a mutation or deletion of one allele of a tumor suppressor gene, and as progeny of that cell proliferate, mutations can occur in the second allele, leading to a loss of control of cellular proliferation. These familial cancers include familial retinoblastoma, familial adenomatous polyps of the colon, and multiple endocrine neoplasia, one form of which involves tumors of the thyroid, parathyroid, and adrenal medulla (MEN type II).

Studies of benign and malignant polyps of the colon show that these tumors have a number of different genetic abnormalities. The incidence of these mutations increases with the level of malignancy. In the early stages, normal cells of the intestinal epithelium proliferate, develop mutations in the APC gene, and polyps develop. This change is associated with a mutation in the *ras* proto-oncogene that converts it to an active oncogene. Progression to the next stage is associated with a deletion or alteration of a tumor suppressor gene on chromosome 5. Subsequently, mutations occur in chromosome 18, inactivating a gene that may be involved in cell adhesion, and in chromosome 17, inactivating the *p53* tumor suppressor gene. The

Nick O'Tyne had been smoking for 40 years before he developed lung cancer. The fact that cancer takes so long to develop has made it difficult to prove that the carcinogens in cigarette smoke cause lung cancer. Studies in England and Wales show that cigarette consumption by men began to increase in the early 1900s. Followed by a 20-year lag, the incidence in lung cancer in men also began to rise. Women began smoking later, in the 1920s. Again the incidence of lung cancer began to increase after a 20-year lag.

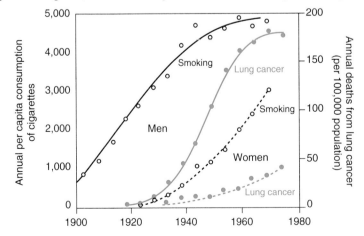

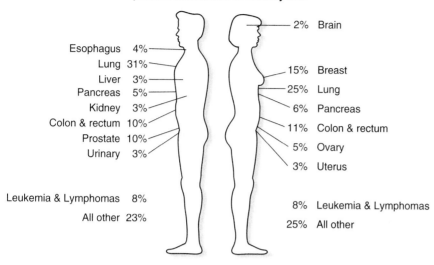

**2003 Estimated cancer deaths, United States
percent distribution of sites by sex**

Esophagus 4%
Lung 31%
Liver 3%
Pancreas 5%
Kidney 3%
Colon & rectum 10%
Prostate 10%
Urinary 3%

Leukemia & Lymphomas 8%
All other 23%

2% Brain
15% Breast
25% Lung
6% Pancreas
11% Colon & rectum
5% Ovary
3% Uterus

8% Leukemia & Lymphomas
25% All other

Fig. 18.18. Estimated cancer deaths by site and sex. Data from The American Cancer Society, Inc: Cancer Facts and Figures, 2003.

cells become malignant, and further mutations result in growth that is more aggressive and metastatic. This sequence of mutations is not always followed precisely, but an accumulation of mutations in these genes is found in a large percentage of colon carcinomas.

VII. AT THE MOLECULAR LEVEL, CANCER IS MANY DIFFERENT DISEASES

More than 20% of the deaths in the United States each year are caused by cancer, with tumors of the lung, large intestine, and the breast being the most common (Fig. 18.18). Different cell types typically use different mechanisms through which they lose the ability to control their own growth. An examination of the genes involved in the development of cancer shows that a particular type of cancer can arise in multiple ways. For example, Patched and Smoothened are the receptor and co-receptor for the signaling peptide, sonic hedgehog. Either mutation of *smoothened*, an oncogene, or inactivation of *patched*, a tumor suppressor gene, can give rise to basal cell carcinoma. Similarly, transforming growth factor β and its signal transduction proteins SMAD4/DPC are part of the same growth-inhibiting pathway, and either may be absent in colon cancer. Thus, treatments which are successful for one patient with colon cancer may not be successful in a second patient with colon cancer because of the differences in the molecular basis of each individual's disease (this now also appears to be the case with breast cancer as well). Medical practice in the future will require identifying the molecular lesions involved in a particular disease and developing appropriate treatments accordingly. The use of gene chip technology (see Chapter 17) to genotype tumor tissues will aid greatly in allowing patient specific treatments to be developed.

 A new treatment for CML based on rational drug design was recently introduced. The fusion protein Bcr-Abl is found only in the transformed cells expressing the Philadelphia chromosome and not in normal cells. Once the structure of Bcr-Abl was determined, the drug Gleevec was designed to specifically bind to and inhibit only the active site of the fusion protein and not the normal protein. Gleevec was successful in blocking Bcr-Abl function, thereby stopping cell proliferation, and in some cells would induce apoptosis, so the cells would die. Because normal cells do not express the hybrid protein, they were not affected by the drug. The problem with this treatment is that some patients suffered relapses, and when their Bcr-Abl proteins were studied it was found in some patients that the fusion protein had a single amino acid substitution near the active site that prevented Gleevec from binding to the protein. Other patients had an amplification of the Bcr-Abl gene product. Thus, Gleevec is a promising first step in designing drugs specifically targeted to tumor cells and is leading the way for rational drug design in the treatment of cancer.

CLINICAL COMMENTS

 Mannie Weitzels. The treatment of a symptomatic patient with CML whose white blood cell count is in excess of 50,000 cells/mL is usually initiated with busulfan. Alkylating agents such as cyclophosphamide have been used alone or in combination with busulfan. Purine and pyrimidine antagonists and hydroxyurea (an inhibitor of the enzyme ribonucleotide reductase, which converts ribonucleotides to deoxyribonucleotides for DNA synthesis) are sometimes effective in CML as well. In addition, trials with both γ- and β-interferon have shown promise in increasing survival in these patients. Interestingly, the latter agents have been associated with the disappearance of the Philadelphia chromosome in dividing marrow cells of some patients treated in this way.

Nick O' Tyne. Surgical resection of the primary lung cancer with an attempt at cure was justified in Nick O'Tyne, who had a good prognosis with a T_1,N_1,M_0 staging classification preoperatively. Without some evidence of spread to the central nervous system at that time, a preoperative CT scan of the brain would not have been justified. This conservative approach would require scanning of all of the potential sites for metastatic disease from a non–small cell cancer of the lung in all patients who present in this way. In an era of runaway costs of health care delivery, such an approach could not be considered cost-effective.

Unfortunately, Mr. O'Tyne developed a metastatic lesion in the right temporal cortex of his brain. Because metastases were almost certainly present in other organs, Mr. O'Tyne's brain tumor was not treated surgically. In spite of palliative radiation therapy to the brain, Mr. O'Tyne succumbed to his disease just 9 months after its discovery, an unusually virulent course for this malignancy. On postmortem examination, it was found that his body was riddled with metastatic disease.

Colin Tuma. Colin Tuma requires yearly colonoscopies to check for new polyps in his intestinal tract. Because the development of a metastatic adenoma requires a number of years (because of the large numbers of mutations that must occur), yearly checks will enable new polyps to be identified and removed before malignant tumors develop.

Mel Anoma. The biopsy of Mel Anoma's excised mole showed that it was not malignant. The most important clinical sign of a malignant melanoma is a change in color in a pigmented lesion. Unlike benign (nondysplastic) nevi, melanomas exhibit striking variations in pigmentation, appearing in shades of black, brown, red, dark blue, and gray. Additional clinical warning signs of a melanoma are: enlargement of a preexisting mole, itching or pain in a preexisting mole, development of a new pigmented lesion during adult life, and irregularity of the borders of a pigmented lesion. **Mel Anoma** was advised to conduct a monthly self-examination, to have a clinical skin examination once or twice yearly, to avoid sunlight, and to use appropriate sunscreens.

The TNM system standardizes the classification of tumors. The T stands for the stage of tumor (the higher the number, the worse the prognosis), the N stands for the number of lymph nodes that are affected by the tumor (again, the higher the number, the worse the prognosis), and M stands for the presence of metastasis (0 for none, 1 for the presence of metastatic cells).

Mutations associated with malignant melanomas include *ras* (gain-of-function in growth signal transduction oncogene), p53 (loss of function of tumor suppressor gene), p16 (loss of function in Cdk inhibitor tumor suppressor gene), Cdk4 (gain of function in a cell cycle progression oncogene) and cadherin/β-catenin regulation (loss of regulation that requires attachment).

BIOCHEMICAL COMMENTS

Viruses and human cancer. Three RNA retroviruses are associated with the development of cancer in humans: HTLV-1, HIV, and hepatitis C. There are also DNA viruses associated with cancer.

HTLV-1. HTLV-1 causes adult T-cell leukemia. The HTLV-1 genome encodes a protein Tax, which is a transcriptional coactivator. The cellular proto-oncogenes c-*sis* and c-*fos* are activated by Tax, thereby altering the normal controls on cellular proliferation and leading to malignancy. Thus, *tax* is a viral oncogene without a counterpart in the host cell genome.

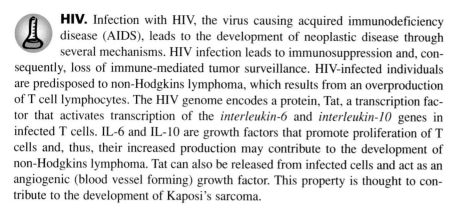

HIV. Infection with HIV, the virus causing acquired immunodeficiency disease (AIDS), leads to the development of neoplastic disease through several mechanisms. HIV infection leads to immunosuppression and, consequently, loss of immune-mediated tumor surveillance. HIV-infected individuals are predisposed to non-Hodgkins lymphoma, which results from an overproduction of T cell lymphocytes. The HIV genome encodes a protein, Tat, a transcription factor that activates transcription of the *interleukin-6* and *interleukin-10* genes in infected T cells. IL-6 and IL-10 are growth factors that promote proliferation of T cells and, thus, their increased production may contribute to the development of non-Hodgkins lymphoma. Tat can also be released from infected cells and act as an angiogenic (blood vessel forming) growth factor. This property is thought to contribute to the development of Kaposi's sarcoma.

DNA viruses. Some DNA viruses also cause human cancer, but by different mechanisms. Three DNA tumor virus families, SV40, papillomavirus, and adenovirus, encode proteins that inactivate pRb and p53. By interfering with the G1/S checkpoint, these oncoproteins increase the probability that mutations in oncogenes and tumor suppressor genes will be incorporated into the genome of infected cells, thereby increasing the probability of transformation. The Epstein-Barr virus encodes a Bcl-2 protein that restricts apoptosis of the infected cell.

Suggested References

Culotta E, Koshland D Jr. Molecule of the year: p53 sweeps through cancer research. Science 1993;262:1958–1959.

Tamm I, Schriever F, and Dorhen B. Apoptosis: implications of basic research for clinical oncology. The Lancet Oncology 2001;2:33–42.

Vogelstein B, Fearon ER, Hamilton SR, et al. Genetic alterations during colorectal tumor development. N Engl J Med 1988;319:525.

Bertram JS. The molecular biology of cancer. Molecular Aspects Med 2000;21:167–223.

Alberts B, Johnson A, Lewis J, Raff M, et al. Cancer. Chapter 23. In Molecular Biology of the Cell, 4th Ed. New York: Garland Scientific, 2002:1313–1362.

Weinberg RA. How cancer arises. Sci Am 1996:275:62–70.

 REVIEW QUESTIONS—CHAPTER 18

1. The *ras* oncogene in Colin Tuma's malignant polyp differs from the *c-ras* proto-oncogene only in the region that encodes the N-terminus of the protein. This portion of the normal and mutant sequences is shown below:

         10   20   30
Normal A T G A C G G A A T A T A A G C T G G T G G T G G T G G G C G C C G G C G G T
Mutant A T G A C G G A A T A T A A G C T G G T G G T G G T G G G C G C C G T C G G T

This mutation is similar to the mutation found in the *ras* oncogene in various tumors. What type of mutation converts the *ras* proto-oncogene to an oncogene?

(A) An insertion that disrupts the reading frame of the protein

(B) A deletion that disrupts the reading frame of the protein

(C) A missense mutation that changes one amino acid within the protein

(D) A silent mutation that has no change in amino acid sequence of the protein

(E) An early termination that creates a stop codon in the reading frame of the protein

2. The mechanism through which Ras becomes an oncogenic protein is which of the following?

    (A) Ras remains bound to GAP.
    (B) Ras can no longer bind cAMP.
    (C) Ras has lost its GTPase activity.
    (D) Ras can no longer bind GTP.
    (E) Ras can no longer be phosphorylated by MAP kinase.

3. Which of the following statements best describes a characteristic of oncogenes?

    (A) All retroviruses contain at least one oncogene.
    (B) Retroviral oncogenes were originally obtained from a cellular host chromosome.
    (C) Proto-oncogenes are genes, found in retroviruses, that have the potential to transform normal cells when inappropriately expressed.
    (D) The oncogenes that lead to human disease are different from those that lead to tumors in animals.
    (E) Oncogenes are mutated versions of normal viral gene products.

4. When p53 increases in response to DNA damage, which of the following events occur?

    (A) p53 induces transcription of cdk4.
    (B) p53 induces transcription of cyclin D.
    (C) p53 binds E2F to activate transcription.
    (D) p53 induces transcription of p21.
    (E) p53 directly phosphorylates the transcription factor jun.

5. A tumor suppressor gene is best described by which of the following?

    (A) A gain-of-function mutation leads to uncontrolled proliferation.
    (B) A loss-of-function mutation leads to uncontrolled proliferation.
    (C) When expressed, the gene suppresses viral genes from being expressed.
    (D) When expressed, the gene specifically blocks the G1/S checkpoint.
    (E) When expressed, the gene induces tumor formation.

Fuel Oxidation and The Generation of ATP

All physiologic processes in living cells require energy transformation. Cells convert the chemical bond energy in foods into other forms, such as an electrochemical gradient across the plasma membrane, or the movement of muscle fibers in an arm, or assembly of complex molecules such as DNA (Fig. 1). These energy transformations can be divided into three principal phases: (1) oxidation of fuels (fat, carbohydrate, and protein), (2) conversion of energy from fuel oxidation into the high-energy phosphate bonds of ATP, and (3) utilization of ATP phosphate bond energy to drive energy-requiring processes.

The first two phases of energy transformation are part of cellular respiration, the overall process of using O_2 and energy derived from oxidizing fuels to generate ATP. We need to breathe principally because our cells require O_2 to generate adequate amounts of ATP from the oxidation of fuels to CO_2. Cellular respiration uses over 90% of the O_2 we inhale.

In phase 1 of respiration, energy is conserved from fuel oxidation by enzymes that transfer electrons from the fuels to the electron-accepting coenzymes NAD^+ and FAD, which are reduced to NADH and FAD(2H), respectively (Fig. 2). The pathways for the oxidation of most fuels (glucose, fatty acids, ketone bodies, and many amino acids) converge in the generation of the activated 2-carbon acetyl group in acetyl CoA. The complete oxidation of the acetyl group to CO_2 occurs in the tricarboxylic acid (TCA) cycle, which collects the energy mostly as NADH and FAD(2H).

In phase 2 of cellular respiration, the energy derived from fuel oxidation is converted to the high-energy phosphate bonds of ATP by the process of oxidative phosphorylation (see Fig. 2). Electrons are transferred from NADH and FAD(2H) to O_2 by the electron transport chain, a series of electron transfer proteins that are located in the inner mitochondrial membrane. Oxidation of NADH and FAD(2H) by O_2 generates an electrochemical potential across the inner mitochondrial membrane in the form of a transmembrane proton gradient (Δp). This electrochemical potential drives the synthesis of ATP form ADP and Pi by a transmembrane enzyme called ATP synthase (or F_0F_1ATPase).

In phase 3 of cellular respiration, the high-energy phosphate bonds of ATP are used for processes such as muscle contraction (mechanical work), maintaining low intracellular Na^+ concentrations (transport work), synthesis of larger molecules such as DNA in anabolic pathways (biosynthetic work), or detoxification (biochemical work). As a consequence of these processes, ATP is either directly or indirectly hydrolyzed to ADP and inorganic phosphate (Pi), or to AMP and pyrophosphate (PPi).

Cellular respiration occurs in mitochondria (Fig. 3). The mitochondrial matrix, which is the compartment enclosed by the inner mitochondrial membrane, contains almost all of the enzymes for the TCA cycle and oxidation of fatty acids,

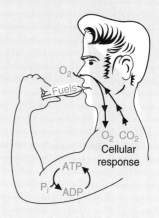

Fig. 1. Energy transformations in fuel metabolism. When ATP energy is transformed into cellular responses, such as muscle contraction, ATP is cleaved to ADP and Pi (inorganic phosphate). In cellular respiration, O_2 is used for regenerating ATP from oxidation of fuels to CO_2.

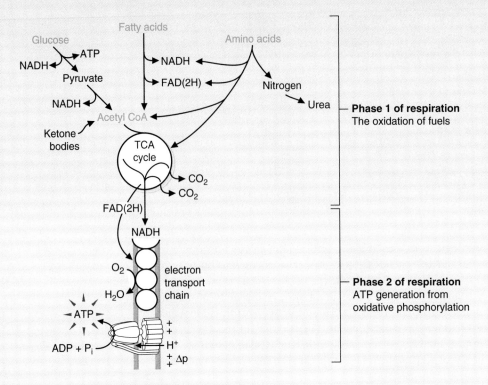

Fig. 2. Cellular respiration. Δp = the proton gradient.

Definitions of prefixes and suffixes used in describing clinical conditions:

an-: Without
-emia: Blood
hyper-: Excessive, above normal
hypo-: Deficient, below normal
-osis: Abnormal or diseased state
-uria: Urine

ketone bodies, and most amino acids. The inner mitochondrial membrane contains the protein complexes of the electron transport chain and ATP synthase, the enzyme complex that generates ATP from ADP and Pi. Some of the subunits of these complexes are encoded by mitochondrial DNA, which resides in the matrix. ATP is generated in the matrix, but most of the energy-using processes in the cell occur outside of the mitochondrion. As a consequence, newly generated ATP must be continuously transported to the cytosol by protein transporters in the impermeable inner mitochondrial membrane and by diffusion through pores in the more permeable outer mitochondrial membrane.

The rates of fuel oxidation and ATP utilization are tightly coordinated through feedback regulation of the electron transport chain and the pathways of fuel oxidation. Thus, if less energy is required for work, more fuel is stored as glycogen or fat in adipose tissue. The basal metabolic rate (BMR), caloric balance, and ΔG (the change in Gibbs free energy, which is the amount of energy available to do useful work) are quantitative ways of describing energy requirements and the energy that can be derived from fuel oxidation. The various types of enzyme regulation described in Chapter 9 are all used to regulate the rate of oxidation of different fuels to meet energy requirements.

Fatty acids are a major fuel in the body. After eating, we store excess fatty acids and carbohydrates that are not oxidized as fat (triacylglycerols) in adipose tissue. Between meals, these fatty acids are released and circulate in blood bound to albumin. In muscle, liver, and other tissues, fatty acids are oxidized to acetyl CoA in the pathway of β-oxidation. NADH and FAD(2H) generated from β-oxidation are reoxidized by O_2 in the electron transport chain, thereby generating ATP (see Fig. 2). Small amounts of certain fatty acids are oxidized through other pathways that convert them to either oxidizable fuels or urinary excretion products (e.g., peroxisomal β-oxidation).

Not all acetyl CoA generated from β-oxidation enters the TCA cycle. In the liver, acetyl CoA generated from β-oxidation of fatty acids can also be converted to the ketone bodies acetoacetate and β-hydroxybutyrate. Ketone bodies are taken up by muscle and other tissues, which convert them back to acetyl CoA for oxidation in the TCA cycle. They become a major fuel for the brain during prolonged fasting.

Amino acids derived from dietary or body proteins are also potential fuels that can be oxidized to acetyl CoA, or converted to glucose and then oxidized (see Fig. 2). These oxidation pathways, like those of fatty acids, generate NADH or FAD(2H). Ammonia, which can be formed during amino acid oxidation, is toxic. It is therefore converted to urea in the liver and excreted in the urine. There are more than 20 different amino acids, each with a somewhat different pathway for oxidation of the carbon skeleton and conversion of its nitrogen to urea. Because of the complexity of amino acid metabolism, use of amino acids as fuels is considered separately in Section Seven, Nitrogen Metabolism.

Glucose is a universal fuel used to generate ATP in every cell type in the body (Fig. 4). In glycolysis, 1 mole of glucose is converted to 2 moles of pyruvate and 2 moles of NADH by cytosolic enzymes. Small amounts of ATP are generated when high-energy pathway intermediates transfer phosphate to ADP in a process termed substrate level phosphorylation. In aerobic glycolysis, the NADH produced from glycolysis is reoxidized by O_2 via the electron transport chain, and pyruvate enters the TCA cycle. In anaerobic glycolysis, the NADH is reoxidized by conversion of pyruvate to lactate, which enters the blood. Although anaerobic glycolysis has a low ATP yield, it is important for tissues with a low oxygen supply and few mitochondria (e.g., the kidney medulla), or tissues experiencing diminished blood flow (ischemia).

All cells continuously use ATP and require a constant supply of fuels to provide energy for the generation of ATP. Chapters 1 through 3 of this text outline the basic patterns of fuel utilization in the human and provide information about dietary components.

The pathologic consequences of metabolic problems in fuel oxidation can be grouped into 2 categories: (1) lack of a required product, or (2) excess of a substrate or pathway intermediate. The product of fuel oxidation is ATP, and an inadequate rate of ATP production occurs under a wide variety of medical conditions. Extreme conditions that interfere with ATP generation from oxidative phosphorylation, such as complete oxygen deprivation (anoxia), or cyanide poisoning, are fatal. A myocardial infarction is caused by a lack of adequate blood flow to regions of the heart (ischemia), thereby depriving cardiomyocytes of oxygen and fuel. Hyperthyroidism is associated with excessive heat generation from fuel oxidation, and in hypothyroidism, ATP generation can decrease to a fatal level. Conditions such as malnutrition, anorexia nervosa, or excessive alcohol consumption may decrease availability of thiamine, Fe^{2+}, and other vitamins and minerals required by the enzymes of fuel oxidation. Mutations in mitochondrial DNA or nuclear DNA result in deficient ATP generation from oxidative metabolism.

In contrast, problems arising from an excess of substrate or fuel are seen in diabetes mellitus, which may result in a potentially fatal ketoacidosis. Lactic acidosis occurs with problems of oxidative metabolism.

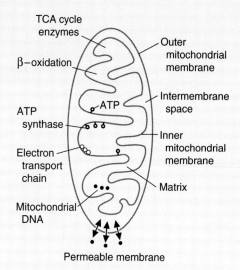

Fig. 3. Oxidative metabolism in mitochondria. The inner mitochondrial membrane forms infoldings, called cristae, which enclose the mitochondrial matrix. Most of the enzymes for the TCA cycle, the β-oxidation of fatty acids, and for mitochondrial DNA synthesis are found in the matrix. ATP synthase and the protein complexes of the electron transport chain are embedded in the inner mitochondrial membrane. The outer mitochondrial membrane is permeable to small ions, but the inner mitochondrial membrane is impermeable.

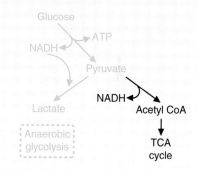

Fig. 4. Glycolysis. In glycolysis, glucose is converted to pyruvate. If the pyruvate is reduced to lactate, the pathway does not require O_2 and is called anaerobic glycolysis. If this pyruvate is converted instead to acetyl CoA and oxidized in the TCA cycle, glycolysis requires O_2 and is aerobic.

19 Cellular Bioenergetics: ATP And O_2

Bioenergetics refers to **cellular energy transformations.**

The ATP-ADP cycle. *In cells, the* **chemical bond energy** *of fuels is transformed into the physiologic responses necessary for life. The central role of the* **high-energy phosphate bonds of ATP** *in these processes is summarized in the* **ATP-ADP cycle** *(Fig. 19.1). To generate ATP through cellular respiration, fuels are degraded by oxidative reactions that transfer most of their* **chemical bond energy** *to* NAD^+ *and FAD to generate the reduced form of these coenzymes,* **NADH** *and* **FAD(2H).** *When NADH and FAD(2H) are oxidized by* O_2 *in the electron transport chain, the energy is used to regenerate ATP in the process of* **oxidative phosphorylation.** *Energy available from cleavage of the high-energy phosphate bonds of ATP can be used directly for* **mechanical work** *(e.g., muscle contraction) or for* **transport work** *(e.g., a* Na^+ *gradient generated by* Na^+*,* K^+*-ATPase). It can also be used for* **biochemical work** *(energy-requiring chemical reactions), such as* **anabolic pathways** *(biosynthesis of large molecules like proteins) or detoxification reactions.* **Phosphoryl transfer** *reactions,* **protein conformational changes,** *and the formation of* **activated intermediates** *containing* **high energy bonds** *(e.g., UDP-sugars) facilitate these energy transformations. Energy released from foods that is not used for work against the environment is transformed into* **heat.**

ATP homeostasis. *Fuel oxidation is regulated to maintain* **ATP homeostasis** *(homeo, same; stasis, state). Regardless of whether the level of cellular fuel utilization is high (with increased ATP consumption), or low (with decreased ATP consumption), the available ATP within the cell is maintained at a constant level by appropriate increases or decreases in the rate of fuel oxidation. Problems in ATP homeostasis and energy balance occur in obesity, hyperthyroidism, and myocardial infarction.*

Energy from Fuel Oxidation. *Fuel oxidation is* **exergonic;** *it releases energy. The maximum quantity of energy released that is available for useful work (e.g., ATP synthesis) is called* $\Delta G^{0\prime}$*, the* **change in Gibbs free energy** *at pH 7.0 under standard conditions. Fuel oxidation has a* **negative** $\Delta G^{0\prime}$*, that is, the products have a lower chemical bond energy than the reactants and their formation is energetically favored. ATP synthesis from ADP and inorganic phosphate is* **endergonic;** *it requires energy and has a positive* $\Delta G^{0\prime}$*. To proceed in our cells, all pathways must have a negative* $\Delta G^{0\prime}$*. How is this accomplished for anabolic pathways such as glycogen synthesis? These metabolic pathways incorporate reactions that expend high-energy bonds to compensate for the energy-requiring steps. Because the* $\Delta G^{0\prime}$*s for a sequence of reactions* **are additive,** *the overall pathway becomes energetically favorable.*

Fuels are oxidized principally by donating electrons to NAD^+ *and FAD, which then donate electrons to* O_2 *in the electron transport chain. The* **caloric value** *of a fuel is related to its* $\Delta G^{0\prime}$ *for transfer of electrons to* O_2*, and its* **reduction potential,** $E^{0\prime}$ *(a measure of its willingness to donate, or accept,*

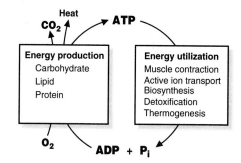

Fig. 19.1. ATP-ADP cycle.

In the thermodynamic perspective of energy expenditure, where energy intake to the body exceeds energy expended, the difference is effectively stored as fat.

Energy intake (food)

Total energy expenditure = Heat produced + work on environment

Metabolism → Energy storage (fat)

- Physical activity variable
- Adaptive thermogenesis
- Obligatory energy expenditure

Cellular and organ functions

The portion of food that is metabolized is regulated to match the total energy expenditure of the body. A certain amount of the energy is obligatory (the amount of energy expended to do the work of the cells, the BMR). Some energy is also expended for adaptive thermogenesis, heat generated in response to cold or diet. An additional amount of energy is used for physical exercise (work against the environment). To voluntarily store less energy as fat, we can vary our caloric intake through dietary changes or our energy expenditure through changes in our physical exercise.

Cora Nari suffered a heart attack 8 months ago and had a significant loss of functional heart muscle. The pain she is experiencing is called angina pectoris, which is a crushing or constricting pain located in the center of the chest, often radiating to the neck or arms (see Ann Jeina, Chapters 6 and 7). The most common cause of angina pectoris is partial blockage of coronary arteries from atherosclerosis. The heart muscle cells beyond the block receive an inadequate blood flow and oxygen, and die when ATP production falls too low.

*electrons). Because fatty acids are more reduced than carbohydrates, they have a higher caloric value. The high affinity of oxygen for electrons (a high positive reduction potential) drives fuel oxidation forward, with release of energy that can be used for ATP synthesis in oxidative phosphorylation. However, smaller amounts of ATP can be generated without the use of O_2 in **anaerobic glycolysis**.*

*Fuel oxidation can also generate **NADPH**, which usually donates electrons to biosynthetic pathways and detoxification reactions. For example, in some reactions catalyzed by **oxygenases**, NADPH is the electron donor and O_2 the electron acceptor.*

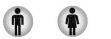

THE WAITING ROOM

Otto Shape is a 26-year old medical student who has completed his first year of medical school. He is 70 inches tall and began medical school weighing 154 lb, within his ideal weight range (see Chapter 1). By the time he finished his last examination in his first year, he weighed 187 lb. He had calculated his BMR at approximately 1,680 kcal, and his energy expenditure for physical exercise equal to 30% of his BMR. He planned on returning to his premedical school weight in 6 weeks over the summer by eating 576 kcal less each day and playing 7 hours of tennis every day. However, he did a summer internship instead of playing tennis. When Otto started his second year of medical school, he weighed 210 lb.

X.S. Teefore (excess T_4) is a 26-year-old man who noted heat intolerance with heavy sweating, heart palpitations, and tremulousness. Over the past 4 months, he has lost weight in spite of a good appetite. He is sleeping poorly and describes himself as feeling "jittery inside."

On physical examination, his heart rate is rapid (116 beats/min) and he appears restless and fidgety. His skin feels warm, and he is perspiring profusely. A fine hand tremor is observed as he extends his arms in front of his chest. His thyroid gland appears to be diffusely enlarged and, on palpation, is approximately 3 times normal size. Thyroid function tests confirm that Mr. Teefore's thyroid gland is secreting excessive amounts of the thyroid hormones T_4 (tetraiodothyronine) and T_3 (triiodothyronine), the major thyroid hormones present in the blood.

Cora Nari is a 64-year-old woman who had a myocardial infarction 8 months ago. Although she managed to lose 6 lb since that time, she remains overweight and has not reduced the fat content of her diet adequately. The graded aerobic exercise program she started 5 weeks after her infarction is now followed irregularly, falling far short of the cardiac conditioning intensity prescribed by her cardiologist. She is readmitted to the hospital cardiac care unit (CCU) after experiencing a severe "viselike pressure" in the mid-chest area while cleaning ice from the windshield of her car. The electrocardiogram (ECG) shows evidence of a new posterior wall myocardial infarction. Signs and symptoms of left ventricular failure are present.

I. ENERGY AVAILABLE TO DO WORK

The basic principle of the ATP-ADP cycle is that fuel oxidation generates ATP, and hydrolysis of ATP to ADP provides the energy to perform most of the work required in the cell. ATP has therefore been called the energy currency of our cells. Like the one dollar bill, it has a defined value, is required to obtain goods and services, and disappears before we know it. To keep up with the demand, we must constantly replenish our ATP supply through the use of O_2 for fuel oxidation.

The amount of energy from ATP cleavage available to do useful work is related to the difference in energy levels between the products and substrates of the reaction and is called the change in Gibbs free energy, ΔG (Δ, difference; G, Gibbs free energy). In cells, the Δ G for energy production from fuel oxidation must be greater than the ΔG of energy-requiring processes, such as protein synthesis and muscle contraction, for life to continue.

The heart is a specialist in the transformation of ATP chemical bond energy into mechanical work. Each single heartbeat uses approximately 2% of the ATP in the heart. If the heart were not able to regenerate ATP, all its ATP would be hydrolyzed in less than 1 minute. Because the amount of ATP required by the heart is so high, it must rely on the pathway of oxidative phosphorylation for generation of this ATP. In **Cora Nari's** heart, hypoxia is affecting her ability to generate ATP.

A. The High-Energy Phosphate Bonds of ATP

The amount of energy released or required by bond cleavage or formation is determined by the chemical properties of the substrates and products. The bonds between the phosphate groups in ATP are called phosphoanhydride bonds (Fig. 19.2). When these bonds are hydrolyzed, energy is released because the products of the reaction (ADP and phosphate) are more stable, with lower bond energies, than the reactants (ATP and H_2O). The instability of the phosphoanhydride bonds arises from their negatively charged phosphate groups, which repel each other and strain the bonds between them. It takes energy to make the phosphate groups stay together. In contrast, there are fewer negative charges in ADP to repel each other. The phosphate group as a free anion is more stable than it is in ATP because of an increase in resonance structures (i.e., the electrons of the oxygen double bond are shared by all the oxygen atoms). As a consequence, ATP hydrolysis is energetically favorable and proceeds with release of energy as heat.

In the cell, ATP is not directly hydrolyzed. Energy released as heat from ATP hydrolysis cannot be transferred efficiently into energy-requiring processes, such as biosynthetic reactions or maintaining an ion gradient. Instead, cellular enzymes directly transfer the phosphate group to a metabolic intermediate or protein that is part of the energy-requiring process (a phosphoryl transfer reaction).

B. Change in Free Energy (ΔG) During a Reaction

How much energy can be obtained from ATP hydrolysis to do the work required in the cell? The maximum amount of useful energy that can be obtained from a

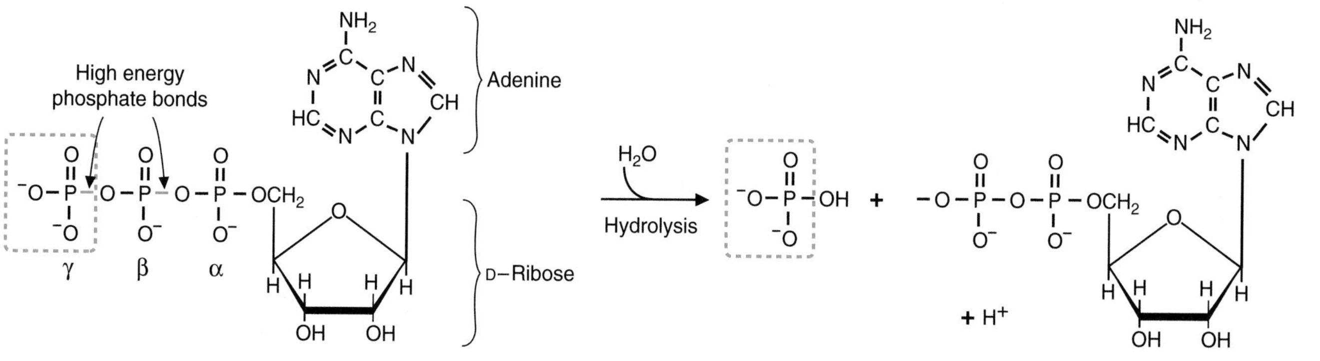

Adenosine 5'-triphosphate
ATP

Phosphate
P_i

Adenosine 5'-diphosphate
ADP

Fig. 19.2. Hydrolysis of ATP to ADP and inorganic phosphate (Pi). Cleavage of the phosphoanhydride bonds between either the β and γ phosphates or the α and β phosphates releases the same amount of energy, approximately −7.3 kcal/mole. However, hydrolysis of the phosphate-adenosine bond (a phosphoester bond) releases less energy (−3.4 kcal/mole), and consequently, this bond is not considered a high-energy phosphate bond. During ATP hydrolysis, the change in disorder during the reaction is small and so ΔG values at physiologic temperature (37°C) are similar to those at standard temperature (25°C). ΔG is affected by pH, which alters the ionization state of the phosphate groups of ATP and by the intracellular concentration of Mg^{2+} ions, which bind to the β and γ phosphate groups of ATP.

reaction is called ΔG, the change in Gibbs free energy. The value of ΔG for a reaction can be influenced by the initial concentration of substrates and products, by temperature, pH, and pressure. The ΔG^0 for a reaction refers to the energy change for a reaction starting at 1 M substrate and product concentrations and proceeding to equilibrium (equilibrium, by definition, occurs when there is no change in substrate and product concentrations with time). $\Delta G^{0\prime}$ is the value for ΔG^0 under standard conditions (pH = 7.0, $[H_2O]$ = 55 M, and 25°C), as well as standard concentrations (Table 19.1).

$\Delta G^{0\prime}$ is equivalent to the chemical bond energy of the products minus that of the reactants, corrected for energy that has gone into entropy (an increase in amount of molecular disorder). This correction for change in entropy is very small for most reactions occurring in cells, and, thus, the $\Delta G^{0\prime}$ for hydrolysis of various chemical bonds reflects the amount of energy available from that bond.

The value of -7.3 kcal/mole (-30.5 kJ/mole) that is generally used for the $\Delta G^{0\prime}$ of ATP hydrolysis is, thus, the amount of energy available from hydrolysis of ATP under standard conditions that can be spent on energy-requiring processes; it defines the "monetary value" of our "ATP currency." Although the difference between cellular conditions (pH 7.3, 37°C) and standard conditions is very small, the difference between cellular concentrations of ATP, ADP, and Pi and the standard 1-M concentrations is huge and greatly affects the availability of energy in the cell.

C. Exothermic and Endothermic Reactions

The value of $\Delta G^{0\prime}$ tells you whether the reaction requires or releases energy, the amount of energy involved, and the ratio of products to substrates at equilibrium. The negative value for the $\Delta G^{0\prime}$ of ATP hydrolysis indicates that, if you begin with equimolar (1 M) concentrations of substrates and products, the reaction proceeds in

Q: The reaction catalyzed by phosphoglucomutase (PGM) is reversible and functions in the synthesis of glycogen from glucose as well as the degradation of glycogen back to glucose. If the $\Delta G^{0\prime}$ for conversion of glucose 6-P to glucose 1-P is +1.65 kcal/mole, what is the $\Delta G^{0\prime}$ of the reverse reaction?

Table 19.1. Thermodynamic Expressions, Laws, and Constants

Definitions

ΔG	Change in free energy, or Gibbs free energy
ΔG^0	Standard free energy change, ΔG at 1 M concentrations of substrates and products
$\Delta G^{0\prime}$	Standard free energy change at 25°C, pH 7.0
ΔH	Change in enthalpy, or heat content
ΔS	Change in entropy, or increase in disorder
$K^{\prime}_{eq}$	Equilibrium constant at 25°C, pH 7.0, incorporating $[H_2O]$ = 55.5 M and $[H+]$ = 10^{-7} M in the constant
$\Delta E^{0\prime}$	Change in reduction potential
~P	Biochemical symbol for a high-energy phosphate bond, i.e., a bond which is hydrolyzed with the release of more than about 7 kcal/mole of heat

Laws of thermodynamics

First law of thermodynamics, the conservation of energy: In any physical or chemical change, the total energy of a system, including its surroundings, remains constant.
Second law of thermodynamics: The universe tends toward disorder. In all natural processes, the total entropy of a system always increases.

Constants

Units of ΔG and ΔH = cal/mole or J/mole: 1 cal = 4.18 J
T, Absolute temperature: K, Kelvin = 273 + °C (25°C = 298° K)
R, Universal gas constant: 1.99 cal/mole·K or 8.31 J/mole·K
F, Faraday constant: F = 23 kcal/mole-volt or 96,500 J/V·mole
Units of $E_0{}^{\prime}$, volts

Formulas

$\Delta G = \Delta H - T\Delta S$
$\Delta G^{0\prime} = -RT\ln K^{\prime}_{eq}$
$\Delta G^{0\prime} = -nF\Delta E^{0\prime}$
$\ln = 2.303 \log_{10}$

Table 19.2. A General Expression for ΔG

To generalize the expression for ΔG, consider a reaction in which
$$aA + bB \rightleftarrows cC + dD$$
The small letters denote a moles of A will combine with b moles of B to produce c moles of C and d moles of D.

$$\Delta G^{0'} = -RT \ln K'_{eq} = -RT \ln \frac{[C]^c_{eq} [D]^d_{eq}}{[A]^a_{eq} [B]^b_{eq}}$$

and

$$\Delta G = \Delta G^{0'} + RT \ln \frac{[C]^c [D]^d}{[A]^a [B]^b}$$

 The ΔG⁰′ for the reverse reaction is −1.65 kcal. The change in free energy is the same for the forward and reverse directions, but has an opposite sign. Because negative ΔG⁰′ values indicate favorable reactions, this reaction under standard conditions favors the conversion of glucose 1-P to glucose 6-P.

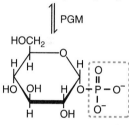

Glucose-6-phosphate (G6P)

↕ PGM

Glucose 1-phosphate (G1P)

For G6P ⟶ G1P:

$\Delta G^{0'} = +1.6 \text{ kcal/mole}$

$\Delta G^{0'} = -RT \ln \dfrac{[G1P]}{[G6P]}$

Fig. 19.3. The phosphoglucomutase reaction. The forward direction is involved in converting glucose to glycogen, and the reverse direction in converting glycogen to glucose 6-P.

the forward direction with the release of energy. From initial concentrations of 1 M, the ATP concentration will decrease, and ADP and Pi will increase until equilibrium is reached.

For a reaction in which a substrate S is converted to a product P, the ratio of the product concentration to the substrate concentration at equilibrium is given by:

Equation 1:

$$\Delta G^{0'} = -RT \ln [P]/[S]$$

(see Table 19.2. for a more general form of this equation; R is equal to the gas constant (1.98 calories/mole-degree Kelvin), and T is equal to the temperature in degrees Kelvin).

Thus, the difference in chemical bond energies of the substrate and product (ΔG⁰′) determines the concentration of each at equilibrium.

Reactions such as ATP hydrolysis are exergonic (release energy) or exothermic (release heat). They have a negative ΔG⁰′ and release energy while proceeding in the forward direction to equilibrium. Endergonic, or endothermic, reactions have a positive ΔG⁰′ for the forward direction (the direction shown), and the backward direction is favored. For example, in the pathway of glycogen synthesis, phosphoglucomutase converts glucose-6-P to glucose-1-P. Glucose-1-P has a higher phosphate bond energy than glucose-6-P because the phosphate is on the aldehyde carbon (Fig 19.3). The ΔG⁰′ for the forward direction (glucose-1-P → glucose-6-P) is, therefore, positive. Beginning at equimolar concentrations of both compounds, there is a net conversion of glucose-1-P back to glucose-6-P and, at equilibrium, the concentration of glucose-6-P is higher than glucose-1-P. The exact ratio is determined by ΔG⁰′ for the reaction.

It is often said that a reaction with a negative ΔG′ proceeds spontaneously in the forward direction, meaning that products accumulate at the expense of reactants. However, ΔG′ is not an indicator of the velocity of the reaction, or the rate at which equilibrium can be reached. In the cell, the velocity of the reaction depends on the efficiency and amount of enzyme available to catalyze the reaction (see Chapter 9), and, therefore, "spontaneously" in this context can be misleading.

Q: The ΔG⁰′ for the conversion of glucose 6-P to glucose 1-P is +1.65 kcal/mole. What is the ratio of [glucose-1-P] to [glucose-6-P] at equilibrium?

II. ENERGY TRANSFORMATIONS TO DO MECHANICAL AND TRANSPORT WORK

To do work in the cell, a mechanism must be available for converting the chemical bond energy of ATP into another form, such as an Na⁺ gradient across a membrane. These energy transformations usually involve intermediate steps in which ATP is bound to a protein, and cleavage of the bound ATP results in a conformational change of the protein.

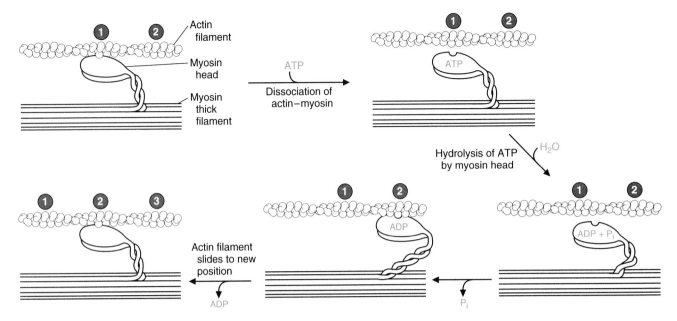

Fig. 19.4. A simplified diagram of myosin ATPase. Muscle fiber is made of thick filaments composed of bundles of the protein myosin, and thin filaments composed of the protein actin (which is activated by Ca^{2+} binding). At many positions along the actin filament, a terminal domain of a myosin molecule, referred to as the "head," binds to a specific site on the actin. The myosin head has an ATP binding site and is an ATPase; it can hydrolyze ATP to ADP and Pi. (1) As ATP binds to myosin, the conformation of myosin changes, and it dissociates from the actin. (2) Myosin hydrolyzes the ATP, again changing conformation. (3) When Pi dissociates, the myosin head reassociates with activated actin at a new position. (4) As ADP dissociates, the myosin again changes conformation, or tightens. This change of conformation at multiple association points between actin and myosin slides the actin filament forward (5).

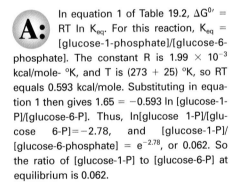

In equation 1 of Table 19.2, $\Delta G^{0\prime} = RT \ln K_{eq}$. For this reaction, $K_{eq} =$ [glucose-1-phosphate]/[glucose-6-phosphate]. The constant R is 1.99×10^{-3} kcal/mole-°K, and T is (273 + 25) °K, so RT equals 0.593 kcal/mole. Substituting in equation 1 then gives $1.65 = -0.593 \ln$ [glucose-1-P]/[glucose-6-P]. Thus, ln[glucose 1-P]/[glucose 6-P]$= -2.78$, and [glucose-1-P]/[glucose-6-phosphate] $= e^{-2.78}$, or 0.062. So the ratio of [glucose-1-P] to [glucose-6-P] at equilibrium is 0.062.

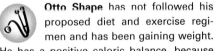

Otto Shape has not followed his proposed diet and exercise regimen and has been gaining weight. He has a positive caloric balance, because his daily energy expenditure is less than his daily energy intake (see Chapter 2). Although the energy expenditure for physical exercise is only approximately 30% of the BMR (basal metabolic rate) in a sedentary individual, it can be 100% or more of the BMR in a person who exercises strenuously for several hours or more. The large increase in ATP utilization for muscle contraction during exercise accounts for its contribution to the daily energy expenditure.

A. Mechanical Work

In mechanical work, the high-energy phosphate bond of ATP is converted into movement by changing the conformation of a protein (Fig.19.4.). For example, in contracting muscle fibers, the hydrolysis of ATP while it is bound to myosin ATPase changes the conformation of myosin so that it is in a "cocked" position ready to associate with the sliding actin filament. Thus, exercising muscle fibers have almost a hundred-fold higher rate of ATP utilization and caloric requirements than resting muscle fibers. Motor proteins, such as kinesins that transport chemicals along fibers, provide another example of mechanical work in a cell.

B. Transport Work

In transport work, called active transport, the high-energy phosphate bond of ATP is used to transport compounds against a concentration gradient (see Chapter10,

The equations for calculating ΔG are based on the first law of thermodynamics (see Table 19.1). The change in chemical bond energy that occurs during a reaction is ΔH, the change in enthalpy of the reaction. At constant temperature and pressure, ΔH is equivalent to the chemical bond energy of the products minus that of the reactants. ΔG, the maximum amount of useful work available from a reaction, is equal to ΔH minus $T\Delta S$. $T\Delta S$ is a correction for the amount of energy that has gone into an increase in the entropy (disorder in arrangement of molecules) of the system.

$$\Delta G = \Delta H - T\Delta S$$

where ΔH = the change in enthalpy, T is the temperature of the system in Kelvin, and ΔS is the change in entropy, or increased disorder of the system. ΔS is often negligible in reactions such as ATP hydrolysis in which the number of substrates (H_2O, ATP) and products (ADP, Pi) are equal and no gas is formed. Under these conditions, the values for ΔG at physiologic temperature (37°C) are similar to those at standard temperature (25°C)

Fig.10.12). In P-ATPases (plasma membrane ATPases) and V-ATPases (vesicular ATPases), the chemical bond energy of ATP is used to reversibly phosphorylate the transport protein and change its conformation. For example, as Na$^+$, K$^+$-ATPase binds and cleaves ATP, it becomes phosphorylated and changes its conformation to release 3 Na$^+$ ions to the outside of the cell, thereby building up a higher extracellular than intra-cellular concentration of Na$^+$. Na$^+$ re-enters the cell on cotransport proteins that drive the uptake of amino acids and many other compounds into the cell. Thus, Na$^+$ must be continuously transported back out. The expenditure of ATP for Na$^+$ transport occurs even while we sleep and is estimated to account for 10 to 30% of our BMR.

A large number of other active transporters also convert ATP chemical bond energy into an ion gradient (membrane potential). Vesicular ATPases pump protons into lyso-somes. Ca^{2+}ATPases in the plasma membrane move Ca^{2+} out of the cell against a con-centration gradient. Similar Ca^{2+}ATPases pump Ca^{2+} into the lumen of the endoplas-mic reticulum and the sarcoplasmic reticulum (in muscle). Thus, a considerable amount of energy is expended in maintaining a low cytoplasmic Ca^{2+} level.

III. BIOCHEMICAL WORK

The high-energy phosphate bonds of ATP are also used for biochemical work. Bio-chemical work occurs in anabolic pathways, which are pathways that synthesize large molecules (e.g., DNA, glycogen, triacylglycerols, and proteins) from smaller compounds. Biochemical work also occurs when toxic compounds are converted to nontoxic compounds that can be excreted (e.g., the liver converts NH$_4^+$ ions to urea in the urea cycle). In general, formation of chemical bonds between two organic molecules (e.g., C-C bonds in fatty acid synthesis or C-N bonds in protein synthe-sis) requires energy and is therefore biochemical work. How do our cells get these necessary energy-requiring reactions to occur?

To answer this question, the next sections consider how energy is used to syn-thesize glycogen from glucose (Fig 19.5). Glycogen is a storage polysaccharide consisting of glucosyl units linked together through glycosidic bonds. If an anabolic pathway, such as glycogen synthesis, were to have an overall positive ΔG$^{0'}$, the cell would be full of glucose and intermediates of the pathway, but very little glycogen would be formed. To avoid this, cells do biochemical work and spend enough of their ATP currency to give anabolic pathways an overall negative ΔG$^{0'}$.

 X.S. Teefore has increased blood levels of thyroid hormones, which accelerate basal metabolic processes that use ATP in our organs (e.g., Na$^+$,K$^+$-ATPase), thereby increasing the BMR. An increased BMR was used for a pre-sumptive diagnosis of hyperthyroidism before development of the tests to measure T3 and T4. Because **X.S. Teefore** did not fully compensate for his increased ATP require-ments with an increased caloric intake, he was in negative caloric balance and lost weight.

Approximately 70% of our resting daily energy requirement arises from work carried out by our largest organs: the heart, brain, kidneys, and liver. Using their rate of oxygen consumption and a P/O ratio of 2.5, it can be estimated that each of these organs is using and producing several times its own weight in ATP each day. The heart, which rhythmically contracts, is using this ATP for mechanical work. In contrast, skeletal muscles in a resting individual use far less ATP per gram of tissue. The kidney has an ATP consumption per gram of tissue similar to that of the heart and is using this ATP largely for transport work to recover usable nutrients and maintain pH and electrolyte balance. The brain, likewise, uses most of its ATP for transport work, main-taining the ion gradients necessary for conduction of the nerve impulse. The liver, in con-trast, has a high rate of ATP consumption and utilization to carry out metabolic work (biosynthesis and detoxification).

Estimated Daily Use of ATP
(g ATP/g tissue)

Heart	16
Brain	6
Kidneys	24
Liver	6
Skeletal Muscle (rest)	0.3
Skeletal Muscle (running)	23.6

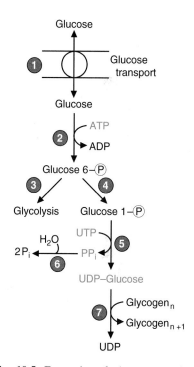

Fig. 19.5. Energetics of glycogen synthesis. Compounds containing high-energy bonds are shown in blue. (1) Glucose is transported into the cell. (2) Glucose phosphorylation uses the high-energy phosphate bond (~P) of ATP in a phosphoryl transfer step. (4) Conversion of glucose 6-phosphate to glucose 1-phosphate by phosphoglucomutase. (5) UDP-Glucose pyrophosphorylase cleaves a ~P bond in UTP, releasing pyrophosphate and forming UDP-glucose, an activated intermediate. (6) The pyrophosphate is hydrolyzed, releasing addi-tional energy. (7) The phosphoester bond of UDP-glucose is cleaved during the addition of a glucosyl unit to the end of a glycogen poly-saccharide chain. The UDP-glucose acts as the leaving group in this reaction. Glucose-6-phosphate also can be metabolized via glycol-ysis (3) when energy is required.

A. ΔG⁰ Values Are Additive

Reactions in which chemical bonds are formed between two organic molecules are usually catalyzed by enzymes that transfer energy from cleavage of ATP in a phosphoryl transfer reaction or by enzymes that cleave a high-energy bond in an activated intermediate of the pathway. Because the $\Delta G^{0\prime}$ values in a reaction sequence are additive, the pathway acquires an overall negative $\Delta G^{0\prime}$, and the reactions in the pathway will occur to move toward an equilibrium state where the concentration of final products is greater than that of the initial reactants.

1. PHOSPHORYL TRANSFER REACTIONS

One of the characteristics of Gibbs free energy is that ΔG^0 values for consecutive steps or reactions in a sequence can be added together to obtain a single value for the overall process. Thus, the high-energy phosphate bonds of ATP can be used to drive a reaction forward that would otherwise be highly unfavorable energetically. Consider, for example, synthesis of glucose 6-P from glucose, the first step in glycolysis and glycogen synthesis (see Fig.19.5, circle 2). If the reaction were to proceed by addition of inorganic phosphate to glucose, glucose-6-P synthesis would have a positive $\Delta G^{0\prime}$ value of 3.3 kcal/mole (Table 19.3). However, when this reaction is coupled to cleavage of the high-energy ATP bond through a phosphoryl transfer reaction, the $\Delta G^{0\prime}$ for glucose-6-P synthesis acquires a net negative value of minus 4.0 kcal/mole, which can be calculated from the sum of the two reactions. Glucose 6-P cannot be transported back out of the cell, and therefore the net negative $\Delta G^{0\prime}$ for glucose 6-P synthesis helps the cell to trap glucose for its own metabolic needs.

The net value for synthesis of glucose 6-P from glucose and ATP would be the same whether or not the two reactions were catalyzed by the same enzyme, were catalyzed by two separate enzymes, or were not catalyzed by an enzyme at all, because it is dictated by the amount of energy in the chemical bonds being broken and formed.

2. ACTIVATED INTERMEDIATES IN GLYCOGEN SYNTHESIS

To synthesize glycogen from glucose, energy is provided by the cleavage of 3 high-energy phosphate bonds in ATP, UTP, and pyrophosphate (PPi)(see Fig. 19.5, Steps 2, 5, and 6). Energy transfer is facilitated by phosphoryl group transfer and by formation of an activated intermediate (UDP-glucose). Step 4, the conversion of glucose 6-phosphate to glucose 1-P, has a positive $\Delta G^{0\prime}$. This step is pulled and pushed in the desired direction by the accumulation of substrate and removal of product in reactions that have a negative $\Delta G^{0\prime}$ from cleavage of high-energy bonds. In Step 5, the UTP high-energy phosphate bond is cleaved to form the activated sugar, UDP-glucose (Fig 19.6). This reaction is further facilitated by cleavage of the high-energy bond in the pyrophosphate (Step 6) that is released in Step 5 (approximately −7.7 kcal). In Step 7, cleavage of the bond between UDP and glucose in the activated intermediate provides the energy for attaching the glucose moiety to the end of the glycogen molecule (approximately −3.3 kcal). In general, the amount of ATP phosphate bond energy used in an anabolic pathway, or detoxification pathway, must provide the pathway with an overall negative $\Delta G^{0\prime}$, so that the concentration of products is favored over that of reactants.

Q: Given a $\Delta G^{0\prime}$ of +1.65 kcal/mole for the conversion of glucose-6-P to glucose-1-P, and a $\Delta G^{0\prime}$ of −4.0 kcal/mole for the conversion of glucose + ATP to glucose-6-P + ADP, what is the value of $\Delta G^{0\prime}$ for the conversion of glucose to glucose-1-P?

Table 19.3. ΔG⁰′ for the Transfer of a Phosphate from ATP to Glucose

Glucose + Pi → glucose-6-P + H_2O	$\Delta G^{0\prime} = +3.3$ kcal/mole
ATP + H_2O → ADP + Pi	$\Delta G^{0\prime} = -7.3$ kcal/mole
Sum: glucose + ATP → glucose-6-P + ADP	$\Delta G^{0\prime} = -4.0$ kcal/mole

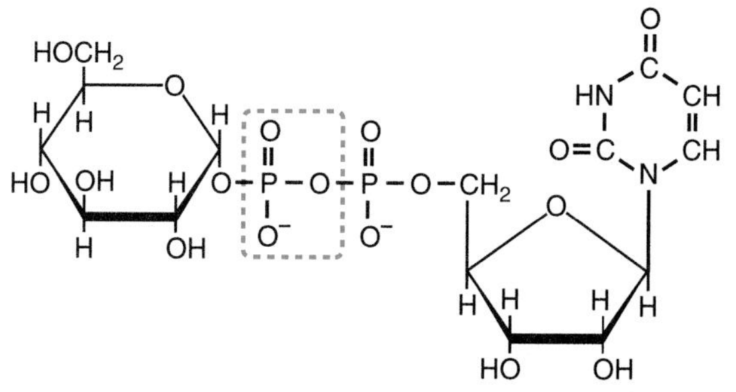

**Uridine diphosphate glucose
(UDP–glucose)**

Fig. 19.6. UDP-glucose contains a high-energy pyrophosphate bond, shown in blue.

B. ΔG Depends on Substrate and Product Concentration

$\Delta G^{0\prime}$ reflects the energy difference between reactants and products at specific concentrations (each at 1 M) and standard conditions (pH 7.0, 25°C). However, these are not the conditions prevailing in cells, where variations from "standard conditions" are relevant to determining actual free energy changes and hence the direction in which reactions are likely to occur. One aspect of free energy changes contributing to the forward direction of anabolic pathways is the dependence of ΔG, the free energy change of a reaction, on the initial substrate and product concentrations. Reactions in the cell with a positive $\Delta G^{0\prime}$ can proceed in the forward direction if the concentration of substrate is raised to high enough levels, or if the concentration of product is decreased to very low levels. Product concentrations can be very low if, for example, the product is rapidly used in a subsequent energetically favorable reaction, or if the product diffuses or is transported away.

1. THE DIFFERENCE BETWEEN ΔG AND ΔG⁰′

The driving force toward equilibrium starting at any concentration of substrate and product is expressed by ΔG, and not by $\Delta G^{0\prime}$, which is the free energy change to reach equilibrium starting with 1 M concentrations of substrate and product. For a reaction in which the substrate S is converted to the product P:

Equation 2

$$\Delta G = \Delta G^{0\prime} + RT \ln [P]/[S]$$

(see Table 19.2, for the general form of this equation).

The expression for ΔG has two terms: $\Delta G^{0\prime}$, the energy change to reach equilibrium starting at equal and 1 M concentrations of substrates and products, and the second term, the energy change to reach equal concentrations of substrate and product starting from any initial concentration. (When [P] = [S] and [P]/[S] = 1, the ln of [P]/[S] is 0, and $\Delta G = \Delta G^{0\prime}$). The second term will be negative for all concentrations of substrate greater than product, and the greater the substrate concentration, the more negative this term will be. Thus, if the substrate concentration is suddenly raised high enough or the product concentration decreased low enough, ΔG (the sum of the first and second terms) will also be negative, and conversion of substrate to product becomes thermodynamically favorable.

2. THE REVERSIBILITY OF THE PHOSPHOGLUCOMUTASE REACTION IN THE CELL

The effect of substrate and product concentration on ΔG and the direction of a reaction in the cell can be illustrated with conversion of glucose-6-P to glucose-1-P, the

A: $\Delta G^{0\prime}$ for the overall reaction is the sum of the individual reactions, and is −2.35 kcal. The individual reactions are:

Glucose + ATP → glucose 6-P + ADP
$\Delta G^{0\prime}$ = −4.0 kcal/mole
Glucose 6-P → glucose 1-P
$\Delta G^{0\prime}$ = +1.65 kcal/mole
Sum: Glucose + ATP → glucose 1-P + ADP
$\Delta G^{0\prime}$ = −2.35 kcal/mole

Thus, the cleavage of ATP has made the synthesis of glucose-1-P from glucose energetically favorable.

reaction catalyzed by phosphoglucomutase in the pathway of glycogen synthesis (see Fig. 19.3). The reaction has a small positive $\Delta G^{0\prime}$ for glucose 1-P synthesis (+1.65.kcal/mole) and at equilibrium, the ratio of [glucose 1-P]/[glucose 6-P] is approximately 6 to 94 (which you calculated in Question 2). However, if another reaction uses glucose 1-P such that this ratio suddenly becomes 3 to 94, there is now a driving force for converting more glucose 6-P to glucose 1-P and restoring the equilibrium ratio. Substitution in equation 2 gives ΔG, the driving force to equilibrium, as $+1.65 + RT \ln [G1P]/[G6P] = 1.65 + (-2.06) = -0.41$, which is a negative value. Thus, a decrease in the ratio of product to substrate has converted the synthesis of glucose 1-P from a thermodynamically unfavorable to a thermodynamically favorable reaction that will proceed in the forward direction until equilibrium is reached.

C. Activated Intermediates with High Energy Bonds

Many biochemical pathways form activated intermediates containing high-energy bonds to facilitate biochemical work. The term "high-energy bond" is a biologic term defined by the $\Delta G^{0\prime}$ for ATP hydrolysis; any bond that can be hydrolyzed with the release of approximately as much, or more, energy than ATP is called a high-energy bond. The high-energy bond in activated intermediates, such as UDP-glucose in glycogen synthesis, facilitate energy transfer.

1. ATP, UTP, GTP, AND CTP

Cells use GTP and CTP, as well as UTP and ATP, to form activated intermediates. Different anabolic pathways generally use different nucleotides as their direct source of high phosphate bond energy: UTP is used for combining sugars, CTP in lipid synthesis, and GTP in protein synthesis.

The high-energy phosphate bonds of UTP, GTP, and CTP are energetically equivalent to ATP and are synthesized from ATP by nucleoside diphosphokinases and nucleoside monophosphokinases. For example, UTP is formed from UDP by a nucleoside diphosphokinase in the reaction:

$$ATP + UDP \leftrightarrow UTP + ADP.$$

ADP is converted back to ATP by the process of oxidative phosphorylation, using energy supplied by fuel oxidation.

Energy-requiring reactions often generate the nucleoside diphosphate ADP. Adenylate kinase, an important enzyme in cellular energy balance, is a nucleoside monophosphate kinase that transfers a phosphate from one ADP to another ADP to form ATP and AMP:

$$ADP + ADP \leftrightarrow AMP + ATP$$

This enzyme, thus, can regenerate ATP under conditions in which ATP utilization is required.

2. OTHER COMPOUNDS WITH HIGH-ENERGY BONDS

In addition to the nucleoside triphosphates, other compounds containing high-energy bonds are formed to facilitate energy transfer in anabolic and catabolic pathways (e.g., 1,3- bisphosphoglycerate in glycolysis and acetyl CoA in the TCA cycle) (Fig.19.7). Creatine phosphate contains a high-energy phosphate bond that allows it to serve as an energy reservoir for ATP synthesis and transport in muscle cells, neurons, and spermatozoa. All of these high-energy bonds are "unstable," and their hydrolysis yields substantial free energy because the products are much more stable, as a result of electron resonance within their structures.

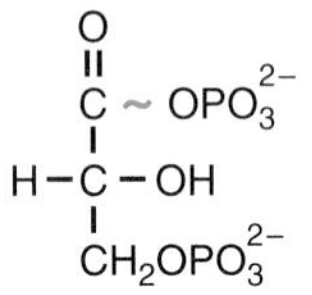

The ΔG of ATP hydrolysis in cells can be very different than $\Delta G^{0\prime}$. The synthesis of ATP rather than its hydrolysis becomes the energetically favorable direction if the [ATP] drops just a little or the [ADP] or [Pi] increase just a little over equilibrium values. Thus, as ATP is hydrolyzed in energy-requiring reactions, the change in the sign of ΔG promotes ATP synthesis.

1,3–Bisphosphoglycerate

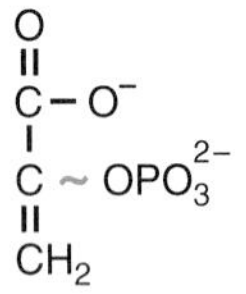

Phosphoenolpyruvate

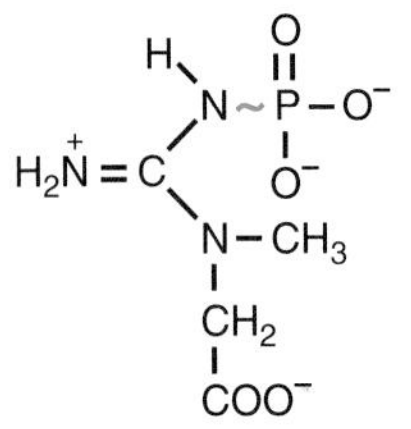

Creatine phosphate

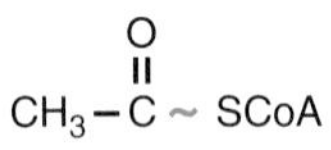

Acetyl CoA

Fig. 19.7. Some compounds with high-energy bonds. 1,3-bisphosphoglycerate and phosphoenolpyruvate are intermediates of glycolysis. Creatine phosphate is a high-energy phosphate reservoir and shuttle in brain, muscle, and spermatozoa. Acetyl CoA is a precursor of the TCA cycle. The high-energy bonds are shown in blue.

IV. THERMOGENESIS

According to the first law of thermodynamics, energy cannot be destroyed. Thus, energy from oxidation of a fuel (its caloric content) must be equal to the amount of heat released, the work performed against the environment, and the increase in order of molecules in our bodies. Some of the energy from fuel oxidation is converted into heat as the fuel is oxidized and some heat is generated as ATP is used to do work. If we become less efficient in converting energy from fuel oxidation into ATP, or if we use an additional amount of ATP for muscular contraction, we will oxidize an additional amount of fuel to maintain ATP homeostasis (constant cellular ATP levels). With the oxidation of additional fuel, we release additional heat. Thus, heat production is a natural consequence of "burning fuel."

Thermogenesis refers to energy expended for the purpose of generating heat in addition to that expended for ATP production. To maintain our body at 37°C, despite changes in environmental temperature, it is necessary to regulate fuel oxidation and its efficiency (as well as heat dissipation). In shivering thermogenesis, we respond to sudden cold with asynchronous muscle contractions (shivers) that increase ATP utilization and, therefore, fuel oxidation and the release of energy as heat. In nonshivering thermogenesis (adaptive thermogenesis), the efficiency of converting energy from fuel oxidation into ATP is decreased. More fuel needs to be oxidized to maintain constant ATP levels and, thus, more heat is generated.

V. ENERGY FROM FUEL OXIDATION

Fuel oxidation provides energy for bodily processes principally through generation of the reduced coenzymes, NADH and FAD(2H). They are used principally to generate ATP in oxidative phosphorylation. However, fuel oxidation also generates NADPH, which is most often used directly in energy-requiring processes. Carbohydrates also may be used to generate ATP through a nonoxidative pathway, called anaerobic glycolysis.

A. Energy Transfer from Fuels through Oxidative Phosphorylation

Fuel oxidation is our major source of ATP and our major means of transferring energy from the chemical bonds of the fuels to cellular energy-requiring processes. The amount of energy available from a fuel is equivalent to the amount of heat that is generated when a fuel is burned. To conserve this energy for the generation of ATP, the process of cellular respiration transforms the energy from the chemical bonds of fuels into the reduction state of electron-accepting coenzymes, NAD^+ and FAD (circle 1, Fig. 19.8). As these compounds transfer electrons to O_2 in the electron transport chain, most of this energy is transformed into an electrochemical gradient across the inner mitochondrial membrane (circle 2, Fig. 19.8). Much of the energy in the electrochemical gradient is used to regenerate ATP from ADP in oxidative phosphorylation (phosphorylation that requires O_2).

1. OXIDATION-REDUCTION REACTIONS

Oxidation-reduction reactions always involve a pair of chemicals: an electron donor, which is oxidized in the reactions, and an electron acceptor, which is reduced in the reaction. In fuel metabolism, the fuel donates electrons, and is oxidized, and NAD^+ and FAD accept electrons, and are reduced.

When is NAD^+, rather than FAD, used in a particular oxidation-reduction reaction? It depends on the chemical properties of the electron donor and the enzyme catalyzing the reaction. In oxidation reactions, NAD^+ accepts two electrons as a hydride ion to form NADH, and a proton (H^+) is released into the medium (Fig 19.9). It is generally used for metabolic reactions involving oxidation of alcohols and aldehydes. In contrast,

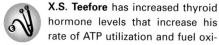

X.S. Teefore has increased thyroid hormone levels that increase his rate of ATP utilization and fuel oxidation. An excess of thyroid hormones also may affect the efficiency of ATP production, resulting in fewer ATP produced for a given O_2 consumption. The increased rate of ATP utilization and diminished efficiency stimulates oxidative metabolism, resulting in a much greater rate of heat production. The hyperthyroid patient, therefore, complains of constantly feeling hot (heat intolerance) and sweaty. (Perspiration allows dissipation of excess heat through evaporation from the skin surface.)

Oxidation is the loss of electrons, and reduction is the gain of electrons. Remember LEO GER:
Loss of Electrons = Oxidation;
Gain of Electrons = Reduction.
Compounds are oxidized in the body in essentially three ways: (1) the transfer of electrons from the compound as a hydrogen atom or a hydride ion, (2) the direct addition of oxygen from O_2, and (3) the direct donation of electrons (e.g., $Fe^{2+} \rightarrow Fe^{3+}$) (see Chapter 5). Fuel oxidation involves the transfer of electrons as a hydrogen atom or a hydride ion and, thus, reduced compounds have more hydrogen relative to oxygen than the oxidized compounds. Consequently, aldehydes are more reduced than acids, and alcohols are more reduced than aldehydes.

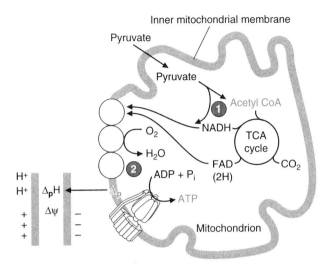

Fig. 19.8. Overview of energy transformations in oxidative phosphorylation. The electrochemical potential gradient across the mitochondrial membrane is represented by ΔpH, the proton gradient, and $\Delta\Psi$, the membrane potential. The role of the electrochemical potential in oxidative phosphorylation is discussed in more depth in Chapter 21.

FAD accepts two electrons as hydrogen atoms, which are donated singly from separate atoms (e.g., formation of a double bond or a disulfide)(Fig. 19.10).

As the reduced coenzymes donate these electrons to O_2 through the electron transport chain, they are reoxidized. The energy derived from reoxidation of NADH and FAD(2H) is available for the generation of ATP by oxidative phosphorylation. In our analogy of ATP as currency, the reduced coenzymes are our "paychecks" for oxidizing fuels. Because our cells spend ATP so fast, we must immediately convert our paychecks into ATP cash.

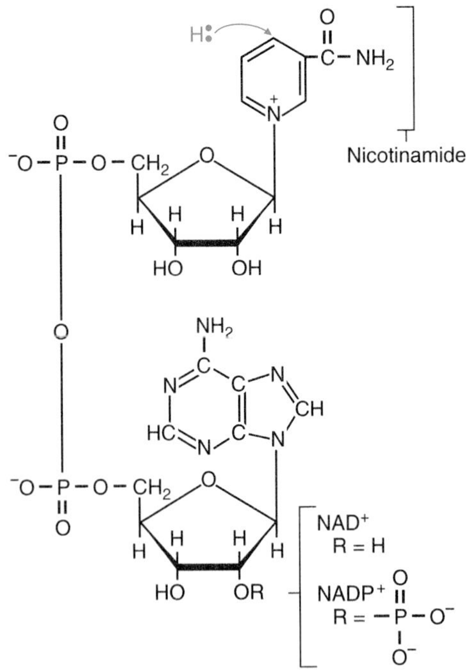

Fig. 19.9. Reduction of NAD$^+$ and NADP$^+$. These structurally related coenzymes are reduced by accepting two electrons as H:$^-$, the hydride ion.

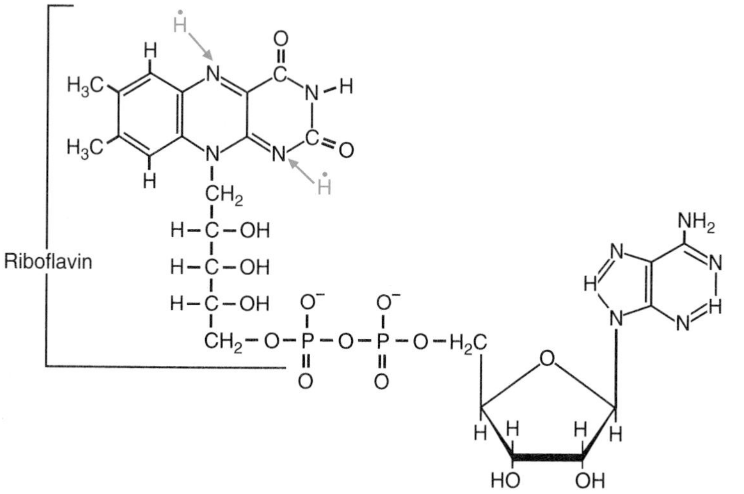

Fig. 19.10. Reduction of FAD. FAD accepts two electrons as two hydrogen atoms and is reduced. The reduced coenzyme is denoted in this text as FAD(2H) because it often accepts a total of two electrons one at a time, never going to the fully reduced form, FADH$_2$. FMN (flavin mononucleotide) consists of riboflavin with one phosphate group attached.

2. REDUCTION POTENTIAL

Each oxidation/reduction reaction makes or takes a fixed amount of energy, ($\Delta G^{0\prime}$), which is directly proportional to the $\Delta E^{\circ\prime}$ (the difference in reduction potentials of the oxidation-reduction pair). The reduction potential of a compound, $E^{\circ\prime}$, is a measure in volts of the energy change when that compound accepts electrons (becomes reduced); minus $E^{\circ\prime}$ is the energy change when the compound donates electrons (becomes oxidized). $E^{\circ\prime}$ can be considered an expression of the willingness of the compound to accept electrons. Some examples of reduction potentials are shown in Table 19.4. Oxygen, which is the best electron acceptor, has the largest positive reduction potential (i.e., is the most willing to accept electrons and be reduced). As a consequence, the transfer of electrons from all compounds to O$_2$ is energetically favorable and occurs with energy release.

The more negative the reduction potential of a compound, the greater is the energy available for ATP generation when that compound passes its electrons to oxygen. The $\Delta G^{0\prime}$ for transfer of electrons from NADH to O$_2$ is greater than the transfer from FAD(2H) to O$_2$ (see the reduction potential values for NADH and FAD(2H) in Table 19.4). Thus, the energy available for ATP synthesis from NADH is approximately -53 kcal, and approximately -41 kcal from the FAD-containing flavoproteins in the electron transport chain.

To calculate the free energy change of an oxidation-reduction reaction, the reduction potential of the electron donor (NADH) is added to that of the acceptor (O$_2$). The $\Delta E^{0\prime}$ for the net reaction is calculated from the sum of the half reactions. For NADH donation of electrons, it is = $+0.320$ volts, opposite of that shown in Table 4 (remember, Table 4 shows the $E^{0\prime}$ for accepting electrons), and for O$_2$ acceptance, it is $+0.816$. The number of electrons being transferred is 2 (so, n = 2). The direct relationship between the energy changes in oxidation-reduction reactions and $\Delta G^{0\prime}$ is expressed by the equation

$$\Delta G^{0\prime} = -n\, F\, \Delta E^{0\prime}$$

where n is the number of electrons transferred and F is Faraday's constant (23 kcal/mole - volt). Thus, a value of approximately -53 kcal/mole is obtained for the energy available for ATP synthesis by transferring two electrons from NADH to oxygen.

Table 19.4. Reduction Potentials of Some Oxidation-Reduction Half-Reactions

Reduction Half-Reactions	E$^{0\prime}$ at pH 7.0
1/2 O$_2$ + 2H$^+$ + 2 e$^-$ → H$_2$O	0.816
Cytochrome a-Fe^{3+} + 1 e$^-$ → cytochrome a-Fe^{2+}	0.290
CoQ + 2H$^+$ + 2 e$^-$ → CoQH$_2$	0.060
Fumarate + 2H$^+$ + 2 e$^-$ → succinate	0.030
Oxalacetate + 2H$^+$ + 2 e$^-$ → malate	−0.102
Acetaldehyde + 2H$^+$ + 2 e$^-$ → ethanol	−0.163
Pyruvate + 2H$^+$ + 2 e$^-$ → lactate	−0.190
Riboflavin + 2H$^+$ + 2 e$^-$ → riboflavin-H$_2$	−0.200
NAD$^+$ + 2H$^+$ + 2 e$^-$ → NADH + H$^+$	−0.320
Acetate + 2H$^+$ + 2 e$^-$ → acetaldehyde	−0.468

Q: **Otto Shape** decided to lose weight by decreasing his intake of fat and alcohol (ethanol), and increasing his content of carbohydrates. Compare the structure of ethanol with that of glucose and fatty acids (below). On the basis of their oxidation state, which compound provides the most energy (calories) per gram?

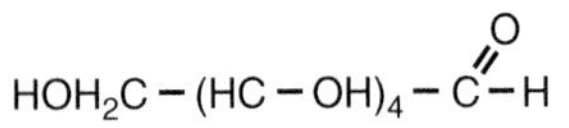

$$HOH_2C-(HC-OH)_4-\overset{\displaystyle O}{\overset{\|}{C}}-H$$

Glucose

$$CH_3CH_2OH$$

Ethanol

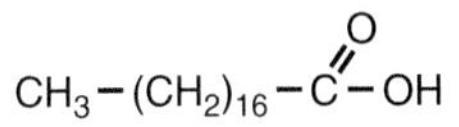

$$CH_3-(CH_2)_{16}-\overset{\displaystyle O}{\overset{\|}{C}}-OH$$

A fatty acid

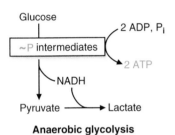

Fig. 19.11. Anaerobic glycolysis. Phosphate is transferred from high-energy intermediates of the pathway to ADP. Because NADH from the pathway is reoxidized by reduction of pyruvate to lactate, no oxygen is required.

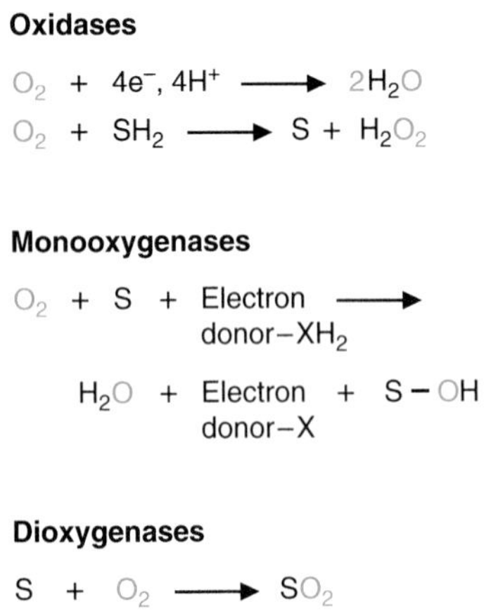

Oxidases

$$O_2 + 4e^-, 4H^+ \longrightarrow 2H_2O$$
$$O_2 + SH_2 \longrightarrow S + H_2O_2$$

Monooxygenases

$$O_2 + S + \text{Electron} \longrightarrow$$
$$\qquad\qquad \text{donor}-XH_2$$
$$H_2O + \text{Electron} + S-OH$$
$$\qquad\qquad \text{donor}-X$$

Dioxygenases

$$S + O_2 \longrightarrow SO_2$$

Fig. 19.12. Oxidases and oxygenases. The fate of O_2 is shown in blue. S represents an organic substrate.

3. CALORIC VALUES OF FUELS

The caloric value of a food is directly related to its oxidation state, which is a measure of $\Delta G^{0\prime}$ for transfer of electrons from that fuel to O_2. The electrons donated by the fuel are from its C-H and C-C bonds. Fatty acids such as palmitate ($CH_3(CH_2)_{14}COOH$) have a caloric value of roughly 9 kcal/g. Glucose is already partially oxidized and has a caloric value of only about 4 kcal/g. The carbons, on an average, contain fewer C-H bonds from which to donate electrons.

The caloric value of a food is applicable in humans only if our cells have enzymes that can oxidize that fuel by transferring electrons from the fuel to NAD^+, $NADP^+$, or FAD. When we burn wood in a fireplace, electrons are transferred from cellulose and other carbohydrates to O_2, releasing energy as heat. However, wood has no caloric content for humans; we cannot digest it and convert cellulose to a form that can be oxidized by our enzymes. Cholesterol, although a lipid, also has no caloric value for us because we cannot oxidize the carbons in its complex ring structure in reactions that generate NADH, FAD(2H), or NADPH.

B. NADPH in Oxidation-Reduction Reactions

$NADP^+$ is similar to NAD^+ and has the same reduction potential. However, $NADP^+$ has an extra phosphate group on the ribose, which affects its enzyme binding (see Fig. 19.9). Consequently, most enzymes use either NAD^+ or $NADP^+$, but seldom both. In certain reactions, fuels are oxidized by transfer of electrons to $NADP^+$ to form NADPH. For example, glucose 6-P dehydrogenase, in the pentose phosphate pathway, transfers electrons from glucose 6-P to $NADP^+$ instead of NAD^+. NADPH usually donates electrons to biosynthetic reactions such as fatty acid synthesis, and to detoxification reactions that use oxygen directly. Consequently, the energy in its reduction potential is usually used in energy-requiring reactions without first being converted to ATP currency.

C. Anaerobic Glycolysis

Not all ATP is generated by fuel oxidation. In anaerobic glycolysis, glucose is degraded in reactions that form high-energy phosphorylated intermediates of the pathway (Fig.19.11). These activated high-energy intermediates provide the energy for the generation of ATP from ADP without involving electron transfer to O_2. Therefore, this pathway is called anaerobic glycolysis, and ATP is generated from substrate level phosphorylation rather than oxidative phosphorylation (see Chapter 22). Anaerobic glycolysis is a critical source of ATP for cells that have a decreased O_2 supply, either because they are physiologically designed that way (e.g., cells in the kidney medulla), or because their supply of O_2 has been pathologically decreased (e.g., coronary artery disease).

VI. OXYGENASES AND OXIDASES NOT INVOLVED IN ATP GENERATION

Approximately 90 to 95% of the oxygen we consume is used by the terminal oxidase in the electron transport chain for ATP generation via oxidative phosphorylation. The remainder of the O_2 is used directly by oxygenases and other oxidases, enzymes that oxidize a compound in the body by transferring electrons directly to O_2 (Fig. 19.12). The large positive reduction potential of O_2 makes all of these reactions extremely favorable thermodynamically, but the electronic structure of O_2 slows the speed of electron transfer. These enzymes, therefore, contain a metal ion that facilitates reduction of O_2.

A. Oxidases

Oxidases transfer electrons from the substrate to O$_2$, which is reduced to water (H$_2$O) or to hydrogen peroxide (H$_2$O$_2$). The terminal protein complex in the electron transport chain, called cytochrome oxidase, is an oxidase because it accepts electrons donated to the chain by NADH and FAD(2H) and uses these to reduce O$_2$ to water. Most of the other oxidases in the cell form hydrogen peroxide (H$_2$O$_2$), instead of H$_2$O, and are called peroxidases. Peroxidases are generally confined to peroxisomes to protect DNA and other cellular components from toxic free radicals (compounds containing single electrons in an outer orbital) generated by hydrogen peroxide.

B. Oxygenases

Oxygenases, in contrast to oxidases, incorporate one or both of the atoms of oxygen into the organic substrate (see Fig 19.12). Monooxygenases, enzymes that incorporate one atom of oxygen into the substrate and the other into H$_2$O, are often named hydroxylases (e.g., phenylalanine hydroxylase, which adds a hydroxyl group to phenylalanine to form tyrosine) or mixed function oxidases. Monooxygenases require an electron donor-substrate, such as NADPH, a coenzyme such as FAD, which can transfer single electrons, and a metal or similar compound that can form a reactive oxygen complex (Fig.19.13). They are usually found in the endoplasmic reticulum, and occasionally in mitochondria. Dioxygenases, enzymes that incorporate both atoms of oxygen into the substrate, are used in the pathways for converting arachidonate into prostaglandins, thromboxanes, and leukotrienes.

VII. ENERGY BALANCE

Our total energy expenditure is equivalent to our oxygen consumption (Fig. 19.14). The resting metabolic rate (energy expenditure of a person at rest, at 25°C, after an overnight fast) accounts for approximately 60 to 70% of our total energy expenditure and O$_2$ consumption, and physical exercise accounts for the

A: In palmitate and other fatty acids, most carbons are more reduced than those in glucose or ethanol (more of the carbons have electrons in carbon–hydrogen bonds). Therefore, fatty acids have the greatest caloric content/gram, 9 kcal. In glucose, the carbons have already formed bonds with oxygen, and fewer electrons in C-H bonds are available to generate energy. Thus, the complete oxidation of glucose gives roughly 4 kcal/g. In ethanol, one carbon is a methyl group with C-H bonds, and one has an OH group. Therefore the oxidation state is intermediate between glucose and fatty acids, and ethanol thus has 7 kcal/g.

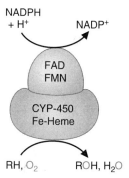

Fig. 19.13. Cytochrome P450 mono-oxygenases. Electrons are donated by NADPH to O$_2$ and the substrate. The flavin coenzymes FAD and FMN in one subunit transfer single electrons to cytochrome P450, which is an Fe-heme containing protein that absorbs light at a wavelength of 450 nm. The enzyme is embedded in a membrane, usually the endoplasmic reticulum.

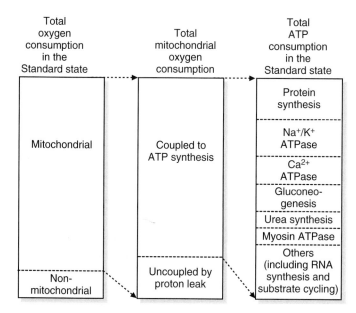

Fig. 19.14. Estimated contribution of processes to energy utilization in standard state. Copied, with permission, from Rolfe DFS, Brown GC. Cellular energy utilization and molecular origin of standard metabolic rate in mammals. Physiol Rev 1997;77:731-758.

remainder. Of the resting metabolic rate, approximately 90 to 95% of O_2 consumption is used by the mitochondrial electron transport chain, and only 5 to 10% is required for nonmitochondrial oxidases and oxygenases and is not related to ATP synthesis. Approximately 20 to 30% of the energy from this mitochondrial O_2 consumption is lost by proton leak back across the mitochondrial membrane, which dissipates the electrochemical gradient without ATP synthesis. The remainder of our O_2 consumption is used for ATPases that maintain ion gradients and for biosynthetic pathways.

ATP homeostasis refers to the ability of our cells to maintain constant levels of ATP despite fluctuations in the rate of utilization. Thus, increased utilization of ATP for exercise or biosynthetic reactions increases the rate of fuel oxidation. The major mechanism employed is feedback regulation; all of the pathways of fuel oxidation leading to generation of ATP are feedback-regulated by ATP levels, or by compounds related to the concentration of ATP. In general, the less ATP used, the less fuel will be oxidized to generate ATP.

According to the first law of thermodynamics, the energy (cal) in our consumed fuel can never be lost. Consumed fuel is either oxidized to meet the energy demands of the basal metabolic rate + exercise, or it is stored as fat. Thus, an intake of calories in excess of those expended results in weight gain. The simple statement, "If you eat too much and don't exercise, you will get fat," is really a summary of the bioenergetics of the ATP-ADP cycle.

CLINICAL COMMENTS

Otto Shape. Otto Shape visited his physician, who noted the increased weight. He recommended several diet modifications to Otto that would decrease the caloric content of his diet and pointed out the importance of exercise for weight reduction. He reminded Otto that the American Heart Association and the American Cancer Society recommended 45 to 60 minutes of moderate-to-vigorous exercise 5 to 7 days per week. He also reminded Otto that he would want to be a role model for his patients. Otto decided to begin an exercise regimen that includes an hour of running each day.

X.S. Teefore. Mr. Teefore exhibited the classical signs and symptoms of hyperthyroidism (increased secretion of the thyroid hormones, T_3 and T_4) including a goiter (enlarged thyroid gland). Thyroid function tests confirmed this diagnosis.

Thyroid hormones (principally T_3) modulate cellular energy production and utilization through their ability to increase the gene transcription of many proteins involved in intermediary metabolism, including enzymes in the TCA cycle and oxidative phosphorylation. They increase the rate of ATP utilization by Na^+, K^+-ATPase, and other enzymes. They also affect the efficiency of energy transformations, so that either more fuel must be oxidized to maintain a given level of ATP, or more ATP must be expended to achieve the desired physiological response. The loss of weight experienced by **X.S. Teefore,** in spite of a very good appetite, reflects his increased caloric requirements and a less efficient utilization of fuels. The result is an enhanced oxidation of adipose tissue stores as well as a catabolic effect on muscle and other protein-containing tissues. Through mechanisms that are not well understood, increased levels of thyroid hormone in the blood also increase the activity or "tone" of the sympathetic (adrenergic) nervous system. An activated sympathetic nervous system leads to a more rapid and forceful heartbeat (tachycardia and palpitations), increased nervousness (anxiety and insomnia), tremulousness (a sense of shakiness or jitteriness), and other symptoms.

The thyroid gland secretes the thyroid hormones tetraiodothyronine (T_4) and triiodothyronine (T_3) (see Fig. 11.8 for the structure of T_3). T_3 is the most active form of the hormone. T_4 is synthesized and secreted in approximately 10 times greater amounts than T_3. Hepatocytes (liver cells) and other cells contain a deiodinase that removes one of the iodines from T_4, converting it to T_3. T_3 exerts its effects on tissues by regulating the transcription of specific genes involved in energy metabolism (see Chapter 16, section III.C.2., Fig. 16.14).

Cora Nari. Cora Nari was in left ventricular heart failure (LVF) when she presented to the hospital with her second heart attack in 8 months. The diagnosis of LVF was based, in part, on her rapid heart rate (104 beats/min) and respiratory rate. On examining her lungs, her physician heard respiratory rales, caused by inspired air bubbling in fluid that had filled her lung air spaces secondary to LVF. This condition is referred to as congestive heart failure.

Cora Nari's rapid heart rate (tachycardia) resulted from a reduced capacity of her ischemic, failing left ventricular muscle to eject a normal amount of blood into the arteries leading away from the heart with each contraction. The resultant drop in intraarterial pressure signaled a reflex response in the central nervous system that, in turn, caused an increase in heart rate in an attempt to bring the total amount of blood leaving the left ventricle each minute (the cardiac output) back toward a more appropriate level to maintain systemic blood pressure.

Treatment of Cora's congestive heart failure will include efforts to reduce the workload of the heart with diuretics and other "load reducers," attempts to improve the force of left ventricular contraction with digitalis and other "inotropes," and the administration of oxygen by nasal cannula to reduce the injury caused by lack of blood flow (ischemia) to the viable heart tissue in the vicinity of the infarction.

BIOCHEMICAL COMMENTS

Active Transport and Cell Death. Most of us cannot remember when we first learned that we would die if we stopped breathing. But exactly how cells die from a lack of oxygen is an intriguing question. Pathologists generally describe two histologically distinct types of cell death: necrosis and apoptosis (programmed cell death). Cell death from a lack of O₂, such as occurs during a myocardial infarction, can be very rapid, and is considered necrosis. The lack of ATP for the active transport of Na⁺ and Ca²⁺ triggers some of the death cascades leading to necrosis (Fig. 19.15).

The influx of Na⁺ and loss of the Na⁺ gradient across the plasma membrane is an early event accompanying ATP depletion during interruption of the O₂ supply. One consequence of the increased intracellular Na⁺ concentration is that other transport processes driven by the Na⁺ gradient are impaired. For example, the Na⁺ / H⁺ exchanger, which normally pumps out H⁺ generated from metabolism in exchange for extracellular Na⁺, can no longer function, and intracellular pH may drop. The increased intracellular H⁺ may impair ATP generation from anaerobic glycolysis. As a consequence of increased intracellular ion concentrations, water enters the cells and hydropic swelling occurs. Swelling is accompanied by the release of creatine kinase MB subunits, troponin I, and troponin C into the blood. These enzymes are measured in the blood as indicators of a myocardial infarction (see Chapters 6 and 7). Swelling is an early event and is considered a reversible stage of cell injury.

Normally, intracellular Ca²⁺ concentration is carefully regulated to fluctuate at low levels (intracellular Ca²⁺ concentration is less than 10⁻⁷ M, compared with approximately 10⁻³ M in extracellular fluid). Fluctuations of Ca²⁺ concentration at these low levels regulate myofibrillar contraction, energy metabolism, and other cellular processes. However, when Ca²⁺ concentration is increased above this normal range, it triggers cell death (necrosis). High Ca²⁺ concentrations activate a phospholipase that increases membrane permeability, resulting in further loss of ion gradients across the cell membrane. They also trigger opening of the mitochondrial permeability transition pore, which results in loss of mitochondrial function and further impairs oxidative phosphorylation.

Intracellular Ca²⁺ levels may increase as a result of cell swelling, the lack of ATP for ATP-dependent Ca²⁺ pumps, or the loss of the Na⁺ gradient. Normally,

Congestive heart failure occurs when the weakened pumping action of the ischemic left ventricular heart muscle causes back pressure to increase in the vessels which bring oxygenated blood from the lungs to the left side of the heart. The pressure inside these pulmonary vessels eventually reaches a critical level above which water from the blood moves down a "pressure gradient" from the capillary lumen into alveolar air spaces of the lung (transudation). The patient experiences shortness of breath as the fluid in the air spaces interferes with oxygen exchange from the inspired air into arterial blood, causing hypoxia. The hypoxia then stimulates the respiratory center in the central nervous system, leading to a more rapid respiratory rate in an effort to increase the oxygen content of the blood. As the patient inhales deeply, the physician hears gurgling sounds (known as inspiratory rales) with a stethoscope placed over the posterior lung bases. These sounds represent the bubbling of inspired air as it enters the fluid-filled pulmonary alveolar air spaces.

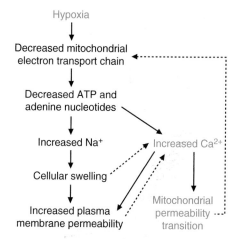

Fig. 19.15. Hypoxia, Ca²⁺, Na⁺, and cell death. Without an adequate O₂ supply, decreased ATP synthesis from oxidative phosphorylation results in an increase of cytoplasmic Na⁺ and Ca²⁺ ions. Increased ions levels can trigger death cascades that involve increased permeability of the plasma membrane, loss of ion gradients, decreased cytosolic pH, mitochondrial Ca²⁺ overload, and a change in mitochondrial permeability called the mitochondrial permeability transition. The solid lines show the first sequence of events; the dashed lines show how these events feedback to accelerate the mitochondrial deterioration, making recovery of oxidative phosphorylation impossible.

Ca^{2+}-ATPases located in the plasma membrane pump Ca^{2+}- out of the cell. Ca^{2+}-ATPases in the endoplasmic reticulum, and in the sarcoplasmic reticulum of heart and other muscles, sequester Ca^{2+} within the membranes, where it is bound by a low-affinity binding protein. Ca^{2+} is released from the sarcoplasmic reticulum in response to a nerve impulse, which signals contraction, and the increase of Ca^{2+} stimulates both muscle contraction and the oxidation of fuels. Within the heart, another Ca^{2+} transporter protein, the Na^+/Ca^{2+} exchange transporter, coordinates the efflux of Ca^{2+} in exchange for Na^+, so that Ca^{2+} is extruded with each contraction.

Suggested References

Nelson DL, Lehninger AL, Cox MM. Lehninger Principles of biochemistry. Chapter 14. In: Principles of Bioenergetics. New York: Worth, 2000:490–526.
Hanson RW. The role of ATP in metabolism. Biochem Educ1989;17:86–92.
Rolfe DES, Brown GC. Cellular energy utilization and molecular origin of standard metabolic rate in mammals. Physiol Rev 1997;77:731–758.

 REVIEW QUESTIONS—CHAPTER 19

1. The highest-energy phosphate bond in ATP is located between which of the following groups?

   (A) Adenosine and phosphate
   (B) Ribose and phosphate
   (C) Ribose and adenine
   (D) Two hydroxyl groups in the ribose ring
   (E) Two phosphate groups

2. Which of the following bioenergetic terms or phrases is correctly defined?

   (A) The first law of thermodynamics states that the universe tends towards a state of increased order.
   (B) The second law of thermodynamics states that the total energy of a system remains constant.
   (C) The change in enthalpy of a reaction is a measure of the total amount of heat that can be released from changes in the chemical bonds.
   (D) $\Delta G^{\circ\prime}$ of a reaction is the standard free energy change measured at 37°C and a pH of 7.4.
   (E) A high-energy bond is a bond that releases more than 3 kcal/mole of heat when it is hydrolyzed.

3. Which statement best describes the direction a chemical reaction will follow?

   (A) A reaction with a positive free energy will proceed in the forward direction if the substrate concentration is raised high enough.
   (B) Under standard conditions, a reaction will proceed in the forward direction if the free energy $\Delta G^{\circ\prime}$ is positive.
   (C) The direction of a reaction is independent of the initial substrate and product concentrations because the direction is determined by the change in free energy.
   (D) The concentration of all of the substrates must be higher than all of the products to proceed in the forward direction.
   (E) The enzyme for the reaction must be working at better than 50% of its maximum efficiency for the reaction to proceed in the forward direction.

4. A patient, Mr. Perkins, has just suffered a heart attack. As a consequence, his heart would display which of the following changes?

   (A) An increased intracellular O_2 concentration
   (B) An increased intracellular ATP concentration
   (C) An increased intracellular H^+ concentration
   (D) A decreased intracellular Ca^{2+} concentration
   (E) A decreased intracellular Na^+ concentration

5. Which of the following statements correctly describes reduction of one of the electron carriers, NAD^+ or FAD?

   (A) NAD^+ accepts two electrons as hydrogen atoms to form $NADH_2$.
   (B) NAD^+ accepts two electrons that are each donated from a separate atom of the substrate.
   (C) NAD^+ accepts two electrons as a hydride ion to form NADH.
   (D) FAD releases a proton as it accepts two electrons.
   (E) FAD must accept two electrons at a time.

20 Tricarboxylic Acid Cycle

The TCA cycle is frequently called the Krebs cycle because Sir Hans Krebs first formulated its reactions into a cycle. It is also called the "citric acid cycle" because citrate was one of the first compounds known to participate. The most common name for this pathway, the tricarboxylic acid or TCA cycle, denotes the involvement of the tricarboxylates citrate and isocitrate.

The major pathways of fuel oxidation generate acetyl CoA, which is the substrate for the TCA cycle. In the first step of the TCA cycle, the acetyl portion of acetyl CoA combines with the 4-carbon intermediate oxaloacetate to form citrate (6 carbons), which is rearranged to form isocitrate. In the next two oxidative decarboxylation reactions, electrons are transferred to NAD^+ to form NADH, and 2 molecules of electron-depleted CO_2 are released. Subsequently, a high-energy phosphate bond in GTP is generated from substrate level phosphorylation. In the remaining portion of the TCA cycle, succinate is oxidized to oxaloacetate with the generation of one FAD(2H) and one NADH. The net reaction of the TCA cycle, which is the sum of the equations for individual steps, shows that the two carbons of the acetyl group have been oxidized to two molecules of CO_2, with conservation of energy as three molecules of NADH, one of FAD(2H), and one of GTP.

*The **TCA cycle** (tricarboxylic acid cycle) accounts for over two thirds of the ATP generated from fuel oxidation. The pathways for oxidation of fatty acids, glucose, amino acids, acetate, and ketone bodies all generate **acetyl CoA**, which is the substrate for the TCA cycle. As the activated 2-carbon acetyl group is oxidized to two molecules of CO_2, energy is conserved as **NADH, FAD(2H),** and **GTP** (Fig. 20.1). NADH and FAD(2H) subsequently donate electrons to O_2 via the electron transport chain, with the generation of ATP from oxidative phosphorylation. Thus, the TCA cycle is central to energy generation from **cellular respiration.***

*Within the TCA cycle, the oxidative decarboxylation of α-ketoglutarate is catalyzed by the multisubunit **α-ketoglutarate dehydrogenase complex,** which contains the coenzymes **thiamine-pyrophosphate, lipoate,** and **FAD.** A similar complex, the **pyruvate dehydrogenase complex (PDC),** catalyzes the oxidation of pyruvate to acetyl CoA, thereby providing a link between the pathways of glycolysis and the TCA cycle (see Fig. 20.1)*

The two-carbon acetyl group is the ultimate source of the electrons that are transferred to NAD^+ and FAD and also the carbon in the two CO_2 molecules that are produced. Oxaloacetate is used and regenerated in each turn of the cycle (see Fig. 20.1). However, when cells use intermediates of the TCA cycle for

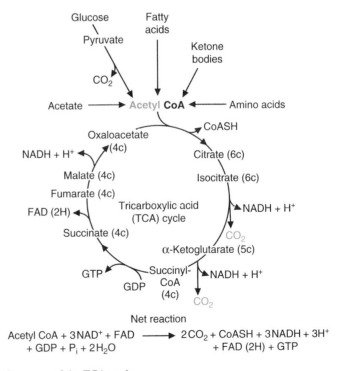

Fig. 20.1. Summary of the TCA cycle.

biosynthetic reactions, the carbons of oxaloacetate must be replaced by **anaplerotic** *(filling up) reactions, such as the* **pyruvate carboxylase reaction.**

The TCA cycle occurs in the mitochondrion, where its flux is tightly coordinated with the rate of the electron transport chain and oxidative phosphorylation through **feedback regulation that reflects the demand for ATP.** The rate of the TCA cycle is increased when ATP utilization in the cell is increased through the response of several enzymes to **ADP levels,** the **NADH/ NAD$^+$ ratio,** the rate of FAD(2H) oxidation or the **Ca^{2+} concentration.** For example, **isocitrate dehydrogenase is allosterically activated by ADP.**

There are two general consequences to impaired functioning of the TCA cycle: (1) an inability to generate ATP from fuel oxidation, and (2) an accumulation of TCA cycle precursors. For example, inhibition of pyruvate oxidation in the TCA cycle results in its reduction to lactate, which can cause a **lactic acidosis.** The most common situation leading to an impaired function of the TCA cycle is a relative lack of oxygen to accept electrons in the electron transport chain.

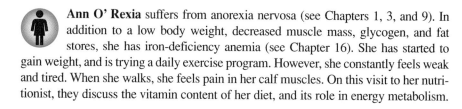

THE WAITING ROOM

 Otto Shape, a 26-year-old medical student, has faithfully followed his diet and aerobic exercise program of daily tennis and jogging (see Chapter 19). He has lost a total of 33 lb and is just 23 lb from his college weight of 154 lb. His exercise capacity has markedly improved; he can run for a longer time at a faster pace before noting shortness of breath or palpitations of his heart. Even his test scores in his medical school classes have improved.

 Ann O' Rexia suffers from anorexia nervosa (see Chapters 1, 3, and 9). In addition to a low body weight, decreased muscle mass, glycogen, and fat stores, she has iron-deficiency anemia (see Chapter 16). She has started to gain weight, and is trying a daily exercise program. However, she constantly feels weak and tired. When she walks, she feels pain in her calf muscles. On this visit to her nutritionist, they discuss the vitamin content of her diet, and its role in energy metabolism.

 Al Martini has been hospitalized for congestive heart failure (see Chapter 8) and for head injuries sustained while driving under the influence of alcohol (Chapters 9 and 10). He completed an alcohol detoxification program, enrolled in a local Alcoholics Anonymous (AA) group, and began seeing a psychologist. During this time, his alcohol-related neurologic and cardiac manifestations of thiamine deficiency partially cleared. However, in spite of the support he was receiving, he began drinking excessive amounts of alcohol again while eating poorly. Three weeks later, he was readmitted with symptoms of "high output" heart failure.

I. REACTIONS OF THE TCA CYCLE

In the TCA cycle, the 2-carbon acetyl group of acetyl CoA is oxidized to 2 CO_2 molecules (see Fig. 20.1). The function of the cycle is to conserve the energy from this oxidation, which it accomplishes principally by transferring electrons from intermediates of the cycle to NAD$^+$ and FAD. The eight electrons donated by the acetyl group eventually end up in three molecules of NADH and one of FAD(2H) (Fig. 20.2). As a consequence, ATP can be generated from oxidative phosphorylation when NADH and FAD(2H) donate these electrons to O_2 via the electron transport chain.

Vitamins and minerals required for the TCA cycle and anaplerotic reactions
Niacin (NAD$^+$)
Riboflavin (FAD)
Pantothenate (CoA)
Thiamine
Biotin
Mg^{2+}
Ca^{2+}
Fe^{2+}
Phosphate

$$H{:}\overset{\displaystyle H}{\underset{\displaystyle H}{C}}{\cdots}\overset{\displaystyle O}{\overset{\|}{C}}\sim SCoA$$

Acetyl CoA

Fig. 20.2. The acetyl group of acetyl CoA. Acetyl CoA donates eight electrons to the TCA cycle, which are shown in blue, and two carbons. The high-energy bond is shown by a ~. The acetyl group is the ultimate source of the carbons in the two molecules of CO_2 that are produced, and the source of electrons in the one molecule of FAD(2H) and 3 molecules NADH, which have each accepted two electrons. However, the same carbon atoms and electrons that enter from one molecule of acetyl CoA do not leave as CO_2, NADH, or FAD(2H) within the same turn of the cycle.

Synthases, such as citrate synthase, catalyze condensation of two organic molecules to form a carbon–carbon bond. Dehydrogenases, such as isocitrate dehydrogenase, are enzymes that remove electron-containing hydrogen or hydride atoms from a substrate and transfer them to electron-accepting coenzymes, such as NAD+ or FAD. Aconitase is an isomerase, an enzyme that catalyzes an internal rearrangement of atoms or electrons. In aconitase, a hydroxyl group is being transferred from one carbon to another. An iron cofactor in the enzyme facilitates this transfer.

Initially, the acetyl group is incorporated into citrate, an intermediate of the TCA cycle (Fig. 20.3). As citrate progresses through the cycle to oxaloacetate, it is oxidized by four dehydrogenases (isocitrate dehydrogenase, α-ketoglutarate dehydrogenase, succinate dehydrogenase, and malate dehydrogenase), which transfer electrons to NAD+ or FAD. The isomerase aconitase rearranges electrons in citrate, thereby forming isocitrate, to facilitate an electron transfer to NAD+.

Although no O_2 is introduced into the TCA cycle, the two molecules of CO_2 produced have more oxygen than the acetyl group. These oxygen atoms are ultimately derived from the carbonyl group of acetyl CoA, two molecules of water added by fumarase and citrate synthase, and the PO_4^{2-} added to GDP.

The overall yield of energy-containing compounds from the TCA cycle is 3 NADH, 1 FAD(2H), and 1 GTP. The high-energy phosphate bond of GTP is generated from substrate level phosphorylation catalyzed by succinate thiokinase (succinyl CoA synthetase). As the NADH and FAD(2H) are reoxidized in the electron transport chain, approximately 2.5 ATP are generated for each NADH, and 1.5 ATP

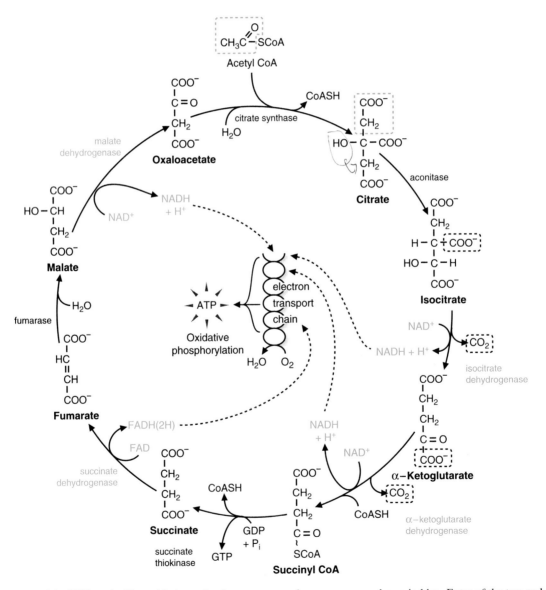

Fig. 20.3. Reactions of the TCA cycle. The oxidation-reduction enzymes and coenzymes are shown in blue. Entry of the two carbons of acetyl CoA into the TCA cycle are indicated with blue dashed boxes. The carbons released as CO_2 are shown with black dashed boxes.

for the FAD(2H). Consequently, the net energy yield from the TCA cycle and oxidative phosphorylation is about 10 high-energy phosphate bonds for each acetyl group oxidized.

A. Formation and Oxidation of Isocitrate

The TCA cycle begins with condensation of the activated acetyl group and oxaloacetate to form the 6-carbon intermediate citrate, a reaction catalyzed by the enzyme citrate synthase (see Fig. 20.3). Because oxaloacetate is regenerated with each turn of the cycle, it is not really considered a substrate of the cycle, or a source of electrons or carbon.

In the next step of the TCA cycle, the hydroxyl (alcohol) group of citrate is moved to an adjacent carbon so that it can be oxidized to form a keto group. The isomerization of citrate to isocitrate is catalyzed by the enzyme aconitase, which is named for an intermediate of the reaction. The enzyme isocitrate dehydrogenase catalyzes the oxidation of the alcohol group and the subsequent cleavage of the carboxyl group to release CO_2 (an oxidative decarboxylation).

B. α-Ketoglutarate to Succinyl CoA

The next step of the TCA cycle is the oxidative decarboxylation of α-ketoglutarate to succinyl CoA, catalyzed by the α-ketoglutarate dehydrogenase complex (see Fig. 20.3). The dehydrogenase complex contains the coenzymes thiamine pyrophosphate, lipoic acid, and FAD.

In this reaction, one of the carboxyl groups of α-ketoglutarate is released as CO_2, and the adjacent keto group is oxidized to the level of an acid, which then combines with CoASH to form succinyl CoA (see Fig. 20.3). Energy from the reaction is conserved principally in the reduction state of NADH, with a smaller amount present in the high-energy thioester bond of succinyl CoA.

C. Generation of GTP

Energy from the succinyl CoA thioester bond is used to generate GTP from GDP and Pi in the reaction catalyzed by succinate thiokinase (see Fig. 20.3). This reaction is an example of substrate level phosphorylation. By definition, substrate level phosphorylation is the formation of a high-energy phosphate bond where none previously existed without the use of molecular O_2 (in other words, NOT oxidative phosphorylation). The high-energy phosphate bond of GTP is energetically equivalent to that of ATP, and can be used directly for energy-requiring reactions like protein synthesis.

D. Oxidation of Succinate to Oxaloacetate

Up to this stage of the TCA cycle, two carbons have been stripped of their available electrons and released as CO_2. Two pairs of these electrons have been transferred to 2 NAD^+, and one GTP has been generated. However, two additional pairs of electrons arising from acetyl CoA still remain in the TCA cycle as part of succinate. The remaining steps of the TCA cycle transfer these two pairs of electrons to FAD and NAD^+ and add H_2O, thereby regenerating oxaloacetate.

The sequence of reactions converting succinate to oxaloacetate begins with the oxidation of succinate to fumarate (see Fig. 20.3). Single electrons are transferred from the two adjacent -CH_2- methylene groups of succinate to an FAD bound to succinate dehydrogenase, thereby forming the double bond of fumarate. From the reduced enzyme-bound FAD, the electrons are passed into the electron transport chain. An OH^- group and a proton from water add to the double bond of fumarate, converting it to malate. In the last reaction of the TCA cycle, the alcohol group of malate is oxidized to a keto group through the donation of electrons to NAD^+.

 Otto Shape's exercise program increases his rate of ATP utilization and his rate of fuel oxidation in the TCA cycle. The TCA cycle generates NADH and FAD(2H), and the electron transport chain transfers electrons from NADH and FAD(2H) to O_2, thereby creating the electrochemical potential that drives ATP synthesis from ADP. As ATP is used in the cell, the rate of the electron transport chain increases. The TCA cycle and other fuel oxidative pathways respond by increasing their rates of NADH and FAD(2H) production.

Succinate thiokinase is also known as succinyl CoA synthetase. Both names refer to the reverse direction of the reaction, i.e., the conversion of succinate to the thioester succinyl CoA, utilizing energy from GTP. Synthases, such as citrate synthase, differ from synthetases in that synthetases cleave a high-energy phosphate bond in ATP, UTP, CTP, or GTP, and synthases do not.

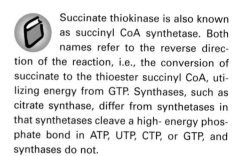 From Figure 20.3, which enzymes in the TCA cycle release CO_2? How many moles of oxaloacetate are consumed in the TCA cycle for each mole of CO_2 produced?

The succinate to oxaloacetate sequence of reactions—oxidation through formation of a double bond, addition of water to the double bond, and oxidation of the resultant alcohol to a ketone is found in many oxidative pathways in the cell, such as the pathways for the oxidation of fatty acids, and oxidation of the branched chain amino acids.

Ann O'Rexia has been malnourished for some time, and has developed subclinical deficiencies of many vitamins, including riboflavin. The coenzymes FAD (flavin adenine dinucleotide) and FMN (flavin mononucleotide) are synthesized from the vitamin riboflavin. Riboflavin is actively transported into cells, where the enzyme flavokinase adds a phosphate to form FMN. FAD synthetase then adds AMP to form FAD. FAD is the major coenzyme in tissues and is generally found tightly bound to proteins, with about 10% being covalently bound. Its turnover in the body is very slow, and people can live for long periods on low intakes without displaying any signs of a riboflavin deficiency.

A: Isocitrate dehydrogenase releases the first CO_2, and α-ketoglutarate dehydrogenase releases the second CO_2. There is no net consumption of oxaloacetate in the TCA cycle—the first step use an oxaloacetate, and the last step produces one. The utilization and regeneration of oxaloacetate is the "cycle" part of the TCA cycle.

Q: One of **Otto Shape's** tennis partners told him that he had heard about a health food designed for athletes that contained succinate. The advertisement made the claim that succinate would provide an excellent source of energy during exercise because it could be metabolized directly without oxygen. Do you see anything wrong with this statement?

With regeneration of oxaloacetate, the TCA cycle is complete; the chemical bond energy, carbon, and electrons donated by the acetyl group have been converted to CO_2, NADH, FAD(2H), GTP, and heat.

II. COENZYMES OF THE TCA CYCLE

The enzymes of the TCA cycle rely heavily on coenzymes for their catalytic function. Isocitrate dehydrogenase and malate dehydrogenase use NAD^+ as a coenzyme, and succinate dehydrogenase uses FAD. Citrate synthase catalyzes a reaction that uses a CoA derivative, acetyl CoA. The α-ketoglutarate dehydrogenase complex uses thiamine pyrophosphate, lipoate and FAD as bound coenzymes, and NAD^+ and CoASH as substrates. Each of these coenzymes has unique structural features that enable it to fulfill its role in the TCA cycle.

A. FAD and NAD^+

Both FAD and NAD^+ are electron-accepting coenzymes. Why is FAD used in some reactions and NAD^+ in others? Their unique structural features enable FAD and NAD^+ to act as electron acceptors in different types of reactions, and play different physiological roles in the cell. FAD is able to accept single electrons (H•), and forms a half-reduced single electron intermediate (Fig. 20.4). It thus participates in reactions in which single electrons are transferred independently from two different atoms, which occurs in double bond formation (e.g., succinate to fumarate) and disulfide bond formation (e.g., lipoate to lipoate disulfide in the α-ketoglutarate

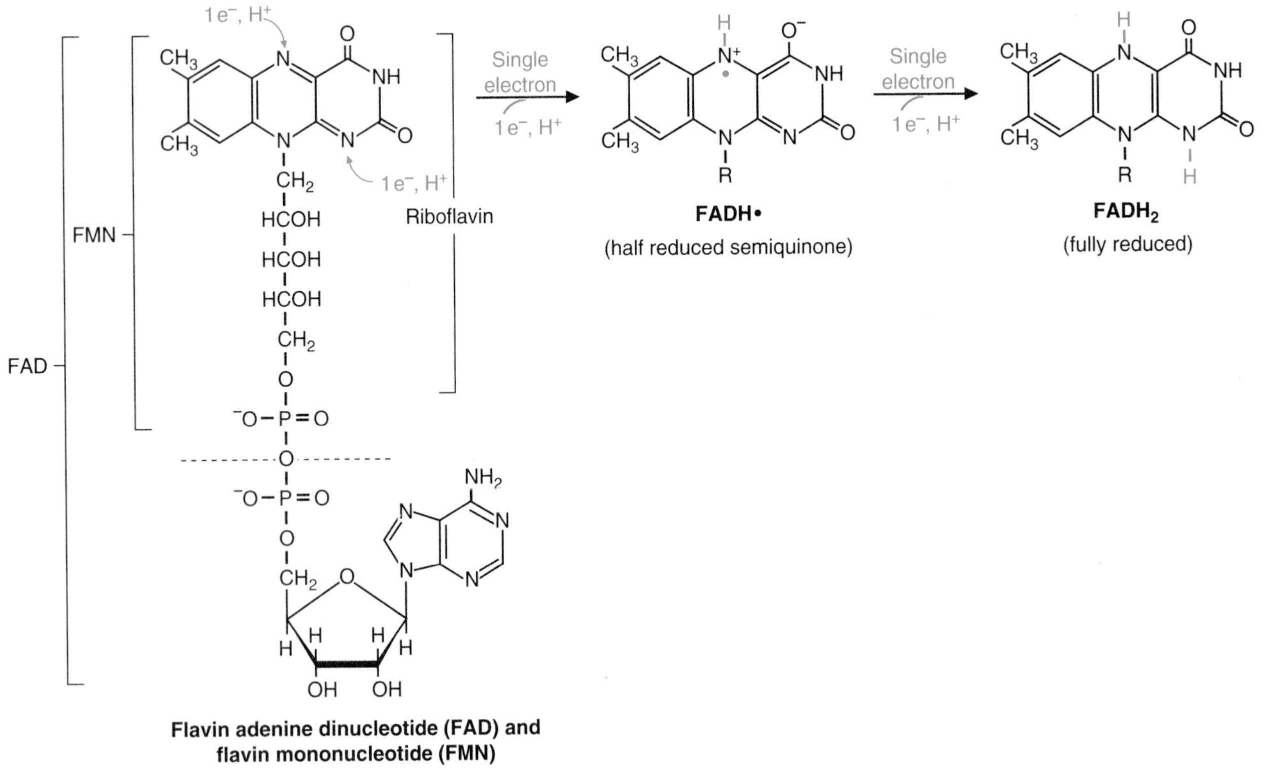

Flavin adenine dinucleotide (FAD) and flavin mononucleotide (FMN)

Fig. 20.4. One-electron steps in the reduction of FAD. When FAD and FMN accept single electrons, they are converted to the half-reduced semiquinone, a semistable free radical form. They can also accept two electrons to form the fully reduced form, $FADH_2$. However, in most dehydrogenases, $FADH_2$ is never formed. Instead, the first electron is shared with a group on the protein as the next electron is transferred. Therefore, in this text, overall acceptance of two electrons by FAD has been denoted by the more general abbreviation, FAD(2H).

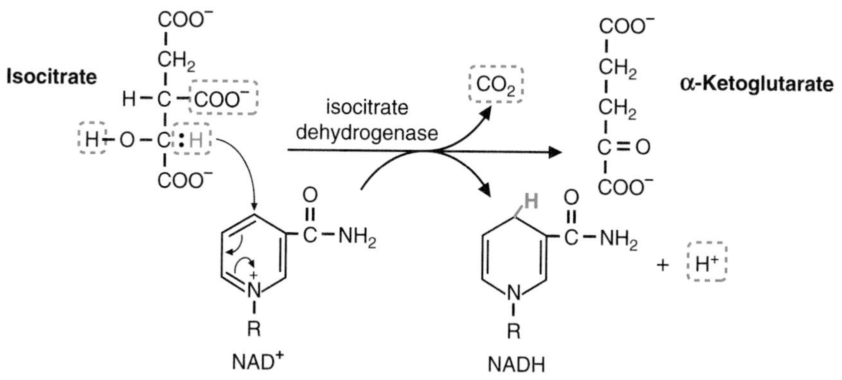

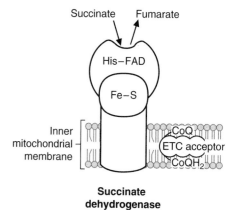

Fig. 20.5. Oxidation and decarboxylation of isocitrate. The alcohol group (C—OH) is oxidized to a ketone, with the C—H electrons donated to NAD$^+$ as the hydride ion. Subsequent electron shifts in the pyridine ring remove the positive charge. The H of the OH group dissociates into water as a proton, H$^+$. NAD$^+$, the electron acceptor, is reduced.

 A: The claim that succinate oxidation could produce energy without oxygen is wrong. It was probably based on the fact that succinate is oxidized to fumarate by the donation of electrons to FAD. However, ATP can only be generated from this process when these electrons are donated to oxygen in the electron transport chain. The energy generated by the electron transport chain is used for ATP synthesis in the process of oxidative phosphorylation. After the covalently bound FAD(2H) is oxidized back to FAD by the electron transport chain, succinate dehydrogenase can oxidize another succinate molecule.

dehydrogenase reaction). In contrast, NAD$^+$ accepts a pair of electrons as the hydride ion (H$^-$), which is attracted to the carbon opposite the positively-charged pyridine ring (Fig. 20.5). This occurs, for example, in the oxidation of alcohols to ketones by malate dehydrogenase and isocitrate dehydrogenase. The nicotinamide ring accepts a hydride ion from the C-H bond, and the alcoholic hydrogen is released into the medium as a positively charged proton, H$^+$.

The free radical, single-electron forms of FAD are very reactive, and FADH can lose its electron through exposure to water or the initiation of chain reactions. As a consequence, FAD must remain very tightly, sometimes covalently, attached to its enzyme while it accepts and transfers electrons to another group bound on the enzyme (Fig 20.6). Because FAD interacts with many functional groups on amino acid side chains in the active site, the E$^{0'}$ for enzyme-bound FAD varies greatly and can be greater or much less than that of NAD$^+$. In contrast, NAD$^+$ and NADH are more like substrate and product than coenzymes.

NADH plays a regulatory role in balancing energy metabolism that FAD(2H) cannot because FAD(2H) remains attached to its enzyme. Free NAD$^+$ binds to a dehydrogenase and is reduced to NADH, which is then released into the medium where it can bind and inhibit a different dehydrogenase. Consequently, oxidative enzymes are controlled by the NADH/NAD$^+$ ratio, and do not generate NADH faster than it can be reoxidized in the electron transport chain. The regulation of the TCA cycle and other pathways of fuel oxidation by the NADH/NAD$^+$ ratio is part of the mechanism for coordinating the rate of fuel oxidation to the rate of ATP utilization.

B. Role of CoA in the TCA Cycle

CoASH, the acylation coenzyme, participates in reactions through the formation of a thioester bond between the sulfur (S) of CoASH and an acyl group (e.g., acetyl

FAD has been referred to as a married coenzyme, and NAD$^+$ is its promiscuous cousin. FAD faithfully accepts only electrons from a substrate that is bound to the same enzyme (or enzyme complex), and donates these without leaving that enzyme. It does this repeatedly while still attached to its enzyme. NAD$^+$, conversely, may accept electrons when bound to any dehydrogenase, and leaves the enzyme immediately afterward. It donates these electrons while bound to a different dehydrogenase, such as NADH dehydrogenase in the electron transport chain. It really gets around!

Fig. 20.6. Succinate dehydrogenase contains covalently bound FAD. As a consequence, succinate dehydrogenase and similar flavoproteins reside in the inner mitochondrial membrane where they can directly transfer electrons into the electron transport chain. The electrons are transferred from the covalently bound FAD to an Fe-S complex on the enzyme, and then to coenzyme Q in the electron transport chain (see Chapter 21). Thus, FAD does not have to dissociate from the enzyme to transfer its electrons. All the other enzymes of the TCA cycle are found in the mitochondrial matrix.

CoASH is synthesized from the vitamin pantothenate in a sequence of reactions which phosphorylate pantothenate, add the sulfhydryl portion of CoA from cysteine, and then add AMP and an additional phosphate group from ATP (see Fig. 8.12). Pantothenate is widely distributed in foods (pantos means everywhere), so it is unlikely that **Ann O'Rexia** has developed a pantothenate deficiency. Although CoA is required in approximately 100 different reactions in mammalian cells, no Recommended Daily Allowance (RDA) has been established for pantothenate, in part because indicators have not yet been found which specifically and sensitively reflect a deficiency of this vitamin in the human. The reported symptoms of pantothenate deficiency (fatigue, nausea, and loss of appetite) are characteristic of vitamin deficiencies in general.

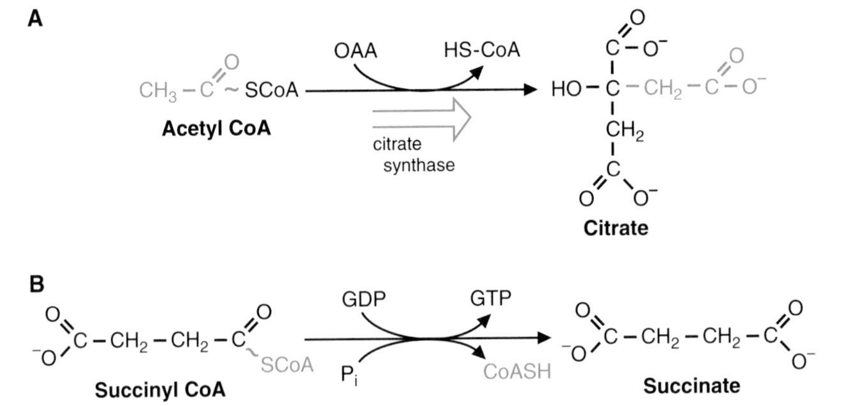

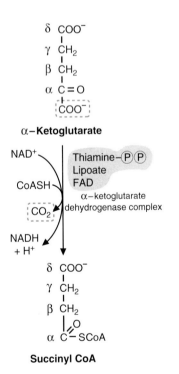

Fig. 20.8. Oxidative decarboxylation of α-ketoglutarate. The α-ketoglutarate dehydrogenase complex oxidizes α-ketoglutarate to succinyl CoA. The carboxyl group is released as CO_2. The keto group on the α-carbon is oxidized, and then forms the acyl CoA thioester, succinyl CoA. The α, β, γ, and δ on succinyl CoA refer to the sequence of atoms in α-ketoglutarate.

A

Acetyl CoA $\xrightarrow[\text{citrate synthase}]{\text{OAA} \quad \text{HS-CoA}}$ Citrate

B

Succinyl CoA $\xrightarrow[\quad P_i \quad \text{CoASH}]{\text{GDP} \quad \text{GTP}}$ Succinate

Fig. 20.7. Utilization of the high-energy thioester bond of acyl CoAs. Energy transformations are shown in blue. **A.** The energy released by hydrolysis of the thioester bond of acetyl CoA in the citrate synthase reaction contributes a large negative $\Delta G^{0\prime}$ to the forward direction of the TCA cycle. **B.** The energy of the succinyl CoA thioester bond is used for the synthesis of the high-energy phosphate bond of GTP.

CoA, succinyl CoA) (Fig. 20.7). The complete structure of CoASH and its vitamin precursor, pantothenate, is shown in Figure 8.12. A thioester bond differs from a typical oxygen ester bond because S, unlike O, does not share its electrons and participate in resonance formations. One of the consequences of this feature of sulfur chemistry is that the carbonyl carbon, the α-carbon and the β-carbon of the acyl group in a CoA thioester can be activated for participation in different types of reactions (e.g., in the citrate synthase reaction, the α-carbon methyl group is activated for condensation with oxaloacetate, see Figs. 20.3 and 20.7A). Another consequence is that the thioester bond is a high-energy bond that has a large negative $\Delta G^{0\prime}$ of hydrolysis (approximately–13 kcal/mole).

The energy from cleavage of the high-energy thioester bonds of succinyl CoA and acetyl CoA is used in two different ways in the TCA cycle. When the succinyl CoA thioester bond is cleaved by succinate thiokinase, the energy is used directly for activating an enzyme-bound phosphate that is transferred to GDP (see Fig. 20.7B). In contrast, when the thioester bond of acetyl CoA is cleaved in the citrate synthase reaction, the energy is released, giving the reaction a large negative $\Delta G^{0\prime}$ of –7.7 kcal/mole. The large negative $\Delta G^{0\prime}$ for citrate formation helps to keep the TCA cycle going in the forward direction.

C. The α-Ketoacid Dehydrogenase Complexes

The α-ketoglutarate dehydrogenase complex is one of a three-member family of similar α-keto acid dehydrogenase complexes. The other members of this family are the pyruvate dehydrogenase complex, and the branched chain amino acid α-keto acid dehydrogenase complex. Each of these complexes is specific for a different α-keto acid structure. In the sequence of reactions catalyzed by the complexes, the α-ketoacid is decarboxylated (i.e., releases the carboxyl group as CO_2) (Fig.20.8). The keto group is oxidized to the level of a carboxylic acid, and then combined with CoASH to form an acyl CoA thioester (e.g., succinyl CoA).

All of the α-ketoacid dehydrogenase complexes are huge enzyme complexes composed of multiple subunits of three different enzymes, E_1, E_2, and E_3 (Fig. 20.9). E_1 is an α-ketoacid decarboxylase which contains thiamine pyrophosphate (TPP); it cleaves off the carboxyl group of the α-keto acid. E_2 is a transacylase containing lipoate; it transfers the acyl portion of the α-keto acid from thiamine to CoASH. E_3 is dihydrolipoyl dehydrogenase, which contains

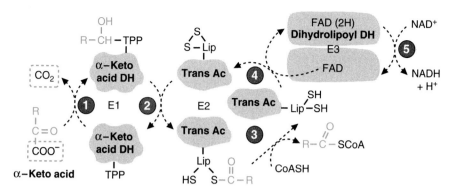

Fig. 20.9. Mechanism of α-keto acid dehydrogenase complexes (including α-ketoglutarate dehydrogenase, pyruvate dehydrogenase and the branched-chain α-keto acid dehydrogenase complex). **R** represents the portion of the α-ketoacid that begins with the β carbon. In α-ketoglutarate, R is CH_2-CH_2-COOH. In pyruvate, R is CH_3. The individual steps in the oxidative decarboxylation of α-keto acids are catalyzed by three different subunits: E_1, α-ketoacid decarboxylase (α-ketoglutarate decarboxylase); E_2, transacylase (trans-succinylase), and E_3, dihydrolipoyl dehydrogenase. Circle 1: Thiamine pyrophosphate (TPP) on E_1 decarboxylates the α-ketoacid and forms a covalent intermediate with the remaining portion. Circle 2: The acyl portion of the α-keto acid is transferred by TPP on E_1 to lipoate on E_2, which is a transacylase. Circle 3: E_2 transfers the acyl group from lipoate to CoASH. This process has reduced the lipoyl disulfide bond to sulfhydryl groups (dihydrolipoyl). Circle 4: E_3, dihydrolipoyl dehydrogenase (DH) transfers the electrons from reduced lipoate to its tightly bound FAD molecule, thereby oxidizing lipoate back to its original disulfide form. Circle 5: The electrons are then transferred from FAD(2H) to NAD$^+$ to form NADH.

FAD; it transfers electrons from reduced lipoate to NAD$^+$. The collection of 3 enzyme activities into one huge complex enables the product of one enzyme to be transferred to the next enzyme without loss of energy. Complex formation also increases the rate of catalysis because the substrates for E_2 and E_3 remain bound to the enzyme complex.

1. THIAMINE PYROPHOSPHATE IN THE α-KETOGLUTARATE DEHYDROGENASE COMPLEX

Thiamine pyrophosphate is synthesized from the vitamin thiamine by the addition of pyrophosphate (see Fig. 8.11). The pyrophosphate group binds magnesium, which binds to amino acid side chains on the enzyme. This binding is relatively weak for a coenzyme, so thiamine turns over rapidly in the body, and a deficiency can develop rapidly in individuals on a thiamine-free or low thiamine diet.

The general function of thiamine pyrophosphate is the cleavage of a carbon-carbon bond next to a keto group. In the α-ketoglutarate, pyruvate, and branched chain α-keto acid dehydrogenase complexes, the functional carbon on the thiazole ring forms a covalent bond with the α-keto carbon, thereby cleaving the bond between the α-keto carbon and the adjacent carboxylic acid group (see Fig. 8.11 for the mechanism of this reaction). Thiamine pyrophosphate is also a coenzyme for transketolase in the pentose phosphate pathway, where it similarly cleaves the carbon-carbon bond next to a keto group. In thiamine deficiency, α-ketoglutarate, pyruvate, and other α-keto acids accumulate in the blood.

2. LIPOATE

Lipoate is a coenzyme found only in α-keto acid dehydrogenase complexes. It is synthesized in the human from carbohydrate and amino acids, and does not require

Q: The E$^{0'}$ for FAD accepting electrons is −0.20 (see Table 19.4). The E$^{0'}$ for NAD$^+$ accepting electrons is −0.32. Thus, transfer of electrons from FAD(2H) to NAD$^+$ is energetically unfavorable. How do the α-keto acid dehydrogenase complexes allow this electron transfer to occur?

In **Al Martini's** heart failure, which is caused by a dietary deficiency of the vitamin thiamine, pyruvate dehydrogenase, α-ketoglutarate dehydrogenase, and the branched chain α-keto acid dehydrogenase complexes are less functional than normal. Because heart muscle, skeletal muscle, and nervous tissue have a high rate of ATP production from the NADH produced by the oxidation of pyruvate to acetyl CoA and of acetyl CoA to CO_2 in the TCA cycle, these tissues present with the most obvious signs of thiamine deficiency.

In Western societies, gross thiamine deficiency is most often associated with alcoholism. The mechanism for active absorption of thiamine is strongly and directly inhibited by alcohol. Subclinical deficiency of thiamine from malnutrition or anorexia may be common in the general population and is usually associated with multiple vitamin deficiencies.

A: The $E^{0'}$ values were calculated in a test tube under standard conditions. When FAD is bound to an enzyme, as it is in the α-keto acid dehydrogenase complexes, amino acid side chains can alter its $E^{0'}$ value. Thus, the transfer of electrons from the bound FAD(2H) to NAD^+ in dihydrolipoyl dehydrogenase is actually energetically favorable.

Arsenic poisoning is caused by the presence of a large number of different arsenious compounds that are effective metabolic inhibitors. Acute accidental or intentional arsenic poisoning requires high doses and involves arsenate (AsO_4^{2-}) and arsenite (AsO^{2-}). Arsenite, which is 10 times more toxic than arsenate, binds to neighboring sulfhydryl groups, such as those in dihydrolipoate and in nearby cysteine pairs (vicinal) found in α-keto acid dehydrogenase complexes and in succinic dehydrogenase. Arsenate weakly inhibits enzymatic reactions involving phosphate, including the enzyme glyceraldehyde 3-P dehydrogenase in glycolysis (see Chapter 22). Thus both aerobic and anaerobic ATP production can be inhibited. The low doses of arsenic compounds found in water supplies are a major public health concern, but are associated with increased risk of cancer rather than direct toxicity.

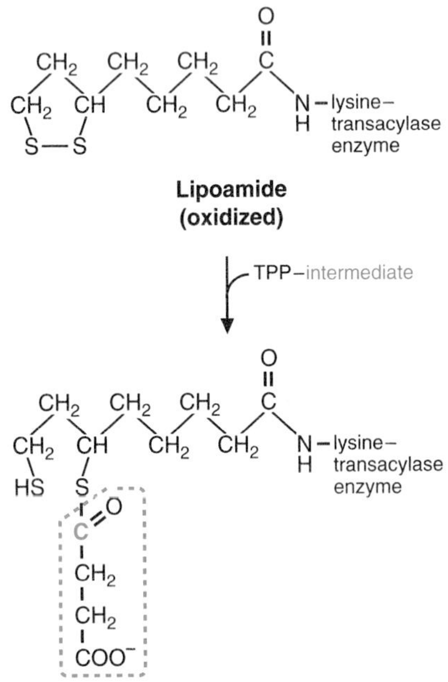

a vitamin precursor. Lipoate is attached to the transacylase enzyme through its carboxyl group, which is covalently bound to the terminal $-NH_2$ of a lysine in the protein (Fig. 20.10). At its functional end, lipoate contains a disulfide group that accepts electrons when it binds the acyl fragment of α-ketoglutarate. It can thus act like a long flexible $-CH_2-$ arm of the enzyme that reaches over to the decarboxylase to pick up the acyl fragment from thiamine and transfer it to the active site containing bound CoASH. It then swings over to dihydrolipoyl dehydrogenase to transfer electrons from the lipoyl sulfhydryl groups to FAD.

3. FAD AND DIHYDROLIPOYL DEHYDROGENASE

FAD on dihydrolipoyl dehydrogenase accepts electrons from the lipoyl sulfhydryl groups and transfers them to bound NAD^+. FAD thus accepts and transfers electrons without leaving its binding site on the enzyme. The direction of the reaction is favored by interactions of FAD with groups on the enzyme, which change its reduction potential and by the overall release of energy from cleavage and oxidation of α-ketoglutarate.

III. ENERGETICS OF THE TCA CYCLE

Like all metabolic pathways, the TCA cycle operates with an overall net negative $\Delta G^{0'}$ (Fig 20.11). The conversion of substrates to products is, therefore, energetically favorable. However, some of the reactions, such as the malate dehydrogenase reaction, have a positive value.

Lipoamide (oxidized)

TPP–intermediate

Fig. 20.10. Function of lipoate. Lipoate is attached to the ε-amino group on the lysine side chain of the tranacylase enzyme (E_2). The oxidized lipoate disulfide form is reduced as it accepts the acyl group from thiamine pyrophosphate (TPP) attached to E_1. The example shown is for the α-ketoglutarate dehydrogenase complex.

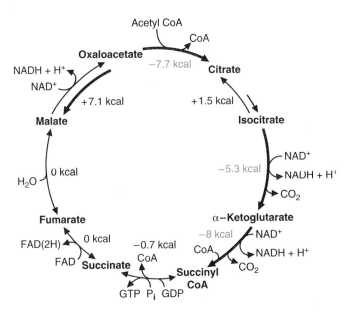

Fig. 20.11. Approximate $\Delta G^{0'}$ values for the reactions in the TCA cycle, given for the forward direction. The reactions with large negative $\Delta G^{0'}$ values are shown in blue. The standard free energy ($\Delta G^{0'}$) refers to the free energy change for conversion of 1 mole of substrate to 1 mole of product under standard conditions (see Chapter 19).

A. Overall Efficiency of the TCA Cycle

The reactions of the TCA cycle are extremely efficient in converting energy in the chemical bonds of the acetyl group to other forms. The total amount of energy available from the acetyl group is about 228 kcal/mole (the amount of energy that could be released from complete combustion of 1 mole of acetyl groups to CO_2 in a bomb calorimeter). The products of the TCA cycle (NADH, FAD(2H), and GTP) contain about 207 kcal (Table 20.1). Thus, the TCA cycle reactions are able to conserve about 90% of the energy available from the oxidation of acetyl CoA.

B. Thermodynamically and Kinetically Reversible and Irreversible reactions

Three reactions in the TCA cycle have large negative values for $\Delta G^{0\prime}$ that strongly favor the forward direction: the reactions catalyzed by citrate synthase, isocitrate dehydrogenase, and α-ketoglutarate dehydrogenase (see Fig. 20.11). Within the TCA cycle, these reactions are physiologically irreversible for two reasons: the products do not rise to high enough concentrations under physiological conditions to overcome the large negative $\Delta G^{0\prime}$ values, and the enzymes involved catalyze the reverse reaction very slowly. These reactions make the major contribution to the overall negative $\Delta G^{0\prime}$ for the TCA cycle, and keep it going in the forward direction.

In contrast to these irreversible reactions, the reactions catalyzed by aconitase and malate dehydrogenase have a positive $\Delta G^{0\prime}$ for the forward direction, and are thermodynamically and kinetically reversible. Because aconitase is rapid in both directions, equilibrium values for the concentration ratio of products to substrates is maintained, and the concentration of citrate is about 20 times that of isocitrate. The accumulation of citrate instead of isocitrate facilitates transport of excess citrate to the cytosol, where it can provide a source of acetyl CoA for pathways like fatty acid and cholesterol synthesis. It also allows citrate to serve as an inhibitor of citrate synthase when flux through isocitrate dehydrogenase is decreased. Likewise, the equilibrium constant of the malate dehydrogenase reaction favors the accumulation of malate over oxaloacetate, resulting in a low oxaloacetate concentration that is influenced by the $NADH/NAD^+$ ratio. Thus, there is a net flux of oxaloacetate towards malate in the liver during fasting (due to fatty acid oxidation, which raises the $NADH/NAD^+$ ratio), and malate can then be transported out of the mitochondria to provide a substrate for gluconeogenesis.

IV. REGULATION OF THE TCA CYCLE

The oxidation of acetyl CoA in the TCA cycle and the conservation of this energy as NADH and FAD(2H) is essential for generation of ATP in almost all tissues in the body. In spite of changes in the supply of fuels, type of fuels in the blood, or rate of ATP utilization, cells maintain ATP homeostasis (a constant level of ATP). The rate of the TCA cycle, like that of all fuel oxidation pathways, is principally regulated to correspond to the rate of the electron transport chain, which is regulated by the ATP/ADP ratio and the rate of ATP utilization (see Chapter 21). The major sites of regulation are shown in Fig 20.12.

Two major messengers feed information on the rate of ATP utilization back to the TCA cycle: (a) the phosphorylation state of ATP, as reflected in ATP and ADP levels, and (b) the reduction state of NAD^+, as reflected in the ratio of $NADH/NAD^+$. Within the cell, even within the mitochondrion, the total adenine nucleotide pool (AMP, ADP, plus ATP) and the total NAD pool (NAD^+ plus NADH) are relatively constant. Thus, an increased rate of ATP utilization results in a small decrease of ATP concentration and an increase of ADP. Likewise, increased NADH oxidation to NAD^+ by the electron transport chain increases the rate of pathways producing NADH. Under normal physiological conditions, the TCA cycle and other

Table 20.1. Energy Yield of the TCA Cycle

kcal/mole	
3 NADH: 3×53	= 159
1 FAD(2H)	= 41
1 GTP	= 7
Sum	= 207

Chapter 19 explains the values given for energy yield from NADH and FAD(2H).

The net standard free energy change for the TCA cycle, $\Delta G^{0\prime}$, can be calculated from the sum of the $\Delta G^{0\prime}$ values for the individual reactions. The $\Delta G^{0\prime}$, -13 kcal, is the amount of energy lost as heat. It can be considered the amount of energy spent to ensure that oxidation of the acetyl group to CO_2 goes to completion. This value is surprisingly small. However, oxidation of NADH and FAD(2H) in the electron transport chain helps to make acetyl oxidation more energetically favorable and pull the TCA cycle forward.

Otto Shape had difficulty losing weight because human fuel utilization is too efficient. His adipose tissue fatty acids are being converted to acetyl CoA, which is being oxidized in the TCA cycle, thereby generating NADH and FAD(2H). The energy in these compounds is used for ATP synthesis from oxidative phosphorylation. If his fuel utilization were less efficient and his ATP yield were lower, he would have to oxidize much greater amounts of fat to get the ATP he needs for exercise.

As **Otto Shape** exercises, his myosin ATPase hydrolyzes ATP to provide the energy for movement of myofibrils. The decrease of ATP and increase of ADP stimulates the electron transport chain to oxidize more NADH and FAD(2H). The TCA cycle is stimulated to provide more NADH and FAD(2H) to the electron transport chain. The activation of the TCA cycle occurs through a decrease of the $NADH/NAD^+$ ratio, an increase of ADP concentration, and an increase of Ca^{2+}. Although regulation of the transcription of genes for TCA cycle enzymes is too slow to respond to changes of ATP demands during exercise, the number and size of mitochondria increase during training. Thus, Otto Shape is increasing his capacity for fuel oxidation as he trains.

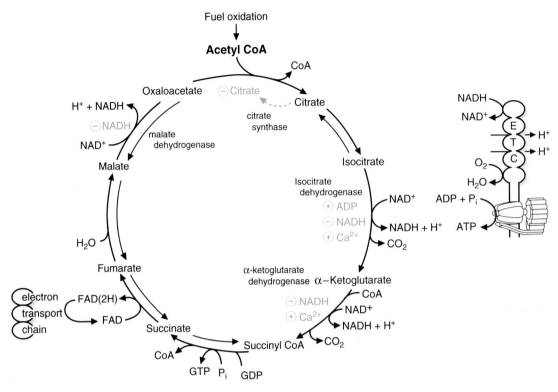

Fig. 20.12. Major regulatory interactions in the TCA cycle. The rate of ATP hydrolysis controls the rate of ATP synthesis, which controls the rate of NADH oxidation in the electron transport chain (ETC). All NADH and FAD(2H) produced by the cycle donate electrons to this chain (shown on the right). Thus, oxidation of acetyl CoA in the TCA cycle can go only as fast as electrons from NADH enter the electron transport chain, which is controlled by the ATP and ADP content of the cells. The ADP and NADH concentrations feed information on the rate of oxidative phosphorylation back to the TCA cycle. Isocitrate dehydrogenase (DH), α-ketoglutarate dehydrogenase (DH), and malate dehydrogenase (DH) are inhibited by increased NADH concentration. The NADH/NAD$^+$ ratio changes the concentration of oxaloacetate. Citrate is a product inhibitor of citrate synthase. ADP is an allosteric activator of isocitrate dehydrogenase. During muscular contraction, increased Ca^{2+} concentrations activate isocitrate DH and α-ketoglutarate dehydrogenase (as well as pyruvate dehydrogenase).

oxidative pathways respond so rapidly to increased ATP demand that the ATP concentration does not significantly change.

A. Regulation of Citrate Synthase

The principles of pathway regulation are summarized in Table 20.2. In pathways subject to feedback regulation, the first step of the pathway must be regulated so that

Table 20.2. Generalizations on the Regulation of Metabolic Pathways

1. Regulation matches function. The type of regulation use depends on the function of the pathway. Tissue-specific isozymes may allow the features of regulatory enzymes to match somewhat different functions of the pathway in different tissues.
2. Regulation of metabolic pathways occurs at rate-limiting steps, the slowest steps, in the pathway. These are reactions in which a small change of rate will affect the flux through the whole pathway.
3. Regulation usually occurs at the first committed step of a pathway or at metabolic branchpoints. In human cells, most pathways are interconnected with other pathways and have regulatory enzymes for every branchpoint.
4. Regulatory enzymes often catalyze physiologically irreversible reactions. These are also the steps that differ in biosynthetic and degradative pathways.
5. Many pathways have "feedback" regulation, that is, the endproduct of the pathway controls the rate of its own synthesis. Feedback regulation may involve inhibition of an early step in the pathway (feedback inhibition) or regulation of gene transcription.
6. Human cells use compartmentation to control access of substrate and activators or inhibitors to different enzymes.
7. Hormonal regulation integrates responses in pathways requiring more than one tissue. Hormones generally regulate fuel metabolism by:
   a. Changing the phosphorylation state of enzymes.
   b. Changing the amount of enzyme present by changing its rate of synthesis (often induction or repression of mRNA synthesis) or degradation.
   c. Changing the concentration of an activator or inhibitor.

precursors flow into alternate pathways if product is not needed. Citrate synthase, which is the first enzyme of the TCA cycle, is a simple enzyme that has no allosteric regulators. Its rate is controlled principally by the concentration of oxaloacetate, its substrate, and the concentration of citrate, a product inhibitor, competitive with oxaloacetate.(see Fig. 20.12). The malate-oxaloacetate equilibrium favors malate, so the oxaloacetate concentration is very low inside the mitochondrion, and is below the $K_{m,app}$ (see Chapter 9, section I.A.4) of citrate synthase. When the NADH/NAD$^+$ ratio decreases, the ratio of oxaloacetate to malate increases. When isocitrate dehydrogenase is activated, the concentration of citrate decreases, thus relieving the product inhibition of citrate synthase. Thus, both increased oxaloacetate and decreased citrate levels regulate the response of citrate synthase to conditions established by the electron transport chain and oxidative phosphorylation. In the liver, the NADH/NAD$^+$ ratio helps determine whether acetyl CoA enters the TCA cycle or goes into the alternate pathway for ketone body synthesis.

B. Allosteric Regulation of Isocitrate Dehydrogenase

Another generalization that can be made about regulation of metabolic pathways is that it occurs at the enzyme that catalyzes the rate-limiting (slowest) step in a pathway (see Table 20.2). Isocitrate dehydrogenase is considered one of the rate-limiting steps of the TCA cycle, and is allosterically activated by ADP and inhibited by NADH (Fig. 20.13). In the absence of ADP, the enzyme exhibits positive cooperativity; as isocitrate binds to one subunit, other subunits are converted to an active conformation (see Chapter 9, section III.A on allosteric enzymes). In the presence of ADP, all of the subunits are in their active conformation, and isocitrate binds more readily. Consequently, the $K_{m,app}$ (the $S_{0.5}$) shifts to a much lower value. Thus, at the concentration of isocitrate found in the mitochondrial matrix, a small change in the concentration of ADP can produce a large change in the rate of the isocitrate dehydrogenase reaction. Small changes in the concentration of the product, NADH, and of the cosubstrate, NAD$^+$, also affect the rate of the enzyme more than they would a nonallosteric enzyme.

C. Regulation of α-Ketoglutarate Dehydrogenase

The α-ketoglutarate dehydrogenase complex, although not an allosteric enzyme, is product-inhibited by NADH and succinyl CoA, and may also be inhibited by GTP (see Fig. 20.12). Thus, both α-ketoglutarate dehydrogenase and isocitrate dehydrogenase respond directly to changes in the relative levels of ADP and hence the rate at which NADH is oxidized by electron transport. Both of these enzymes are also activated by Ca^{2+}. In contracting heart muscle, and possibly other muscle tissues, the release of Ca^{2+} from the sarcoplasmic reticulum during muscle contraction may provide an additional activation of these enzymes when ATP is being rapidly hydrolyzed.

D. Regulation of TCA Cycle Intermediates

Regulation of the TCA cycle serves two functions: it ensures that NADH is generated fast enough to maintain ATP homeostasis and it regulates the concentration of TCA cycle intermediates. For example, in the liver, a decreased rate of isocitrate dehydrogenase increases citrate concentration, which stimulates citrate efflux to the cytosol. A number of regulatory interactions occur in the TCA cycle, in addition to those mentioned above, that control the levels of TCA intermediates and their flux into pathways that adjoin the TCA cycle.

V. PRECURSORS OF ACETYL CoA

Compounds enter the TCA cycle as acetyl CoA or as an intermediate that can be converted to malate or oxaloacetate. Compounds that enter as acetyl CoA are

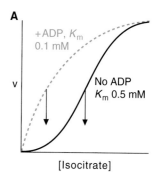

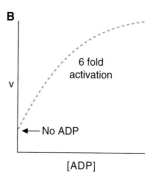

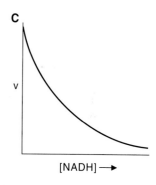

Fig. 20.13. Allosteric regulation of isocitrate dehydrogenase (ICDH). Isocitrate dehydrogenase has eight subunits, and two active sites. Isocitrate, NAD$^+$, and NADH bind in the active site; ADP and Ca^{2+} are activators and bind to separate allosteric sites. **A.** A graph of velocity versus isocitrate concentration shows positive cooperativity (sigmoid curve) in the absence of ADP. The allosteric activator ADP changes the curve into one closer to a rectangular hyperbola, and decreases the K_m ($S_{0.5}$) for isocitrate. **B.** The allosteric activation by ADP is not an all-or-nothing response. The extent of activation by ADP depends on its concentration. **C.** Increases in the concentration of product, NADH, decrease the velocity of the enzyme through effects on the allosteric activation.

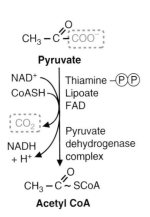

Acetate (acetic acid) is present in the diet, and can be produced from the oxidation of ethanol. Roman soldiers carried vinegar, a dilute solution of acetic acid. The acidity of the vinegar made it a relatively safe source of drinking water because many kinds of pathogenic bacteria do not grow well in acid solutions. The acetate, which is activated to acetyl CoA, provided an excellent fuel for muscular exercise.

oxidized to CO_2. Compounds that enter as TCA cycle intermediates replenish intermediates that have been used in biosynthetic pathways, such as gluconeogenesis or heme synthesis, but cannot be fully oxidized to CO_2.

A. Sources of Acetyl CoA

Acetyl CoA serves as a common point of convergence for the major pathways of fuel oxidation. It is generated directly from the β-oxidation of fatty acids and degradation of the ketone bodies β-hydroxybutyrate and acetoacetate (Fig. 20.14). It is also formed from acetate, which can arise from the diet or from ethanol oxidation. Glucose and other carbohydrates enter glycolysis, a pathway common to all cells, and are oxidized to pyruvate. The amino acids alanine and serine are also converted to pyruvate. Pyruvate is oxidized to acetyl CoA by the pyruvate dehydrogenase complex. A number of amino acids, such as leucine and isoleucine are also oxidized to acetyl CoA. Thus, the final oxidation of acetyl CoA to CO_2 in the TCA cycle is the last step in all the major pathways of fuel oxidation.

B. Pyruvate Dehydrogenase Complex

The pyruvate dehydrogenase complex (PDC) oxidizes pyruvate to acetyl CoA, thus linking glycolysis and the TCA cycle. In the brain, which is dependent on the oxidation of glucose to CO_2 to fulfill its ATP needs, regulation of the PDC is a life and death matter.

1.   STRUCTURE OF PDC

PDC belongs to the α-ketoacid dehydrogenase complex family and, thus, shares structural and catalytic features with the α-ketoglutarate dehydrogenase complex and the branched chain α-ketoacid dehydrogenase complex (Fig. 20.15). It contains the same three basic types of catalytic subunits: (1) pyruvate decarboxylase subunits that bind thiamine-pyrophosphate (E_1); (2) transacetylase subunits that bind lipoate (E_2), and (3) dihyrolipoyl dehydrogenase subunits that bind FAD (E_3) (see Fig. 20.9). Although the E_1 and E_2 enzymes in PDC are relatively specific for pyruvate, the same dihydrolipoyl dehydrogenase participates in all of the α-ketoacid dehydrogenase

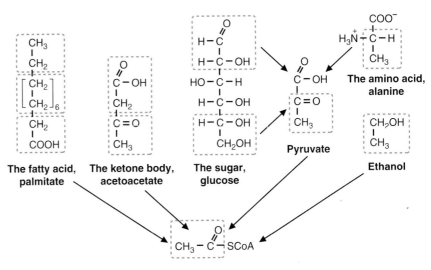

Fig. 20.14. Origin of the acetyl group from various fuels. Acetyl CoA is derived from the oxidation of fuels. The portions of fatty acids, ketone bodies, glucose, pyruvate, the amino acid alanine, and ethanol that are converted to the acetyl group of acetyl CoA are shown in blue.

Fig. 20.15. Pyruvate dehydrogenase complex (PDC) catalyzes oxidation of the α-ketoacid pyruvate to acetyl CoA.

complexes. In addition to these three types of subunits, the PDC complex contains one additional catalytic subunit, protein X, which is a transacetylase. Each functional component of the PDC complex is present in multiple copies (e.g., bovine heart PDC has 30 subunits of E_1, 60 subunits of E_2, and 6 subunits each of E_3 and X). The E_1 enzyme is itself a tetramer of two different types of subunits, α and β.

2. REGULATION OF PDC

PDC activity is controlled principally through phosphorylation by pyruvate dehydrogenase kinase, which inhibits the enzyme, and dephosphorylation by pyruvate dehydrogenase phosphatase, which activates it (Fig. 20.16). Pyruvate dehydrogenase kinase and pyruvate dehydrogenase phosphatase are regulatory subunits within the PDC complex and act only on the complex. PDC kinase transfers a phosphate from ATP to specific serine hydroxyl (ser-OH) groups on pyruvate decarboxylase (E_1). PDC phosphatase removes these phosphate groups by hydrolysis. Phosphorylation of just one serine on the PDC E_1 α subunit can decrease its activity by over 99%. PDC kinase is present in complexes as tissue-specific isozymes that vary in their regulatory properties.

PDC kinase is, itself, inhibited by ADP and pyruvate. Thus, when rapid ATP utilization results in an increase of ADP, or when activation of glycolysis increases pyruvate levels, PDC kinase is inhibited, and PDC remains in an active, nonphosphorylated form. PDC phosphatase requires Ca^{2+} for full activity. In the heart, increased intramitochondrial Ca^{2+} during rapid contraction activates the phosphatase, thereby increasing the amount of active, nonphosphorylated PDC.

PDC is also regulated through inhibition by its products, acetyl CoA and NADH. This inhibition is stronger than regular product inhibition because their binding to

 Deficiencies of the pyruvate dehydrogenase complex (PDC) are among the most common inherited diseases leading to lacticacidemia and, like pyruvate carboxylase deficiency, are grouped into the category of Leigh's disease. In its severe form, PDC deficiency presents with overwhelming lactic acidosis at birth, with death in the neonatal period. In a second form of presentation, the lactic academia is moderate, but there is profound psychomotor retardation with increasing age. In many cases, concomitant damage to the brain stem and basal ganglia lead to death in infancy. The neurological symptoms arise because the brain has a very limited ability to use fatty acids as a fuel, and is, therefore, dependent on glucose metabolism for its energy supply.

The most common PDC genetic defects are in the gene for the α subunit of E_1. The E_1 α-gene is X-linked. Because of its importance in central nervous system metabolism, pyruvate dehydrogenase deficiency is a problem in both males and females, even if the female is a carrier. For this reason, it is classified as an X-linked dominant disorder.

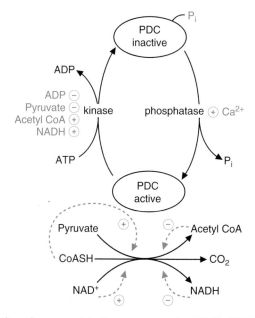

Fig. 20.16. Regulation of pyruvate dehydrogenase complex (PDC). PDC kinase, a subunit of the enzyme, phosphorylates PDC at a specific serine residue, thereby converting PDC to an inactive form. The kinase is inhibited by ADP and pyruvate. PDC phosphatase, another subunit of the enzyme, removes the phosphate, thereby activating PDC. The phosphatase is activated by Ca^{2+}. When the substrates, pyruvate and CoASH, are bound to PDC, the kinase activity is inhibited and PDC is active. When the products acetyl CoA and NADH bind to PDC, the kinase activity is stimulated, and the enzyme is phosphorylated to the inactive form. E_1 and the kinase exist as tissue-specific isozymes with overlapping tissue specificity, and somewhat different regulatory properties.

PDC stimulates its phosphorylation to the inactive form. The substrates of the enzyme, CoASH and NAD^+, antagonize this product inhibition. Thus, when an ample supply of acetyl CoA for the TCA cycle is already available from fatty acid oxidation, acetyl CoA and NADH build up and dramatically decrease their own further synthesis by PDC.

PDC can also be rapidly activated through a mechanism involving insulin, which plays a prominent role in adipocytes. In many tissues, insulin may, slowly over time, increase the amount of pyruvate dehydrogenase complex present.

The rate of other fuel oxidation pathways that feed into the TCA cycle is also increased when ATP utilization increases. Insulin, other hormones and diet control the availability of fuels for these oxidative pathways.

VI. TCA CYCLE INTERMEDIATES AND ANAPLEROTIC REACTIONS

A. TCA Cycle Intermediates are Precursors for Biosynthetic Pathways

 Pyruvate, citrate, α-ketoglutarate and malate, ADP, ATP, and phosphate (as well as many other compounds) have specific transporters in the inner mitochondrial membrane that transport compounds between the mitochondrial matrix and cytosol in exchange for a compound of similar charge. In contrast, CoASH, acetyl CoA, other CoA derivatives, NAD^+ and NADH, and oxaloacetate, are not transported at a metabolically significant rate. To obtain cytosolic acetyl CoA, many cells transport citrate to the cytosol, where it is cleaved to acetyl CoA and oxaloacetate by citrate lyase.

The intermediates of the TCA cycle serve as precursors for a variety of different pathways present in different cell types (Fig. 20.17). This is particularly important in the central metabolic role of the liver. The TCA cycle in the liver is often called an "open cycle" because there is such a high efflux of intermediates. After a high carbohydrate meal, citrate efflux and cleavage to acetyl CoA provides acetyl units for cytosolic fatty acid synthesis. During fasting, gluconeogenic precursors are converted to malate, which leaves the mitochondria for cytosolic gluconeogenesis. The liver also uses TCA cycle intermediates to synthesize carbon skeletons of amino acids. Succinyl CoA may be removed from the TCA cycle to form heme in cells of the liver and bone marrow. In the brain, α-ketoglutarate is converted to glutamate and then to γ-aminobutyric acid (GABA), a neurotransmitter. In skeletal muscle, α-ketoglutarate is converted to glutamine, which is transported through the blood to other tissues.

B. Anaplerotic Reactions

Removal of any of the intermediates from the TCA cycle removes the 4 carbons that are used to regenerate oxaloacetate during each turn of the cycle. With depletion of oxaloacetate, it is impossible to continue oxidizing acetyl CoA. To enable the TCA

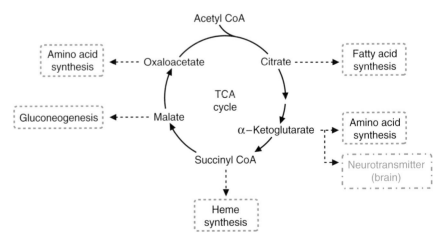

Fig. 20.17. Efflux of intermediates from the TCA cycle. In the liver, TCA cycle intermediates are continuously withdrawn into the pathways of fatty acid synthesis, amino acid synthesis, gluconeogenesis, and heme synthesis. In brain, α-ketoglutarate is converted to glutamate and GABA, both neurotransmitters.

cycle to keep running, cells have to supply enough four-carbon intermediates from degradation of carbohydrate or certain amino acids to compensate for the rate of removal. Pathways or reactions that replenish the intermediates of the TCA cycle are referred to as anaplerotic ("filling up").

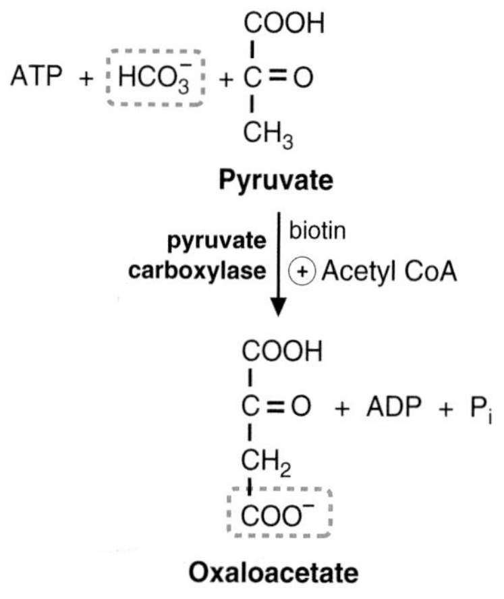

1. PYRUVATE CARBOXYLASE IS A MAJOR ANAPLEROTIC ENZYME

Pyruvate carboxylase is one of the major anaplerotic enzymes in the cell. It catalyzes the addition of CO_2 to pyruvate to form oxaloacetate (Fig. 20.18). Like most carboxylases, pyruvate carboxylase contains biotin, which forms a covalent intermediate with CO_2 in a reaction requiring ATP and Mg^{2+} (see Fig. 8.12, Chap. 8). The activated CO_2 is then transferred to pyruvate to form the carboxyl group of oxaloacetate.

Pyruvate carboxylase is found in many tissues, such as liver, brain, adipocytes, and fibroblasts, where its function is anaplerotic. Its concentration is high in liver and kidney cortex, where there is a continuous removal of oxaloacetate and malate from the TCA cycle to enter the gluconeogenic pathway.

Pyruvate carboxylase is activated by acetyl CoA and inhibited by high concentrations of many acyl CoA derivatives. As the concentration of oxaloacetate is depleted through the efflux of TCA cycle intermediates, the rate of the citrate synthase reaction decreases and acetyl CoA concentration rises. The acetyl CoA then activates pyruvate carboxylase to synthesize more oxaloacetate.

2. AMINO ACID DEGRADATION FORMS TCA CYCLE INTERMEDIATES

The pathways for oxidation of many amino acids convert their carbon skeletons into 5- and 4-carbon intermediates of the TCA cycle that can regenerate oxaloacetate (Fig 20.19). Alanine and serine carbons can enter through pyruvate carboxylase (see Fig.20.19, circle 1). In all tissues with mitochondria (except for, surprisingly, the liver), oxidation of the two branched chain amino acids isoleucine and valine to succinyl CoA forms a major anaplerotic route (see Fig.20.19, circle 3). In the liver, other compounds forming propionyl CoA (e.g., methionine, thymine and odd-chain length or branched fatty acids) also enter the TCA cycle as succinyl CoA. In most tissues, glutamine is taken up from the blood, converted to glutamate, and then oxidized to α-ketoglutarate, forming another major anaplerotic route (see Fig.20.19, circle 2). However, the TCA cycle cannot be resupplied with intermediates by even chain length fatty acid oxidation, or ketone body oxidation, which forms only acetyl CoA. In the TCA cycle, two carbons are lost from citrate before succinyl CoA is formed, and, therefore, there is no net conversion of acetyl carbon to oxaloacetate.

Fig. 20.18. Pyruvate carboxylase reaction. Pyruvate carboxylase adds a carboxyl group from bicarbonate (which is in equilibrium with CO_2) to pyruvate to form oxaloacetate. Biotin is used to activate and transfer the CO_2. The energy to form the covalent biotin–CO_2 complex is provided by the high-energy phosphate bond of ATP, which is cleaved in the reaction. The enzyme is activated by acetyl CoA.

Biotin is a vitamin. A deficiency of biotin is very rare in humans because it is required in such small amounts and is synthesized by intestinal bacteria. However, an interesting case of biotin deficiency arose in a man eating a diet composed principally of peanuts and raw egg whites. Egg whites contain a biotin binding protein, avidin. Since he did not denature avidin by cooking the egg whites, it depleted his diet of biotin.

Pyruvate carboxylase deficiency is one of the genetic diseases grouped together under the clinical manifestations of Leigh's disease (subacute necrotizing encephalopathy). In the mild form, the patient presents early in life with delayed development and a mild-to-moderate lactic acidemia. Patients who survive are severely mentally retarded, and there is a loss of cerebral neurons. In the brain, pyruvate carboxylase is present in the astrocytes, which use TCA cycle intermediates to synthesize glutamine. This pathway is essential for neuronal survival. The major cause of the lactic acidemia is that cells dependent on pyruvate carboxylase for an anaplerotic supply of oxaloacetate cannot oxidize pyruvate in the TCA cycle (because of low oxaloacetate levels), and the liver cannot convert pyruvate to glucose (because the pyruvate carboxylase reaction is required for this pathway to occur), so the excess pyruvate is converted to lactate.

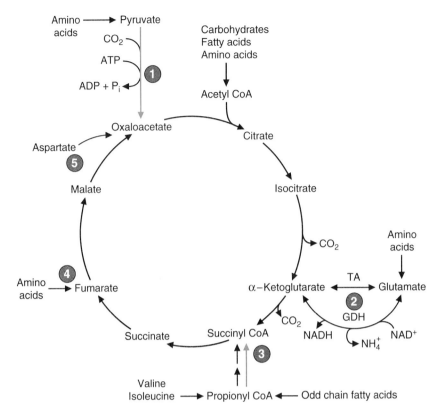

Fig. 20.19. Major anaplerotic pathways of the TCA cycle. 1 and 3 (blue arrows) are the two major anabolic pathways. (1) Pyruvate carboxylase (2) Glutamate is reversibly converted to α-ketoglutarate by transaminases (TA) and glutamate dehydrogenase (GDH) in many tissues. (3) The carbon skeletons of valine and isoleucine, a 3-carbon unit from odd chain fatty acid oxidation, and a number of other compounds enter the TCA cycle at the level of succinyl CoA. Other amino acids are also degraded to fumarate (4) and oxaloacetate (5), principally in the liver.

CLINICAL COMMENTS

Otto Shape. Otto Shape is experiencing the benefits of physical conditioning. A variety of functional adaptations in the heart, lungs, vascular system, and skeletal muscle occur in response to regular graded exercise. The pumping efficiency of the heart increases, allowing a greater cardiac output with fewer beats per minute and at a lower rate of oxygen utilization. The lungs extract a greater percentage of oxygen from the inspired air, allowing fewer respirations per unit of activity. The vasodilatory capacity of the arterial beds in skeletal muscle increases, promoting greater delivery of oxygen and fuels to exercising muscle. Concurrently, the venous drainage capacity in muscle is enhanced, ensuring that lactic acid will not accumulate in contracting tissues. These adaptive changes in physiological responses are accompanied by increases in the number, size, and activity of skeletal muscle mitochondria, along with the content of TCA cycle enzymes and components of the electron transport chain. These changes markedly enhance the oxidative capacity of exercising muscle.

Ann O'Rexia. Ann O'Rexia is experiencing fatigue for a number of reasons. She has iron deficiency anemia, which affects both iron-containing hemoglobin in her red blood cells, iron in aconitase and succinic dehydrogenase, as well as iron in the heme proteins of the electron

In skeletal muscle and other tissues, ATP is generated by anaerobic glycolysis when the rate of aerobic respiration is inadequate to meet the rate of ATP utilization. Under these circumstances, the rate of pyruvate production exceeds the cell's capacity to oxidize NADH in the electron transport chain, and hence, to oxidize pyruvate in the TCA cycle. The excess pyruvate is reduced to lactate. Because lactate is an acid, its accumulation affects the muscle and causes pain and swelling.

transport chain. She may also be experiencing the consequences of multiple vitamin deficiencies, including thiamine, riboflavin, and niacin (the vitamin precursor of NAD^+). It is less likely, but possible, that she also has subclinical deficiencies of pantothenate (the precursor of CoA) or biotin. Because of this, Ann's muscle must use glycolysis as their primary source of energy, which results in sore muscles.

Riboflavin deficiency generally occurs in conjunction with other water-soluble vitamin deficiencies. The classic deficiency symptoms are cheilosis (inflammation of the corners of the mouth), glossitis (magenta tongue), and seborrheic ("greasy") dermatitis. It is also characterized by sore throat, edema of the pharyngeal and oral mucus membranes, and normochromic, normocytic anemia associated with pure red cell cytoplasia of the bone marrow. However, it is not known whether the glossitis and dermatitis are actually due to multiple vitamin deficiencies.

Al Martini. Al Martini presents a second time with an alcohol-related high output form of heart failure sometimes referred to as "wet" beriberi, or as the "beriberi heart" (see Chapter 9). The term "wet" refers to the fluid retention which may eventually occur when left ventricular contractility is so compromised that cardiac output, although initially relatively "high," cannot meet the "demands" of the peripheral vascular beds, which have dilated in response to the thiamine deficiency.

The cardiomyopathy is directly related to a reduction in the normal biochemical function of the vitamin thiamine in heart muscle. Inhibition of the α-keto acid dehydrogenase complexes causes accumulation of α-keto acids in heart muscle (and in blood), resulting in a chemically-induced cardiomyopathy. Impairment of two other functions of thiamine may also contribute to the cardiomyopathy. Thiamine pyrophosphate serves as the coenzyme for transketolase in the pentose phosphate pathway, and pentose phosphates accumulate in thiamine deficiency. In addition, thiamine triphosphate (a different coenzyme form) may function in Na^+ conductance channels.

Immediate treatment with large doses (50–100 mg) of intravenous thiamine may produce a measurable decrease in cardiac output and increase in peripheral vascular resistance as early as 30 minutes after the initial injection. Dietary supplementation of thiamine is not as effective because ethanol consumption interferes with thiamine absorption. Because ethanol also affects the absorption of most water-soluble vitamins, or their conversion to the coenzyme form, **Al Martini** was also given a bolus containing a multivitamin supplement.

BIOCHEMICAL COMMENTS

Compartmentation of Mitochondrial Enzymes. The mitochondrion forms a structural, functional, and regulatory compartment within the cell. The inner mitochondrial membrane is impermeable to anions and cations, and compounds can cross the membrane only on specific transport proteins. The enzymes of the TCA cycle, therefore, have more direct access to products of the previous reaction in the pathway than they would if these products were able to diffuse throughout the cell. Complex formation between enzymes also restricts access to pathway intermediates. Malate dehydrogenase and citrate synthase may form a loosely associated complex. The multienzyme pyruvate dehydrogenase and α-ketoglutarate dehydrogenase complexes are examples of substrate channeling by tightly bound enzymes; only the transacylase enzyme has access to the thiamine-bound intermediate of the reaction, and only lipoamide dehydrogenase has access to reduced lipoic acid.

Riboflavin has a wide distribution in foods, and small amounts are present as coenzymes in most plant and animal tissues. Eggs, lean meats, milk, broccoli, and enriched breads and cereals are especially good sources. A portion of our niacin requirement can be met by synthesis from tryptophan. Meat (especially red meat), liver, legumes, milk, eggs, alfalfa, cereal grains, yeast, and fish are good sources of niacin and tryptophan.

Beri-beri, now known to be caused by thiamine deficiency, was attributed to lack of a nitrogenous component in food by Takaki, a Japanese surgeon, in 1884. In 1890, Eijkman, a Dutch physician working in Java, noted that the polyneuritis associated with beri-beri could be prevented by rice bran that had been removed during polishing. Thiamine is present in the bran portion of grains, and abundant in pork and legumes. In contrast to most vitamins, milk and milk products, seafood, fruits, and vegetables are NOT good sources of thiamine.

Thiamine
"Now polished rice isn't nice",
Said the Dutchman Eijkman.
Whole grains are a far better
Source of thiamine.
For beri-beri is very, very
Hard on your nerves, you see.
Polyneuritis and an enlarged heart
May both accompany
A very bad diet, a very sad diet
A diet thiamine-free.
And many who dine, only on wine
Or consume brandy, whiskey or gin
May never recover, if you don't discover
They can't absorb thiamine.
Wernicke-Korsakoff describe the signs
And the confusion in the minds
Of patients with this deficiency.
So good doctors remember, try to recall
Before you charge your fee,
To give an injection, *im* or *iv*
Of this vitamin B.

—revised from an anonymous author

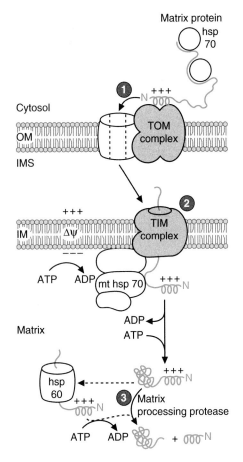

Fig. 20.20. Model for the import of nuclear-encoded proteins into the mitochondrial matrix. The matrix preprotein with its positively charged N-terminal presequence is shown in blue. Abbreviations: OM, outer mitochondrial membrane; IMS, intramembrane space; IM, inner mitochondrial membrane; TOM, translocases of the outer mitochondrial membrane; TIM, translocases of the inner mitochondrial membrane; mthsp70, mitochondrial heat shock protein 70.

Compartmentation plays an important role in regulation. The close association between the rate of the electron transport chain and the rate of the TCA cycle is maintained by their mutual access to the same pool of NADH and NAD$^+$ in the mitochondrial matrix. NAD$^+$, NADH, CoASH, and acyl CoA derivatives have no transport proteins and cannot cross the mitochondrial membrane. Thus, all of the dehydrogenases compete for the same NAD$^+$ molecules, and are inhibited when NADH rises. Likewise, accumulation of acyl CoA derivatives (e.g., acetyl CoA) within the mitochondrial matrix affects other CoA-utilizing reactions, either by competing at the active site or limiting CoASH availability.

 Import of Nuclear Encoded Proteins. All mitochondrial matrix proteins, such as the TCA cycle enzymes, are encoded by the nuclear genome. They are imported into the mitochondrial matrix as unfolded proteins that are pushed and pulled through channels in the outer and inner mitochondrial membranes (Fig. 20.20). Proteins destined for the mitochondrial matrix have a targeting N-terminal presequence of about 20 amino acids that includes several positively charged amino acid residues. They are synthesized on free ribosomes in the cytosol and maintain an unfolded conformation by binding to hsp70 chaperonins. This basic presequence binds to a receptor in a TOM complex (**t**ranslocators of the **o**uter **m**embrane) (see Fig. 20.20, step 1). The TOM complexes consist of channel proteins, assembly proteins and receptor proteins with different specificities (e.g., TOM20 binds the matrix protein presequence). Negatively charged acidic residues on the receptors and in the channel pore assist in translocation of the matrix protein through the channel, presequence first.

The matrix preprotein is translocated across the inner membrane through a TIM complex (**t**ranslocases of the **i**nner **m**embrane) (see Fig. 20.20, step 2). Insertion of the preprotein into the TIM channel is driven by the potential difference across the membrane, $\Delta\psi$. Mitochondrial hsp70 (mthsp70), which is bound to the matrix side of the TIM complex, binds the incoming preprotein and may "ratchet" it through the membrane. ATP is required for binding of mthsp70 to the TIM complex and again for the subsequent dissociation of the mthsp70 and the matrix preprotein. In the matrix, the preprotein may require another heat shock protein, hsp60, for proper folding. The final step in the import process is cleavage of the signal sequence by a matrix processing protease (see Fig. 20.20, step 3).

Proteins of the inner mitochondrial membrane are imported through a similar process, using TOM and TIM complexes containing different protein components.

Suggested References

Robinson, BH. Lactic acidemia: Disorders of pyruvate carboxylase and pyruvate dehydrogenase. In: Scriver CR, Beudet AL, Sly WS, Valle D, eds: The Metabolic and Molecular Bases of Inherited Disease. Vol. I. 8th Ed. New York: McGraw-Hill, 2001:4451–4480.

REVIEW QUESTIONS—CHAPTER 20

1. Which of the following coenzymes is unique to α-ketoacid dehydrogenase complexes?

   (A) NAD$^+$
   (B) FAD
   (C) GDP
   (D) H$_2$O
   (E) Lipoic acid

2. A patient diagnosed with thiamine deficiency exhibited fatigue and muscle cramps. The muscle cramps have been related to an accumulation of metabolic acids. Which of the following metabolic acids is most likely to accumulate in a thiamine deficiency?

   (A) Isocitric acid
   (B) Pyruvic acid
   (C) Succinic acid
   (D) Malic acid
   (E) Oxaloacetic acid

3. Succinate dehydrogenase differs from all other enzymes in the TCA cycle in that it is the only enzyme that displays which of the following characteristics?

   (A) It is embedded in the inner mitochondrial membrane.
   (B) It is inhibited by NADH.
   (C) It contains bound FAD.
   (D) It contains Fe-S centers.
   (E) It is regulated by a kinase.

4. During exercise, stimulation of the tricarboxylic acid cycle results principally from which of the following?

   (A) Allosteric activation of isocitrate dehydrogenase by increased NADH
   (B) Allosteric activation of fumarase by increased ADP
   (C) A rapid decrease in the concentration of four carbon intermediates
   (D) Product inhibition of citrate synthase
   (E) Stimulation of the flux through a number of enzymes by a decreased $NADH/NAD^+$ ratio

5. Coenzyme A is synthesized from which of the following vitamins?

   (A) Niacin
   (B) Riboflavin
   (C) Vitamin A
   (D) Pantothenate
   (E) Vitamin C

21 Oxidative Phosphorylation and Mitochondrial Function

Energy from fuel oxidation is converted to the high-energy phosphate bonds of adenosine triphosphate (ATP) by the process of **oxidative phosphorylation.** *Most of the energy from oxidation of fuels in the TCA cycle and other pathways is conserved in the form of the reduced electron-accepting coenzymes, NADH and FAD(2H). The* **electron transport chain** *oxidizes* **NADH** *and* **FAD(2H),** *and donates the electrons to* O_2, *which is reduced to* H_2O *(Fig. 21.1). Energy from reduction of* O_2 *is used for phosphorylation of adenosine diphosphate (ADP) to ATP by* **ATP synthase** *($F_0 F_1$ATPase). The net yield of oxidative phosphorylation is approximately 2.5 moles of ATP per mole of NADH oxidized, or 1.5 moles of ATP per mole of FAD(2H) oxidized.*

Most cells are dependent on oxidative phosphorylation for ATP homeostasis. The ability to generate ATP depends on O_2 and an intact inner mitochondrial membrane. During oxygen deprivation from ischemia (a low blood flow), an inability to generate energy from the electron transport chain results in an increased permeability of this membrane and mitochondrial swelling. Mitochondrial swelling is a key element in the pathogenesis of irreversible cell injury leading to cell lysis and death (necrosis).

***Chemiosmotic model of ATP synthesis.** The* **chemiosmotic model** *explains how energy from transport of electrons to* O_2 *is transformed into the high-energy phosphate bond of ATP (see Fig. 21.1). Basically, the electron transport chain contains three large* **protein complexes (I, III, and IV)** *that span the inner mitochondrial membrane. As electrons pass through these complexes in a series of oxidation–reduction reactions, protons are transferred from the mitochondrial matrix to the cytosolic side of the inner mitochondrial membrane. The pumping of protons generates an* **electrochemical gradient** *(Δp) across the membrane composed of the membrane potential and the proton gradient. ATP synthase contains a proton pore through the inner mitochondrial membrane and a catalytic headpiece that protrudes into the matrix. As protons are driven*

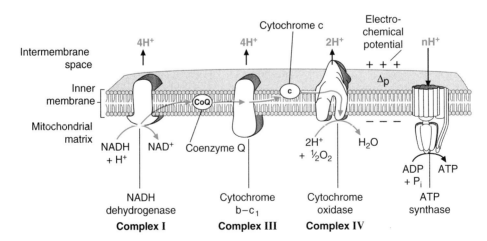

Fig. 21.1. Oxidative phosphorylation. Blue arrows show the path of electron transport from NADH to O_2. As electrons pass through the chain, protons are pumped from the mitochondrial matrix to the intermembrane space, thereby establishing an electochemical potential gradient, Δp, across the inner mitochondrial membrane. The positive and negative charges on the membrane denote the membrane potential ($\Delta\psi$). Δp drives protons into the matrix through a pore in ATP synthase, which uses the energy to form ATP from ADP and Pi.

into the matrix through the pore, they change the conformation of the head-piece, which releases ATP from one site and catalyzes formation of ATP from ADP and Pi at another site.

Deficiencies of electron transport. *In cells, complete transfer of electrons from NADH and FAD(2H) through the chain to O_2 is necessary for ATP generation. Impaired transfer through any complex can have pathologic consequences. Fatigue can result from iron-defeciency* **anemia,** *which decreases* **Fe** *for* **Fe-S centers** *and* **cytochromes. Cytochrome c_1 oxidase,** *which contains the* **O_2 binding site,** *is inhibited by* **cyanide. Mitochondrial DNA (mtDNA),** *which is maternally inherited, encodes some of the subunits of the electron transport chain complexes and ATP synthase.* **Oxphos diseases** *are caused by* **mutations** *in* **nuclear DNA** *or* **mt DNA** *that decrease mitochondrial capacity for oxidative phosphorylation.*

Regulation of oxidative phosphorylation. *The rate of the electron transport chain is* **coupled** *to the rate of ATP synthesis by the transmembrane electochemical gradient. As ATP is used for energy-requiring processes and ADP levels increase, proton influx through the ATP synthase pore generates more ATP, and the electron transport chain responds to restore Δp. In* **uncoupling,** *protons return to the matrix by a mechanism that bypasses the ATP synthase pore, and the energy is released as heat.* **Proton leakage,** **chemical uncouplers,** *and regulated* **uncoupling proteins** *increase our metabolic rate and heat generation.*

Mitochondria and cell death. *Although oxidative phosphorylation is a mitochondrial process, most ATP utilization occurs outside of the mitochondrion. ATP synthesized from oxidative phosphorylation is actively transported from the matrix to the intermembrane space by* **adenine nucleotide translocase (ANT).** **Porins form voltage-dependent anion channels (VDAC)** *through the outer mitochondrial membrane for the diffusion of H_2O, ATP metabolites, and other ions. Under certain types of stress, ANT, VDAC, and other proteins form a nonspecific open channel known as the* **mitochondrial permeability transition pore.** *This pore is associated with events that lead rapidly to* **necrotic cell death.**

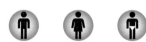

THE WAITING ROOM

Cora Nari was recovering uneventfully from her heart attack 1 month earlier (see Chapter 19), when she won the Georgia State lottery. When she heard her number announced over television, she experienced crushing chest pain, grew short of breath, and passed out. She regained consciousness as she was being rushed to the hospital emergency room.

On initial examination, her blood pressure was extremely high and her heart rhythm irregular. Her blood levels of CK-MB and TnI (troponin I) were elevated. An electrocardiogram showed unequivocal evidence of severe lack of oxygen (ischemia) in the muscles of the anterior and lateral walls of her heart. Life support measures including nasal oxygen were initiated. An intravenous drip of nitroprusside, a vasodilating agent, was started in an effort to reduce her hypertension. After her blood pressure was well controlled, a decision was made to administer intravenous tissue plasminogen activator (TPA) in an attempt to break up any intracoronary artery blood clots in vessels supplying the ischemic myocardium (thrombolytic therapy).

Cora Nari is experiencing a second myocardial infarction. Ischemia (a low blood flow) has caused hypoxia (low levels of oxygen) in her heart muscle, resulting in inadequate generation of ATP for the maintenance of low intracellular Na^+ and Ca^{2+} levels (see Chapter 19). As a consequence, cells have become swollen and the cytosolic proteins creatine kinase (MB isoform) and troponin (heart isoform) have leaked into the blood. (See Ann Jeina, Chapters 6 and 7).

An ^{123}I thyroid uptake and scan performed on **X.S. Teefore** confirmed that his hyperthyroidism was the result of Graves disease (see Chapter 19). Graves disease, also known as diffuse toxic goiter, is an autoimmune genetic disorder caused by the generation of human thyroid-stimulating immunoglobulins. These immunoglobulins stimulate enlargement of the thyroid gland (goiter) and excess secretion of the thyroid hormones, T_3 and T_4. As a consequence, Mr. Teefore's heat intolerance and sweating were growing worse with time.

Ivy Sharer, an intravenous drug abuser, appeared to be responding well to her multidrug regimens to treat pulmonary tuberculosis and AIDS (see Chapters 11, 12, 15, and 16). In the past 6 weeks, however, she has developed increasing weakness in her extremities to the point that she has difficulty carrying light objects or walking. Physical examination indicates a diffuse proximal and distal muscle weakness associated with muscle atrophy. The muscles are neither painful on motion nor tender to compression. The blood level of the muscle enzymes, creatine phosphokinase (CK) and aldolase, are normal. An electromyogram (EMG) revealed a generalized reduction in the muscle action potentials, suggestive of a primary myopathic process. Proton spectroscopy of her brain and upper spinal cord showed no anatomic or biochemical abnormalities. The diffuse and progressive skeletal muscle weakness was out of proportion to that expected from her AIDS or her tuberculosis. This information led her physicians to consider the possibility that her skeletal muscle dysfunction might be drug induced.

I. OXIDATIVE PHOSPHORYLATION

Generation of ATP from oxidative phosphorylation requires an electron donor (NADH or FAD(2H)), an electron acceptor (O_2), an intact inner mitochondrial membrane that is impermeable to protons, all the components of the electron transport chain, and ATP synthase. It is regulated by the rate of ATP utilization.

A. Overview of Oxidative Phosphorylation

Our understanding of oxidative phosphorylation is based on the chemiosmotic hypothesis, which proposes that the energy for ATP synthesis is provided by an electrochemical gradient across the inner mitochondrial membrane. This electrochemical gradient is generated by the components of the electron transport chain, which pump protons across the inner mitochondrial membrane as they sequentially accept and donate electrons (see Fig. 21.1). The final acceptor is O_2, which is reduced to H_2O.

1. ELECTRON TRANSFER FROM NADH TO O_2

In the electron transport chain, electrons donated by NADH or FAD(2H) are passed sequentially through a series of electron carriers embedded in the inner mitochondrial membrane. Each of the components of the electron transfer chain is oxidized as it accepts an electron, and then reduced as it passes the electrons to the next member of the chain. From NADH, electrons are transferred sequentially through NADH dehydrogenase (complex I), CoQ (coenzyme Q), the cytochrome b-c_1 complex (complex III), cytochrome c, and finally cytochrome c oxidase (complex IV). NADH dehydrogenase, the cytochrome b-c_1 complex and cytochrome c oxidase are each multisubunit protein complexes that span the inner mitochondrial membrane. CoQ is a lipid soluble quinone that is not protein-bound and is free to diffuse in the lipid membrane. It transports electrons from complex I to complex III and is an intrinsic part of the proton pumps for each of these complexes. Cytochome c is a small protein in the inner membrane space that transfers electrons from the b–c_1

Arlyn Foma, who has a follicular type non-Hodgkin's lymphoma, was being treated with the anthracycline drug doxorubicin (see Chapter 16). During the course of his treatment, he developed biventricular heart failure. Although doxorubicin is a highly effective anticancer agent against a wide variety of human tumors, its clinical use is limited by a specific, cumulative, dose-dependent cardiotoxicity. Impairment of mitochondrial function may play a major role in this toxicity. Doxorubicin binds to cardiolipin, a lipid component of the inner membrane of mitochondria, where it might directly affect components of oxidative phosphorylation. Doxorubicin inhibits succinate oxidation, inactivates cytochrome oxidase, interacts with CoQ, affects ion pumps, and inhibits ATP synthase, resulting in decreased ATP levels and mildly swollen mitochondria. It decreases the ability of the mitochondria to sequester Ca^{2+} and increases free radicals (highly reactive single-electron forms) leading to damage of the mitochondrial membrane (see Chapter 24). It also might affect heart function indirectly through other mechanisms.

complex to cytochrome oxidase. The terminal complex, cytochrome c oxidase, contains the binding site for O_2. As O_2 accepts electrons from the chain, it is reduced to H_2O.

2. THE ELECTROCHEMICAL POTENTIAL GRADIENT

At each of the three large membrane-spanning complexes in the chain, electron transfer is accompanied by proton pumping across the membrane. There is an energy drop of approximately 16 kcal in reduction potential as electrons pass through each of these complexes, which provides the energy required to move protons against a concentration gradient. The membrane is impermeable to protons, so they cannot diffuse through the lipid bilayer back into the matrix. Thus, in actively respiring mitochondria, the intermembrane space and cytosol may be approximately 0.75 pH units lower than the matrix.

The transmembrane movement of protons generates an electrochemical gradient with two components: the membrane potential (the external face of the membrane is charged positive relative to the matrix side) and the proton gradient (the inter membrane space has a higher proton concentration and is therefore more acidic than the matrix) (Fig. 21.2). The electrochemical gradient is sometimes called the proton motive force because it is the energy pushing the protons to re-enter the matrix to equilibrate on both sides of the membrane. The protons are attracted to the more negatively charged matrix side of the membrane, where the pH is more alkaline.

3. ATP SYNTHASE

ATP synthase (F_0F_1ATPase), the enzyme that generates ATP, is a multisubunit enzyme containing an inner membrane portion (F_0) and a stalk and headpiece (F_1) that project into the matrix (Fig. 21.3). The 12 **c** subunits in the membrane form a rotor that is attached to a central asymmetric shaft composed of the ε and γ subunits. The headpiece is composed of three $\alpha\beta$ subunit pairs. Each β subunit contains a catalytic site for ATP synthesis. The headpiece is held stationary by a δ subunit attached to a long **b** subunit connected to subunit **a** in the membrane.

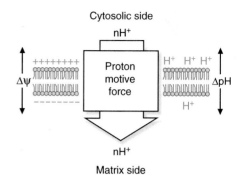

Fig. 21.2. Proton motive force (electrochemical gradient) across the inner mitochondrial membrane. The proton motive force consists of a membrane potential, $\Delta\psi$, and a proton gradient, denoted by ΔpH for the difference in pH across the membrane. The electrochemical potential is called the proton motive force because it represents the potential energy driving protons to return to the more negatively charged alkaline matrix.

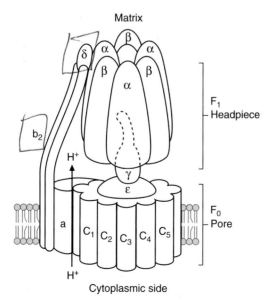

Fig. 21.3. ATP synthase (F_0F_1ATPase).

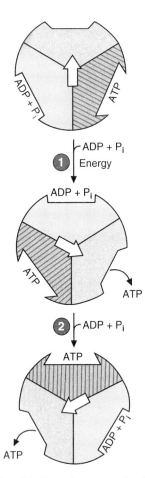

Fig. 21.4. Binding change mechanism for ATP synthesis. The three αβ subunit pairs of the ATP synthase headpiece have binding sites that can exist in three different conformations, depending on the position of the γ stalk subunit. Step 1: When ADP + Pi bind to an open site and the proton influx rotates the γ spindle (represented by the arrow), the conformation of the subunits change and ATP is released from one site. (ATP dissociation is, thus, the energy-requiring step). Bound ADP and Pi combine to form ATP at another site. Step 2: As the ADP + Pi bind to the new open site, and the γ shaft rotates, the conformations of the sites change again, and ATP is released. ADP and Pi combine to form another ATP.

FMN, like FAD, is synthesized from the vitamin riboflavin. It contains the electron-accepting flavin ring structure, but not the adenosine monophosphate (AMP) portion of FAD (see Fig. 19.10). Severe riboflavin deficiency decreases the ability of mitochondria to generate ATP from oxidative phosphorylation due to the lack of FMN in the electron carriers.

The influx of protons through the proton channel turns the rotor. The proton channel is formed by the **c** subunits on one side and the **a** subunit on the other side. Although continuous, it has two offset portions, one portion directly open to the intermembrane space and one portion directly open to the matrix. In the current model, each **c** subunit contains a glutamyl carboxyl group that extends into the proton channel. As this carboxyl group accepts a proton from the intermembrane space, the **c** subunit rotates into the hydrophobic lipid membrane. The rotation exposes a different proton-containing **c** subunit to the portion of the channel directly open to the matrix side. Because the matrix has a lower proton concentration, the glutamyl carboxylic acid group releases a proton into the matrix portion of the channel. Rotation is completed by an attraction between the negatively charged glutamyl residue and a positively charged arginyl group on the **a** subunit.

According to the binding change mechanism, as the asymmetric shaft rotates to a new position, it forms different binding associations with the αβ subunits (Fig. 21.4). The new position of the shaft alters the conformation of one β subunit so that it releases a molecule of ATP and another subunit spontaneously catalyzes synthesis of ATP from inorganic phosphate, one proton, and ADP. Thus, energy from the electrochemical gradient is used to change the conformation of the ATP synthase subunits so that the newly synthesized ATP is released. Twelve **c** subunits are hypothesized, and it takes 12 protons to complete one turn of the rotor and synthesize three ATP.

B. Oxidation–Reduction Components of the Electron Transport Chain

Electron transport to O_2 occurs via a series of oxidation–reduction steps in which each successive component of the chain is reduced as it accepts electrons and oxidized as it passes electrons to the next component of the chain. The oxidation–reduction components of the chain include flavin mononucleotide (FMN), Fe-S centers, CoQ, and Fe in the cytochromes b, c_1, c, a, and a_3. Cu is also a component of cytochromes a and a_3 (Fig. 21.5). With the exception of CoQ, all of these electron acceptors are tightly bound to the protein subunits of the carriers.

The reduction potential of each complex of the chain is at a lower energy level than the previous complex, so that energy is released as electrons pass through each complex. This energy is used to move protons against their concentration gradient, so that they become concentrated on the cytosolic side of the inner membrane.

1.   NADH DEHYDROGENASE

NADH dehydrogenase is an enormous 42-subunit complex that contains a binding site for NADH, several FMN and iron-sulfur (Fe-S) center binding proteins, and binding sites for CoQ (see Fig 21.5). An FMN accepts two electrons from NADH and is able to pass single electrons to the Fe-S centers (Fig. 21.6). Fe-S centers, which are able to delocalize single electrons into large orbitals, transfer electrons to and from CoQ. Fe-S centers are also present in other enzyme systems, such as other proteins, which transfer electrons to CoQ, in the cytochrome b–c_1 complex, and in aconitase in the TCA cycle.

2.   SUCCINATE DEHYDROGENASE AND OTHER FLAVOPROTEINS

In addition to NADH dehydrogenase, succinic dehydrogenase and other flavoproteins in the inner mitochondrial membrane also pass electrons to CoQ (see Fig. 21.5). Succinate dehydrogenase is part of the TCA cycle. ETF-CoQ oxidoreductase accepts electrons from ETF (**e**lectron **t**ransferring **f**lavoprotein), which acquires them from fatty acid oxidation and other pathways. Both of these flavoproteins have Fe-S centers. α-Glycerophosphate dehydrogenase is a flavoprotein that is part of a shuttle for reoxidizing cytosolic NADH.

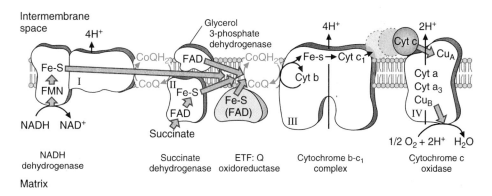

Fig. 21.5. Components of the electron transfer chain. NADH dehydrogenase (complex I) spans the membrane and has a proton pumping mechanism involving CoQ. The electrons go from CoQ to cytochrome b–c1 complex (complex III), and electron transfer does NOT involve complex II. Succinate dehydrogenase (complex II), glycerol 3-phosphate dehydrogenase, and ETF:Q oxidoreductase (shown in blue) all transfer electrons to CoQ, but do not span the membrane and do not have a proton pumping mechanism. As CoQ accepts protons from the matrix side, it is converted to QH_2. Electrons are transferred from complex III to complex IV (cytochrome c oxidase) by cytochrome c, a small cytochrome in the intermembrane space that has reversible binding sites on the b–c_1 complex and cytochrome c oxidase.

The free energy drop between NADH and CoQ of approximately -13 to -14 kcal is able to support movement of four protons. However, the FAD in succinate dehydrogenase (as well as ETF-CoQ oxidoreductase and α-glycerophosphate dehydrogenase) is at roughly the same energy level as CoQ, and there is no energy released as they transfer electrons to CoQ. These proteins do not span the membrane and consequently do not have a proton pumping mechanism.

3.   COENZYME Q

CoQ is the only component of the electron transport chain that is not protein bound. The large hydrophobic side chain of 10 isoprenoid units (50 carbons) confers lipid solubility, and CoQ is able to diffuse through the lipids of the inner mitochondrial membrane (Fig. 21.7). When the oxidized quinone form accepts a single electron, it forms a free radical (a compound with a single electron in an orbital). The transfer of single electrons makes it the major site for generation of toxic oxygen free radicals in the body (see Chapter 24).

The long side chain of CoQ has 10 of the 5-carbon isoprenoid units, and is sometimes called CoQ_{10}. It is also called ubiquinone (the quinone found everywhere) because quinones with similar structures are found in all plants and animals. CoQ can be synthesized in the human from precursors derived from carbohydrates and fat. The long isoprenoid side chain is formed in the pathway that produces the isoprenoid precursors of cholesterol. CoQ_{10} is sometimes prescribed for patients recovering from a myocardial infarction, in an effort to increase their exercise capacity.

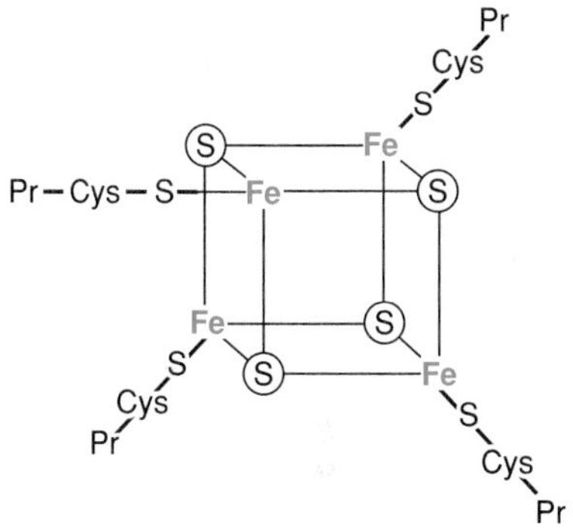

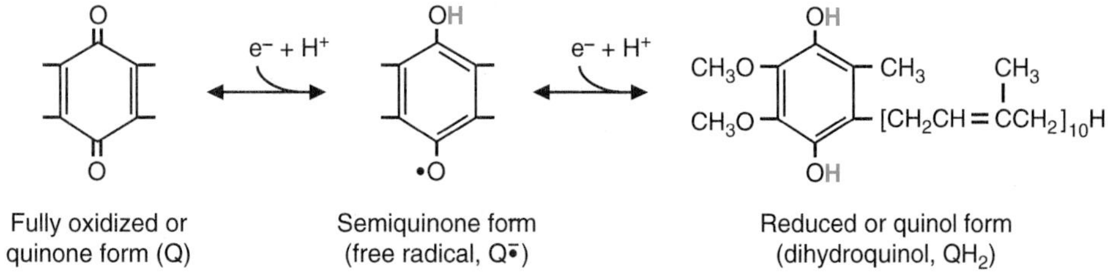

Fig. 21.6. Fe_4S_4 center. In Fe-S centers, the Fe is chelated to free sulfur (S) atoms, and to cysteine sulfhydryl groups on proteins. Other Fe-S centers contain Fe_2S_2. The protein subunits are sometimes called non-heme iron proteins. When these proteins are treated with acid, the free sulfur produces hydrogen sulfide (H_2S)—the familiar smell of rotten eggs.

Fig. 21.7. Coenzyme Q contains a quinone with a long lipophilic side chain comprising 10 isoprenoid units (thus, it is sometimes called CoQ_{10}.) CoQ can accept one electron (e^-) to become the half-reduced form, or 2 e^- to become fully reduced.

The semiquinone can accept a second electron and two protons from the matrix side of the membrane to form the fully reduced quinone. The mobility of CoQ in the membrane, its ability to accept one or two electrons, and its ability to accept and donate protons enable it to participate in the proton pumps for both complexes I and III as it shuttles electrons between them (see Section I.C.).

4. CYTOCHROMES

The remainder of the components in the electron transport chain are cytochromes (see Fig. 21.5). Each cytochrome is a protein that contains a bound heme (i.e., an Fe atom bound to a porphyrin nucleus similar in structure to the heme in hemoglobin) (Fig. 21.8).

Because of differences in the protein component of the cytochromes and small differences in the heme structure, each heme has a different reduction potential. The cytochromes of the b-c_1 complex have a higher energy level than those of cytochrome oxidase (a and a_3). Thus, energy is released by electron transfer between complexes III and IV. The iron atoms in the cytochromes are in the Fe^{3+} state. As they accept an electron, they are reduced to Fe^{2+}. As they are reoxidized to Fe^{3+}, the electrons pass to the next component of the electron transport chain.

5. COPPER (Cu^+) AND THE REDUCTION OF OXYGEN

The last cytochrome complex is cytochrome oxidase, which passes electrons from cytochrome c to O_2 (see Fig. 21.5). It contains cytochromes a and a_3 and the oxygen binding site. A whole oxygen molecule, O_2, must accept four electrons to be reduced to 2 H_2O. Bound copper (Cu^+) ions in the cytochrome oxidase complex facilitate the collection of the four electrons and the reduction of O_2.

Cytochrome oxidase has a much lower K_m for O_2 than myoglobin (the heme-containing intracellular oxygen carrier) or hemoglobin (the heme-containing oxygen transporter in the blood). Thus, O_2 is "pulled" from the erythrocyte to myoglobin, and from myoglobin to cytochrome oxidase, where it is reduced to H_2O.

Although iron deficiency anemia is characterized by decreased levels of hemoglobin and other iron-containing proteins in the blood, the iron-containing cytochromes and Fe-S centers of the electron transport chain in tissues such as skeletal muscle are affected as rapidly. Fatigue in iron deficiency anemia, in patients such as **Ann O'Rexia** (see Chapter 16), results, in part, from the lack of electron transport for ATP production.

The iron in the heme in hemoglobin, unlike the iron in the heme of cytochromes, never changes its oxidation state (it is Fe^{2+} in hemoglobin). If the iron in hemoglobin were to become oxidized (Fe^{3+}), the oxygen-binding capacity of the molecule would be lost. Normally, the protein structures binding the heme either protect the iron from oxidation (such as the globin proteins), or allow oxidation to occur (such as happens in the cytochromes). However, in hemoglobin M, a rare hemoglobin variant found in the human population, a tyrosine is substituted for the histidine at position F8 in the normal hemoglobin A. This tyrosine stabilizes the Fe^{3+} form of heme, and these subunits cannot bind oxygen. This is a lethal condition if homozygous.

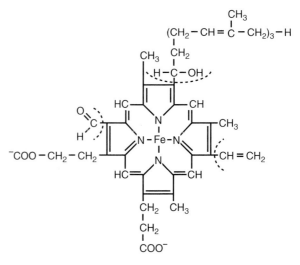

Fig. 21.8. Heme A. Heme A is found in cytochromes a and a_3. Cytochromes are proteins containing a heme chelated with an iron atom. Hemes are derivatives of protoporphyrin IX. Each cytochrome has a heme with different modifications of the side chains (indicated with dashed lines), resulting in a slightly different reduction potential and, consequently, a different position in the sequence of electron transfer.

C. Pumping of Protons

One of the tenets of the chemiosmotic theory is that energy from the oxidation–reduction reactions of the electron transport chain is used to transport protons from the matrix to the intermembrane space. This proton pumping is generally facilitated by the vectorial arrangement of the membrane spanning complexes. Their structure allows them to pick up electrons and protons on one side of the membrane and release protons on the other side of the membrane as they transfer an electron to the next component of the chain. The direct physical link between proton movement and electron transfer can be illustrated by an examination of the Q cycle for the b-c_1 complex (Fig. 21.9). The Q cycle involves a double cycle of CoQ reduction and oxidation. CoQ accepts two protons at the matrix side together with two electrons; it then releases protons into the intermembrane space while donating one electron back to another component of the cytochrome b-c_1 complex and one to cytochrome c.

The mechanism for pumping protons at the NADH dehydrogenase complex is not well understood, but it involves a Q cycle in which the Fe-S centers and FMN might participate. However, transmembrane proton movement at cytochrome c oxidase probably involves direct transport of the proton through a series of bound water molecules or amino acid side chains in the protein, a mechanism that has been described as a "proton wire."

The significance of the direct link between the electron transfer and proton movement is that one cannot occur without the other. Thus, when protons are not being used for ATP synthesis, the proton gradient and the membrane potential build up. This "proton back-pressure" controls the rate of proton pumping, which controls electron transport and O_2 consumption.

D. Energy Yield from the Electron Transport Chain

The overall free energy release from oxidation of NADH by O_2 is approximately −53 kcal, and from FAD(2H), it is approximately −41 kcal. This $\Delta G^{0'}$ is so negative

Electron Transport Chain
Transferring 2 electrons
To Coenzyme Q
Takes Fe-S proteins
And riboflavin, too.

Transferring an electron
Down the E.T. chain
Takes Fe 3 to Fe 2
And back to 3 again.

Transferring 4 electrons
To an oxygen
Takes some Cu^{++} ions
And Fe porphyrin.

Transferring 2 electrons
From NADH to O_2
Pumps just 10 protons
That's the best that it can do

Transferring 2 electrons
From reduced FAD
Pumps only 6 protons
And makes less ATP.
— C.M. Smith

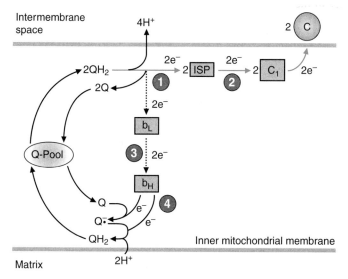

Fig. 21.9. The proton motive Q cycle for the b–c_1 complex. (1) From 2 QH_2, electrons go down two different paths: one path is through an FeS center protein (ISP) toward cytochrome c (shown with blue arrows). Another path is "backward" to one of the b cytochromes, shown with dashed arrows. (2) Electrons are transferred from ISP through cytochrome c_1. Cytochrome c, which is in the intermembrane space, binds to the b–c_1 complex to accept an electron. (3) Returning electrons go through another b cytochrome and are directed toward the matrix. (4) At the matrix side, electrons and $2H^+$ are accepted by Q. Q, Coenzyme Q; Q•⁻, CoQ semiquinone; QH_2, CoQ hydroquinone.

Cora Nari has a lack of oxygen in the anterior and lateral walls of her heart caused by severe ischemia (lack of blood flow) resulting from clots formed at the site of ruptured atherosclerotic plaques. The limited availability of O_2 to act as an electron acceptor will decrease proton pumping and generation of an electrochemical potential gradient across the inner mitochondrial membrane. As a consequence, the rate of ATP generation in her heart will decrease, thereby triggering events that lead to irreversible cell injury.

Intravenous nitroprusside rapidly lowers elevated blood pressure through its direct vasodilating action. Fortunately, it was only required in **Cora Nari**'s case for several hours. During prolonged infusions of 24 to 48 hours or more, nitroprusside is converted to cyanide, an inhibitor of the cytochrome c oxidase complex. Because small amounts of cyanide are detoxified in the liver by conversion to thiocyanate, which is excreted in the urine, the conversion of nitroprusside to cyanide can be monitored by following blood thiocyanate levels.

that the chain is never reversible; we never synthesize oxygen from H_2O. It is so negative that it drives NADH and FAD(2H) formation from the pathways of fuel oxidation, such as the TCA cycle and glycolysis, to completion.

Overall, each NADH donates two electrons, equivalent to the reduction of ½ of an O_2 molecule. A generally (but not universally) accepted estimate of the stoichiometry of ATP synthesis is that four protons are pumped at complex I, four protons at complex III, and two at complex IV. With four protons translocated for each ATP synthesized, an estimated 2.5 ATPs are formed for each NADH oxidized and 1.5 ATPs for each of the other FAD(2H)-containing flavoproteins that donate electrons to CoQ. (This calculation neglects proton requirements for the transport of phosphate and substrates from the cytosol, as well as the basal proton leak.) Thus, only approximately 30% of the energy available from NADH and FAD(2H) oxidation by O_2 is used for ATP synthesis. Some of the remaining energy in the electrochemical potential is used for the transport of anions and Ca^{2+} into the mitochondrion. The remainder of the energy is released as heat. Consequently, the electron transport chain is also our major source of heat.

E. Respiratory Chain Inhibition and Sequential Transfer

In the cell, electron flow in the electron transport chain must be sequential from NADH or a flavoprotein all the way to O_2 to generate ATP (see Fig. 21.5). In the absence of O_2, there is no ATP generated from oxidative phosphorylation because electrons back up in the chain. Even complex I cannot pump protons to generate the electrochemical gradient, because every molecule of CoQ already has electrons that it cannot pass down the chain without an O_2 to accept them at the end. The action of the respiratory chain inhibitor cyanide, which binds to cytochrome oxidase, is similar to that of anoxia; it prevents proton pumping by all three complexes. Complete inhibition of the b-c_1 complex prevents pumping at cytochrome

Cyanide binds to the Fe^{3+} in the heme of the cytochrome aa_3 component of cytochrome c oxidase and prevents electron transport to O_2. Mitochondrial respiration and energy production cease, and cell death rapidly occurs. The central nervous system is the primary target for cyanide toxicity. Acute inhalation of high concentrations of cyanide (e.g., smoke inhalation during a fire) provokes a brief central nervous system stimulation rapidly followed by convulsion, coma, and death. Acute exposure to lower amounts can cause lightheadedness, breathlessness, dizziness, numbness, and headaches.

Cyanide is present in the air as hydrogen cyanide (HCN), in soil and water as cyanide salts (e.g., NaCN), and in foods as cyanoglycosides. Most of the cyanide in the air usually comes from automobile exhaust. Examples of populations with potentially high exposures include active and passive smokers, people who are exposed to house or other building fires, residents who live near cyanide- or thiocyanate-containing hazardous waste sites, and workers involved in a number of manufacturing processes (e.g., photography or pesticide application.)

Cyanoglycosides such as amygdalin are present in edible plants such as almonds, pits from stone fruits (e.g., apricots, peaches, plums, cherries), sorghum, cassava, soybeans, spinach, lima beans, sweet potatoes, maize, millet, sugar cane, and bamboo shoots.

Amygdalin, a cyanoglycoside

HCN is released from cyanoglycosides by β-glucosidases present in the plant or in intestinal bacteria. Small amounts are inactivated in the liver principally by rhodanase, which converts it to thiocyanate.

In the United States, toxic amounts have been ingested as ground apricot pits, either due to health food promotion or as a treatment for cancer. The drug Laetrile (amygdalin) was used as a cancer therapeutic agent, although it was banned in the United States because it was ineffective and potentially toxic. Commercial fruit juices made from unpitted fruit could provide toxic amounts of cyanide, particularly in infants or children. In countries in which cassava is a dietary staple, improper processing results in retention of its high cyanide content at potentially toxic levels.

oxidase because there is no donor of electrons; it prevents pumping at complex I because there is no electron acceptor. Although complete inhibition of any one complex inhibits proton pumping at all of the complexes, partial inhibition of proton pumping can occur when only a fraction of the molecules of a complex contain bound inhibitor. The partial inhibition results in a partial decrease of the maximal rate of ATP synthesis.

II. OXPHOS DISEASES

Clinical diseases involving components of oxidative phosphorylation (referred to as OXPHOS diseases) are among the most commonly encountered degenerative diseases. The clinical pathology may be caused by gene mutations in either mitochondrial DNA (mtDNA) or nuclear DNA (nDNA) that encode proteins required for normal oxidative phosphorylation.

A. Mitochondrial DNA and OXPHOS Diseases

The mtDNA is a small 16,569 nucleotide pair, double-stranded, circular DNA. It encodes 13 subunits of the complexes involved in oxidative phosphorylation: 7 of the 42 subunits of complex I (NADH dehydrogenase complex), 1 of the 11 subunits of complex III (cytochrome b-c_1 complex), 3 of 13 of the subunits of complex IV (cytochrome oxidase), and two subunits of the F_0 portion ATP–synthase complex. In addition, mtDNA encodes the necessary components for translation of its mRNA: a large and small rRNA and 22 tRNAs. Mutations in mtDNA have been identified as deletions, duplications, or point mutations (Table 21.1).

The genetics of mutations in mtDNA are defined by *maternal inheritance, replicative segregation, threshold expression, a high mtDNA mutation rate*, and the *accumulation of somatic mutations with age*. The *maternal inheritance* pattern reflects the exclusive transmission of mtDNA from the mother to her children. The egg contains approximately 300,000 molecules of mtDNA packaged into mitochondria. These are

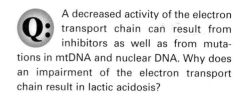

A decreased activity of the electron transport chain can result from inhibitors as well as from mutations in mtDNA and nuclear DNA. Why does an impairment of the electron transport chain result in lactic acidosis?

Oxidative phosphorylation (OXPHOS) is responsible for producing most of the ATP that our cells require. The genes responsible for the polypeptides that comprise the OXPHOS complexes within the mitochondria are located within either the nuclear DNA (nDNA) or the mitochondrial DNA (mtDNA). A broad spectrum of human disorders (the OXPHOS diseases) may result from genetic mutations or nongenetic alterations (spontaneous mutations) in either the nDNA or the mtDNA. Increasingly, such changes appear to be responsible for at least some aspects of common disorders, such as Parkinson's disease, dilated and hypertrophic cardiomyopathies, diabetes mellitus, Alzheimer disease, depressive disorders, and a host of less well-known clinical entities.

Table 21.1 Examples of OXPHOS Diseases Arising from mtDNA Mutations

Syndrome	Characteristic Symptoms	mtDNA Mutation
I. mtDNA rearrangements in which genes are deleted or duplicated.		
Kearns-Sayre syndrome	Onset before 20 years of age, characterized by opthalmoplegia, atypical retinitis pigmentosa, mitochondrial myopathy, and one of the following: cardiac conduction defect, cerebellar syndrome, or elevated CSF proteins.	Deletion of contiguous segments of tRNA and OXPHOS polypeptides, or duplication mutations consisting of tandemly arranged normal mtDNA and an mtDNA with a deletion mutation.
Pearson syndrome	Systemic disorder of oxidative phosphorylation that predominantly affects bone marrow	(same as above)
II. mtDNA point mutations in tRNA or ribosomal RNA genes		
MERRF (**m**yoclonic **e**pilepsy and **r**agged-**r**ed **f**iber disease)	Progressive myoclonic epilepsy, a mitochondrial myopathy with ragged-red fibers, and a slowly progressive dementia. Onset of symptoms: late childhood to adult	tRNA[lys]
MELAS (mitochondrial **m**yopathy, **e**ncephalo-myopathy, **l**actic **a**cidosis, and **s**troke-like episodes)	Progressive neurodengenerative disease characterized by stoke-like episodes first occurring between 5 and 15 years of age and a mitochondrial myopathy	80-90% mutations in tRNA[leu]
III. mtDNA missense mutations in OXPHOS polypeptides		
Leigh disease (subacute necrotizing encephaolpathy)	Mean age of onset, 1.5–5 years; clinical manifestations included optic atrophy, opththalmoplegia, nystagmus, respiratory abnormalities, ataxia, hypotonia, spasticity, and developmental delay or regression.	7–20 % of cases have mutations in Fo subunits of F_0-F_1-ATPase.
LHON (**L**eber **h**ereditary **o**ptic **n**europathy)	Late onset, acute optic atrophy.	90% of European and Asian cases result from mutation in NADH dehydrogenase.

The effect of inhibition of electron transport is an impaired oxidation of pyruvate, fatty acids, and other fuels. In many cases, the inhibition of mitochondrial electron transport results in higher than normal levels of lactate and pyruvate in the blood and an increased lactate/pyruvate ratio. NADH oxidation requires the completed transfer of electrons from NADH to O_2, and a defect anywhere along the chain will result in the accumulation of NADH and decrease of NAD^+. The increase in $NADH/NAD^+$ inhibits pyruvate dehydrogenase and causes the accumulation of pyruvate. It also increases the conversion of pyruvate to lactate, and elevated levels of lactate appear in the blood. A large number of genetic defects of the proteins in respiratory chain complexes have, therefore, been classified together as "congenital lactic acidosis."

A patient experienced spontaneous muscle jerking (myoclonus) in her mid-teens, and her condition progressed over 10 years to include debilitating myoclonus, neurosensory hearing loss, dementia, hypoventilation, and mild cardiomyopathy. Energy metabolism was affected in the central nervous system, heart, and skeletal muscle, resulting in lactic acidosis. A history indicated that the patient's mother, her grandmother, and two maternal aunts had symptoms involving either nervous or muscular tissue (clearly a case of maternal inheritance). However, no other relative had identical symptoms. The symptoms and history of the patient are those of myoclonic epileptic ragged red fiber disease (MERRF). The affected tissues (central nervous system and muscle) are two of the tissues with the highest ATP requirements. Most cases of MERRF are caused by a point mutation in mitochondrial $tRNA^{lys}$ ($mtRNA^{lys}$). The mitochondria, obtained by muscle biopsy, are enlarged and show abnormal patterns of cristae. The muscle tissue also shows ragged red fibers.

Q: How does shivering generate heat?

retained during fertilization, whereas those of the sperm do not enter the egg or are lost. Usually, some mitochondria are present with the mutant mtDNA and some with normal (wild-type) DNA. As cells divide during mitosis and meiosis mitochondria replicate by fission, but various amounts of mitochondria with mutant and wild-type DNA are distributed to each daughter cell (*replicative segregation*). Thus, any cell can have a mixture of mitochondria, each with mutant or wild-type mtDNAs (heteroplasmy). The mitotic and meiotic segregation of the heteroplasmic mtDNA mutation results in variable oxidative phosphorylation deficiencies between patients with the same mutation, and even among a patient's own tissues.

The disease pathology usually becomes worse with age, because a small amount of normal mitochondria might confer normal function and exercise capacity while the patient is young. As the patient ages, somatic (spontaneous) mutations in mtDNA accumulate from the generation of free radicals within the mitochondria (see Chapter 24). These mutations frequently become permanent, partly because mtDNA does not have access to the same repair mechanisms available for nuclear DNA (*high mutation rate*). Even in normal individuals, somatic mutations result in a decline of oxidative phosphorylation capacity with age (*accumulation of somatic mutations with age*). At some stage, the ATP-generating capacity of a tissue falls below the tissue-specific threshold for normal function (*threshhold expression*). In general, symptoms of these defects would appear in one or more of the tissues with the highest ATP demands: nervous tissue, heart, skeletal muscle, and kidney.

B. Other Genetic Disorders of Oxidative Phosphorylation

Genetic mutations also have been reported for mitochondrial proteins encoded by nuclear DNA. Most of the estimated 1,000 proteins required for oxidative phosphorylation are encoded by nuclear DNA, whereas mtDNA encodes only 13 subunits of the oxidative phosphorylation complexes (including ATP synthase). Nuclear DNA encodes the additional 70 or more subunits of the oxidative phosphorylation complexes, as well as adenine nucleotide translocase (ANT) and other anion translocators. Coordinate regulation of expression of nuclear and mtDNA, import of proteins into the mitochondria, assembly of the complexes, and regulation of mitochondrial fission are nuclear encoded.

Nuclear DNA mutations differ from mtDNA mutations in several important respects. These mutations do not show a pattern of maternal inheritance but are usually autosomal recessive. The mutations are uniformly distributed to daughter cells and therefore are expressed in all tissues containing the allele for a particular tissue-specific isoform. However, phenotypic expression still will be most apparent in tissues with high ATP requirements.

III. COUPLING OF ELECTRON TRANSPORT AND ATP SYNTHESIS

The electrochemical gradient couples the rate of the electron transport chain to the rate of ATP synthesis. Because electron flow requires proton pumping, electron flow cannot occur faster than protons are used for ATP synthesis (coupled oxidative phosphorylation) or returned to the matrix by a mechanism that short circuits the ATP synthase pore (uncoupling).

The nuclear respiratory factors (NRF-1 and NRF-2) are nuclear transcription factors that bind to and activate promotor regions of the nuclear genes encoding subunits of the respiratory chain complexes, including cytochrome c. They also activate the transcription of the nuclear gene for the mitochondrial transcription factor (mTF)-A. The protein product of this gene translocates into the mitochondrial matrix, where it stimulates transcription and replication of the mitochondrial genome.

A. Regulation through Coupling

As ATP chemical bond energy is used by energy-requiring reactions, ADP and Pi concentrations increase. The more ADP present to bind to the ATP synthase, the greater will be proton flow through the ATP synthase pore, from the intermembrane space to the matrix. Thus, as ADP levels rise, proton influx increases, and the electrochemical gradient decreases (Fig 21.10). The proton pumps of the electron transport chain respond with increased proton pumping and electron flow to maintain the electrochemical gradient. The result is increased O_2 consumption. The increased oxidation of NADH in the electron transport chain and the increased concentration of ADP stimulate the pathways of fuel oxidation, such as the TCA cycle, to supply more NADH and FAD(2H) to the electron transport chain. For example, during exercise, we use more ATP for muscle contraction, consume more oxygen, oxidize more fuel (which means burn more calories), and generate more heat from the electron transport chain. If we rest, and the rate of ATP utilization decreases, proton influx decreases, the electrochemical gradient increases, and proton "back-pressure" decreases the rate of the electron transport chain. NADH and FAD(2H) cannot be oxidized as rapidly in the electron transport chain, and consequently, their build-up inhibits the enzymes that generate them.

The system is poised to maintain very high levels of ATP at all times. In most tissues, the rate of ATP utilization is nearly constant over time. However, in skeletal muscles, the rates of ATP hydrolysis change dramatically as the muscle goes from rest to rapid contraction. Even under these circumstances, ATP concentration decreases by only approximately 20% because it is so rapidly regenerated. In the heart, Ca^{2+} activation of TCA cycle enzymes provides an extra push to NADH generation, so that neither ATP nor NADH levels fall as ATP demand is increased. The electron transport chain has a very high capacity and can respond very rapidly to any increase in ATP utilization.

B. Uncoupling ATP Synthesis from Electron Transport

When protons leak back into the matrix without going through the ATP synthase pore, they dissipate the electrochemical gradient across the membrane without generating ATP. This phenomenon is called "uncoupling" oxidative phosphorylation. It occurs with chemical compounds, known as uncouplers, and it occurs physiologically with uncoupling proteins that form proton conductance channels through the membrane. Uncoupling of oxidative phosphorylation results in increased oxygen consumption and heat production as electron flow and proton pumping attempt to maintain the electrochemical gradient.

1. CHEMICAL UNCOUPLERS OF OXIDATIVE PHOSPHORYLATION

Chemical uncouplers, also known as proton ionophores, are lipid-soluble compounds that rapidly transport protons from the cytosolic to the matrix side of the inner mitochondrial membrane (Fig. 21.11). Because the proton concentration is higher in the intermembrane space than in the matrix, uncouplers pick up protons from the intermembrane space. Their lipid solubility enables them to diffuse through the inner mitochondrial membrane while carrying protons and release these

A: Shivering results from muscular contraction, which increases the rate of ATP hydrolysis. As a consequence of proton entry for ATP synthesis, the electron transport chain is stimulated. Oxygen consumption increases, as does the amount of energy lost as heat by the electron transport chain.

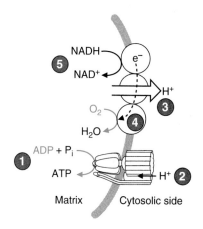

Fig. 21.10. The concentration of ADP (or the phosphate potential -[ATP]/[ADP][P_i]) controls the rate of oxygen consumption. (1) ADP is phosphorylated to ATP by ATP synthase. (2) The release of the ATP requires proton flow through ATP synthase into the matrix. (3) The use of protons from the intermembrane space for ATP synthesis decreases the proton gradient. (4) As a result, the electron transport chain pumps more protons, and oxygen is reduced to H_2O. (5) As NADH donates electrons to the electron transport chain, NAD^+ is regenerated and returns to the TCA cycle or other NADH-producing pathways.

A skeletal muscle biopsy performed on **Ivy Sharer** indicated proliferation of subsarcolemmal mitochondria with degeneration of muscle fibers (ragged-red fibers) in approximately 55% of the total fibers observed. An analysis of mitochondrial (mtDNA) indicated no genetic mutations but did show a moderate quantitative depletion of mtDNA.

Ivy Sharer's AIDS was being treated with zidovudine (AZT), which also can act as an inhibitor of the mitochondrial DNA polymerase (polymerase γ). A review of the drugs' potential adverse effects showed that, rarely, it may cause varying degrees of mtDNA depletion in different tissues, including skeletal muscle. The depletion may cause a severe mitochondrial myopathy, including "ragged-red fiber" accumulation within the skeletal muscle cells associated with ultrastructural abnormalities in their mitochondria.

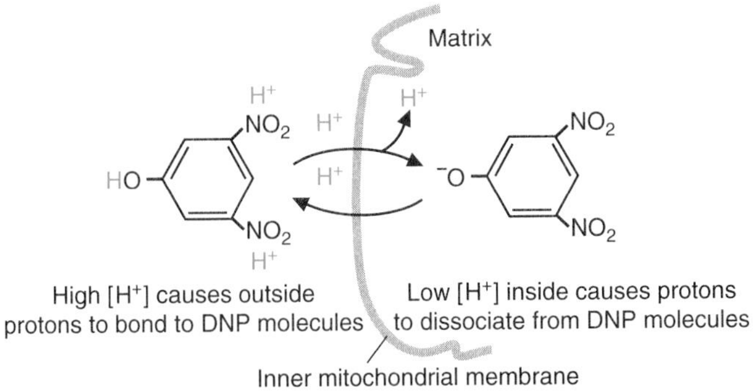

High [H⁺] causes outside protons to bond to DNP molecules

Low [H⁺] inside causes protons to dissociate from DNP molecules

Inner mitochondrial membrane

Fig. 21.11. Dinitrophenol (DNP) is lipid soluble and can therefore diffuse across the membrane. It has a dissociable proton with a pK_a near 7.2. Thus, in the intermembrane space where [H⁺] is high (pH low), DNP picks up a proton, which it carries across the membrane. At the lower proton concentration of the matrix, the H⁺ dissociates. As a consequence, cells cannot maintain their electrochemical gradient or synthesize ATP. DNP was once recommended in the United States as a weight loss drug, based on the principle that decreased [ATP] and increased electron transport stimulate fuel oxidation. However, several deaths resulted from its use.

protons on the matrix side. The rapid influx of protons dissipates the electrochemical potential gradient; therefore, the mitochondria are unable to synthesize ATP. Eventually, mitochondrial integrity and function are lost.

2. UNCOUPLING PROTEINS AND THERMOGENESIS

Uncoupling proteins (UCPs) form channels through the inner mitochondrial membrane that are able to conduct protons from the intermembrane space to the matrix, thereby short-circuiting ATP synthase.

UCP1 (thermogenin) is associated with heat production in brown adipose tissue. The major function of brown adipose tissue is nonshivering thermogenesis, whereas the major function of white adipose tissue is the storage of triacylglycerols in white lipid droplets. The brown color arises from the large number of mitochondria that participate. Human infants, who have little voluntary control over their environment and may kick their blankets off at night, have brown fat deposits along the neck, the breastplate, between the scapulae, and around the kidneys to protect them from cold. However, there is very little brown fat in most adults.

In response to cold, sympathetic nerve endings release norepinephrine, which activates a lipase in brown adipose tissue that releases fatty acids from triacylglycerols (Fig 21.12). Fatty acids serve as a fuel for the tissue (i.e., are oxidized to generate the electrochemical potential gradient and ATP) and participate directly in the proton conductance channel by activating UCP1 along with reduced CoQ. When UCP1 is activated by purine nucleotides, fatty acids, and CoQ, it transports protons from the cytosolic side of the inner mitochondrial membrane back into the mitochondrial matrix without ATP generation. Thus, it partially uncouples oxidative phosphorylation and generates additional heat.

The uncoupling proteins exist as a family of proteins: UCP1 (thermogenin) is expressed in brown adipose tissue; UCP2 is found in most cells, UCP3 is found principally in skeletal muscle; UCP4 and UCP5 are found in the brain. These are highly regulated proteins that, when activated, increase the amount of energy from fuel oxidation that is being released as heat. Because they affect metabolic efficiency, differences in the level of UCPs (particularly skeletal muscle UCP3) may contribute to the tendency toward obesity in some individuals or populations. UCPs also may decrease the amount of reduced CoQ available to form oxygen free radicals, thereby decreasing mitochondrial and cell injury.

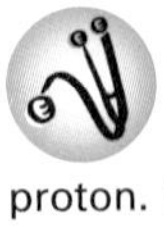

Salicylate, which is a degradation product of aspirin in the human, is lipid soluble and has a dissociable proton. In high concentrations, as in salicylate poisoning, salicylate is able to partially uncouple mitochondria. The decline of ATP concentration in the cell and consequent increase of AMP in the cytosol stimulates glycolysis. The overstimulation of the glycolytic pathway (see Chapter 22) results in increased levels of lactic acid in the blood and a metabolic acidosis. Fortunately, **Dennis Veere** did not develop this consequence of aspirin poisoning (see Chapter 4).

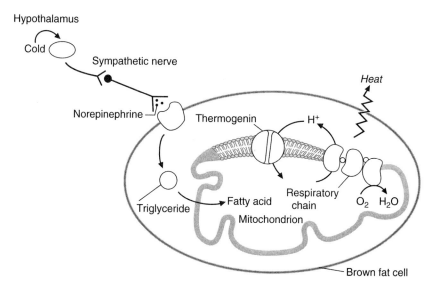

Fig. 21.12. Brown fat is a tissue specialized for nonshivering thermogenesis. Cold or excessive food intake stimulates the release of norepinephrine from the sympathetic nerve endings. As a result, a lipase is activated that releases fatty acids for oxidation. The proton conductance protein, thermogenin, is activated, and protons are brought into the matrix. This stimulates the electron transport chain, which increases its rate of NADH and FAD(2H) oxidation and produces more heat.

3.   PROTON LEAK AND RESTING METABOLIC RATE

A low level of proton leak across the inner mitochondrial membrane occurs in our mitochondria all of the time, and our mitochondria thus are normally partially uncoupled. It has been estimated that more than 20% of our resting metabolic rate is the energy expended to maintain the electrochemical gradient dissipated by our basal proton leak (also referred to as global proton leak). Some of the proton leak results from permeability of the membrane associated with proteins embedded in the lipid bilayer. An unknown amount may result from uncoupling proteins.

IV. TRANSPORT THROUGH INNER AND OUTER MITOCHONDRIAL MEMBRANES

Most of the newly synthesized ATP that is released into the mitochondrial matrix must be transported out of the mitochondria, where it is used for energy-requiring processes such as active ion transport, muscle contraction, or biosynthetic reactions. Likewise, ADP, phosphate, pyruvate, and other metabolites must be transported into the matrix. This requires transport of compounds through both the inner and outer mitochondrial membranes.

A. Transport through the Inner Mitochondrial Membrane

The inner mitochondrial membrane forms a tight permeability barrier to all polar molecules, including ATP, ADP, P_i, anions such as pyruvate, and cations such as Ca^{2+}, H^+, and K^+. Yet the process of oxidative phosphorylation depends on rapid and continuous transport of many of these molecules across the inner mitochondrial membrane (Fig. 21.13). Ions and other polar molecules are transported across the inner mitochondrial membrane by specific protein translocases that nearly balance charge during the transport process. Most of the exchange transport is a form of active transport that generally uses energy from the electrochemical potential gradient, either the membrane potential or the proton gradient.

The inner and outer membranes differ substantially in their lipid content. The inner mitochondrial membrane is 22% cardiolipin and contains almost no cholesterol. The outer membrane resembles the cell membrane; it is less than 3% cardiolipin and approximately 45% cholesterol.

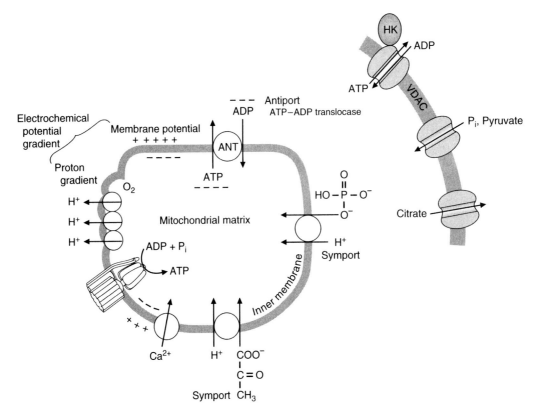

Fig. 21.13. Transport of compounds across the inner and outer mitochondrial membranes. The electrochemical potential gradient drives the transport of ions across the inner mitochondrial membrane on specific translocases. Each translocase is composed of specific membrane-spanning helices that bind only specific compounds (ANT; adenine nucleotide translocase). In contrast, the outer membrane contains relatively large unspecific pores called VDAC (voltage-dependent anion channels) through which a wide range of ions diffuse. These bind cytosolic proteins such as hexokinase (HK), which enables HK to have access to newly exported ATP.

ANT is an antiport, an exchange protein that translocates one ion in exchange for a molecule of similar charge. In contrast, the phosphate transporter and the pyruvate transporter are symports, which are translocases that co-transport two molecules of opposite charge. The Ca^{2+} channel is called a uniporter because no other ions are involved. All of the metabolites entering or leaving the TCA cycle are transported across the inner mitochondrial membrane by specific transport proteins. This includes the dicarboxylate transporter (phosphate–malate exchange), the tricarboxylate transporter (citrate–malate exchange), the aspartate-glutamate transporter, and the malate-α-ketoglutarate transporter.

Investigators reported finding antibodies against cardiac ATP-ADP translocase in an individual who died of a viral cardiomyopathy. How could these antibodies result in death?

ATP-ADP translocase (also called ANT for **a**denine **n**ucleotide **t**ranslocase) transports ATP formed in the mitochondrial matrix to the intermembrane space in a specific 1:1 exchange for ADP produced from energy-requiring reactions outside of the mitochondria (see Fig. 21.13). Because ATP contains four negative charges and ADP only three, the exchange is promoted by the electrochemical potential gradient, because the net effect is the transport of one negative charge from the matrix to the cytosol. Similar antiports exist for most metabolic anions. In contrast, inorganic phosphate and pyruvate are transported into the mitochondrial matrix on specific transporters called symports together with a proton. A specific transport protein for Ca^{2+} uptake, called the Ca^{2+} uniporter, is driven by the electrochemical potential gradient, which is negatively charged on the matrix side of the membrane relative to the cytosolic side.

B. Transport through the Outer Mitochondrial Membrane

Whereas the inner mitochondrial membrane is highly impermeable, the outer mitochondrial membrane is permeable to compounds with a molecular weight up to approximately 6,000 daltons because it contains large nonspecific pores called voltage-dependent anion channels (VDAC) that are formed by mitochondrial porins (see Fig. 21.13). Unlike most transport proteins, which are membrane-spanning helices with specific binding sites, VDACs are composed of porin homodimers that form a β-barrel with a relatively large nonspecific water-filled pore through the center. These channels are "open" at low transmembrane potential, with a preference for anions such as phosphate, chloride, pyruvate, citrate, and adenine nucleotides.

A: As ATP is hydrolyzed during muscular contraction, ADP is formed. This ADP must exchange into the mitochondria on ATP-ADP translocase to be converted back to ATP. Inhibition of ATP-ADP translocase results in rapid depletion of the cytosol ATP levels and loss of cardiac contractility.

VDACs thus facilitate translocation of these anions between the intermembrane space and the cytosol. A number of cytosolic kinases, such as the hexokinase that initiates glycolysis, bind to the cytosolic side of the channel, where they have ready access to newly synthesized ATP.

C. The Mitochondrial Permeability Transition Pore

The mitochondrial permeability transition involves the opening of a large nonspecific pore (called MPTP, the **m**itochondrial **p**ermeability **t**ransition **p**ore) through the inner mitochondrial membrane and outer membranes at sites where they form a junction (Fig. 21.14). The basic components of the mitochondrial permeability transition pore are adenine nucleotide translocase (ANT), the voltage-dependant anion channel (VDAC), and cyclophilin D (which is a cis-trans isomerase for the proline peptide bond). Normally ANT is a closed pore that functions specifically in a 1:1 exchange of matrix ATP for ADP in the intermembrane space. However, increased mitochondrial matrix Ca^{2+}, excess phosphate, or ROS (reactive oxygen species that form oxygen or oxygen–nitrogen radicals) can activate opening of the pore. Conversely, ATP on the cytosolic side of the pore (and possibly a pH below 7.0) and a membrane potential across the inner membrane protect against pore opening. Opening of the MPTP can be triggered by ischemia (hypoxia), which results in a temporary lack of O_2 for maintaining the proton gradient and ATP synthesis. When the proton gradient is not being generated by the electron transport chain, ATP synthase runs backward and hydrolyzes ATP in an attempt to restore the gradient, thus rapidly depleting cellular levels of ATP. As ATP is hydrolyzed to ADP, the ADP is converted to adenine, and the nucleotide pool is no longer able to protect against pore opening. This can lead to a downward spiral of cellular events. A lack of ATP for maintaining the low intracellular Ca^{2+} can contribute to pore opening. When the MPTP pore opens, protons will flood in, and maintaining a proton gradient becomes impossible. Anions and cations enter the matrix, mitochondrial swelling ensues, and the mitochondria become irreversibly damaged. The result is cell lysis and death (necrosis).

In addition to a normal role in movement of molecules across the mitochondrial outer membrane, VDACs appear to have roles in processes leading to cell death. These roles are influenced by proteins that bind to the VDACs. By forming a component of the mitochondrial permeability transition pore, VDACs may contribute to events leading to cell necrosis. Alternatively, binding of pro-apoptotic or anti-apoptotic members of the Bcl-2 family may change the permeability of the outer membrane so as to either favor or block events leading to programmed cell death (apoptosis).

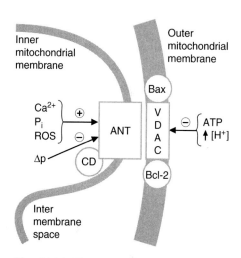

Fig. 21.14. The mitochondrial permeability transition pore (MPTP). In the MPTP, ANT is thought to complex with VDAC. The conformation of ANT is regulated by cyclophilin D (CD), and Ca^{2+}. VDACs bind a number of proteins, including Bcl2 and Bax, which regulate apoptosis. The change to an open pore is activated by Ca^{2+}, depletion of adenine nucleotides, and oxygen radicals (ROS) that alter SH groups. It is inhibited by the electrochemical potential gradient (Δp), by cytosolic ATP, and by a low cytosolic pH.

CLINICAL COMMENTS

Cora Nari. Thrombolysis stimulated by intravenous recombinant tissue plasminogen activator (TPA) restored O_2 to **Cora Nari's** heart muscle and successfully decreased the extent of ischemic damage. The rationale for the use of TPA within 4 to 6 hours after the onset of a myocardial infarction relates

As infusion of TPA lysed the clot blocking blood flow to **Cora Nari's** heart, oxygenated blood was reintroduced into the ischemic heart. Although oxygen may rapidly restore the capacity to generate ATP, it often increases cell death, a phenomenon called ischemia–reperfusion injury.

During ischemia, a number of factors may protect heart cells against irreversible injury and cell death until oxygen is reintroduced. The stimulation of anaerobic glycolysis in the cytosol generates ATP without oxygen as glucose is converted to lactic acid. Lactic acid decreases cytosolic pH. Both cytosolic ATP and a lowering of the pH protect against opening of the MPTP. In addition, Ca^{2+} uptake by mitochondria requires a membrane potential, and it is matrix Ca^{2+} that activates opening of the MPTP. Thus, depending on the severity of the ischemic insult, the MPTP may not open, or may open and reseal, until oxygen is reintroduced. Then, depending on the sequence of events, reestablishment of the proton gradient, mitochondrial uptake of Ca^{2+}, or an increase of pH above 7.0 may activate the MPTP before the cell has recovered. In addition, the reintroduction of O_2 generates oxygen free radicals, particularly through free radical forms of CoQ in the electron transport chain. These also may open the MPTP. The role of free radicals in ischemia–reperfusion injury is covered in more detail in Chapter 24.

to the function of the normal intrinsic fibrinolytic system (see Chapter 45). This system is designed to dissolve unwanted intravascular clots through the action of the enzyme plasmin, a protease that digests the fibrin matrix within the clot. TPA stimulates the conversion of plasminogen to its active form, plasmin. The result is a lysis of the thrombus and improved blood flow through the previously obstructed vessel, allowing fuels and oxygen to reach the heart cells. The human TPA protein used in Mrs. Nari is produced by recombinant DNA technology (see Chapter 17). This treatment rapidly restored oxygen supply to the heart.

In addition to increased transcription of genes encoding TCA cycle enzymes and certain other enzymes of fuel oxidation, thyroid hormones increase the level of UCP2 and UCP3. In hyperthyroidism, the efficiency with which energy is derived from the oxidation of these fuels is significantly less than normal. As a consequence of the increased rate of the electron transport chain, hyperthyroidism results in increased heat production. Patients with hyperthyroidism, such as **X.S. Teefore,** complain of constantly feeling hot and sweaty.

X.S. Teefore. Mr. Teefore could be treated with antithyroid drugs, by subtotal resection of the thyroid gland, or with radioactive iodine. Successful treatment normalizes thyroid hormone secretion, and all of the signs, symptoms, and metabolic alterations of hyperthyroidism quickly subside.

Ivy Sharer. In the case of **Ivy Sharer,** a diffuse myopathic process was superimposed on her AIDS and her pulmonary tuberculosis, either of which could have caused progressive weakness. In addition, she could have been suffering from a congenital mtDNA myopathy, symptomatic only as she ages. A systematic diagnostic process, however, finally led her physician to conclude that her myopathy was caused by a disorder of oxidative phosphorylation induced by her treatment with zidovudine (AZT). Fortunately, when AZT was discontinued, Ivy's myopathic symptoms gradually subsided. A repeat skeletal muscle biopsy performed 4 months later showed that her skeletal muscle cell mtDNA had been restored to normal and that she had experienced a reversible drug-induced disorder of oxidative phosphorylation.

BIOCHEMICAL COMMENTS

Mitochondria and Apoptosis The loss of mitochondrial integrity is a major route initiating apoptosis (see Chapter 18, section V). The intermembrane space contains procaspases -2, -3, and -9, which are proteolytic enzymes that are in the zymogen form (i.e., must be proteolytically cleaved to be active). It also contains apoptosis initiating factor (AIF) and caspase-activated DNAase (CAD). Cytochrome c, which is loosely bound to the outer mitochondrial membrane, may also enter the intermembrane space when the electrochemical potential gradient is lost. The release of cytochrome c and the other proteins into the cytosol initiates apoptosis.

Cytochrome c allosterically activates cytosolic apoptosis activating factor (Apaf-1), which activates the initiator caspase-9. Caspase-9, in turn, activates effector caspases-3, -6, and -7 through proteolytic cleavage, which then degrade cytoplasmic proteins. AIF, which has a nuclear targeting sequence, is transported into the nucleus, where it initiates chromatin condensation and degradation. Caspase-2 and caspase-9 also activate CAD, which migrates to the nucleus and hydrolyzes bonds in nuclear DNA.

But how are cytochrome c and the other proteins released? The VDAC pore is not large enough to allow the passage of proteins. A number of theories have been proposed, each supported and contradicted by experimental evidence. One is that Bax (a member of the Bcl-2 family of proteins that forms an ion channel in the outer mitochondrial membrane) allows the entry of ions into the intermembrane space, causing swelling of this space and rupture of the outer mitochondrial membrane. Another theory is that Bax and VDAC (which is known to bind Bax and other Bcl-2 family members) combine to form an extremely large pore, much larger than formed by either alone. Finally, it is possible that the MPTP or ANT participate in rupture of the outer membrane, but close in a way that still provides the energy for apoptosis.

Suggested References

Boyer PD. A perspective of the binding change mechanism for ATP synthesis. FASEB J 1989;3:2164–2178.

Brown GC. Control of respiration and ATP synthesis in mammalian mitochondria and cells. Biochem J 1992;284:1–11.

Lactic acidosis and mitochondrial myopathy in a young woman. Nutr Rev 1988;46:157–163.

Halestrap AP. The mitochondrial permeability transition: its molecular mechanism and role in reperfusion injury. Biochem Soc Symp 1999;66:181–203.

Lowell BB, Spiegelman BM. Towards a molecular understanding of adaptive thermogenesis. Nature 2000;404:652–660.

Olson RD, Mushlin PS. Doxorubicin cardiotoxicity: analysis of prevailing hypotheses. FASEB J 1990;4:3076–3086.

Shoffner JM. Oxidative phosphorylation diseases. In: Scriver CR, Beaudet AL, Sly WS, Valle D, eds. The Metabolic and Molecular Bases of Inherited Disease, vol II. 8th Ed. New York: McGraw-Hill, 2001:2367–2424.

 REVIEW QUESTIONS—CHAPTER 21

1. Consider the following experiment. Carefully isolated liver mitochondria are incubated in the presence of a limiting amount of malate. Three minutes after adding the substrate, cyanide is added, and the reaction is allowed to proceed for another 7 minutes. At this point, which of the following components of the electron transfer chain will be in an oxidized state?

    (A) Complex I
    (B) Complex II
    (C) Complex III
    (D) Coenzyme Q
    (E) Cytochrome C

2. Consider the following experiment. Carefully isolated liver mitochondria are placed in a weakly buffered solution. Malate is added as an energy source, and an increase in oxygen consumption confirms that the electron transfer chain is functioning properly within these organelles. Valinomycin and potassium are then added to the mitochondrial suspension. Valinomycin is a drug that allows potassium ions to freely cross the inner mitochondrial membrane. What is the effect of valinomycin on the proton motive force that had been generated by the oxidation of malate?

    (A) The proton motive force will be reduced to a value of zero
    (B) There will be no change in the proton motive force
    (C) The proton motive force will be increased
    (D) The proton motive force will be decreased, but to a value greater than zero
    (E) The proton motive force will be decreased to a value less than zero

3. Dinitrophenol acts as an uncoupler of oxidative phosphorylation by which of the following mechanisms?

    (A) Activating the H^+-ATPase
    (B) Activating coenzyme Q
    (C) Blocking proton transport across the inner mitochondrial membrane
    (D) Allowing for proton exchange across the inner mitochondrial membrane
    (E) Enhancing oxygen transport across the inner mitochondrial membrane

4. A 25-year-old female presents with chronic fatigue. A series of blood tests are ordered, and the results suggest that her red blood cell count is low because of iron deficiency anemia. Such a deficiency would lead to fatigue because of which of the following?

    (A) Her decrease in Fe-S centers is impairing the transfer of electrons in the electron transport chain.
    (B) She is not producing as much H_2O in the electron transport chain, leading to dehydration, which has resulted in fatigue.
    (C) Iron forms a chelate with NADH and FAD(2H) that is necessary for them to donate their electrons to the electron transport chain.
    (D) Iron acts as a cofactor for α-ketoglutarate DH in the TCA cycle, a reaction required for the flow of electrons through the electron transport chain.
    (E) Iron accompanies the protons that are pumped from the mitochondrial matrix to the cytosolic side of the inner mitochondrial membrane. Without iron, the proton gradient cannot be maintained to produce adequate ATP.

5. Which of the following would be expected for a patient with an OXPHOS disease?

    (A) A high ATP:ADP ratio in the mitochondria
    (B) A high NADH:NAD$^+$ ratio in the mitochondria
    (C) A deletion on the X chromosome
    (D) A high activity of complex II of the electron transport chain
    (E) A defect in the integrity of the inner mitochondrial membrane

22 Generation of ATP from Glucose: Glycolysis

Glucose is the universal fuel for human cells. Every cell type in the human is able to generate adenosine triphosphate (ATP) from glycolysis, the pathway in which glucose is oxidized and cleaved to form pyruvate. The importance of glycolysis in our fuel economy is related to the availability of glucose in the blood, as well as the ability of glycolysis to generate ATP in both the presence and absence of O_2. Glucose is the major sugar in our diet and the sugar that circulates in the blood to ensure that all cells have a continuous fuel supply. The brain uses glucose almost exclusively as a fuel.

*Glycolysis begins with the phosphorylation of glucose to glucose 6-phosphate (**glucose-6-P**) by **hexokinase** (HK). In subsequent steps of the pathway, one glucose-6-P molecule is oxidized to two **pyruvate** molecules with generation of two molecules of **NADH** (Fig. 22.1). A net generation of two molecules of ATP occurs through direct transfer of **high-energy phosphate** from intermediates of the pathway to ADP (**substrate level phosphorylation**).*

*Glycolysis occurs in the **cytosol** and generates cytosolic NADH. Because NADH cannot cross the inner mitochondrial membrane, its reducing equivalents are transferred to the electron transport chain by either the **malate-aspartate shuttle** or the **glycerol 3-phosphate shuttle** (see Fig. 22.1). Pyruvate is then oxidized completely to CO_2 by pyruvate dehydrogenase and the TCA cycle. Complete **aerobic oxidation** of glucose to CO_2 can generate approximately **30 to 32 moles of ATP per mole of glucose**.*

*When cells have a limited supply of oxygen (e.g., kidney medulla), or few or no mitochondria (e.g., the red cell), or greatly increased demands for ATP (e.g., skeletal muscle during high-intensity exercise), they rely on **anaerobic glycolysis** for generation of ATP. In anaerobic glycolysis, **lactate dehydrogenase** oxidizes the NADH generated from glycolysis by reducing pyruvate to **lactate** (Fig. 22.2). Because O_2 is not required to reoxidize the NADH, the pathway is referred to as anaerobic. The energy yield from anaerobic glycolysis (2 moles of ATP per mole of glucose) is much lower than the yield from aerobic oxidation. The lactate (lactic acid) is released into the blood. Under pathologic conditions that cause **hypoxia**, tissues may generate enough lactic acid to cause **lactic acidemia**.*

*In each cell, glycolysis is regulated to ensure that **ATP homeostasis** is maintained, without using more glucose than necessary. In most cell types, **hexokinase (HK)**, the first enzyme of glycolysis, is inhibited by glucose 6-phosphate (see Fig. 22.1). Thus, glucose is not taken up and phosphorylated by a cell unless glucose-6-P enters a metabolic pathway, such as glycolysis or glycogen synthesis. The control of glucose-6-P entry into glycolysis occurs at phosphofructokinase-1 (**PFK-1**), the rate-limiting enzyme of the pathway. PFK-1 is **allosterically inhibited by ATP** and **allosterically activated by AMP**. AMP increases in the cytosol as ATP is hydrolyzed by energy-requiring reactions.*

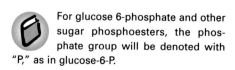 For glucose 6-phosphate and other sugar phosphoesters, the phosphate group will be denoted with "P," as in glucose-6-P.

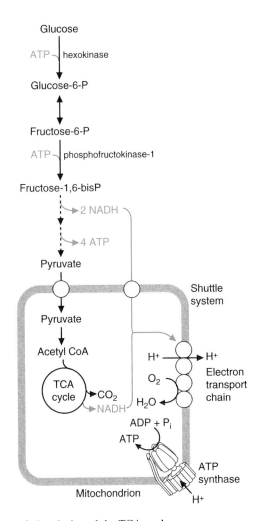

Fig. 22.1. Overview of glycolysis and the TCA cycle.

*Glycolysis has functions in addition to ATP production. For example, in liver and adipose tissue, this pathway generates pyruvate as a precursor for **fatty acid biosynthesis**. Glycolysis also provides precursors for the synthesis of compounds such as amino acids and 5-carbon sugar phosphates.*

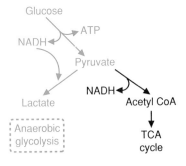

Fig. 22.2. Anaerobic glycolysis (shown in blue). The conversion of glucose to lactate generates 2 ATP from substrate-level phosphorylation. Because there is no net generation of NADH, there is no need for O_2, and, thus, the pathway is anaerobic.

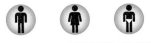

THE WAITING ROOM

Lopa Fusor is a 68-year-old woman who is admitted to the hospital emergency room with very low blood pressure (80/40 mm Hg) caused by an acute hemorrhage from a previously diagnosed ulcer of the stomach. Lopa's bleeding stomach ulcer has reduced her effective blood volume severely enough to compromise her ability to perfuse (deliver blood to) her tissues. She is, therefore, a "low perfuser." She is also known to have chronic obstructive pulmonary disease (COPD) as a result of 42 years of smoking two packs of cigarettes per day. Her respiratory rate is rapid and labored, her skin is cold and clammy, and her lips are slightly blue (cyanotic). She appears anxious and moderately confused.

As appropriate emergency measures are taken to stabilize her and elevate her blood pressure, blood is sent for immediate blood typing and cross-matching, so that blood transfusions can be started. A battery of laboratory tests are ordered, including venous hemoglobin, hematocrit, and lactate levels, and arterial blood pH, partial pressures of oxygen (pO_2) and carbon dioxide (pCO_2), bicarbonate, and oxygen saturation. Results show that the hemorrhaging and COPD have resulted in hypoxemia, with decreased oxygen delivery to her tissues, and both a respiratory and metabolic acidosis.

Otto Shape, a 26-year-old medical student, had gained weight during his first sedentary year in medical school. During his second year, he began watching his diet, jogging for an hour 4 times each week, and playing tennis twice a week. He has decided to compete in a 5-km race. To prepare for the race, he begins training with wind sprints, bouts of alternately running and walking.

Ivan Applebod is a 56-year-old morbidly obese accountant (see Chapters 1–3). He decided to see his dentist because he felt excruciating pain in his teeth when he ate ice cream. He really likes sweets and keeps hard candy in his pocket. The dentist noted from Mr. Applebod's history that he had numerous cavities as a child in his baby teeth. At this visit, the dentist found cavities in two of Mr. Applebod's teeth.

The hematocrit (the percentage of the volume of blood occupied by packed red blood cells) and hemoglobin content (g hemoglobin in 100 mL blood) are measured to determine whether the oxygen-carrying capacity of the blood is adequate. They can be decreased by conditions that interfere with erythropoiesis (synthesis of red blood cells in bone marrow), such as iron deficiency. They also can be decreased during chronic bleeding, but not during immediate acute hemorrhage, if interstitial fluid replaces the lost blood volume and dilutes out the red blood cells. The pCO_2 and pO_2 are the partial pressures of CO_2 and O_2 in the blood. The pO_2 and oxygen saturation determine whether adequate oxygen is available for tissues. Measurement of the pCO_2 and bicarbonate can distinguish between a metabolic and a respiratory acidosis (see Chapter 4).

I. GLYCOLYSIS

Glycolysis is one of the principle pathways for generating ATP in cells and is present in all cell types. The central role of glycolysis in fuel metabolism is related to its ability to generate ATP with, and without, oxygen. The oxidation of glucose to pyruvate generates ATP from substrate-level phosphorylation (the transfer of phosphate from high-energy intermediates of the pathway to ADP) and NADH. Subsequently, the pyruvate may be oxidized to CO_2 in the TCA cycle and ATP generated from electron transfer to oxygen in oxidative phosphorylation. However, if the pyruvate and NADH from glycolysis are converted to lactate (anaerobic glycolysis), ATP can be generated in the absence of oxygen, via substrate-level phosphorylation.

Glucose is readily available from our diet, internal glycogen stores, and the blood. Carbohydrate provides 50% or more of the calories in most diets, and glucose is the major carbohydrate. Other dietary sugars, such as fructose and galactose, are oxidized by conversion to intermediates of glycolysis. Glucose is stored in cells as glycogen, which can provide an internal source of fuel for glycolysis in emergency situations (e.g., decreased supply of fuels and oxygen during ischemia, a low blood flow). Insulin and other hormones maintain blood glucose at a constant level (glucose homeostasis), thereby ensuring that glucose is always available to cells that depend on glycolysis for generation of ATP.

In addition to serving as an anaerobic and aerobic source of ATP, glycolysis is an anabolic pathway that provides biosynthetic precursors. For example, in liver and adipose tissue, this pathway generates pyruvate as a precursor for fatty acid biosynthesis. Glycolysis also provides precursors for the synthesis of compounds such as amino acids and ribose-5-phosphate, the precursor of nucleotides. The integration of glycolysis with other anabolic pathways is discussed in Chapter 36.

After a high-carbohydrate meal, glucose is the major fuel for almost all tissues. Exceptions include intestinal mucosal cells, which transport glucose from the gut into the blood, and cells in the proximal convoluted tubule of the kidney, which return glucose from the renal filtrate to the blood. During fasting, the brain continues to oxidize glucose because it has a limited capacity for the oxidation of fatty acids or other fuels. Cells also continue to use glucose for the portion of their ATP generation that must be met by anaerobic glycolysis, due to either a limited oxygen supply or a limited capacity for oxidative phosphorylation (e.g., the red blood cell).

A. The Reactions of Glycolysis

The glycolytic pathway, which cleaves 1 mole of glucose to 2 moles of the 3-carbon compound pyruvate, consists of a preparative phase and an ATP-generating phase. In the initial preparative phase of glycolysis, glucose is phosphorylated

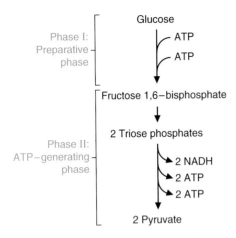

Fig. 22.3. Phases of the glycolytic pathway.

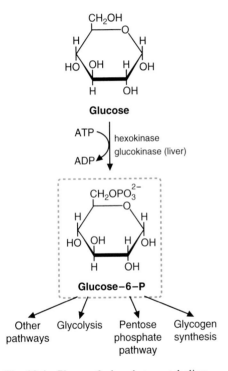

Fig. 22.4. Glucose 6-phosphate metabolism.

Hexokinases, other kinases, and many other enzymes that catalyze reactions involving the hydrolysis of ATP require Mg^{2+}. The Mg^{2+} forms a complex with the phosphate groups of ATP. Kinases also require K^+.

twice by ATP and cleaved into two triose phosphates (Fig. 22.3). The ATP expenditure in the beginning of the preparative phase is sometimes called "priming the pump," because this initial utilization of 2 moles of ATP/ mole of glucose results in the production of 4 moles of ATP/mole of glucose in the ATP-generating phase.

In the ATP-generating phase, glyceraldehyde 3-phosphate (a triose phosphate) is oxidized by NAD^+ and phosphorylated using inorganic phosphate. The high-energy phosphate bond generated in this step is transferred to ADP to form ATP. The remaining phosphate is also rearranged to form another high-energy phosphate bond that is transferred to ADP. Because there were 2 moles of triose phosphate formed, the yield from the ATP-generating phase is 4 ATP and 2 NADH. The result is a net yield of 2 moles of ATP, 2 moles of NADH, and 2 moles of pyruvate per mole of glucose.

1. CONVERSION OF GLUCOSE TO GLUCOSE 6-PHOSPHATE

Glucose metabolism begins with transfer of a phosphate from ATP to glucose to form glucose-6-P (Fig. 22.4). Phosphorylation of glucose commits it to metabolism within the cell because glucose-6-P cannot be transported back across the plasma membrane. The phosphorylation reaction is irreversible under physiologic conditions because the reaction has a high negative $\Delta G^{0\prime}$. Phosphorylation does not, however, commit glucose to glycolysis.

Glucose-6-P is a branchpoint in carbohydrate metabolism. It is a precursor for almost every pathway that uses glucose, including glycolysis, the pentose phosphate pathway, and glycogen synthesis. From the opposite point of view, it also can be generated from other pathways of carbohydrate metabolism, such as glycogenolysis (breakdown of glycogen), the pentose phosphate pathway, and gluconeogenesis (the synthesis of glucose from non-carbohydrate sources).

Hexokinases, the enzymes that catalyze the phosphorylation of glucose, are a family of tissue-specific isoenzymes that differ in their kinetic properties. The isoenzyme found in liver and β cells of the pancreas has a much higher K_m than other hexokinases and is called glucokinase. In many cells, some of the hexokinase is bound to porins in the outer mitochondrial membrane (voltage-dependent anion channels; see Chapter 21), which gives these enzymes first access to newly synthesized ATP as it exits the mitochondria.

2. CONVERSION OF GLUCOSE-6-P TO THE TRIOSE PHOSPHATES

In the remainder of the preparative phase of glycolysis, glucose-6-P is isomerized to fructose 6-phosphate (fructose-6-P), again phosphorylated, and subsequently cleaved into two 3-carbon fragments (Fig 22.5). The isomerization, which positions a keto group next to carbon 3, is essential for the subsequent cleavage of the bond between carbons 3 and 4.

The next step of glycolysis, phosphorylation of fructose-6-P to fructose 1,6-bisphosphate (fructose-1,6-bisP) by phosphofructokinase-1 (PFK-1), is generally considered the first committed step of the pathway. This phosphorylation requires ATP and is thermodynamically and kinetically irreversible. Therefore, PFK-1 irrevocably commits glucose to the glycolytic pathway. PFK-1 is a regulated enzyme in cells, and its regulation controls the entry of glucose into glycolysis. Like hexokinase, it exists as tissue-specific isoenzymes whose regulatory properties match variations in the role of glycolysis in different tissues.

Fructose-1,6-bisP is cleaved into two phosphorylated 3-carbon compounds (triose phosphates) by aldolase (see Fig. 22.5). Dihydroxyacetone phosphate (DHAP) is isomerized to glyceraldehyde 3-phosphate (glyceraldehyde-3-P), which is a triose phosphate. Thus, for every mole of glucose entering glycolysis, 2 moles of glyceraldehyde-3-P continue through the pathway.

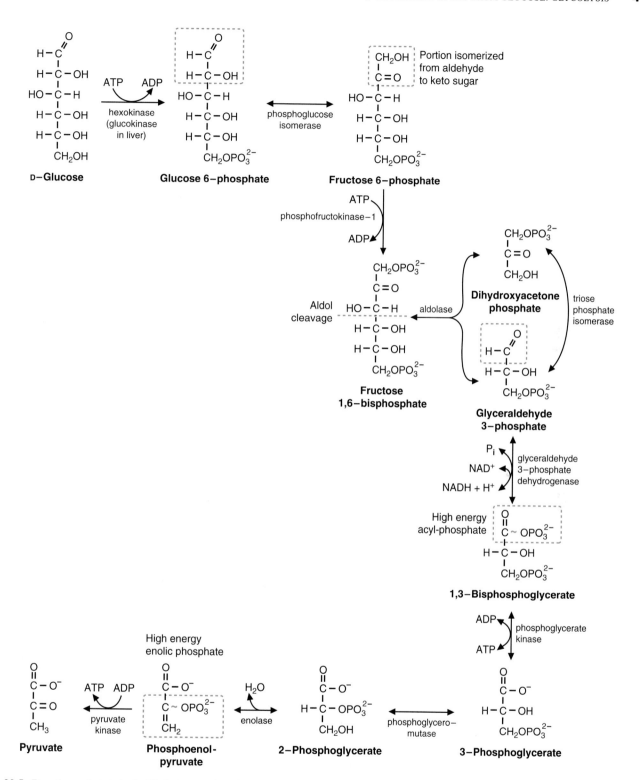

Fig. 22.5. Reactions of glycolysis. High-energy phosphates are shown in blue.

Aldolase is named for the mechanism of the forward reaction, which is an aldol cleavage, and the mechanism of the reverse reaction, which is an aldol condensation. The enzyme exists as tissue-specific isoenzymes, which all catalyze the cleavage of fructose 1,6-bisphosphate but differ in their specificities for fructose 1-P. The enzyme uses a lysine residue at the active site to form a covalent bond with the substrate during the course of the reaction. Inability to form this covalent linkage inactivates the enzyme.

3.   OXIDATION AND SUBSTRATE LEVEL PHOSPHORYLATION

In the next part of the glycolytic pathway, glyceraldehyde-3-P is oxidized and phosphorylated so that subsequent intermediates of glycolysis can donate phosphate to ADP to generate ATP. The first reaction in this sequence, catalyzed by glyceraldehyde-3-P dehydrogenase, is really the key to the pathway (see Fig. 22.5). This enzyme oxidizes the aldehyde group of glyceraldehyde-3-P to an enzyme-bound carboxyl group and transfers the electrons to NAD^+ to form NADH. The oxidation step is dependent on a cysteine residue at the active site of the enzyme, which forms a high-energy thioester bond during the course of the reaction. The high-energy intermediate immediately accepts an inorganic phosphate to form the high-energy acyl phosphate bond in 1,3-bisphosphoglycerate, releasing the product from the cysteine residue on the enzyme. This high-energy phosphate bond is the start of substrate-level phosphorylation (the formation of a high-energy phosphate bond where none previously existed, without the utilization of oxygen).

In the next reaction, the phosphate in this bond is transferred to ADP to form ATP by 3-phosphoglycerate kinase. The energy of the acyl phosphate bond is high enough (~13 kcal/mole) so that transfer to ADP is an energetically favorable process. 3-phosphoglycerate is also a product of this reaction.

To transfer the remaining low-energy phosphoester on 3-phosphoglycerate to ADP, it must be converted into a high-energy bond. This conversion is accomplished by moving the phosphate to the second carbon (forming 2-phosphoglycerate) and then removing water to form phosphoenolpyruvate (PEP). The enolphosphate bond is a high-energy bond (its hydrolysis releases approximately 14 kcal/mole of energy), so the transfer of phosphate to ADP by pyruvate kinase is energetically favorable (see Fig. 22.5). This final reaction converts PEP to pyruvate.

4.   SUMMARY OF THE GLYCOLYTIC PATHWAY

The overall net reaction in the glycolytic pathway is:

$$Glucose + 2NAD^+ + 2P_i + 2ADP \rightarrow 2Pyruvate + 2NADH + 4H^+ + 2ATP + 2H_2O$$

The pathway occurs with an overall negative $\Delta G^{0'}$ of approximately –22 kcal. Therefore, it cannot be reversed without the expenditure of energy.

B. Oxidative Fates of Pyruvate and NADH

The NADH produced from glycolysis must be continuously reoxidized back to NAD^+ to provide an electron acceptor for the glyceraldehyde-3-P dehydrogenase reaction and prevent product inhibition. Without oxidation of this NADH, glycolysis cannot continue. There are two alternate routes for oxidation of cytosolic NADH (Fig. 22.6). One route is aerobic, involving shuttles that transfer reducing equivalents across the mitochondrial membrane and ultimately to the electron transport chain and oxygen (see Fig. 22.6A). The other route is anaerobic (without the use of oxygen). In anaerobic glycolysis, NADH is reoxidized in the cytosol by lactate dehydrogenase, which reduces pyruvate to lactate (see Fig. 22.6B).

The fate of pyruvate depends on the route used for NADH oxidation. If NADH is reoxidized in a shuttle system, pyruvate can be used for other pathways, one of which is oxidation to acetyl-CoA and entry into the TCA cycle for complete oxidation. Alternatively, in anaerobic glycolysis, pyruvate is reduced to lactate and diverted away from other potential pathways. Thus, the use of the shuttle systems allows for more ATP to be generated than by anaerobic glycolysis by both oxidizing the cytoplasmically derived NADH in the electron transport chain and by allowing pyruvate to be oxidized completely to CO_2.

The reason that shuttles are required for the oxidation of cytosolic NADH by the electron transport chain is that the inner mitochondrial membrane is impermeable

Kinases transfer a phosphate from ATP to another compound. Hexokinase transfers a phosphate to glucose or another hexose to form a hexose phosphate. 3-Phosphoglycerate kinase is named for the reaction that is the reverse of glycolysis, transfer of phosphate from ATP to 3-phosphoglycerate to form 1,3-bisphosphoglycerate. Pyruvate kinase is also named for the reverse reaction (phosphorylation of pyruvate by ATP), although this direction does not occur under physiologic conditions.

The confusion experienced by **Lopa Fusor** in the emergency room is caused by an inadequate delivery of oxygen to the brain. Neurons have very high ATP requirements, and most of this ATP is provided by aerobic oxidation of glucose to pyruvate in glycolysis, and pyruvate oxidation to CO_2 in the TCA cycle. The brain has little or no capacity to oxidize fatty acids, and, therefore, its glucose consumption is high (approximately 125–150 g/day in the adult). Its oxygen demands are also high. If cerebral oxygen supply were completely interrupted, the brain would last only 10 seconds. The only reason consciousness lasts longer during anoxia or asphyxia is that there is still some oxygen in the lungs and in circulating blood. A decrease of blood flow to approximately ½ of the normal rate results in a loss of consciousness.

A. Aerobic glycolysis

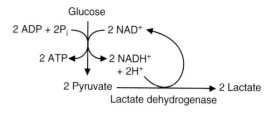

B. Anaerobic glycolysis

Fig. 22.6. Alternate fates of pyruvate. **A.** The pyruvate produced by glycolysis enters mitochondria and is oxidized to CO_2 and H_2O. The reducing equivalents in NADH enter mitochondria via a shuttle system. **B.** Pyruvate is reduced to lactate in the cytosol, thereby using the reducing equivalents in NADH.

to NADH, and no transport protein exists that can directly translocate NADH across this membrane. Consequently, NADH is reoxidized to NAD^+ in the cytosol by a reaction that transfers the electrons to DHAP in the glycerol 3-phosphate (glycerol-3-P) shuttle and oxaloacetate in the malate–aspartate shuttle. The NAD^+ that is formed in the cytosol returns to glycolysis while glycerol-3-P or malate carry the reducing equivalents that are ultimately transferred across the inner mitochondrial membrane. Thus, these shuttles transfer electrons and not NADH per se.

1. GLYCEROL 3–PHOSPHATE SHUTTLE

The glycerol 3–phosphate shuttle is the major shuttle in most tissues. In this shuttle, cytosolic NAD^+ is regenerated by cytoplasmic glycerol 3-phosphate dehydrogenase, which transfers electrons from NADH to DHAP to form glycerol 3-phosphate (Fig. 22.7). Glycerol 3-phosphate then diffuses through the outer mitochondrial membrane to the inner mitochondrial membrane, where the electrons are donated to a membrane-bound flavin adenive dinucleotide (FAD)-containing glycerophosphate dehydrogenase. This enzyme, like succinate dehydrogenase, ultimately donates electrons to CoQ, resulting in an energy yield of approximately 1.5 ATP from oxidative phosphorylation. Dihydroxyacetone phosphate returns to the cytosol to continue the shuttle. The sum of the reactions in this shuttle system is simply:

$$NADH_{cytosol} + H^+ + FAD_{mitochondria} \rightarrow NAD^+_{cytosol} + FAD(2H)_{mitochondria}$$

2. MALATE–ASPARTATE SHUTTLE

Many tissues contain both the glycerol-3-P shuttle and the malate–aspartate shuttle. In the malate–aspartate shuttle (Fig. 22.8), cytosolic NAD^+ is regenerated by cytosolic malate dehydrogenase, which transfers electrons from NADH to cytosolic oxaloacetate to form malate. Malate is transported across the inner mitochondrial membrane by a specific translocase, which exchanges malate for α-ketoglutarate. In the matrix, malate is oxidized back to oxaloacetate by mitochondrial malate dehydrogenase, and NADH is generated. This NADH can donate electrons to the electron transport chain with generation of approximately 2.5 moles of ATP per mole of NADH. The newly formed oxaloacetate cannot pass back through the inner mitochondrial membrane under physiologic conditions, so aspartate is used to

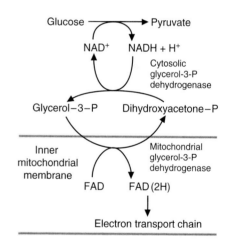

Fig. 22.7. Glycerol 3-phosphate shuttle. Because NAD^+ and NADH cannot cross the mitochondrial membrane, shuttles transfer the reducing equivalents into mitochondria. Dihydroxyacetone phosphate (DHAP) is reduced to glycerol-3-P by cytosolic glycerol 3-P dehydrogenase, using cytosolic NADH produced in glycolysis. Glycerol-3-P then reacts in the inner mitochondrial membrane with mitochondrial glycerol-3-P dehydrogenase, which transfers the electrons to FAD and regenerates DHAP, which returns to the cytosol. The electron transport chain transfers the electrons to O_2, which generates approximately 1.5 ATP for each FAD(2H) that is oxidized.

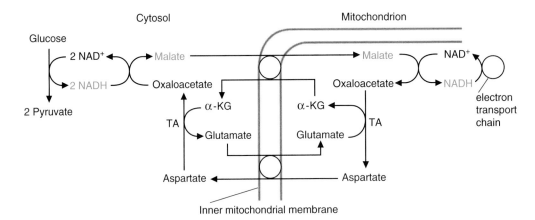

Fig. 22.8. Malate–aspartate shuttle. NADH produced by glycolysis reduces oxaloacetate (OAA) to malate, which crosses the mitochondrial membrane and is reoxidized to OAA. The mitochondrial NADH donates electrons to the electron transport chain, with 2.5 ATPs generated for each NADH. To complete the shuttle, oxaloacetate must return to the cytosol, although it cannot be directly transported on a translocase. Instead, it is transaminated to aspartate, which is then transported out to the cytosol, where it is transaminated back to oxaloacetate. The translocators exchange compounds in such a way that the shuttle is completely balanced. TA = transamination reaction. α-KG = α-ketoglutarate.

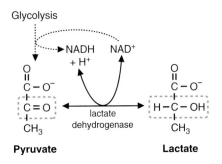

Fig. 22.9. Lactate dehydrogenase reaction. Pyruvate, which may be produced by glycolysis, is reduced to lactate. The reaction, which occurs in the cytosol, requires NADH and is catalyzed by lactate dehydrogenase. This reaction is readily reversible.

Q: What are the energy-generating steps as pyruvate is completely oxidized to carbon dioxide to generate 12.5 molecules of ATP per pyruvate?

return the oxaloacetate carbon skeleton to the cytosol. In the matrix, transamination reactions transfer an amino group to oxaloacetate to form aspartate, which is transported out to the cytosol (using an aspartate/glutamate exchange translocase) and converted back to oxaloacetate through another transamination reaction. The sum of all the reactions of this shuttle system is simply:

$$NADH_{cytosol} + NAD^+_{matrix} \rightarrow NAD^+_{cytosol} + NADH_{matrix}.$$

C. Anaerobic Glycolysis

When the oxidative capacity of a cell is limited (e.g., the red blood cell, which has no mitochondria), the pyruvate and NADH produced from glycolysis cannot be oxidized aerobically. The NADH is therefore oxidized to NAD^+ in the cytosol by reduction of pyruvate to lactate. This reaction is catalyzed by lactate dehydrogenase (LDH) (Fig. 22.9). The net reaction for anaerobic glycolysis is:

$$Glucose + 2\ ADP + 2\ P_i \rightarrow 2\ Lactate + 2\ ATP + 2\ H_2O + 2\ H^+$$

1. ENERGY YIELD OF AEROBIC VERSUS ANAEROBIC GLYCOLYSIS

In both aerobic and anaerobic glycolysis, each mole of glucose generates 2 moles of ATP, 2 of NADH and 2 of pyruvate. The energy yield from anaerobic glycolysis (glucose to 2 lactate) is only 2 moles of ATP per mole of glucose, as the NADH is recycled to NAD^+ by reducing pyruvate to lactate. Neither the NADH nor pyruvate produced is thus used for further energy generation. However, when oxygen is available, and cytosolic NADH can be oxidized via a shuttle system, pyruvate can also enter the mitochondria and be completely oxidized to CO_2 via PDH and the TCA cycle. The oxidation of pyruvate via this route generates roughly 12.5 moles of ATP per mole of pyruvate. If the cytosolic NADH is oxidized by the glycerol 3-P shuttle, approximately 1.5 moles of ATP are produced per NADH. If, instead, the NADH is oxidized by the malate–aspartate shuttle, approximately 2.5 moles are produced. Thus, the two NADH molecules produced during glycolysis can lead to 3 to 5 molecules of ATP being produced, depending on which shuttle system is used to transfer the reducing equivalents. Because each pyruvate produced can give rise to 12.5 molecules of ATP, altogether 30 to 32 molecules of ATP can be produced from one mole of glucose oxidized to carbon dioxide.

In response to the hypoxemia caused by **Lopa Fusor's** COPD, she has increased hypoxia-inducible factor-1 (HIF-1) in her tissues. HIF-1 is a gene transcription factor found in tissues throughout the body (including brain, heart, kidney, lung, liver, pancreas, skeletal muscle, and white blood cells) that plays a homeostatic role in coordinating tissue responses to hypoxia. Each tissue will respond with a subset of the following changes. HIF-1 increases transcription of the genes for many of the glycolytic enzymes, including PFK-1, enolase, phosphoglycerate kinase, and lactate dehydrogenase. HIF-1 also increases synthesis of a number of proteins that enhance oxygen delivery to tissues, including erythropoietin, which increases the generation of red blood cells in bone marrow; vascular endothelial growth factor, which regulates angiogenesis (formation of blood vessels); and inducible nitric oxide synthase, which synthesizes nitric oxide, a vasodilator. As a consequence, Mrs. Fusor was able to maintain hematocrit and hemoglobin levels that were on the high side of the normal range, and her tissues had an increased capacity for anaerobic glycolysis.

To produce the same amount of ATP per unit time from anaerobic glycolysis as from the complete aerobic oxidation of glucose to CO_2, anaerobic glycolysis must occur approximately 15 times faster, and use approximately 15 times more glucose. Cells achieve this high rate of glycolysis by expressing high levels of glycolytic enzymes. In certain skeletal muscles and in most cells during hypoxic crises, high rates of glycolysis are associated with rapid degradation of internal glycogen stores to supply the required glucose-6-P.

2. ACID PRODUCTION IN ANAEROBIC GLYCOLYSIS

Anaerobic glycolysis results in acid production in the form of H^+. Glycolysis forms pyruvic acid, which is reduced to lactic acid. At an intracellular pH of 7.35, lactic acid dissociates to form the carboxylate anion, lactate, and H^+ (the pKa for lactic acid is 3.85). Lactate and the H^+ are both transported out of the cell into interstitial fluid by a transporter on the plasma membrane and eventually diffuse into the blood. If the amount of lactate generated exceeds the buffering capacity of the blood, the pH drops below the normal range, resulting in lacticacidosis (see Chapter 4).

3. TISSUES DEPENDENT ON ANAEROBIC GLYCOLYSIS

Many tissues, including red and white blood cells, the kidney medulla, the tissues of the eye, and skeletal muscles, rely on anaerobic glycolysis for at least a portion of their ATP requirements (Table 22.1). Tissues (or cells) that are heavily dependent on anaerobic glycolysis usually have a low ATP demand, high levels of glycolytic enzymes, and few capillaries, such that oxygen must diffuse over a greater distance to reach target cells. The lack of mitochondria, or the increased rate of glycolysis, is often related to some aspect of cell function. For example, the mature red blood cell has no mitochondria because oxidative metabolism might interfere with its function in transporting oxygen bound to hemoglobin. Some of the lactic acid generated by anaerobic glycolysis in skin is secreted in sweat, where it acts as an antibacterial agent. Many large tumors use anaerobic glycolysis for ATP production, and lack capillaries in their core.

In tissues with some mitochondria, both aerobic and anaerobic glycolysis occur simultaneously. The relative proportion of the two pathways depends on the mitochondrial oxidative capacity of the tissue and its oxygen supply and may vary between cell types within the same tissue because of cell distance from the capillaries. When a cell's energy demand exceeds the capacity of the rate of the electron transport chain and oxidative phosphorylation to produce ATP, glycolysis is activated, and the increased NADH/NAD$^+$ ratio will direct excess pyruvate into lactate. Because under these conditions pyruvate dehydrogenase, the TCA cycle, and the electron transport chain are operating as fast as they can, anaerobic glycolysis is meeting the need for additional ATP.

The dental caries in **Ivan Applebod's** mouth were caused principally by the low pH generated from lactic acid production by oral bacteria. Below a pH of 5.5, decalcification of tooth enamel and dentine occurs. Lactobacilli and *S. mutans* are major contributors to this process because almost all of their energy is derived from the conversion of glucose or fructose to lactic acid, and they are able to grow well at the low pH generated by this process. Mr. Applebod's dentist explained that bacteria in his dental plaque could convert all the sugar in his candy into acid in less than 20 minutes. The acid is buffered by bicarbonate and other buffers in saliva, but saliva production decreases in the evening. Thus, the acid could dissolve the hydroxyapatite in his tooth enamel during the night.

Table 22.1. Major Tissue Sites of Lactate Production in a Resting Man. An average 70-kg man consumes about 300 g of carbohydrate per day.

Daily Lactate Production (g/day)	
Total lactate production	115
Red blood cells	29
Skin	20
Brain	17
Skeletal muscle	16
Renal medulla	15
Intestinal muscosa	8
Other tissues	10

A: In the complete oxidation of pyruvate to carbon dioxide, four steps generate NADH (pyruvate dehydrogenase, isocitrate dehydrogenase, α-ketoglutarate dehydrogenase, and malate dehydrogenase). One step generates FAD(2H) (succinate dehydrogenase), and one substrate level phosphorylation (succinate thiokinase). Thus, because each NADH generates 2.5 ATPs, the overall contribution by NADH is 10 ATP molecules. The FAD(2H) generates an additional 1.5 ATP, and the substrate-level phosphorylation provides one more. Therefore, 10 + 1.5 + 1 = 12.5 molecules of ATP.

The tissues of the eye are also partially dependent on anaerobic glycolysis.

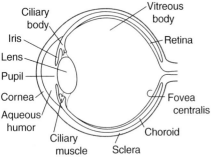

The eye contains cells that transmit or focus light, and these cells cannot, therefore, be filled with opaque structures such as mitochondria, or densely packed capillary beds. The corneal epithelium generates most of its ATP aerobically from its few mitochondria but still metabolizes some glucose anaerobically. Oxygen is supplied by diffusion from the air. The lens of the eye is composed of fibers that must remain birefringent to transmit and focus light, so mitochondria are nearly absent. The small amount of ATP required (principally for ion balance) can readily be generated from anaerobic glycolysis even though the energy yield is low. The lens is able to pick up glucose and release lactate into the vitreous body and aqueous humor. It does not need oxygen and has no use for capillaries.

 Lactate dehydrogenase (LDH) is a tetramer composed of A subunits (also called M for skeletal muscle form) and B subunits (also called H for heart). Different tissues produce different amounts of the two subunits, which then combine randomly to form five different tetramers (M_4, M_3H_1, M_2H_2, M_1H_3, and H_4). These isoenzymes differ only slightly in their properties, with the kinetic properties of the M_4 form facilitating conversion of pyruvate to lactate in skeletal muscle and the H_4 form facilitating conversion of lactate to pyruvate in the heart.

4. FATE OF LACTATE

Lactate released from cells undergoing anaerobic glycolysis is taken up by other tissues (primarily the liver, heart, and skeletal muscle) and oxidized back to pyruvate. In the liver, the pyruvate is used to synthesize glucose (gluconeogenesis), which is returned to the blood. The cycling of lactate and glucose between peripheral tissues and liver is called the Cori cycle (Fig. 22.10).

In many other tissues, lactate is oxidized to pyruvate, which is then oxidized to CO_2 in the TCA cycle. Although the equilibrium of the lactate dehydrogenase reaction favors lactate production, flux occurs in the opposite direction if NADH is being rapidly oxidized in the electron transport chain (or being used for gluconeogenesis):

$$Lactate + NAD^+ \rightarrow Pyruvate + NADH + H^+$$

The heart, with its huge mitochondrial content and oxidative capacity, is able to use lactate released from other tissues as a fuel. During an exercise such as bicycle riding, lactate released into the blood from skeletal muscles in the leg might be used by resting skeletal muscles in the arm. In the brain, glial cells and astrocytes produce lactate, which is used by neurons or released into the blood.

II. OTHER FUNCTIONS OF GLYCOLYSIS

Glycolysis, in addition to providing ATP, generates precursors for biosynthetic pathways (Fig. 22.11). Intermediates of the pathway can be converted to ribose 5-phosphate, the sugar incorporated into nucleotides such as ATP. Other sugars, such as UDP-glucose, mannose, and sialic acid, are also formed from intermediates of glycolysis. Serine is synthesized from 3-phosphoglycerate, and alanine from pyruvate. The backbone of triacylglycerols, glycerol 3-phosphate, is derived from dihydroxyacetone phosphate in the glycolytic pathway.

The liver is the major site of biosynthetic reactions in the body. In addition to those pathways mentioned previously, the liver synthesizes fatty acids from the pyruvate generated by glycolysis. It also synthesizes glucose from lactate, glycerol 3-phosphate, and amino acids in the gluconeogenic pathway, which is principally a reversal of glycolysis. Consequently, in liver, many of the glycolytic enzymes exist as isoenzymes with properties suited for these functions.

The bisphosphoglycerate shunt is a "side reaction" of the glycolytic pathway in which 1,3-bis-phosphoglycerate is converted to 2,3-bis-phosphoglycerate (2,3-BPG). Red blood cells form 2,3-BPG to serve as an allosteric inhibitor of oxygen binding to heme (see Chapter 44). 2,3-BPG reenters the glycolytic pathway via dephosphorylation to 3-phosphoglycerate. 2,3-BPG also functions as a coenzyme in the conversion of 3-phosphoglycerate to 2-phosphoglycerate by the glycolytic

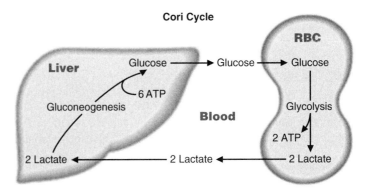

Fig. 22.10. Cori cycle. Glucose, produced in the liver by gluconeogenesis, is converted by glycolysis in muscle, red blood cells, and many other cells, to lactate. Lactate returns to the liver and is reconverted to glucose by gluconeogenesis.

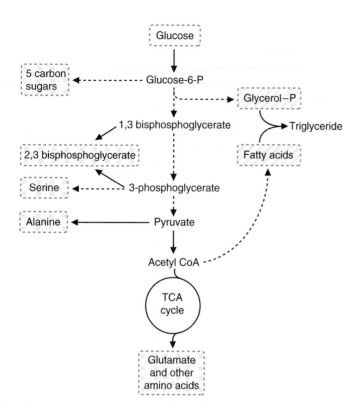

Fig. 22.11. Biosynthetic functions of glycolysis. Compounds formed from intermediates of glycolysis are shown in blue. These pathways are discussed in subsequent chapters of the book. Dotted lines indicate that more than one step is required for the conversion shown in the figure.

enzyme phosphoglyceromutase. Because 2,3-BPG is not depleted by its role in this catalytic process, most cells need only very small amounts.

III. REGULATION OF GLYCOLYSIS BY THE NEED FOR ATP

One of the major functions of glycolysis is the generation of ATP, and, therefore, the pathway is regulated to maintain ATP homeostasis in all cells. Phosphofructokinase-1 (PFK-1) and pyruvate dehydrogenase (PDH), which links glycolysis and the TCA cycle, are both major regulatory sites that respond to feedback indicators of the rate of ATP utilization (Fig. 22.12). The supply of glucose-6-P for glycolysis is tissue dependent and can be regulated at the steps of glucose transport into cells, glycogenolysis (the degradation of glycogen to form glucose), or the rate of glucose phosphorylation by hexokinase isoenzymes. Other regulatory mechanisms integrate the ATP-generating role of glycolysis with its anabolic roles.

All of the regulatory enzymes of glycolysis exist as tissue-specific isoenzymes, which alter the regulation of the pathway to match variations in conditions and needs in different tissues. For example, in the liver, an isoenzyme of pyruvate kinase introduces an additional regulatory site in glycolysis that contributes to the inhibition of glycolysis when the reverse pathway, gluconeogenesis, is activated.

A. Relationship between ATP, ADP, and AMP Concentrations

The AMP levels within the cytosol provide a better indicator of the rate of ATP utilization than the ATP concentration itself (Fig. 22.13). The concentration of AMP

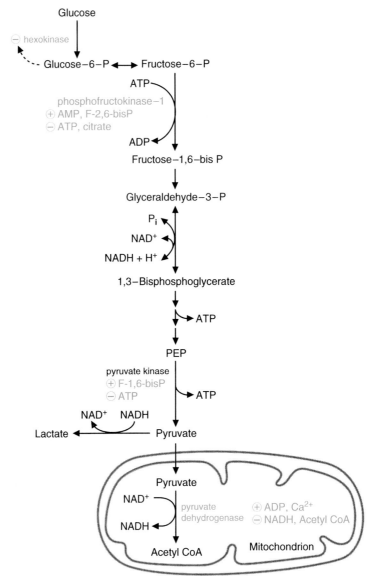

Fig. 22.12. Major sites of regulation in the glycolytic pathway. Hexokinase and phosphofructokinase-1 are the major regulatory enzymes in skeletal muscle. The activity of pyruvate dehydrogenase in the mitochondrion determines whether pyruvate is converted to lactate or to acetyl CoA. The regulation shown for pyruvate kinase only occurs for the liver (L) isoenzyme.

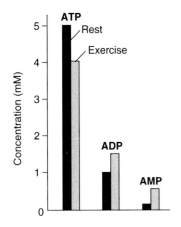

Fig. 22.13. Changes in ATP, ADP, and AMP concentrations in skeletal muscle during exercise. The concentration of ATP decreases by only approximately 20% during exercise, and the concentration of ADP rises. The concentration of AMP, produced by the adenylate kinase reaction, increases manyfold and serves as a sensitive indicator of decreasing ATP levels.

in the cytosol is determined by the equilibrium position of the adenylate kinase reaction.

adenylate kinase
$$2\ ADP \leftrightarrow AMP + ATP$$

The equilibrium is such that hydrolysis of ATP to ADP in energy-requiring reactions increases both the ADP and AMP contents of the cytosol. However, ATP is present in much higher quantities than AMP or ADP, so that a small decrease of ATP concentration in the cytosol causes a much larger percentage increase in the small AMP pool. In skeletal muscles, for instance, ATP levels are approximately 5 mM and decrease by no more than 20% during strenuous exercise (see Fig. 22.13). At the same time, ADP levels may increase by 50%, and AMP levels, which are in the micromolar range, increase by 300%. AMP activates a number of metabolic pathways, including glycolysis, glycogenolysis, and fatty acid oxidation (particularly in muscle tissues), to ensure that ATP homeostasis is maintained.

B. Regulation of Hexokinases

Hexokinases exist as tissue-specific isoenzymes whose regulatory properties reflect the role of glycolysis in different tissues. In most tissues, hexokinase is a low-K_m enzyme with a high affinity for glucose (see Chapter 9). It is inhibited by physiologic concentrations of its product, glucose-6-P (see Fig. 22.12). If glucose-6-P does not enter glycolysis or another pathway, it accumulates and decreases the activity of hexokinase. In the liver, the isoenzyme glucokinase is a high-K_m enzyme that is not readily inhibited by glucose-6-P. Thus, glycolysis can continue in liver even when energy levels are high so that anabolic pathways, such as the synthesis of the major energy storage compounds, glycogen and fatty acids, can occur.

C. Regulation of PFK-1

Phosphofructokinase-1 (PFK-1) is the rate-limiting enzyme of glycolysis and controls the rate of glucose-6-P entry into glycolysis in most tissues. PFK-1 is an allosteric enzyme that has a total of six binding sites: two are for substrates (Mg-ATP and fructose-6-P) and four are allosteric regulatory sites (see Fig. 22.12). The allosteric regulatory sites occupy a physically different domain on the enzyme than the catalytic site. When an allosteric effector binds, it changes the conformation at the active site and may activate or inhibit the enzyme (see also Chapter 9). The allosteric sites for PFK-1 include an inhibitory site for MgATP, an inhibitory site for citrate and other anions, an allosteric activation site for AMP, and an allosteric activation site for fructose 2,6-bisphosphate (fructose-2,6-bisP) and other bisphosphates. Several different tissue-specific isoforms of PFK-1 are affected in different ways by the concentration of these substrates and allosteric effectors, but all contain these four allosteric sites.

1. ALLOSTERIC REGULATION OF PFK-1 BY AMP AND ATP

ATP binds to two different sites on the enzyme, the substrate binding site and an allosteric inhibitory site. Under physiologic conditions in the cell, the ATP concentration is usually high enough to saturate the substrate binding site and inhibit the enzyme by binding to the ATP allosteric site. This effect of ATP is opposed by AMP, which binds to a separate allosteric activator site (Figure 22.14). For most of the PFK-1 isoenzymes, the binding of AMP increases the affinity of the enzyme for fructose 6-P (e.g., shifts the kinetic curve to the left). Thus, increases in AMP concentration can greatly increase the rate of the enzyme (see Fig. 22.14), particularly when fructose-6-P concentrations are low.

2. REGULATION OF PFK-1 BY FRUCTOSE 2,6-BISPHOSPHATE

Fructose-2,6-bisP is also an allosteric activator of PFK-1 that opposes the ATP inhibition. Its effect on the rate of activity of PFK-1 is qualitatively similar to that of AMP, but it has a separate binding site. Fructose-2,6-bisP is NOT an intermediate

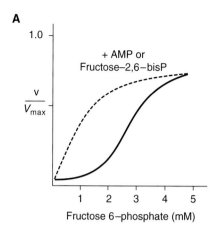

A

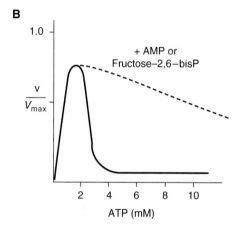

B

Fig. 22.14. Regulation of PFK-1 by AMP, ATP and fructose-2,6-bisP. **A.** AMP and fructose 2,6-bisphosphate activate PFK-1. **B.** ATP increases the rate of the reaction at low concentrations, but allosterically inhibits the enzyme at high concentrations.

Otto Shape has started high-intensity exercise that will increase the production of lactate in his exercising skeletal muscles. In skeletal muscles, the amount of aerobic versus anaerobic glycolysis that occurs varies with intensity of the exercise, with duration of the exercise, with the type of skeletal muscle fiber involved, and with the level of training. Human skeletal muscles are usually combinations of type I fibers (called fast glycolytic fibers, or white muscle fibers) and type IIb fibers (called slow oxidative fibers, or red muscle fibers). The designation of fast or slow refers to their rate of shortening, which is determined by the isoenzyme of myosin ATPase present. Compared with glycolytic fibers, oxidative fibers have a higher content of mitochondria and myoglobin, which gives them a red color. The gastrocnemius, a muscle in the leg used for running, has a high content of type IIb fibers. However, these fibers will still produce lactate during sprints when the ATP demand exceeds their oxidative capacity.

[handwritten annotation at top: PFK-2 domains: kinase: F6P → F2,6 biP / phosphatase: F2,6biP → F6P]

PFK-1 exists as a group of tissue-specific isoenzymes whose regulatory features match the role of glycolysis in different tissues. Three different types of PFK-1 isoenzyme subunits exist: M (muscle), L (liver), and C. The three subunits show variable expression in different tissues, with some tissues having more than one type. For example, mature human muscle expresses only the M subunit, the liver expresses principally the L subunit, and erythrocytes express both the M and the L subunits. The C subunit is present in highest levels in platelets, placenta, kidney, and fibroblasts but is relatively common to most tissues. Both the M and L subunits are sensitive to AMP and ATP regulation, but the C subunits are much less so. Active PFK-1 is a tetramer, composed of four subunits. Within muscle, the M4 form predominates but within tissues that express multiple isoenzymes of PFK-1 heterotetramers can form that have full activity.

Under ischemic conditions, AMP levels within the heart rapidly increase because of the lack of ATP production via oxidative phosphorylation. The increase in AMP levels activates an AMP-dependent protein kinase (protein kinase B), which phosphorylates the heart isoenzyme of PFK-2 to activate its kinase activity. This results in increased levels of fructose-2,6-bisP, which activates PFK-1 along with AMP such that the rate of glycolysis can increase to compensate for the lack of ATP production via aerobic means.

During **Cora Nari**'s myocardial infarction (see Chapter 20), her heart had a limited supply of oxygen and blood-borne fuels. The absence of oxygen for oxidative phosphorylation would decrease the levels of ATP and increase those of AMP, an activator of PFK-1 and the AMP-dependent protein kinase, resulting in a compensatory increase of anaerobic glycolysis and lactate production. However, obstruction of a vessel leading to her heart would decrease lactate removal, resulting in a decrease of intracellular pH. Under these conditions, at very low pH levels, glycolysis is inhibited and unable to compensate for the lack of oxidative phosphorylation.

of glycolysis but is synthesized by an enzyme that phosphorylates fructose 6-phosphate at the 2 position. The enzyme is therefore named phosphofructokinase-2 (PFK-2); it is a bifunctional enzyme with two separate domains, a kinase domain and a phosphatase domain. At the kinase domain, fructose-6-P is phosphorylated to fructose-2,6-bisP and at the phosphatase domain, fructose-2,6-bisP is hydrolyzed back to fructose-6-P. PFK-2 is regulated through changes in the ratio of activity of the two domains. For example, in skeletal muscles, high concentrations of fructose-6-P activate the kinase and inhibit the phosphatase, thereby increasing the concentration of fructose-2,6-bisP and activating glycolysis.

PFK-2 also can be regulated through phosphorylation by serine/threonine protein kinases. The liver isoenzyme contains a phosphorylation site near the amino terminal that decreases the activity of the kinase and increases the phosphatase activity. This site is phosphorylated by the cAMP-dependent protein kinase (protein kinase A) and is responsible for decreased levels of liver fructose-2,6-bisP during fasting conditions (as modulated by circulating glucagon levels, which is discussed in detail in Chapters 26 and 31). The cardiac isoenzyme contains a phosphorylation site near the carboxy terminal that can be phosphorylated in response to adrenergic activators of contraction (such as norepinephrine) and by increased AMP levels. Phosphorylation at this site increases the kinase activity and increases fructose-2,6-bisP levels, thereby contributing to the activation of glycolysis.

3. ALLOSTERIC INHIBITION OF PFK-1 AT THE CITRATE SITE

The function of the citrate–anion allosteric site is to integrate glycolysis with other pathways. For example, the inhibition of PFK-1 by citrate may play a role in decreasing glycolytic flux in the heart during the oxidation of fatty acids.

D. Regulation of Pyruvate Kinase

Pyruvate kinase exists as tissue-specific isoenzymes. The form present in brain and muscle contains no allosteric sites, and pyruvate kinase does not contribute to the regulation of glycolysis in these tissues. However, the liver isoenzyme can be inhibited through phosphorylation by the cAMP-dependent protein kinase, and by a number of allosteric effectors that contribute to the inhibition of glycolysis during fasting conditions. These allosteric effectors include activation by fructose-1,6-bisP, which ties the rate of pyruvate kinase to that of PFK-1, and inhibition by ATP, which signifies high energy levels.

E. Pyruvate Dehydrogenase Regulation and Glycolysis

Pyruvate dehydrogenase is also regulated principally by the rate of ATP utilization (see Chapter 20) through rapid phosphorylation to an inactive form. Thus, in a normal respiring cell, with an adequate supply of O_2, glycolysis and the TCA cycle are activated together, and glucose can be completely oxidized to CO_2. However, when tissues do not have an adequate supply of O_2 to meet their ATP demands, the increased NADH/NAD$^+$ ratio inhibits pyruvate dehydrogenase, but AMP activates glycolysis. A proportion of the pyruvate will then be reduced to lactate to allow glycolysis to continue.

IV. LACTIC ACIDEMIA

Lactate production is a normal part of metabolism. In the absence of disease, elevated lactate levels in the blood are associated with anaerobic glycolysis during exercise. In lactic acidosis, lactic acid accumulates in blood to levels that significantly affect the pH (lactate levels greater than 5 mM and a decrease of blood pH below 7.2).

Lactic acidosis generally results from a greatly increased NADH/NAD$^+$ ratio in tissues (Fig.22.15). The increased NADH concentration prevents pyruvate oxidation in the TCA cycle and directs pyruvate to lactate. To compensate for the decreased ATP production from oxidative metabolism, PFK-1, and, therefore, the entire glycolytic pathway is activated. For example, consumption of high amounts of alcohol, which is rapidly oxidized in the liver and increases NADH levels, can result in a lactic acidosis. Hypoxia in any tissue increases lactate production as cells attempt to compensate for a lack of O_2 for oxidative phosphorylation.

A number of other problems that interfere either with the electron transport chain or pyruvate oxidation in the TCA cycle result in lactic acidemia (see Fig.22.15). For example, OXPHOS diseases (inherited deficiencies in subunits of complexes in the electron transport chain, such as MERFF) increase the NADH/NAD$^+$ ratio and

Q: Lactate and pyruvate are in equilibrium in the cell, and the ratio of lactate to pyruvate reflects the NADH/NAD$^+$ ratio. Both acids are released into blood, and the normal ratio of lactate to pyruvate in blood is approximately 25:1. This ratio can provide a useful clinical diagnostic tool. Because lactic acidemia can be the result of a number of problems, such as hypoxia, MERFF, thiamine deficiency, and pyruvate dehydrogenase deficiency, under which of these conditions would you expect the *lactate/pyruvate ratio* in blood to be much greater than normal?

Lopa Fusor had a decreased arterial pO_2 and elevated arterial pCO_2 caused by underperfusion of her lungs. The elevated CO_2 content resulted in an increase of H_2CO_3 and acidity of the blood (see Chapter 4). The decreased O_2 delivery to tissues resulted in increased lactate production from anaerobic glycolysis, and an elevation of serum lactate to 10 times normal levels. The reduction in her arterial pH to 7.18 (reference range, 7.35–7.45) resulted, therefore, from both a mild respiratory acidosis (elevated pCO_2) and a more profound metabolic acidosis (elevated serum lactate level).

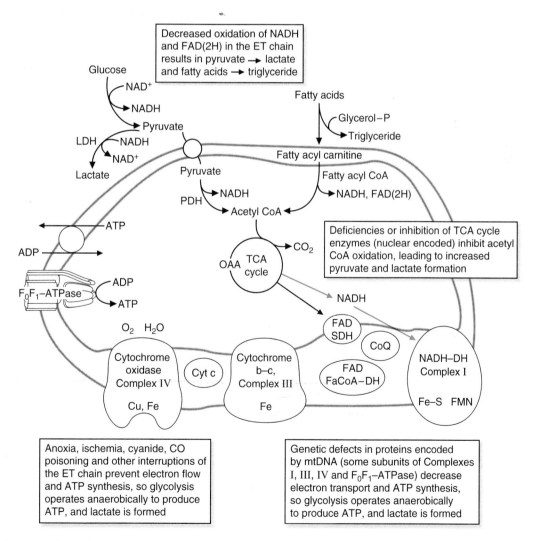

Fig. 22.15. Pathways leading to lactic acidemia.

A: Hypoxia and inherited deficiencies of subunits in the electron transport chain impair NADH oxidation, resulting in a higher NADH/NAD$^+$ ratio in the cell, and, therefore, a higher lactate/pyruvate ratio in blood. In contrast, conditions that cause lactic acidemia as a result of defects in the enzymes of pyruvate metabolism (thiamine deficiency or pyruvate dehydrogenase deficiency) would increase both pyruvate and lactate in the blood and have little effect on the ratio.

inhibit PDH (see Chapter 21). Impaired PDH activity from an inherited deficiency of E$_1$ (the decarboxylase subunit of the complex), or from severe thiamine deficiency, increases blood lactate levels (see Chapter 20). Pyruvate carboxylase deficiency also can result in lactic acidosis (see Chapter 20), because of an accumulation of pyruvate.

Lactic acidosis can also result from inhibition of lactate utilization in gluconeogenesis (e.g., hereditary fructose intolerance, which is due to a defective aldolase gene). If other pathways that use glucose-6-P are blocked, glucose-6-P can be shunted into glycolysis and lactate production (e.g., glucose 6-phosphatase deficiency).

CLINICAL COMMENTS

Lopa Fusor was admitted to he hospital with severe hypotension caused by an acute hemorrhage. Her plasma lactic acid level was elevated and her arterial pH was low. The underlying mechanism for Ms. Fusor's derangement in acid-base balance is a severe reduction in the amount of oxygen delivered to her tissues for cellular respiration (hypoxemia). Several concurrent processes contributed to this oxygen lack. The first was her severely reduced blood pressure caused by a brisk hemorrhage from a bleeding gastric ulcer. The blood loss led to hypoperfusion and, therefore, reduced delivery of oxygen to her tissues. The marked reduction in the number of red blood cells in her circulation caused by blood loss further compromised oxygen delivery. The preexisting chronic obstructive pulmonary disease (COPD) added to her hypoxemia by decreasing her ventilation, and, therefore, the transfer of oxygen to blood (low pO$_2$). In addition, her COPD led to retention of carbon dioxide (high pCO$_2$), which caused a respiratory acidosis because the retained CO$_2$ interacted with water to form carbonic acid (H$_2$CO$_3$), which dissociates to H$^+$ and bicarbonate.

In skeletal muscles, lactate production occurs when the need for ATP exceeds the capacity of the mitochondria for oxidative phosphorylation. Thus, increased lactate production accompanies an increased rate of the TCA cycle. The extent to which skeletal muscles use aerobic versus anaerobic glycolysis to supply ATP varies with the intensity of exercise. At low-intensity exercise, the rate of ATP utilization is lower, and fibers can generate this ATP from oxidative phosphorylation, with the complete oxidation of glucose to CO$_2$. However, when **Otto Shape** sprints, a high-intensity exercise, the ATP demand exceeds the rate at which the electron transport chain and TCA cycle can generate ATP from oxidative phosphorylation. The increased AMP level signals the need for additional ATP and stimulates PFK-1. The NADH/NAD$^+$ ratio directs the increase in pyruvate production toward lactate. The fall in pH causes muscle fatigue and pain. As he trains, the amount of mitochondria and myoglobin will increase in his skeletal muscle fibers, and these fibers will rely less on anaerobic glycolysis.

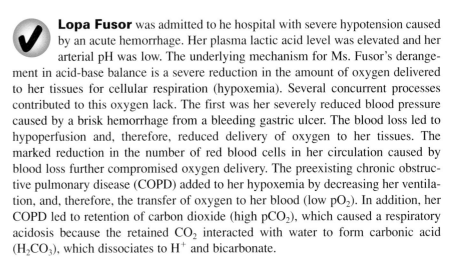

Fig. 22.16. General structure of dextran. Glucosyl residues are linked by α-1,3, α-1,6, and some α-1,4 bonds.

Ivan Applebod had two sites of dental caries: one on a smooth surface and one in a fissure. The decreased pH resulting from lactic acid production by lactobacilli, which grow anaerobically within the fissure, is a major cause of fissure caries. *Streptococs mutans (S. mutans)* plays a major role in smooth surface caries because it secretes dextran, an insoluble polysaccharide, which forms the base for plaque. *S. mutans* contains dextran-sucrase, a glucosyltransferase that transfers glucosyl units from dietary sucrose (the glucose-fructose disaccharide in sugar and sweets) to form the α(1→6) and α(1→3) linkages between the glucosyl units in dextran (Fig. 22.16). Dextran-sucrase is specific for sucrose and does not catalyze the polymerization of free glucose, or glucose from other disaccharides or polysaccharides. Thus sucrose is responsible for the cariogenic potential of candy. The sticky water-insoluble dextran mediates the attachment of *S. mutans* and other bacteria to the tooth surface. This also keeps the acids produced from these bacteria close to the enamel surface. Fructose from sucrose is converted to intermediates of glycolysis and is rapidly metabolized to lactic acid. Other bacteria present in the plaque produce different acids from anaerobic metabolism, such as acetic acid and formic acid. The decrease in pH that results initiates demineralization of the hydroxyapatite of the tooth enamel. **Ivan Applebod's** caries in his baby teeth could have been caused by sucking on bottles containing fruit juice. The sugar in fruit juice is also sucrose, and babies who fall asleep with a bottle of fruit juice in their mouth may develop caries. Rapid decay of these baby teeth can harm the development of their permanent teeth.

BIOCHEMICAL COMMENTS

How is the first high-energy bond created in the glycolytic pathway? This is the work of the glyceraldehyde 3-phosphate dehydrogenase reaction, which converts glyceraldehyde-3-P to 1,3 bisphosphglycerate. This reaction can be considered to be two separate half reactions, the first being the oxidation of glyceraldehyde-3-P to 3-phosphoglycerate, and the second the addition of inorganic phosphate to 3-phosphoglycerate to produce 1,3 bisphosphoglycerate. The $\Delta G^{0'}$ for the first reaction is approximately -12 kcal/mole; for the second reaction, it is approximately $+12$ kcal/mole. Thus, although the first half reaction is extremely favorable, the second half reaction is unfavorable and would not proceed under cellular conditions. So how does the enzyme help this reaction to proceed? This is accomplished through the enzyme forming a covalent bond with the substrate, using an essential cysteine residue at the active site to form a high-energy thioester linkage during the course of the reaction

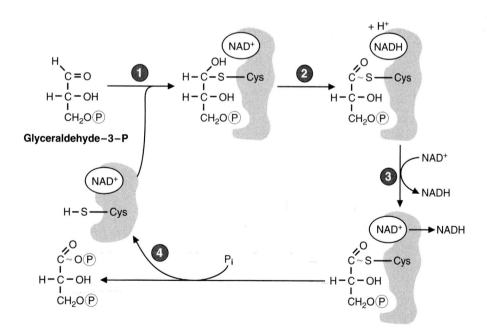

Fig. 22.17. Mechanism of the glyceraldehyde 3-phosphate dehydrogenase reaction. 1. The enzyme forms a covalent linkage with the substrate, using a cysteine group at the active site. The enzyme also contains bound NAD$^+$ close to the active site. 2. The substrate is oxidized, forming a high-energy thioester linkage (in blue), and NADH. 3. NADH has a low affinity for the enzyme and is replaced by a new molecule of NAD$^+$. 4. Inorganic phosphate attacks the thioester linkage, releasing the product 1,3 bisphosphoglycerate, and regenerating the active enzyme in a form ready to initiate another reaction.

(Fig. 22.17). Thus, the energy that would be released as heat in the oxidation of glyceraldehyde-3-P to 3-phosphoglycerate is conserved in the thioester linkage that is formed (such that the $\Delta G^{0\prime}$ of the formation of the thioester intermediate from glyceraldehyde-3-P is close to zero). Then, replacement of the sulfur with inorganic phosphate to form the final product, 1,3 bisphosphoglycerate, is relatively straightforward, as the $\Delta G^{0\prime}$ for that conversion is also close to zero, and the acylphosphate bond retains the energy from the oxidation of the aldehyde. This is one example of how covalent catalysis by an enzyme can result in the conservation of energy between different bond types.

Suggested References

Cole AS, Eastoe JE. Biochemistry and Oral Biology. 2nd Ed. Boston: Butterworth, 1988:490–519.

Robinson BH. Lacticacidemia: Disorders of pyruvate carboxylase and pyruvate dehydrogenase. In: Scriver CR, Beudet AL, Sly WS, Valle D, eds. The Metabolic and Molecular Bases of Inherited Disease, vol. 1. 8th Ed. New York: McGraw-Hill, 2001: 4451–4480.

 REVIEW QUESTIONS—CHAPTER 22

1. A major role of glycolysis is which of the following?

   (A) To synthesize glucose
   (B) To generate energy
   (C) To produce FAD(2H)
   (D) To synthesize glycogen
   (E) To use ATP to generate heat

2. Starting with glyceraldehyde 3-phosphate and synthesizing one molecule of pyruvate, the net yield of ATP and NADH would be which of the following?

   (A) 1 ATP, 1 NADH
   (B) 1 ATP, 2 NADH
   (C) 1 ATP, 4 NADH
   (D) 2 ATP, 1 NADH
   (E) 2 ATP, 2 NADH
   (F) 2 ATP, 4 NADH
   (G) 3 ATP, 1 NADH
   (H) 3 ATP, 2 NADH
   (I) 3 ATP, 4 NADH

3. When glycogen is degraded, glucose 1-phosphate is formed. Glucose 1-phosphate can then be isomerized to glucose 6-phosphate. Starting with glucose 1-phosphate, and ending with 2 molecules of pyruvate, what is the net yield of glycolysis, in terms of ATP and NADH formed?

   (A) 1 ATP, 1 NADH
   (B) 1 ATP, 2 NADH
   (C) 1 ATP, 3 NADH
   (D) 2 ATP, 1 NADH
   (E) 2 ATP, 2 NADH
   (F) 2 ATP, 3 NADH
   (G) 3 ATP, 1 NADH
   (H) 3 ATP, 2 NADH
   (I) 3 ATP, 3 NADH

4. Which of the following statements correctly describes an aspect of glycolysis?

    (A) ATP is formed by oxidative phosphorylation.
    (B) 2 ATP are used in the beginning of the pathway.
    (C) Pyruvate kinase is the rate-limiting enzyme.
    (D) One pyruvate and three CO_2 are formed from the oxidation of one glucose molecule.
    (E) The reactions take place in the matrix of the mitochondria.

5. How many moles of ATP are generated by the complete aerobic oxidation of 1 mole of glucose to 6 moles of CO_2?

    (A) 2–4
    (B) 10–12
    (C) 18–22
    (D) 30–32
    (E) 60–64

23 Oxidation of Fatty Acids and Ketone Bodies

Fatty acids are a major fuel for humans and supply our energy needs between meals and during periods of increased demand, such as exercise. During overnight fasting, fatty acids become the major fuel for cardiac muscle, skeletal muscle, and liver. The liver converts fatty acids to ketone bodies (acetoacetate and β-hydroxybutyrate), which also serve as major fuels for tissues (e.g., the gut). The brain, which does not have a significant capacity for fatty acid oxidation, can use ketone bodies as a fuel during prolonged fasting.

*The route of metabolism for a fatty acid depends somewhat on its chain length. Fatty acids are generally classified as **very-long-chain length fatty acids** (greater than C20), **long-chain fatty acids** (C12–C20), **medium-chain fatty acids** (C6–C12), and **short-chain fatty acids** (C4).*

*ATP is generated from oxidation of fatty acids in the pathway of **β-oxidation**. Between meals and during overnight fasting, **long-chain fatty acids** are released from adipose tissue triacylglycerols. They circulate through blood bound to **albumin** (Fig. 23.1). In cells, they are converted to **fatty acyl CoA** derivatives by **acyl CoA synthetases**. The activated acyl group is transported into the mitochondrial matrix bound to **carnitine**, where fatty acyl CoA is regenerated. In the pathway of **β-oxidation**, the fatty acyl group is sequentially oxidized to yield FAD(2H), NADH, and acetyl CoA. Subsequent oxidation of NADH and FAD(2H) in the electron transport chain, and oxidation of acetyl CoA to CO_2 in the TCA cycle, generates ATP from oxidative phosphorylation.*

*Many fatty acids have structures that require variations of this basic pattern. Long-chain fatty acids that are **unsaturated fatty acids** generally require additional isomerization and oxidation–reduction reactions to rearrange their double bonds during β-oxidation. Metabolism of water-soluble **medium-chain-length fatty acids** does not require carnitine and occurs only in liver. **Odd-chain-length fatty acids** undergo β-oxidation to the terminal three-carbon **propionyl CoA**, which enters the TCA cycle as succinyl CoA.*

*Fatty acids that do not readily undergo mitochondrial β-oxidation are oxidized first by alternate routes that convert them to more suitable substrates or to urinary excretion products. **Excess fatty acids** may undergo microsomal ω-**oxidation**, which converts them to **dicarboxylic acids** that appear in urine. **Very-long-chain fatty acids** (both straight chain and **branched fatty acids** such as phytanic acid) are whittled down to size in peroxisomes. **Peroxisomal α- and β-oxidiation** generates hydrogen peroxide (H_2O_2), NADH, acetyl CoA, or propionyl CoA and a short- to medium-chain-length acyl CoA. The acyl CoA products are transferred to mitochondria to complete their metabolism.*

*In the liver, much of the acetyl CoA generated from fatty acid oxidation is converted to the ketone bodies, **acetoacetate** and **β-hydroxybutyrate,** which enter the blood (see Fig. 23.1). In other tissues, these ketone bodies are converted to acetyl*

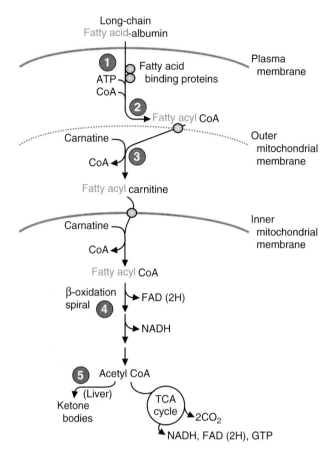

Fig. 23.1. Overview of mitochondrial long-chain fatty acid metabolism. (1) Fatty acid binding proteins (FaBP) transport fatty acids across the plasma membrane and bind them in the cytosol. (2) Fatty acyl CoA synthetase activates fatty acids to fatty acyl CoAs. (3) Carnitine transports the activated fatty acyl group into mitochondria. (4) β-oxidation generates NADH, FAD(2H), and acetyl CoA (5) In the liver, acetyl CoA is converted to ketone bodies

CoA, which is oxidized in the TCA cycle. The liver synthesizes ketone bodies but cannot use them as a fuel.

*The **rate of fatty acid oxidation** is linked to the rate of NADH, FAD(2H), and acetyl CoA oxidation, and, thus, to the rate of oxidative phosphorylation and **ATP utilization**. Additional regulation occurs through **malonyl CoA**, which inhibits formation of the fatty acyl carnitine derivatives. Fatty acids and ketone bodies are used as a fuel when their level increases in the blood, which is determined by hormonal regulation of adipose tissue lipolysis.*

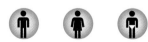

THE WAITING ROOM

Otto Shape was disappointed that he did not place in his 5-km race and has decided that short-distance running is probably not right for him. After careful consideration, he decides to train for the marathon by running 12 miles three times per week. He is now 13 pounds over his ideal weight, and he plans on losing this weight while studying for his Pharmacology finals. He considers a variety of dietary supplements to increase his endurance and selects one containing carnitine, CoQ, pantothenate, riboflavin, and creatine.

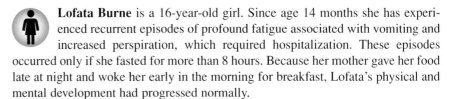

Lofata Burne is a 16-year-old girl. Since age 14 months she has experienced recurrent episodes of profound fatigue associated with vomiting and increased perspiration, which required hospitalization. These episodes occurred only if she fasted for more than 8 hours. Because her mother gave her food late at night and woke her early in the morning for breakfast, Lofata's physical and mental development had progressed normally.

On the day of admission for this episode, Lofata had missed breakfast, and by noon she was extremely fatigued, nauseated, sweaty, and limp. She was unable to hold any food in her stomach and was rushed to the hospital, where an infusion of glucose was started intravenously. Her symptoms responded dramatically to this therapy.

Her initial serum glucose level was low at 38 mg/dL (reference range for fasting serum glucose levels = 70–100). Her blood urea nitrogen (BUN) level was slightly elevated at 26 mg/dL (reference range = 8–25) as a result of vomiting, which led to a degree of dehydration. Her blood levels of liver transaminases were slightly elevated, although her liver was not palpably enlarged. Despite elevated levels of free fatty acids (4.3 mM) in the blood, blood ketone bodies were below normal.

Di Abietes, a 27-year-old woman with type 1 diabetes mellitus, had been admitted to the hospital in a ketoacidotic coma a year ago (see Chapter 4). She had been feeling drowsy and had been vomiting for 24 hours before that admission. At the time of admission, she was clinically dehydrated, her blood pressure was low, and her breathing was deep and rapid (Kussmaul breathing). Her pulse was rapid, and her breath had the odor of acetone. Her arterial blood pH was 7.08 (reference range, 7.36–7.44), and her blood ketone body levels were 15 mM (normal is approximately 0.2 mM for a person on a normal diet).

During Otto's distance running (a moderate-intensity exercise), decreases in insulin and increases in insulin counterregulatory hormones, such as epinephrine and norepinephrine, increase adipose tissue lipolysis. Thus, his muscles are being provided with a supply of fatty acids in the blood that they can use as a fuel.

Lofata Burne developed symptoms during fasting, when adipose tissue lipolysis was elevated. Under these circumstances, muscle tissue, liver, and many other tissues are oxidizing fatty acids as a fuel. After overnight fasting, approximately 60 to 70% of our energy supply is derived from the oxidation of fatty acids.

I.   FATTY ACIDS AS FUELS

The fatty acids oxidized as fuels are principally long-chain fatty acids released from adipose tissue triacylglycerol stores between meals, during overnight fasting, and during periods of increased fuel demand (e.g., during exercise). Adipose tissue triacylglycerols are derived from two sources; dietary lipids and triacylglycerols synthesized in the liver. The major fatty acids oxidized are the long-chain fatty acids, palmitate, oleate, and stearate, because they are highest in dietary lipids and are also synthesized in the human.

Between meals, a decreased insulin level and increased levels of insulin counterregulatory hormones (e.g., glucagon) activate lipolysis, and free fatty acids are transported to tissues bound to serum albumin. Within tissues, energy is derived from oxidation of fatty acids to acetyl CoA in the pathway of β-oxidation. Most of the enzymes involved in fatty acid oxidation are present as 2-3 isoenzymes, which have different but overlapping specificities for the chain length of the fatty acid. Metabolism of unsaturated fatty acids, odd-chain-length fatty acids, and medium-chain-length fatty acids requires variations of this basic pattern. The acetyl CoA produced from fatty acid oxidation is principally oxidized in the TCA cycle or converted to ketone bodies in the liver.

A.   Characteristics of Fatty Acids Used as Fuels

Fat constitutes approximately 38% of the calories in the average North American diet. Of this, more than 95% of the calories are present as triacylglycerols (3 fatty acids esterified to a glycerol backbone). During ingestion and absorption, dietary triacylglycerols are broken down into their constituents and then reassembled for transport to adipose tissue in chylomicrons (see Chapter 2). Thus, the fatty acid composition of adipose triacylglycerols varies with the type of food consumed.

The most common dietary fatty acids are the saturated long-chain fatty acids palmitate (C16) and stearate (C18), the monounsaturated fatty acid oleate (C18:1), and the polyunsaturated essential fatty acid, linoleate (C18:2) (To review fatty acid nomenclature, consult Chapter 5). Animal fat contains principally saturated and monounsaturated long-chain fatty acids, whereas vegetable oils contain linoleate and some longer-chain and polyunsaturated fatty acids. They also contain smaller amounts of branched-chain and odd-chain-length fatty acids. Medium-chain-length fatty acids are present principally in dairy fat (e.g., milk and butter), maternal milk, and vegetable oils.

Adipose tissue triacylglycerols also contain fatty acids synthesized in the liver, principally from excess calories ingested as glucose. The pathway of fatty acid synthesis generates palmitate, which can be elongated to form stearate, and unsaturated to form oleate. These fatty acids are assembled into triacylglycerols and transported to adipose tissue as the lipoprotein VLDL (very-low-density lipoprotein).

B. Transport and Activation of Long-Chain Fatty Acids

Long-chain fatty acids are hydrophobic and water insoluble. In addition, they are toxic to cells because they can disrupt the hydrophobic bonding between amino acid side chains in proteins. Consequently, they are transported in the blood and in cells bound to proteins.

1. CELLULAR UPTAKE OF LONG-CHAIN FATTY ACIDS

During fasting and other conditions of metabolic need, long-chain fatty acids are released from adipose tissue triacylglycerols by lipases. They travel in the blood bound in the hydrophobic binding pocket of albumin, the major serum protein (see Fig. 23.1).

Fatty acids enter cells both by a saturable transport process and by diffusion through the lipid plasma membrane. A fatty acid binding protein in the plasma membrane facilitates transport. An additional fatty acid binding protein binds the fatty acid intracellularly and may facilitate its transport to the mitochondrion. The free fatty acid concentration in cells is, therefore, extremely low.

2. ACTIVATION OF LONG-CHAIN FATTY ACIDS

Fatty acids must be activated to acyl CoA derivatives before they can participate in β-oxidation and other metabolic pathways (Fig. 23.2). The process of activation involves an acyl CoA synthetase (also called a thiokinase) that uses ATP energy to form the fatty acyl CoA thioester bond. In this reaction, the β bond of ATP is cleaved to form a fatty acyl AMP intermediate and pyrophosphate (PPi). Subsequent cleavage of PPi helps to drive the reaction.

The acyl CoA synthetase that activates long-chain fatty acids, 12 to 20 carbons in length, is present in three locations in the cell: the endoplasmic reticulum, outer mitochondrial membranes, and peroxisomal membranes (Table 23.1). This enzyme has no activity toward C22 or longer fatty acids, and little activity below C12. In contrast, the synthetase for activation of very-long-chain fatty acids is present in peroxisomes, and the medium-chain-length fatty acid activating enzyme is present only in the mitochondrial matrix of liver and kidney cells.

3. FATES OF FATTY ACYL COAS

Fatty acyl CoA formation, like the phosphorylation of glucose, is a prerequisite to metabolism of the fatty acid in the cell (Fig. 23.3). The multiple locations of the long-chain acyl CoA synthetase reflects the location of different metabolic routes taken by fatty acyl CoA derivatives in the cell (e.g., triacylglycerol and phospholipid synthesis

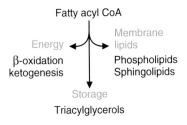

Fig. 23.3. Major metabolic routes for long-chain fatty acyl CoAs. Fatty acids are activated to acyl CoA compounds for degradation in mitochondrial β-oxidation, or incorporation into triacylglycerols or membrane lipids. When β-oxidation is blocked through an inherited enzyme deficiency, or metabolic regulation, excess fatty acids are diverted into triacylglycerol synthesis.

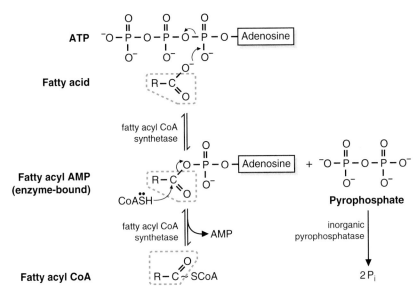

Fig. 23.2. Activation of a fatty acid by a fatty acyl CoA synthetase. The fatty acid is activated by reacting with ATP to form a high-energy fatty acyl AMP and pyrophosphate. The AMP is then exchanged for CoA. Pyrophosphate is cleaved by a pyrophosphatase.

Table 23.1. Chain-Length Specificity of Fatty Acid Activation and Oxidation Enzymes

Enzyme	Chain Length	Comments
Acyl CoA synthetases		
Very Long Chain	14–26	Only found in peroxisomes
Long Chain	12–20	Enzyme present in membranes of ER, mitochondria, and peroxisomes to facilitate different metabolic routes of acyl CoAs.
Medium Chain	6–12	Exists as many variants, present only in mitochondrial matrix of kidney and liver. Also involved in xenobiotic metabolism.
Acetyl	2–4	Present in cytoplasm and possibly mitochondrial matrix
Acyltransferases		
CPTI	12–16	Although maximum activity is for fatty acids 12–16 carbons long, it also acts on many smaller acyl CoA derivatives
Medium Chain (Octanoylcarnitine transferase)	6–12	Substrate is medium-chain acyl CoA derivatives generated during peroxisomal oxidation.
Carnitine:acetyl transferase	2	High level in skeletal muscle and heart to facilitate use of acetate as a fuel
Acyl CoA Dehydrogenases		
VLCAD	14–20	Present in inner mitochondrial membrane
LCAD	12–18	Members of same enzyme family, which also includes acyl CoA dehydrogenases for carbon skeleton of branched-chain amino acids.
MCAD	4–12	
SCAD	4–6	
Other enzymes		
Enoyl CoA hydratase, Short-chain	>4	Also called crotonase. Activity decreases with increasing chain length.
L-3-Hydroxyacyl CoA dehydrogenase, Short-Chain	4–16	Activity decreases with increasing chain length
Acetoacetyl CoA thiolase	4	Specific for acetoacetyl CoA
Trifunctional Protein	12–16	Complex of long-chain enoyl hydratase, acyl CoA dehydrogenase and a thiolase with broad specificity. Most active with longer chains.

in the endoplasmic reticulum, oxidation and plasmalogen synthesis in the peroxisome, and β-oxidation in mitochondria). In the liver and some other tissues, fatty acids that are not being used for energy generation are re-incorporated (re-esterified) into triacylglycerols.

4. TRANSPORT OF LONG-CHAIN FATTY ACIDS INTO MITOCHONDRIA

Carnitine serves as the carrier that transports activated long chain fatty acyl groups across the inner mitochondrial membrane (Fig. 23.4). Carnitine acyl transferases are able to reversibly transfer an activated fatty acyl group from CoA to the hydroxyl group of carnitine to form an acylcarnitine ester. The reaction is reversible, so that the fatty acyl CoA derivative can be regenerated from the carnitine ester.

Carnitine:palmitoyltransferase I (CPTI; also called carnitine acyltransferase I, CATI), the enzyme that transfers long-chain fatty acyl groups from CoA to carnitine, is located on the outer mitochondrial membrane (Fig. 23.5). Fatty acylcarnitine crosses the inner mitochondrial membrane with the aid of a translocase. The fatty acyl group is transferred back to CoA by a second enzyme, carnitine:palmitoyltransferase II (CPTII or CATII). The carnitine released in this reaction returns to the cytosolic side of the mitochondrial membrane by the same translocase that brings fatty acylcarnitine to the matrix side. Long-chain fatty acyl CoA, now located within the mitochondrial matrix, is a substrate for β-oxidation.

Carnitine is obtained from the diet or synthesized from the side chain of lysine by a pathway that begins in skeletal muscle, and is completed in the liver. The reactions use S-adenosylmethionine to donate methyl groups, and vitamin C (ascorbic acid) is also required for these reactions. Skeletal muscles have a

 A number of inherited diseases in the metabolism of carnitine or acylcarnitines have been described. These include defects in the following enzymes or systems: the transporter for carnitine uptake into muscle; CPT I; carnitine-acylcarnitine translocase; and CPTII. Classical CPTII deficiency, the most common of these diseases, is characterized by adolescent to adult onset of recurrent episodes of acute myoglobinuria precipitated by prolonged exercise or fasting. During these episodes, the patient is weak, and may be somewhat hypoglycemic with diminished ketosis (hypoketosis), but metabolic decompensation is not severe. Lipid deposits are found in skeletal muscles. CPK levels, and long-chain acylcarnitines are elevated in the blood. CPTII levels in fibroblasts are approximately 25% of normal. The remaining CPTII activity probably accounts for the mild effect on liver metabolism. In contrast, when CPTII deficiency has presented in infants, CPT II levels are below 10% of normal, the hypoglycemia and hypoketosis are severe, hepatomegaly occurs from the triacylglycerol deposits, and cardiomyopathy is also present.

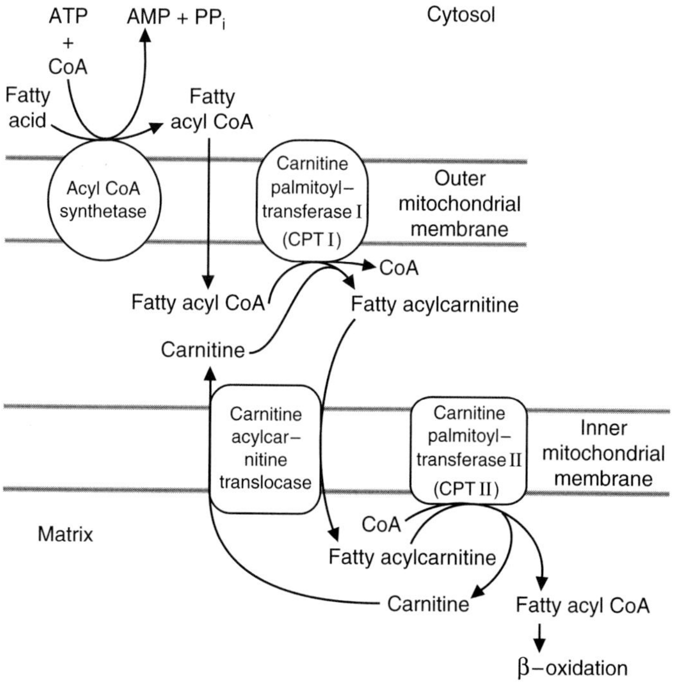

Fig. 23.5. Transport of long-chain fatty acids into mitochondria. The fatty acyl CoA crosses the outer mitochondrial membrane. Carnitine palmitoyl transferase I in the outer mitochondrial membrane transfers the fatty acyl group to carnitine and releases CoASH. The fatty acyl carnitine is translocated into the mitochondrial matrix as carnitine moves out. Carnitine palmitoyl transferase II on the inner mitochondrial membrane transfers the fatty acyl group back to CoASH, to form fatty acyl CoA in the matrix.

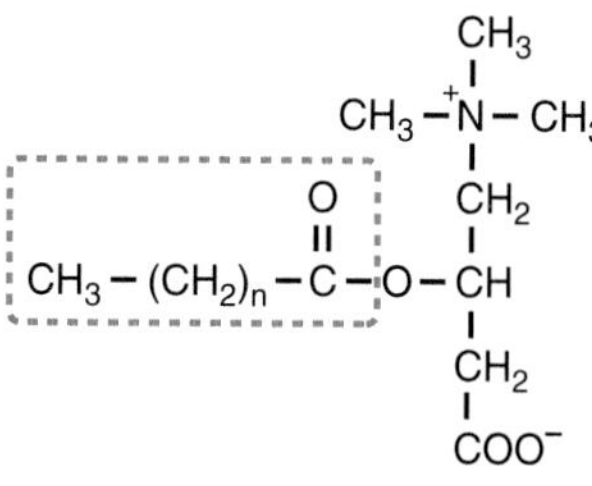

Fig. 23.4. Structure of fatty acylcarnitine. Carnitine: palmitoyl transferases catalyze the reversible transfer of a long-chain fatty acyl group from the fatty acyl CoA to the hydroxyl group of carnitine. The atoms in the dashed box originate from the fatty acyl CoA.

Fatty acylcarnitine

Otto Shape's power supplement contains carnitine. However, his body can synthesize enough carnitine to meet his needs, and his diet contains carnitine. Carnitine deficiency has been found only in infants fed a soy-based formula that was not supplemented with carnitine. His other supplements likewise probably provide no benefit, but are designed to facilitate fatty acid oxidation during exercise. Riboflavin is the vitamin precursor of FAD, which is required for acyl CoA dehydrogenases and ETFs. CoQ is synthesized in the body, but it is the recipient in the electron transport chain for electrons passed from complexes I and II and the ETFs. Some reports suggest that supplementation with pantothenate, the precursor of CoA, improves performance.

high-affinity uptake system for carnitine, and most of the carnitine in the body is stored in skeletal muscle.

C. β-Oxidation of Long-Chain Fatty Acids

The oxidation of fatty acids to acetyl CoA in the β-oxidation spiral conserves energy as FAD(2H) and NADH. FAD(2H) and NADH are oxidized in the electron transport chain, generating ATP from oxidative phosphorylation. Acetyl CoA is oxidized in the TCA cycle or converted to ketone bodies.

1.   THE β-OXIDATION SPIRAL

The fatty acid β-oxidation pathway sequentially cleaves the fatty acyl group into 2-carbon acetyl CoA units, beginning with the carboxyl end attached to CoA (Fig. 23.6). Before cleavage, the β-carbon is oxidized to a keto group in two reactions that generate NADH and FAD(2H); thus, the pathway is called β-oxidation. As each acetyl group is released, the cycle of β-oxidation and cleavage begins again, but each time the fatty acyl group is 2 carbons shorter.

There are four types of reactions in the β-oxidation pathway (Fig. 23.7). In the first step, a double bond is formed between the β- and α-carbons by an acyl CoA dehydrogenase that transfers electrons to FAD. The double bond is in the trans

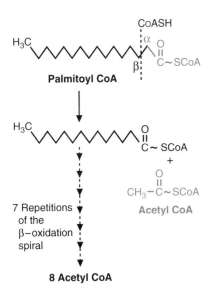

Fig. 23.6. Overview of β-oxidation. Oxidation at the β-carbon is followed by cleavage of the α—β bond, releasing acetyl CoA and a fatty acyl CoA that is two carbons shorter than the original. The carbons cleaved to form acetyl CoA are shown in blue. Successive spirals of β-oxidation completely cleave an even-chain fatty acyl CoA to acetyl CoA.

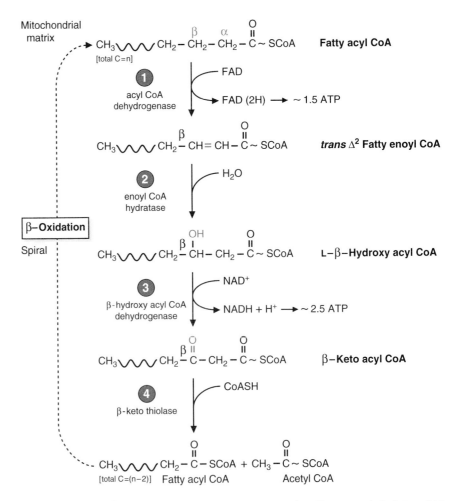

Fig. 23.7. Steps of β-oxidation . The four steps are repeated until an even-chain fatty acid is completely converted to acetyl CoA. The FAD(2H) and NADH are reoxidized by the electron transport chain, producing ATP.

configuration (a Δ^2-*trans* double bond). In the next step, an OH from water is added to the β-carbon, and an H from water is added to the β-carbon. The enzyme is called an enoyl hydratase (hydratases add the elements of water, and "ene" in a name denotes a double bond). In the third step of β-oxidation, the hydroxyl group on the β-carbon is oxidized to a ketone by a hydroxyacyl CoA dehydrogenase. In this reaction, as in the conversion of most alcohols to ketones, the electrons are transferred to NAD^+ to form NADH. In the last reaction of the sequence, the bond between the β- and α-carbons is cleaved by a reaction that attaches CoASH to the β-carbon, and acetyl CoA is released. This is a thiolytic reaction (lysis refers to breakage of the bond, and thio refers to the sulfur), catalyzed by enzymes called β-ketothiolases. The release of two carbons from the carboxyl end of the original fatty acyl CoA produces acetyl CoA and a fatty acyl CoA that is two carbons shorter than the original.

The shortened fatty acyl CoA repeats these four steps until all of its carbons are converted to acetyl CoA. β-Oxidation is, thus, a spiral rather than a cycle. In the last spiral, cleavage of the four-carbon fatty acyl CoA (butyryl CoA) produces two acetyl CoA. Thus, an even chain fatty acid such as palmitoyl CoA, which has 16 carbons, is cleaved seven times, producing 7 FAD(2H), 7 NADH, and 8 acetyl CoA.

2. ENERGY YIELD OF β-OXIDATION

Like the FAD in all flavoproteins, FAD(2H) bound to the acyl CoA dehydrogenases is oxidized back to FAD without dissociating from the protein (Fig. 23.8). Electron transfer flavoproteins (ETF) in the mitochondrial matrix accept electrons from the enzyme-bound FAD(2H) and transfer these electrons to ETF-QO (**electron transfer flavoprotein -CoQ oxidoreductase**) in the inner mitochondrial membrane. ETF-QO, also a flavoprotein, transfers the electrons to CoQ in the electron transport chain. Oxidative phosphorylation thus generates approximately 1.5 ATP for each FAD(2H) produced in the β-oxidation spiral.

The total energy yield from the oxidation of 1 mole of palmityl CoA to 8 moles of acetyl CoA is therefore 28 moles of ATP: 1.5 for each of the 7 FAD(2H), and 2.5 for each of the 7 NADH. To calculate the energy yield from oxidation of 1 mole of palmitate, two ATP need to be subtracted from the total because two high-energy phosphate bonds are cleaved when palmitate is activated to palmityl CoA.

3. CHAIN LENGTH SPECIFITY IN β-OXIDATION

The four reactions of β-oxidation are catalyzed by sets of enzymes that are each specific for fatty acids with different chain lengths (see Table 23.1). The acyl dehydrogenases, which catalyze the first step of the pathway, are part of an enzyme family that have four different ranges of specificity. The subsequent steps of the spiral use enzymes specific for long- or short-chain enoyl CoAs. Although these enzymes are structurally distinct, their specificity overlaps to some extent.

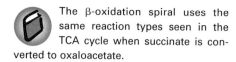

The β-oxidation spiral uses the same reaction types seen in the TCA cycle when succinate is converted to oxaloacetate.

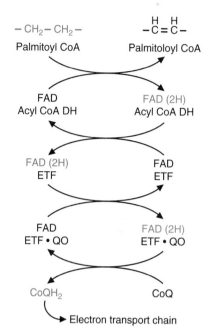

Fig. 23.8. Transfer of electrons from acyl CoA dehydrogenase to the electron transport chain. Abbreviations: ETF, electron-transferring flavoprotein; ETF-QO, electron-transferring flavoprotein–Coenzyme Q oxidoreductase.

What is the total ATP yield for the oxidation of 1 mole of palmitic acid to carbon dioxide and water?

After reviewing **Lofata Burne's** previous hospital records, a specialist suspected that Lofata's medical problems were caused by a disorder in fatty acid metabolism. A battery of tests showed that Lofata's blood contained elevated levels of several partially oxidized medium-chain fatty acids, such as octanoic acid (8:0) and 4-decenoic acid (10:1, Δ4). A urine specimen showed an increase in organic acid metabolites of medium-chain fatty acids containing 6 to 10 carbons, including medium-chain acylcarnitine derivatives. The profile of acylcarnitine species in the urine was characteristic of a genetically determined medium-chain acyl CoA dehydrogenase (MCAD) deficiency. In this disease, long-chain fatty acids are metabolized by β-oxidation to a medium-chain-length acyl CoA, such as octanoyl CoA. Because further oxidation of this compound is blocked in MCAD deficiency, the medium chain acyl group is transferred back to carnitine. These acylcarnitines are water soluble and appear in blood and urine. The specific enzyme deficiency was demonstrated in cultured fibroblasts from Lofata's skin as well as in her circulating monocytic leukocytes.

In LCAD deficiency, fatty acylcarnitines accumulate in the blood. Those containing 14 carbons predominate. However, these do not appear in the urine.

A: Palmitic acid is 16 carbons long, with no double bonds, so it requires 7 oxidation spirals to be completely converted to acetyl-CoA. After 7 spirals, there are 7 FAD(2H), 7 NADH, and 8 acetyl-CoA. Each NADH yields 2.5 ATP, each FAD(2H) yields 1.5 ATP, and each acetyl-CoA yields 10 ATP as it is processed around the TCA cycle. This then yields 17.5 + 10.5 + 80.5 = 108 ATP. However, activation of palmitic acid to palmityl-CoA requires two high-energy bonds, so the net yield is 108 − 2, or 106 moles of ATP.

Linoleate, although high in the diet, cannot be synthesized in the human and is an essential fatty acid. It is required for formation of arachidonate, which is present in plasma lipids, and is used for eicosanoid synthesis. Therefore, only a portion of the linoleate pool is rapidly oxidized.

The medium-chain-length acyl CoA synthetase has a broad range of specificity for compounds of approximately the same size that contain a carboxyl group, such as drugs (salicylate, from aspirin metabolism, and valproate, which is used to treat epileptic seizures), or benzoate, a common component of plants. Once the drug acyl CoA is formed, the acyl group is conjugated with glycine to form a urinary excretion product. With certain disorders of fatty acid oxidation, medium- and short-chain fatty acylglycines may appear in the urine, together with acylcarnitines or dicarboxylic acids.

As the fatty acyl chains are shortened by consecutive cleavage of two acetyl units, they are transferred from enzymes that act on longer chains to those that act on shorter chains. Medium- or short-chain fatty acyl CoAs that may be formed from dietary fatty acids, or transferred from peroxisomes, enter the spiral at the enzyme most active for fatty acids of their chain length

4. OXIDATION OF UNSATURATED FATTY ACIDS

Approximately one half of the fatty acids in the human diet are unsaturated, containing cis double bonds, with oleate (C18:1, Δ^9) and linoleate ($18:2,\Delta^{9,12}$) being the most common. In β-oxidation of saturated fatty acids, a trans double bond is created between the 2nd and 3rd (α and β) carbons. For unsaturated fatty acids to undergo the β-oxidation spiral, their *cis* double bonds must be isomerized to *trans* double bonds that will end up between the 2nd and 3rd carbons during β-oxidation, or the double bond must be reduced. The process is illustrated for the polyunsaturated fatty acid linoleate in Fig. 23.9. Linoleate undergoes β-oxidation until one double bond is between carbons 3 and 4 near the carboxyl end of the fatty acyl chain, and the other is between carbons 6 and 7. An isomerase moves the double bond from the 3,4 position so that it is *trans* and in the 2,3 position, and β-oxidation continues. When a conjugated pair of double bonds is formed (two double bonds separated by one single bond) at positions 2 and 4, an NADPH-dependent reductase reduces the pair to one trans double bond at position 3. Then isomerization and β-oxidation resume.

In oleate (C18:1, Δ^9), there is only one double bond between carbons 9 and 10. It is handled by an isomerization reaction similar to that shown for the double bond at position 9 of linoleate.

5. ODD-CHAIN-LENGTH FATTY ACIDS

Fatty acids containing an odd number of carbon atoms undergo β-oxidation, producing acetyl CoA, until the last spiral, when five carbons remain in the fatty acyl CoA. In this case, cleavage by thiolase produces acetyl CoA and a three-carbon fatty acyl CoA, propionyl CoA (Fig. 23.10). Carboxylation of propionyl CoA yields methylmalonyl CoA, which is ultimately converted to succinyl CoA in a vitamin B12–dependent reaction (Fig. 23.11). Propionyl CoA also arises from the oxidation of branched chain amino acids.

The propionyl CoA to succinyl CoA pathway is a major anaplerotic route for the TCA cycle and is used in the degradation of valine, isoleucine, and a number of other compounds. In the liver, this route provides precursors of oxaloacetate, which is converted to glucose. Thus, this small proportion of the odd-carbon-number fatty acid chain can be converted to glucose. In contrast, the acetyl CoA formed from β-oxidation of even-chain number fatty acids in the liver either enters the TCA cycle, where it is principally oxidized to CO_2, or is converted to ketone bodies.

D. Oxidation of Medium-Chain-Length Fatty Acids

Dietary medium-chain-length fatty acids are more water soluble than long-chain fatty acids and are not stored in adipose triacylglyce. After a meal, they enter the blood and pass into the portal vein to the liver. In the liver, they enter the mitochondrial matrix by the monocarboxylate transporter and are activated to acyl CoA derivatives in the mitochondrial matrix (see Fig. 23.1). Medium-chain-length acyl CoAs, like long-chain acyl CoAs, are oxidized to acetyl CoA via the β-oxidation spiral. Medium-chain acyl CoAs also can arise from the peroxisomal oxidation pathway.

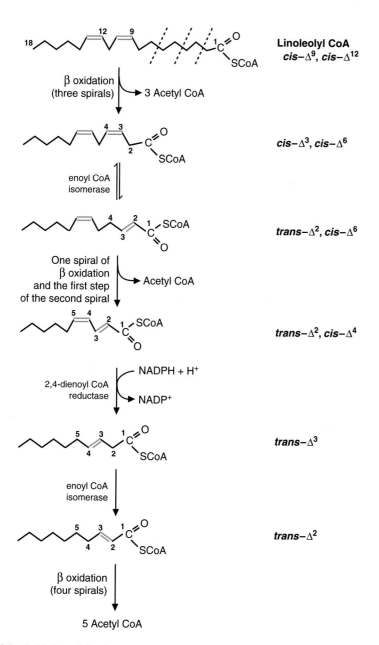

Fig. 23.9. Oxidation of linoleate. After three spirals of β-oxidation (dashed lines), there is now a 3,4 cis double bond and a 6,7 cis double bond. The 3,4 cis double bond is isomerized to a 2,3-trans double bond, which is in the proper configuration for the normal enzymes to act. One spiral of β-oxidation occurs, plus the first step of a second spiral. A reductase that uses NADPH now converts these two double bonds (between carbons 2 and 3 and carbons 4 and 5) to one double bond between carbons 3 and 4 in a trans configuration. The isomerase (which can act on double bonds that are in either the cis or the trans configuration) moves this double bond to the 2,3-trans position, and β-oxidation can resume.

E. Regulation of β-Oxidation

Fatty acids are used as fuels principally when they are released from adipose tissue triacylglycerols in response to hormones that signal fasting or increased demand. Many tissues, such as muscle and kidney, oxidize fatty acids completely to CO_2 and H_2O. In these tissues, the acetyl CoA produced by β-oxidation enters the TCA cycle. The FAD(2H) and the NADH from β-oxidation and the TCA cycle are

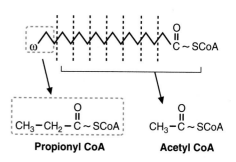

Fig. 23.10. Formation of propionyl CoA from odd-chain fatty acids. Successive spirals of β-oxidation cleave each of the bonds marked with dashed lines, producing acetyl CoA except for the three carbons at the ω-end, which produce propionyl CoA.

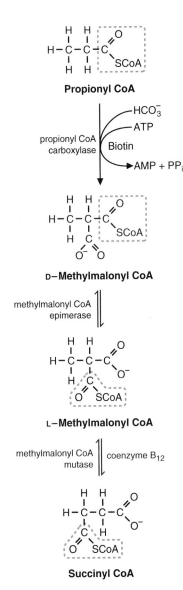

Fig. 23.11. Conversion of propionyl CoA to succinyl CoA. Succinyl CoA, an intermediate of the TCA cycle, can form malate, which can be converted to glucose in the liver through the process of gluconeogenesis. Certain amino acids also form glucose by this route (see Chapter 39).

 As **Otto Shape** runs, his skeletal muscles increase their use of ATP and their rate of fuel oxidation. Fatty acid oxidation is accelerated by the increased rate of the electron transport chain. As ATP is used and AMP increases, an AMP-dependent protein kinase acts to facilitate fuel utilization and maintain ATP homeostasis. Phosphorylation of acetyl CoA carboxylase results in a decreased level of malonyl CoA and increased activity of carnitine: palmitoyl CoA transferase I. At the same time, AMP-dependent protein kinase facilitates the recruitment of glucose transporters into the plasma membrane of skeletal muscle, thereby increasing the rate of glucose uptake. AMP and hormonal signals also increase the supply of glucose 6-P from glycogenolysis. Thus, his muscles are supplied with more fuel, and all the oxidative pathways are accelerated.

reoxidized by the electron transport chain, and ATP is generated. The process of β-oxidation is regulated by the cells' requirements for energy (i.e., by the levels of ATP and NADH), because fatty acids cannot be oxidized any faster than NADH and FAD(2H) are reoxidized in the electron transport chain.

Fatty acid oxidation also may be restricted by the mitochondrial CoASH pool size. Acetyl CoASH units must enter the TCA cycle or another metabolic pathway to regenerate CoASH required for formation of the fatty acyl CoA derivative from fatty acyl carnitine.

An additional type of regulation occurs at carnitine:palmitoyltransferase I (CPTI). Carnitine:palmitoyltransferase I is inhibited by malonyl CoA, which is synthesized in the cytosol of many tissues by acetyl CoA carboxylase (Fig. 23.12). Acetyl CoA carboxylase is regulated by a number of different mechanisms, some of which are tissue dependent. In skeletal muscles and liver, it is inhibited when phosphorylated by protein kinase B, an AMP-dependent protein kinase. Thus, during exercise when AMP levels increase, AMP-dependent protein kinase phosphorylates acetyl CoA carboxylase, which becomes inactive. Consequently, malonyl CoA levels decrease, carnitine:palmitoyltransferase I is activated, and the β-oxidation of fatty acids is able to restore ATP homeostasis and decrease AMP levels. In liver, in addition to the regulation by the AMP-dependent protein kinase acetyl CoA carboxylase is activated by insulin-dependent mechanisms, which promotes the conversion of malonyl CoA to palmitate in the fatty acid synthesis pathway. Thus, in the liver, malonyl CoA inhibition of CPTI prevents newly synthesized fatty acids from being oxidized.

β-oxidation is strictly an aerobic pathway, dependent on oxygen, a good blood supply, and adequate levels of mitochondria. Tissues that lack mitochondria, such

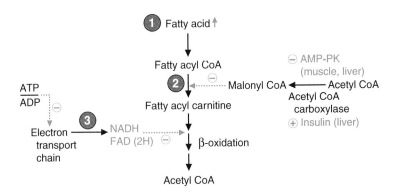

Fig. 23.12. Regulation of β-oxidation. (1) Hormones control the supply of fatty acids in the blood. (2) Carnitine:palmitoyl transferase I is inhibited by malonyl CoA, which is synthesized by acetyl CoA carboxylase (ACC). AMP-PK is the AMP-dependent protein kinase. (3) The rate of ATP utilization controls the rate of the electron transport chain, which regulates the oxidative enzymes of β-oxidation and the TCA cycle.

as red blood cells, cannot oxidize fatty acids by β-oxidation. Fatty acids also do not serve as a significant fuel for the brain. They are not used by adipocytes, whose function is to store triacylglycerols to provide a fuel for other tissues. Those tissues that do not use fatty acids as a fuel, or use them only to a limited extent, are able to use ketone bodies instead.

II. ALTERNATE ROUTES OF FATTY ACID OXIDATION

Fatty acids that are not readily oxidized by the enzymes of β-oxidation enter alternate pathways of oxidation, including peroxisomal β- and α-oxidation and microsomal ω-oxidation. The function of these pathways is to convert as much as possible of the unusual fatty acids to compounds that can be used as fuels or biosynthetic precursors, and to convert the remainder to compounds that can be excreted in bile or urine. During prolonged fasting, fatty acids released from adipose triacylglycerols may enter the ω-oxidation or peroxisomal β-oxidation pathway, even though they have a normal composition. These pathways not only use fatty acids, but they act on xenobiotic carboxylic acids that are large hydrophobic molecules resembling fatty acids.

A. Peroxisomal Oxidation of Fatty Acids

A small proportion of our diet consists of very-long-chain fatty acids (20 or more carbons) or branched-chain fatty acids arising from degradative products of chlorophyll. Very-long-chain fatty acid synthesis also occurs within the body, especially in cells of the brain and nervous system, which incorporate them into the sphingolipids of myelin. These fatty acids are oxidized by peroxisomal β- and α-oxidation pathways, which are essentially chain-shortening pathways.

1. VERY-LONG-CHAIN FATTY ACIDS

Very-long-chain fatty acids of 24 to 26 carbons are oxidized exclusively in peroxisomes by a sequence of reactions similar to mitochondrial β-oxidation in that they generate acetyl CoA and NADH. However, the peroxisomal oxidation of straight-chain fatty acids stops when the chain reaches 4 to 6 carbons in length. Some of the long-chain fatty acids also may be oxidized by this route.

The long-chain fatty acyl CoA synthetase is present in the peroxisomal membrane, and the acyl CoA derivatives enter the peroxisome by a transporter that does not require carnitine. The first enzyme of peroxisomal β-oxidation is an oxidase, which donates electrons directly to molecular oxygen and produces hydrogen peroxide (H_2O_2) (Fig.23.13). (In contrast, the first enzyme of mitochondrial β-oxidation is a dehydrogenase that contains FAD and transfers the electrons to the electron transport chain via ETF.) Thus, the first enzyme of peroxisomal oxidation is not linked to energy production. The three remaining steps of β-oxidation are catalyzed by enoyl-CoA hydratase, hydroxyacyl CoA dehydrogenase, and thiolase, enzymes with activities similar to those found in mitochondrial β-oxidation, but coded for by different genes. Thus, one NADH and one acetyl CoA are generated for each turn of the spiral. The peroxisomal β-oxidation spiral continues generating acetyl CoA until a medium-chain acyl CoA, which may be as short as butyryl CoA, is produced (Fig. 23.14).

Within the peroxisome, the acetyl groups can be transferred from CoA to carnitine by an acetylcarnitine transferase, or they can enter the cytosol. A similar reaction converts medium-chain-length acyl CoAs and the short-chain butyryl CoA to acyl carnitine derivatives. These acylcarnitines diffuse from the peroxisome to the mitochondria, pass through the outer mitochondrial membrane, and are transported through the inner mitochondrial membrane via the carnitine translocase system.

Xenobiotic: a term used to cover all organic compounds that are foreign to an organism. This can also include naturally occurring compounds that are administered by alternate routes or at unusual concentrations. Drugs can be considered xenobiotics.

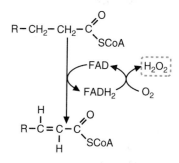

Fig. 23.13. Oxidation of fatty acids in peroxisomes. The first step of β-oxidation is catalyzed by an FAD-containing oxidase. The electrons are transferred from FAD(2H) to O_2, which is reduced to hydrogen peroxide (H_2O_2).

A number of inherited deficiencies of peroxisomal enzymes have been described. Zellweger's syndrome, which results from defective peroxisomal biogenesis, leads to complex developmental and metabolic phenotypes affecting principally the liver and the brain. One of the metabolic characteristics of these diseases is an elevation of C26:0, and C26:1 fatty acid levels in plasma. Refsum's disease is caused by a deficiency in a single peroxisomal enzyme, the phytanoyl CoA hydroxylase that carries out α-oxidation of phytanic acid. Symptoms include retinitis pigmentosa, cerebellar ataxia, and chronic polyneuropathy. Because phytanic acid is obtained solely from the diet, placing patients on a low–phytanic acid diet has resulted in marked improvement.

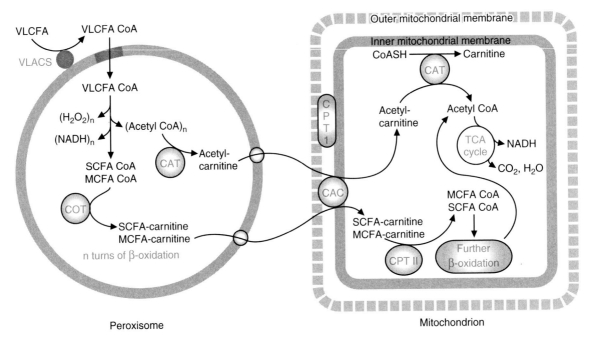

Fig. 23.14. Chain-shortening by peroxisomal β-oxidation. Abbreviations: VLCFA, very-long-chain fatty acyl; VLACS, very-long-chain acyl-CoA synthetase; MCFA, medium-chain fatty acyl; SCFA, short-chain fatty acyl; CAT, carnitine:acetyltransferase; COT, carnitine:octanoyltransferase; CAC: carnitine:acylcarnitine carrier; CPT1, carnitine: palmitoyltransferase 1; CPT2, carnitine: palmityltransferase 2; OMM, outer mitochondrial membrane; IMM, inner mitochondrial membrane. Very-long-chain fatty acyl CoAs and some long-chain fatty acyl CoAs are oxidized in peroxisomes through n cycles of β-oxidation to the stage of a short- to medium-chain fatty acyl CoA. These short to medium fatty acyl CoAs are converted to carnitine derivatives by COT or CAT in the peroxisomes. In the mitochondria, SCFA-carnitine are converted back to acyl CoA derivatives by either CPT2 or CAT.

They are converted back to acyl CoAs by carnitine: acyltransferases appropriate for their chain length and enter the normal pathways for β-oxidation and acetyl CoA metabolism. The electrons from NADH and acetyl CoA can also pass from the peroxisome to the cytosol. The export of NADH-containing electrons occurs through use of a shuttle system similar to those described for NADH electron transfer into the mitochondria.

Peroxisomes are present in almost every cell type and contain many degradative enzymes, in addition to fatty acyl CoA oxidase, that generate hydrogen peroxide. H_2O_2 can generate toxic free radicals. Thus, these enzymes are confined to peroxisomes, where the H_2O_2 can be neutralized by the free radical defense enzyme, catalase. Catalase converts H_2O_2 to water and O_2.

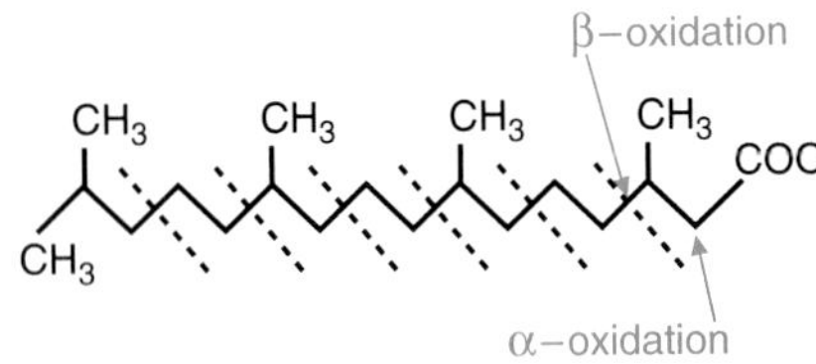

2. LONG-CHAIN BRANCHED-CHAIN FATTY ACIDS

Two of the most common branched-chain fatty acids in the diet are phytanic acid and pristanic acid, which are degradation products of chlorophyll and thus are consumed in green vegetables (Fig.23.15). Animals do not synthesize branched-chain fatty acids. These two multi-methylated fatty acids are oxidized in peroxisomes to the level of a branched C8 fatty acid, which is then transferred to mitochondria. The pathway thus is similar to that for the oxidation of straight very-long-chain fatty acids.

Phytanic acid, a multi-methylated C20 fatty acid, is first oxidized to pristanic acid using the α-oxidation pathway (see Fig.23.15). Phytanic acid hydroxylase introduces a hydroxyl group on the α-carbon, which is then oxidized to a carboxyl group with release of the original carboxyl group as CO_2. By shortening the fatty acid by one carbon, the methyl groups will appear on the α-carbon rather than the

Fig. 23.15. Oxidation of phytanic acid. A peroxisomal α-hydroxylase oxidizes the α-carbon, and its subsequent oxidation to a carboxyl group releases the carboxyl carbon as CO_2. Subsequent spirals of peroxisomal β-oxidation alternately release propionyl and acetyl CoA. At a chain length of approximately 8 carbons, the remaining branched fatty acid is transferred to mitochondria as a medium-chain carnitine derivative.

β-carbon during the β-oxidation spiral, and can no longer interfere with oxidation of the β-carbon. Peroxisomal β-oxidation thus can proceed normally, releasing propionyl CoA and acetyl CoA with alternate turns of the spiral. When a medium chain length of approximately eight carbons is reached, the fatty acid is transferred to the mitochondrion as a carnitine derivative, and β-oxidation is resumed.

B. ω-Oxidation of Fatty Acids

Fatty acids also may be oxidized at the ω-carbon of the chain (the terminal methyl group) by enzymes in the endoplasmic reticulum (Fig. 23.16). The ω-methyl group is first oxidized to an alcohol by an enzyme that uses cytochrome P450, molecular oxygen, and NADPH. Dehydrogenases convert the alcohol group to a carboxylic acid. The dicarboxylic acids produced by ω-oxidation can undergo β-oxidation, forming compounds with 6 to 10 carbons that are water-soluble. Such compounds may then enter blood, be oxidized as medium-chain fatty acids, or be excreted in urine as medium-chain dicarboxylic acids.

The pathways of peroxisomal α and β-oxidation, and microsomal ω-oxidation, are not feedback regulated. These pathways function to decrease levels of water-insoluble fatty acids or of xenobiotic compounds with a fatty acid–like structure that would become toxic to cells at high concentrations. Thus, their rate is regulated by the availability of substrate.

III. METABOLISM OF KETONE BODIES

Overall, fatty acids released from adipose triacylglycerols serve as the major fuel for the body during fasting. These fatty acids are completely oxidized to CO_2 and H_2O by some tissues. In the liver, much of the acetyl CoA generated from β-oxidation of fatty acids is used for synthesis of the ketone bodies acetoacetate and β-hydroxybutyrate, which enter the blood (Fig. 23.17). In skeletal muscles and other

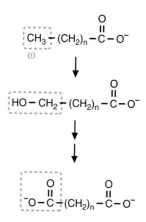

Fig. 23.16. ω-Oxidation of fatty acids converts them to dicarboxylic acids.

Normally, ω-oxidation is a minor process. However, in conditions that interfere with β-oxidation (such as carnitine deficiency or deficiency in an enzyme of β-oxidation), ω-oxidation produces dicarboxylic acids in increased amounts. These dicarboxylic acids are excreted in the urine.

Lofata Burne was excreting dicarboxylic acids in her urine, particularly adipic acid (which has 6 carbons) and suberic acid (which has 8 carbons).

-OOC—CH2—CH2—CH2—CH2—COO-
Adipic acid
-OOC—CH2—CH2—CH2—CH2—CH2—CH2—COO-Suberic acid

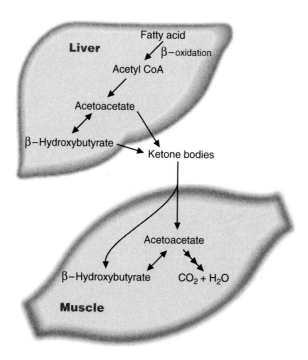

Fig. 23.17. The ketone bodies, acetoacetate and β-hydroxybutyrate, are synthesized in the liver. Their principle fate is conversion back to acetyl CoA and oxidation in the TCA cycle in other tissues.

tissues, these ketone bodies are converted back to acetyl CoA, which is oxidized in the TCA cycle with generation of ATP. An alternate fate of acetoacetate in tissues is the formation of cytosolic acetyl CoA.

A. Synthesis of Ketone Bodies

In the liver, ketone bodies are synthesized in the mitochondrial matrix from acetyl CoA generated from fatty acid oxidation (Fig. 23.18). The thiolase reaction of fatty acid oxidation, which converts acetoacetyl CoA to two molecules of acetyl CoA, is a reversible reaction, although formation of acetoacetyl-CoA is not the favored direction. It can, thus, when acetyl-CoA levels are high, generate acetoacetyl CoA

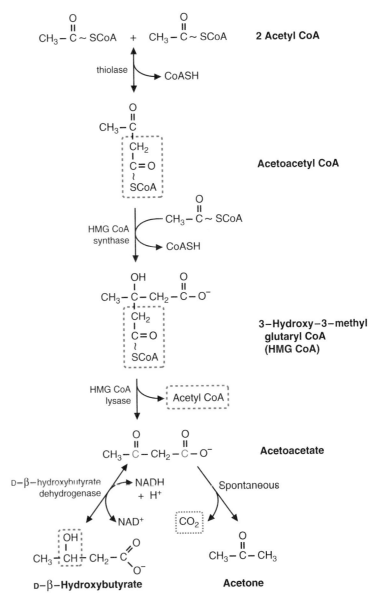

Fig. 23.18. Synthesis of the ketone bodies acetoacetate, β-hydroxybutyrate, and acetone. The portion of HMG-CoA shown in blue is released as acetyl CoA, and the remainder of the molecule forms acetoacetate. Acetoacetate is reduced to β-hydroxybutyrate or decarboxylated to acetone. Note that the dehydrogenase that interconverts acetoacetate and β-hydroxybutyrate is specific for the D-isomer. Thus, it differs from the dehydrogenases of β-oxidation, which act on 3-hydroxy acyl CoA derivatives and is specific for the L-isomer.

for ketone body synthesis. The acetoacetyl CoA will react with acetyl CoA to produce 3-hydroxy-3-methylglutaryl CoA (HMG-CoA). The enzyme that catalyzes this reaction is HMG-CoA synthase. In the next reaction of the pathway, HMG-CoA lyase catalyzes the cleavage of HMG-CoA to form acetyl CoA and acetoacetate.

Acetoacetate can directly enter the blood or it can be reduced by β-hydroxybutyrate dehydrogenase to β-hydroxybutyrate, which enters the blood (see Fig. 23.18). This dehydrogenase reaction is readily reversible and interconverts these two ketone bodies, which exist in an equilibrium ratio determined by the NADH/NAD$^+$ ratio of the mitochondrial matrix. Under normal conditions, the ratio of β-hydroxybutyrate to acetoacetate in the blood is approximately 1:1.

An alternate fate of acetoacetate is spontaneous decarboxylation, a nonenzymatic reaction that cleaves acetoacetate into CO2 and acetone (see Fig. 23.18). Because acetone is volatile, it is expired by the lungs. A small amount of acetone may be further metabolized in the body.

B. Oxidation of Ketone Bodies as Fuels

Acetoacetate and β-hydroxybutyrate can be oxidized as fuels in most tissues, including skeletal muscle, brain, certain cells of the kidney, and cells of the intestinal mucosa. Cells transport both acetoacetate and β-hydroxybutyrate from the circulating blood into the cytosol, and into the mitochondrial matrix. Here β-hydroxybutyrate is oxidized back to acetoacetate by β-hydroxybutyrate dehydrogenase. This reaction produces NADH. Subsequent steps convert acetoacetate to acetyl CoA (Fig. 23.19).

In mitochondria, acetoacetate is activated to acetoacetyl CoA by succinyl CoA:acetoacetate CoA transferase. As the name suggests, CoA is transferred from succinyl CoA, a TCA cycle intermediate, to acetoacetate. Although the liver produces ketone bodies, it does not use them, because this thiotransferase enzyme is not present in sufficient quantity.

Acetoacetyl CoA is cleaved to two molecules of acetyl CoA by acetoacetyl CoA thiolase, the same enzyme involved in β-oxidation. The principal fate of this acetyl CoA is oxidation in the TCA cycle.

The energy yield from oxidation of acetoacetate is equivalent to the yield for oxidation of 2 acetyl CoA in the TCA cycle (20 ATP) minus the energy for activation of acetoacetate (1 ATP). The energy of activation is calculated at one high-energy phosphate bond, because succinyl CoA is normally converted to succinate in the TCA cycle, with generation of one molecule of GTP (the energy equivalent of ATP). However, when the high-energy thioester bond of succinyl CoA is transferred to acetoacetate, succinate is produced without the generation of this GTP. Oxidation of β-hydroxybutyrate generates one additional NADH. Therefore the net energy yield from one molecule of β-hydroxybutyrate is approximately 21.5 molecules of ATP.

C. Alternate Pathways of Ketone Body Metabolism

Although fatty acid oxidation is usually the major source of ketone bodies, they also can be generated from the catabolism of certain amino acids: leucine, isoleucine, lysine, tryptophan, phenylalanine, and tyrosine. These amino acids are called ketogenic amino acids because their carbon skeleton is catabolized to acetyl CoA or acetoacetyl CoA, which may enter the pathway of ketone body synthesis in liver. Leucine and isoleucine also form acetyl CoA and acetoacetyl CoA in other tissues, as well as the liver.

Acetoacetate can be activated to acetoacetyl CoA in the cytosol by an enzyme similar to the acyl CoA synthetases. This acetoacetyl CoA can be used directly in cholesterol synthesis. It also can be cleaved to two molecules of acetyl CoA by a cytosolic thiolase. Cytosolic acetyl CoA is required for processes such as acetylcholine synthesis in neuronal cells.

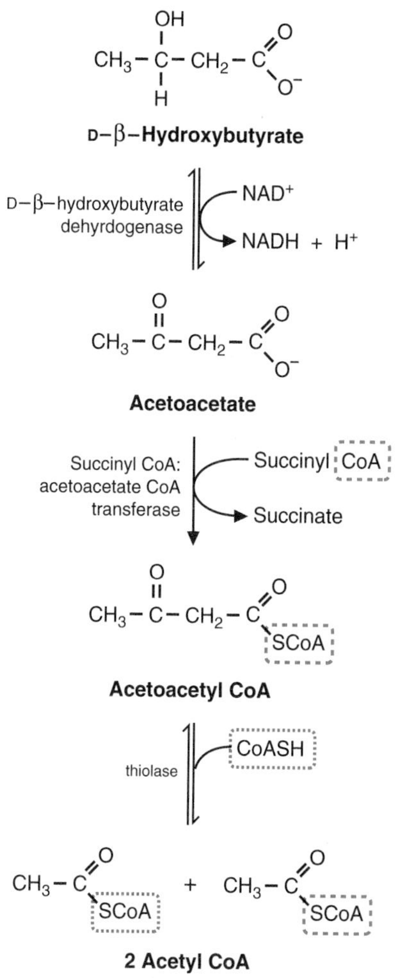

Fig. 23.19. Oxidation of ketone bodies. β-Hydroxybutyrate is oxidized to acetoacetate, which is activated by accepting a CoA group from succinyl CoA. Acetoacetyl CoA is cleaved to two acetyl CoA, which enter the TCA cycle and are oxidized.

Ketogenic diets, which are high-fat diets with a 3:1 ratio of lipid to carbohydrate, are being used to reduce the frequency of epileptic seizures in children. The reason for its effectiveness in the treatment of epilepsy is not known. Ketogenic diets are also used to treat children with pyruvate dehydrogenase deficiency. Ketone bodies can be used as a fuel by the brain in the absence of pyruvate dehydrogenase. They also can provide a source of cytosolic acetyl CoA for acetylcholine synthesis. They often contain medium-chain triglycerides, which induce ketosis more effectively than long-chain triglycerides.

IV. THE ROLE OF FATTY ACIDS AND KETONE BODIES IN FUEL HOMEOSTASIS

Fatty acids are used as fuels whenever fatty acid levels are elevated in the blood, that is, during fasting, starvation, as a result of a high-fat, low-carbohydrate diet, or during long-term low- to mild-intensity exercise. Under these conditions, a decrease in insulin and increased levels of glucagon, epinephrine, or other hormones stimulate adipose tissue lipolysis. Fatty acids begin to increase in the blood approximately 3 to 4 hours after a meal and progressively increase with time of fasting up to approximately 2 to 3 days (Fig. 23.20). In the liver, the rate of ketone body synthesis increases as the supply of fatty acids increases. However, the blood level of ketone bodies continues to increase, presumably because their utilization by skeletal muscles decreases.

After 2 to 3 days of starvation, ketone bodies rise to a level in the blood that enables them to enter brain cells, where they are oxidized, thereby reducing the amount of glucose required by the brain. During prolonged fasting, they may supply as much as two thirds of the energy requirements of the brain. The reduction in glucose requirements spares skeletal muscle protein, which is a major source of amino acid precursors for hepatic glucose synthesis from gluconeogenesis.

A. Preferential Utilization of Fatty Acids

As fatty acids increase in the blood, they are used by skeletal muscles and certain other tissues in preference to glucose. Fatty acid oxidation generates NADH and FAD(2H) through both β-oxidation and the TCA cycle, resulting in relatively high NADH/NAD$^+$ ratios, acetyl CoA concentration, and ATP/ADP or ATP/AMP levels. In skeletal muscles, AMP-dependent protein kinase (see Section I.E.) adjusts the concentration of malonyl CoA so that CPT1 and β-oxidation operate at a rate that is able to sustain ATP homeostasis. With adequate levels of ATP obtained from fatty acid (or ketone body) oxidation, the rate of glycolysis is decreased. The activity of the regulatory enzymes in glycolysis and the TCA cycle (pyruvate dehydrogenase and PFK-1) are decreased by the changes in concentration of their allosteric regulators (ADP, an activator of PDH,

Children are more prone to ketosis than adults because their body enters the fasting state more rapidly. Their bodies use more energy per unit mass (because their muscle-to-adipose-tissue ratio is higher), and liver glycogen stores are depleted faster (the ratio of their brain mass to liver mass is higher). In children, blood ketone body levels reach 2 mM in 24 hours; in adults, it takes more than 3 days to reach this level. Mild pediatric infections causing anorexia and vomiting are the commonest cause of ketosis in children. Mild ketosis is observed in children after prolonged exercise, perhaps attributable to an abrupt decrease in muscular use of fatty acids liberated during exercise. The liver then oxidizes these fatty acids and produces ketone bodies.

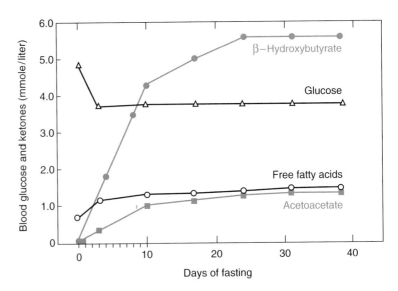

Fig. 23.20. Levels of ketone bodies in the blood at various times during fasting. Glucose levels remain relatively constant, as do levels of fatty acids. Ketone body levels, however, increase markedly, rising to levels at which they can be used by the brain and other nervous tissue. From Cahill GF Jr, Aoki TT. Med Times 1970;98:109.

decreases in concentration; NADH, and acetyl CoA, inhibitors of PDH, are increased in concentration under these conditions; and ATP and citrate, inhibitors of PFK-1, are increased in concentration). As a consequence, glucose-6-P accumulates. Glucose-6-P inhibits hexokinase, thereby decreasing the rate of entry of glucose into glycolysis, and its uptake from the blood. In skeletal muscles, this pattern of fuel metabolism is facilitated by the decrease in insulin concentration (see Chapter 36). Preferential utilization of fatty acids does not, however, restrict the ability of glycolysis to respond to an increase in AMP or ADP levels, such as might occur during exercise or oxygen limitation.

B. Tissues That Use Ketone Bodies

Skeletal muscles, the heart, the liver, and many other tissues use fatty acids as their major fuel during fasting and other conditions that increase fatty acids in the blood. However, a number of other tissues (or cell types), such as the brain, use ketone bodies to a greater extent. For example, cells of the intestinal muscosa, which transport fatty acids from the intestine to the blood, use ketone bodies and amino acids during starvation, rather than fatty acids. Adipocytes, which store fatty acids in triacylglycerols, do not use fatty acids as a fuel during fasting but can use ketone bodies. Ketone bodies cross the placenta, and can be used by the fetus. Almost all tissues and cell types, with the exception of liver and red blood cells, are able to use ketone bodies as fuels.

C. Regulation of Ketone Body Synthesis

A number of events, in addition to the increased supply of fatty acids from adipose triacylglycerols, promote hepatic ketone body synthesis during fasting. The decreased insulin/glucagon ratio results in inhibition of acetyl CoA carboxylase and decreased malonyl CoA levels, which activates CPTI, thereby allowing fatty acyl CoA to enter the pathway of β-oxidation. (Fig. 23.21). When oxidation of fatty acyl CoA to acetyl CoA generates enough NADH and FAD(2H) to supply the ATP needs of the liver, acetyl CoA is diverted from the TCA cycle into ketogenesis and oxaloacetate in the TCA cycle is diverted toward malate and into glucose synthesis (gluconeogenesis). This pattern is regulated by the NADH/NAD$^+$ ratio, which is relatively high during β-oxidation. As the length of time of fasting continues, increased transcription of the gene for mitochondrial HMG-CoA synthase facilitates high rates of ketone body production. Although the liver has been described as "altruistic" because it provides ketone bodies for other tissues, it is simply getting rid of fuel that it does not need.

 The level of total ketone bodies in **Lofata Burne's** blood greatly exceeds normal fasting levels and the mild ketosis produced during exercise. In a person on a normal mealtime schedule, total blood ketone bodies rarely exceed 0.2 mM. During prolonged fasting, they may rise to 4 to 5 mM. Levels above 7 mM are considered evidence of ketoacidosis, because the acid produced must reach this level to exceed the bicarbonate buffer system in the blood and compensatory respiration (Kussmaul's respiration) (see Chapter 4).

 Why can't red blood cells use ketone bodies for energy?

CLINICAL COMMENTS

As **Otto Shape** runs, he increases the rate at which his muscles oxidize all fuels. The increased rate of ATP utilization stimulates the electron transport chain, which oxidizes NADH and FAD(2H) much faster, thereby increasing the rate at which fatty acids are oxidized. During exercise, he also uses muscle glycogen stores, which contribute glucose to glycolysis. In some of the fibers, the glucose is used anaerobically, thereby producing lactate. Some of the lactate will be used by his heart, and some will be taken up by the liver to be converted to glucose. As he trains, he increases his mitochondrial capacity, as well as his oxygen delivery, resulting in an increased ability to oxidize fatty acids and ketone bodies. As he runs, he increases fatty acid release from adipose tissue triacylglycerols. In the liver, fatty acids are being converted to ketone bodies, providing his muscles with another fuel. As a consequence, he experiences mild ketosis after his 12-mile run.

A: Red blood cells lack mitochondria, which is the site of ketone body utilization.

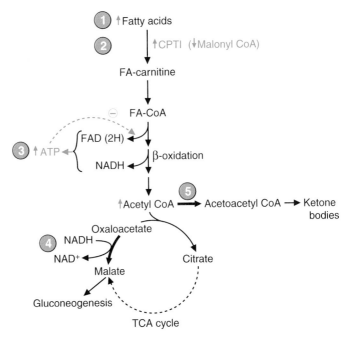

Fig. 23.21. Regulation of ketone body synthesis. (1) The supply of fatty acids is increased. (2) The malonyl CoA inhibition of CPTI is lifted by inactivation of acetyl CoA carboxylase. (3) β-Oxidation supplies NADH and FAD(2H), which are used by the electron transport chain for oxidative phosphorylation. As ATP levels increase, less NADH is oxidized, and the NADH/NAD$^+$ ratio is increased. (4) Oxaloacetate is converted into malate because of the high NADH levels, and the malate enters the cytoplasm for gluconeogenesis,. (5) Acetyl CoA is diverted from the TCA cycle into ketogenesis, in part because of low oxaloacetate levels, which reduces the rate of the citrate synthase reaction.

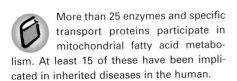 More than 25 enzymes and specific transport proteins participate in mitochondrial fatty acid metabolism. At least 15 of these have been implicated in inherited diseases in the human.

Recently, medium-chain acyl-CoA dehydrogenase (MCAD) deficiency, the cause of **Lofata Burne's** problems, has emerged as one of the most common of the inborn errors of metabolism, with a carrier frequency ranging from 1 in 40 in northern European populations to less than 1 in 100 in Asians. Overall, the predicted disease frequency for MCAD deficiency is 1 in 15,000 persons.

MCAD deficiency is an autosomal recessive disorder caused by the substitution of a T for an A at position 985 of the MCAD gene. This mutation causes a lysine to replace a glutamate residue in the protein, resulting in the production of an unstable dehydrogenase.

The most frequent manifestation of MCAD deficiency is intermittent hypoketotic hypoglycemia during fasting (low levels of ketone bodies and low levels of glucose in the blood). Fatty acids normally would be oxidized to CO_2 and H_2O under these conditions. In MCAD deficiency, however, fatty acids are oxidized only until they reach medium-chain length As a result, the body must rely to a greater extent on oxidation of blood glucose to meet its energy needs.

However, hepatic gluconeogenesis appears to be impaired in MCAD. Inhibition of gluconeogenesis may be caused by the lack of hepatic fatty acid oxidation to supply the energy required for gluconeogenesis, or by the accumulation of unoxidized fatty acid metabolites that inhibit gluconeogenic enzymes. As a consequence, liver glycogen stores are depleted more rapidly, and hypoglycemia results. The decrease in hepatic fatty acid oxidation results in less acetyl CoA for ketone body synthesis, and consequently a hypoketotic hypoglycemia develops.

Some of the symptoms once ascribed to hypoglycemia are now believed to be caused by the accumulation of toxic fatty acid intermediates, especially in those patients with only mild reductions in blood glucose levels. **Lofata Burne's** mild elevation in the blood of liver transaminases may reflect an infiltration of her liver cells with unoxidized medium-chain fatty acids.

The management of MCAD-deficient patients includes the intake of a relatively high-carbohydrate diet and the avoidance of prolonged fasting.

 Di Abietes, a 26-year-old woman with type 1 diabetes mellitus, was admitted to the hospital in diabetic ketoacidosis. In this complication of diabetes mellitus, an acute deficiency of insulin, coupled with a relative excess of glucagon, results in a rapid mobilization of fuel stores from muscle (amino acids) and adipose tissue (fatty acids). Some of the amino acids are converted to glucose, and fatty acids are converted to ketones (acetoacetate, β-hydroxybutyrate, and acetone). The high glucagon: insulin ratio promotes the hepatic production of ketones. In response to the metabolic "stress," the levels of insulin-antagonistic hormones, such as catecholamines, glucocorticoids, and growth hormone, are increased in the blood. The insulin deficiency further reduces the peripheral utilization of glucose and ketones. As a result of this interrelated dysmetabolism, plasma glucose levels reach 500 mg/dL (27.8 mmol/L) or more (normal fasting levels are 70–100 mg/dL, or 3.9–5.5 mmol/L), and plasma ketones rise to levels of 8 to 15 mmol/L or more (normal is in the range of 0.2–2 mmol/L, depending on the fed state of the individual).

The increased glucose presented to the renal glomeruli induces an osmotic diuresis, which further depletes intravascular volume, further reducing the renal excretion of hydrogen ions and glucose. As a result, the metabolic acidosis worsens, and the hyperosmolarity of the blood increases, at times exceeding 330 mOsm/kg (normal is in the range of 285–295 mOsm/kg). The severity of the hyperosmolar state correlates closely with the degree of central nervous system dysfunction and may end in coma and even death if left untreated.

BIOCHEMICAL COMMENTS

 The unripe fruit of the akee tree produces a toxin, hypoglycin, which causes a condition known as Jamaican vomiting sickness. The victims of the toxin are usually unwary children who eat this unripe fruit and develop a severe hypoglycemia, which is often fatal.

Although hypoglycin causes hypoglycemia, it acts by inhibiting an acyl CoA dehydrogenase involved in β-oxidation that has specificity for short- and medium-chain fatty acids. Because more glucose must be oxidized to compensate for the decreased ability of fatty acids to serve as fuel, blood glucose levels may fall to extremely low levels. Fatty acid levels, however, rise because of decreased β-oxidation. As a result of the increased fatty acid levels, α-oxidation increases, and dicarboxylic acids are excreted in the urine. The diminished capacity to oxidize fatty acids in liver mitochondria results in decreased levels of acetyl CoA, the substrate for ketone body synthesis.

Suggested References

Laffel L. Ketone bodies: a review of physiology, pathophysiology and application of monitoring to diabetes. Diabetes Metab Rev 1999;15:412–426.
Roe CR, Ding J. Mitochondrial fatty acid oxidation disorders. In: Scriver CR, Beudet AL, Sly WS, Valle D, eds. The Metabolic and Molecular Bases of Inherited Disease, vol 1, 8th Ed. New York: McGraw-Hill, 2001: 2297–2326.

Wanders JA, Jakobs C, Skjeldal OH. Refsum disease. In: Scriver CR, Beudet AL, Sly WS, Valle D, eds. The Metabolic and Molecular Bases of Inherited Disease, vol 1, 8th Ed. New York: McGraw-Hill, 2001: 3303–3321.

Ronald JA, Tein I. Metabolic myopathies. Seminars in Pediatric Neurology 1996;3:59–98.

 REVIEW QUESTIONS—CHAPTER 23

1. A lack of the enzyme ETF:CoQ oxidoreductase leads to death. This is due to which of the following reasons?

   (A) The energy yield from glucose utilization is dramatically reduced.
   (B) The energy yield from alcohol utilization is dramatically reduced.
   (C) The energy yield from ketone body utilization is dramatically reduced.
   (D) The energy yield from fatty acid utilization is dramatically reduced.
   (E) The energy yield from glycogen utilization is dramatically reduced.

2. The ATP yield from the complete oxidation of 1 mole of a $C_{18:0}$ fatty acid to carbon dioxide and water would be closest to which **ONE** of the following?

   (A) 105
   (B) 115
   (C) 120
   (D) 125
   (E) 130

3. The oxidation of fatty acids is best described by which of the following sets of reactions?

   (A) Oxidation, hydration, oxidation, carbon-carbon bond breaking
   (B) Oxidation, dehydration, oxidation, carbon-carbon bond breaking
   (C) Oxidation, hydration, reduction, carbon-carbon bond breaking
   (D) Oxidation, dehydration, reduction, oxidation, carbon-carbon bond breaking
   (E) Reduction, hydration, oxidation, carbon-carbon bond breaking

4. An individual with a deficiency of an enzyme in the pathway for carnitine synthesis is not eating adequate amounts of carnitine in the diet. Which of the following effects would you expect during fasting as compared with an individual with an adequate intake and synthesis of carnitine?

   (A) Fatty acid oxidation is increased.
   (B) Ketone body synthesis is increased.
   (C) Blood glucose levels are increased.
   (D) The levels of dicarboxylic acids in the blood would be increased.
   (E) The levels of very-long-chain fatty acids in the blood would be increased.

5. At which one of the periods listed below will fatty acids be the major source of fuel for the tissues of the body?

   (A) Immediately after breakfast
   (B) Minutes after a snack
   (C) Immediately after dinner
   (D) While running the first mile of a marathon
   (E) While running the last mile of a marathon

24 Oxygen Toxicity and Free Radical Injury

*O_2 is both essential to human life and **toxic**. We are dependent on O_2 for oxidation reactions in the pathways of adenosine triphosphate (ATP) generation, detoxification, and biosynthesis. However, when O_2 accepts single electrons, it is transformed into highly reactive **oxygen radicals** that damage cellular lipids, proteins, and DNA. Damage by reactive oxygen radicals contributes to cellular death and degeneration in a wide range of diseases (Table 24.1).*

***Radicals** are compounds that contain a single electron, usually in an outside orbital. Oxygen is a **biradical**, a molecule that has two unpaired electrons in separate orbitals (Fig. 24.1). Through a number of enzymatic and nonenzymatic processes that routinely occur in cells, O_2 accepts **single electrons** to form **reactive oxygen species (ROS)**. ROS are highly reactive oxygen radicals, or compounds that are readily converted in cells to these reactive radicals. The ROS formed by reduction of O_2 are the radical **superoxide (O_2^-)**, the nonradical **hydrogen peroxide (H_2O_2)**, and the **hydroxyl radical (OH•)**.*

*ROS may be generated nonenzymatically, or enzymatically as accidental byproducts or major products of reactions. Superoxide may be generated nonenzymatically from CoQ, or from metal-containing enzymes (e.g., **cytochrome P450, xanthine oxidase, and NADPH oxidase**). The highly toxic hydroxyl radical is formed nonenzymatically from superoxide in the presence of Fe^{3+} or Cu^+ by the **Fenton reaction**, and from hydrogen peroxide in the **Haber–Weiss reaction**.*

*Oxygen radicals and their derivatives can be deadly to cells. The hydroxyl radical causes oxidative damage to proteins and DNA. It also forms **lipid peroxides** and **malondialdehyde** from membrane lipids containing **polyunsaturated fatty acids**. In some cases, free radical damage is the direct cause of a disease state (e.g., tissue damage initiated by exposure to ionizing radiation). In **neurodegenerative diseases,** such as Parkinson's disease, or in ischemia-reperfusion injury, ROS may perpetuate the cellular damage caused by another process.*

*Oxygen radicals are joined in their destructive damage by the free radical nitric oxide (NO) and the reactive oxygen species **hypochlorous acid (HOCl)**. NO*

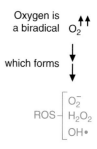

Fig 24.1. O_2 is a biradical. It has two antibonding electrons with parallel spins, denoted by the parallel arrows. It has a tendency to form toxic reactive oxygen species (ROS), such as superoxide (O_2^-), the nonradical hydrogen peroxide (H_2O_2), and the hydroxyl radical (OH•).

Table 24.1. Some Disease States Associated with Free Radical Injury

Atherogenesis	Cerebrovascular disorders
Emphysema bronchitis	Ischemia/reperfusion injury
Duchenne-type muscular dystrophy	Neurodegenerative disorders
	Amyotrophic lateral sclerosis (Lou Gehrig's disease)
Pregnancy/preeclampsia	Alzheimer's disease
Cervical cancer	Down's syndrome
Alcohol-induced liver disease	Ischemia/reperfusion injury following stroke
Hemodialysis	Oxphos diseases (Mitochondrial DNA disorders)
Diabetes	Multiple sclerosis
Acute renal failure	Parkinson's disease
Aging	
Retrolental fibroplasia	

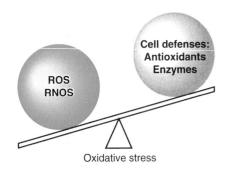

Fig 24.2. Oxidative stress. Oxidative stress occurs when the rate of ROS and RNOS production overbalances the rate of their removal by cellular defense mechanisms. These defense mechanisms include a number of enzymes and antioxidants. Antioxidants usually react nonenzymatically with ROS.

The basal ganglia are part of a neuronal feedback loop that modulates and integrates the flow of information from the cerebral cortex to the motor neurons of the spinal cord. The neostriatum is the major input structure from the cerebral cortex. The substantia nigra pars compacta consists of neurons that provide integrative input to the neostriatum through pigmented neurons that use dopamine as a neurotransmitter (the nigrastriatal pathway). Integrated information feeds back to the basal ganglia and to the cerebral cortex to control voluntary movement. In Parkinson's disease, a decrease in the amount of dopamine reaching the basal ganglia results in the movement disorder.

In ventricular fibrillation, rapid premature beats from an irritative focus in ventricular muscle occur in runs of varying duration. Persistent fibrillation compromises cardiac output, leading to death. This arrythmia can result from severe ischemia (lack of blood flow) in the ventricular muscle of the heart caused by clots forming at the site of a ruptured atherosclerotic plaque. However, **Cora Nari's** rapid beats began during the infusion of TPA as the clot was lysed. Thus, they probably resulted from reperfusing a previously ischemic area of her heart with oxygenated blood. This phenomenon is known as ischemia–reperfusion injury, and it is caused by cytotoxic ROS derived from oxygen in the blood that reperfuses previously hypoxic cells. Ischemic–reperfusion injury also may occur when tissue oxygenation is interrupted during surgery or transplantation.

combines with O_2 or superoxide to form reactive **nitrogen oxygen species (RNOS),** such as the nonradical peroxynitrite or the radical **nitrogen dioxide.** RNOS are present in the environment (e.g., cigarette smoke) and generated in cells. During phagocytosis of invading microorganisms, cells of the immune system produce O_2^-, HOCl, and NO through the actions of **NADPH oxidase, myeloperoxidase, and inducible nitric oxide synthase,** respectively. In addition to killing phagocytosed invading microorganisms, these toxic metabolites may damage surrounding tissue components.

Cells **protect** themselves against damage by ROS and other radicals through **repair processes, compartmentalization** of free radical production, **defense enzymes,** and **endogenous and exogenous antioxidants (free radical scavengers).** The defense enzyme **superoxide dismutase (SOD)** removes the superoxide free radical. Catalase and glutathione peroxidase remove hydrogen peroxide and lipid peroxides. **Vitamin E, vitamin C,** and **plant flavonoids** act as **antioxidants. Oxidative stress** occurs when the rate of ROS generation exceeds the capacity of the cell for their removal (Fig. 24.2).

THE WAITING ROOM

Two years ago, **Les Dopaman** (less dopamine), a 62-year-old man, noted an increasing tremor of his right hand when sitting quietly (resting tremor). The tremor disappeared if he actively used this hand to do purposeful movement. As this symptom progressed, he also complained of stiffness in his muscles that slowed his movements (bradykinesia). His wife noticed a change in his gait; he had begun taking short, shuffling steps and leaned forward as he walked (postural imbalance). He often appeared to be staring ahead with a rather immobile facial expression. She noted a tremor of his eyelids when he was asleep and, recently, a tremor of his legs when he was at rest. Because of these progressive symptoms and some subtle personality changes (anxiety and emotional lability), she convinced Les to see their family doctor.

The doctor suspected that her patient probably had primary or idiopathic parkinsonism (Parkinson's disease) and referred Mr. Dopaman to a neurologist. In Parkinson's disease, neurons of the substantia nigra pars compacta, containing the pigment melanin and the neurotransmitter dopamine, degenerate.

Cora Nari had done well since the successful lysis of blood clots in her coronary arteries with the use of intravenous recombinant tissue plasminogen activator (TPA)(see Chapters 19 and 21). This therapy had quickly relieved the crushing chest pain (angina) she experienced when she won the lottery. At her first office visit after discharge from the hospital, Cora's cardiologist told her she had developed multiple premature contractions of the ventricular muscle of her heart as the clots were being lysed. This process could have led to a life-threatening arrhythmia known as ventricular fibrillation. However, Cora's arrhythmia responded quickly to pharmacologic suppression and did not recur during the remainder of her hospitalization.

I. O_2 AND THE GENERATION OF ROS

The generation of reactive oxygen species from O_2 in our cells is a natural everyday occurrence. They are formed as accidental products of nonenzymatic and enzymatic reactions. Occasionally, they are deliberately synthesized in enzyme-catalyzed reactions. Ultraviolet radiation and pollutants in the air can increase formation of toxic oxygen-containing compounds.

A. The Radical Nature of O_2

A radical, by definition, is a molecule that has a single unpaired electron in an orbital. A free radical is a radical capable of independent existence. (Radicals formed in an enzyme active site during a reaction, for example, are not considered free radicals unless they can dissociate from the protein to interact with other molecules.) Radicals are highly reactive and initiate chain reactions by extracting an electron from a neighboring molecule to complete their own orbitals. Although the transition metals (e.g., Fe, Cu, and Mo) have single electrons in orbitals, they are not usually considered free radicals because they are relatively stable, do not initiate chain reactions, and are bound to proteins in the cell.

The oxygen atom is a biradical, which means it has two single electrons in different orbitals. These electrons cannot both travel in the same orbital because they have parallel spins (spin in the same direction). Although oxygen is very reactive from a thermodynamic standpoint, its single electrons cannot react rapidly with the paired electrons found in the covalent bonds of organic molecules. As a consequence, O_2 reacts slowly through the acceptance of single electrons in reactions that require a catalyst (such as a metal-containing enzyme).

O_2 is capable of accepting a total of four electrons, which reduces it to water (Fig. 24.3). When O_2 accepts one electron, superoxide is formed. Superoxide is still a radical because it has one unpaired electron remaining. This reaction is not thermodynamically favorable and requires a moderately strong reducing agent that can donate single electrons (e.g., CoQH· in the electron transport chain). When superoxide accepts an electron, it is reduced to hydrogen peroxide, which is not a radical. The hydroxyl radical is formed in the next one-electron reduction step in the reduction sequence. Finally, acceptance of the last electron reduces the hydroxyl radical to H_2O.

B. Characteristics of Reactive Oxygen Species

Reactive oxygen species (ROS) are oxygen-containing compounds that are highly reactive free radicals, or compounds readily converted to these oxygen free radicals in the cell. The major oxygen metabolites produced by one-electron reduction of oxygen (superoxide, hydrogen peroxide, and the hydroxyl radical) are classified as ROS (Table 24.2).

Reactive free radicals extract electrons (usually as hydrogen atoms) from other compounds to complete their own orbitals, thereby initiating free radical chain reactions. The hydroxyl radical is probably the most potent of the ROS. It initiates chain reactions that form lipid peroxides and organic radicals and adds directly to compounds. The superoxide anion is also highly reactive, but has limited lipid solubility and cannot diffuse far. However, it can generate the more reactive hydroxyl and hydroperoxy radicals by reacting nonenzymatically with hydrogen peroxide in the Haber–Weiss reaction (Fig 24.4).

Hydrogen peroxide, although not actually a radical, is a weak oxidizing agent that is classified as an ROS because it can generate the hydroxyl radical (OH•). Transition metals, such as Fe^{2+} or Cu^+, catalyze formation of the hydroxyl radical from hydrogen peroxide in the nonenzymatic Fenton reaction (see Fig. 24.4.).

The two unpaired electrons in oxygen have the same (parallel) spin and are called antibonding electrons. In contrast, carbon–carbon and carbon–hydrogen bonds each contain two electrons, which have antiparallel spins and form a thermodynamically stable pair. As a consequence, O_2 cannot readily oxidize a covalent bond because one of its electrons would have to flip its spin around to make new pairs. The difficulty in changing spins is called the **spin restriction.** Without the spin restriction, organic life forms could not have developed in the oxygen atmosphere on earth because they would be spontaneously oxidized by O_2. Instead, O_2 is confined to slower one-electron reactions catalyzed by metals (or metalloenzymes).

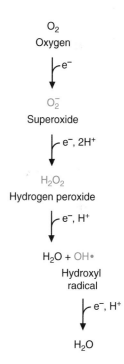

Fig 24.3. Reduction of oxygen by four one-electron steps. The four one-electron reduction steps for O_2 progressively generate superoxide, hydrogen peroxide, and the hydroxyl radical plus water. Superoxide is sometimes written O_2⁻· to better illustrate its single unpaired electron. H_2O_2, the half-reduced form of O_2, has accepted two electrons and is, therefore, not an oxygen radical.

To decrease occurrence of the Fenton reaction, accessibility to transition metals, such as Fe^{2+} and Cu^+, are highly restricted in cells, or in the body as a whole. Events that release iron from cellular storage sites, such as a crushing injury, are associated with increased free radical injury.

Table 24.2. Reactive Oxygen Species (ROS) and Reactive Nitrogen–Oxygen Species (RNOS)

Reactive Species	Properties
O_2^- Superoxide anion	Produced by the electron transport chain and at other sites. Cannot diffuse far from the site of origin. Generates other ROS.
H_2O_2 Hydrogen peroxide	Not a free radical, but can generate free radicals by reaction with a transition metal (e.g., Fe^{2+}). Can diffuse into and through cell membranes.
OH• Hydroxyl radical	The most reactive species in attacking biologic molecules. Produced from H_2O_2 in the Fenton reaction in the presence of Fe^{2+} or Cu^+.
RO•, R•, R-S• Organic radicals	Organic free radicals (R denotes remainder of the compound.) Produced from ROH, RH (e.g., at the carbon of a double bond in a fatty acid) or RSH by OH• attack.
RCOO• Peroxyl radical	An organic peroxyl radical, such as occurs during lipid degradation (also denoted LOO•)
HOCl Hypochlorous acid	Produced in neutrophils during the respiratory burst to destroy invading organisms. Toxicity is through halogenation and oxidation reactions. Attacking species is OCl^-
$O_2^{\downarrow\uparrow}$ Singlet oxygen	Oxygen with antiparallel spins. Produced at high oxygen tensions from absorption of *uv* light. Decays so fast that it is probably not a significant in vivo source of toxicity.
NO Nitric oxide	RNOS. A free radical produced endogenously by nitric oxide synthase. Binds to metal ions. Combines with O_2 or other oxygen-containing radicals to produce additional RNOS.
$ONOO^-$ Peroxynitrite	RNOS. A strong oxidizing agent that is not a free radical. It can generate NO_2 (nitrogen dioxide), which is a radical.

The Haber–Weiss reaction

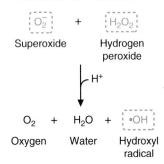

The Fenton reaction

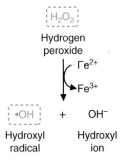

Fig 24.4. Generation of the hydroxyl radical by the nonenzymatic Haber–Weiss and Fenton reactions. In the simplified versions of these reactions shown here, the transfer of single electrons generates the hydroxyl radical. ROS are shown in blue. In addition to Fe^{2+}, Cu^+ and many other metals can also serve as single-electron donors in the Fenton reaction.

Because hydrogen peroxide is lipid soluble, it can diffuse through membranes and generate OH• at localized Fe^{2+}- or Cu^+-containing sites, such as the mitochondria. Hydrogen peroxide is also the precursor of hypochlorous acid (HOCl), a powerful oxidizing agent that is produced endogenously and enzymatically by phagocytic cells.

Organic radicals are generated when superoxide or the hydroxyl radical indiscriminately extract electrons from other molecules. Organic peroxy radicals are intermediates of chain reactions, such as lipid peroxidation. Other organic radicals, such as the ethoxy radical, are intermediates of enzymatic reactions that escape into solution (see Table 24.2).

An additional group of oxygen-containing radicals, termed RNOS, contain nitrogen as well as oxygen. These are derived principally from the free radical nitric oxide (NO), which is produced endogenously by the enzyme nitric oxide synthase. Nitric oxide combines with O_2 or superoxide to produce additional RNOS.

C. Major Sources of Primary Reactive Oxygen Species in the Cell

ROS are constantly being formed in the cell; approximately 3 to 5% of the oxygen we consume is converted to oxygen free radicals. Some are produced as accidental by-products of normal enzymatic reactions that escape from the active site of metal-containing enzymes during oxidation reactions. Others, such as hydrogen peroxide, are physiologic products of oxidases in peroxisomes. Deliberate production of toxic free radicals occurs in the inflammatory response. Drugs, natural radiation, air pollutants, and other chemicals also can increase formation of free radicals in cells.

1. CoQ GENERATES SUPEROXIDE

One of the major sites of superoxide generation is Coenzyme Q (CoQ) in the mitochondrial electron transport chain (Fig. 24.5). The one-electron reduced form of CoQ (CoQH•) is free within the membrane and can accidentally transfer an electron to dissolved O_2, thereby forming superoxide. In contrast, when O_2 binds to cytochrome oxidase and accepts electrons, none of the O_2 radical intermediates are released from the enzyme, and no ROS are generated.

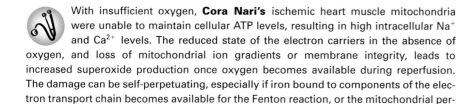 With insufficient oxygen, **Cora Nari's** ischemic heart muscle mitochondria were unable to maintain cellular ATP levels, resulting in high intracellular Na^+ and Ca^{2+} levels. The reduced state of the electron carriers in the absence of oxygen, and loss of mitochondrial ion gradients or membrane integrity, leads to increased superoxide production once oxygen becomes available during reperfusion. The damage can be self-perpetuating, especially if iron bound to components of the electron transport chain becomes available for the Fenton reaction, or the mitochondrial permeability transition is activated.

2. OXIDASES, OXYGENASES, AND PEROXIDASES

Most of the oxidases, peroxidases, and oxygenases in the cell bind O_2 and transfer single electrons to it via a metal. Free radical intermediates of these reactions may be accidentally released before the reduction is complete.

Cytochrome P450 enzymes are a major source of free radicals "leaked" from reactions.

Because these enzymes catalyze reactions in which single electrons are transferred to O_2 and an organic substrate, the possibility of accidentally generating and releasing free radical intermediates is high (see Chapters 19 and 25). Induction of P450 enzymes by alcohol, drugs, or chemical toxicants leads to increased cellular injury. When substrates for cytochrome P450 enzymes are not present, its potential for destructive damage is diminished by repression of gene transcription.

Hydrogen peroxide and lipid peroxides are generated enzymatically as major reaction products by a number of oxidases present in peroxisomes, mitochondria, and the endoplasmic reticulum. For example, monoamine oxidase, which oxidatively degrades the neurotransmitter dopamine, generates H_2O_2 at the mitochondrial membrane of certain neurons. Peroxisomal fatty acid oxidase generates H_2O_2 rather than FAD(2H) during the oxidation of very-long-chain fatty acids (see Chapter 23). Xanthine oxidase, an enzyme of purine degradation that can reduce O_2 to O_2^- or H_2O_2 in the cytosol, is thought to be a major contributor to ischemia–reperfusion injury, especially in intestinal mucosal and endothelial cells. Lipid peroxides are also formed enzymatically as intermediates in the pathways for synthesis of many eicosanoids, including leukotrienes and prostaglandins.

3. IONIZING RADIATION

Cosmic rays that continuously bombard the earth, radioactive chemicals, and x-rays are forms of ionizing radiation. Ionizing radiation has a high enough energy level that it can split water into the hydroxyl and hydrogen radicals, thus leading to radiation damage to the skin, mutations, cancer, and cell death (Fig. 24.6). It also may generate organic radicals through direct collision with organic cellular components.

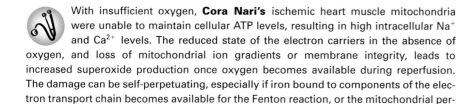 Production of ROS by xanthine oxidase in endothelial cells may be enhanced during ischemia–reperfusion in **Cora Nari's** heart. In undamaged tissues, xanthine oxidase exists as a dehydrogenase that uses NAD^+ rather than O_2 as an electron acceptor in the pathway for degradation of purines (hypoxanthine ↔ xanthine ↔ uric acid (see Chapter 41). When O_2 levels decrease, phosphorylation of ADP to ATP decreases, and degradation of ADP and adenine through xanthine oxidase increases. In the process, xanthine dehydrogenase is converted to an oxidase. As long as O_2 levels are below the high K_m of the enzyme for O_2, little damage is done. However, during reperfusion when O_2 levels return to normal, xanthine oxidase generates H_2O_2 and O_2^- at the site of injury.

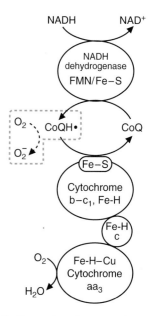

Fig 24.5. Generation of superoxide by CoQ in the electron transport chain. In the process of transporting electrons to O_2, some of the electrons escape when CoQH• accidentally interacts with O_2 to form superoxide. Fe-H represents the Fe-heme center of the cytochromes.

Carbon tetrachloride (CCl_4), which is used as a solvent in the dry-cleaning industry, is converted by cytochrome P450 to a highly reactive free radical that has caused hepatocellular necrosis in workers. When the enzyme-bound CCl_4 accepts an electron, it dissociates into CCl_3• and Cl•. The CCl_3• radical, which cannot continue through the P450 reaction sequence, "leaks" from the enzyme active site and initiates chain reactions in the surrounding polyunsaturated lipids of the endoplasmic reticulum. These reactions spread into the plasma membrane and to proteins, eventually resulting in cell swelling, accumulation of lipids, and cell death.

Les Dopaman, who is in the early stages of Parkinson's disease, is treated with a monoamine oxidase B inhibitor. Monoamine oxidase is a copper-containing enzyme that inactivates dopamine in neurons, producing H_2O_2. The drug was originally administered to inhibit dopamine degradation. However, current theory suggests that the effectiveness of the drug is also related to decrease of free radical formation within the cells of the basal ganglia. The dopaminergic neurons involved are particularly susceptible to the cytotoxic effects of ROS and RNOS that may arise from H_2O_2.

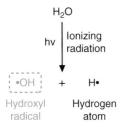

Fig 24.6. Generation of free radicals from radiation.

II. OXYGEN RADICAL REACTIONS WITH CELLULAR COMPONENTS

Oxygen radicals produce cellular dysfunction by reacting with lipids, proteins, carbohydrates, and DNA to extract electrons (summarized in Fig. 24.7). Evidence of free radical damage has been described in over 100 disease states. In some of these diseases, free radical damage is the primary cause of the disease; in others, it enhances complications of the disease.

A. Membrane Attack: Formation of Lipid and Lipid Peroxy Radicals

Chain reactions that form lipid free radicals and lipid peroxides in membranes make a major contribution to ROS-induced injury (Fig. 24.8). An initiator (such as a hydroxyl radical produced locally in the Fenton reaction) begins the chain reaction. It extracts a hydrogen atom, preferably from the double bond of a polyunsaturated fatty acid in a membrane lipid. The chain reaction is propagated when O_2 adds to form lipid peroxyl radicals and lipid peroxides. Eventually lipid degradation occurs, forming such products as malondialdehyde (from fatty acids with three or more double bonds), and ethane and pentane (from the ω-terminal carbons of 3 and 6 fatty acids, respectively). Malondialdehyde appears in the blood and urine and is used as an indicator of free radical damage.

Peroxidation of lipid molecules invariably changes or damages lipid molecular structure. In addition to the self-destructive nature of membrane lipid peroxidation, the aldehydes that are formed can cross-link proteins. When the damaged lipids are the constituents of biologic membranes, the cohesive lipid bilayer arrangement and stable structural organization is disrupted (see Fig. 24.7). Disruption of mitochondrial membrane integrity may result in further free radical production.

The appearance of lipofuscin granules in many tissues increases during aging. The pigment lipofuscin (from the Greek "lipos" for lipids and the Latin "fuscus" for dark) consists of a heterogeneous mixture of cross-linked polymerized lipids and protein formed by reactions between amino acid residues and lipid peroxidation products, such as malondialdehyde. These cross-linked products are probably derived from peroxidatively damaged cell organelles that were autophagocytized by lysosomes but could not be digested. When these dark pigments appear on the skin of the hands in aged individuals, they are referred to as "liver spots," a traditional hallmark of aging. In **Les Dopaman** and other patients with Parkinson's disease, lipofuscin appears as Lewy bodies in degenerating neurons.

Evidence of protein damage shows up in many diseases, particularly those associated with aging. In patients with cataracts, proteins in the lens of the eye exhibit free radical damage and contain methionine sulfoxide residues and tryptophan degradation products.

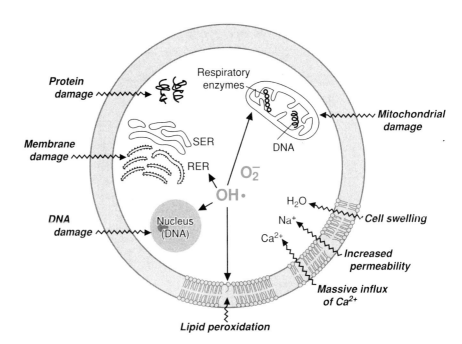

Fig 24.7. Free radical–mediated cellular injury. Superoxide and the hydroxyl radical initiate lipid peroxidation in the cellular, mitochondrial, nuclear, and endoplasmic reticulum membranes. The increase in cellular permeability results in an influx of Ca^{2+}, which causes further mitochondrial damage. The cysteine sulfhydryl groups and other amino acid residues on proteins are oxidized and degraded. Nuclear and mitochondrial DNA can be oxidized, resulting in strand breaks and other types of damage. RNOS (NO, NO_2, and peroxynitrite) have similar effects.

B. Proteins and Peptides

In proteins, the amino acids proline, histidine, arginine, cysteine, and methionine are particularity susceptible to hydroxyl radical attack and oxidative damage. As a consequence of oxidative damage, the protein may fragment or residues cross-link with other residues. Free radical attack on protein cysteine residues can result in cross-linking and formation of aggregates that prevents their degradation. However, oxidative damage increases the susceptibility of other proteins to proteolytic digestion.

Free radical attack and oxidation of the cytseine sulfhydryl residues of the tripeptide glutathione (γ-glutamyl-cysteinyl-glycine; see section V.A.3.) increases oxidative damage throughout the cell. Glutathione is a major component of cellular defense against free radical injury, and its oxidation reduces its protective effects.

C. DNA

Oxygen-derived free radicals are also a major source of DNA damage. Approximately 20 types of oxidatively altered DNA molecules have been identified. The nonspecific binding of Fe^{2+} to DNA facilitates localized production of the hydroxyl radical, which can cause base alterations in the DNA (Fig. 24.9). It also can attack the deoxyribose backbone and cause strand breaks. This DNA damage can be repaired to some extent by the cell (see Chapter 12), or minimized by apoptosis of the cell.

III. NITRIC OXIDE AND REACTIVE NITROGEN-OXYGEN SPECIES (RNOS)

Nitric oxide (NO) is an oxygen-containing free radical which, like O_2, is both essential to life and toxic. NO has a single electron, and therefore binds to other compounds containing single electrons, such as Fe^{3+}. As a gas, it diffuses through the cytosol and lipid membranes and into cells. At low concentrations, it functions physiologically as a neurotransmitter and a hormone that causes vasodilation. However, at high concentrations, it combines with O_2 or with superoxide to form additional reactive and toxic species containing both nitrogen and oxygen (RNOS). RNOS are involved in neurodegenerative diseases, such as Parkinson's disease, and in chronic inflammatory diseases, such as rheumatoid arthritis.

A. Nitric Oxide Synthase

At low concentrations, nitric oxide serves as a neurotransmitter or a hormone. It is synthesized from arginine by nitric oxide synthases (Fig 24.10). As a gas, it is able to diffuse through water and lipid membranes, and into target cells. In the target cell, it exerts its physiologic effects by high-affinity binding to Fe-heme in the enzyme guanylyl cyclase, thereby activating a signal transduction cascade. However, NO is rapidly inactivated by nonspecific binding to many molecules, and therefore cells that produce NO need to be close to the target cells.

The body has three different tissue-specific isoforms of NO synthase, each encoded by a different gene: neuronal nitric oxide synthase (nNOS, isoform I), inducible nitric oxide synthase (iNOS, isoform II), and endothelial nitric oxide synthase (eNOS, isoform III). nNOS and eNOS are tightly regulated by Ca^{2+} concentration to produce the small amounts of NO required for its role as a neurotransmitter and hormone. In contrast, iNOS is present in many cells of the immune system and cell types with a similar lineage, such as macrophages and

Nitroglycerin, in tablet form, is often given to patients with coronary artery disease who experience ischemia-induced chest pain (angina). The nitroglycerin decomposes in the blood, forming NO, a potent vasodilator, which increases blood flow to the heart and relieves the angina.

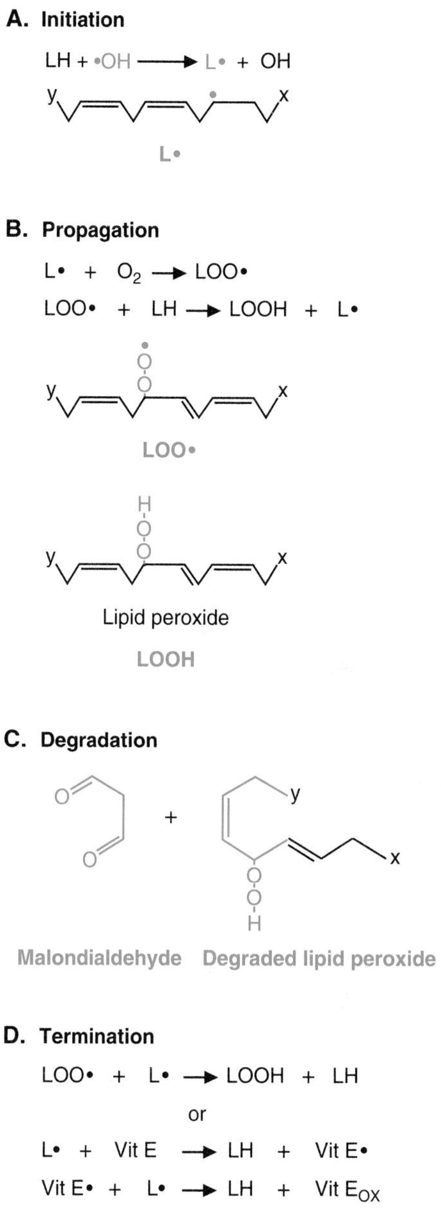

A. Initiation

$$LH + \cdot OH \longrightarrow L\cdot + OH$$

B. Propagation

$$L\cdot + O_2 \longrightarrow LOO\cdot$$
$$LOO\cdot + LH \longrightarrow LOOH + L\cdot$$

LOO•

Lipid peroxide

LOOH

C. Degradation

Malondialdehyde   Degraded lipid peroxide

D. Termination

$$LOO\cdot + L\cdot \longrightarrow LOOH + LH$$

or

$$L\cdot + Vit\ E \longrightarrow LH + Vit\ E\cdot$$
$$Vit\ E\cdot + L\cdot \longrightarrow LH + Vit\ E_{OX}$$

Fig 24.8. Lipid peroxidation: a free radical chain reaction. **A.** Lipid peroxidation is initiated by a hydroxyl or other radical that extracts a hydrogen atom from a polyunsaturated lipid (LH), thereby forming a lipid radical (L•). **B.** The free radical chain reaction is propagated by reaction with O_2, forming the lipid peroxy radical (LOO•) and lipid peroxide (LOOH). **C.** Rearrangements of the single electron result in degradation of the lipid. Malondialdehyde, one of the compounds formed, is soluble and appears in blood. **D.** The chain reaction can be terminated by vitamin E and other lipid-soluble antioxidants that donate single electrons. Two subsequent reduction steps form a stable, oxidized antioxidant.

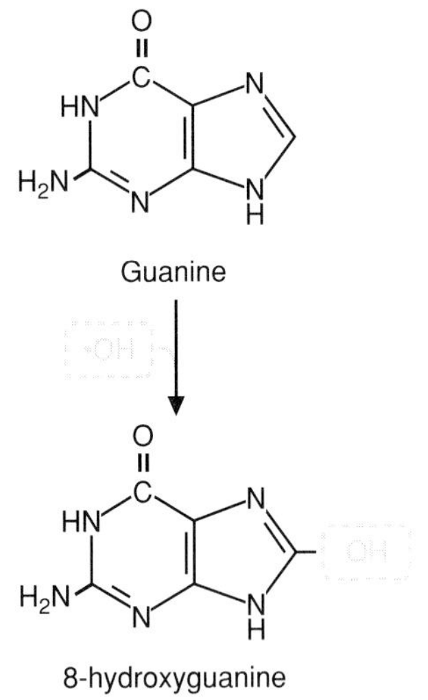

Fig 24.9. Conversion of guanine to 8-hydroxyguanine by the hydroxy radical. The amount of 8-hydroxyguanosine present in cells can be used to estimate the amount of oxidative damage they have sustained. The addition of the hydroxyl group to guanine allows it to mispair with T residues, leading to the creation of a daughter molecule with an A-T base pair in this position.

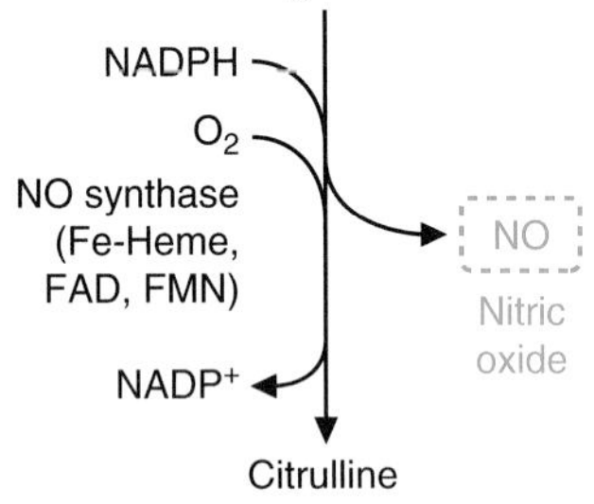

brain astroglia. This isoenzyme of nitric oxide synthase is regulated principally by induction of gene transcription, and not by changes in Ca^{2+} concentration. It produces high and toxic levels of NO to assist in killing invading microorganisms. It is these very high levels of NO that are associated with generation of RNOS and NO toxicity.

B. NO Toxicity

The toxic actions of NO can be divided into two categories: direct toxic effects resulting from binding to Fe-containing proteins, and indirect effects mediated by compounds formed when NO combines with O_2 or with superoxide to form RNOS.

1. DIRECT TOXIC EFFECTS OF NO

NO, as a radical, exerts direct toxic effects by combining with Fe-containing compounds that also have single electrons. Major destructive sites of attack include Fe-S centers (e.g., electron transport chain complexes I-III, aconitase) and Fe-heme proteins (e.g., hemoglobin and electron transport chain cytochromes). However, there is usually little damage because NO is present in low concentrations and Fe-heme compounds are present in excess capacity. NO can cause serious damage, however, through direct inhibition of respiration in cells that are already compromised through oxidative phosphorylation diseases or ischemia.

2. RNOS TOXICITY

When present in very high concentrations (e.g., during inflammation), NO combines nonenzymatically with superoxide to form peroxynitrite ($ONOO^-$), or with O_2 to form N_2O_3 (Fig. 24.11). Peroxynitrite, although not a free radical, is a strong

Fig 24.10. Nitric oxide synthase synthesizes the free radical NO. Like cytochrome P450 enzymes, NO synthase uses Fe-heme, FAD, and FMN to transfer single electrons from NADPH to O_2.

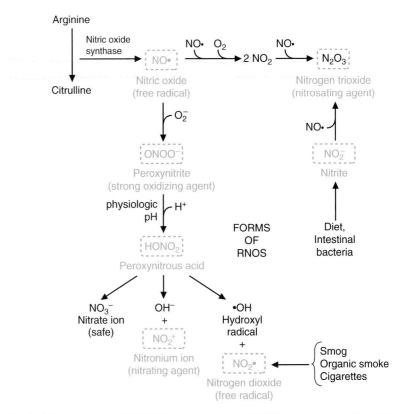

Fig 24.11. Formation of RNOS from nitric oxide. RNOS are shown in blue. The type of damage caused by each RNOS is shown in parentheses. Of all the nitrogen–oxygen-containing compounds shown, only nitrate is relatively nontoxic.

oxidizing agent that is stable and directly toxic. It can diffuse through the cell and lipid membranes to interact with a wide range of targets, including protein methionine and -SH groups (e.g., Fe-S centers in the electron transport chain). It also breaks down to form additional RNOS, including the free radical nitrogen dioxide (NO_2), an effective initiator of lipid peroxidation. Peroxynitrite products also nitrate aromatic rings, forming compounds such as nitrotyrosine or nitroguanosine. N_2O_3, which can be derived either from NO_2 or nitrite, is the agent of nitrosative stress, and nitrosylates sulfhydryl and similarily reactive groups in the cell. Nitrosylation will usually interefere with the proper functioning of the protein or lipid that has been modified. Thus, RNOS can do as much oxidative and free radical damage as non–nitrogen-containing ROS, as well as nitrating and nitrosylating compounds. The result is widespread and includes inhibition of a large number of enzymes; mitochondrial lipid peroxidation; inhibition of the electron transport chain and energy depletion; single-stranded or double-stranded breaks in DNA; and modification of bases in DNA.

 NO_2 is one of the toxic agents present in smog, automobile exhaust, gas ranges, pilot lights, cigarette smoke, and smoke from forest fires or burning buildings.

IV. FORMATION OF FREE RADICALS DURING PHAGOCYTOSIS AND INFLAMMATION

In response to infectious agents and other stimuli, phagocytic cells of the immune system (neutrophils, eosinophils, and monocytes/macrophages) exhibit a rapid consumption of O_2 called the respiratory burst. The respiratory burst is a major source of superoxide, hydrogen peroxide, the hydroxyl radical, hypochlorous acid (HOCl), and RNOS. The generation of free radicals is part of the human antimicrobial defense system and is intended to destroy invading microorganisms, tumor cells, and other cells targeted for removal.

A. NADPH Oxidase

The respiratory burst results from the activity of NADPH oxidase, which catalyzes the transfer of an electron from NADPH to O_2 to form superoxide (Fig. 24.12). NADPH oxidase is assembled from cytosol and membranous proteins recruited into the phagolysosome membrane as it surrounds an invading microorganism.

Superoxide is released into the intramembranous space of the phagolysosome, where it is generally converted to hydrogen peroxide and other ROS that are effective against bacteria and fungal pathogens. Hydrogen peroxide is formed by superoxide dismutase, which may come from the phagocytic cell or the invading microorganism.

B. Myeloperoxidase and HOCl

The formation of hypochlorous acid from H_2O_2 is catalyzed by myeloperoxidase, a heme-containing enzyme that is present only in phagocytic cells of the immune system (predominantly neutrophils).

Myeloperoxidase   **Dissociation**
$$H_2O_2 + Cl^- + H^+ \rightarrow HOCl + H_2O \rightarrow {}^-OCl + H^+ + H_2O$$

Myeloperoxidase contains two Fe heme-like centers, which give it the green color seen in pus. Hypochlorous acid is a powerful toxin that destroys bacteria within seconds through halogenation and oxidation reactions. It oxidizes many Fe and S-containing groups (e.g., sulfhydryl groups, iron-sulfur centers, ferredoxin, heme-proteins, methionine), oxidatively decarboxylates and deaminates proteins, and cleaves peptide bonds. Aerobic bacteria under attack rapidly lose membrane

In patients with chronic granulomatous disease, phagocytes have genetic defects in NADPH oxidase. NADPH oxidase has four different subunits (two in the cell membrane and two recruited from the cytosol), and the genetic defect may be in any of the genes that encode these subunits. The membrane catalytic subunit β of NADPH oxidase is a 91-kDa flavocytochrome glycoprotein. It transfers electrons from bound NADPH to FAD, which transfers them to the Fe–heme components. The membranous α-subunit (p22) is required for stabilization. Two additional cytosolic proteins (p47phox and p67phox) are also required for assembly of the complex. Rac, a monomeric GTPase in the Ras subfamily of the Rho superfamily (see Chapter 9), is also required for assembly. The 91-kDa subunit is affected most often in X-linked chronic granulatomous disease, whereas the α-subunit is affected in a rare autosomal recessive form. The cytosolic subunits are affected most often in patients with the autosomal recessive form of granulomatous disease. In addition to their enhanced susceptibility to bacterial and fungal infections, these patients suffer from an apparent dysregulation of normal inflammatory responses.

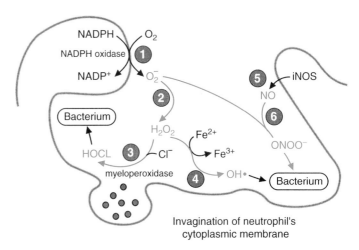

Fig 24.12. Production of reactive oxygen species during the phagocytic respiratory burst by activated neutrophils. (1) Activation of NADPH oxidase on the outer side of the plasma membrane initiates the respiratory burst with the generation of superoxide. During phagocytosis, the plasma membrane invaginates, so superoxide is released into the vacuole space. (2) Superoxide (either spontaneously or enzymatically via superoxide dismutase [SOD]) generates H_2O_2. (3) Granules containing myeloperoxidase are secreted into the phagosome, where myeloperoxidase generates HOCl and other halides. (4) H_2O_2 can also generate the hydroxyl radical from the Fenton reaction. (5) Inducible nitric oxide synthase may be activated and generate NO. (6) Nitric oxide combines with superoxide to form peroxynitrite, which may generate additional RNOS. The result is an attack on the membranes and other components of phagocytosed cells, and eventual lysis. The whole process is referred to as the respiratory burst because it lasts only 30 to 60 minutes and consumes O_2.

transport, possibly because of damage to ATP synthase or electron transport chain components (which reside in the plasma membrane of bacteria).

C. RNOS and Inflammation

When human neutrophils of the immune system are activated to produce NO, NADPH oxidase is also activated. NO reacts rapidly with superoxide to generate peroxynitrite, which forms additional RNOS. NO also may be released into the surrounding medium, to combine with superoxide in target cells.

In a number of disease states, free radical release by neutrophils or macrophages during an inflammation contributes to injury in the surrounding tissues. During stroke or myocardial infarction, phagocytic cells that move into the ischemic area to remove dead cells may increase the area and extent of damage. The self-perpetuating mechanism of radical release by neutrophils during inflammation and immune complex formation may explain some of the features of chronic inflammation in patients with rheumatoid arthritis. As a result of free radical release, the immunoglobulin G (IgG) proteins present in the synovial fluid are partially oxidized, which improves their binding with the rheumatoid factor antibody. This binding, in turn, stimulates the neutrophils to release more free radicals.

V. CELLULAR DEFENSES AGAINST OXYGEN TOXICITY

Our defenses against oxygen toxicity fall into the categories of antioxidant defense enzymes, dietary and endogenous antioxidants (free radical scavengers), cellular compartmentation, metal sequestration, and repair of damaged cellular components. The antioxidant defense enzymes react with ROS and cellular products of free radical chain reactions to convert them to nontoxic products. Dietary antioxidants, such as vitamin E and flavonoids, and endogenous antioxidants, such as urate, can

During **Cora Nari's** ischemia (decreased blood flow), the ability of her heart to generate ATP from oxidative phosphorylation was compromised. The damage appeared to accelerate when oxygen was first reintroduced (reperfused) into the tissue. During ischemia, CoQ and the other single-electron components of the electron transport chain become saturated with electrons. When oxygen is reintroduced (reperfusion), electron donation to O_2 to form superoxide is increased. The increase of superoxide results in enhanced formation of hydrogen peroxide and the hydroxyl radical. Macrophages in the area to clean up cell debris from ischemic injury produce nitric oxide, which may further damage mitochondria by generating RNOS that attack Fe-S centers and cytochromes in the electron transport chain membrane lipids. Thus, the RNOS may increase the infarct size.

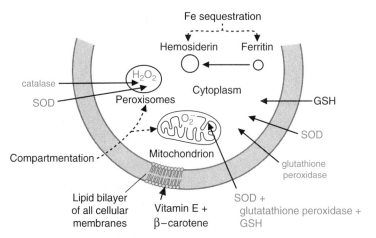

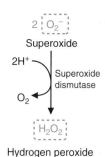

Fig 24.13 Compartmentation of free radical defenses. Various defenses against ROS are found in the different subcellular compartments of the cell. The location of free radical defense enzymes (shown in blue) matches the type and amount of ROS generated in each subcellular compartment. The highest activities of these enzymes are found in the liver, adrenal gland, and kidney, where mitochondrial and peroxisomal contents are high, and cytochrome P450 enzymes are found in abundance in the smooth ER. The enzymes superoxide dismutase (SOD) and glutathione peroxidase are present as isozymes in the different compartments. Another form of compartmentation involves the sequestration of Fe, which is stored as mobilizable Fe in ferritin. Excess Fe is stored in nonmobilizable hemosiderin deposits. Glutathione (GSH) is a nonenzymatic antioxidant.

Fig 24.14. Superoxide dismutase converts superoxide to hydrogen peroxide, which is nontoxic unless converted to other ROS.

terminate free radical chain reactions. Defense through compartmentation refers to separation of species and sites involved in ROS generation from the rest of the cell (Fig. 24.13). For example, many of the enzymes that produce hydrogen peroxide are sequestered in peroxisomes with a high content of antioxidant enzymes. Metals are bound to a wide range of proteins within the blood and in cells, preventing their participation in the Fenton reaction. Iron, for example, is tightly bound to its storage protein, ferritin and cannot react with hydrogen peroxide. Repair mechanisms for DNA, and for removal of oxidized fatty acids from membrane lipids, are available to the cell. Oxidized amino acids on proteins are continuously repaired through protein degradation and resynthesis of new proteins.

A. Antioxidant Scavenging Enzymes

The enzymatic defense against ROS includes superoxide dismutase, catalase, and glutathione peroxidase.

1. SUPEROXIDE DISMUTASE (SOD)

Conversion of superoxide anion to hydrogen peroxide and O_2 (dismutation) by superoxide dismutase (SOD) is often called the primary defense against oxidative stress because superoxide is such a strong initiator of chain reactions (Fig 24.14). SOD exists as three isoenzyme forms, a Cu^+-Zn^{2+} form present in the cytosol, a Mn^{2+} form present in mitochondria, and a Cu^+-Zn^{2+} form found extracellularly. The activity of Cu^+-Zn^{2+} SOD is increased by chemicals or conditions (such as hyperbaric oxygen) that increase the production of superoxide.

In the body, iron and other metals are sequestered from interaction with ROS or O_2 by their binding to transport proteins (haptoglobin, hemoglobin, transferrin, ceruloplasmin, and metallothionein) in the blood, and to intracellular storage proteins (ferritin, hemosiderin). Metals also are found bound to many enzymes, particularly those that react with O_2. Usually, these enzymes have reaction mechanisms that minimize nonspecific single-electron transfer from the metal to other compounds.

The intracellular form of the Cu^+–Zn^{2+} superoxide dismutase is encoded by the SOD1 gene. To date, 58 mutations in this gene have been discovered in individuals affected by familial amyotrophic lateral sclerosis (Lou Gehrig's disease). How a mutation in this gene leads to the symptoms of this disease has yet to be understood. It is important to note that only 5 to 10% of the total cases of diagnosed amyotrophic lateral sclerosis are caused by the familial form.

Q: Why does the cell need such a high content of SOD in mitochondria?

Premature infants with low levels of lung surfactant (see Chapter 33) require oxygen therapy. The level of oxygen must be closely monitored to prevent retinopathy and subsequent blindness (the retinopathy of prematurity) and to prevent bronchial pulmonary dysplasia. The tendency for these complications to develop is enhanced by the possibility of low levels of SOD and vitamin E in the premature infant.

Mitochondria are major sites for generation of superoxide from the interaction of CoQ and O_2. The Mn^{2+} superoxide dismutase present in mitochondria is not regulated through induction/repression of gene transcription, presumably because the rate of superoxide generation is always high. Mitochondria also have a high content of glutathione and glutathione peroxidase, and can thus convert H_2O_2 to H_2O and prevent lipid peroxidation.

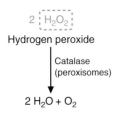

Fig 24.15. Catalase reduces hydrogen peroxide. (ROS is shown in a blue box).

Selenium (Se) is present in human proteins principally as selenocysteine (cysteine with the sulfur group replaced by Se, abbreviated sec). This amino acid functions in catalysis, and has been found in 11 or more human enzymes, including the four enzymes of the glutathione peroxidase family. Selenium is supplied in the diet as selenomethionine from plants (methionine with the Se replacing the sulfur), selenocysteine from animal foods, and inorganic selenium. Se from all of these sources can be converted to selenophosphate. Selenophosphate reacts with a unique tRNA containing bound serine to form a selenocysteine-tRNA, which incorporates selenocystiene into the appropriate protein as it is being synthesized. Se homeostasis in the body is controlled principally through regulation of its secretion as methylated Se. The current dietary requirement is approximately 70 μg/day for adult males and 55 μg for females. Deficiency symptoms reflect diminished antioxidant defenses and include symptoms of vitamin E deficiency.

2. CATALASE

Hydrogen peroxide, once formed, must be reduced to water to prevent it from forming the hydroxyl radical in the Fenton reaction or Haber–Weiss reactions (see Fig. 24.4) One of the enzymes capable of reducing hydrogen peroxide is catalase (Fig.24.15). Catalase is found principally in peroxisomes, and to a lesser extent in the cytosol and microsomal fraction of the cell. The highest activities are found in tissues with a high peroxisomal content (kidney and liver). In cells of the immune system, catalase serves to protect the cell against its own respiratory burst.

3. GLUTATHIONE PEROXIDASE AND GLUTATHIONE REDUCTASE

Glutathione (γ-glutamylcysteinylglycine) is one of the body's principal means of protecting against oxidative damage (see also Chapter 29). Glutathione is a tripeptide composed of glutamate, cysteine, and glycine, with the amino group of cysteine joined in peptide linkage to the γ-carboxyl group of glutamate (Fig. 24.16). In reactions catalyzed by glutathione peroxidases, the reactive sulfhydryl groups reduce hydrogen peroxide to water and lipid peroxides to nontoxic alcohols. In these reactions, two glutathione molecules are oxidized to form a single molecule, glutathione disulfide. The sulfhydryl groups are also oxidized in nonenzymatic chain terminating reactions with organic radicals.

Glutathione peroxidases exist as a family of selenium enzymes with somewhat different properties and tissue locations. Within cells, they are found principally in the cytosol and mitochondria, and are the major means for removing H_2O_2 produced outside of peroxisomes. They contribute to our dietary requirement for selenium and account for the protective effect of selenium in the prevention of free radical injury.

Once oxidized glutathione (GSSG) is formed, it must be reduced back to the sulfhydryl form by glutathione reductase in a redox cycle (Fig. 24.17). Glutathione reductase contains an FAD, and catalyzes transfer of electrons from NADPH to the disulfide bond of GSSG. NADPH is, thus, essential for protection against free radical injury. The major source of NADPH for this reaction is the pentose phosphate pathway (see Chapter 29).

B. Nonenzymatic Antioxidants (Free Radical Scavengers)

Free radical scavengers convert free radicals to a nonradical nontoxic form in nonenzymatic reactions. Most free radical scavengers are antioxidants, compounds

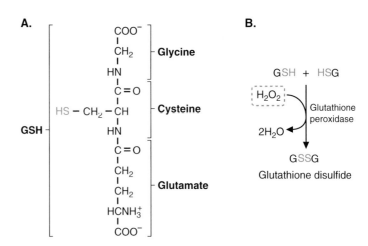

Fig 24.16. Glutathione peroxidase reduces hydrogen peroxide to water. A. The structure of glutathione. The sulfhydryl group of glutathione, which is oxidized to a disulfide, is shown in blue. B. Glutathione peroxidase transfer electrons from glutathione (GSH) to hydrogen peroxide.

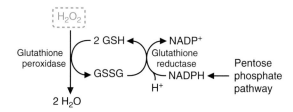

Fig 24.17. Glutathione redox cycle. Glutathione reductase regenerates reduced glutathione. (ROS is shown in the blue box).

that neutralize free radicals by donating a hydrogen atom (with its one electron) to the radical. Antioxidants, therefore, reduce free radicals and are themselves oxidized in the reaction. Dietary free radical scavengers (e.g., vitamin E, ascorbic acid, carotenoids, and flavonoids) as well as endogenously produced free radical scavengers (e.g., urate and melatonin) have a common structural feature, a conjugated double bond system that may be an aromatic ring.

1. VITAMIN E

Vitamin E (α-tocopherol), the most widely distributed antioxidant in nature, is a lipid-soluble antioxidant vitamin that functions principally to protect against lipid peroxidation in membranes (see Fig. 24.13). Vitamin E comprises a number of tocopherols that differ in their methylation pattern. Among these, α-tocopherol is the most potent antioxidant and present in the highest amount in our diet (Fig. 24.18).

Vitamin E is an efficient antioxidant and nonenzymatic terminator of free radical chain reactions, and has little pro-oxidant activity. When Vitamin E donates an electron to a lipid peroxy radical, it is converted to a free radical form that is stabilized by resonance. If this free radical form were to act as a pro-oxidant and abstract an electron from a polyunsaturated lipid, it would be oxidizing that lipid and actually propagate the free radical chain reaction. The chemistry of vitamin E is such that it has a much greater tendency to donate a second electron and go to the fully oxidized form.

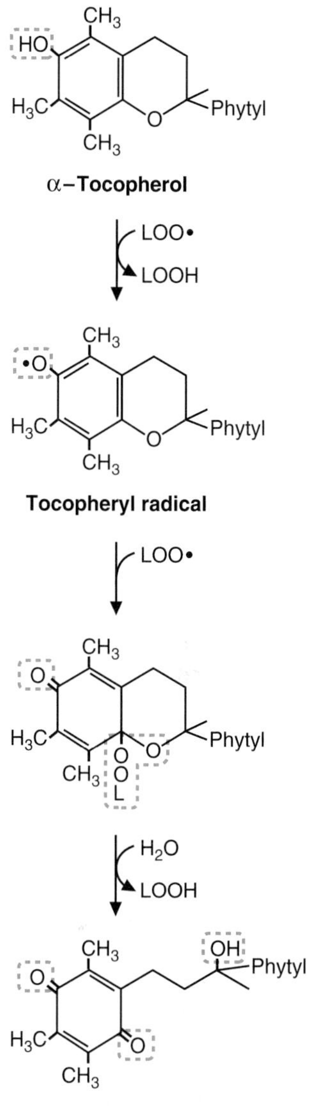

2. ASCORBIC ACID

Although ascorbate (vitamin C) is an oxidation-reduction coenzyme that functions in collagen synthesis and other reactions, it also plays a role in free radical defense. Reduced ascorbate can regenerate the reduced form of vitamin E through donating electrons in a redox cycle (Fig. 24.19). It is water-soluble and circulates unbound in blood and extracellular fluid, where it has access to the lipid-soluble vitamin E present in membranes and lipoprotein particles.

3. CAROTENOIDS

Carotenoids is a term applied to β-carotene (the precursor of vitamin A) and similar compounds with functional oxygen-containing substituents on the rings, such as zeaxanthin and lutein (Fig. 24.20). These compounds can exert antioxidant effects, as well as quench singlet O_2 (singlet oxygen is a highly reactive oxygen species in which there are no unpaired electrons in the outer orbitals, but there is one orbital that is completely empty). Epidemiologic studies have shown a correlation between diets high in fruits and vegetables and health benefits, leading to the hypothesis that carotenoids might slow the progression of cancer, atherosclerosis, and other degenerative diseases by acting as chain-breaking antioxidants. However, in clinical

α–Tocopherol

Tocopheryl radical

Tocopheryl quinone

Fig 24.18. Vitamin E (α-tocopherol) terminates free radical lipid peroxidation by donating single electrons to lipid peroxyl radicals (LOO•) to form the more stable lipid peroxide, LOOH. In so doing, the α-tocopherol is converted to the fully oxidized tocopheryl quinone.

Vitamin E is found in the diet in the lipid fractions of some vegetable oils and in liver, egg yolks, and cereals. It is absorbed together with lipids, and fat malabsorption results in symptomatic deficiencies. Vitamin E circulates in the blood in lipoprotein particles. Its deficiency causes neurologic symptoms, probably because the polyunsaturated lipids in myelin and other membranes of the nervous system are particularly sensitive to free radical injury.

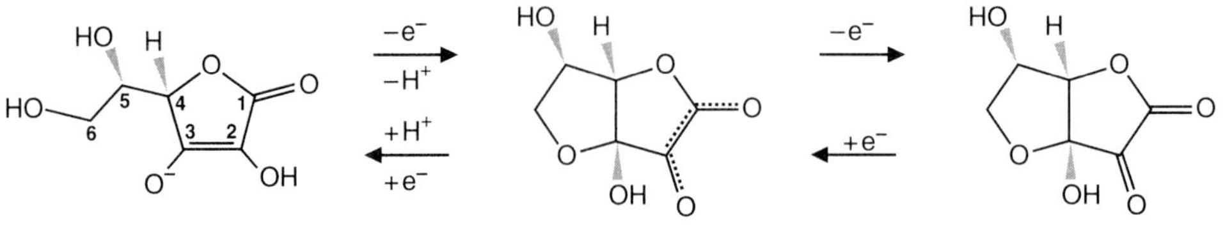

Fig 24.19. L-Ascorbate (the reduced form) donates single electrons to free radicals or disulfides in two steps as it is oxidized to dehydro-L-ascorbic acid. Its principle role in free radical defense is probably regeneration of vitamin E. However, it also may react with superoxide, hydrogen peroxide, hypochlorite, the hydroxyl and peroxyl radicals, and NO_2.

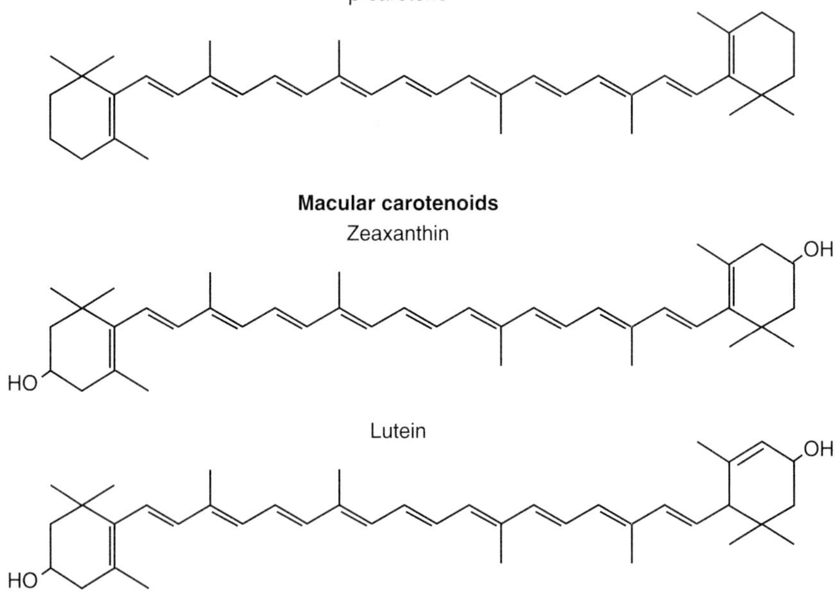

Fig 24.20. Carotenoids are compounds related in structure to β-carotene. Lutein and zeaxanthin (the macular carotenoids) are analogs containing hydroxyl groups.

Epidemiologic evidence suggests that individuals with a higher intake of foods containing vitamin E, β-carotene, and vitamin C have a somewhat lower risk of cancer and certain other ROS-related diseases than do individuals on diets deficient in these vitamins. However, studies in which well-nourished populations were given supplements of these antioxidant vitamins found either no effects or harmful effects compared with the beneficial effects from eating foods containing a wide variety of antioxidant compounds. Of the pure chemical supplements tested, there is evidence only for the efficacy of vitamin E. In two clinical trials, β-carotene (or β-carotene + vitamin A) was associated with a higher incidence of lung cancer among smokers and higher mortality rates. In one study, vitamin E intake was associated with a higher incidence of hemorrhagic stroke (possibly because of vitamin K mimicry).

trials, β-carotene supplements had either no effect or an undesirable effect. Its ineffectiveness may be due to the pro-oxidant activity of the free radical form.

In contrast, epidemiologic studies relating the intake of lutein and zeoxanthin with decreased incidence of age-related macular degeneration have received progressive support. These two carotenoids are concentrated in the macula (the central portion of the retina) and are called the macular carotenoids.

Age-related macular degeneration (AMD) is the leading cause of blindness in the United States among persons older than 50 years of age, and it affects 1.7 million people worldwide. In AMD, visual loss is related to oxidative damage to the retinal pigment epithelium (RPE) and the choriocapillaris epithelium. The photoreceptor/retinal pigment complex is exposed to sunlight, it is bathed in near arterial levels of oxygen, and the membranes contain high concentrations of polyunsaturated fatty acids, all of which are conducive to oxidative damage. Lipofuscin granules, which accumulate in the RPE throughout life, may serve as photosensitizers, initiating damage by absorbing blue light and generating singlet oxygen that forms other radicals. Dark sunglasses are protective. Epidemiologic studies showed that the intake of lutein and zeanthin in dark green leafy vegetables (e.g., spinach and collard greens) also may be protective. Lutein and zeaxanthein accumulate in the macula and protect against free radical damage by absorbing blue light and quenching singlet oxygen.

4. OTHER DIETARY ANTIOXIDANTS

Flavonoids are a group of structurally similar compounds containing two spatially separate aromatic rings that are found in red wine, green tea, chocolate, and other plant-derived foods (Fig. 24.21). Flavonoids have been hypothesized to contribute to our free radical defenses in a number of ways. Some flavonoids inhibit enzymes responsible for superoxide anion production, such as xanthine oxidase. Others efficiently chelate Fe and Cu, making it impossible for these metals to participate in the Fenton reaction. They also may act as free radical scavengers by donating electrons to superoxide or lipid peroxy radicals, or stabilize free radicals by complexing with them.

It is difficult to tell how much dietary flavonoids contribute to our free radical defense system; they have a high pro-oxidant activity and are poorly absorbed. Nonetheless, we generally consume large amounts of flavonoids (approximately 800 mg/day), and there is evidence that they can contribute to the maintenance of vitamin E as an antioxidant.

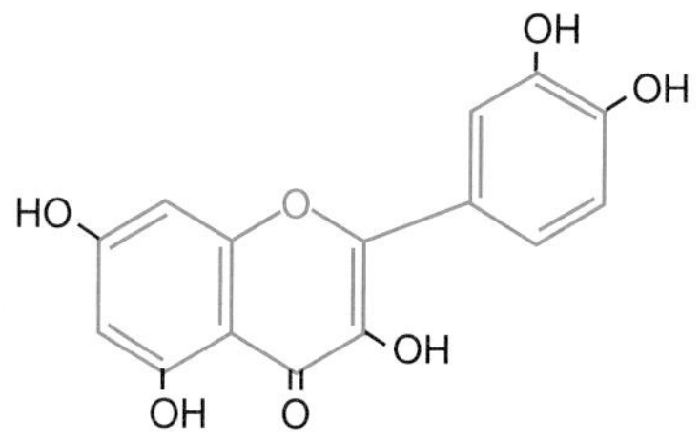

5. ENDOGENOUS ANTIOXIDANTS

A number of compounds synthesized endogenously for other functions, or as urinary excretion products, also function nonenzymatically as free radical antioxidants. Uric acid is formed from the degradation of purines and is released into extracellular fluids, including blood, saliva, and lung lining fluid (Fig. 24.22). Together with protein thiols, it accounts for the major free radical trapping capacity of plasma. It is particularly important in the upper airways, where there are few other antioxidants. It can directly scavenge hydroxyl radicals, oxyheme oxidants formed between the reaction of hemoglobin and peroxy radicals, and peroxyl radicals themselves. Having acted as a scavenger, uric acid produces a range of oxidation products that are subsequently excreted.

Melatonin, which is a secretory product of the pineal gland, is a neurohormone that functions in regulation of our circadian rhythm, light–dark signal transduction, and sleep induction. In addition to these receptor-mediated functions, it functions as a nonenzymatic free radical scavenger that donates an electron (as hydrogen) to "neutralize" free radicals. It also can react with ROS and RNOS to form addition products, thereby undergoing suicidal transformations. Its effectiveness is related to both its lack of pro-oxidant activity and its joint hydrophilic/hydrophobic nature that allows it to pass through membranes and the blood-brain barrier.

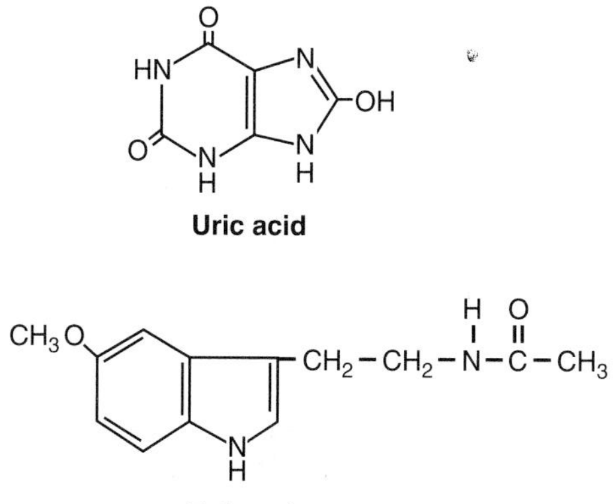

A flavonoid

Fig 24.21. The flavonoid quercetin. All flavonoids have the same ring structure, shown in blue. They differ in ring substituents (=O, -OH, and OCH_3). Quercetin is effective in Fe chelation and antioxidant activity. It is widely distributed in fruits (principally in the skins) and in vegetables (e.g., onions).

Uric acid

Melatonin

Fig 24.22. Endogenous antioxidants. Uric acid and melatonin both act to successively neutralize several molecules of ROS.

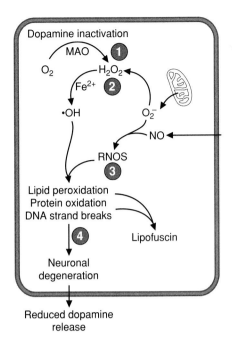

Fig 24.23. A model for the role of ROS and RNOS in neuronal degradation in Parkinson's disease. 1. Dopamine levels are reduced by monoamine oxidase, which generates H_2O_2. 2. Superoxide also can be produced by mitochondria, which SOD will convert to H_2O_2. Iron levels increase, which allows the Fenton reaction to proceed, generating hydroxyl radicals. 3. NO, produced by inducible nitric oxide synthase, reacts with superoxide to form RNOS. 4. The RNOS and hydroxyl radical lead to radical chain reactions that result in lipid peroxidation, protein oxidation, the formation of lipofuscin, and neuronal degeneration. The end result is a reduced production and release of dopamine, which leads to the clinical symptoms observed.

CLINICAL COMMENTS

Les Dopaman has "primary" parkinsonism. The pathogenesis of this disease is not well established and may be multifactorial (Fig. 24.23). The major clinical disturbances in Parkinson's disease are a result of dopamine depletion in the neostriatum, resulting from degeneration of dopaminergic neurons whose cell bodies reside in the substantia nigra pars compacta. The decrease in dopamine production is the result of severe degeneration of these nigrostriatal neurons. Although the agent that initiates the disease is unknown, a variety of studies support a role for free radicals in Parkinson's disease. Within these neurons, dopamine turnover is increased, dopamine levels are lower, glutathione is decreased, and lipofuscin (Lewy bodies) is increased. Iron levels are higher, and ferritin, the storage form of iron, is lower. Furthermore, the disease is mimicked by the compound 1-methyl-4-phenylpyridinium (MPP^+), an inhibitor of NADH dehydrogenase that increases superoxide production in these neurons. Even so, it is not known whether oxidative stress makes a primary or secondary contribution to the disease process.

Drug therapy is based on the severity of the disease. In the early phases of the disease, a monoamine oxidase B-inhibitor is used that inhibits dopamine degradation and decreases hydrogen peroxide formation. In later stages of the disease, patients are treated with levodopa (L-dopa), a precursor of dopamine.

Cora Nari experienced angina caused by severe ischemia in the ventricular muscle of her heart. The ischemia was caused by clots that formed at the site of atherosclerotic plaques within the lumen of the coronary arteries. When TPA was infused to dissolve the clots, the ischemic area of her heart was reperfused with oxygenated blood, resulting in ischemic–reperfusion injury. In her case, the reperfusion injury resulted in ventricular fibrillation.

During ischemia, several events occur simultaneously in cardiomyocytes. A decreased O_2 supply results in decreased ATP generation from mitochondrial oxidative phosphorylation and inhibition of cardiac muscle contraction. As a consequence, cytosolic AMP concentration increases, activating anaerobic glycolysis and lactic acid production. If ATP levels are inadequate to maintain Na^+, K^+-ATPase activity, intracellular Na^+ increases, resulting in cellular swelling, a further increase in H^+ concentration, and increases of cytosolic and subsequently mitochondrial Ca^{2+} levels. The decrease in ATP and increase in Ca^{2+} may open the mitochondrial permeability transition pore, resulting in permanent inhibition of oxidative phosphorylation. Damage to lipid membranes is further enhanced by Ca^{2+} activation of phospholipases.

Reperfusion with O_2 allows recovery of oxidative phosphorylation, provided that the mitochondrial membrane has maintained some integrity and the mitochondrial transition pore can close. However, it also increases generation of free radicals. The transfer of electrons from CoQ• to O_2 to generate superoxide is increased. Endothelial production of superoxide by xanthine oxidase also may increase. These radicals may go on to form the hydroxyl radical, which can enhance the damage to components of the electron transport chain and mitochondrial lipids, as well as activate the

Currently, an intense study of ischemic insults to a variety of animal organs is underway, in an effort to discover ways of preventing reperfusion injury. These include methods designed to increase endogenous antioxidant activity, to reduce the generation of free radicals, and, finally, to develop exogenous antioxidants that, when administered before reperfusion, would prevent its injurious effects. Each of these approaches has met with some success, but their clinical application awaits further refinement. With the growing number of invasive procedures aimed at restoring arterial blood flow through partially obstructed coronary vessels, such as clot lysis, balloon or laser angioplasty, and coronary artery bypass grafting, development of methods to prevent ischemia–reperfusion injury will become increasingly urgent.

mitochondrial permeability transition. As macrophages move into the area to clean up cellular debris, they may generate NO and superoxide, thus introducing peroxynitrite and other free radicals into the area. Depending on the route and timing involved, the acute results may be cell death through necrosis, with slower cell death through apoptosis in the surrounding tissue.

In **Cora Nari's** case, oxygen was restored before permanent impairment of oxidative phosphorylation had occurred and the stage of irreversible injury was reached. However, reintroduction of oxygen induced ventricular fibrillation, from which she recovered.

BIOCHEMICAL COMMENTS

Protection Against Ozone in Lung Lining Fluid The lung lining fluid, a thin fluid layer extending from the nasal cavity to the most distal lung alveoli, protects the epithelial cells lining our airways from ozone and other pollutants. Although ozone is not a radical species, many of its toxic effects are mediated through generation of the classical ROS, as well as generation of aldehydes and ozonides. Polyunsaturated fatty acids represent the primary target for ozone, and peroxidation of membrane lipids is the most important mechanism of ozone-induced injury. However, ozone also oxidizes proteins.

The lung lining fluid has two phases; a gel-phase that traps microorganisms and large particles, and a sol (soluble) phase containing a variety of ROS defense mechanisms that prevent pollutants from reaching the underlying lung epithelial cells (Fig. 24.24). When the ozone level of inspired air is low, ozone is neutralized principally by uric acid (UA) present in the fluid lining the nasal cavity. In the proximal and distal regions of the respiratory tract, glutathione (GSH) and ascorbic acid (AA), in addition to UA, react directly with ozone. Ozone that escapes this antioxidant screen may react directly with proteins, lipids, and carbohydrates (CHO) to generate secondary oxidants, such as lipid peroxides, that can initiate chain reactions. A second layer of defense protects against these oxidation and peroxidation products: β-tocopherol (vitamin E) and glutathione react directly with lipid radicals; glutathione peroxidase reacts with hydrogen peroxide and lipid peroxides, and

Although most individuals are able to protect against small amounts of ozone in the atmosphere, even slightly elevated ozone concentrations produce respiratory symptoms in 10 to 20% of the healthy population.

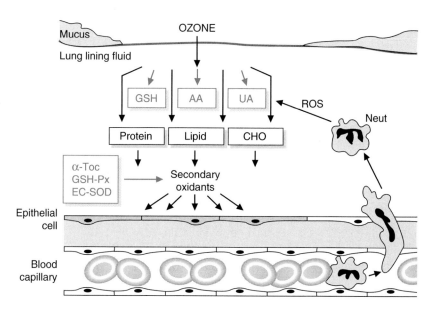

Fig 24.24. Protection against ozone in the lung lining fluid. GSH, glutathione; AA, ascorbic acid (vitamin C); UA, uric acid; CHO, carbohydrate; α-TOC, vitamin E; GSH-Px, glutathione peroxidase; ED-SOD, extracellular superoxide dismutase; *Neut*, neutrophil.

extracellular superoxide dismutase (EC-SOD) converts superoxide to hydrogen peroxide. However, oxidative stress may still overwhelm even this extensive defense network because ozone also promotes neutrophil migration into the lung lining fluid. Once activated, the neutrophils (Neut) produce a second wave of ROS (superoxide, HOCl, and NO).

Suggested References

Gutteridge JMC, Halliwell B. Antioxidants in Nutrition, Health and Disease. Oxford: Oxford University Press, 1994.

Halestrap AP. The mitochondrial permeability transition: its molecular mechanism and role in reperfusion injury. Biochem Soc Symp 1999;66:181–203.

Mudway IS, Kelly FJ. Ozone and the lung: a sensitive issue. Mol Aspects Med 2000;21:1–48.

Pietta P-G. Flavonoids as antioxidants. J Nat Prod 2000;63:1035–1042.

Reiter RJ, Tan D-X, Wenbo A, Manchester LC, Karownik M, Calvo JR. Pharmacology and physiology of melatonin in the reduction of oxidative stress in vivo. Biol Signals Recept 2000;9:160–171.

Shigenaga MK, Hagen TM, Ames BN. Oxidative damage and mitochondrial decay in aging. Proc Natl Acad Sci USA 1994;92:10771–10778.

Winkler BS, Boulton ME, Gottsch JD, Sternberg P. Oxidative damage and age-related macular degeneration. Molecular Vision 1999;5:32.

Zhang Y, Dawson, VL, Dawson, TM. Oxidative stress and genetics in the pathogenesis of Parkinson's disease. Neurobiol Dis 2000;7:240–250.

 REVIEW QUESTIONS—CHAPTER 24

1. Which of the following vitamins or enzymes is unable to protect against free radical damage?

   (A) β-Carotene
   (B) Glutathione peroxidase
   (C) Superoxide dismutase
   (D) Vitamin B6
   (E) Vitamin C
   (F) Vitamin E

2. Superoxide dismutase catalyzes which of the following reactions?

   (A) $O_2^- + e^- + 2H^+$ yields H_2O_2
   (B) $2\ O_2^- + 2H^+$ yields $H_2O_2 + O_2$
   (C) $O_2^- + HO\cdot + H^+$ yields $CO_2 + H_2O$
   (D) $H_2O_2 + O_2$ yields $4\ H_2O$
   (E) $O_2^- + H_2O_2 + H^+$ yields $2\ H_2O + O_2$

3. The mechanism of vitamin E as an antioxidant is best described by which of the following?

   (A) Vitamin E binds to free radicals and sequesters them from the contents of the cell.
   (B) Vitamin E participates in the oxidation of the radicals.
   (C) Vitamin E participates in the reduction of the radicals.
   (D) Vitamin E forms a covalent bond with the radicals, thereby stabilizing the radical state.
   (E) Vitamin E inhibits enzymes that produce free radicals.

4. An accumulation of hydrogen peroxide in a cellular compartment can be converted to dangerous radical forms in the presence of which metal?

    (A) Se
    (B) Fe
    (C) Mn
    (D) Mg
    (E) Mb

5. The level of oxidative damage to mitochondrial DNA is 10 times greater than that to nuclear DNA. This could be due, in part, to which of the following?

    (A) Superoxide dismutase is present in the mitochondria.
    (B) The nucleus lacks glutathione.
    (C) The nuclear membrane presents a barrier to reactive oxygen species.
    (D) The mitochondrial membrane is permeable to reactive oxygen species.
    (E) Mitochondrial DNA lacks histones.

25 Metabolism of Ethanol

*Ethanol is a **dietary fuel** that is metabolized to acetate principally in the liver, with the generation of NADH. The principal route for metabolism of ethanol is through hepatic **alcohol dehydrogenases**, which oxidize ethanol to **acetaldehyde** in the cytosol (Fig. 25.1). Acetaldehyde is further oxidized by **acetaldehyde dehydrogenases** to **acetate**, principally **in mitochondria**. Acetaldehyde, which is toxic, also may enter the blood. **NADH** produced by these reactions is used for adenosine triphosphate (ATP) generation through oxidative phosphorylation. Most of the acetate enters the blood and is taken up by skeletal muscles and other tissues, where it is activated to **acetyl CoA** and is oxidized in the TCA cycle.*

*Approximately 10 to 20% of ingested ethanol is oxidized through a microsomal oxidizing system (**MEOS**), comprising **cytochrome P450** enzymes in the endoplasmic reticulum (especially **CYP2E1**). CYP2E1 has a high K_m for ethanol and is inducible by ethanol. Therefore, the proportion of ethanol metabolized through this route is greater at high ethanol concentrations, and greater after chronic consumption of ethanol.*

*Acute effects of alcohol ingestion arise principally from the generation of NADH, which greatly increases the **NADH/NAD$^+$** ratio of the liver. As a consequence, **fatty acid oxidation is inhibited**, and **ketogenesis** may occur. The elevated **NADH/NAD$^+$** ratio may also cause **lactic acidosis** and inhibit **gluconeogenesis**.*

*Ethanol metabolism may result in **alchohol-induced liver disease**, including **hepatic steatosis** (fatty liver), **alcohol-induced hepatitis**, and **cirrhosis**. The principal toxic products of ethanol metabolism include **acetaldehyde** and **free radicals**. Acetaldehyde forms **adducts** with proteins and other compounds. The **hydroxyethyl radical** produced by MEOS and other radicals produced during*

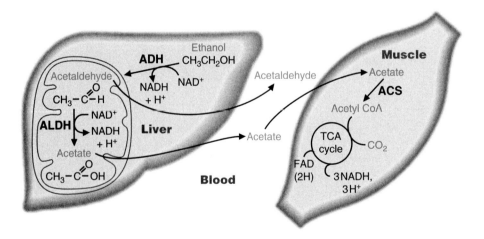

Fig. 25.1. The major route for metabolism of ethanol and use of acetate by the muscle. (ADH, alcohol dehydrogenase; ALDH, acetaldehyde dehydrogenase; ACS, acetyl-CoA synthetase).

*inflammation cause irreversible damage to the liver. Many other tissues are adversely affected by ethanol, acetaldehyde, or by the consequences of **hepatic dysmetabolism** and injury. **Genetic polymorphisms** in the enzymes of ethanol metabolism may be responsible for individual variations in the development of alcoholism or the development of liver cirrhosis.*

THE WAITING ROOM

A dietary history for **Ivan Applebod** showed that he had continued his habit of drinking scotch and soda each evening while watching TV, but he did not add the ethanol calories to his dietary intake. He justifies this calculation on the basis of a comment he heard on a radio program that calories from alcohol ingestion "don't count" because they are empty calories that do not cause weight gain.

Al Martini was found lying semiconscious at the bottom of the stairs by his landlady when she returned from an overnight visit with friends. His face had multiple bruises and his right forearm was grotesquely angulated. Nonbloody dried vomitus stained his clothing. Mr. Martini was rushed by ambulance to the emergency room at the nearest hospital. In addition to multiple bruises and the compound fracture of his right forearm, he had deep and rapid (Kussmaul) respirations and was moderately dehydrated.

Initial laboratory studies showed a relatively large anion gap of 34 mmol/L (reference range = 9–15 mmol/L). An arterial blood gas analysis confirmed the presence of a metabolic acidosis. Mr. Martini's blood alcohol level was only slightly elevated. His serum glucose was 68 mg/dL (low normal).

The anion gap is calculated by subtracting the sum of the value for serum chloride and for the serum HCO_3^- content from the serum sodium concentration. If the gap is greater than normal, it suggests that acids such as the ketone bodies acetoacetate and β-hydroxybutyrate are present in the blood in increased amounts.

Jean Ann Tonich, a 46-year-old commercial artist, recently lost her job because of absenteeism. Her husband of 24 years had left her 10 months earlier. She complains of loss of appetite, fatigue, muscle weakness, and emotional depression. She has had occasional pain in the area of her liver, at times accompanied by nausea and vomiting.

On physical examination she appears disheveled and pale. The physician notes tenderness to light percussion over her liver and detects a small amount of ascites (fluid within the peritoneal cavity around the abdominal organs). The lower edge of her liver is palpable about 2 inches below the lower margin of her right rib cage, suggesting liver enlargement, and feels somewhat more firm and nodular than normal. Jean Ann's spleen is not palpably enlarged. There is a suggestion of mild jaundice. No obvious neurologic or cognitive abnormalities are present.

After detecting a hint of alcohol on Jean Ann's breath, the physician questions her about possible alcohol abuse, which she denies. With more intensive questioning, however, Jean Ann admits that for the last 5 or 6 years she began drinking gin on a daily basis (approximately 4–5 drinks, or 68–85 g ethanol) and eating infrequently. Laboratory tests showed that her serum ethanol level on the initial office visit was 245 mg/dL (0.245%). A serum ethanol level above 150 mg/dL (0.15%) is considered indicative of inebriation.

Jaundice is a yellow discoloration involving the sclerae (the "whites"' of the eyes) and skin. It is caused by the deposition of bilirubin, a yellow degradation product of heme. Bilirubin accumulates in the blood under conditions of liver injury, bile duct obstruction, and excessive degradation of heme.

Jean Ann Tonich's admitted ethanol consumption exceeds the definition of moderate drinking. Moderate drinking is now defined as not more than two drinks per day for men, but only one drink per day for women. A drink is defined as 12 oz of regular beer, 5 oz of wine, or 1.5 oz distilled spirits (80 proof).

I. ETHANOL METABOLISM

Ethanol is a small molecule that is both lipid and water soluble. It is, therefore, readily absorbed from the intestine by passive diffusion. A small percentage of ingested ethanol (0-5%) enters the gastric mucosal cells of the upper GI tract (tongue, mouth,

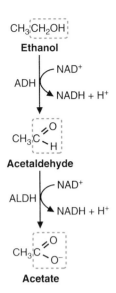

Fig. 25.2. The pathway of ethanol metabolism (ADH, alcohol dehydrogenase; ALDH, acetaldehyde dehydrogenase).

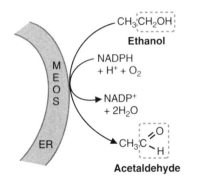

Fig. 25.3. The reaction catalyzed by MEOS (which includes CYP2E1) in the endoplasmic reticulum.

esophagus, and stomach), where it is metabolized. The remainder enters the blood. Of this, 85 to 98% is metabolized in the liver, and only 2 to 10% is excreted through the lungs or kidneys.

The major route of ethanol metabolism in the liver is through liver alcohol dehydrogenase, a cytosolic enzyme that oxidizes ethanol to acetaldehyde with reduction of NAD^+ to NADH (Fig.25.2). If it is not removed by metabolism, acetaldehyde exerts toxic actions in the liver and can enter the blood and exert toxic effects in other tissues.

Approximately 90% of the acetaldehyde that is generated is further metabolized to acetate in the liver. The major enzyme involved is a low K_m mitochondrial acetaldehyde dehydrogenase (ALDH), which oxidizes acetaldehyde to acetate with generation of NADH (see Fig. 25.2). Acetate, which has no toxic effects, may be activated to acetyl CoA in the liver (where it can enter either the TCA cycle or the pathway for fatty acid synthesis). However, most of the acetate that is generated enters the blood and is activated to acetyl CoA in skeletal muscles and other tissues (see Fig. 25.1). Acetate is generally considered nontoxic and is a normal constituent of the diet.

The other principal route of ethanol oxidation in the liver is the microsomal ethanol oxidizing system (MEOS), which also oxidizes ethanol to acetaldehyde (Fig. 25.3). The principal microsomal enzyme involved is a cytochrome P450 mixed-function oxidase isozyme (CYP2E1), which uses NADPH as an additional electron donor and O_2 as an electron acceptor. This route accounts for only 10 to 20% of ethanol oxidation in a moderate drinker.

Each of the enzyme activities involved in ethanol metabolism (alcohol dehydrogenase, acetaldehyde dehydrogenase, and CYP2E1) exist as a family of isoenzymes. Individual variations in the quantity of these isoenzymes influence a number of factors, such as the rate of ethanol clearance from the blood, the degree of inebriation exhibited by an individual, and differences in individual susceptibility to the development of alcohol-induced liver disease.

A. Alcohol Dehydrogenase

Alcohol dehydrogenase (ADH) exists as a family of isoenzymes with varying specificity for chain length of the alcohol substrate (Table 25.1). Ethanol is a small molecule that does not exhibit much in the way of unique structural characteristics and, at high concentrations, is nonspecifically metabolized by many members of the ADH family. The alcohol dehydrogenases that exhibit the highest specificity for ethanol are the class I alcohol dehydrogenases. We have three genes for class I alcohol dehydrogenases, each of which exists as allelic variants (polymorphisms).

Table 25.1. Isozymes of Medium-Chain-Length Alcohol Dehydrogenases

Class	Gene	Sub-Unit	Tissue Distribution	Properties
I	ADH 1 ADH 2 ADH 3	α β γ	Most abundant in liver and adrenal glands. Much lower levels in kidney, lung, colon, small intestine, eye, ovary, blood vessels. None in brain or heart	K_m of 0.05–4 mM for ethanol. Active only with ethanol. High tissue capacity.
II	ADH 4	π	Primarily liver, lower levels in GI tract	K_m of 34 mM for ethanol.
III	ADH 5	χ	Ubiquitously expressed, but at higher levels in liver. The only isozyme present in germinal cells.	Relatively inactive toward ethanol. Active mainly toward long-chain alcohols, and ω-OH fatty acids.
IV	ADH 7	σ	Present in highest levels in upper GI tract, gingiva and mouth, esophagus, down to the stomach. Not present in liver.	K_m of 28 mM. It is the most active of medium-chain alcohol DH toward retinal.
V	ADH 6	-	May be highest in fetal liver.	Some activity toward ethanol

The class I alcohol dehydrogenases are present in high quantities in the liver, representing approximately 3% of all soluble protein. These alcohol dehydrogenases, commonly referred to collectively as liver alcohol dehydrogenase, have low K_ms for ethanol between 0.05 and 4 mM (high affinities). Thus, the liver is the major site of ethanol metabolism and the major site at which the toxic metabolite acetaldehyde is generated.

Although the class IV and class II enzymes make minor contributions to ethanol metabolism, they may contribute to its toxic effects. Ethanol concentrations can be quite high in the upper GI tract (e.g., beer is approximately 0.8 M ethanol), and acetaldehyde generated here by class IV enzymes (gastric ADH) might contribute to the risk for cancer associated with heavy drinking. Class II ADH genes are expressed primarily in the liver and at lower levels in the lower gastrointestinal tract.

B. Acetaldehyde Dehydrogenases

Acetaldehyde is oxidized to acetate, with the generation of NADH, by acetaldehyde dehydrogenases (see Fig. 25.2). More than 80% of acetaldehyde oxidation in the human liver is normally catalyzed by mitochondrial acetaldehyde dehydrogenase (ALDH2), which has a high affinity for acetaldehyde and is highly specific. However, individuals with a common allelic variant of ALDH2 have a greatly decreased capacity for acetaldehyde metabolism

Most of the remainder of acetaldehyde oxidation occurs through a cytosolic acetaldehyde dehydrogenase (ALDH1). Additional aldehyde dehydrogenases act on a variety of organic alcohols, toxins, and pollutants.

C. Fate of Acetate

Metabolism of acetate requires activation to acetyl CoA by acetyl CoA synthetase in a reaction similar to that catalyzed by fatty acyl CoA synthetases (Fig. 25.4). In liver, the principle isoform of acetyl CoA synthetase (ACS I) is a cytosolic enzyme that generates acetyl CoA for the cytosolic pathways of cholesterol and fatty acid synthesis. Acetate entry into these pathways is under regulatory control by mechanisms involving cholesterol or insulin. Thus, most of the acetate generated enters the blood.

Acetate is taken up and oxidized by other tissues, notably heart and skeletal muscle, which have a high concentration of the mitochondrial acetyl CoA synthetase isoform (ACSII). This enzyme is present in the mitochondrial matrix. It therefore generates acetyl CoA that can directly enter the TCA cycle and be oxidized to CO_2.

D. Microsomal Ethanol Oxidizing System

Ethanol is also oxidized to acetaldehyde in the liver by the microsomal ethanol oxidizing system, which comprises members of the cytochrome P450 superfamily of enzymes. Ethanol and NADPH both donate electrons in the reaction, which reduces O_2 to $2H_2O$ (Fig. 25.5). The cytochrome P450 enzymes all have two

The human has at least seven, and possibly more, genes that code for specific isoenzymes of medium-chain-length alcohol dehydrogenases, the major enzyme responsible for the oxidation of ethanol to acetaldehyde in the human. These different alcohol dehydrogenases have an approximately 60 to 70% identity and are assumed to have arisen from a common ancestral gene similar to the class III isoenzyme many millions of years ago. The class I alcohol dehydrogenases (ADH 1, ADH 2, and ADH 3) are all present in high concentration in the liver, and have a relatively high affinity and capacity for ethanol at low concentrations. (These properties are quantitatively reflected by their low K_m, a parameter discussed in Chapter 9). They have a 90 to 94% sequence identity and are able to form both homo- and hetero-dimers, among themselves (e.g., ββ or βγ). However, none of the ADHs can form dimers with an ADH from another class. The three genes for class I alcohol dehydrogenases are arranged in tandem, head to tail, on chromosome 4. The genes for the other classes of alcohol dehydrogenase are also on chromosome 4 in nearby locations.

ADH 2 and ADH 3 are present as functional polymorphisms that differ in their properties. Genetic polymorphisms for ADH partially account for the observed differences in ethanol elimination rates among various individuals or populations. Although susceptibility to alcoholism is a complex function of genetics and socioeconomic factors, possession of the ADH 2*2 allele, which encodes a relatively fast ADH (high V_{max}), is associated with a decreased susceptibility to alcoholism—presumably because of nausea and flushing caused by acetaldehyde accumulation (because the aldehyde dehydrogenase gene cannot keep up with the amount of acetaldehyde produced). This particular allele has a relatively high frequency in the East Asian population and a low frequency among white Europeans. In contrast, the ADH 2*1/2*1 genotype (homozygous for allele 1 of the ADH 2 gene) is a risk factor for the development of Wernicke-Korsakoff syndrome, a neuropsychiatric syndrome commonly associated with alcoholism.

The accumulation of acetaldehyde causes nausea and vomiting, and, therefore, inactive acetaldehyde dehydrogenases are associated with a distaste for alcoholic beverages and protection against alcoholism. In one of the common allelic variants of ALDH2 (ALDH2*2), a single substitution increases the K_m for acetaldehyde 260-fold (lowers the affinity) and decreases the V_{max} 10-fold, resulting in a very inactive enzyme. Homozygosity for the ALDH2*2 allele affords absolute protection against alcoholism; no individual with this genotype has been found among alcoholics. Alcoholics are frequently treated with acetaldehyde dehydrogenase inhibitors (e.g., disulfiram) to help them abstain from alcohol intake. Unfortunately, alcoholics who continue to drink while taking this drug are exposed to the toxic effects of elevated acetaldehyde levels.

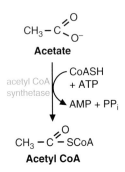

Fig. 25.4. The activation of acetate to acetyl CoA

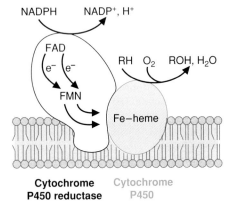

Fig. 25.5. General structure of cytochrome P450 enzymes. O_2 binds to the P450 Fe-heme in the active site and is activated to a reactive form by accepting electrons. The electrons are donated by the cytochrome P450 reductase, which contains an FAD plus an FMN or Fe-S center to facilitate the transfer of single electrons from NADPH to O_2. The P450 enzymes involved in steroidogenesis have a somewhat different structure. For CYP2E1, RH is ethanol (CH_3CH_2OH) and ROH is acetaldehyde (CH_3COH).

CYP represents **cy**tochrome **P**450. P450 is an Fe-heme similar to that found in the cytochromes of the electron transport chain ("P" denotes the heme **p**igment, and 450 is the wavelength of visible light absorbed by the pigment). In CYP2E1, the "2" refers to the gene family, which comprises isoenzymes with greater than 40% amino acid sequence identity. The "E" refers to the subfamily, a grouping of isoenzymes with greater than 55 to 60% sequence identity, and the "1" refers to the individual enzymes within this subfamily.

major catalytic protein components: an electron-donating reductase system that transfers electrons from NADPH (cytochrome P450 reductase) and a cytochrome P450. The cytochrome P450 protein contains the binding sites for O_2 and the substrate (e.g., ethanol) and carries out the reaction. The enzymes are present in the endoplasmic reticulum, which on isolation from disrupted cells forms a membrane fraction after centrifugation that was formerly called "microsomes" by biochemists.

1. CYP2E1

MEOS is part of the superfamily of cytochrome P450 enzymes, all of which catalyze similar oxidative reactions. Within the superfamily, at least 10 distinct gene families are found in mammals. More than 100 different cytochrome P450 isozymes exist within these 10 gene families. Each isoenzyme has a distinct classification according to its structural relationship with other isoenzymes. The isoenzyme that has the highest activity toward ethanol is called CYP2E1. A great deal of overlapping specificity exists among the various P450 isoenzymes, and ethanol is also oxidized by several other P450 isoenzymes. "MEOS" refers to the combined ethanol oxidizing activity of all the P450 enzymes.

CYP2E1 has a much higher K_m for ethanol than the class I alcohol dehydrogenases (11 mM [51 mg/dL] compared with 0.05–4 mM [0.23 to 18.4 mg/dL]). Thus, a greater proportion of ingested ethanol is metabolized through CYP2E1 at high levels of ethanol consumption than at low levels.

2. INDUCTION OF P450 ENZYMES

The P450 enzymes are inducible both by their most specific substrate and by substrates for some of the other cytochrome P450 enzymes. Chronic consumption of ethanol increases hepatic CYP2E1 levels approximately 5- to 10-fold. However, it also causes a twofold to fourfold increase in some of the other P450s from the same subfamily, from different subfamilies, and even from different gene families. The endoplasmic reticulum undergoes proliferation, with a general increase in the content of microsomal enzymes, including those that are not directly involved in ethanol metabolism.

The increase in CYP2E1 with ethanol consumption occurs through transcriptional, post-transcriptional, and post-translational regulation. Increased levels of mRNA, resulting from induction of gene transcription or stabilization of message, are found in actively drinking patients. The protein is also stabilized against degradation. In general, the mechanism for induction of P450 enzymes by their substrates occurs through the binding of the substrate (or related compound) to an intracellular receptor protein, followed by binding of the activated receptor to a response element in the target gene. Whether ethanol induction of CYP2E1 follows this general pattern has not yet been shown.

Overlapping specificity in the catalytic activity of P450 enzymes and in their inducers is responsible for several types of drug interactions. For example, phenobarbital, a barbiturate long used as a sleeping pill or for treatment of epilepsy, is converted to an inactive metabolite by cytochrome P450 monooxygenases CYP2B1 and CYP2B2. After treatment with phenobarbital, CYP2B2 is increased 50- to 100-fold. Individuals who take phenobarbital for prolonged periods develop a drug tolerance as CYP2B2 is induced, and the drug is metabolized to an inactive metabolite more rapidly. Consequently, these individuals use progressively higher doses of phenobarbital.

Ethanol is an inhibitor of the phenobarbital-oxidizing P450 system. When large amounts of ethanol are consumed, the inactivation of phenobarbital is directly or indirectly inhibited. Therefore, when high doses of phenobarbital and ethanol are consumed at the same time, toxic levels of the barbiturate can accumulate in the blood.

Although induction of CYP2E1 increases ethanol clearance from the blood, it has negative consequences. Acetaldehyde may be produced faster than it can be metabolized by acetaldehyde dehydrogenases, thereby increasing the risk of hepatic injury. An increased amount of acetaldehyde can enter the blood and can damage other tissues. In addition, cytochrome P450 enzymes are capable of generating free radicals, which also may lead to increased hepatic injury and cirrhosis (see Chapter 24).

E. Variations in the Pattern of Ethanol Metabolism

The routes and rates of ethanol oxidation vary from individual to individual. Differences in ethanol metabolism may influence whether an individual becomes a chronic alcoholic, develops alcohol-induced liver disease, or develops other diseases associated with increased alcohol consumption (such as hepatocarcinogenesis, lung cancer, or breast cancer). Factors that determine the rate and route of ethanol oxidation in individuals include:

- Genotype—Polymorphic forms of alcohol dehydrogenases and acetaldehyde dehydrogenases can greatly affect the rate of ethanol oxidation and the accumulation of acetaldehyde. CYP2E1 activity may vary as much as 20-fold between individuals, partly because of differences in the inducibility of different allelic variants.
- Drinking history—The level of gastric alcohol dehydrogenase (ADH) decreases and CYP2E1 increases with the progression from a naïve, to a moderate, and to a heavy and chronic consumer of alcohol.
- Gender—Blood levels of ethanol after consuming a drink are normally higher for women than for men, partly because of lower levels of gastric ADH activity in women. After chronic consumption of ethanol, gastric ADH decreases in both men and women, but the gender differences become even greater. Gender differences in blood alcohol levels also occur because women are normally smaller. Furthermore, in females, alcohol is distributed in a 12% smaller water space because a woman's body composition consists of more fat and less water than that of a man.
- Quantity—The amount of ethanol an individual consumes over a small amount of time determines its metabolic route. Small amounts of ethanol are metabolized most efficiently through the low K_m pathway of class I ADH and class II ALDH. Little accumulation of NADH occurs to inhibit ethanol metabolism via these dehydrogenases. However, when higher amounts of ethanol are consumed in a short period, a disproportionately greater amount is metabolized through MEOS. MEOS, which has a much higher K_m for ethanol, functions principally at high concentrations of ethanol. A higher activity of MEOS would be expected to correlate with tendency to develop alcohol-induced liver disease, because both acetaldehyde and free radical levels would be increased.

F. The Energy Yield of Ethanol Oxidation

The ATP yield from ethanol oxidation to acetate varies with the route of ethanol metabolism. If ethanol is oxidized by the major route of cytosolic ADH and mitochondrial ALDH, one cytosolic and one mitochondrial NADH are generated with a maximum yield of 5 ATP. Oxidation of acetyl CoA in the TCA cycle and electron transport chain leads to the generation of 10 high-energy phosphate bonds. However, activation of acetate to acetyl CoA requires two high-energy phosphate bonds (one in the cleavage of ATP to AMP+ pyrophosphate and one in the cleavage of pyrophosphate to phosphate), which must be subtracted. Thus the maximum total energy yield is 13 moles of ATP per mole of ethanol.

In contrast, oxidation of ethanol to acetaldehyde by CYP2E1 consumes energy in the form of NADPH, which is equivalent to 2.5 ATP. Thus, for every mole of

As blood ethanol concentration rises above 18 mM (the legal intoxication limit is now defined as 0.08% in most states of the United States, which is approximately 18 mM), the brain and central nervous system are affected. Induction of CYP2E1 increases the rate of ethanol clearance from the blood, thereby contributing to increased alcohol tolerance. However, the apparent ability of a chronic alcoholic to drink without appearing inebriated is partly a learned behavior.

At **Ivan Applebod's** low level of ethanol consumption, ethanol is oxidized to acetate via ADH and ALDH in the liver and the acetate is activated to acetyl CoA and oxidized to CO$_2$ in skeletal muscle and other tissues. The overall energy yield of 13 ATP per ethanol molecule accounts for the caloric value of ethanol, approximately 7 Cal/g. However, chronic consumption of substantial amounts of alcohol does not have the effect on body weight expected from the caloric intake. This is partly attributable to induction of MEOS, resulting in a proportionately greater metabolism of ethanol through MEOS with its lower energy yield (only approximately 8 ATP). In general, weight loss diets recommend no, or low, alcohol consumption because ethanol calories are "empty" in the sense that alcoholic beverages are generally low in vitamins, essential amino acids, and other required nutrients, but not empty of calories.

ethanol metabolized by this route, only a maximum of 8.0 moles of ATP can be generated (10 ATP from acetylCoA oxidation through the TCA cycle, minus 2 for acetate activation; the NADH generated by aldehyde dehydrogenase is balanced by the loss of NADPH in the MEOS step).

II. TOXIC EFFECTS OF ETHANOL METABOLISM

Alcohol-induced liver disease, a common and sometimes fatal consequence of chronic ethanol abuse, may manifest itself in three forms: fatty liver, alcohol-induced hepatitis, and cirrhosis. Each may occur alone, or they may be present in any combination in a given patient. Alcohol-induced cirrhosis is discovered in up to 9% of all autopsies performed in the United States, with a peak incidence in patients 40 to 55 years of age.

However, ethanol ingestion also has acute effects on liver metabolism, including inhibition of fatty acid oxidation and stimulation of triacylglycerol synthesis, leading to a fatty liver. It also can result in ketoacidosis or lactic acidosis and cause hypoglycemia or hyperglycemia, depending on the dietary state. These effects are considered reversible.

In contrast, acetaldehyde and free radicals generated from ethanol metabolism can result in alcohol-induced hepatitis, a condition in which the liver is inflamed and cells become necrotic and die. Diffuse damage to hepatocytes results in cirrhosis, characterized by fibrosis (scarring), disturbance of the normal architecture and blood flow, loss of liver function and, ultimately, hepatic failure.

A. Acute Effects of Ethanol Arising from the Increased NADH /NAD$^+$ Ratio

Many of the acute effects of ethanol ingestion arise from the increased NADH/NAD$^+$ ratio in the liver (Fig. 25.6). At lower levels of ethanol intake, the rate of ethanol oxidation is regulated by the supply of ethanol (usually determined by how much ethanol we consume) and the rate at which NADH is reoxidized in the electron transport chain. NADH is not a very effective product inhibitor of ADH or ALDH, and there is no other feedback regulation by ATP, ADP, or AMP. As a consequence, NADH generated in the cytosol and mitochondria tends to accumulate, increasing the NADH/NAD$^+$ ratio to high levels (see Fig. 25.6, circle 1). The increase is even greater as the mitochondria become damaged from acetaldehyde or free radical injury.

1. CHANGES IN FATTY ACID METABOLISM

The high NADH/NAD$^+$ ratio generated from ethanol oxidation inhibits the oxidation of fatty acids, which accumulate in the liver (see Fig. 25.6, circles 2 and 3) These fatty acids are re-esterified into triacylglycerols by combining with glycerol 3-P. The increased NADH/NAD$^+$ ratio increases the availability of glycerol 3-P by promoting its synthesis from intermediates of glycolysis. The triacylglycerols are incorporated into VLDL (very-low-density lipoproteins), which accumulate in the liver and enter the blood, resulting in an ethanol-induced hyperlipidemia.

Although just a few drinks may result in hepatic fat accumulation, chronic consumption of alcohol greatly enhances the development of a fatty liver. Re-esterification of fatty acids into triacylglycerols by fatty acyl CoA transferases in the ER is enhanced (see Fig. 25.6). Because the transferases are microsomal enzymes, they are induced by ethanol consumption just as MEOS is induced. The result is a fatty liver (hepatic steatosis).

The source of the fatty acids can be dietary fat, fatty acids synthesized in the liver, or fatty acids released from adipose tissue stores. Adipose tissue lipolysis increases after ethanol consumption, possibly because of a release of epinephrine.

The hyperlipidemia is greatly enhanced if fat is ingested with ethanol. Thus, "happy hour" foods (e.g., pizza, fried potato skins with sour cream, nachos, and deep-fried peppers stuffed with cream cheese and wrapped in bacon) are exactly the wrong things to eat while drinking. Steamed vegetables or salads with your beer would be much better for your liver.

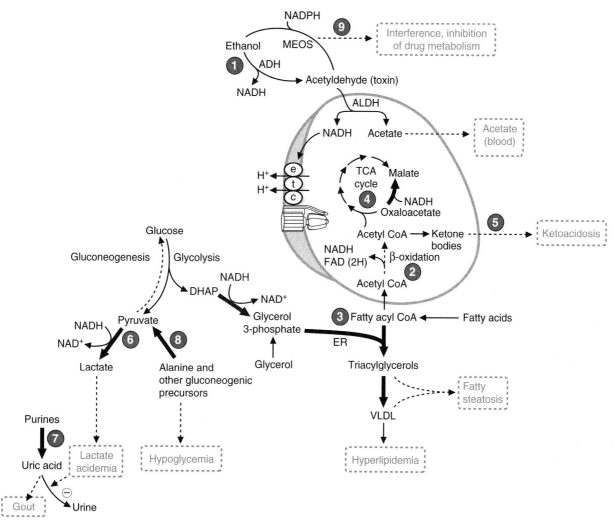

Fig. 25.6. Acute effects of ethanol metabolism on lipid metabolism in the liver. (1) Metabolism of ethanol generates a high NADH/NAD$^+$ ratio. (2) The high NADH/NAD$^+$ ratio inhibits fatty acid oxidation and the TCA cycle, resulting in accumulation of fatty acids. (3) Fatty acids are re-esterified to glycerol 3-P by acyltransferases in the endoplasmic reticulum. Glycerol 3-P levels are increased because a high NADH/NAD$^+$ ratio favors its formation from dihydroxyacetone phosphate (an intermediate of glycolysis). Ethanol-stimulated increases of endoplasmic reticulum enzymes also favors triacylglycerol formation. (4) NADH generated from ethanol oxidation can meet the requirements of the cell for ATP generation from oxidative phosphorylation. Thus, acetyl CoA oxidation in the TCA cycle is inhibited. (5) The high NADH/NAD$^+$ ratio shifts oxaloacetate (OAA) toward malate, and acetyl CoA is directed into ketone body synthesis. Options 6–8 are discussed in the text.

2. ALCOHOL-INDUCED KETOACIDOSIS.

Fatty acids that are oxidized are converted to acetyl CoA and subsequently to ketone bodies (acetoacetate and β-hydroxybutyrate). Enough NADH is generated from oxidation of ethanol and fatty acids that there is no need to oxidize acetyl CoA in the TCA cycle. The very high NADH/NAD$^+$ ratio shifts all of the oxaloacetate in the TCA cycle to malate, leaving the oxaloacetate levels too low for citrate synthase to synhesize citrate (see Fig. 25.6, circle 4). The acetyl CoA enters the pathway for ketone body synthesis instead of the TCA cycle.

Although ketone bodies are being produced at a high rate, their metabolism in other tissues is restricted by the supply of acetate, which is the preferred fuel. Thus, the blood concentration of ketone bodies may be much higher than found under normal fasting conditions.

 Al Martini's admitting physician suspected an alcohol-induced ketoacidosis superimposed on a starvation ketoacidosis. Tests showed that his plasma free fatty acid level was elevated, and his plasma β-hydroxybutyrate level was 40 times the upper limit of normal. The increased NADH/NAD$^-$ ratio from ethanol consumption inhibited the TCA cycle and shifted acetyl CoA from fatty acid oxidation into the pathway of ketone body synthesis.

3. LACTIC ACIDOSIS, HYPERURICEMIA, AND HYPOGLYCEMIA

Another consequence of the very high $NADH/NAD^+$ ratio is that the balance in the lactate dehydrogenase reaction is shifted toward lactate, resulting in a lacticacidosis (see Fig. 25.6, circle 6). The elevation of blood lactate may decrease excretion of uric acid (see Fig. 25.6, circle 7) by the kidney. Consequently patients with gout (which results from precipitated uric acid crystals in the joints) are advised not to drink excessive amounts of ethanol. Increased degradation of purines also may contribute to hyperuricemia.

The increased $NADH/NAD^+$ ratio also can cause hypoglycemia in a fasting individual who has been drinking and is dependent on gluconeogenesis to maintain blood glucose levels (Fig. 25.6, circles 6 and 8). Alanine and lactate are major gluconeogenic precursors that enter gluconeogenesis as pyruvate. The high $NADH/NAD^+$ ratio shifts the lactate dehydrogenase equilibrium to lactate, so that pyruvate formed from alanine is converted to lactate and cannot enter gluconeogenesis. The high $NADH/NAD^+$ ratio also prevents other major gluconeogenic precursors, such as oxaloacetate and glycerol, from entering the gluconeogenic pathway.

In contrast, ethanol consumption with a meal may result in a transient hyperglycemia, possibly because the high $NADH/NAD^+$ ratio inhibits glycolysis at the glyceraldehyde-3-P dehydrogenase step.

B. Acetaldehyde Toxicity

Many of the toxic effects of chronic ethanol consumption result from accumulation of acetaldehyde, which is produced from ethanol both by alcohol dehydrogenases and MEOS. Acetaldehyde accumulates in the liver and is released into the blood after heavy doses of ethanol (Fig. 25.7). It is highly reactive and binds covalently to amino groups, sulfhydryl groups, nucleotides, and phospholipids to form "adducts."

1. ACETALDEHYDE AND ALCOHOL-INDUCED HEPATITIS

One of the results of acetaldehyde-adduct formation with amino acids is a general decrease in hepatic protein synthesis (see Fig. 25.7, circle 1). Calmodulin, ribonuclease, and tubulin are some of the proteins affected. Proteins in the heart and other tissues also may be affected by acetaldehyde that appears in the blood.

As a consequence of forming acetaldehyde adducts of tubulin, there is a diminished secretion of serum proteins and VLDL lipoproteins from the liver. The liver synthesizes many blood proteins, including serum albumin, blood coagulation factors, and transport proteins for vitamins, steroids, and iron. These proteins accumulate in the liver, together with lipid. The accumulation of proteins results in an influx of water (see Fig. 25.7, circle 6) within the hepatocytes and a swelling of the liver that contributes to portal hypertension and a disruption of hepatic architecture.

2. ACETALDEHYDE AND FREE RADICAL DAMAGE

Acetaldehyde adduct formation enhances free radical damage. Acetaldehyde binds directly to glutathione and diminishes its ability to protect against H_2O_2 and prevent lipid peroxidation (see Fig. 25.7, circle 2). It also binds to free radical defense enzymes.

Damage to mitochondria from acetaldehyde and free radicals perpetuates a cycle of toxicity (see Fig. 25.7, circles 3 and 4). With chronic consumption of ethanol, mitochondria become damaged, the rate of electron transport is inhibited, and oxidative phosphorylation tends to become uncoupled. Fatty acid

The noncaloric effect of heavy and chronic ethanol ingestion that led **Ivan Applebod** to believe ethanol has no calories may be partly attributable to uncoupling of oxidative phosphorylation. The hepatic mitochondria from tissues of chronic alcoholics may be partially uncoupled and unable to maintain the transmembrane proton gradient necessary for normal rates of ATP synthesis. Consequently, a greater proportion of the energy in ethanol would be converted to heat. Metabolic disturbances such as the loss of ketone bodies in urine, or futile cycling of glucose, also might contribute to a dimished energy value for ethanol.

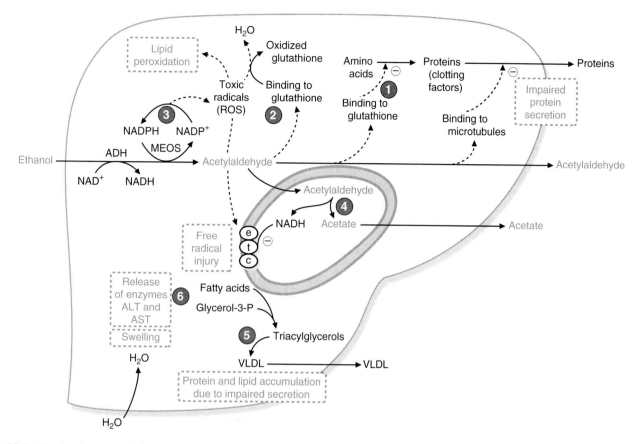

Fig. 25.7. The development of alcohol-induced hepatitis. (1) Acetaldehyde adduct formation decreases protein synthesis and impairs protein secretion. (2) Free radical injury results partly from acetaldehyde adduct formation with glutathione. (3) Induction of MEOS increases formation of free radicals, which leads to lipid peroxidation and cell damage. (4) Mitochondrial damage inhibits the electron transport chain, which decreases acetaldehyde oxidation. (5) Microtubule damage increases VLDL and protein accumulation. (6) Cell damage leads to release of the hepatic enzymes alanine aminotransferase (ALT) and aspartate aminotransferase (AST).

oxidation is decreased even further, thereby enhancing lipid accumulation (see Fig. 25.7, circle 5). The mitochondrial changes further impair mitochondrial acetaldehyde oxidation, thereby initiating a cycle of progressively increasing acetaldehyde damage.

C. Ethanol and Free Radical Formation

Increased oxidative stress in the liver during chronic ethanol intoxication arises from increased production of free radicals, principally by CYP2E1. FAD and FMN in the reductase and heme in the cytochrome P450 system transfer single electrons, thus operating through a mechanism that can generate free radicals. The hydroxyethyl radical ($CH_3CH_2O\cdot$) is produced during ethanol metabolism and can be released as a free radical. Induction of CYP2E1, as well as other cytochrome P450 enzymes, can increase the generation of free radicals from drug metabolism and from the activation of toxins and carcinogens (see Fig. 25.7, circle 3). These effects are enhanced by acetaldehyde-adduct damage.

Phospholipids, the major lipid in cellular membranes, are a primary target of peroxidation caused by free radical release. Peroxidation of lipids in the inner mitochondrial membrane may contribute to the inhibition of electron transport and uncoupling of mitochondria, leading to inflammation and cellular necrosis. Induction of CYP2E1 and other P450 cytochromes also increases formation of other radicals and the activation of hepatocarcinogens.

Because of the possibility of mild alcoholic hepatitis and perhaps chronic alcohol-induced cirrhosis, the physician ordered liver function studies on **Jean Ann Tonich**. The tests indicated an alanine aminotransferase (ALT) level of 46 units/L (reference range = 5–30) and an aspartate aminotransferase (AST) level of 98 units/L (reference range = 10–30). The concentration of these enzymes is high in hepatocytes. When hepatocellular membranes are damaged in any way, these enzymes are released into the blood. Jean Ann Tonich's serum alkaline phosphatase level was 151 units/L (reference range = 56–155 for an adult female). The serum total bilirubin level was 2.4 mg/dL (reference range = 0.2–1.0). These tests show impaired capacity for normal liver function. Her blood hemoglobin and hematocrit levels were slightly below the normal range, consistent with a toxic effect of ethanol on red blood cell production by bone marrow. Serum folate, vitamin B12 and iron levels were also slightly suppressed. Folate is dependent on the liver for its activation and recovery from the enterohepatic circulation. Vitamin B12 and iron are dependent on the liver for synthesis of their blood carrier proteins. Thus, **Jean Ann Tonich** shows many of the consequences of hepatic damage.

In liver fibrosis, disruption of the normal liver architecture, including sinusoids, impairs blood from the portal vein. Increased portal vein pressure (portal hypertension) causes capillaries to anastomose (to meet and unite or run into each other) and form thin-walled dilated esophageal venous conduits known as esophageal varices. When these burst, there is hemorrhaging into the gastrointestinal tract. The bleeding can be very profuse because of the high venous pressure within these varices in addition to the adverse effect of impaired hepatic function on the production of blood clotting proteins.

D. Hepatic Cirrhosis and Loss of Liver Function

Liver injury is irreversible at the stage that hepatic cirrhosis develops. Initially the liver may be enlarged, full of fat, crossed with collagen fibers (fibrosis), and have nodules of regenerating hepatocytes ballooning between the fibers. As liver function is lost, the liver becomes shrunken (Laennec's cirrhosis). During the development of cirrhosis, many of the normal metabolic functions of the liver are lost, including biosynthetic and detoxification pathways. Synthesis of blood proteins, including blood coagulation factors and serum albumin, is decreased. The capacity to incorporate amino groups into urea is decreased, resulting in the accumulation of toxic levels of ammonia in the blood. Conjugation and excretion of the yellow pigment bilirubin (a product of heme degradation) is diminished, and bilirubin accumulates in the blood. It is deposited in many tissues, including the skin and sclerae of the eyes, causing the patient to become visibly yellow. Such a patient is said to be jaundiced.

CLINICAL COMMENTS

Ivan Applebod. When ethanol consumption is low (less than 15% of the calories in the diet), it is efficiently used to produce ATP, thereby contributing to **Ivan Applebod's** weight gain. However, in individuals with chronic consumption of large amounts of ethanol, the caloric content of ethanol is not converted to ATP as effectively. Some of the factors that may contribute to this decreased efficiency include mitochondrial damage (inhibition of oxidative phosphorylation and uncoupling) resulting in the loss of calories as heat, increased recycling of metabolites such as ketone bodies, and inhibition of the normal pathways of fatty acid and glucose oxidation. In addition, heavier drinkers metabolize an increased amount of alcohol through MEOS, which generates less ATP.

Al Martini. Al Martini was suffering from acute effects of high ethanol ingestion in the absence of food intake. Both heavy ethanol consumption and low caloric intake increase adipose tissue lipolysis and elevate blood fatty acids. As a consequence of his elevated hepatic NADH/NAD$^+$ ratio, acetyl CoA produced from fatty acid oxidation was diverted from the TCA cycle into the pathway of ketone body synthesis. Because his skeletal muscles were using acetate as a fuel, ketone body utilization was diminished, resulting in ketoacidosis. **Al Martini's** moderately low blood glucose level also suggests that his high hepatic NADH level prevented pyruvate and glycerol from entering the gluconeogenic pathway. Pyruvate is diverted to lactate, which may have contributed to his metabolic acidosis and anion gap.

Rehydration with intravenous fluids containing glucose and potassium was initiated. His initial potassium was low, possibly secondary to vomiting. An orthopedic surgeon was consulted regarding the compound fracture of his right forearm.

Jean Ann Tonich. Jean Ann Tonich's signs and symptoms, as well as her laboratory profile, were consistent with the presence of mild reversible alcohol-induced hepatocellular inflammation (alcohol-induced hepatitis) superimposed on a degree of irreversible scarring of liver tissues known as chronic alcoholic (Laennec's) cirrhosis of the liver. The chronic inflammatory process associated with long-term ethanol abuse in patients such as **Jean Ann Tonich** is accompanied by increases in the levels of serum alanine aminotransferase (ALT) and aspartate aminotransferase (AST). Her elevated bilirubin and alkaline phosphatase were consistent with hepatic damage. Her values for ALT and

AST were significantly below those seen in acute viral hepatitis. In addition, the ratio of the absolute values for serum ALT and AST often differ in the two diseases, tending to be greater than 1 in acute viral hepatitis and less than 1 in chronic alcohol-induced cirrhosis. The reason for the difference in ratio of enzyme activities released is not understood, but a lower level of ALT in the serum may be attributable to an alcohol-induced deficiency of pyridoxal phosphate. In addition, serologic tests for viral hepatitis were nonreactive. Her serum folate, vitamin B12, and iron levels were also slightly suppressed, indicating impaired nutritional status.

Jean Ann Tonich was strongly cautioned to abstain from alcohol immediately and to improve her nutritional status. In addition, Jean Ann was referred to the hospital drug and alcohol rehabilitation unit for appropriate psychological therapy and supportive social counseling. The physician also arranged for a follow-up office visit in 2 weeks.

Although the full spectrum of alcohol-induced liver disease may be present in a well-nourished individual, the presence of nutritional deficiencies enhances the progression of the disease. Ethanol creates nutritional deficiencies in a number of different ways. The ingestion of ethanol reduces the gastrointestinal absorption of foods containing essential nutrients, including vitamins, essential fatty acids, and essential amino acids. For example, ethanol interferes with absorption of folate, thiamine, and other nutrients. Secondary malabsorption can occur through gastrointestinal complications, pancreatic insufficiency, and impaired hepatic metabolism or impaired hepatic storage of nutrients, such as vitamin A. Changes in the level of transport proteins produced by the liver also strongly affect nutrient status.

BIOCHEMICAL COMMENTS

Fibrosis in Chronic Alcohol-Induced Liver Disease Fibrosis is the excessive accumulation of connective tissue in parenchymal organs. In the liver, it is a frequent event following a repeated or chronic insult of sufficient intensity (such as chronic ethanol intoxication or infection by a hepatitis virus) to trigger a "wound healing–like" reaction. Regardless of the insult, the events are similar: an overproduction of extracellular matrix components occurs, with the tendency to progress into sclerosis, accompanied by a degenerative alteration in the composition of matrix components. (Table 25.2) Some individuals (fewer than 20% of those who chronically consume alcohol) go on to develop cirrhosis.

The development of hepatic fibrosis after ethanol consumption is related to stimulation of the mitogenic development of stellate (Ito) cells into myofibroblasts, and stimulation of the production of collagen type I and fibronectin by these cells. The stellate cells are perisinusoidal cells lodged in the space of Disse that produce extracellular matrix protein. Normally the space of Disse contains basement membrane—like collagen (collagen type IV) and laminin. As the stellate cells are activated, they change from a resting cell filled with lipids and vitamin A to one that proliferates, loses its vitamin A content, and secretes large quantities of extracellular matrix components.

One of the initial events in the activation and proliferation of stellate cells is the activation of Kupffer cells, which are macrophages resident in the liver sinusoids

Table 25.2. Hepatic Injury

Stage of Injury	Main Features
Fibrosis: Increase of connective tissue	
	Accumulation of both fibrillar and basement membrane–like collagens
	Increase of laminen and fibronectin
	Thickening of connective tissue septae
	Capillarization of the sinusoids
Sclerosis: Aging of fibrotic tissue	
	Decrease of hyaluronic acid and heparan sulfate proteoglycans
	Increase of chondroitin sulfate proteoglycans
	Progressive fragmentation and disappearance of elastic fibers
	Distortion of sinusoidal architecture and parenchymal damage
Cirrhosis: End-stage process of liver fibrotic degeneration	
	Whole liver heavily distorted by thick bands of collagen surrounding nodules of hepatocytes with regenerative foci

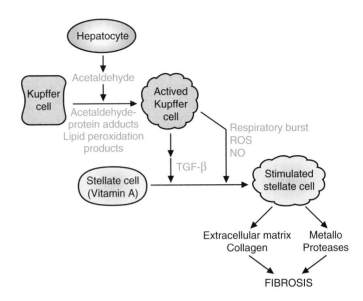

Fig. 25.8. Proposed model for the development of hepatic fibrosis involving hepatocytes, Kupffer cells, and stellate (Ito) cells. ROS, reactive oxygen species; NO, nitric oxide: TGFβ1, transforming growth factor β1.

 Cytokines are proteins produced by inflammatory cells that serve as communicators with other cells. Chemokines are even smaller proteins produced by inflammatory cells that promote migration of other inflammatory cells (e.g., from the blood into the site of injury).

(Fig.25.8). The Kupffer cells are probably activated by a product of the damaged hepatocytes, such as necrotic debris, iron, ROS, acetaldehyde, or aldehyde products of lipid peroxidation. Kupffer cells also may produce acetaldehyde from ethanol internally through their own MEOS pathway.

Activated Kupffer cells produce a number of products that contribute to activation of stellate cells. They generate additional ROS through NADPH oxidase during the oxidative burst and NOS through inducible NO synthase (see Chapter 24). In addition, they secrete an impressive array of growth factors, such as cytokines, chemokines, prostaglandins, and other reactive molecules. The cytokine transforming growth factor β1 (TGFβ1), produced by both Kupffer cells and sinusoidal endothelial cells, is a major player in the activation of stellate cells. Once activated, the stellate cells produce collagen and proteases, leading to an enhanced fibrotic network within the liver.

Suggested References

Lieber CS. Medical disorders of alcoholism. New England J Med 1995;33:1058–1065.

Lieber CS. Cytochrome P-4502E1: Its physiological and pathological role. Physiol Rev 1997;77:517–544.

Mezey E. Metabolic effects of alcohol. Fed Proc 1985;44:134–138.

Poli G. Pathogenesis of liver fibrosis: Role of oxidative stress. Mol Aspects Med 2000;21:49–98.

REVIEW QUESTIONS—CHAPTER 25

1. The fate of acetate, the product of ethanol metabolism, is which of the following?

   (A) It is taken up by other tissues and activated to acetyl CoA.
   (B) It is toxic to the tissues of the body and can lead to hepatic necrosis.
   (C) It is excreted in bile.
   (D) It enters the TCA cycle directly to be oxidized.
   (E) It is converted into NADH by alcohol dehydrogenase.

2. Which of the following would be expected to occur after acute alcohol ingestion?

    (A) The activation of fatty acid oxidation
    (B) Lactic acidosis
    (C) The inhibition of ketogenesis
    (D) An increase in the $NAD^+/NADH$ ratio
    (E) An increase in gluconeogenesis

3. A chronic alcoholic is in treatment for alcohol abuse. The drug disulfiram is prescribed for the patient. This drug deters the consumption of alcohol by which of the following mechanisms?

    (A) Inhibiting the absorption of ethanol so that an individual cannot become intoxicated, regardless of how much he drinks
    (B) Inhibiting the conversion of ethanol to acetaldehyde, which would cause the excretion of unmetabolized ethanol
    (C) Blocking the conversion of acetaldehyde to acetate, which causes the accumulation of acetaldehyde
    (D) Activating the excessive metabolism of ethanol to acetate, which causes inebriation with consumption of a small amount of alcohol
    (E) Preventing the excretion of acetate, which causes nausea and vomiting

4. Induction of CYP2E1 would result in which of the following?

    (A) A decreased clearance of ethanol from the blood
    (B) A decrease in the rate of acetaldehyde production
    (C) A low possibility of the generation of free radicals
    (D) Protection from hepatic damage
    (E) An increase of one's alcohol tolerance level

5. Which one of the following consequences of chronic alcohol consumption is irreversible?

    (A) Inhibition of fatty acid oxidation
    (B) Activation of triacylglycerol synthesis
    (C) Ketoacidosis
    (D) Lactic acidosis
    (E) Liver cirrhosis

Carbohydrate Metabolism

Glucose is central to all of metabolism. It is the universal fuel for human cells and the source of carbon for the synthesis of most other compounds. Every human cell type uses glucose to obtain energy. The release of insulin and glucagon by the pancreas aids in the body's use and storage of glucose. Other dietary sugars (mainly fructose and galactose) are converted to glucose or to intermediates of glucose metabolism.

Glucose is the precursor for the synthesis of an array of other sugars required for the production of specialized compounds, such as lactose, cell surface antigens, nucleotides, or glycosaminoglycans. Glucose is also the fundamental precursor of noncarbohydrate compounds; it can be converted to lipids (including fatty acids, cholesterol, and steroid hormones), amino acids, and nucleic acids. Only those compounds that are synthesized from vitamins, essential amino acids, and essential fatty acids cannot be synthesized from glucose in humans.

More than 40% of the calories in the typical diet in the United States are obtained from starch, sucrose, and lactose. These dietary carbohydrates are converted to glucose, galactose, and fructose in the digestive tract (Fig. 1). Monosaccharides are absorbed from the intestine, enter the blood, and travel to the tissues where they are metabolized.

After glucose is transported into cells, it is phosphorylated by a hexokinase to form glucose 6-phosphate. Glucose 6-phosphate can then enter a number of metabolic pathways. The three that are common to all cell types are glycolysis, the pentose phosphate pathway, and glycogen synthesis (Fig. 2). In tissues, fructose and galactose are converted to intermediates of glucose metabolism. Thus, the fate of these sugars parallels that of glucose (Fig. 3).

The major fate of glucose 6-phosphate is oxidation via the pathway of glycolysis (see Chapter 22), which provides a source of ATP for all cell types. Cells that lack mitochondria cannot oxidize other fuels. They produce ATP from anaerobic glycolysis (the conversion of glucose to lactic acid). Cells that contain mitochondria

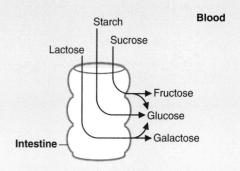

Fig 1. Overview of carbohydrate digestion. The major carbohydrates of the diet (starch, lactose, and sucrose) are digested to produce monosaccharides (glucose, fructose, and galactose), which enter the blood.

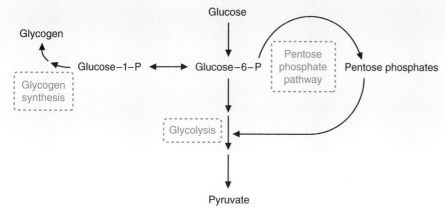

Fig 2. Major pathways of glucose metabolism.

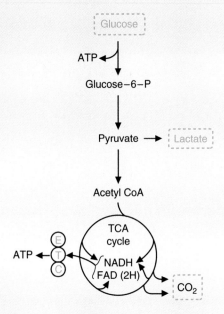

Fig 4. Conversion of glucose to lactate or to CO_2. ETC = electron transport chain.

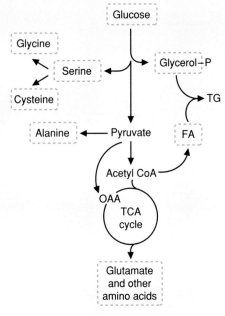

Fig 5. Conversion of glucose to amino acids and to the glycerol and fatty acid (FA) moieties of triacylglycerols (TG). OAA = oxaloacetate.

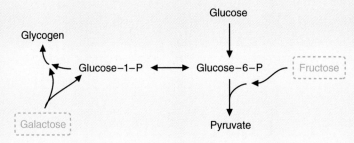

Fig 3. Overview of fructose and galactose metabolism. Fructose and galactose are converted to intermediates of glucose metabolism.

oxidize glucose to CO_2 and H_2O via glycolysis and the TCA cycle (Fig. 4). Some tissues, such as the brain, depend on the oxidation of glucose to CO_2 and H_2O for energy because they have a limited capacity to use other fuels.

Glucose produces the intermediates of glycolysis and the TCA cycle that are used for the synthesis of amino acids and both the glycerol and fatty acid moieties of triacylglycerols (Fig. 5).

Another important fate of glucose 6-phosphate is oxidation via the pentose phosphate pathway, which generates NADPH. The reducing equivalents of NADPH are used for biosynthetic reactions and for the prevention of oxidative damage to cells (see Chapter 24). In this pathway, glucose is oxidatively decarboxylated to 5-carbon sugars (pentoses), which may reenter the glycolytic pathway. They also may be used for nucleotide synthesis (Fig. 6). There are also non-oxidative reactions, which can convert six- and five-carbon sugars.

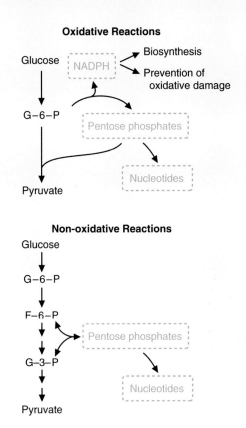

Fig 6. Overview of the pentose phosphate pathway. The oxidative reactions generate both NADPH and pentose phosphates. The non-oxidative reactions only generate pentose phosphates.

474

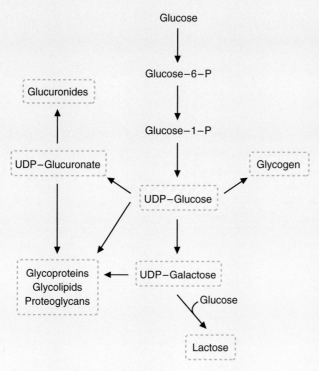

Fig 7. Products derived from UDP-glucose.

Glucose 6-phosphate is also converted to UDP-glucose, which has many functions in the cell (Fig. 7). The major fate of UDP-glucose is the synthesis of glycogen, the storage polymer of glucose. Although most cells have glycogen to provide emergency supplies of glucose, the largest stores are in muscle and liver. Muscle glycogen is used to generate ATP during muscle contraction. Liver glycogen is used to maintain blood glucose during fasting and during exercise or periods of enhanced need. UDP-Glucose is also used for the formation of other sugars, and galactose and glucose are interconverted while attached to UDP. UDP-Galactose is used for lactose synthesis in the mammary gland. In the liver, UDP-glucose is oxidized to UDP-glucuronate, which is used to convert bilirubin and other toxic compounds to glucuronides for excretion (see Fig. 7).

Nucleotide sugars are also used for the synthesis of proteoglycans, glycoproteins, and glycolipids (see Fig. 7). Proteoglycans are major carbohydrate components of the extracellular matrix, cartilage, and extracellular fluids (such as the synovial fluid of joints), and they are discussed in more detail in Chapter 49. Most extracellular proteins are glycoproteins, i.e., they contain covalently attached carbohydrates. For both cell membrane glycoproteins and glycolipids, the carbohydrate portion extends into the extracellular space.

All cells are continuously supplied with glucose under normal circumstances; the body maintains a relatively narrow range of glucose concentration in the blood (approximately 80-100 mg/dL) in spite of the changes in dietary supply and tissue demand as we sleep and exercise. This process is called glucose homeostasis. Low blood glucose levels (hypoglycemia) are prevented by a release of glucose from the large glycogen stores in the liver (glycogenolysis); by synthesis of glucose from lactate, glycerol, and amino acids in liver (gluconeogenesis) (Fig. 8); and to a limited extent by a release of fatty acids from adipose tissue stores (lipolysis) to provide an alternate fuel when glucose is in short supply. High blood glucose levels (hyperglycemia) are prevented both by the conversion of glucose to glycogen and by its conversion to triacylglycerols in liver and adipose tissue. Thus, the pathways for glucose utilization as a fuel cannot be considered as totally separate from pathways involving amino acid and fatty acid metabolism (Fig. 9).

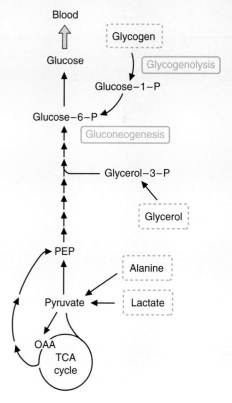

Fig 8. Production of blood glucose from glycogen (by glycogenolysis) and from alanine, lactate, and glycerol (by gluconeogenesis). PEP = phosphoenolpyruvate; OAA = oxaloacetate.

475

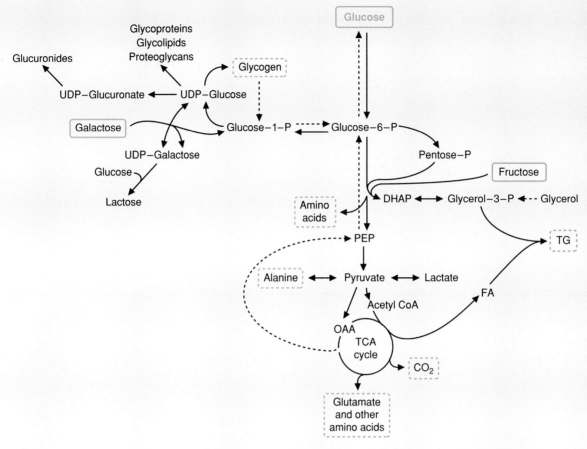

Fig 9. Overview of the major pathways of glucose metabolism. Pathways for production of blood glucose are shown by dashed lines. FA = fatty acids; TG = triacylglycerols; OAA = oxaloacetate; PEP = phosphoenolpyruvate; UDP-G = UDP-glucose; DHAP = dihydroxyacetone phosphate.

Intertissue balance in the utilization and storage of glucose during fasting and feeding is accomplished principally by the actions of the hormones of metabolic homeostasis—insulin and glucagon (Fig. 10). However, cortisol, epinephrine, norepinephrine, and other hormones are also involved in intertissue adjustments of supply and demand in response to changes of physiologic state.

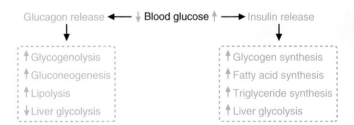

Fig 10. Pathways regulated by the release of glucagon (in response to a lowering of blood glucose levels) and insulin (released in response to an elevation of blood glucose levels). Tissue-specific differences occur in the response to these hormones, as detailed in the subsequent chapters of this section.

26 Basic Concepts in the Regulation of Fuel Metabolism by Insulin, Glucagon, and Other Hormones

*All cells continuously use adenosine triphosphate (ATP) and require a constant supply of fuels to provide energy for ATP generation. **Insulin** and **glucagon** are the two major hormones that regulate fuel mobilization and storage. Their function is to ensure that cells have a constant source of glucose, fatty acids, and amino acids for ATP generation and for cellular maintenance (Fig. 26.1).*

*Because most tissues are partially or totally dependent on glucose for ATP generation and for production of precursors of other pathways, insulin and glucagon **maintain blood glucose** levels near 80 to 100 mg/dL (90 mg/dL is the same as 5 mM), despite the fact that carbohydrate intake varies considerably over the course of a day. The maintenance of constant blood glucose levels (**glucose homeostasis**) requires these two hormones to regulate **carbohydrate**, **lipid**, and **amino acid metabolism** in accordance with the needs and capacities of individual tissues. Basically, the dietary intake of all fuels in excess of immediate need is stored, and the appropriate fuel is mobilized when a demand occurs. For example, when dietary glucose is not available in sufficient quantities that all tissues can use it, fatty acids are mobilized and made available to skeletal muscle for use as a fuel (see Chapters 2 and 23), and the liver can convert fatty acids to ketone bodies for use by the brain. Fatty acids spare glucose for use by the brain and other glucose-dependent tissues (such as the red blood cell).*

*The concentrations of insulin and glucagon in the blood regulate fuel storage and mobilization (Fig. 26.2). Insulin, released in response to carbohydrate ingestion, promotes glucose utilization as a fuel and glucose storage as fat and glycogen. **Insulin is also the major anabolic hormone of the body**. It increases protein synthesis and cell growth in addition to fuel storage. Blood insulin levels decrease as glucose is taken up by tissues and used. Glucagon, the major **counterregulatory hormone** of insulin, is decreased in response to a carbohydrate meal and elevated during fasting. Its concentration in the blood signals the absence of dietary glucose, and it promotes glucose production via **glycogenolysis** (glycogen degradation) and **gluconeogenesis** (glucose synthesis from amino acids and other noncarbohydrate precursors). Increased levels of glucagon relative to insulin also stimulate the **mobilization of fatty acids** from adipose tissue. **Epinephrine** (the fight or flight hormone) and cortisol (a glucocorticoid released from the adrenal cortex in response to fasting and chronic stress) have effects on fuel metabolism that oppose those of insulin. These two hormones are therefore also considered insulin counterregulatory hormones.*

*Insulin and glucagon are polypeptide hormones synthesized as **prohormones** in the β and α cells, respectively, in the islets of Langerhans in the pancreas. **Proinsulin** is cleaved into mature insulin and **C-peptide** in vesicles and precipitated*

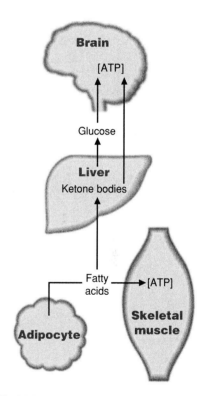

Fig 26.1. Maintenance of fuel supplies to tissues. Glucagon release activates the pathways shown.

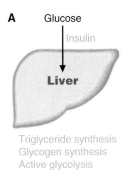

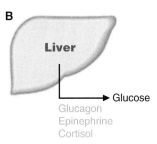

Fig 26.2. Insulin and the insulin counterregulatory hormones. (A) Insulin promotes glucose storage, as triglyceride (TG) or glycogen. (B) Glucagon, epinephrine, and cortisol promote glucose release from the liver, activating glycogenolysis and gluconeogenesis.

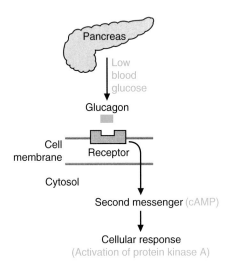

Fig 26.3. Cellular response to glucagon, which is released from the pancreas in response to a decrease in blood glucose levels.

with Zn^{2+}. Insulin secretion is regulated principally by blood glucose levels. Glucagon is also synthesized as a prohormone and cleaved into mature glucagon within storage vesicles. Its release is regulated principally through suppression by glucose and by insulin.

*Glucagon exerts its effects on cells by binding to a receptor on the cell surface, which stimulates the synthesis of the intracellular second messenger, cyclic adenosine monophosphate (**cAMP**) (Fig. 26.3). cAMP activates **protein kinase A**, which phosphorylates key regulatory enzymes, activating some and inhibiting others. Changes of cAMP levels also induce or repress the synthesis of a number of enzymes. Insulin promotes the dephosphorylation of these key enzymes.*

*Insulin binds to a receptor on the cell surface, but the postreceptor events that follow differ from those stimulated by glucagon. Insulin binding activates both autophosphorylation of the receptor and the phosphorylation of other enzymes by the receptor's **tyrosine kinase** domain (see Chapter 11, section III.B.3). The complete routes for **signal transduction** between this point and the final effects of insulin on the regulatory enzymes of fuel metabolism have not yet been fully established.*

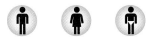

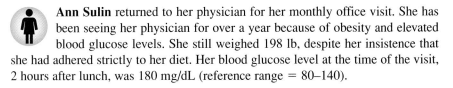

T H E   W A I T I N G   R O O M

Ann Sulin returned to her physician for her monthly office visit. She has been seeing her physician for over a year because of obesity and elevated blood glucose levels. She still weighed 198 lb, despite her insistence that she had adhered strictly to her diet. Her blood glucose level at the time of the visit, 2 hours after lunch, was 180 mg/dL (reference range = 80–140).

Bea Selmass is a 46-year-old woman who 6 months earlier began noting episodes of fatigue and confusion as she finished her daily pre-breakfast jog. These episodes were occasionally accompanied by blurred vision and an unusually urgent hunger. The ingestion of food relieved all of her symptoms within 25 to 30 minutes. In the last month, these attacks have occurred more frequently throughout the day, and she has learned to diminish their occurrence by eating between meals. As a result, she has recently gained 8 lb.

A random serum glucose level done at 4:30 PM during her first office visit was subnormal at 46 mg/dL. Her physician, suspecting she had a form of fasting hypoglycemia, ordered a series of fasting serum glucose levels. In addition, he asked Bea to keep a careful daily diary of all of the symptoms that she experienced when her attacks were most severe.

I.   METABOLIC HOMEOSTASIS

Living cells require a constant source of fuels from which to derive ATP for the maintenance of normal cell function and growth. Therefore, a balance must be achieved between carbohydrate, fat, and protein intake, their storage when present in excess of immediate need, and their mobilization and synthesis when in demand. The balance between need and availability is referred to as metabolic homeostasis (Fig. 26.4). The intertissue integration required for metabolic homeostasis is achieved in three principal ways:

- The concentration of nutrients or metabolites in the blood affects the rate at which they are used and stored in different tissues;

- Hormones carry messages to individual tissues about the physiologic state of the body and nutrient supply or demand;
- The central nervous system uses neural signals to control tissue metabolism, directly or through the release of hormones.

Insulin and glucagon are the two major hormones that regulate fuel storage and mobilization (see Fig. 26.2). Insulin is the major anabolic hormone of the body. It promotes the storage of fuels and the utilization of fuels for growth. Glucagon is the major hormone of fuel mobilization. Other hormones, such as epinephrine, are released as a response of the central nervous system to hypoglycemia, exercise, or other types of physiologic stress. Epinephrine and other stress hormones also increase the availability of fuels (Fig. 26.5).

The special role of glucose in metabolic homeostasis is dictated by the fact that many tissues (e.g., the brain, red blood cells, the lens of the eye, the kidney medulla, exercising skeletal muscle) are dependent on glycolysis for all or a portion of their energy needs and require uninterrupted access to glucose on a second-to-second basis to meet their rapid rate of ATP utilization. In the adult, a minimum of 190 g glucose is required per day; approximately 150 g for the brain and 40 g for other tissues. Significant decreases of blood glucose below 60 mg/dL limit glucose metabolism in the brain and elicit hypoglycemic symptoms (as experienced by **Bea Selmass**), presumably because the overall process of glucose flux through the blood-brain barrier, into the interstitial fluid, and subsequently into the neuronal cells, is slow at low blood glucose levels because of the K_m values of the glucose transporters required for this to occur (see Chapter 27)

The continuous movement of fuels into and out of storage depots is necessitated by the high amounts of fuel required each day to meet the need for ATP. Disastrous results would occur if even a day's supply of glucose, amino acids, and fatty acids were left circulating in the blood. Glucose and amino acids would be at such high concentrations that the hyperosmolar effect would cause progressively severe neurologic deficits and even coma. The concentration of glucose and amino acids would be above the renal tubular threshold for these substances (the maximal concentration in the blood at which the kidney can completely resorb metabolites), and some of these compounds would be wasted as they spilled over into the urine. Nonenzymatic glycosylation of proteins would increase at higher blood glucose

Fatty acids provide an example of the influence that the level of a compound in the blood has on its own rate of metabolism. The concentration of fatty acids in the blood is the major factor determining whether skeletal muscles will use fatty acids or glucose as a fuel (see Chapter 23). In contrast, hormones are (by definition) carriers of messages between tissues. Insulin and glucagon, for example, are two hormonal messengers that participate in the regulation of fuel metabolism by carrying messages that reflect the timing and composition of our dietary intake of fuels. Epinephrine, however, is a flight-or-flight hormone that signals an immediate need for increased fuel availability. Its level is regulated principally through the activation of the sympathetic nervous system.

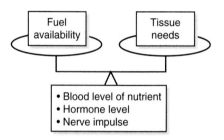

Fig 26.4. Metabolic homeostasis. The balance between fuel availability and the needs of tissues for different fuels is achieved by three types of messages: the level of the fuel or nutrients in the blood, the level of one of the hormones of metabolic homeostasis, or nerve impulses that affect tissue metabolism or the release of hormones.

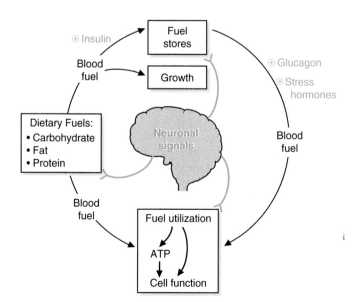

Fig 26.5. Signals that regulate metabolic homeostasis. The major stress hormones are epinephrine and cortisol.

Hyperglycemia may cause a constellation of symptoms such as polyuria and subsequent polydipsia (increased thirst). The inability to move glucose into cells necessitates the oxidation of lipids as an alternative fuel. As a result adipose stores are used, and the patient with poorly controlled diabetes mellitus loses weight in spite of a good appetite. Extremely high levels of serum glucose can cause nonketotic hyperosmolar coma in patients with type 2 diabetes mellitus. Such patients usually have sufficient insulin responsiveness to block fatty acid release and ketone body formation, but they are unable to significantly stimulate glucose entry into peripheral tissues. The severely elevated levels of glucose in the blood compared with inside the cell leads to an osmotic effect that causes water to leave the cells and enter the blood. Because of the osmotic diuretic effect of hyperglycemia, the kidney produces more urine, leading to dehydration, which in turn may lead to even higher levels of blood glucose. If dehydration becomes severe, further cerebral dysfunction occurs and the patient may become comatose. Chronic hyperglycemia also produces pathologic effects through the nonenzymatic glycosylation of a variety of proteins. Hemoglobin A (HbA), one of the proteins that becomes glycosylated, forms HbA$_{1c}$ (see Chapter 7). **Ann Sulin's** high levels of HbA$_{1c}$ (14% of the total HbA, compared with the reference range of 4.7–6.4%) indicate that her blood glucose has been significantly elevated over the last 12 to 14 weeks, the half-life of hemoglobin in the bloodstream.

All membrane and serum proteins exposed to high levels of glucose in the blood or interstitial fluid are candidates for nonenzymatic glycosylation. This process distorts protein structure and slows protein degradation, which leads to an accumulation of these products in various organs, thereby adversely affecting organ function. These events contribute to the long-term microvascular and macrovascular complications of diabetes mellitus, which include diabetic retinopathy, nephropathy, and neuropathy (microvascular), in addition to coronary artery, cerebral artery, and peripheral artery insufficiency (macrovascular).

levels. Triacylglycerols circulate in cholesterol-containing lipoproteins, and the levels of these lipoproteins would be chronically elevated, increasing the likelihood of atherosclerotic vascular disease. Consequently, glucose and other fuels are continuously moved in and out of storage depots as needed.

II. MAJOR HORMONES OF METABOLIC HOMEOSTASIS

The hormones that contribute to metabolic homeostasis respond to changes in the circulating levels of fuels that, in part, are determined by the timing and composition of our diet. Insulin and glucagon are considered the major hormones of metabolic homeostasis because they continuously fluctuate in response to our daily eating pattern. They provide good examples of the basic concepts of hormonal regulation. Certain features of the release and action of other insulin counterregulatory hormones, such as epinephrine, norepinephrine, and cortisol, will be described and compared with insulin and glucagon.

Insulin is the major anabolic hormone that promotes the storage of nutrients: glucose storage as glycogen in liver and muscle, conversion of glucose to triacylglycerols in liver and their storage in adipose tissue, and amino acid uptake and protein synthesis in skeletal muscle (Fig. 26.6). It also increases the synthesis of albumin and other blood proteins by the liver. Insulin promotes the utilization of glucose as a fuel by stimulating its transport into muscle and adipose tissue. At the same time, insulin acts to inhibit fuel mobilization.

Glucagon acts to maintain fuel availability in the absence of dietary glucose by stimulating the release of glucose from liver glycogen (see Chapter 28), by stimulating gluconeogenesis from lactate, glycerol, and amino acids (see Chapter 31), and, in conjunction with decreased insulin, by mobilizing fatty acids from adipose triacylglycerols to provide an alternate source of fuel (see Chapter 23 and Fig. 26.7). Its sites of action are principally the liver and adipose tissue; it has no influence on skeletal muscle metabolism because muscle cells lack glucagon receptors.

The release of insulin from the beta cells of the pancreas is dictated primarily by the blood glucose level. The highest levels of insulin occur approximately 30 to 45 minutes after a high-carbohydrate meal (Fig. 26.8). They return to basal levels as the blood glucose concentration falls, approximately 120 minutes after the meal. The release of glucagon from the alpha cells of the pancreas, conversely, is controlled principally through suppression by glucose and insulin. Therefore, the lowest levels of glucagon occur after a high-carbohydrate meal. Because all of the effects of glucagon are opposed by insulin, the simultaneous stimulation of insulin release and suppression of glucagon secretion by a high-carbohydrate meal provides an integrated control of carbohydrate, fat, and protein metabolism.

Bea Selmass's studies confirmed that her fasting serum glucose levels were below normal. She continued to experience the fatigue, confusion, and blurred vision she had described on her first office visit. These symptoms are called neuroglycopenic (neurologic symptoms resulting from an inadequate supply of glucose to the brain for the generation of ATP).

Bea also noted the symptoms that are part of the adrenergic response to hypoglycemic stress. Stimulation of the sympathetic nervous system (because of the low levels of glucose reaching the brain) results in the release of epinephrine, a stress hormone, from the adrenal medulla. Elevated epinephrine levels cause tachycardia, palpitations, anxiety, tremulousness, pallor, and sweating.

In addition to the symptoms described by **Bea Selmass**, individuals may experience confusion, lightheadedness, headache, aberrant behavior, blurred vision, loss of consciousness, or seizures.

Ms. Selmass's doctor explained that the general diagnosis of "fasting" hypoglycemia was now established and that a specific cause for this disorder must be found.

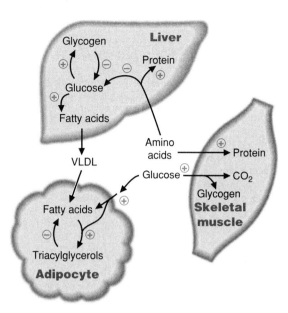

Fig 26.6. Major sites of insulin action on fuel metabolism. + = stimulated by insulin; − = inhibited by insulin.

Insulin and glucagon are not the only regulators of fuel metabolism. The intertissue balance between the utilization and storage of glucose, fat, and protein is also accomplished by the circulating levels of metabolites in the blood, by neuronal signals, and by the other hormones of metabolic homeostasis (epinephrine, norepinephrine, cortisol, and others) (Table 26.1). These hormones oppose the actions of insulin by mobilizing fuels. Like glucagon, they are called insulin counterregulatory hormones (Fig. 26.9). Of all these hormones, only insulin and glucagon are synthe-

The message carried by glucagon is that "glucose is gone"; i.e., the current supply of glucose is inadequate to meet the immediate fuel requirements of the body.

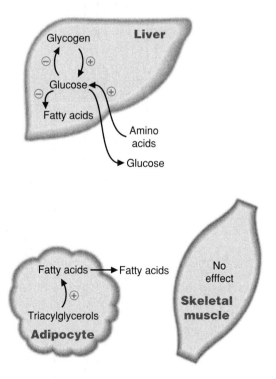

Fig 26.7. Major sites of glucagon action in fuel metabolism. + = pathways stimulated by glucagon; − = pathways inhibited by glucagon.

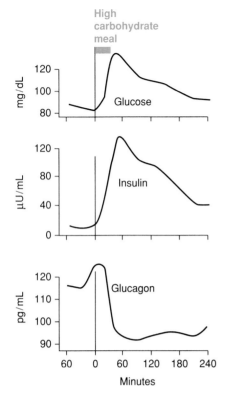

Fig 26.8. Blood glucose, insulin, and glucagon levels after a high-carbohydrate meal.

Table 26.1. Physiologic Actions of Insulin and Insulin Counterregulatory Hormones

Hormone	Function	Major Metabolic Pathways Affected
Insulin	• Promotes fuel storage after a meal • Promotes growth	• Stimulates glucose storage as glycogen (muscle and liver) • Stimulates fatty acid synthesis and storage after a high-carbohydrate meal • Stimulates amino acid uptake and protein synthesis
Glucagon	• Mobilizes fuels • Maintains blood glucose levels during fasting	• Activates gluconeogenesis and glycogenolysis (liver) during fasting • Activates fatty acid release from adipose tissue
Epinephrine	• Mobilizes fuels during acute stress	• Stimulates glucose production from glycogen (muscle and liver) • Stimulates fatty acid release from adipose issue
Cortisol	• Provides for changing requirements over the long-term	• Stimulates amino acid mobilization from muscle protein • Stimulates gluconeogenesis • Stimulates fatty acid release from adipose issue

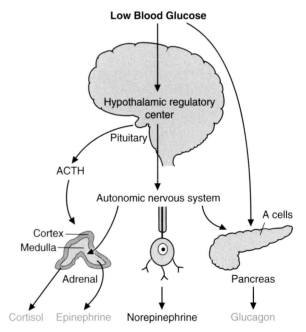

Fig 26.9. Major insulin counterregulatory hormones. The stress of a low blood glucose level mediates the release of the major insulin counterregulatory hormones through neuronal signals. Hypoglycemia is one of the stress signals that stimulates the release of cortisol, epinephrine, and norepinephrine. Adrenocorticotropic hormone (ACTH) is released from the pituitary and stimulates the release of cortisol (a glucocorticoid) from the adrenal cortex. Neuronal signals stimulate the release of epinephrine from the adrenal medulla and norepinephrine from nerve endings. Neuronal signals also play a minor role in the release of glucagon. Although norepinephrine has counterregulatory actions, it is not a major counterregulatory hormone.

sized and released in direct response to changing levels of fuels in the blood. The release of cortisol, epinephrine, and norepinephrine is mediated by neuronal signals. Rising levels of the insulin counterregulatory hormones in the blood, reflect, for the most part, a current increase in the demand for fuel.

III. SYNTHESIS AND RELEASE OF INSULIN AND GLUCAGON

A. Endocrine Pancreas

Insulin and glucagon are synthesized in different cell types of the endocrine pancreas, which consists of microscopic clusters of small glands, the islets of Langerhans, scattered among the cells of the exocrine pancreas. The α cells secrete glucagon, and the β cells secrete insulin into the hepatic portal vein via the pancreatic veins.

B. Synthesis and Secretion of Insulin

Insulin is a polypeptide hormone. The active form of insulin is composed of two polypeptide chains (the A-chain and the B-chain) linked by two interchain disulfide bonds. The A-chain has an additional intrachain disulfide bond (Fig. 26.10).

Insulin, like many other polypeptide hormones, is synthesized as a preprohormone that is converted in the rough endoplasmic reticulum (RER) to proinsulin. The "pre" sequence, a short hydrophobic signal sequence at the N-terminal end, is cleaved as it enters the lumen of the RER. Proinsulin folds into the proper conformation, and disulfide bonds are formed between the cysteine residues. It is then transported in microvesicles to the Golgi complex. It leaves the Golgi complex in storage vesicles, where a protease removes the C-peptide (a fragment with no hormonal activity) and a few small remnants, resulting in the formation of biologically active insulin (see Fig. 26.10). Zinc ions are also transported in these storage vesicles. Cleavage of the C-peptide decreases the solubility of the resulting insulin, which then coprecipitates with zinc. Exocytosis of the insulin storage vesicles from the cytosol of the β cell into the blood is stimulated by rising levels of glucose in the blood bathing the β cells.

Glucose enters the β cell via specific glucose transporter proteins known as GLUT2 (see Chapter 27). Glucose is phosphorylated through the action of glucokinase to form glucose 6-phosphate, which is metabolized through glycolysis, the TCA cycle, and oxidative phosphorylation. These reactions result in an increase in ATP levels within the β cell (circle 1 in Fig. 26.11). As the β cell [ATP]/[ADP] ratio increases, the activity of a membrane-bound, ATP-dependent K^+ channel (K^+_{ATP}) is inhibited (i.e., the channel is closed)(circle 2 in Fig. 26.11). The closing of this channel leads to a membrane depolarization (circle 3, Fig. 26.11), which activates a voltage-gated Ca^{2+} channel that allows Ca^{2+} to enter the β cell such that intracellular Ca^{2+} levels increase significantly (circle 4, Fig. 26.11). The increase in intracellular Ca^{2+} stimulates the fusion of insulin containing exocytotic vesicles with the plasma membrane, resulting in insulin secretion (circle 5, Fig. 26.11). Thus, an increase in glucose levels within the β cells initiates insulin release.

 A form of diabetes known as MODY (maturity onset diabetes of the young) results from mutations in either pancreatic glucokinase or specific nuclear transcription factors. MODY type 2 is due to a glucokinase mutation that results in an enzyme with reduced activity, either due to an elevated K_m for glucose or a reduced V_{max} for the reaction. Because insulin release is dependent on normal glucose metabolism within the β cell that yields a critical [ATP]/[ADP] ratio in the β cell, individuals with this glucokinase mutation cannot significantly metabolize glucose unless glucose levels are higher than normal. Thus, although these patients can release insulin, they do so at higher than normal glucose levels, and are therefore almost always in a hyperglycemic state. Interestingly, however, these patients are somewhat resistant to the long-term complications of chronic hyperglycemia.

 The message that insulin carries to tissues is that glucose is plentiful and it can be used as an immediate fuel or can be converted to storage forms such as triacylglycerol in adipocytes or glycogen in liver and muscle.

Because insulin stimulates the uptake of glucose into tissues where it may be immediately oxidized or stored for later oxidation, this regulatory hormone lowers blood glucose levels. Therefore, one of the possible causes of **Bea Selmass's** hypoglycemia is an insulinoma, a tumor that produces excessive insulin.

 Whenever an endocrine gland continues to release its hormone in spite of the presence of signals that normally would suppress its secretion, this persistent inappropriate release is said to be "autonomous." Secretory neoplasms of endocrine glands generally produce their hormonal product autonomously in a chronic fashion.

Autonomous hypersecretion of insulin from a suspected pancreatic β-cell tumor (an insulinoma) can be demonstrated in several ways. The simplest test is to simultaneously draw blood for the measurement of both glucose and insulin at a time when the patient is spontaneously experiencing the characteristic adrenergic or neuroglycopenic symptoms of hypoglycemia. During such a test, **Bea Selmass's** glucose levels fell to 45 mg/dL (normal = 80–100), and her ratio of insulin to glucose was far higher than normal. The elevated insulin levels markedly increased glucose uptake by the peripheral tissues, resulting in a dramatic lowering of blood glucose levels. In normal individuals, as blood glucose levels drop, insulin levels also drop.

Di Abietes has type 1 diabetes mellitus, formerly known as insulin-dependent diabetes mellitus (IDDM). This metabolic disorder is usually caused by antibody-mediated (autoimmune) destruction of the β cells of the pancreas. Susceptibility to type 1 diabetes mellitus is, in part, conferred by a genetic defect in the human leukocyte antigen (HLA) region of β cells which codes for the major histocompatibility complex II (MHC II). This protein presents an intracellular antigen to the cell surface for "self-recognition" by the cells involved in the immune response. Because of this defective protein, a cell-mediated immune response leads to varying degrees of β cell destruction and eventually to dependence on exogenous insulin administration to control the levels of glucose in the blood.

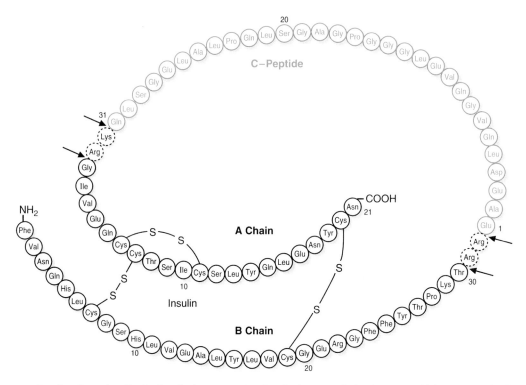

Fig 26.10. Cleavage of proinsulin to insulin. Proinsulin is converted to insulin by proteolytic cleavage, which removes the C-peptide and a few additional amino acid residues. Cleavage occurs at the arrows. From Murray RK, et al. Harper's Biochemistry, 23rd Ed. Stanford, CT: Appleton & Lange, 1993:560.

C. Stimulation and Inhibition of Insulin Release

The release of insulin occurs within minutes after the pancreas is exposed to a high glucose concentration. The threshold for insulin release is approximately 80 mg glucose/dL. Above 80 mg/dL, the rate of insulin release is not an all-or-nothing response but is proportional to the glucose concentration up to approximately 300 mg/dL glucose. As insulin is secreted, the synthesis of new insulin molecules is stimulated, so that secretion is maintained until blood glucose levels fall. Insulin is rapidly removed from the circulation and degraded by the liver (and, to a lesser

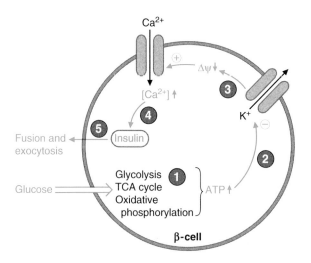

Fig 26.11. Release of insulin by the β-cells. Details are provided in the text.

Table 26.2. Regulators of Insulin Release[a]

Major Regulators	Effect
Glucose	+
Minor regulators	
Amino acids	+
Neural input	+
Gut hormones[b]	+
Epinephrine (adrenergic)	−

[a] + = stimulates
 − = inhibits
[b] gut hormones that regulate fuel metabolism are discussed in Chapter 43.

extent, by kidney and skeletal muscle), so that blood insulin levels decrease rapidly once the rate of secretion slows.

A number of factors other than the blood glucose concentration can modulate insulin release (Table 26.2). The pancreatic islets are innervated by the autonomic nervous system, including a branch of the vagus nerve. These neural signals help to coordinate insulin release with the secretory signals initiated by the ingestion of fuels. However, signals from the central nervous system are not required for insulin secretion. Certain amino acids also can stimulate insulin secretion, although the amount of insulin released during a high-protein meal is very much lower than that released by a high-carbohydrate meal. Gastric inhibitory polypeptide (GIP, a gut hormone released after the ingestion of food) also aids in the onset of insulin release. Epinephrine, secreted in response to fasting, stress, trauma, and vigorous exercise, decreases the release of insulin. Epinephrine release signals energy utilization, which indicates that less insulin needs to be secreted, as insulin stimulates energy storage.

D. Synthesis and Secretion of Glucagon

Glucagon, a polypeptide hormone, is synthesized in the α cells of the pancreas by cleavage of the much larger preproglucagon, a 160–amino acid peptide. Like insulin, preproglucagon is produced on the rough endoplasmic reticulum and is converted to proglucagon as it enters the ER lumen. Proteolytic cleavage at various sites produces the mature 29–amino acid glucagon (molecular weight 3,500) and larger glucagon-containing fragments (named glucagon-like peptides 1 and 2). Glucagon is rapidly metabolized, primarily in the liver and kidneys. Its plasma half-life is only about 3 to 5 minutes.

Glucagon secretion is regulated principally by circulating levels of glucose and insulin. Increasing levels of each inhibit glucagon release. Glucose probably has both a direct suppressive effect on secretion of glucagon from the α cell as well as an indirect effect, the latter being mediated by its ability to stimulate the release of insulin. The direction of blood flow in the islets of the pancreas carries insulin from the β cells in the center of the islets to the peripheral α cells, where it suppresses glucagon secretion.

 Ann Sulin is taking a sulfonylurea compound known as glipizide to treat her diabetes. The sulfonylureas act on the K^+_{ATP} channels on the surface of the pancreatic β cells. The binding of the drug to these channels closes K^+ channels (as do elevated ATP levels), which, in turn, increases Ca^{2+} movement into the interior of the β cell. This influx of calcium modulates the interaction of the insulin storage vesicles with the plasma membrane of the β cell, resulting in the release of insulin into the circulation.

 Measurements of proinsulin and the connecting peptide between the α and β chains of insulin (C-peptide) in **Bea Selmass's** blood during her hospital fast provided confirmation that she had an insulinoma. Insulin and C-peptide are secreted in approximately equal proportions from the β cell, but C-peptide is not cleared from the blood as rapidly as insulin. Therefore, it provides a reasonably accurate estimate of the rate of insulin secretion. Plasma C-peptide measurements are also potentially useful in treating patients with diabetes mellitus because they provide a way to estimate the degree of endogenous insulin secretion in patients who are receiving exogenous insulin, which lacks the C-peptide.

Patients with type 1 diabetes mellitus, such as **Di Abietes**, have almost undetectable levels of insulin in their blood. Patients with type 2 diabetes mellitus, such as **Ann Sulin**, conversely, have normal or even elevated levels of insulin in their blood; however, the level of insulin in their blood is inappropriately low relative to their elevated blood glucose concentration. In type 2 diabetes mellitus, skeletal muscle, liver, and other tissues exhibit a resistance to the actions of insulin. As a result, insulin has a smaller than normal effect on glucose and fat metabolism in such patients. Levels of insulin in the blood must be higher than normal to maintain normal blood glucose levels. In the early stages of type 2 diabetes mellitus, these compensatory adjustments in insulin release may keep the blood glucose levels near the normal range. Over time, as the β cells capacity to secrete high levels of insulin declines, blood glucose levels increase, and exogenous insulin becomes necessary.

Table 26.3 Regulators of Glucagon Release[a]

Major Regulators	Effect
Glucose	−
Insulin	−
Amino acids	+
Minor regulators	
Cortisol	+
Neural (stress)	+
Epinephrine	+
Gut hormones	+

[a] + = stimulates
  − = inhibits

Amino acids induce both insulin and glucagon secretion. Although this may seem paradoxical, it actually makes good sense. Insulin release stimulates amino acid uptake by tissues and enhances protein synthesis. However, because glucagon levels also increase in response to a protein meal, gluconeogenesis is enhanced (at the expense of protein synthesis), and the amino acids that are taken up by the tissues serve as a substrate for gluconeogenesis. The synthesis of glycogen and triglycerides is also reduced when glucagon levels rise in the blood.

In fasting subjects, the average level of immunoreactive glucagon in the blood is 75 pg/mL and does not vary as much as insulin during the daily fasting–feeding cycle. However, only 30 to 40% of the measured immunoreactive glucagon is mature pancreatic glucagon. The rest is composed of larger immunoreactive fragments also produced in the pancreas or in the intestinal L cells.

The physiologic importance of insulin's usual action of mediating the suppressive effect of glucose on glucagon secretion is apparent in patients with types 1 and 2 diabetes mellitus. Despite the presence of hyperglycemia, glucagon levels in such patients initially remain elevated (near fasting levels) either because of the absence of insulin's suppressive effect or because of the resistance of the α cells to insulin's suppressive effect even in the face of adequate insulin levels in type 2 patients. Thus, these patients have inappropriately high glucagon levels, leading to the suggestion that diabetes mellitus is actually a "bi-hormonal" disorder.

Certain hormones stimulate glucagon secretion. Among these are the catecholamines (including epinephrine), cortisol, and certain gastrointestinal (gut) hormones (Table 26.3).

Many amino acids also stimulate glucagon release (Fig. 26.12). Thus, the high levels of glucagon that would be expected in the fasting state do not decrease after a high-protein meal. In fact, glucagon levels may increase, stimulating gluconeogenesis in the absence of dietary glucose. The relative amounts of insulin and glucagon in the blood after a mixed meal are dependent on the composition of the meal, because glucose stimulates insulin release, and amino acids stimulate glucagon release.

IV. MECHANISMS OF HORMONE ACTION

For a hormone to affect the flux of substrates through a metabolic pathway, it must be able to change the rate at which that pathway proceeds by increasing or decreasing the rate of the slowest step(s). Either directly or indirectly, hormones affect the

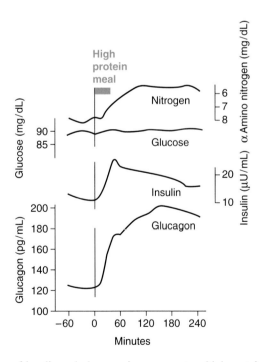

Fig 26.12. Release of insulin and glucagon in response to a high-protein meal. This figure shows the increase in the release of insulin and glucagon into the blood after an overnight fast followed by the ingestion of 100 g protein (equivalent to a slice of roast beef). Insulin levels do not increase nearly as much as they do after a high-carbohydrate meal (see Fig. 26.8). The levels of glucagon, however, significantly increase above those present in the fasting state.

activity of specific enzymes or transport proteins that regulate the flux through a pathway. Thus, ultimately, the hormone must either cause the amount of the substrate for the enzyme to increase (if substrate supply is a rate-limiting factor), change the conformation at the active site by phosphorylating the enzyme, change the concentration of an allosteric effector of the enzyme, or change the amount of the protein by inducing or repressing its synthesis or by changing its turnover rate or location. Insulin, glucagon, and other hormones use all of these regulatory mechanisms to regulate the rate of flux in metabolic pathways. The effects mediated by phosphorylation or changes in the kinetic properties of an enzyme occur rapidly, within minutes. In contrast, it may take hours for induction or repression of enzyme synthesis to change the amount of an enzyme in the cell.

The details of hormone action were previously described in Chapter 11 and are only summarized here.

A. Signal Transduction by Hormones That Bind to Plasma Membrane Receptors

Hormones initiate their actions on target cells by binding to specific receptors or binding proteins. In the case of polypeptide hormones (such as insulin and glucagon), and catecholamines (epinephrine and norepinephrine), the action of the hormone is mediated through binding to a specific receptor on the plasma membrane (see Chapter 11, section III). The first message of the hormone is transmitted to intracellular enzymes by the activated receptor and an intracellular second messenger; the hormone does not need to enter the cell to exert its effects. (In contrast, steroid hormones such as cortisol and the thyroid hormone triiodothyronine [T_3] enter the cytosol and eventually move into the cell nucleus to exert their effects.)

The mechanism by which the message carried by the hormone ultimately affects the rate of the regulatory enzyme in the target cell is called signal transduction. The three basic types of signal transduction for hormones binding to receptors on the plasma membrane are (*a*) receptor coupling to adenylate cyclase which produces cAMP, (*b*) receptor kinase activity, and (*c*) receptor coupling to hydrolysis of phosphatidylinositol bisphosphate (PIP_2). The hormones of metabolic homeostasis each use one of these mechanisms to carry out their physiologic effect. In addition, some hormones and neurotransmitters act through receptor coupling to gated ion channels (previously described in Chapter 11).

1. SIGNAL TRANSDUCTION BY INSULIN

Insulin initiates its action by binding to a receptor on the plasma membrane of insulin's many target cells (see Fig. 11.13). The insulin receptor has two types of subunits, the α-subunits to which insulin binds, and the β-subunits, which span the membrane and protrude into the cytosol. The cytosolic portion of the β-subunit has tyrosine kinase activity. On binding of insulin, the tyrosine kinase phosphorylates tyrosine residues on the β-subunit (autophosphorylation) as well as on several other enzymes within the cytosol. A principal substrate for phosphorylation by the receptor, insulin receptor substrate (IRS-1), then recognizes and binds to various signal transduction proteins in regions referred to as SH_2 domains. IRS-1 is involved in many of the physiologic responses to insulin through complex mechanisms that are the subject of intensive investigation. The basic tissue-specific cellular responses to insulin, however, can be grouped into five major categories: (*a*) insulin reverses glucagon-stimulated phosphorylation, (*b*) insulin works through a phosphorylation cascade that stimulates the phosphorylation of several enzymes, (*c*) insulin induces and represses the synthesis of specific enzymes, (*d*) insulin acts as a growth factor and has a general stimulatory effect on protein synthesis, and (*e*) insulin stimulates glucose and amino acid transport into cells (see Fig. 10 of section introduction, p. 484).

During the "stress" of hypoglycemia, the autonomic nervous system stimulates the pancreas to secrete glucagon, which tends to restore the serum glucose level to normal. The increased activity of the adrenergic nervous system (through epinephrine) also alerts a patient, such as **Bea Selmass**, to the presence of increasingly severe hypoglycemia. Hopefully, this will induce the patient to ingest simple sugars or other carbohydrates, which, in turn, will also increase glucose levels in the blood. **Bea Selmass** gained 8 lb before resection of her pancreatic insulin-secreting adenoma through this mechanism.

A number of mechanisms have been proposed for the action of insulin in reversing glucagon-stimulated phosphorylation of the enzymes of carbohydrate metabolism. From the student's point of view, the ability of insulin to reverse glucagon-stimulated phosphorylation occurs as if it were lowering cAMP and stimulating phosphatases that could remove those phosphates added by protein kinase A. In reality, the mechanism is more complex and still not fully understood.

2. SIGNAL TRANSDUCTION BY GLUCAGON

The pathway for signal transduction by glucagon is one common to a number of hormones; the glucagon receptor is coupled to adenylate cyclase and cAMP production (see Fig. 11.11). Glucagon, through G proteins, activates the membrane-bound adenylate cyclase, increasing the synthesis of the intracellular second messenger 3′,5′-cyclic AMP (cAMP) (see Fig. 9.10). cAMP activates protein kinase A (cAMP-dependent protein kinase), which changes the activity of enzymes by phosphorylating them at specific serine residues. Phosphorylation activates some enzymes and inhibits others.

The G proteins, which couple the glucagon receptor to adenylate cyclase, are proteins in the plasma membrane that bind guanosine triphosphate (GTP) and have dissociable subunits that interact with both the receptor and adenylate cyclase. In the absence of glucagon, the stimulatory G_s protein complex binds guanosine diphosphate (GDP) but cannot bind to the unoccupied receptor or adenylate cyclase (see Fig. 11.17). Once glucagon binds to the receptor, the receptor also binds the G_s complex, which then releases GDP and binds GTP. The α-subunit then dissociates from the βγ-subunits and binds to adenylate cyclase, thereby activating it. As the GTP on the α-subunit is hydrolyzed to GDP, the subunit dissociates and recomplexes with the β- and γ-subunits. Only continued occupancy of the glucagon receptor can keep adenylate cyclase active.

Although glucagon works by activating adenylate cyclase, a few hormones inhibit adenylate cyclase. In this case, the inhibitory G protein complex is called a G_i complex.

cAMP is very rapidly degraded to AMP by a membrane-bound phosphodiesterase. The concentration of cAMP is thus very low in the cell so that changes in its concentration can occur rapidly in response to changes in the rate of synthesis. The amount of cAMP present at any time is a direct reflection of hormone binding and the activity of adenylate cyclase. It is not affected by ATP, ADP, or AMP levels in the cell.

cAMP transmits the hormone signal to the cell by activating protein kinase A (cAMP-dependent protein kinase). As cAMP binds to the regulatory subunits of protein kinase A, these subunits dissociate from the catalytic subunits, which are thereby activated (see Figs. 9.9 and 9.11). Activated protein kinase A phosphorylates serine residues of key regulatory enzymes in the pathways of carbohydrate and fat metabolism. Some enzymes are activated and others are inhibited by this change in phosphorylation state. The message of the hormone is terminated by the action of semispecific protein phosphatases that remove phosphate groups from the enzymes. The activity of the protein phosphatases is also controlled through hormonal regulation.

Changes in the phosphorylation state of proteins that bind to cAMP response elements (CREs) in the promoter region of genes contribute to the regulation of gene transcription by a number of cAMP-coupled hormones (see Chapter 16). For instance, cAMP response element binding protein (CREB) is directly phosphorylated by protein kinase A, a step essential for the initiation of transcription. Phosphorylation at other sites on CREB, by a variety of kinases, also may play a role in regulating transcription.

cAMP is the intracellular second messenger for a number of hormones that regulate fuel metabolism. The specificity of the physiologic response to each hormone results from the presence of specific receptors for that hormone in target tissues. For example, glucagon activates glucose production from glycogen in liver, but not in skeletal muscle because glucagon receptors are present in liver but absent in skeletal muscle. However, skeletal muscle has adenylate cyclase, cAMP, and protein kinase A, which can be activated by epinephrine binding to the β_2 receptors in the membrane of muscle cells. Liver cells also have epinephrine receptors.

Phosphodiesterase is inhibited by methylxanthines, a class of compounds that includes caffeine. Would the effect of a methylxanthine on fuel metabolism be similar to fasting or to a high-carbohydrate meal?

The mechanism for signal transduction by glucagon illustrates some of the important principles of hormonal signaling mechanisms. The first principle is that specificity of action in tissues is conferred by the receptor on a target cell for glucagon. In general, the major actions of glucagon occur in liver, adipose tissue, and certain cells of the kidney that contain glucagon receptors. The second principle is that signal transduction involves amplification of the first message. Glucagon and other hormones are present in the blood in very low concentrations. However, these minute concentrations of hormone are adequate to initiate a cellular response because the binding of one molecule of glucagon to one receptor ultimately activates many protein kinase A molecules, each of which phosphorylates hundreds of downstream enzymes. The third principle involves integration of metabolic responses. For instance, the glucagon-stimulated phosphorylation of enzymes simultaneously activates glycogen degradation, inhibits glycogen synthesis, and inhibits glycolysis in the liver (see Fig. 10 in section introduction, p. 484.). The fourth principle involves augmentation and antagonism of signals. An example of augmentation involves the actions of glucagon and epinephrine (which is released during exercise). Although these hormones bind to different receptors, each can increase cAMP and stimulate glycogen degradation. A fifth principle is that of rapid signal termination. In the case of glucagon, both the termination of the G_s protein activation and the rapid degradation of cAMP contribute to signal termination.

B. Signal Transduction by Cortisol and Other Hormones That Interact with Intracellular Receptors

Signal transduction by the glucocorticoid cortisol and other steroids and by thyroid hormone involves hormone binding to intracellular (cytosolic) receptors or binding proteins, after which this hormone–binding protein complex moves into the nucleus, where it interacts with chromatin. This interaction changes the rate of gene transcription in the target cells (see Chapter 16). The cellular responses to these hormones will continue as long as the target cell is exposed to the specific hormones. Thus, disorders that cause a chronic excess in their secretion will result in an equally persistent influence on fuel metabolism. For example, chronic stress such as that seen in prolonged sepsis may lead to varying degrees of glucose intolerance if high levels of epinephrine and cortisol persist.

The effects of cortisol on gene transcription are usually synergistic to those of certain other hormones. For instance, the rates of gene transcription for some of the enzymes in the pathway for glucose synthesis from amino acids (gluconeogenesis) are induced by glucagon as well as by cortisol.

C. Signal Transduction by Epinephrine and Norepinephrine

Epinephrine and norepinephrine are catecholamines (Fig. 26.13). They can act as neurotransmitters or as hormones. A neurotransmitter allows a neural signal to be transmitted across the juncture or synapse between the nerve terminal of a proximal nerve axon and the cell body of a distal neuron. A hormone, conversely, is released into the blood and travels in the circulation to interact with specific receptors on the plasma membrane or cytosol of the target organ. The general effect of these catecholamines is to prepare us for fight or flight. Under these acutely stressful circumstances, these "stress" hormones increase fuel mobilization, cardiac output, blood flow, etc., which enable us to meet these stresses. The catecholamines bind to adrenergic receptors (the term *adrenergic* refers to nerve cells or fibers that are part of the involuntary or autonomic nervous system, a system that employs norepinephrine as a neurotransmitter).

 Inhibition of phosphodiesterase by methylxanthine would increase cAMP and have the same effects on fuel metabolism as would an increase of glucagon and epinephrine, in the fasted state. Increased fuel mobilization would occur through glycogenolysis (the release of glucose from glycogen), and through lipolysis (the release of fatty acids from triacylglycerols).

 Protein kinases are a class of enzymes that change the activity of other enzymes by phosphorylating them at serine or tyrosine residues and are referred to as serine or tyrosine kinases, respectively. Serine kinases also phosphorylate some enzymes at threonine residues. Protein kinase A (a serine kinase) phosphorylates many of the enzymes in the pathways of fuel metabolism.

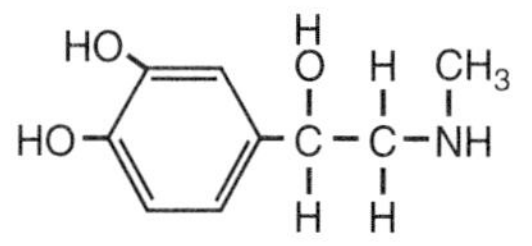

Epinephrine

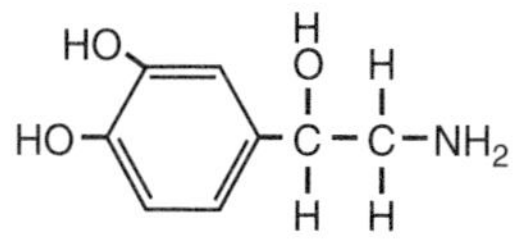

Norepinephrine

Fig 26.13. Structure of epinephrine and norepinephrine. Epinephrine and norepinephrine are synthesized from tyrosine and act as both hormones and neurotransmitters. They are catecholamines, the term *catechol* referring to a ring structure containing two hydroxyl groups.

There are nine different types of adrenergic receptors: α_{1A}, α_{1B}, α_{1D}, α_{2A}, α_{2B}, α_{2C}, β_1, β_2, and β_3. Only the three β and α_1 receptors are discussed here. The three β receptors work through the adenylate cyclase–cAMP system, activating a G_s protein, which activates adenylate cyclase, and eventually protein kinase A. The β_1 receptor is the major adrenergic receptor in the human heart and is primarily stimulated by norepinephrine. On activation, the β_1 receptor increases the rate of muscle contraction, in part because of PKA-mediated phosphorylation of phospholamban (see Chapter 47). The β_2 receptor is present in liver, skeletal muscle, and other tissues and is involved in the mobilization of fuels (such as the release of glucose through glycogenolysis). It also mediates vascular, bronchial, and uterine smooth muscle contraction. Epinephrine is a much more potent agonist for this receptor than norepinephrine, whose major action is neurotransmission. The β_3 receptor is found predominantly in adipose tissue and to a lesser extent in skeletal muscle. Activation of this receptor stimulates fatty acid oxidation and thermogenesis, and agonists for this receptor may prove to be beneficial weight loss agents. The α_1 receptors, which are postsynaptic receptors, mediate vascular and smooth muscle contraction. They work through the phosphatidylinositol bisphosphate system (see Chapter 11, section III.B.2) through activation of a G_q protein, and phospholipase C-β. This receptor also mediates glycogenolysis in liver.

CLINICAL COMMENTS

 Di Abietes has type 1 diabetes mellitus (formally designated insulin-dependent diabetes mellitus, IDDM) whereas **Ann Sulin** has type 2 diabetes mellitus (formally called non–insulin-dependent diabetes mellitus). Although the pathogenesis differs for these major forms of diabetes mellitus, both cause varying degrees of hyperglycemia. In type 1, the pancreatic β cells are gradually destroyed by antibodies directed at a variety of proteins within the β cells. As insulin secretory capacity by the β cells gradually diminishes below a critical level, the symptoms of chronic hyperglycemia develop rapidly. In type 2 diabetes mellitus, these symptoms develop more subtly and gradually over the course of months or years. Eighty-five percent or more of type 2 patients are obese and, like **Ivan Applebod,** have a high waist–hip ratio with regard to adipose tissue disposition. This abnormal distribution of fat in the visceral (peri-intestinal) adipocytes is associated with reduced sensitivity of fat cells, muscle cells, and liver cells to the actions of insulin outlined above. This insulin resistance can be diminished through weight loss, specifically in the visceral depots.

 Bea Selmass underwent a high-resolution ultrasonographic (ultrasound) study of her upper abdomen, which showed a 2.6-cm mass in the midportion of her pancreas. With this finding, her physicians decided that further noninvasive studies would not be necessary before surgical exploration of her upper abdomen was performed. At the time of surgery, a yellow-white 2.8-cm mass consisting primarily of insulin-rich β cells was resected from her pancreas. No cytologic changes of malignancy were seen on cytologic examination of the surgical specimen, and no gross evidence of malignant behavior by the tumor (such as local metastases) was found. Bea had an uneventful postoperative recovery and no longer experienced the signs and symptoms of insulin-induced hypoglycemia.

BIOCHEMICAL COMMENTS

 One of the important cellular responses to insulin is the reversal of glucagon-stimulated phosphorylation of enzymes. Mechanisms proposed for this action include the inhibition of adenylate cyclase, a reduction of

Ann O'Rexia, to stay thin, frequently fasts for prolonged periods, but jogs every morning (see Chapter 2). The release of epinephrine and norepinephrine and the increase of glucagon and fall of insulin during her exercise provide coordinated and augmented signals that stimulate the release of fuels above the fasting levels. Fuel mobilization will occur, of course, only as long as she has fuel stored as triacylglycerols.

Ann Sulin, a patient with type 2 diabetes mellitus, is experiencing insulin resistance. Her levels of circulating insulin are normal to high, although inappropriately low for her elevated level of blood glucose. However, her insulin target cells, such as muscle and fat, do not respond as those of a nondiabetic subject would to this level of insulin. For most type 2 patients, the site of insulin resistance is subsequent to binding of insulin to its receptor; i.e., the number of receptors and their affinity for insulin is near normal. However, the binding of insulin at these receptors does not elicit most of the normal intracellular effects of insulin discussed earlier. Consequently, there is little stimulation of glucose metabolism and storage after a high-carbohydrate meal and little inhibition of hepatic gluconeogenesis.

cAMP levels, the stimulation of phosphodiesterase, the production of a specific protein (insulin factor), the release of a second messenger from a bound glycosylated phosphatidylinositol, and the phosphorylation of enzymes at a site that antagonizes protein kinase A phosphorylation. Not all of these physiologic actions of insulin occur in each of the insulin-sensitive organs of the body.

Insulin is also able to antagonize the actions of glucagon at the level of specific induction or repression of key regulatory enzymes of carbohydrate metabolism. For instance, the rate of synthesis of mRNA for phosphoenolpyruvate carboxykinase, a key enzyme of the gluconeogenic pathway, is increased severalfold by glucagon (via cAMP) and decreased by insulin. Thus, all of the effects of glucagon, even the induction of certain enzymes, can be reversed by insulin. This antagonism is exerted through an insulin-sensitive hormone response element (IRE) in the promoter region of the genes. Insulin causes repression of the synthesis of enzymes that are induced by glucagon.

The general stimulation of protein synthesis by insulin (its mitogenic or growth-promoting effect) appears to occur through both a general increase in rates of mRNA translation for a broad spectrum of structural proteins. These actions result from a phosphorylation cascade initiated by autophosphorylation of the insulin receptor and ending in the phosphorylation of subunits of proteins that bind to and inhibit eukaryotic protein synthesis initiation factors (eIFs). When phosphorylated, the inhibitory proteins are released from the eIFs, allowing translation of mRNA to be stimulated. In this respect, the actions of insulin are similar to those of hormones that act as growth factors and also have receptors with tyrosine kinase activity.

In addition to signal transduction, activation of the insulin receptor mediates the internalization of receptor-bound insulin molecules increasing their subsequent degradation. Although unoccupied receptors can be internalized and eventually recycled to the plasma membrane, the receptor can be irreversibly degraded after prolonged occupation by insulin. The result of this process, referred to as receptor downregulation, is an attenuation of the insulin signal. The physiologic importance of receptor internalization on insulin sensitivity is poorly understood but could eventually lead to chronic hyperglycemia.

Suggested References

- Kahn SE, Porte D Jr. β-cell dysfunction in type 2 diabetes. In: Scriver CR, Beaudet AL, Sly WS, Valle D, eds. The Metabolic and Molecular Bases of Inherited Disease, 8th Ed. New York: McGraw-Hill, 2001:1407–1431.
- O'Brien C. Missing link in insulin's path to protein production. Science 1994;266:542–543.
- Saltiel AR, Pessin JE. Insulin signalling pathways in time and space. Trends Cell Biol. 2002;12:65–71.
- Stride A, Hattersley AT. Different genes, different diabetes: lessons from maturity-onset diabetes of the young. Ann Med 2002;34:207–216.
- White MF, Kahn CR. The insulin signalling system. J Biol Chem 1994;269:1–4.

REVIEW QUESTIONS—CHAPTER 26

1. A patient with type I diabetes mellitus takes an insulin injection before eating dinner but then gets distracted and does not eat. Approximately 3 hours later, the patient becomes shaky, sweaty, and confused. These symptoms have occurred because of which of the following?

    (A) Increased glucagon release from the pancreas
    (B) Decreased glucagon release from the pancreas
    (C) High blood glucose levels
    (D) Low blood glucose levels
    (E) Elevated ketone body levels

2. Caffeine is a potent inhibitor of the enzyme cAMP phosphodiesterase. Which of the following consequences would you expect to occur in the liver after drinking two cups of strong expresso coffee?

    (A) A prolonged response to insulin
    (B) A prolonged response to glucagon
    (C) An inhibition of protein kinase A
    (D) An enhancement of glycolytic activity
    (E) A reduced rate of glucose export to the circulation

3. Assume that an increase in blood glucose concentration from 5 to 10 mM would result in insulin release by the pancreas. A mutation in pancreatic glucokinase can lead to MODY because of which of the following within the pancreatic β-cell?

    (A) An inability to raise cAMP levels
    (B) An inability to raise ATP levels
    (C) An inability to stimulate gene transcription
    (D) An inability to activate glycogen degradation
    (E) An inability to raise intracellular lactate levels

4. Which one of the following organs has the highest demand for glucose as a fuel?

    (A) Brain
    (B) Muscle (skeletal)
    (C) Heart
    (D) Liver
    (E) Pancreas

5. Glucagon release does not alter muscle metabolism because of which of the following?

    (A) Muscle cells lack adenylate cyclase.
    (B) Muscle cells lack protein kinase A.
    (C) Muscle cells lack G proteins.
    (D) Muscle cells lack GTP.
    (E) Muscle cells lack the glucagon receptor.

27 Digestion, Absorption, and Transport of Carbohydrates

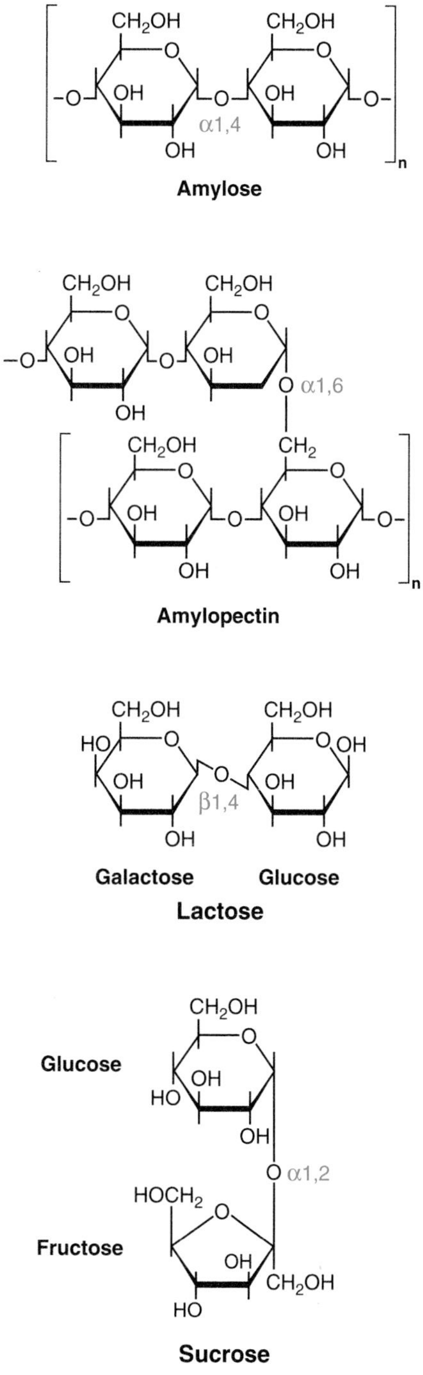

Amylose

Amylopectin

Galactose   Glucose

Lactose

Glucose

Fructose

Sucrose

Carbohydrates are the largest source of dietary calories for most of the world's population. The major carbohydrates in the American diet are starch, lactose, and sucrose. The **starches amylose** *and* **amylopectin** *are polysaccharides composed of hundreds to millions of glucosyl units linked together through α-1,4 and α-1,6 glycosidic bonds (Fig. 27.1).* **Lactose** *is a disaccharide composed of glucose and galactose, linked together through a β-1,4 glycosidic bond.* **Sucrose** *is a disaccharide composed of glucose and fructose, linked through an α-1,2 glycosidic bond. The digestive processes convert all of these dietary carbohydrates to their constituent monosaccharides by* **hydrolyzing glycosidic bonds** *between the sugars.*

The digestion of starch begins in the mouth (Fig. 27.2). The **salivary** *gland releases* **a-amylase,** *which converts starch to smaller polysaccharides called* **α-dextrins.** *Salivary α-amylase is inactivated by the acidity of the stomach (HCl).* **Pancreatic α-amylase** *and bicarbonate are secreted by the exocrine pancreas into the lumen of the small intestine, where bicarbonate neutralizes the gastric secretions. Pancreatic α-amylase continues the digestion of α-dextrins, converting them to disaccharides (***maltose***), trisaccharides (***maltotriose***), and oligosaccharides called* **limit dextrins.** *Limit dextrins usually contain four to nine glucosyl residues and an* **isomaltose** *branch (two glucosyl residues attached through an α-1,6 glycosidic bond).*

The digestion of the disaccharides lactose and sucrose, as well as further digestion of maltose, maltotriose and limit dextrins, occurs through **disacchari- dases** *attached to the membrane surface of the* **brush border (microvilli)** *of intestinal epithelial cells.* **Glucoamylase** *hydrolyzes the α-1,4 bonds of dextrins. The* **sucrase–isomaltase complex** *hydrolyzes sucrose, most of maltose, and almost all of the isomaltose formed by glucoamylase from limit dextrins.* **Lactase- glycosylceramidase** *(β-glycosidase) hydrolyzes the β-glycosidic bonds in* **lactose** *and* **glycolipids.** *A fourth disaccharidase complex,* **trehalase,** *hydrolyzes the bond (an α-1,1 glycosidic bond) between two glucosyl units in the sugar trehalose. The monosaccharides produced by these hydrolases (glucose, fructose, and galactose) are then transported into the intestinal epithelial cells.*

Fig. 27.1. The structures of common dietary carbohydrates. For disaccharides and greater, the sugars are linked through glycosidic bonds between the anomeric carbon of one sugar and a hydroxyl group on another sugar. The glycosidic bond may be either α or β, depending on its position above or below the plane of the sugar containing the anomeric carbon. (see Chapter 5, Section II.A, to review terms used in the description of sugars). The starch amylose is a polysaccharide of glucose residues linked with α-1,4 glycosidic bonds. Amylopectin is amylase with the addition of α-1,6 glycosidic branchpoints. Dietary sugars may be monosaccharides (single sugar residues), disaccharides (two sugar residues), oligosaccharides (several sugar residues) or polysaccharides (hundreds of sugar residues).

A common malabsorption syndrome, **lactose intolerance,** is characterized by nausea, diarrhea, and flatulence after ingesting dairy products or other foods containing lactose. One of the causes of lactose intolerance is a low level of lactase, which decreases after infancy in most of the world's population (**nonpersistant lactase** or **adult hypolactasia).** However, lactase activity remains high in some populations (**persistent lactase),** including Northwestern Europeans and their descendants.

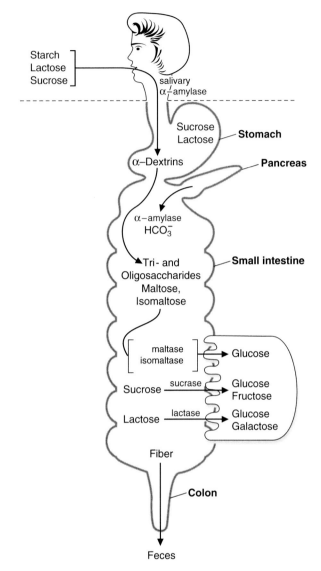

Fig. 27.2. Overview of carbohydrate digestion. **Digestion** of the carbohydrates occurs first, followed by **absorption** of monosaccharides. Subsequent **metabolic** reactions occur after the sugars are absorbed.

Dietary fiber, composed principally of polysaccharides, cannot be digested by human enzymes in the intestinal tract. In the colon, dietary fiber and other nondigested carbohydrates may be converted to gases (H_2, CO_2, and methane) and short-chain fatty acids (principally acetic acid, propionic acid, and butyric acid) by bacteria in the colon.

Glucose, galactose, and fructose formed by the digestive enzymes are transported into the absorptive epithelial cells of the small intestine by protein-mediated Na$^+$-dependent active transport and facilitative diffusion. Monosaccharides are transported from these cells into the blood and circulate to the liver and peripheral tissues, where they are taken up by facilitative transporters. Facilitative transport of glucose across epithelial cells and other cell membranes is mediated by a family of tissue-specific glucose transport proteins (GLUT I–V). The type of transporter found in each cell reflects the role of glucose metabolism in that cell.

THE WAITING ROOM

Deria Voider is a 20-year-old exchange student from Nigeria who has noted gastrointestinal bloating, abdominal cramps, and intermittent diarrhea ever since arriving in the United States 6 months earlier. A careful history shows that these symptoms occur most commonly about 45 minutes to 1 hour after eating breakfast but may occur after other meals as well. Dairy products, not a part of Deria's diet in Nigeria, were identified as the probable offending agent because her gastrointestinal symptoms disappeared when milk and milk products were eliminated from her diet.

Ann Sulin's fasting and postprandial blood glucose levels are frequently above the normal range in spite of good compliance with insulin therapy. Her physician has referred her to a dietician skilled in training diabetic patients in the successful application of an appropriate American Diabetes Association diet. As part of the program, Ms. Sulin is asked to incorporate foods containing fiber into her diet, such as whole grains (e.g., wheat, oats, corn), legumes (e.g., peas, beans, lentils), tubers (e.g., potatoes, peanuts), and fruits.

Nona Melos (no sweets) is a 7-month-old baby girl, the second child born to unrelated parents. Her mother had a healthy, full-term pregnancy, and Nona's birth weight was normal. She did not respond well to breastfeeding and was changed entirely to a formula based on cow's milk at 4 weeks. Between 7 and 12 weeks of age, she was admitted to the hospital twice with a history of screaming after feeding but was discharged after observation without a specific diagnosis. Elimination of cow's milk from her diet did not relieve her symptoms; Nona's mother reported that the screaming bouts were worse after Nona drank juice and that Nona frequently had gas and a distended abdomen. At 7 months she was still thriving (weight above 97th percentile) with no abnormal findings on physical examination. A stool sample was taken.

The dietary sugar in fruit juice and other sweets is sucrose, a disaccharide composed of glucose and fructose joined through their anomeric carbons. **Nona Melos'** symptoms of pain and abdominal distension are caused by an inability to digest sucrose or absorb fructose, which are converted to gas by colonic bacteria. "Melos" is Latin for sweets, and her name means "no sweets." Nona Melos's stool sample had a pH of 5 and gave a positive test for sugar. The possibility of carbohydrate malabsorption was considered, and a hydrogen breath test was recommended.

I. DIETARY CARBOHYDRATES

Carbohydrates are the largest source of calories in the average American diet and usually constitute 40 to 45% of our caloric intake. The plant starches amylopectin and amylose, which are present in grains, tubers, and vegetables, constitute approximately 50 to 60% of the carbohydrate calories consumed. These starches are polysaccharides, containing 10,000 to 1 million glucosyl units. In amylose, the glucosyl residues form a straight chain linked via α-1,4 glycosidic bonds; in amylopectin, the α-1,4 chains contain branches connected via α-1,6 glycosidic bonds (see Fig. 27.1). The other major sugar found in fruits and vegetables is sucrose, a disaccharide of glucose and fructose (see Fig. 27.1). Sucrose and small amounts of the monosaccharides glucose and fructose are the major natural sweeteners found in fruit, honey, and vegetables. Dietary fiber, that portion of the diet that cannot be digested by human enzymes of the intestinal tract, is also composed principally of plant polysaccharides and a polymer called lignan.

Most foods derived from animals, such as meat or fish, contain very little carbohydrate except for small amounts of glycogen (which has a structure similar to amylopectin) and glycolipids. The major dietary carbohydrate of animal origin is lactose, a disaccharide composed of glucose and galactose found exclusively in milk and milk products (see Fig. 27.1).

Sweeteners, in the form of sucrose and high-fructose corn syrup (starch, partly hydrolyzed and isomerized to fructose), also appear in the diet as additives to processed foods. On average, a person in the United States consumes 65 lb added sucrose and 40 lb high-fructose corn syrup solids per year.

Starch blockers had been marketed many years ago as a means of losing weight without having to exercise or reduce your daily caloric intake. Starch blockers were based on a protein found in beans, which blocked the action of amylase. Thus, as the advertisements proclaimed, one could eat a large amount of starch during a meal, and as long as you took the starch blocker, the starch would pass through the digestive track without being metabolized. Unfortunately, this was too good to be true, and starch blockers were never shown to be effective in aiding weight loss. This was probably because of a combination of factors, such as inactivation of the inhibitor by the low pH in the stomach, and an excess of amylase activity as compared with the amount of starch blocker ingested. Recently this issue has been revisited, as a starch blocker from wheat has been developed that may work as advertised, although much more work is required to determine whether this amylase inhibitor will be safe and effective in humans.

Although all cells require glucose for metabolic functions, neither glucose nor other sugars are specifically required in the diet. Glucose can be synthesized from many amino acids found in dietary protein. Fructose, galactose, xylose, and all the other sugars required for metabolic processes in the human can be synthesized from glucose.

II. DIGESTION OF DIETARY CARBOHYDRATES

In the digestive tract, dietary polysaccharides and disaccharides are converted to monosaccharides by glycosidases, enzymes that hydrolyze the glycosidic bonds between the sugars. All of these enzymes exhibit some specificity for the sugar, the glycosidic bond (α or β), and the number of saccharide units in the chain. The monosaccharides formed by glycosidases are transported across the intestinal mucosal cells into the interstitial fluid and subsequently enter the bloodstream. Undigested carbohydrates enter the colon, where they may be fermented by bacteria.

A. Salivary and Pancreatic α-Amylase

The digestion of starch (amylopectin and amylose) begins in the mouth, where chewing mixes the food with saliva. The salivary glands secrete approximately 1 liter of liquid per day into the mouth, containing salivary α-amylase and other components. α-Amylase is an endoglucosidase, which means that it hydrolyzes internal α-1,4 bonds between glucosyl residues at random intervals in the polysaccharide chains (Fig. 27.3). The shortened polysaccharide chains that are formed are called α-dextrins. Salivary α-amylase may be largely inactivated by the acidity of the stomach contents, which contain HCl secreted by the peptic cells.

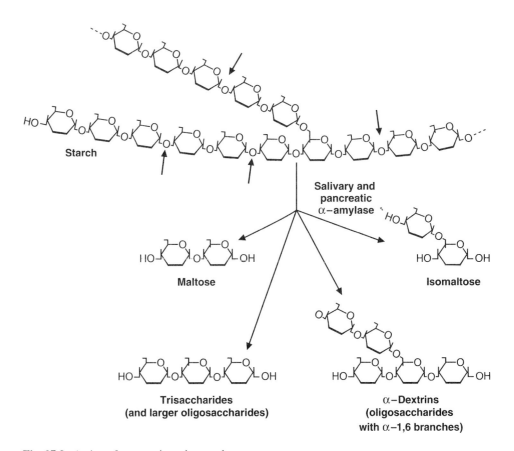

Fig. 27.3. Action of pancreatic and α-amylase.

The acidic gastric juice enters the duodenum, the upper part of the small intestine, where digestion continues. Secretions from the exocrine pancreas (approximately 1.5 liters/day) flow down the pancreatic duct and also enter the duodenum. These secretions contain bicarbonate (HCO_3^-), which neutralizes the acidic pH of stomach contents, and digestive enzymes, including pancreatic α-amylase.

Pancreatic α-amylase continues to hydrolyze the starches and glycogen, forming the disaccharide maltose, the trisaccharide maltotriose, and oligosaccharides. These oligosaccharides, called limit dextrins, are usually four to nine glucosyl units long and contain one or more α-1,6 branches. The two glucosyl residues that contain the α-1,6 glycosidic bond will eventually become the disaccharide isomaltose, but α-amylase does not cleave these branched oligosaccharides all the way down to isomaltose.

α-Amylase has no activity toward sugar containing polymers other than glucose linked by α-1,4 bonds. α-Amylase displays no activity toward the α-1,6- bond at branchpoints and has little activity for the α-1,4 bond at the nonreducing end of a chain.

B. Disaccharidases of the Intestinal Brush-Border Membrane

The dietary disaccharides lactose and sucrose, as well as the products of starch digestion, are converted to monosaccharides by glycosidases attached to the membrane in the brush-border of absorptive cells (Fig. 27.4). The different glycosidase activities are found in four glycoproteins: glucoamylase, the sucrase–maltase complex, the smaller glycoprotein trehalase, and lactase-glucosylceramidase (Table 27.1). These glycosidases are collectively called the small intestinal disaccharidases, although glucoamylase is really an oligosaccharidase.

1. GLUCOAMYLASE

Glucoamylase and the sucrase–isomaltase complex have similar structures and exhibit a great deal of sequence homogeneity (Fig. 27.5). A membrane-spanning domain near the N-terminal attaches the protein to the luminal membrane. The long polypeptide chain forms two globular domains, each with a catalytic site. In glucoamylase, the two catalytic sites have similar activities, with only small differences in substrate specificity. The protein is heavily glycosylated with oligosaccharides that protect it from digestive proteases.

Glucoamylase is an exoglucosidase that is specific for the α–1,4 bonds between glucosyl residues (Fig. 27.6). It begins at the nonreducing end of a polysaccharide or limit dextrin, and sequentially hydrolyzes the bonds to release glucose monosaccharides. It will digest a limit dextrin down to isomaltose, the glucosyl disaccharide with an α–1,6-branch, that is subsequently hydrolyzed principally by the isomaltase activity in the sucrase–isomaltase complex.

2. SUCRASE–ISOMALTASE COMPLEX

The structure of the sucrase–isomaltase complex is very similar to that of glucoamylase, and these two proteins have a high degree of sequence homology. However, after the single polypeptide chain of sucrase–isomaltase is inserted through the membrane and the protein protrudes into the intestinal lumen, an intestinal protease clips it into two separate subunits that remain attached to each other. Each subunit has a catalytic site that differs in substrate specificity from the other through noncovalent interactions. The sucrase–maltase site accounts for approximately 100% of the intestine's ability to hydrolyze sucrose in addition to maltase activity; the isomaltase–maltase site accounts for almost all of the intestine's ability to hydrolyze α-1,6-bonds (Fig. 27.7), in addition to maltase activity. Together, these sites account for approximately 80% of the maltase activity of the small intestine. The remainder of the maltase activity is found in the glucoamylase complex.

Amylase activity in the gut is abundant and is not normally rate limiting for the process of digestion. Alcohol-induced pancreatitis or surgical removal of part of the pancreas can decrease pancreatic secretion. Pancreatic exocrine secretion into the intestine also can be decreased through cystic fibrosis, in which mucus blocks the pancreatic duct, which eventually degenerates. However, pancreatic exocrine secretion can be decreased to 10% of normal and still not affect the rate of starch digestion, because amylases are secreted in the saliva and pancreatic fluid in excessive amounts. In contrast, protein and fat digestion is more strongly affected in cystic fibrosis.

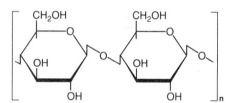

Can the glycosidic bonds of the structure shown above be hydrolyzed by α-amylose?

Individuals with genetic deficiencies of the sucrase-isomaltase complex show symptoms of sucrose intolerance but are able to digest normal amounts of starch in a meal, without problems. The maltase activity in the glucoamylase complex, and residual activity in the sucrase-isomaltase complex (which is normally present in excess of need) is apparently sufficient to digest normal amounts of dietary starch.

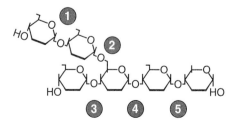

Which of the bonds in the structure above are hydrolyzed by the sucrase–isomaltase complex? Which by glucoamylase?

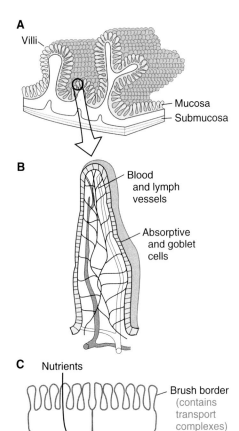

Fig. 27.4. Location of disaccharide complexes in intestinal villi.

Table 27.1. The Different Forms of the Brush Border Glycosidases

Complex	Catalytic Sites	Principal Activities
β-Glucoamylase	α-Glucosidase	Split α-1,4 glycosidic bonds between glucosyl units, beginning sequentially with the residue at the tail end (nonreducing end) of the chain. This is an exoglycosidase. Substrates include amylase, amylopectin, glycogen and maltose.
	α-Glucosidase	Same as above, but with slightly different specificity and affinities for the substrates
Sucrase–Isomaltase	Sucrase–maltase	Splits sucrose, maltose, and maltotriose
	Isomaltase–maltase	Splits α-1, 6 bonds in a number of limit dextrins, as well as the α-1,4 bonds in maltose and maltotriose.
β-Glycosidase	Glucosyl–ceramidase (Phlorizin hydrolase)	Splits β-glycosidic bonds between glucose or galactose and hydrophobic residues, such as the glycolipids glucosylceramide and galactosylceramide
	Lactase	Splits the β-1,4 bond between glucose and galactose. To a lesser extent also splits the β-1,4 bond between some cellulose disaccharides.
Trehalase	Trehalase	Splits bond in trehalose, which is 2 glucosyl units linked α-1,1 through their anomeric carbons.

3.   TREHALASE

Trehalase is only half as long as the other disaccharidases and has only one catalytic site. It hydrolyzes the glycosidic bond in trehalose, a disaccharide composed of two glucosyl units linked by an α-bond between their anomeric carbons (Fig. 27.8). Trehalose, which is found in insects, algae, mushrooms, and other fungi, is not currently a major dietary component in the United States. However, unwitting consumption of trehalose can cause nausea, vomiting, and other symptoms of severe gastrointestinal distress if consumed by an individual deficient in the enzyme. Trehalase deficiency was discovered when a woman became very sick after eating mushrooms and was initially thought to have α-amanitin poisoning.

4.   β-GLYCOSIDASE COMPLEX (LACTASE-GLUCOSYLCERAMIDASE)

The β-glycosidase complex is another large glycoprotein found in the brush border that has two catalytic sites extending in the lumen of the intestine. However, its primary structure is very different from the other enzymes, and it is attached to the membrane through its carboxyl end by a phosphatidylglycan anchor (see Fig.10.7). The lactase catalytic site hydrolyzes the β-bond connecting glucose and galactose in lactose (a β-galactosidase activity; Fig. 27.9). The major activity of the other catalytic site in humans is the β-bond between glucose or galactose and ceramide in glycolipids (this catalytic site is sometimes called phlorizin hydrolase, named for its ability to hydrolyze an artificial substrate).

5.   LOCATION WITHIN THE INTESTINE

The production of maltose, maltotriose, and limit dextrins by pancreatic α-amylase occurs in the duodenum, the most proximal portion of the small intestine. Sucrase–isomaltase activity is highest in the jejunum, where the enzymes can hydrolyze sucrose and the products of starch digestion. β-Glycosidase activity is also highest in the jejenum. Glucoamylase activity progressively increases along the length of the small intestine, and its activity is highest in the ileum. Thus, it

 No. This polysaccharide is cellulose, which contains β-1,4 glycosidic bonds. Pancreatic and salivary α-amylase cleave only α-1,4 bonds between glucosyl units.

 Bonds (1) and (3) would first be hydrolyzed by glucoamylase. Bond (2) would require isomaltase. Bonds (4) and (5) could then be hydrolyzed by the sucrase–isomaltase complex, or by the glucoamylase complex, all of which can convert maltotriose and maltose to glucose.

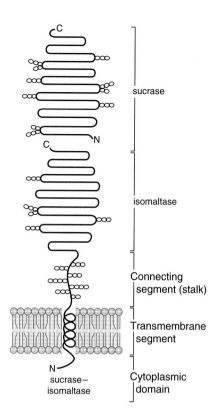

Fig. 27.5. The major portion of the sucrase-isomaltase complex, containing the catalytic sites, protrudes from the absorptive cells into the lumen of the intestine. Other domains of the protein form a connecting segment (stalk), and an anchoring segment that extends through the membrane into the cell. The complex is synthesized as a single polypeptide chain that is split into its two enzyme subunits extracellularly. Each subunit is a domain with a catalytic site (sucrase-maltase) and isomaltase-maltase sites. In spite of their maltase activity, these catalytic sites are often called just sucrase and isomaltase.

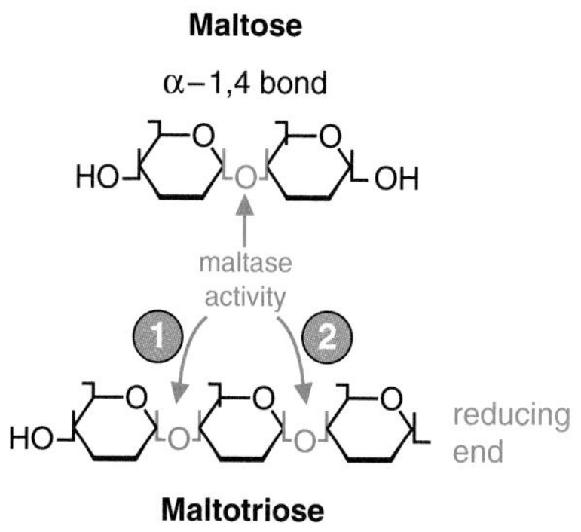

Maltose

α–1,4 bond

Fig. 27.6. Glucoamylase activity. Glucoamylase is an α-1,4 exoglycosidase, which initiates cleavage at the nonreducing end of the sugar. Thus, for malotriose, the bond labeled 1 will be hydrolyzed first, which frees up the bond at position 2 to be the next one hydrolyzed.

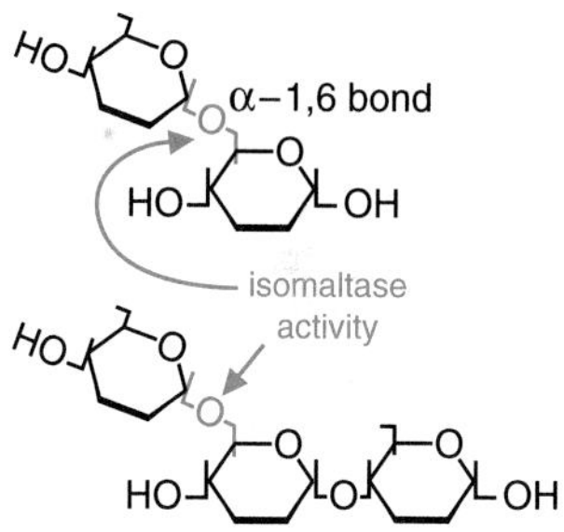

Fig. 27.7. Isomaltase activity. Arrows indicate the α-1,6 bonds that are cleaved.

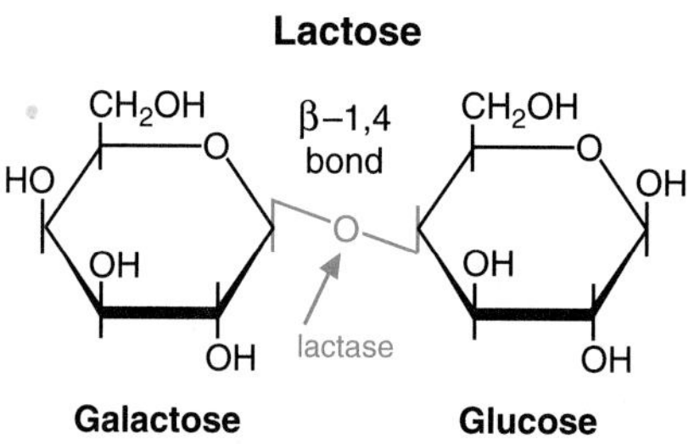

Lactose

Fig. 27.9. Lactase activity. Lactase is a β-galactosidase. It cleaves the β-galactoside lactose, the major sugar in milk, forming galactose and glucose.

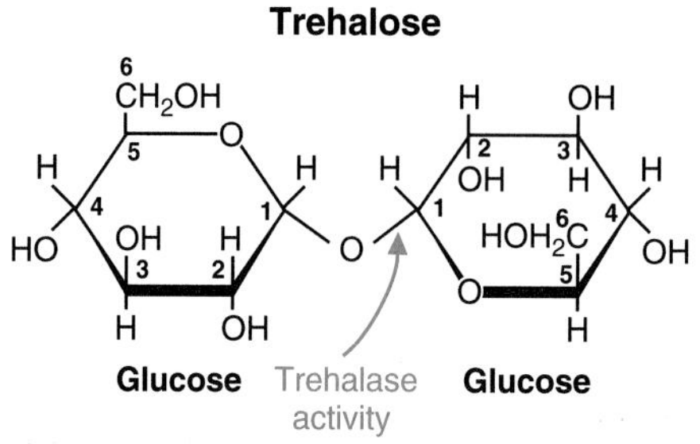

Trehalose

Fig. 27.8. Trehalose. This disaccharide contains two glucose moieties linked by an unusual bond that joins their anomeric carbons. It is cleaved by trehalase.

presents a final opportunity for digestion of starch oligomers that have escaped amylase and disaccharidase activities at the more proximal regions of the intestine.

C. Metabolism of Sugars by Colonic Bacteria

Not all of the starch ingested as part of foods is normally digested in the small intestine (Fig. 27.10). Starches high in amylose, or less well hydrated (e.g., starch in dried beans), are resistant to digestion and enter the colon. Dietary fiber and undigested sugars also enter the colon. Here colonic bacteria rapidly metabolize the saccharides, forming gases, short-chain fatty acids, and lactate. The major short-chain fatty acids formed are acetic acid (two carbon), propionic acid (three carbon), and butyric acid (four carbon). The short-chain fatty acids are absorbed by the colonic mucosal cells and can provide a substantial source of energy for these cells. The major gases formed are hydrogen gas (H_2), carbon dioxide (CO_2), and methane (CH_4). These gases are released through the colon, resulting in flatulence, or in the breath. Incomplete products of digestion in the intestines increase the retention of water in the colon, resulting in diarrhea.

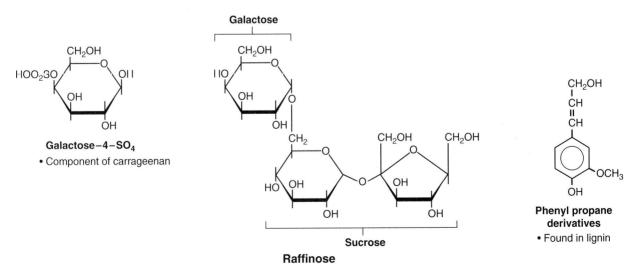

Fig. 27.10. Some indigestible carbohydrates. These compounds are components of dietary fiber.

Nona Melos was given a hydrogen breath test, a test measuring the amount of hydrogen gas released after consuming a test dose of sugar. The association of **Nona Melos's** symptoms with her ingestion of fruit juices suggests that she might have a problem resulting from a low sucrase activity or an inability to absorb fructose. Her ability to thrive and her adequate weight gain suggest that any deficiencies of the sucrase–isomaltase complex must be partial and do not result in a functionally important reduction in maltase activity (maltase activity is also present in the glucoamylase complex). Her urine tested negative for sugar, suggesting the problem is in digestion or absorption, because only sugars that are absorbed and enter the blood can be found in urine. The basis of the hydrogen breath test is that if a sugar is not absorbed, it is metabolized in the intestinal lumen by bacteria that produce various gases, including hydrogen. The test is often accompanied by measurements of the amount of sugar appearing in the blood or feces, and acidity of the feces.

Q: Beans, peas, soybeans, and other leguminous plants contain oligosaccharides with (1,6)-linked galactose residues that cannot be hydrolyzed for absorption, including sucrose with 1, 2, or 3 galactose residues attached (see Fig. 27.10). What is the fate of these polysaccharides in the intestine?

D. Lactose Intolerance

Lactose intolerance refers to a condition of pain, nausea, and flatulence after the ingestion of foods containing lactose, most notably dairy products. Although it is often caused by low levels of lactase, it also can be caused by intestinal injury (defined below).

1. NONPERSISTENT AND PERSISTANT LACTASE

Lactase activity increases in the human from about 6 to 8 weeks of gestation, and it rises during the late gestational period (27–32 weeks) through full term. It remains high for about 1 month after birth and then begins to decline. For most of the world's population, lactase activity decreases to adult levels at approximately 5 to 7 years of age. Adult levels are less than 10% of that present in infants. These populations have adult hypolactasia (formerly called adult lactase deficiency) and exhibit the lactase nonpersistence phenotype. In people who are derived mainly from western Northern Europeans, and milk-dependent Nomadic tribes of Saharan Africa, the levels of lactase remain at, or only slightly below, infant levels throughout adulthood (lactase persistence phenotype). Thus, adult hypolactasia is the normal condition for most of the world's population. (Table 27.2).

2. INTESTINAL INJURY

Intestinal diseases that injure the absorptive cells of the intestinal villi diminish lactase activity along the intestine, producing a condition known as secondary lactase deficiency. Kwashiorkor (protein malnutrition), colitis, gastroenteritis, tropical and

 Lactose intolerance can either be the result of a primary deficiency of lactase production in the small bowel (as is the case for **Deria Voider**) or it can be secondary to an injury to the intestinal mucosa, where lactase is normally produced. The lactose that is not absorbed is converted by colonic bacteria to lactic acid, methane gas (CH_4), and H_2 gas (see figure on left). The osmotic effect of the lactose and lactic acid in the bowel lumen is responsible for the diarrhea often seen as part of this syndrome. Similar symptoms can result from sensitivity to milk proteins (milk intolerance) or from the malabsorption of other dietary sugars.

In adults suspected of having a lactase deficiency, the diagnosis is usually made inferentially when avoidance of all dairy products results in relief of symptoms and a rechallenge with these foods reproduces the characteristic syndrome. If the results of these measures are equivocal, however, the malabsorption of lactose can be more specifically determined by measuring the H_2 content of the patient's breath after a test dose of lactose has been consumed.

Deria Voider's symptoms did not appear if she took tablets containing lactase when she ate dairy products.

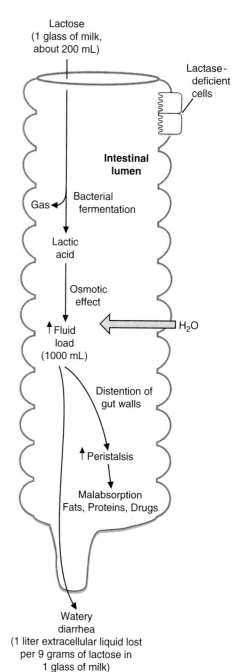

Lactose
(1 glass of milk,
about 200 mL)

Lactase-
deficient
cells

**Intestinal
lumen**

Gas ◄ Bacterial
fermentation

Lactic
acid

Osmotic
effect

↑Fluid
load
(1000 mL)   ◄ H_2O

Distention of
gut walls

↑Peristalsis

Malabsorption
Fats, Proteins, Drugs

Watery
diarrhea
(1 liter extracellular liquid lost
per 9 grams of lactose in
1 glass of milk)

A: These sugars are not digested well by the human intestine but form good sources of energy for the bacteria of the gut. These bacteria convert the sugars to H_2, lactic acid and short-chain fatty acids. The amount of gas released after a meal containing beans is especially notorious.

Table 27.2. Prevalence of Late-Onset Lactase Deficiency

Group	Prevalence (%)
U.S. population	
Asians	100
American Indians (Oklahoma)	95
Black Americans	81
Mexican Americans	56
White Americans	24
Other Populations	
Ibo, Yoruba (Nigeria)	89
Italians	71
Aborigines (Australia)	67
Greeks	53
Danes	3
Dutch	0

Reproduced with permission from Annu Rev Med 1990;41:145. © 1990 by Annual Reviews, Inc.

nontropical sprue, and excessive alcohol consumption fall into this category. These diseases also affect other disaccharidases, but sucrase, maltase, isomaltase, and glucoamylase activities are usually present at such excessive levels that there are no pathologic effects. Lactase is usually the first activity lost and the last to recover.

III. DIETARY FIBER

Dietary fiber is the portion of the diet resistant to digestion by human digestive enzymes. It consists principally of plant materials that are polysaccharide derivatives and lignan (see Fig.27.10). The components of fiber are often divided into the categories of soluble and insoluble fiber, according to their ability to dissolve in water. Insoluble fiber consists of three major categories; cellulose, hemicellulose, and lignins. Soluble fiber categories include pectins, mucilages, and gums (Table 27.3). Although human enzymes cannot digest fiber, the bacterial flora in the normal human gut may metabolize the more soluble dietary fibers to gases and short-chain fatty acids, much as they do undigested starch and sugars. Some of these

Table 27.3 Types of Fiber in the Diet

Classical Nomenclature	Classes of compounds	Dietary Sources
Insoluble Fiber		
Cellulose	Polysaccharide composed of glucosyl residues linked β-1,4.	Whole wheat flour, unprocessed bran, cabbage, peas, green beans, wax beans, broccoli, brussel sprouts, cucumber with skin, green peppers, apples, carrots
Hemicelluloses	Polymers of arabinoxylans or galactomannans	Bran cereals, whole grains, brussel sprouts, mustard beans, beet root
Lignin	Noncarbohydrate, polymeric derivatives of phenylpropane	Bran cereals, unprocessed bran, strawberries, eggplant, peas, green beans, radishes
Water Soluble Fiber (or dispersable)		
Pectic Substances	Galactouranans, arabinoglactans, β-glucans, arabinoxylans	Squash, apples, citrus fruits
Gums	Galactomannans, arabinogalactans	Oatmeal, dried beans, cauliflower, green beans, cabbage, carrots, dried peas, potatoes, strawberries
Mucilages	Wide range of branched and substituted galactans	Flax seed, psyllium, mustard seed

fatty acids may be absorbed and used by the colonic epithelial cells of the gut, and some may travel to the liver through the hepatic portal vein. We may obtain as much as 10% of our total calories from compounds produced by bacterial digestion of substances in our digestive tract.

In 2002, the Committee on Dietary Reference Intakes issued new guidelines for fiber ingestion; anywhere from 19 to 38 g/day, depending on age and sex of the individual. No distinction was made between soluble and insoluble fibers. Adult males between the ages of 14 and 50 years require 38 grams of fiber per day. Females from ages 4 to 8 years require 25 g/day; from ages 9 to 16 years, 26 g/day; and from ages 19 to 30, 25 g/day. These numbers are increased during pregnancy and lactation. One beneficial effect of fiber is seen in diverticular disease, in which sacs or pouches may develop in the colon because of a weakening of the muscle and submucosal structures. Fiber is thought to "soften" the stool, thereby reducing pressure on the colonic wall and enhancing expulsion of feces.

Certain types of soluble fiber have been associated with disease prevention. For example, pectins may lower blood cholesterol levels by binding bile acids. β-glucan (obtained from oats) has also been shown, in some studies, to reduce cholesterol levels through a reduction in bile acid resorption in the intestine (see Chapter 34). Pectins also may have a beneficial effect in the diet of individuals with diabetes mellitus by slowing the rate of absorption of simple sugars and preventing high blood glucose levels after meals. However, each of the beneficial effects which have been related to "fiber" are relatively specific for the type of fiber, and the physical form of food which contains the fiber. This factor, along with many others, has made it difficult to obtain conclusive results from studies of the effects of fiber on human health.

IV. ABSORPTION OF SUGARS

Once the carbohydrates have been split into monosaccharides, the sugars are transported across the intestinal epithelial cells and into the blood for distribution to all tissues. Not all complex carbohydrates are digested at the same rate within the intestine, and some carbohydrate sources lead to a near-immediate rise in blood glucose levels after ingestion, whereas others slowly raise blood glucose levels over an extended period after ingestion. The glycemic index of a food is an indication of how rapidly blood glucose levels rise after consumption. Glucose and maltose have the highest glycemic indices (142, with white bread defined as an index of 100). Table 27.4 indicates the glycemic index for a variety of food types. Although there is no need to memorize this table, note that cornflakes and potatoes have high glycemic indices, whereas yogurt and skim milk have particularly low glycemic indices.

A. Absorption by the Intestinal Epithelium

Glucose is transported through the absorptive cells of the intestine by facilitated diffusion and by Na^+-dependent facilitated transport. (See Chapter 10 for a description of transport mechanisms.) Glucose, therefore, enters the absorptive cells by binding

Pectins are found in fruits, such as apples. Could this be the basis for the saying "An apple a day keeps the doctor away"?

Carrageenan is a type of fiber derived from seaweed. It is composed of sulfated galactose and galacturonic acid derivatives (see Fig. 27.10). The negatively charged sulfate groups form hydrogen bonds with water and convert the polysaccharide into a gel-like substance. It is added to many foods, such as ice cream and McDonald's McLean burger.

The glycemic response to ingested foods depends not only on the glycemic index of the foods, but also on the fiber and fat content of the food, as well as its method of preparation. Highly glycemic carbohydrates can be consumed before and after exercise, as their metabolism results in a rapid entry of glucose into the blood, where it is then immediately available for muscle use. Low glycemic carbohydrates enter the circulation slowly and can be used to best advantage if consumed before exercise, such that as exercise progresses glucose is slowly being absorbed from the intestine into the circulation, where it can be used to maintain blood glucose levels during the exercise period.

The dietician explained to **Ann Sulin** the rationale for a person with diabetes to watch their diet. It is important for Ann to add a variety of fibers to her diet. The gel-forming, water-retaining pectins and gums delay gastric emptying and retard the rate of absorption of disaccharides and monosaccharides, thus reducing the rate at which blood glucose levels rise. The glycemic index of foods also needs to be considered for appropriate maintenance of blood glucose levels in diabetic patients. Consumption of a low glycemic index diet results in a lower rise in blood glucose levels after eating, which can be more easily controlled by exogenous insulin. For example, Ms. Sulin is advised to eat pasta and rice (glycemic index of 67 and 65, respectively) instead of potatoes (glycemic index of 80–120, depending on the method of preparation), and to incorporate breakfast cereals composed of wheat bran, barley, and oats into her morning routine.

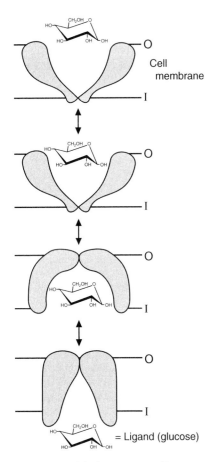

Fig. 27.11. Facilitative transport. Transport of glucose occurs without rotation of the glucose molecule. Multiple groups on the protein bind the hydroxyl groups of glucose and close behind it as it is released into the cell (i.e., the transporter acts like a "gated pore"). O = outside; I = inside.

The glucose molecule is extremely polar and cannot diffuse through the hydrophobic phospholipid bilayer of the cell membrane. Each hydroxyl group of the glucose molecule forms at least two hydrogen bonds with water molecules, and random movement would require energy to dislodge the polar hydroxyl groups from their hydrogen bonds and to disrupt the Van der Waals' forces between the hydrocarbon tails of the fatty acids in the membrane phospholipid.

The epithelial cells of the kidney, which reabsorb glucose into the blood, have Na⁺-dependent glucose transporters similar to those of intestinal epithelial cells. They are thus also able to transport glucose against its concentration gradient. Other types of cells use mainly facilitative glucose transporters that carry glucose down its concentration gradient.

Table 27.4 Glycemic Index of Selected Foods, with Values Adjusted to White Bread of 100

Breads		Legumes	
Whole wheat	100	Baked beans (canned)	70
Pumpernickel (whole grain rye)	88	Butter beans	46
Pasta		Garden peas (frozen)	85
Spaghetti, white, boiled	67		
		Kidney beans (dried)	43
Cereal grains		Kidney beans (canned)	74
Barley (pearled)	36	Peanuts	15
Rice (instant, boiled 1 min)	65	Fruit	
Rice, polished (boiled 10–25 min)	81	Apple	52
Sweet corn	80	Apple juice	45
Breakfast cereals		Orange	59
All bran	74	Raisins	93
Cornflakes	121	Sugars	
Muesli	96	Fructose	27
Cookies		Glucose	142
Oatmeal	78	Lactose	57
Plain water crackers	100	Sucrose	83
Root vegetables		Dairy Products	
Potatoes (instant)	120	Ice cream	69
Potato (new,white, boiled)	80	Whole milk	44
Potato chips	77	Skim milk	46
Yam	74	Yogurt	52

to transport proteins, membrane-spanning proteins that bind the glucose molecule on one side of the membrane and release it on the opposite side (Fig. 27.11). Two types of glucose transport proteins are present in the intestinal absorptive cells: the Na⁺-dependent glucose transporters and the facilitative glucose transporters (Fig. 27.12).

1. NA⁺-DEPENDENT TRANSPORTERS

Na⁺-dependent glucose transporters, which are located on the luminal side of the absorptive cells, enable these cells to concentrate glucose from the intestinal lumen. A low intracellular Na⁺ concentration is maintained by a Na⁺,K⁺-ATPase on the serosal (blood) side of the cell that uses the energy from ATP cleavage to pump Na⁺ out of the cell into the blood. Thus, the transport of glucose from a low concentration in the lumen to a high concentration in the cell is promoted by the cotransport of Na⁺ from a high concentration in the lumen to a low concentration in the cell (secondary active transport).

2. FACILITATIVE GLUCOSE TRANSPORTERS

Facilitative glucose transporters, which do not bind Na⁺, are located on the serosal side of the cells. Glucose moves via the facilitative transporters from the high concentration inside the cell to the lower concentration in the blood without the expenditure of energy. In addition to the Na⁺-dependent glucose transporters, facilitative transporters for glucose also exist on the luminal side of the absorptive cells. The various types of facilitative glucose transporters found in the plasma membranes of cells (referred to as GLUT 1 to GLUT 5), are described in Table 27.5. One common structural theme to these proteins is that they all contain 12 membrane-spanning domains. Note that the sodium-linked transporter on the luminal side of the intestinal epithelial cell is not a member of the GLUT family.

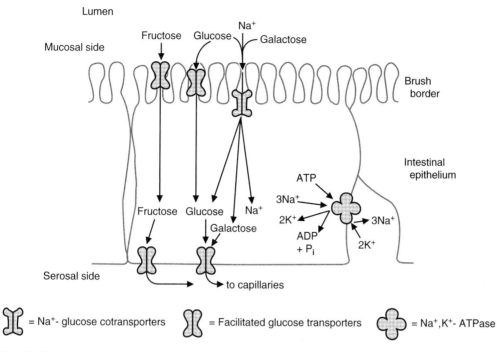

Fig. 27.12. Na$^+$-dependent and facilitative transporters in the intestinal epithelial cells. Both glucose and fructose are transported by the facilitated glucose transporters on the luminal and serosal sides of the absorptive cells. Glucose and galactose are transported by the Na$^+$-glucose cotransporters on the luminal (mucosal) side of the absorptive cells.

Table 27.5. Properties of the GLUT 1-GLUT 5 Isoforms of the Glucose Transport Proteins

Transporter	Tissue Distribution	Comments
GLUT 1	Human erythrocyte Blood-brain barrier Blood-retinal barrier Blood-placental barrier Blood-testis barrier	Expressed in cell types with barrier functions; a high-affinity glucose transport system

GLUT 2	Liver
	Kidney
	Pancreatic β-cell
	Serosal surface of Intestinal
	  mucosa cells
		A high capacity, low affinity transporter.
		  May be used as the glucose sensor in the
		  pancreas.

GLUT 3	Brain (neurons)	Major transporter in the central nervous system. A high-affinity system.

GLUT 4	Adipose tissue
	Skeletal muscle
	Heart muscle
		Insulin-sensitive transporter. In the presence
		  of insulin the number of GLUT 4
		  transporters increases on the cell surface.
		  A high-affinity system

GLUT 5	Intestinal epithelium Spermatozoa	This is actually a fructose transporter.

Genetic techniques have identified additional GLUT transporters (GLUT 7-12), but the role of these transporters has not yet been fully described.

3. GALACTOSE AND FRUCTOSE ABSORPTION THROUGH GLUCOSE TRANSPORTERS

Galactose is absorbed through the same mechanisms as glucose. It enters the absorptive cells on the luminal side via the Na^+-dependent glucose transporters and facilitative glucose transporters and is transported through the serosal side on the facilitative glucose transporters.

Fructose both enters and leaves absorptive epithelial cells by facilitated diffusion, apparently via transport proteins that are part of the GLUT family. The transporter on the luminal side has been identified as GLUT 5. Although this transporter can transport glucose, it has a much higher activity with fructose (see Fig. 27.12). Other fructose transport proteins also may be present. For reasons as yet unknown, fructose is absorbed at a much more rapid rate when it is ingested as sucrose than when it is ingested as a monosaccharide.

B. Transport of Monosaccharides into Tissues

The properties of the GLUT transport proteins differ between tissues, reflecting the function of glucose metabolism in each tissue. In most cell types, the rate of glucose transport across the cell membrane is not rate-limiting for glucose metabolism. This is because the isoform of transporter present in these cell types has a relatively low K_m for glucose (that is, a low concentration of glucose will result in half the maximal rate of glucose transport) or is present in relatively high concentration in the cell membrane so that the intracellular glucose concentration reflects that in the blood. Because the hexokinase isozyme present in these cells has an even lower K_m for glucose (0.05–0.10 mM), variations in blood glucose levels do not affect the intracellular rate of glucose phosphorylation. However, in several tissues, the rate of transport becomes rate limiting when the serum level of glucose is low or when low levels of insulin signal the absence of dietary glucose.

In the liver, the K_m for the glucose transporter (GLUT 2) is relatively high compared with that of other tissues, probably 15 mM or above. This is in keeping with the liver's role as the organ that maintains blood glucose levels. As such, the liver will only convert glucose into other energy storage molecules when the blood glucose levels are high, such as the time immediately after ingestion of a meal. In muscle and adipose tissue, the transport of glucose is greatly stimulated by insulin. The mechanism involves the recruitment of glucose transporters (specifically, GLUT 4) from intracellular vesicles into the plasma membrane (Fig. 27.13). In adipose tissue, the stimulation of glucose transport across the plasma membrane by insulin increases its availability for the synthesis of fatty acids and glycerol from the glycolytic pathway. In skeletal muscle, the stimulation of glucose transport by insulin increases its availability for glycolysis and glycogen synthesis.

V. GLUCOSE TRANSPORT THROUGH THE BLOOD-BRAIN BARRIER AND INTO NEURONS

A hypoglycemic response is elicited by a decrease of blood glucose concentration to some point between 18 and 54 mg/dL (1 and 3 mM). The hypoglycemic response is a result of a decreased supply of glucose to the brain and starts with light-headedness and dizziness and may progress to coma. The slow rate of transport of glucose through the blood-brain barrier (from the blood into the cerebrospinal fluid) at low levels of glucose is thought to be responsible for this neuroglycopenic response. Glucose transport from the cerebrospinal fluid across the plasma membranes of neurons is rapid and is not rate limiting for ATP generation from glycolysis.

The erythrocyte (red blood cell) is an example of a tissue in which glucose transport is not rate-limiting. Although the glucose transporter (GLUT 1) has a K_m of 1 to 7 mM, it is present in extremely high concentrations, constituting approximately 5% of all membrane proteins. Consequently, as the blood glucose levels fall from a postprandial level of 140 mg/dL (7.5 mM) to the normal fasting level of 80 mg/dL (4.5 mM), or even the hypoglycemic level of 40 mg/dL (2.2 mM), the supply of glucose is still adequate for the rates at which glycolysis and the pentose phosphate pathway operate.

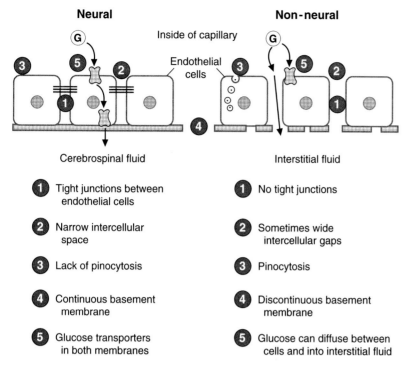

Fig. 27.14. Glucose transport through the capillary endothelium in neural and nonneural tissues. Characteristics of transport in each type of tissue are listed by numbers that refer to the numbers in the drawing. G = glucose.

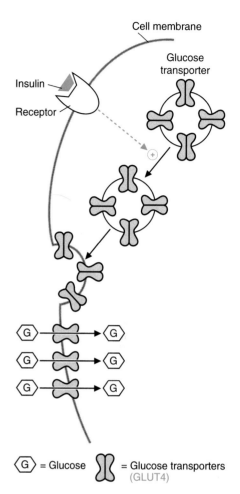

Fig. 27.13. Stimulation by insulin of glucose transport into muscle and adipose cells. Binding of insulin to its cell membrane receptor causes vesicles containing glucose transport proteins to move from inside the cell to the cell membrane.

In the brain, the endothelial cells of the capillaries have extremely tight junctions, and glucose must pass from the blood into the extracellular cerebrospinal fluid by GLUT 1 transporters in the endothelial cell membranes (Fig. 27.14), and then through the basement membrane. Measurements of the overall process of glucose transport from the blood into the brain (mediated by GLUT 3 on neural cells) show a $K_{m,app}$ of 7 to 11 mM, and a maximal velocity not much greater than the rate of glucose utilization by the brain. Thus, decreases of blood glucose below the fasting level of 80 to 90 mg/dL (approximately 5 mM) are likely to significantly affect the rate of glucose metabolism in the brain, because of reduced glucose transport into the brain.

CLINICAL COMMENTS

One of five Americans experiences some form of gastrointestinal discomfort from 30 minutes to 12 hours after ingesting lactose-rich foods. Most become symptomatic when they consume more than 25 g lactose at one time (e.g., 1 pint of milk or its equivalent). **Deria Voider's** symptoms were caused by her "new" diet in this country, which included a glass of milk in addition to the milk she used on her cereal with breakfast each morning.

Management of lactose intolerance includes a reduction or avoidance of lactose-containing foods depending on the severity of the deficiency of intestinal lactase. Hard cheeses (cheddar, Swiss, Jarlsberg) are low in lactose and may be tolerated by patients with only moderate lactase deficiency. Yogurt with "live and active cultures" printed on the package contain bacteria that release free lactases when the bacteria are lysed by gastric acid and proteolytic enzymes. The free lactases then digest the lactose. Commercially available milk products that have been hydrolyzed with a lactase enzyme provide a 70% reduction in total lactose content, which may be adequate to prevent digestive symptoms in mildly affected patients. Tablets and capsules containing lactase are also available and should be taken one-half hour before meals.

Many adults who have a lactase deficiency develop the ability to ingest small amounts of lactose in dairy products without experiencing symptoms. This adaptation probably involves an increase in the population of colonic bacteria that can cleave lactose and not a recovery or induction of human lactase synthesis. For many individuals, dairy products are the major dietary source of calcium, and their complete elimination from the diet can lead to osteoporosis.

Lactose, however, is used as a "filler" or carrying agent in more than 1,000 prescription and over-the-counter drugs in this country. People with lactose intolerance often unwittingly ingest lactose with their medications.

Poorly controlled diabetic patients such as **Ann Sulin** frequently have elevations in serum glucose levels (hyperglycemia). This is often attributable to a lack of circulating, active insulin, which will stimulate glucose uptake (through the recruitment of GLUT 4 transporters from the endoplasmic reticulum to the plasma membrane) by the peripheral tissues (heart, muscle, and adipose tissue). Without uptake by these tissues, glucose tends to accumulate within the bloodstream, leading to hyperglycemia.

The large amount of H_2 produced on fructose ingestion suggested that **Nona Melos's** problem was one of a deficiency in fructose transport into the absorptive cells of the intestinal villi. If fructose were being absorbed properly, the fructose would not have traveled to the colonic bacteria, which metabolized the fructose to generate the hydrogen gas. To confirm the diagnosis, a jejunal biopsy was taken; lactase, sucrase, maltase, and trehalase activities were normal in the jejunal cells. The tissue was also tested for the enzymes of fructose metabolism; these were in the normal range as well. Although Nona had no sugar in her urine, malabsorption of disaccharides can result in their appearance in the urine if damage to the intestinal mucosal cells allows their passage into the interstitial fluid. When Nona was placed on a diet free of fruit juices and other foods containing fructose, she did well and could tolerate small amounts of pure sucrose.

More than 50% of the adult population are estimated to be unable to absorb fructose in high doses (50 g), and more than 10% cannot completely absorb 25 g fructose. These individuals, like those with other disorders of fructose metabolism, must avoid fruits and other foods containing high concentrations of fructose.

BIOCHEMICAL COMMENTS

Cholera is an acute watery diarrheal disorder caused by the water-borne, Gram-negative bacterium *Vibrio cholerae*. It is a disease of antiquity; descriptions of epidemics of the disease date to before 500 BC. During epidemics, the infection is spread by large numbers of vibrio that enter water sources from the voluminous liquid stools and contaminate the environment, particularly in areas of extreme poverty where plumbing and modern waste-disposal systems are primitive or nonexistent.

After being ingested, the *V. cholerae* organisms attach to the brush border of the intestinal epithelium and secrete an exotoxin that binds irreversibly to a specific chemical receptor (G_{M1} ganglioside) on the cell surface. This exotoxin catalyzes an ADP-ribosylation reaction that increases adenylate cyclase activity and thus cAMP levels in the enterocyte. As a result, the normal absorption of sodium, anions, and water from the gut lumen into the intestinal cell is markedly diminished. The exotoxin also stimulates the crypt cells to secrete chloride, accompanied by cations and water, from the bloodstream into the lumen of the gut. The resulting loss of solute-rich diarrheal fluid may, in severe cases, exceed 1 liter/hour, leading to rapid dehydration and even death.

The therapeutic approach to cholera takes advantage of the fact that the Na^+-dependent transporters for glucose and amino acids are not affected by the cholera exotoxin. As a result, coadministration of glucose and Na^+ by mouth results in the uptake of glucose and Na^+, accompanied by chloride and water, thereby partially correcting the ion deficits and fluid loss. Amino acids and small peptides are also adsorbed by Na^+-dependent cotransport involving transport proteins distinct from the Na^+-dependent glucose transporters. Therefore, addition of protein to the glucose–sodium replacement solution enhances its effectiveness and markedly decreases the severity of the diarrhea. Adjunctive antibiotic therapy also shortens the diarrheal phase of cholera but does not decrease the need for the oral replacement therapy outlined earlier.

Suggested Readings

Bell GJ, Burant CF, Takeda J, Gould GW. Structure and function of mammalian facilitative sugar transporters. J Biol Chem 1993;278:19161–19164.

Brown GK. Glucose transporters: structure, function and consequences of deficiency. J Inherit Metab Dis 2000;23:237–246.

Buller HA, Grand RJ. Lactose intolerance. Annu Rev Med 1990;41:141–148.

Linder MC, ed. Nutrition and metabolism of carbohydrates. In: Nutritional Biochemistry and Metabolism with Clinical Applications, 2nd Ed. New York: Elsevier, 1991:21–50.

Semenza G, Auricchio S, Mantei, N. Small-intestinal disaccharidases. In: Scriver CR, Beaudet AL, Sly WS, Valle D, eds. The metabolic and molecular bases of inherited disease, 8th Ed. New York: McGraw-Hill, 2001:1623–1650.

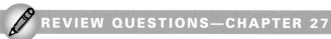 **REVIEW QUESTIONS—CHAPTER 27**

1. The facilitative transporter most responsible for transporting fructose from the blood into cells is which of the following?

    (A) GLUT 1
    (B) GLUT 2
    (C) GLUT 3
    (D) GLUT 4
    (E) GLUT 5

2. An alcoholic patient developed a pancreatitis that affected his exocrine pancreatic function. He exhibited discomfort after eating a high-carbohydrate meal. The patient most likely had a reduced ability to digest which of the following?

    (A) Starch
    (B) Lactose
    (C) Fiber
    (D) Sucrose
    (E) Maltose

3. A type I diabetic neglects to take his insulin injections while on a weekend vacation. Cells of which tissue would be most greatly affected by this mistake?

    (A) Brain
    (B) Liver
    (C) Muscle
    (D) Red blood cells
    (E) Pancreas

4. After digestion of a piece of cake that contains flour, milk, and sucrose as its primary ingredients, the major carbohydrate products entering the blood are which of the following?

   (A) Glucose
   (B) Fructose and galactose
   (C) Galactose and glucose
   (D) Fructose and glucose
   (E) Glucose, galactose and fructose

5. A patient has a genetic defect that causes intestinal epithelial cells to produce disaccharidases of much lower activity than normal. Compared with a normal person, after eating a bowl of milk and oatmeal sweetened with table sugar, this patient will exhibit higher levels of which of the following?

   (A) Maltose, sucrose, and lactose in the stool
   (B) Starch in the stool
   (C) Galactose and fructose in the blood
   (D) Glycogen in the muscles
   (E) Insulin in the blood

28 Formation and Degradation of Glycogen

Glycogen is the storage form of glucose found in most types of cells. It is composed of glucosyl units linked by **α-1,4 glycosidic bonds**, *with* **α-1,6 branches** *occurring roughly every 8 to 10 glucosyl units (Fig. 28.1). The liver and skeletal muscle contain the largest glycogen stores.*

The formation of glycogen from glucose is an energy-requiring pathway that begins, like most of glucose metabolism, with the phosphorylation of glucose to **glucose 6-phosphate***. Glycogen synthesis from glucose 6-phosphate involves the formation of uridine diphosphate glucose (***UDP-glucose***) and the transfer of glucosyl units from UDP-glucose to the ends of the glycogen chains by the enzyme* **glycogen synthase***. Once the chains reach approximately 11 glucosyl units, a* **branching enzyme** *moves six to eight units to form an α (1,6) branch.*

Glycogenolysis, the pathway for glycogen degradation, is not the reverse of the biosynthetic pathway. The degradative enzyme **glycogen phosphorylase** *removes glucosyl units one at a time from the ends of the glycogen chains, converting them to* **glucose 1-phosphate** *without resynthesizing UDP-glucose or UTP. A* **debranching enzyme** *removes the glucosyl residues near each branchpoint.*

Liver glycogen serves as a source of **blood glucose***. To generate glucose, the glucose 1-phosphate produced from glycogen degradation is converted to*

Glycogen degradation is a phosphorolysis reaction (breaking of a bond using a phosphate ion as a nucleophile). Enzymes that catalyze phosphorolysis reactions are named phosphorylase. Because more than one type of phosphorylase exists, the substrate usually is included in the name of the enzyme, such as glycogen phosphorylase or purine nucleoside phosphorylase.

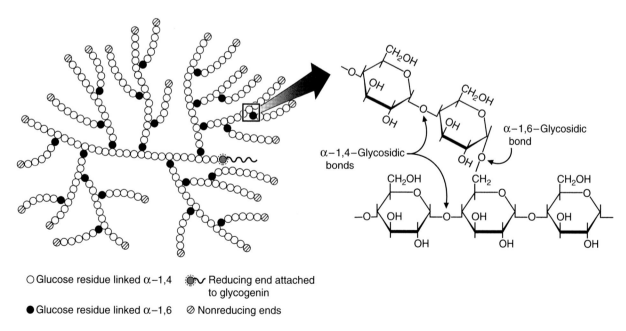

○ Glucose residue linked α–1,4   ◉〜 Reducing end attached to glycogenin

● Glucose residue linked α–1,6   ⊘ Nonreducing ends

Fig. 28.1. Glycogen structure. Glycogen is composed of glucosyl units linked by α-1,4-glycosidic bonds and α-1,6-glycosidic bonds. The branches occur more frequently in the center of the molecule, and less frequently in the periphery. The anomeric carbon that is not attached to another glucosyl residue (the reducing end) is attached to the protein glycogenin by a glycosidic bond.

glucose 6-phosphate. **Glucose 6-phosphatase**, *an enzyme found only in liver and kidney, converts glucose 6-phosphate to free glucose, which then enters the blood.*

Glycogen synthesis and degradation are regulated in liver by **hormonal changes** *that signal the need for blood glucose (see Chapter 26). The body maintains fasting blood glucose levels at approximately 80 mg/dL to ensure that the brain and other tissues that are dependent on glucose for the generation of adenosine triphosphate (ATP) have a continuous supply. The lack of dietary glucose, signaled by a decrease of the* **insulin/glucagon ratio**, *activates liver glycogenolysis and inhibits glycogen synthesis.* **Epinephrine**, *which signals an increased utilization of blood glucose and other fuels for exercise or emergency situations, also activates liver glycogenolysis. The hormones that regulate liver glycogen metabolism work principally through changes in the* **phosphorylation** *state of glycogen synthase in the biosynthetic pathway and glycogen phosphorylase in the degradative pathway.*

In skeletal muscle, glycogen supplies glucose 6-phosphate for ATP synthesis in the glycolytic pathway. Muscle glycogen phosphorylase is stimulated during exercise by the increase of adenosine monophosphate (AMP), an **allosteric activator** *of the enzyme, and also by phosphorylation. The phosphorylation is stimulated by* **calcium** *released during contraction, and by the "fight-or-flight" hormone epinephrine. Glycogen synthesis is activated in resting muscles by the elevation of insulin after carbohydrate ingestion.*

The neonate must rapidly adapt to an intermittent fuel supply after birth. Once the umbilical cord is clamped, the supply of glucose from the maternal circulation is interrupted. The combined effect of epinephrine and glucagon on the liver glycogen stores of the neonate rapidly restore glucose levels to normal.

THE WAITING ROOM

A newborn baby girl, **Getta Carbo,** was born after a 38-week gestation. Her mother, a 36-year-old woman, had moderate hypertension during the last trimester of pregnancy related to a recurrent urinary tract infection that resulted in a severe loss of appetite and recurrent vomiting in the month preceding delivery. Fetal bradycardia (slower than normal fetal heart rate) was detected with each uterine contraction of labor, a sign of possible fetal distress.

At birth Getta was cyanotic (a bluish discoloration caused by a lack of adequate oxygenation of tissues) and limp. She responded to several minutes of assisted ventilation. Her Apgar score of 3 was low at 1 minute after birth, but improved to a score of 7 at 5 minutes.

Physical examination in the nursery at 10 minutes showed a thin, malnourished female newborn. Her body temperature was slightly low, her heart rate was rapid, and her respiratory rate of 35 breaths/minute was elevated. Getta's birth weight was only 2,100 g, compared with a normal value of 3,300 g. Her length was 47 cm, and her head circumference was 33 cm (low normal). The laboratory reported that Getta's serum glucose level when she was unresponsive was 14 mg/dL. A glucose value below 40 mg/dL (2.5 mM) is considered to be abnormal in newborn infants.

At 5 hours of age, she was apneic (not breathing) and unresponsive. Ventilatory resuscitation was initiated and a cannula placed in the umbilical vein. Blood for a glucose level was drawn through this cannula, and 5 mL of a 20% glucose solution was injected. Getta slowly responded to this therapy.

The Apgar score is an objective estimate of the overall condition of the newborn, determined at both 1 and 5 minutes after birth. The best score is 10 (normal in all respects).

Jim Bodie, a 19-year-old body builder, was rushed to the hospital emergency room in a coma. One-half hour earlier, his mother had heard a loud crashing sound in the basement where Jim had been lifting weights and completing his daily workout on the treadmill. She found her son on the floor having severe jerking movements of all muscles (a grand mal seizure).

In the emergency room, the doctors learned that despite the objections of his family and friends, Jim regularly used androgens and other anabolic steroids in an effort to bulk up his muscle mass.

On initial physical examination, he was comatose with occasional involuntary jerking movements of his extremities. Foamy saliva dripped from his mouth. He had bitten his tongue and had lost bowel and bladder control at the height of the seizure.

The laboratory reported a serum glucose level of 18 mg/dL (extremely low). The intravenous infusion of 5% glucose (5 g of glucose per 100 mL of solution), which had been started earlier, was increased to 10%. In addition, 50 g glucose was given over 30 seconds through the intravenous tubing.

Jim Bodie's treadmill exercise and most other types of moderate exercise involving whole body movement (running, skiing, dancing, tennis) increase the utilization of blood glucose and other fuels by skeletal muscles. The blood glucose is normally supplied by the stimulation of liver glycogenolysis and gluconeogenesis.

I. STRUCTURE OF GLYCOGEN

Glycogen, the storage form of glucose, is a branched glucose polysaccharide composed of chains of glucosyl units linked by α-1,4 bonds with α-1,6 branches every 8 to 10 residues (see Fig. 28.1). In a molecule of this highly branched structure, only one glucosyl residue has an anomeric carbon that is not linked to another glucose residue. This anomeric carbon at the beginning of the chain is attached to the protein glycogenin. The other ends of the chains are called nonreducing ends (see Chapter 5). The branched structure permits rapid degradation and rapid synthesis of glycogen because enzymes can work on several chains simultaneously from the multiple nonreducing ends.

Glycogen is present in tissues as polymers of very high molecular weight (10^7–10^8) collected together in glycogen particles. The enzymes involved in glycogen synthesis and degradation, and some of the regulatory enzymes, are bound to the surface of the glycogen particles.

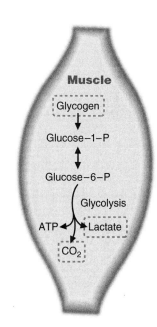

II. FUNCTION OF GLYCOGEN IN SKELETAL MUSCLE AND LIVER

Glycogen is found in most cell types, where it serves as a reservoir of glucosyl units for ATP generation from glycolysis.

Glycogen is degraded mainly to glucose 1-phosphate, which is converted to glucose 6-phosphate. In skeletal muscle and other cell types, the glucose 6-phosphate enters the glycolytic pathway (Fig. 28.2). Glycogen is an extremely important fuel source for skeletal muscle when ATP demands are high and when glucose 6-phosphate is used rapidly in anaerobic glycolysis. In many other cell types, the small glycogen reservoir serves a similar purpose; it is an emergency fuel source that supplies glucose for the generation of ATP in the absence of oxygen or during restricted blood flow. In general, glycogenolysis and glycolysis are activated together in these cells.

Glycogen serves a very different purpose in liver than in skeletal muscle and other tissues (see Fig. 28.2). Liver glycogen is the first and immediate source of glucose for the maintenance of blood glucose levels. In the liver, the glucose 6-phosphate that is generated from glycogen degradation is hydrolyzed to glucose by glucose 6-phosphatase, an enzyme present only in the liver and kidneys. Glycogen degradation thus provides a readily mobilized source of blood glucose as dietary glucose decreases, or as exercise increases the utilization of blood glucose by muscles.

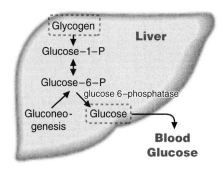

Fig. 28.2. Glycogenolysis in skeletal muscle and liver. Glycogen stores serve different functions in muscle cells and liver. In the muscle and most other cell types, glycogen stores serve as a fuel source for the generation of ATP. In the liver, glycogen stores serve as a source of blood glucose.

Regulation of glycogen synthesis serves to prevent futile cycling and waste of ATP. Futile cycling refers to a situation in which a substrate is converted to a product through one pathway, and the product converted back to the substrate through another pathway. Because the biosynthetic pathway is energy-requiring, futile cycling results in a waste of high-energy phosphate bonds. Thus, glycogen synthesis is activated when glycogen degradation is inhibited, and vice versa.

The pathways of glycogenolysis and gluconeogenesis in the liver both supply blood glucose, and, consequently, these two pathways are activated together by glucagon. Gluconeogenesis, the synthesis of glucose from amino acids and other gluconeogenic precursors (discussed in detail in Chapter 31), also forms glucose 6-phosphate, so that glucose 6-phosphatase serves as a "gateway" to the blood for both pathways (see Fig. 28.2).

III. SYNTHESIS AND DEGRADATION OF GLYCOGEN

Glycogen synthesis, like almost all the pathways of glucose metabolism, begins with the phosphorylation of glucose to glucose 6-phosphate by hexokinase or, in the liver, glucokinase (Fig. 28.3). Glucose 6-phosphate is the precursor of glycolysis, the pentose phosphate pathway, and of pathways for the synthesis of other sugars. In the pathway for glycogen synthesis, glucose 6-phosphate is converted to glucose 1-phosphate by phosphoglucomutase, a reversible reaction.

Glycogen is both formed from and degraded to glucose 1-phosphate, but the biosynthetic and degradative pathways are separate and involve different enzymes (see Fig. 28.3). The biosynthetic pathway is an energy-requiring pathway; high-energy phosphate from UTP is used to activate the glucosyl residues to UDP-glucose (Fig. 28.4). In the degradative pathway, the glycosidic bonds between the glucosyl residues in glycogen are simply cleaved by the addition of phosphate to produce glucose 1-phosphate (or water to produce free glucose), and UDP-glucose is not resynthesized. The existence of separate pathways for the formation and degradation of important compounds is a common theme in metabolism. Because

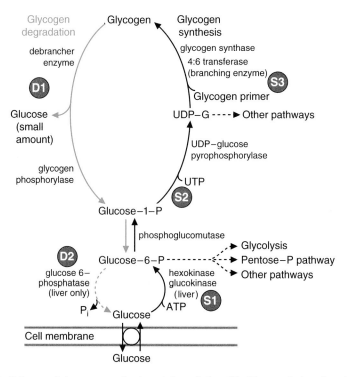

Fig. 28.3. Scheme of glycogen synthesis and degradation. **S1.** Glucose 6-phosphate is formed from glucose by hexokinase in most cells, and glucokinase in the liver. It is a metabolic branch-point for the pathways of glycolysis, the pentose phosphate pathway, and glycogen synthesis. **S2.** UDP-Glucose (UDP-G) is synthesized from glucose 1-phosphate. UDP-Glucose is the branchpoint for glycogen synthesis and other pathways requiring the addition of carbohydrate units. **S3.** Glycogen synthesis is catalyzed by glycogen synthase and the branching enzyme. **D1.** Glycogen degradation is catalyzed by glycogen phosphorylase and a debrancher enzyme. **D2.** Glucose 6-phosphatase in the liver generates free glucose from glucose 6-phosphate.

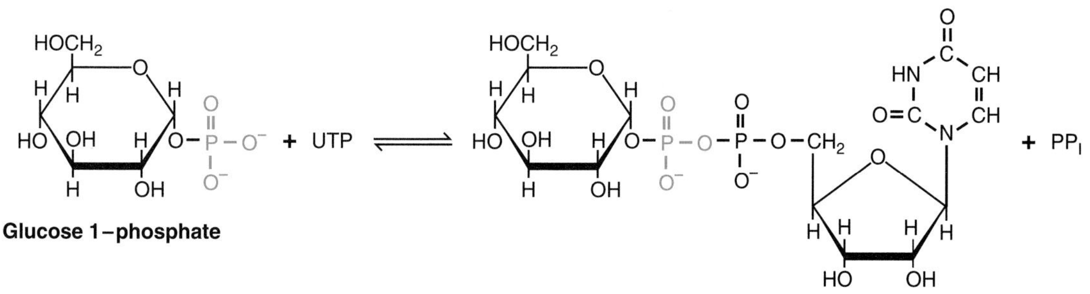

Glucose 1–phosphate

**Uridine diphosphate glucose
(UDP–Glucose)**

Fig. 28.4. Formation of UDP-glucose. The high-energy phosphate bond of UTP provides the energy for the formation of a high-energy bond in UDP-glucose. Pyrophosphate (PP_i), released by the reaction, is cleaved to 2 P_i.

the synthesis and degradation pathways use different enzymes, one can be activated while the other is inhibited.

A. Glycogen Synthesis

Glycogen synthesis requires the formation of α-1,4-glycosidic bonds to link glucosyl residues in long chains and the formation of an α-1,6 branch every 8 to 10 residues (Fig. 28.5). Most of glycogen synthesis occurs through the lengthening of the polysaccharide chains of a preexisting glycogen molecule (a glycogen primer) in which the reducing end of the glycogen is attached to the protein glycogenin. To lengthen the glycogen chains, glucosyl residues are added from UDP-glucose to the nonreducing ends of the chain by glycogen synthase. The anomeric carbon of each glucosyl residue is attached in an α-1,4 bond to the hydroxyl on carbon 4 of the terminal glucosyl residue. When the chain reaches 11 residues in length, a 6- to 8-residue piece is cleaved by amylo-4:6-transferase and reattached to a glucosyl unit by an α-1,6 bond. Both chains continue to lengthen until they are long enough to produce two new branches. This process continues, producing highly branched molecules. Glycogen synthase, the enzyme that attaches the glucosyl residues in 1,4-bonds, is the regulated step in the pathway.

The synthesis of new glycogen primer molecules also occurs. Glycogenin, the protein to which glycogen is attached, glycosylates itself (autoglycosylation) by attaching the glucosyl residue of UDP-glucose to the hydroxyl side chain of a serine residue in the protein. The protein then extends the carbohydrate chain (using UDP-glucose as the substrate) until the glucosyl chain is long enough to serve as a substrate for glycogen synthase.

B. Degradation of Glycogen

Glycogen is degraded by two enzymes, glycogen phosphorylase and the debrancher enzyme (Fig. 28.6). The enzyme glycogen phosphorylase starts at the end of a chain and successively cleaves glucosyl residues by adding phosphate to the terminal glycosidic bond, thereby releasing glucose 1-phosphate. However, glycogen phosphorylase cannot act on the glycosidic bonds of the four glucosyl residues closest to a branchpoint because the branching chain sterically hinders a proper fit into the catalytic site of the enzyme. The debrancher enzyme, which catalyzes the removal of the four residues closest to the branchpoint, has two catalytic activities: it acts as a transferase and as an α 1,6-glucosidase. As a transferase, the debrancher first removes a unit containing three glucose residues, and adds it to the end of a longer chain by an α-1,4 bond. The one glucosyl residue remaining at the 1,6-branch is hydrolyzed by the amylo-1,6-glucosidase activity of the debrancher, resulting in the release of free glucose. Thus, one glucose and approximately 7 to 9 glucose 1-phosphate residues are released for every branchpoint.

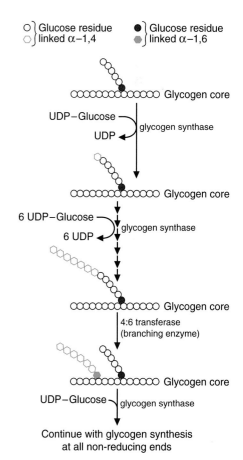

Continue with glycogen synthesis
at all non-reducing ends

Fig. 28.5. Glycogen synthesis. See text for details.

Branching of glycogen serves two major roles; increased sites for synthesis and degradation, and enhancing the solubility of the molecule.

A genetic defect of lysosomal glucosidase, called type II glycogen storage disease, leads to the accumulation of glycogen particles in large, membrane-enclosed residual bodies, which disrupt the function of liver and muscle cells. Children with this disease usually die of heart failure at a few months of age.

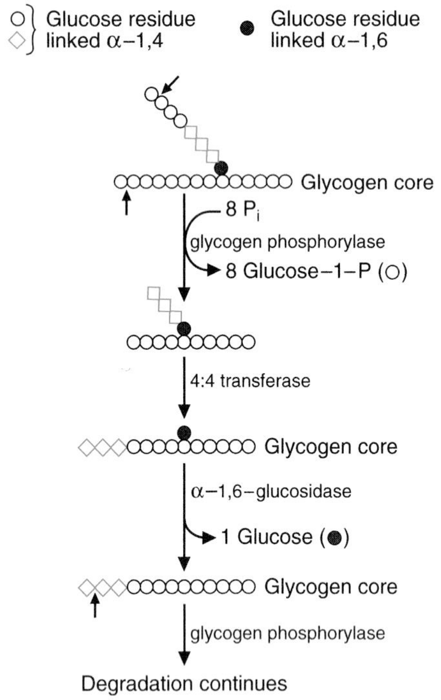

Fig. 28.6. Glycogen degradation. See text for details.

Q: A series of inborn errors of metabolism, the glycogen storage diseases, result from deficiencies in the enzymes of glycogenolysis (see Table 28.1). Muscle glycogen phosphorylase, the key regulatory enzyme of glycogen degradation, is genetically different from liver glycogen phosphorylase, and thus a person may have a defect in one and not the other. Why do you think that a genetic deficiency in muscle glycogen phosphorylase (McArdle's disease) is a mere inconvenience, whereas a deficiency of liver glycogen phosphorylase (Hers' disease) can be lethal?

Some degradation of glycogen also occurs within lysosomes when glycogen particles become surrounded by membranes that then fuse with the lysosomal membranes. A lysosomal glucosidase hydrolyzes this glycogen to glucose.

IV. REGULATION OF GLYCOGEN SYNTHESIS AND DEGRADATION

The regulation of glycogen synthesis in different tissues matches the function of glycogen in each tissue. Liver glycogen serves principally for the support of blood glucose during fasting or during extreme need (e.g., exercise), and the degradative and biosynthetic pathways are regulated principally by changes in

Table 28.1. Glycogen Storage Diseases

Type	Enzyme Affected	Primary Organ Involved	Manifestations[a]
O	Glycogen synthase	Liver	Hypoglycemia, hyperketonemia, FTT[b] early death
I[c]	Glucose 6-phosphatase (Von Gierke's disease)	Liver	Enlarged liver and kidney, growth failure, fasting hypoglycemia, acidosis, lipemia, thrombocyte dysfunction. Hypoglycemia is the most severe.
II	Lysosomal α-glucosidase	All organs with lysosomes	Infantile form: early-onset progressive muscle hypotonia, cardiac failure, death before 2 years; juvenile form: later-onset myopathy with variable cardiac involvement, adult form: limb-girdle muscular dystrophy-like features. Glycogen deposits accumulate in lysosomes.
III	Amylo-1,6-glucosidase (debrancher)	Liver, skeletal muscle, heart	Fasting hypoglycemia; hepatomegaly in infancy in some. myopathic features. Glycogen deposits have short outer branches.
IV	Amylo-4,6-glucosidase (branching enzyme)	Liver	Hepatosplenomegaly; symptoms may arise from a hepatic reaction to the presence of a foreign body (glycogen with long outer branches). Usually fatal.
V	Muscle glycogen phosphorylase (McArdle's disease)	Skeletal muscle	Exercise-induced muscular pain, cramps, and progressive weakness, sometimes with myoglobinuria
VI	Liver glycogen phosphorylase	Liver	Hepatomegaly, mild hypoglycemia, good prognosis
VII	Phosphofructokinase-I	Muscle, red blood cells	As in type V, in addition, enzymopathic hemolysis
IX[d]	Phosphorylase kinase	Liver	As in VI. Hepatomegaly.
X	cAMP-dependant Protein kinase A	Liver	Hepatomegaly.

Reproduced with permission, from Annu Rev Nutr 1993; 13:85. © 1993 by Annual Reviews, Inc.
[a] All of these diseases but type O are characterized by increased glycogen deposits.
[b] FTT = failure to thrive
[c] Glucose 6-phosphatase is composed of several subunits that also transport glucose, glucose 6-phosphate, phosphate, and pyrophosphate across the endoplasmic reticulum membranes. Therefore, there are several subtypes of this disease, corresponding to defects in the different subunits.
[d] There are several subtypes of this disease, corresponding to different mutations and patterns of inheritance.

Table 28.2. Regulation of Liver and Muscle Glycogen Stores[a]

State	Regulators	Response of Tissue
	Liver	
Fasting	Blood: Glucagon ↑ Insulin ↓ Tissue: cAMP ↑	Glycogen degradation ↑ Glycogen synthesis ↓
Carbohydrate meal	Blood: Glucagon ↓ Insulin ↑ Glucose ↑ Tissue: cAMP ↓ Glucose ↑	Glycogen degradation ↓ Glycogen synthesis ↑
Exercise and stress	Blood: Epinephrine ↑ Tissue: cAMP ↑ Ca²⁺-calmodulin ↑	Glycogen degradation ↑ Glycogen synthesis ↓
	Muscle	
Fasting (rest)	Blood: Insulin ↓	Glycogen synthesis ↓ Glucose transport ↓
Carbohydrate meal (rest)	Blood: Insulin ↑	Glycogen synthesis ↑ Glucose transport ↑
Exercise	Blood: Epinephrine ↑ Tissue: AMP ↑ Ca²⁺-calmodulin ↑ cAMP ↑	Glycogen synthesis ↓ Glycogen degradation ↑ Glycolysis ↑

[a]↑ = increased compared with other physiologic states; ↓ = decreased compared with other physiologic states.

the insulin/glucagon ratio and by blood glucose levels, which reflect the availability of dietary glucose (Table 28.2). Degradation of liver glycogen is also activated by epinephrine, which is released in response to exercise, hypoglycemia, or other stress situations in which there is an immediate demand for blood glucose. In contrast, in skeletal muscles, glycogen is a reservoir of glucosyl units for the generation of ATP from glycolysis and glucose oxidation. As a consequence, muscle glycogenolysis is regulated principally by AMP, which signals a lack of ATP, and by Ca²⁺ released during contraction. Epinephrine, which is released in response to exercise and other stress situations, also activates skeletal muscle glycogenolysis. The glycogen stores of resting muscle decrease very little during fasting.

A. Regulation of Glycogen Metabolism in Liver

Liver glycogen is synthesized after a carbohydrate meal when blood glucose levels are elevated, and degraded as blood glucose levels decrease. When an individual eats a carbohydrate-containing meal, blood glucose levels immediately increase, insulin levels increase, and glucagon levels decrease (see Fig. 26.8). The increase of blood glucose levels and the rise of the insulin/glucagon ratio inhibit glycogen degradation and stimulate glycogen synthesis. The immediate increased transport of glucose into peripheral tissues, and storage of blood glucose as glycogen, helps to bring circulating blood glucose levels back to the normal 80- to 100-mg/dL range of the fasted state. As the length of time after a carbohydrate-containing meal increases, insulin levels decrease, and glucagon levels increase. The fall of the insulin/glucagon ratio results in inhibition of the biosynthetic pathway and

 Muscle glycogen is used within the muscle to support exercise. Thus, an individual with McArdle's disease (type V glycogen storage disease) experiences no other symptoms but unusual fatigue and muscle cramps during exercise. These symptoms may be accompanied by myoglobinuria and release of muscle creatine kinase into the blood.

Liver glycogen is the first reservoir for the support of blood glucose levels, and a deficiency in glycogen phosphorylase or any of the other enzymes of liver glycogen degradation can result in fasting hypoglycemia. The hypoglycemia is usually mild because patients can still synthesize glucose from gluconeogenesis (see Table 28.1).

 Maternal blood glucose readily crosses the placenta to enter the fetal circulation. During the last 9 or 10 weeks of gestation, glycogen formed from maternal glucose is deposited in the fetal liver under the influence of the insulin-dominated hormonal milieu of that period. At birth, maternal glucose supplies cease, causing a temporary physiologic drop in glucose levels in the newborn's blood, even in normal healthy infants. This drop serves as one of the signals for glucagon release from the newborn's pancreas, which, in turn, stimulates glycogenolysis. As a result, the glucose levels in the newborn return to normal.

Healthy full-term babies have adequate stores of liver glycogen to survive short (12 hours) periods of caloric deprivation provided other aspects of fuel metabolism are normal. Because **Getta Carbo's** mother was markedly anorexic during the critical period when the fetal liver is normally synthesizing glycogen from glucose supplied in the maternal blood, Getta's liver glycogen stores were below normal. Thus, because fetal glycogen is the major source of fuel for the newborn in the early hours of life, Getta became profoundly hypoglycemic within 5 hours of birth because of her low levels of stored carbohydrate.

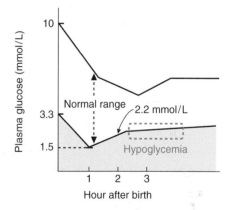

Plasma glucose levels in the neonate. The normal range of blood glucose levels in the neonate lies between the two black lines. The stippled blue area represents the range of hypoglycemia in the neonate that should be treated. Treatment of neonates with blood glucose levels that fall within the dashed blue box, the zone of clinical uncertainty, is controversial. The units of plasma glucose are given in millimoles/L. Both milligrams/dL (milligrams/100 mL) and millimoles/L are used clinically for the values of blood glucose: 80 mg/dL glucose is equivalent to 5 mmol/L (5 mM). From Mehta A. Arch Dis Child 1994;70:F54.

A patient was diagnosed as an infant with type III glycogen storage disease, a deficiency of debrancher enzyme (see Table 28.1). The patient had hepatomegaly (an enlarged liver) and experienced bouts of mild hypoglycemia. To diagnose the disease, glycogen was obtained from the patient's liver by biopsy after the patient had fasted overnight and compared with normal glycogen. The glycogen samples were treated with a preparation of commercial glycogen phosphorylase and commerical debrancher enzyme. The amounts of glucose 1-phosphate and glucose produced in the assay were then measured. The ratio of glucose 1-phosphate to glucose for the normal glycogen sample was 9:1, and the ratio for the patient was 3:1. Can you explain these results?

Table 28.3. Effect of Fasting on Liver Glycogen Content in the Human

Length of Fast (hours)	Glycogen Content (μmol/g liver)	Rate of Glycogenolysis (μmol/kg-min)
0	300	—
2	260	4.3
4	216	4.3
24	42	1.7
64	16	0.3

activation of the degradative pathway. As a result, liver glycogen is rapidly degraded to glucose, which is released into the blood.

Although glycogenolysis and gluconeogenesis are activated together by the same regulatory mechanisms, glycogenolysis responds more rapidly, with a greater outpouring of glucose. A substantial proportion of liver glycogen is degraded within the first few hours after eating (Table 28.3). The rate of glycogenolysis is fairly constant for the first 22 hours, but in a prolonged fast the rate decreases significantly as the liver glycogen supplies dwindle. Liver glycogen stores are, therefore, a rapidly rebuilt and degraded store of glucose, ever responsive to small and rapid changes of blood glucose levels.

1. NOMENCLATURE CONCERNS WITH ENZYMES METABOLIZING GLYCOGEN

Both glycogen phosphorylase and glycogen synthase will be covalently modified to regulate their activity (Fig. 28.7). When activated by covalent modification, glycogen phosphorylase is referred to as glycogen phosphorylase **a** (remember **a** for active); when the covalent modification is removed, and the enzyme is inactive, it is referred to as glycogen phosphorylase **b**. Glycogen synthase, when not covalently modified is active, and can be designated glycogen synthase **a** or glycogen synthase **I** (the I stands for *independent* of modifiers for activity). When glycogen synthase is covalently modified, it is inactive, in the form of glycogen synthase **b** or glycogen synthase **D** (for *dependent* on a modifier for activity).

2. REGULATION OF LIVER GLYCOGEN METABOLISM BY INSULIN AND GLUCAGON

Insulin and glucagon regulate liver glycogen metabolism by changing the phosphorylation state of glycogen phosphorylase in the degradative pathway and glycogen synthase in the biosynthetic pathway. An increase of glucagon and decrease of insulin during the fasting state initiates a cAMP-directed phosphorylation cascade, which results in the phosphorylation of glycogen phosphorylase to an active enzyme, and the

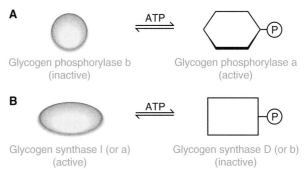

Fig. 28.7. The conversion of active and inactive forms of glycogen phosphorylase (**A**) and glycogen synthase (**B**). Note how the nomenclature changes depending on the phosphorylation and activity state of the enzyme.

phosphorylation of glycogen synthase to an inactive enzyme (Fig. 28.8). As a consequence, glycogen degradation is stimulated, and glycogen synthesis is inhibited.

3. GLUCAGON ACTIVATES A PHOSPHORYLATION CASCADE THAT CONVERTS GLYCOGEN PHOSPHORYLASE b TO GLYCOGEN PHOSPHORYLASE a

Glucagon regulates glycogen metabolism through its intracellular second messenger cAMP and protein kinase A (see Chapter 26). Glucagon, by binding to its cell membrane receptor, transmits a signal through G proteins that activates adenylate cyclase, causing cAMP levels to increase (see Fig. 28.8). cAMP binds to the regulatory subunits of protein kinase A, which dissociate from the catalytic subunits. The catalytic subunits of protein kinase A are activated by the dissociation and phosphorylate the enzyme phosphorylase kinase, activating it. Phosphorylase kinase is the protein kinase that converts the inactive liver glycogen phosphorylase b conformer to the active glycogen phosphorylase a conformer by transferring a phosphate from ATP to a specific serine residue on the

 With a deficiency of debrancher enzyme, but normal levels of glycogen phosphorylase, the glycogen chains of the patient could be degraded in vivo only to within 4 residues of the branchpoint. When the glycogen samples were treated with the commercial preparation containing normal enzymes, one glucose residue was released for each α-1,6 branch. However, in the patient's glycogen sample, with the short outer branches, three glucose 1-phosphates and one glucose residue were obtained for each α-1,6 branch. Normal glycogen has 8-10 glucosyl residues per branch, and thus gives a ratio of approximately 9 moles of glucose 1-phosphate to 1 mole of glucose.

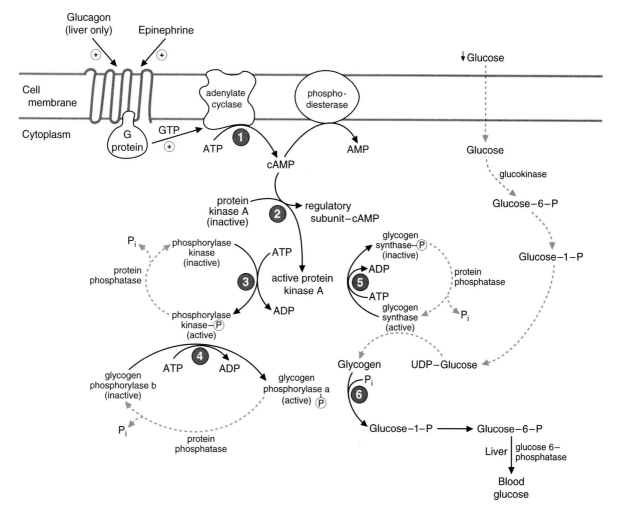

Fig. 28.8. Regulation of glycogen synthesis and degradation in the liver. 1. Glucagon binding to the glucagon receptor or epinephrine binding to a β receptor in the liver activates adenylate cyclase, via G proteins, which synthesizes cAMP from ATP. 2. cAMP binds to protein kinase A (cAMP-dependent protein kinase), thereby activating the catalytic subunits. 3. Protein kinase A activates phosphorylase kinase by phosphorylation. 4. Phosphorylase kinase adds a phosphate to specific serine residues on glycogen phosphorylase b, thereby converting it to the active glycogen phosphorylase a. 5. Protein kinase A also phosphorylates glycogen synthase, thereby decreasing its activity. 6. As a result of the inhibition of glycogen synthase and the activation of glycogen phosphorylase, glycogen is degraded to glucose 1-phosphate. The blue dashed lines denote reactions that are decreased in the livers of fasting individuals.

To remember whether a particular enzyme has been activated or inhibited by cAMP-dependent phosphorylation, consider whether it makes sense for the enzyme to be active or inhibited under fasting conditions (In a **PHast, PHosphorylate**).

Most of the enzymes that are regulated by phosphorylation have multiple phosphorylation sites. Glycogen phosphorylase, which has only one serine per subunit, and can be phosphorylated only by phosphorylase kinase, is the exception. For some enzymes, the phosphorylation sites are antagonistic, and phosphorylation initiated by one hormone counteracts the effects of other hormones. For other enzymes, the phosphorylation sites are synergistic, and phosphorylation at one site stimulated by one hormone can act synergistically with phosphorylation at another site.

Most of the enzymes that are regulated by phosphorylation also can be converted to the active conformation by allosteric effectors. Glycogen synthase b, the less active form of glycogen synthase, can be activated by the accumulation of glucose 6-phosphate above physiologic levels. The activation of glycogen synthase by glucose 6-phosphate may be important in individuals with glucose 6-phosphatase deficiency, a disorder known as type I or von Gierke's glycogen storage disease. When glucose 6-phosphate produced from gluconeogenesis accumulates in the liver, it activates glycogen synthesis even though the individual may be hypoglycemic and have low insulin levels. Glucose 1-phosphate is also elevated, resulting in the inhibition of glycogen phosphorylase. As a consequence, large glycogen deposits accumulate, and hepatomegaly occurs.

phosphorylase subunits. As a result of the activation of glycogen phosphorylase, glycogenolysis is stimulated.

4. INHIBITION OF GLYCOGEN SYNTHASE BY GLUCAGON-DIRECTED PHOSPHORYLATION

When glycogen degradation is activated by the cAMP-stimulated phosphorylation cascade, glycogen synthesis is simultaneously inhibited. The enzyme glycogen synthase is also phosphorylated by protein kinase A, but this phosphorylation results in a less active form, glycogen synthase b.

The phosphorylation of glycogen synthase is far more complex than glycogen phosphorylase. Glycogen synthase has multiple phosphorylation sites and is acted on by up to 10 different protein kinases. Phosphorylation by protein kinase A does not, by itself, inactivate glycogen synthase. Instead, phosphorylation by protein kinase A facilitates the subsequent addition of phosphate groups by other kinases, and these inactivate the enzyme. A term that has been applied to changes of activity resulting from multiple phosphorylation is hierarchical or synergistic phosphorylation-the phosphorylation of one site makes another site more reactive and easier to phosphorylate by a different protein kinase

5. REGULATION OF PROTEIN PHOSPHATASES

At the same time that protein kinase A and phosphorylase kinase are adding phosphate groups to enzymes, the protein phosphatases that remove this phosphate are inhibited. Protein phosphatases remove the phosphate groups, bound to serine or other residues of enzymes, by hydrolysis. Hepatic protein phosphatase-1 (hepatic PP-1), one of the major protein phosphatases involved in glycogen metabolism, removes phosphate groups from phosphorylase kinase, glycogen phosphorylase, and glycogen synthase. During fasting, hepatic PP-1 is inactivated by a number of mechanisms. One is dissociation from the glycogen particle, such that the substrates are no longer available to the phosphatase. A second is the binding of inhibitor proteins, such as the protein called inhibitor-1, which, when phosphorylated by a glucagon (or epinephrine)-directed mechanism, binds to and inhibits phosphatase action. Insulin indirectly activates hepatic PP-1 through its own signal transduction cascade initiated at the insulin receptor tyrosine kinase.

6. INSULIN IN LIVER GLYCOGEN METABOLISM

Insulin is antagonistic to glucagon in the degradation and synthesis of glycogen. The glucose level in the blood is the signal controlling the secretion of insulin and glucagon. Glucose stimulates insulin release and suppresses glucagon release; one increases while the other decreases after a high carbohydrate meal. However, insulin levels in the blood change to a greater degree with the fasting-feeding cycle than the glucagon levels, and thus insulin is considered the principal regulator of glycogen synthesis and degradation. The role of insulin in glycogen metabolism is often overlooked because the mechanisms by which insulin reverses all of the effects of glucagon on individual metabolic enzymes is still under investigation. In addition to the activation of hepatic PP-1 through the insulin receptor tyrosine kinase phosphorylation cascade, insulin may activate the phosphodiesterase that converts cAMP to AMP, thereby decreasing cAMP levels and inactivating protein kinase A. Regardless of the mechanisms involved, insulin is able to reverse all of the effects of glucagon and is the most important hormonal regulator of blood glucose levels.

7. BLOOD GLUCOSE LEVELS AND GLYCOGEN SYNTHESIS AND DEGRADATION

When an individual eats a high-carbohydrate meal, glycogen degradation immediately stops. Although the changes in insulin and glucagon levels are relatively rapid (10–15 minutes), the direct inhibitory effect of rising glucose levels on glycogen degradation is even more rapid. Glucose, as an allosteric effector, inhibits liver glycogen phosphorylase a by stimulating dephosphorylation of this enzyme. As insulin levels rise and glucagon levels fall, cAMP levels decrease and protein kinase A reassociates with its inhibitory subunits and becomes inactive. The protein phosphatases are activated, and phosphorylase a and glycogen synthase b are dephosphorylated. The collective result of these effects is rapid inhibition of glycogen degradation, and rapid activation of glycogen synthesis.

8. EPINEPHRINE AND CALCIUM IN THE REGULATION OF LIVER GLYCOGEN

Epinephrine, the "fight-or-flight" hormone, is released from the adrenal medulla in response to neural signals reflecting an increased demand for glucose. To flee from a dangerous situation, skeletal muscles use increased amounts of blood glucose to generate ATP. As a result, liver glycogenolysis must be stimulated. In the liver, epinephrine stimulates glycogenolysis through two different types of receptors, the α- and β-agonist receptors.

a. EPINEPHRINE ACTING AT THE β-RECEPTORS

Epinephrine, acting at the β-receptors, transmits a signal through G proteins to adenylate cyclase, which increases cAMP and activates protein kinase A. Hence, regulation of glycogen degradation and synthesis in liver by epinephrine and glucagon are similar (see Fig. 28.8).

b. EPINEPHRINE ACTING AT α-RECEPTORS

Epinephrine also binds to α-receptors in the liver. This binding activates glycogenolysis and inhibits glycogen synthesis principally by increasing the Ca^{2+} levels in the liver. The effects of epinephrine at the α-agonist receptor are mediated by the phosphatidylinositol bisphosphate (PIP_2)-Ca^{2+} signal transduction system, one of the principal intracellular second messenger systems employed by many hormones (Fig. 28.9) (see Chapter 11).

In the PIP_2-Ca^{2+} signal transduction system, the signal is transferred from the epinephrine receptor to membrane-bound phospholipase C by G proteins. Phospholipase C hydrolyzes PIP_2 to form diacylglycerol (DAG) and inositol trisphosphate (IP_3). IP_3 stimulates the release of Ca^{2+} from the endoplasmic reticulum. Ca^{2+} and DAG activate protein kinase C. The amount of calcium bound to one of the calcium-binding proteins, calmodulin, is also increased.

Calcium/calmodulin associates as a subunit with a number of enzymes and modifies their activities. It binds to inactive phosphorylase kinase, thereby partially activating this enzyme. (The fully activated enzyme is both bound to the calcium/calmodulin subunit and phosphorylated.) Phosphorylase kinase then phosphorylates glycogen phosphorylase b, thereby activating glycogen degradation. Calcium/calmodulin is also a modifier protein that activates one of the glycogen synthase kinases (calcium/calmodulin synthase kinase). Protein kinase C, calcium/calmodulin synthase kinase, and phosphorylase kinase all phosphorylate glycogen synthase at different serine residues on the enzyme, thereby inhibiting glycogen synthase and thus glycogen synthesis.

An inability of liver and muscle to store glucose as glycogen contributes to the hyperglycemia in patients, such as **Di Abietes,** with type 1 diabetes mellitus and in patients, such as **Ann Sulin,** with type 2 diabetes mellitus. The absence of insulin in type 1 diabetes mellitus patients and the high levels of glucagon result in decreased activity of glycogen synthase. Glycogen synthesis in skeletal muscles of type 1 patients is also limited by the lack of insulin-stimulated glucose transport. Insulin resistance in type 2 patients has the same effect.

An injection of insulin suppresses glucagon release and alters the insulin/glucagon ratio. The result is rapid uptake of glucose into skeletal muscle and rapid conversion of glucose to glycogen in skeletal muscle and liver.

In the neonate, the release of epinephrine during labor and birth normally contributes to restoring blood glucose levels. Unfortunately, **Getta Carbo** did not have adequate liver glycogen stores to support a rise in her blood glucose levels.

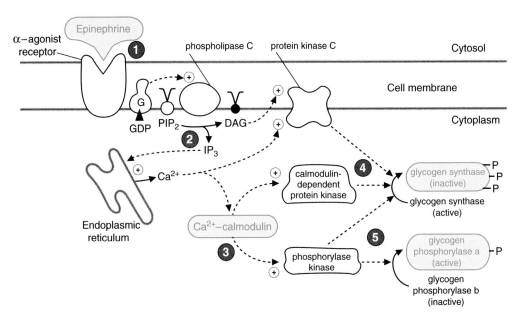

Fig. 28.9. Regulation of glycogen synthesis and degradation by epinephrine and Ca^{2+}. 1. The effect of epinephrine binding to α-agonist receptors in liver transmits a signal via G proteins to phospholipase C, which hydrolyzes PIP_2 to DAG and IP_3. 2. IP_3 stimulates the release of Ca^{2+} from the endoplasmic reticulum. 3. Ca^{2+} binds to the modifier protein calmodulin, which activates calmodulin-dependent protein kinase and phosphorylase kinase. Both Ca^{2+} and DAG activate protein kinase C. 4. These three kinases phosphorylate glycogen synthase at different sites and decrease its activity. 5. Phosphorylase kinase phosphorylates glycogen phosphorylase b to the active form. It therefore activates glycogenolysis as well as inhibiting glycogen synthesis.

The effect of epinephrine in the liver, therefore, enhances or is synergistic with the effects of glucagon. Epinephrine release during bouts of hypoglycemia or during exercise can stimulate hepatic glycogenolysis and inhibit glycogen synthesis very rapidly.

B. Regulation of Glycogen Synthesis and Degradation in Skeletal Muscle

The regulation of glycogenolysis in skeletal muscle is related to the availability of ATP for muscular contraction. Skeletal muscle glycogen produces glucose

Jim Bodie gradually regained consciousness with continued infusions of high-concentration glucose titrated to keep his serum glucose level between 120 and 160 mg/dL. Although he remained somnolent and moderately confused over the next 12 hours, he was eventually able to tell his physicians that he had self-injected approximately 80 units of regular (short-acting) insulin every 6 hours while eating a high-carbohydrate diet for the last 2 days preceding his seizure. Normal subjects under basal conditions secrete an average of 40 units of insulin daily. He had last injected insulin just before exercising. An article in a body-building magazine that he had recently read cited the anabolic effects of insulin on increasing muscle mass. He had purchased the insulin and necessary syringes from the same underground drug source from whom he regularly bought his anabolic steroids.

Normally, muscle glycogenolysis supplies the glucose required for the kinds of high-intensity exercise that require anaerobic glycolysis, such as weight-lifting. Jim's treadmill exercise also uses blood glucose, which is supplied by liver glycogenolysis. The high serum insulin levels, resulting from the injection he gave himself just before his workout, activated both glucose transport into skeletal muscle and glycogen synthesis, while inhibiting glycogen degradation. His exercise, which would continue to use blood glucose, could normally be supported by breakdown of liver glycogen. However, glycogen synthesis in his liver was activated, and glycogen degradation was inhibited by the insulin injection.

1-phosphate and a small amount of free glucose. Glucose 1-phosphate is converted to glucose 6-phosphate, which is committed to the glycolytic pathway; the absence of glucose 6-phosphatase in skeletal muscle prevents conversion of the glucosyl units from glycogen to blood glucose. Skeletal muscle glycogen is therefore degraded only when the demand for ATP generation from glycolysis is high. The highest demands occur during anaerobic glycolysis, which requires more moles of glucose for each ATP produced than oxidation of glucose to CO_2 (see Chapter 22). Anaerobic glycolysis occurs in tissues that have fewer mitochondria, a higher content of glycolytic enzymes, and higher levels of glycogen, or fast-twitch glycolytic fibers. It occurs most frequently at the onset of exercise–before vasodilation occurs to bring in blood-borne fuels. The regulation of skeletal muscle glycogen degradation therefore must respond very rapidly to the need for ATP, indicated by the increase in AMP.

The regulation of skeletal muscle glycogen synthesis and degradation differs from that in liver in several important respects: (*a*) glucagon has no effect on muscle, and thus glycogen levels in muscle do not vary with the fasting/feeding state; (*b*) AMP is an allosteric activator of the muscle isozyme of glycogen phosphorylase, but not liver glycogen phosphorylase (Fig. 28.10); (*c*) the effects of Ca^{2+} in muscle result principally from the release of Ca^{2+} from the sarcoplasmic reticulum after neural stimulation, and not from epinephrine-stimulated uptake; (*d*) glucose is not a physiologic inhibitor of glycogen phosphorylase a in muscle; (*e*) glycogen is a stronger feedback inhibitor of muscle glycogen synthase than of liver glycogen synthase, resulting in a smaller amount of stored glycogen per gram weight of muscle tissue. However, the effects of epinephrine-stimulated phosphorylation by protein kinase A on skeletal muscle glycogen degradation and glycogen synthesis are similar to those occurring in liver (see Fig. 28.8).

Muscle glycogen phosphorylase is a genetically distinct isoenzyme of liver glycogen phosphorylase and contains an amino acid sequence that has a purine nucleotide

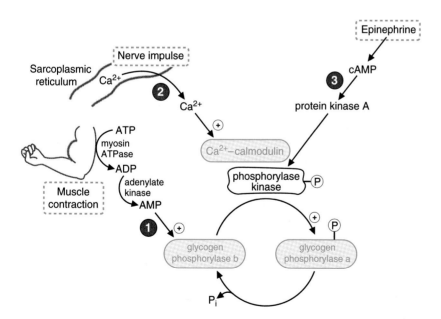

Fig. 28.10. Activation of muscle glycogen phosphorylase during exercise. Glycogenolysis in skeletal muscle is initiated by muscle contraction, neural impulses, and epinephrine. 1. AMP produced from the degradation of ATP during muscular contraction allosterically activates glycogen phosphorylase b. 2. The neural impulses that initiate contraction release Ca^{2+} from the sarcoplasmic reticulum. The Ca^{2+} binds to calmodulin, which is a modifier protein that activates phosphorylase kinase. 3. Phosphorylase kinase is also activated through phosphorylation by protein kinase A. The formation of cAMP and the resultant activation of protein kinase A are initiated by the binding of epinephrine to plasma membrane receptors.

binding site. When AMP binds to this site, it changes the conformation at the catalytic site to a structure very similar to that in the phosphorylated enzyme (see Fig. 9.9). Thus, hydrolysis of ATP to ADP and the consequent increase of AMP generated by adenylate kinase during muscular contraction can directly stimulate glycogenolysis to provide fuel for the glycolytic pathway. AMP also stimulates glycolysis by activating phosphofructokinase-1, so this one effector activates both glycogenolysis and glycolysis. The activation of the calcium/calmodulin subunit of phosphorylase kinase by the Ca^{2+} released from the sarcoplasmic reticulum during muscle contraction also provides a direct and rapid means of stimulating glycogen degradation.

CLINICAL COMMENTS

Getta Carbo's hypoglycemia illustrates the importance of glycogen stores in the neonate. At birth, the fetus must make two major adjustments in the way fuels are used: it must adapt to using a greater variety of fuels than were available in utero, and it must adjust to intermittent feeding. In utero, the fetus receives a relatively constant supply of glucose from the maternal circulation through the placenta, producing a level of glucose in the fetus that approximates 75% of maternal blood levels. With regard to the hormonal regulation of fuel utilization in utero, fetal tissues function in an environment dominated by insulin, which promotes growth. During the last 10 weeks of gestation, this hormonal milieu leads to glycogen formation and storage. At birth, the infant's diet changes to one containing greater amounts of fat and lactose (galactose and glucose in equal ratio), presented at intervals rather than in a constant fashion. At the same time, the neonate's need for glucose will be relatively larger than that of the adult because the newborn's ratio of brain to liver weight is greater. Thus, the infant has even greater difficulty in maintaining glucose homeostasis than the adult.

At the moment that the umbilical cord is clamped, the normal neonate is faced with a metabolic problem: the high insulin levels of late fetal existence must be quickly reversed to prevent hypoglycemia. This reversal is accomplished through the secretion of the counterregulatory hormones epinephrine and glucagon. Glucagon release is triggered by the normal decline of blood glucose after birth. The neural response that stimulates the release of both glucagon and epinephrine is activated by the anoxia, cord clamping, and tactile stimulation that are part of a normal delivery. These responses have been referred to as the "normal sensor function" of the neonate.

Within 3 to 4 hours of birth, these counterregulatory hormones reestablish normal serum glucose levels in the newborn's blood through their glycogenolytic and gluconeogenic actions. The failure of Getta's normal "sensor function" was partly the result of maternal malnutrition, which resulted in an inadequate deposition of glycogen in Getta's liver before birth. The consequence was a serious degree of postnatal hypoglycemia.

The ability to maintain glucose homeostasis during the first few days of life also depends on the activation of gluconeogenesis and the mobilization of fatty acids. Fatty acid oxidation in the liver not only promotes gluconeogenesis (see Chapter 31) but generates ketone bodies. The neonatal brain has an enhanced capacity to use ketone bodies relative to that of infants (fourfold) and adults (40-fold). This ability is consistent with the relatively high fat content of breast milk.

Jim Bodie attempted to build up his muscle mass with androgens and with insulin. The anabolic (nitrogen-retaining) effects of androgens on skeletal muscle cells enhance muscle mass by increasing amino acid flux into muscle and by stimulating protein synthesis. Exogenous insulin has the potential to increase muscle mass by similar actions and also by increasing the content of muscle glycogen.

The most serious side effect of exogenous insulin administration is the development of severe hypoglycemia, such as occurred in **Jim Bodie**. The immediate adverse effect relates to an inadequate flow of fuel (glucose) to the metabolizing brain. When hypoglycemia is extreme, the patient may suffer a seizure and, if the hypoglycemia worsens, may lapse into a coma and die. If untreated, irreversible brain damage occurs in those who survive.

BIOCHEMICAL COMMENTS

The regulatory effect of insulin is frequently described as one of activating protein phosphatases. The effects of insulin on the regulation of hepatic and skeletal PP-1 are complex and not yet fully understood.

PP-1 is targeted to glycogen particles by four tissue-specific targeting factors: G_M is found in striated muscle; G_L is found in liver; PTG (protein targeting to glycogen) is found in almost all tissues; and R6 is also found in most tissues. The targeting factors bind to PP-1 and glycogen and localize the PP-1 to the glycogen particles, where the enzyme will be physically close to the regulated enzymes of glycogen metabolism, phosphorylase kinase, glycogen phosphorylase, and glycogen synthase. Regulation of the phosphatase will involve complex interactions between the target enzymes, the targeting subunit, the phosphatase, and protein inhibitor I. The interactions are also tissue specific in the case of G_M and G_L.

A simplistic view of hepatic PP-1 regulation is as follows. PP-1 is bound to G_L and the glycogen particle. Glycogen phosphorylase a binds to the complex, and in so doing alters the conformation of PP-1, rendering it inactive. When glucose levels rise in the blood (for example, after eating a meal), the glucose is transported into the liver cells via GLUT 2 transporters, and the intracellular glucose level increases. Glucose can bind to glycogen phosphorylase a, which relieves the inhibition of PP-1, and glycogen phosphorylase a will be converted to glycogen phosphorylase b by active PP-1. Additionally, as the intracellular glucose is converted to glucose 6-phosphate by glucokinase, the increase in glucose-6-P levels activates PP-1 to dephosphorylate glycogen synthase, thereby activating the glycogen synthesizing enzyme. The complicated view of hepatic PP-1 regulation also must take into account the PTG-PP-1 interactions (PTG is also expressed in the liver) and the kinases that are activated by either insulin or glucagon/epinephrine, which lead to alterations in glycogen metabolizing enzyme activities.

In contrast to hepatic regulation, muscle regulation of PP-1 activity via G_M is directly responsive to phosphorylation by kinases. A phosphorylation event that appears to be critical is that of ser-67 in G_M. Phosphorylation of ser-67 by the cAMP-dependent protein kinase leads to a dissociation of PP-1 from G_M, and, therefore, the phosphatase is removed from its substrates and cannot reverse the phosphorylation of the target enzymes. If ser-67 is altered to a threonine, the phosphorylation at that site is blocked, and PP-1 does not dissociate from G_M. This indicates the importance of the phosphorylation event in regulating PP-1 action in the muscle.

Future work will be needed before a complete understanding of how insulin reverses glucagon/epinephrine stimulation of glycogenolysis is obtained.

Suggested Readings

Chen YT. Glycogen storage diseases. In: Scriver CR, Beaudet AL, Valle D, Sly WS, et al., eds. The Metabolic and Molecular Bases of Inherited Disease, vol I, 8th Ed. New York: McGraw-Hill, 2001:1521–1551.

Parker PH, Ballew M, Greene HL. Nutritional management of glycogen storage disease. Annu Rev Nutr 1993;13:83–109.

Roach, P. Glycogen and its metabolism. Current Mol Med 2002;2:101–120.

Skurat AV, Roach PJ. Regulation of glycogen synthesis. In: LeRoith D, Taylor SI, Olefsky JM, eds. Diabetes Mellitus: A Fundamental and Clinical Text, 2nd Ed. New York: Lippincott, Williams & Wilkins, 2000:251–264.

 REVIEW QUESTIONS—CHAPTER 28

1. The degradation of glycogen normally produces which of the following?

   (A) More glucose than glucose 1-phosphate
   (B) More glucose 1-phosphate than glucose
   (C) Equal amounts of glucose and glucose 1-phosphate
   (D) Neither glucose or glucose 1-phosphate
   (E) Only glucose 1-phosphate

2. A patient has large deposits of liver glycogen, which, after an overnight fast, had shorter than normal branches. This abnormality could be caused by a defective form of which of the following proteins or activities?

   (A) Glycogen phosphorylase
   (B) Glucagon receptor
   (C) Glycogenin
   (D) Amylo 1,6 glucosidase
   (E) Amylo 4,6 transferase

3. An adolescent patient with a deficiency of muscle phosphorylase was examined while exercising her forearm by squeezing a rubber ball. Compared with a normal person performing the same exercise, this patient would exhibit which of the following?

   (A) Exercise for a longer time without fatigue
   (B) Have increased glucose levels in blood drawn from her forearm
   (C) Have decreased lactate levels in blood drawn from her forearm
   (D) Have lower levels of glycogen in biopsy specimens from her forearm muscle
   (E) Hyperglycemia

4. In a glucose tolerance test, an individual in the basal metabolic state ingests a large amount of glucose. If the individual is normal, this ingestion should result in which of the following?

   (A) An enhanced glycogen synthase activity in the liver
   (B) An increased ratio of glycogen phosphorylase a to glycogen phosphorylase b in the liver
   (C) An increased rate of lactate formation by red blood cells
   (D) An inhibition of protein phosphatase I activity in the liver
   (E) An increase of cAMP levels in the liver

5. Consider a type 1 diabetic who has neglected to take insulin for the past 72 hours and has not eaten much as well. Which of the following best describes the activity level of hepatic enzymes involved in glycogen metabolism under these conditions?

	Glycogen Synthase	Phosphorylase Kinase	Glycogen Phosphorylase
(A)	Active	Active	Active
(B)	Active	Active	Inactive
(C)	Active	Inactive	Inactive
(D)	Inactive	Inactive	Inactive
(E)	Inactive	Active	Inactive
(F)	Inactive	Active	Active

29 Pathways of Sugar Metabolism: Pentose Phosphate Pathway, Fructose, and Galactose Metabolism

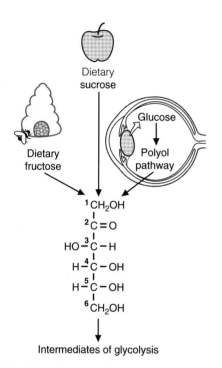

Fig. 29.1. Fructose. The sugar fructose is found in the diet as the free sugar in foods such as honey or as a component of the disaccharide sucrose in fruits and sweets. It also can be synthesized from glucose via the polyol pathway. In the lens of the eye, the polyol pathway contributes to the formation of cataracts. Fructose is metabolized by conversion to intermediates of glycolysis.

Enzymes can generally use either NADPH or NADH, but not both. Reactions requiring the input of electrons as hydride ions are usually catalyzed by enzymes specific for NADPH.

Glucose is at the center of carbohydrate metabolism and is the major dietary sugar. Other sugars in the diet are converted to intermediates of glucose metabolism, and their fates parallel that of glucose. When carbohydrates other than glucose are required for the synthesis of diverse compounds such as lactose, glycoproteins, or glycolipids, they are synthesized from glucose.

*Fructose, the second most common sugar in the adult diet, is ingested principally as the monosaccharide or as part of **sucrose** (Fig. 29.1). It is metabolized principally in the liver (and to a lesser extent in the small intestine and kidney) by phosphorylation at the 1-position to form **fructose 1-P**, followed by conversion to intermediates of the glycolytic pathway. The major products of its metabolism in liver are, therefore, the same as glucose (including lactate, blood glucose, and glycogen). **Essential fructosuria (fructokinase deficiency)** and **hereditary fructose intolerance** (a deficiency of the fructose 1-phosphate cleavage by **aldolase B**) are inherited disorders of fructose metabolism.*

*Fructose synthesis from glucose in the **polyol pathway** occurs in seminal vesicles and other tissues. **Aldose reductase** converts glucose to the sugar alcohol sorbitol (a polyol), which is then oxidized to fructose. In the lens of the eye, elevated levels of **sorbitol** in diabetes mellitus may contribute to **cataract** formation.*

*Galactose is ingested principally as **lactose,** which is converted to galactose and glucose in the intestine. **Galactose** is converted to glucose principally in the liver. It is phosphorylated to galactose 1-phosphate by **galactokinase** and activated to a UDP-sugar by **galactosyl uridylyltransferase**. The metabolic pathway subsequently generates glucose 1-phosphate. **Classical galactosemia**, a deficiency of galactosyl uridylyltransferase, results in the accumulation of galactose 1-phosphate in the liver and the inhibition of hepatic glycogen metabolism and other pathways that require UDP sugars. Cataracts can occur from accumulation of galactose in the blood, which is converted to **galactitol** (the sugar alcohol of galactose) in the lens of the eye.*

*The **pentose phosphate pathway** consists of both **oxidative** and **nonoxidative** components (Fig. 29.2). In the oxidative pathway, glucose 6-phosphate is oxidized to **ribulose 5-phosphate**, CO_2, and **NADPH**. Ribulose 5-phosphate, a pentose, can be converted to **ribose 5-phosphate** for nucleotide biosynthesis. The NADPH is used for reductive pathways, such as **fatty acid biosynthesis**, **detoxification** of drugs by monooxygenases, and the **glutathione defense system** against injury by reactive oxygen species (ROS).*

In the nonoxidative phase of the pathway, ribulose 5-phosphate is converted to ribose 5-phosphate and to intermediates of the glycolytic pathway. This portion of

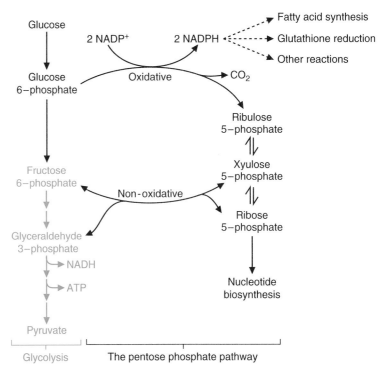

Fig. 29.2. Overview of the pentose phosphate pathway. The pentose phosphate pathway generates NADPH for reactions requiring reducing equivalents (electrons) or ribose 5-phosphate for nucleotide biosynthesis. Glucose 6-phosphate is a substrate for both the pentose phosphate pathway and glycolysis. The 5-carbon sugar intermediates of the pentose phosphate pathway are reversibly interconverted to intermediates of glycolysis. The portion of glycolysis that is not part of the pentose phosphate pathway is shown in blue.

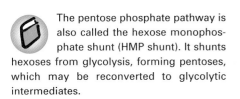

The pentose phosphate pathway is also called the hexose monophosphate shunt (HMP shunt). It shunts hexoses from glycolysis, forming pentoses, which may be reconverted to glycolytic intermediates.

the pathway is reversible; therefore, ribose 5-phosphate can also be formed from intermediates of glycolysis. One of the enzymes involved in these sugar interconversions, **transketolase,** *uses* **thiamine pyrophosphate** *as a coenzyme.*

The sugars produced by the pentose phosphate pathway enter glycolysis as fructose 6-phosphate and glyceraldehyde 3-phosphate, and their further metabolism in the glycolytic pathway generates NADH, adenosine triphsphate (ATP), and pyruvate. The overall equation for the conversion of glucose 6-phosphate to fructose 6-phosphate and glyceraldehyde 3-phosphate through both the oxidative and nonoxidative reactions of the pentose phosphate pathway is:

$$3 \text{ glucose-6-P} + 6 \text{ NADP}^+ \rightarrow 3 \text{ } CO_2 + 6 \text{ NADPH} + 6 \text{ } H^+ + 2 \text{ fructose-6-P} + \text{glyceraldehyde-3-P.}$$

THE WAITING ROOM

Candice Sucher is an 18-year-old girl who presented to her physician for a precollege physical examination. While taking her medical history, the doctor learned that she carefully avoided eating all fruits and any foods that contained table sugar. She related that, from a very early age, she had learned that these foods caused severe weakness and symptoms suggestive of low blood sugar, such as tremulousness and sweating. Her medical history also indicated that her mother had described her as having been a very irritable baby who often cried incessantly, especially after meals, and vomited frequently. At these times, Candice's abdomen had become distended, and she became drowsy and apathetic. Her mother had intuitively eliminated certain foods from Candice's diet, after which the severity and frequency of these symptoms diminished.

Erin Galway is a 3-week-old female infant who began vomiting 3 days after birth, usually within 30 minutes after breastfeeding. Her abdomen became distended at these times, and she became irritable and cried frequently. When her mother noted that the whites of Erin's eyes were yellow, she took her to a pediatrician. The doctor agreed that Erin was slightly jaundiced. He also noted an enlargement of her liver and questioned the possibility of early cataract formation in the lenses of Erin's eyes. He ordered liver and kidney function tests and did two separate dipstick urine tests in his office, one designed to measure only glucose in the urine and the other capable of detecting any of the reducing sugars.

Al Martini developed a fever of 101.5°F on the second day of his hospitalization for acute alcoholism. He had a cough productive of gray sputum. A chest x-ray showed right lower lobe pneumonia. A stain of his sputum showed many small pleomorphic Gram-negative bacilli. Sputum was sent for culture and a determination of which antibiotics would be effective in treating the causative organism (sensitivity testing). Because his landlady stated that he had an allergy to penicillin, he was started on a course of the antibiotic combination of trimethoprim and sulfamethoxazole (TMP/sulfa). To his landlady's knowledge, he had never been treated with a sulfa drug previously.

On the third day of therapy with TMP/sulfa for his pneumonia, **Al Martini** was slightly jaundiced. His hemoglobin level had fallen by 3.5 g/dL from the value on admission, and his urine was red-brown because of the presence of free hemoglobin. Mr. Martini had apparently suffered acute hemolysis (lysis or destruction of some of his red blood cells) induced by his infection and exposure to the sulfa drug.

I. FRUCTOSE

Fructose is found in the diet as a component of sucrose in fruit, as a free sugar in honey, and in high-fructose corn syrup (see Fig. 29.1). Fructose enters epithelial cells and other types of cells by facilitated diffusion on the GLUT V transporter. It is metabolized to intermediates of glycolysis. Problems with fructose absorption and metabolism are relatively more common than with other sugars.

A. Fructose Metabolism

Fructose is metabolized by conversion to glyceraldehyde-3-P and dihydroxyacetone phosphate, which are intermediates of glycolysis (Fig. 29.3). The steps parallel those of glycolysis. The first step in the metabolism of fructose, as with glucose, is phosphorylation. Fructokinase, the major kinase involved, phosphorylates fructose in the 1-position. Fructokinase has a high V_{max}, and rapidly phosphorylates fructose as it enters the cell. The fructose 1-phosphate formed is not an intermediate of glycolysis but rather is cleaved by aldolase B to dihydroxyacetone phosphate (an intermediate of glycolysis) and glyceraldehyde. Glyceraldehyde is then phosphorylated to glyceraldehyde-3-P by triose kinase. Dihydroxyacetone phosphate and glyceraldehyde 3-phosphate are intermediates of the glycolytic pathway and can proceed through it to pyruvate, the TCA cycle, and fatty acid synthesis. Alternately, these intermediates can also be converted to glucose by gluconeogenesis. In other words, the fate of fructose parallels that of glucose.

When individuals with defects of aldolase B ingest fructose, the extremely high levels of fructose 1-phosphate that accumulate in the liver and kidney cause a number of adverse effects. Hypoglycemia results from inhibition of glycogenolysis and gluconeogenesis. Glycogen phosphorylase (and possibly phosphoglucomutase and other enzymes of glycogen metabolism) are inhibited by the accumulated fructose 1-phosphate. Aldolase B is required for glucose synthesis from glyceraldehyde 3-phosphate and dihydroxyacetone phosphate, and its low activity in aldolase B–deficient individuals is further decreased by the accumulated fructose 1-phosphate. The inhibition of gluconeogenesis results in lactic acidosis.

The accumulation of fructose 1-phosphate also substantially depletes the phosphate pools. The fructokinase reaction uses ATP at a rapid rate such that the mitochondria regenerate ATP rapidly, which leads to a drop in free phosphate levels. The low levels of phosphate release inhibition of AMP deaminase, which converts AMP to inosine monophosphate (IMP). The nitrogenous base of IMP (hypoxanthine) is degraded to uric acid. The lack of phosphate and depletion of adenine nucleotides lead to a loss of ATP, further contributing to the inhibition of biosynthetic pathways, including gluconeogenesis.

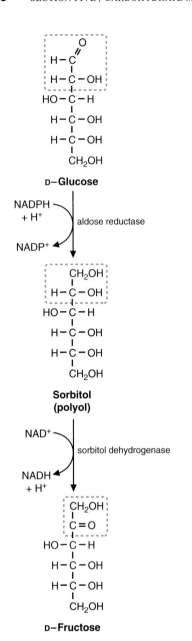

Fig. 29.4. The polyol pathway converts glucose to fructose.

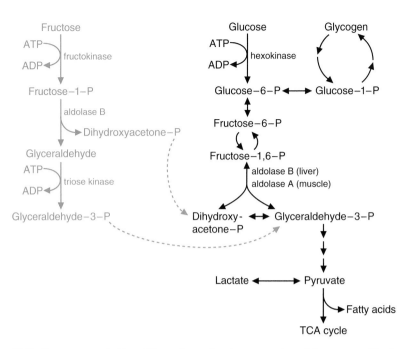

Fig. 29.3. Fructose metabolism. The pathway for the conversion of fructose to dihydroxy-acetone phosphate and glyceraldehyde 3-phosphate is shown in blue. These two compounds are intermediates of glycolysis and are converted in the liver principally to glucose, glycogen, or fatty acids. In the liver, aldolase B cleaves both fructose 1-phosphate in the pathway for fructose metabolism, and fructose 1,6-bisphosphate in the pathway for glycolysis.

The metabolism of fructose occurs principally in the liver and to a lesser extent in the small intestinal mucosa and proximal epithelium of the renal tubule, because these tissues have both fructokinase and aldolase B. Aldolase exists as several isoforms: aldolases A, B, C, and fetal aldolase. Although all of these aldolase isoforms can cleave fructose 1,6-bisphosphate, the intermediate of glycolysis, only aldolase B can also cleave fructose 1-phosphate. Aldolase A, present in muscle and most other tissues, and aldolase C, present in brain, have almost no ability to cleave fructose 1-phosphate. Fetal aldolase, present in the liver before birth, is similar to aldolase C.

Aldolase B is the rate-limiting enzyme of fructose metabolism, although it is not a rate-limiting enzyme of glycolysis. It has a much lower affinity for fructose 1-phosphate than fructose 1,6-bisphosphate (although the k_{cat} is the same) and is very slow at physiologic levels of fructose 1-phosphate. As a consequence, after ingesting a high dose of fructose, normal individuals accumulate fructose 1-phosphate in the liver while it is slowly converted to glycolytic intermediates. Individuals with hereditary fructose intolerance (a deficiency of aldolase B) accumulate much higher amounts of fructose 1-phosphate in their livers.

Other tissues also have the capacity to metabolize fructose but do so much more slowly. The hexokinase isoforms present in muscle, adipose tissue, and other tissues can convert fructose to fructose 6-phosphate, but react so much more efficiently with glucose. As a result, fructose phosphorylation is very slow in the presence of physiologic levels of intracellular glucose and glucose 6-phosphate.

Q: Essential fructosuria is a rare and benign genetic disorder caused by a deficiency of the enzyme fructokinase. Why is this disease benign, when a deficiency of aldolase B (hereditary fructose intolerance) can be fatal? Could **Candice Sucher** have essential fructosuria?

B. Synthesis of Fructose in the Polyol Pathway

Fructose can be synthesized from glucose in the polyol pathway. The polyol pathway is named for the first step of the pathway in which sugars are reduced to the sugar alcohol by the enzyme aldose reductase (Fig. 29.4) Glucose is reduced to the sugar alcohol sorbitol, and sorbitol is then oxidized to fructose.

This pathway is present in seminal vesicles, which synthesize fructose for the seminal fluid. Spermatozoa use fructose as a major fuel source while in the seminal fluid and then switch to glucose once in the female reproductive tract. Utilization of fructose is thought to prevent acrosomal breakdown of the plasma membrane (and consequent activation) while the spermatozoa are still in the seminal fluid.

The polyol pathway is present in many tissues, but its function in all tissues is not understood. Aldose reductase is relatively nonspecific, and its major function may be the metabolism of an aldehyde sugar other than glucose. The activity of this enzyme can lead to major problems in the lens of the eye, where it is responsible for the production of sorbitol from glucose and galactitol from galactose. When the concentration of glucose or galactose is elevated in the blood, their respective sugar alcohols are synthesized in the lens more rapidly than they are removed, resulting in increased osmotic pressure within the lens.

II. GALACTOSE METABOLISM—METABOLISM TO GLUCOSE-1-P

Dietary galactose is metabolized principally by phosphorylation to galactose 1-phosphate, and then conversion to UDP-galactose and glucose 1-phosphate (Fig. 29.5). The phosphorylation of galactose, again an important first step in the pathway, is carried out by a specific kinase, galactokinase. The formation of UDP-galactose is accomplished by attack of the phosphate oxygen on galactose 1-phosphate on the α phosphate of UDP-glucose, releasing glucose 1-phosphate while forming UDP-galactose. The enzyme that catalyzes this reaction is galactose 1-phosphate uridylyltransferase. The UDP-galactose is then converted to UDP-glucose by the reversible UDP-glucose epimerase (the configuration of the hydroxyl group on carbon four is reversed in this reaction). The net result of this sequence of reactions is that galactose is converted to glucose 1-phosphate, at the expense of 1 high-energy bond of ATP. The sum of these reactions is indicated in the equations that follow:

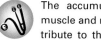

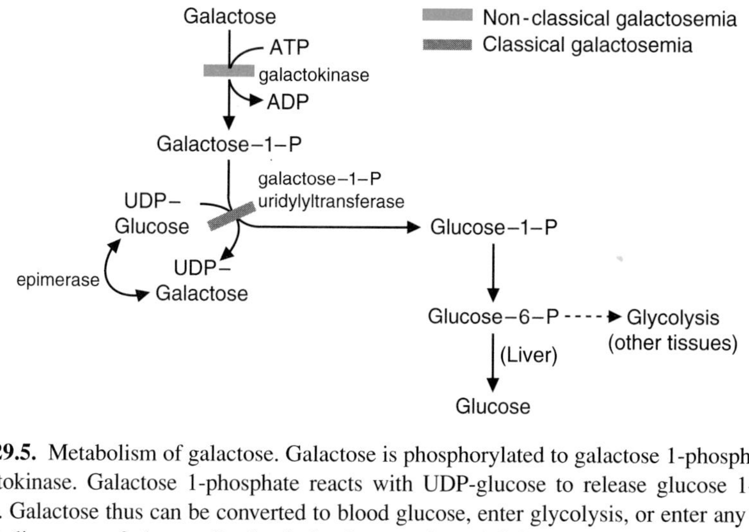

The accumulation of sorbitol in muscle and nerve tissues may contribute to the peripheral neuropathy characteristic of patients with poorly controlled diabetes mellitus. This is one of the reasons it is so important for **Di Abietes** (who has type 1 diabetes mellitus) and **Ann Sulin** (who has type 2 diabetes mellitus) to achieve good glycemic control.

The accumulation of sugars and sugar alcohols in the lens of patients with hyperglycemia (e.g., diabetes mellitus) results in the formation of cataracts. Glucose levels are elevated and increase the synthesis of sorbitol and fructose. As a consequence, a high osmotic pressure is created in the lens. The high glucose and fructose levels also result in nonenzymatic glycosylation of lens proteins. The result of the increased osmotic pressure and the glycosylation of the lens protein is an opaque cloudiness of the lens known as a cataract. **Erin Galway** seemed to have an early cataract, probably caused by the accumulation of galactose and its sugar alcohol galactitol.

Fig. 29.5. Metabolism of galactose. Galactose is phosphorylated to galactose 1-phosphate by galactokinase. Galactose 1-phosphate reacts with UDP-glucose to release glucose 1-phosphate. Galactose thus can be converted to blood glucose, enter glycolysis, or enter any of the metabolic routes of glucose. In classical galactosemia, a deficiency of galactose 1-phosphate uridylyltransferase (shown in grey) results in the accumulation of galactose 1-phosphate in tissues and the appearance of galactose in the blood and urine. In nonclassical galactosemia, a deficiency of galactokinase results in the accumulation of galactose.

In essential fructosuria, fructose cannot be converted to fructose 1-phosphate. This condition is benign because no toxic metabolites of fructose accumulate in the liver, and the patient remains nearly asymptomatic. Some of the ingested fructose is slowly phosphorylated by hexokinase in nonhepatic tissues and metabolized by glycolysis, and some appears in the urine. There is no renal threshold for fructose; the appearance of fructose in the urine (fructosuria) does not require a high fructose concentration in the blood.

Hereditary fructose intolerance, conversely, results in the accumulation of fructose 1-phosphate and fructose. By inhibiting glycogenolysis and gluconeogenesis, the high levels of fructose 1-phosphate caused the hypoglycemia that **Candice Sucher** experienced as an infant when she became apathetic and drowsy, and as an adult when she experienced sweating and tremulousness.

Erin Galway's urine was negative for glucose when measured with the glucose oxidase strip but was positive for the presence of a reducing sugar. The reducing sugar was identified as galactose. Her liver function tests showed an increase in serum bilirubin and in several liver enzymes. Albumin was present in her urine. These findings and the clinical history increased her physician's suspicion that Erin had classical galactosemia.

Classical galactosemia is caused by a deficiency of galactose 1-phosphate uridylyltransferase. In this disease, galactose 1-phosphate accumulates in tissues, and galactose is elevated in the blood and urine. This condition differs from the rarer deficiency of galactokinase (nonclassical galactosemia), in which galactosemia and galactosuria occur but galactose 1-phosphate is not formed. Both enzyme defects result in cataracts from galactitol formation by aldose reductase in the polyol pathway. Aldose reductase has a relatively high K_m for galactose, approximately 12 to 20 mM, so that galactitol is formed only in galactosemic patients who have eaten galactose. Galactitol is not further metabolized and diffuses out of the lens very slowly. Thus, hypergalactosemia is even more likely to cause cataracts than hyperglycemia. **Erin Galway**, although only 3 weeks old, appeared to have early cataracts forming in the lens of her eyes.

One of the most serious problems of classical galactosemia is an irreversible mental retardation. Realizing this problem, **Erin Galway's** physician wanted to begin immediate dietary therapy. A test that measures galactose 1-phosphate uridylyltransferase in erythrocytes was ordered. The enzyme activity was virtually absent, confirming the diagnosis of classical galactosemia.

(1) Galactose + ATP $\xrightarrow{\text{galactokinase}}$ Galactose-1-P + ADP

(2) Galactose-1-P + UDP-glucose $\xrightarrow[\text{uridylyltransferase}]{\text{galactose-1-P}}$ UDP-galactose + glucose-1-P

(3) UDP-galactose $\xrightarrow{\text{UDP-glucose epimerase}}$ UDP-glucose

Net Equation: Galactose + ATP $\longrightarrow$ Glucose-1-P + ADP

The enzymes for galactose conversion to glucose 1-phosphate are present in many tissues, including the adult erythrocyte, fibroblasts, and fetal tissues. The liver has a high activity of these enzymes, and can convert dietary galactose to blood glucose and glycogen. The fate of dietary galactose, like that of fructose, therefore, parallels that of glucose. The ability to metabolize galactose is even higher in infants than in adults. Newborn infants ingest up to 1 g galactose per kg per feeding (as lactose). Yet the rate of metabolism is so high that the blood level in the systemic circulation is less than 3 mg/dL, and none of the galactose is lost in the urine.

III. THE PENTOSE PHOSPHATE PATHWAY

The pentose phosphate pathway is essentially a scenic bypass route around the first stage of glycolysis that generates NADPH and ribose-5-P (as well as other pentose sugars). Glucose 6-phosphate is the common precursor for both pathways. The oxidative first stage of the pentose phosphate pathway generates two moles of NADPH per glucose 6-phosphate oxidized. The second stage of the pentose phosphate pathway generates ribose-5-P and converts unused intermediates to fructose-6-P and glyceraldehyde-3-P in the glycolytic pathway (see Fig. 29.2). All cells require NADPH for reductive detoxification, and most cells require ribose-5-P for nucleotide synthesis. Consequently, the pathway is present in all cells. The enzymes reside in the cytosol, as do the enzymes of glycolysis.

A. Oxidative Phase of the Pentose Phosphate Pathway

1. NADPH PRODUCTION

In the oxidative first phase of the pentose phosphate pathway, glucose 6-phosphate is oxidatively decarboxylated to a pentose sugar, ribulose 5-phosphate (Fig. 29.6). The first enzyme of this pathway, glucose 6-phosphate dehydrogenase, oxidizes the aldehyde at C1 and reduces NADP$^+$ to NADPH. The gluconolactone that is formed is rapidly hydrolyzed to 6-phosphogluconate, a sugar acid with a carboxylic acid group at C1. The next oxidation step releases this carboxyl group as CO_2, with the electrons being transferred to NADP$^+$. This reaction is mechanistically very similar to the one catalyzed by isocitrate dehydrogenase in the TCA cycle. Thus, two moles of NADPH per mole of glucose 6-phosphate are formed from this portion of the pathway.

NADPH, rather than NADH, is generally used in the cell for pathways that require the input of electrons for reductive reactions because the ratio of NADPH/NADP$^+$ is much greater than the NADH/NAD$^+$ ratio. The NADH generated from fuel oxidation is rapidly oxidized back to NAD$^+$ by NADH dehydrogenase in the electron transport chain, so the level of NADH is very low in the cell.

NADPH can be generated from a number of reactions in the liver and other tissues, but not the red blood cell. For example, in tissues with mitochondria, an energy-requiring transhydrogenase located near the complexes of the electron transport chain can transfer reducing equivalents from NADH to NADP$^+$ to generate NADPH.

NADPH, however, cannot be directly oxidized by the electron transport chain, and the ratio of NADPH to NADP$^+$ in cells is greater than one. The reduction potential of NADPH therefore can contribute to the energy needed for biosynthetic processes and provide a constant source of reducing power for detoxification reactions.

2. RIBOSE 5-PHOSPHATE FROM THE OXIDATIVE ARM OF THE PATHWAY

To generate ribose 5-phosphate from the oxidative pathway, the ribulose 5-phosphate formed from the action of the two oxidative steps is isomerized to produce ribose 5-phosphate (a ketose-to-aldose conversion, similar to fructose 6-phosphate being isomerized to glucose 6-phosphate; see section III.B.1 below). The ribose 5-phosphate can then enter the pathway for nucleotide synthesis, if needed, or can be converted to glycolytic intermediates, as described below for the nonoxidative phase of the pentose phosphate pathway. The pathway through which the ribose 5-phosphate travels is determined by the needs of the cell at the time of its synthesis.

B. The Nonoxidative Phase of the Pentose Phosphate Pathway

The nonoxidative reactions of this pathway are reversible reactions that allow intermediates of glycolysis (specifically glyceraldehyde-3-P and fructose-6-P) to be converted to five-carbon sugars (such as ribose-5-P), and vice versa. The needs of the cell will determine in which direction this pathway proceeds. If the cell has produced ribose-5-P, but does not need to synthesize nucleotides, then the ribose-5-P will be converted to glycolytic intermediates. If the cell still requires NADPH, the ribose-5-P will be converted back into glucose-6-P using nonoxidative reactions (see below). And finally, if the cell already has a high level of NADPH, but needs to produce nucleotides, the oxidative reactions of the pentose phosphate pathway will be inhibited, and the glycolytic intermediates fructose-6-P and glyceraldehyde-3-P will be used to produce the five carbon sugars using exclusively the nonoxidative phase of the pentose phosphate pathway.

1. THE CONVERSION OF RIBOSE 5-PHOSPHATE TO GLYCOLYTIC INTERMEDIATES

The nonoxidative portion of the pentose phosphate pathway consists of a series of rearrangement and transfer reactions that first convert ribulose 5-phosphate to ribose 5-phosphate and xylulose 5-phosphate, and then the ribose 5-phosphate and xyulose 5-phosphate are converted to intermediates of the glycolytic pathway. The enzymes involved are an epimerase, an isomerase, transketolase, and transaldolase.

The epimerase and isomerase convert ribulose 5-phosphate to two other 5-carbon sugars (Fig. 29.7). The isomerase converts ribulose 5-phosphate to ribose 5-phosphate. The epimerase changes the stereochemical position of one hydroxyl group (at carbon 3), converting ribulose 5-phosphate to xylulose 5-phosphate.

Transketolase transfers 2-carbon fragments of keto sugars (sugars with a keto group at C2) to other sugars. Transketolase picks up a 2-carbon fragment from xylulose 5-phosphate by cleaving the carbon–carbon bond between the keto group and the adjacent carbon, thereby releasing glyceraldehyde 3-phosphate (Fig. 29.8). The 2-carbon fragment is covalently bound to thiamine pyrophosphate, which transfers

Xyulose 5-phosphate has recently been identified as an activator of protein phosphatase 2A (PP2A). PP2A removes phosphates from PFK-2 and from a transcription factor that binds to carbohydrate response elements in promoters of genes such as pyruvate kinase. The hydrolysis of the phosphates activates both proteins, such that xyulose 5-phosphate can regulate pathways relating to both carbohydrate and fat metabolism.

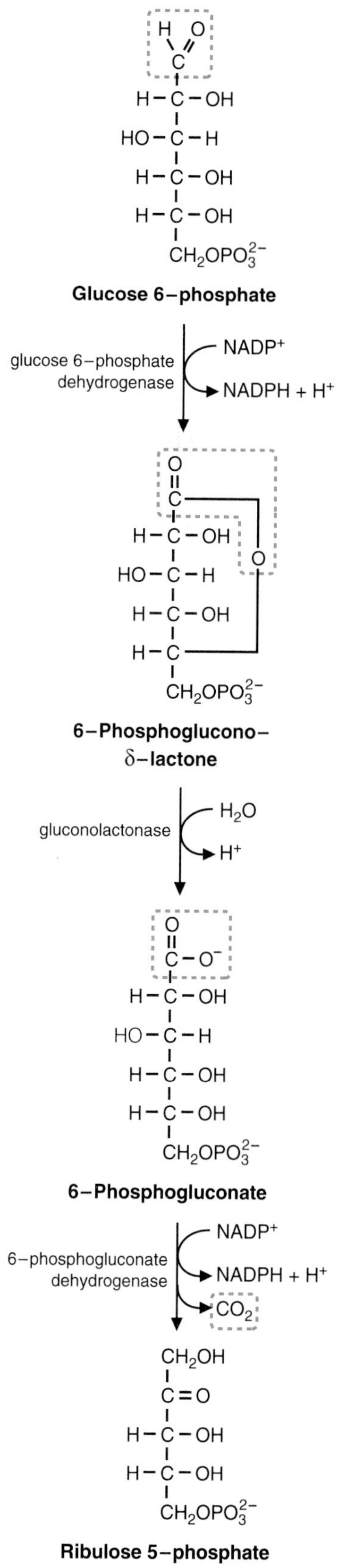

Glucose 6–phosphate

glucose 6–phosphate dehydrogenase — NADP⁺ ↘ NADPH + H⁺

6–Phosphoglucono- δ–lactone

gluconolactonase — H₂O ↘ H⁺

6–Phosphogluconate

6–phosphogluconate dehydrogenase — NADP⁺ ↘ NADPH + H⁺ ↘ CO₂

Ribulose 5–phosphate

Fig. 29.6. Oxidative portion of the pentose phosphate pathway. Carbon 1 of glucose 6-phosphate is oxidized to an acid and then released as CO_2 in an oxidative decarboxylation reaction. Each oxidation step generates an NADPH.

Doctors suspected that the underlying factor in the destruction of **Al Martini's** red blood cells was an X-linked defect in the gene that codes for glucose 6-phosphate dehydrogenase. The red blood cell is dependent on this enzyme for a source of NADPH to maintain reduced levels of glutathione, one of its major defenses against oxidative stress (see Chapter 24). Glucose 6-phosphate dehydrogenase deficiency is the most common known enzymopathy, and affects approximately 7% of the world's population and about 2% of the U.S. population. Most glucose 6-phosphate dehydrogenase–deficient individuals are asymptomatic but can undergo an episode of hemolytic anemia if exposed to certain drugs, to certain types of infections, or if they ingest fava beans. When questioned, Al Martini replied that he did not know what a fava bean was and had no idea whether he was sensitive to them.

it to the aldehyde carbon of another sugar, forming a new ketose. The role of thiamine-pyrophosphate here is thus very similar to its role in the oxidative decarboxylation of pyruvate and α-ketoglutarate (see Chapter 20, section I.B). Two reactions in the pentose phosphate pathway use transketolase; in the first, the 2-carbon keto fragment from xylulose 5-phosphate is transferred to ribose 5-phosphate to form sedoheptulose 7-phosphate, and in the other, a 2-carbon keto fragment (usually derived from xylulose 5-phosphate) is transferred to erythrose 4-phosphate to form fructose 6-phosphate.

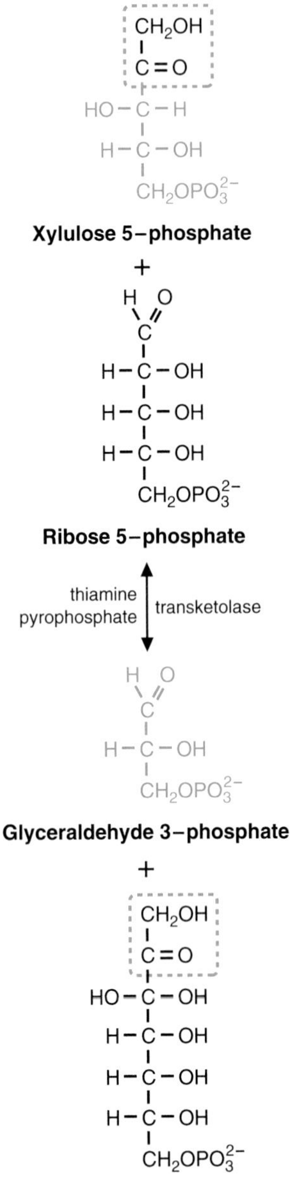

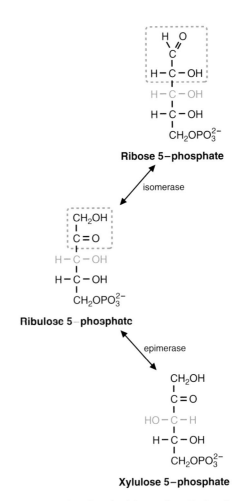

Fig. 29.7. Ribulose 5-phosphate is epimerized (to xyulose 5-phosphate) and isomerized (to ribose 5-phosphate).

Fig. 29.8. Two-carbon unit transferred by transketolase. Transketolase cleaves the bond next to the keto group and transfers the 2-carbon keto fragment to an aldehyde. Thiamine pyrophosphate carries the 2-carbon fragment, forming a covalent bond with the carbon of the keto group.

Transaldolase transfers a 3-carbon keto fragment from sedoheptulose 7-phosphate to glyceraldehyde 3-phosphate to form erythrose 4-phosphate and fructose 6-phosphate (Fig. 29.9). The aldol cleavage occurs between the two hydroxyl carbons adjacent to the keto group (on carbons 3 and 4 of the sugar). This reaction is similar to the aldolase reaction in glycolysis, and the enzyme uses an active amino group, from the side chain of lysine, to catalyze the reaction.

The net result of the metabolism of 3 moles of ribulose 5-phosphate in the pentose phosphate pathway is the formation of 2 moles of fructose 6-phosphate and 1 mole of glyceraldehyde 3-phosphate, which then continue through the glycolytic pathway with the production of NADH, ATP, and pyruvate. Because the pentose phosphate pathway begins with glucose 6-phosphate, and feeds back into the

 The transketolase activity of red blood cells is used to measure thiamine nutritional status and diagnose the presence of thiamine deficiency. The activity of transketolase is measured in the presence and absence of added thiamine pyrophosphate. If the thiamine intake of a patient is adequate, the addition of thiamine pyrophosphate does not increase the activity of transketolase because it already contains bound thiamine pyrophosphate. If the patient is thiamine deficient, transketolase activity will be low, and adding thiamine pyrophosphate will greatly stimulate the reaction. **Al Martini** was diagnosed in Chapter 19 as having beriberi heart disease resulting from thiamine deficiency. The diagnosis was based on laboratory tests confirming the thiamine deficiency.

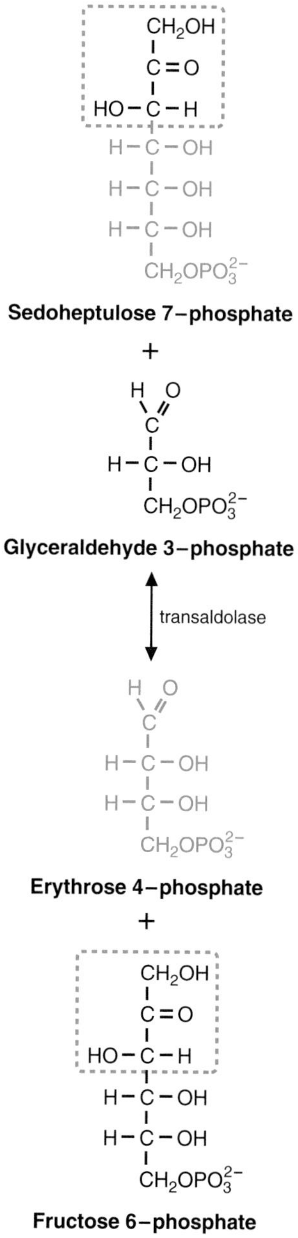

$$CH_2OH$$
$$|$$
$$C=O$$
$$|$$
$$HO-C-H$$
$$|$$
$$H-C-OH$$
$$|$$
$$H-C-OH$$
$$|$$
$$H-C-OH$$
$$|$$
$$CH_2OPO_3^{2-}$$

Sedoheptulose 7–phosphate

+

$$\begin{array}{c} H \quad O \\ \backslash \quad \! / \! / \\ C \\ | \\ H-C-OH \\ | \\ CH_2OPO_3^{2-} \end{array}$$

Glyceraldehyde 3–phosphate

↕ transaldolase

$$\begin{array}{c} H \quad O \\ \backslash \quad \! / \! / \\ C \\ | \\ H-C-OH \\ | \\ H-C-OH \\ | \\ CH_2OPO_3^{2-} \end{array}$$

Erythrose 4–phosphate

+

$$CH_2OH$$
$$|$$
$$C=O$$
$$|$$
$$HO-C-H$$
$$|$$
$$H-C-OH$$
$$|$$
$$H-C-OH$$
$$|$$
$$CH_2OPO_3^{2-}$$

Fructose 6–phosphate

Fig. 29.9. Transaldolase transfers a 3-carbon fragment that contains an alcohol group next to a keto group.

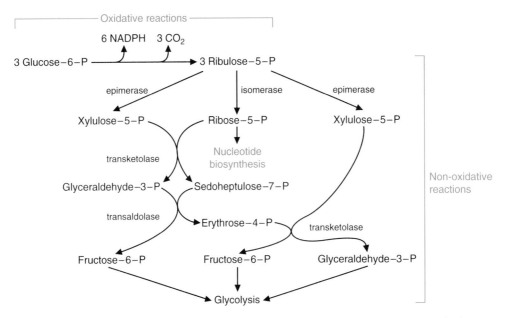

Fig. 29.10. A balanced sequence of reactions in the pentose phosphate pathway. The interconversion of sugars in the pentose phosphate pathway results in conversion of 3 glucose 6-phosphate to 6 NADPH, 3 CO_2, 2 fructose 6-phosphate, and one glyceraldehyde 3-phosphate.

glycolytic pathway, it is sometimes called the hexose monophosphate shunt (a shunt or a pathway for glucose 6-phosphate). The reaction sequence starting from glucose-6-P, and involving both the oxidative and nonoxidative phases of the pathway, is shown in Figure 29.10.

2. GENERATION OF RIBOSE 5-PHOSPHATE FROM INTERMEDIATES OF GLYCOLYSIS

The reactions catalyzed by the epimerase, isomerase, transketolase, and transaldolase are all reversible reactions under physiologic conditions. Thus, ribose 5-phosphate required for purine and pyrimidine synthesis can be generated from intermediates of the glycolytic pathway, as well as from the oxidative phase of the pentose phosphate pathway. The sequence of reactions that generate ribose 5-phosphate from intermediates of glycolysis is indicated below.

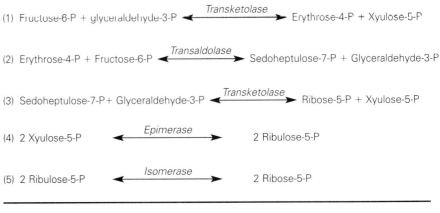

C. Role of the Pentose Phosphate Pathway in the Generation of NADPH

In general, the oxidative phase of the pentose phosphate pathway is the major source of NADPH in cells. NADPH provides the reducing equivalents for biosynthetic reactions and for oxidation–reduction reactions involved in protection against the toxicity of ROS (see Chapter 24). The glutathione-mediated defense against oxidative stress is common to all cell types (including the red blood cell), and the requirement for NADPH to maintain levels of reduced glutathione probably accounts for the universal distribution of the pentose phosphate pathway among different types of cells. Fig. 29.11 illustrates the importance of this pathway in maintaining the membrane integrity of the red blood cell. NADPH is also used for anabolic pathways, such as fatty acid synthesis, cholesterol synthesis, and fatty acid chain elongation (Table 29.1). It is the source of reducing equivalents for cytochrome P450 hydroxylation of aromatic compounds, steroids, alcohols, and drugs. The highest concentrations of glucose 6-phosphate dehydrogenase are found in phagocytic cells, where NADPH oxidase uses NADPH to form superoxide from molecular oxygen. The superoxide then generates hydrogen peroxide, which kills the microorganisms taken up by the phagocytic cells (see Chapter 24).

The entry of glucose 6-phosphate into the pentose phosphate pathway is controlled by the cellular concentration of NADPH. NADPH is a strong product inhibitor of glucose 6-phosphate dehydrogenase, the first enzyme of the pathway. As NADPH is oxidized in other pathways, the product inhibition of glucose 6-phosphate dehydrogenase is relieved, and the rate of the enzyme is accelerated to produce more NADPH.

Table 29.1. Pathways That Require NADPH

Detoxification
- Reduction of oxidized glutathione
- Cytochrome P450 monooxygenases

Reductive synthesis
- Fatty acid synthesis
- Fatty acid chain elongation
- Cholesterol synthesis
- Neurotransmitter synthesis
- Nucleotide synthesis
- Superoxide synthesis

Q: How does the net energy yield from the metabolism of 3 moles of glucose 6-phosphate through the pentose phosphate pathway to pyruvate compare with the yield of 3 moles of glucose 6-phosphate through glycolysis?

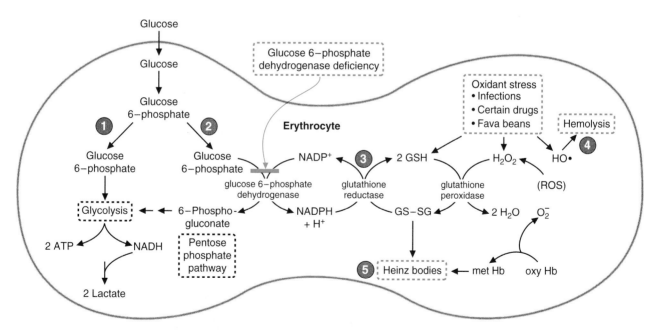

Fig. 29.11. Hemolysis caused by reactive oxygen species. **1.** Maintenance of the integrity of the erythrocyte membrane depends on its ability to generate ATP and NADH from glycolysis. **2.** NADPH is generated by the pentose phosphate pathway. **3.** NADPH is used for the reduction of oxidized glutathione to reduced glutathione. Glutathione is necessary for the removal of H_2O_2 and lipid peroxides generated by reactive oxygen species (ROS). **4.** In the erythrocytes of healthy individuals, the continuous generation of superoxide ion from the nonenzymatic oxidation of hemoglobin provides a source of reactive oxygen species. The glutathione defense system is compromised by glucose 6-phosphate dehydrogenase deficiency, infections, certain drugs, and the purine glycosides of fava beans. **5.** As a consequence, Heinz bodies, aggregates of cross-linked hemoglobin, form on the cell membranes and subject the cell to mechanical stress as it tries to go through small capillaries. The action of the ROS on the cell membrane as well as mechanical stress from the lack of deformability result in hemolysis.

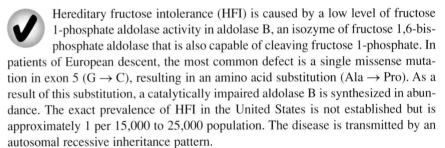

A: The net energy yield from 3 moles of glucose 6-phosphate metabolized through the pentose phosphate pathway and then the last portion of the glycolytic pathway is 6 moles of NADPH, 3 moles of CO_2, 5 moles of NADH, 8 moles of ATP, and 5 moles of pyruvate. In contrast, the metabolism of 3 moles of glucose 6-phosphate through glycolysis is 6 moles of NADH, 9 moles of ATP, and 6 moles of pyruvate.

Table 29.2. Cellular Needs Dictate the Direction of the Pentose Phosphate Pathway Reactions

Cellular Need	Direction of Pathway
NADPH only	Oxidative reactions produce NADPH; nonoxidative reactions convert ribulose-5-P to glucose-6-P to produce more NADPH
NADPH + ribose-5-P	Oxidative reactions produce NADPH and ribulose-5-P; the isomerase converts ribulose-5-P to ribose-5-P.
Ribose-5-P only	Only the nonoxidative reactions. High NADPH inhibits glucose-6-P dehydrogenase, so transketolase and transaldolase will be used to convert fructose-6-P and glyceraldehyde-3-P to ribose-5-P.
NADPH and pyruvate	Both the oxidative and nonoxidative reactions are used. The oxidative reactions generate NADPH and ribulose-5-P. The nonoxidative reactions convert the ribulose-5-P to fructose-6-P and glyceraldehyde-3-P, and glycolysis will convert these intermediates to pyruvate.

In the liver, the synthesis of fatty acids from glucose is a major route of NADPH reoxidation. The synthesis of liver glucose 6-phosphate dehydrogenase, like the key enzymes of glycolysis and fatty acid synthesis, is induced by the increased insulin/glucagon ratio after a high-carbohydrate meal. A summary of the possible routes glucose-6-P may follow using the pentose phosphate pathway is presented in Table 29.2.

CLINICAL COMMENTS

Hereditary fructose intolerance (HFI) is caused by a low level of fructose 1-phosphate aldolase activity in aldolase B, an isozyme of fructose 1,6-bisphosphate aldolase that is also capable of cleaving fructose 1-phosphate. In patients of European descent, the most common defect is a single missense mutation in exon 5 (G → C), resulting in an amino acid substitution (Ala → Pro). As a result of this substitution, a catalytically impaired aldolase B is synthesized in abundance. The exact prevalence of HFI in the United States is not established but is approximately 1 per 15,000 to 25,000 population. The disease is transmitted by an autosomal recessive inheritance pattern.

When affected patients such as **Candice Sucher** ingest fructose, fructose is converted to fructose 1-phosphate. Because of the deficiency of aldolase B, fructose 1-phosphate cannot be further metabolized to dihydroxyacetone phosphate and glyceraldehyde and accumulates in those tissues that have fructokinase (liver, kidney, and small intestine). Fructose is detected in the urine with the reducing sugar test (see Chapter 5). A DNA screening test (based on the generation of a new restriction site by the mutation) now provides a safe method to confirm a diagnosis of hereditary fructose intolerance.

In the infant and small child, the major symptoms include poor feeding, vomiting, intestinal discomfort, and failure to thrive. The greater the ingestion of dietary fructose, the more severe the clinical reaction. The result of prolonged ingestion of fructose is ultrastructural changes in the liver and kidney resulting in hepatic and renal failure. Hereditary fructose intolerance is usually a disease of infancy, because adults with fructose intolerance who have survived avoid the ingestion of fruits, table sugar, and other sweets.

Erin Galway has galactosemia, which is caused by a deficiency of galactose 1-phosphate uridylyltransferase; it is one of the most common genetic diseases. Galactosemia is an autosomal recessive disorder of galactose metabolism that occurs in about 1 in 60,000 newborns. Approximately two thirds of the states in the United States screen newborns for this disease because failure to begin immediate treatment results in mental retardation. Failure to thrive is the most common initial clinical symptom. Vomiting or diarrhea is found in most patients, usually starting within a few days of milk ingestion. Signs of deranged liver function, either jaundice or hepatomegaly, are present almost as frequently after the first week of life. The jaundice of intrinsic liver disease may be accentuated by the severe hemolysis in some patients. Cataracts have been observed within a few days of birth.

Management of patients requires elimination of galactose from the diet. Failure to eliminate this sugar results in progressive liver failure and death. In infants, artificial milk made from casein or soybean hydrolysate is used.

Al Martini's sputum culture sent on the second day of his admission for acute alcoholism and pneumonia grew out *Haemophilus influenzae*. This organism is sensitive to a variety of antibiotics, including TMP/sulfa. Unfortunately, it appeared that Mr. Martini had suffered an acute hemolysis (lysis or destruction of some of his red blood cells), probably induced by exposure to the sulfa drug and his infection with *H. influenzae*. The hemoglobin that escaped from the lysed red blood cells was filtered by his kidneys and appeared in his urine.

By mechanisms that are not fully delineated, certain drugs (such as sulfa drugs and antimalarials), a variety of infectious agents, and exposure to fava beans can cause red blood cell destruction in individuals with a genetic deficiency of glucose 6-phosphate dehydrogenase. Presumably, these patients cannot generate enough reduced NADPH to defend against the ROS. Although erythrocytes lack most of the other enzymatic sources of NADPH for the glutathione antioxidant system, they do have the defense mechanisms provided by the antioxidant vitamins E and C and catalase. Thus, individuals who are not totally deficient in glucose 6-phosphate dehydrogenase remain asymptomatic unless an additional oxidative stress, such as an infection, generates additional oxygen radicals.

Some drugs, such as the antimalarial primaquine and the sulfonamide which Al Martini is taking, affect the ability of red blood cells to defend against oxidative stress. Fava beans, which look like fat string beans and are sometimes called broad beans, contain the purine glycosides vicine and isouramil. These compounds react with glutathione. It has been suggested that cellular levels of reduced glutathione (GSH) decrease to such an extent that critical sulfhydryl groups in some key proteins cannot be maintained in reduced form.

The highest prevalence rates for glucose 6-phosphate dehydrogenase deficiency are found in tropical Africa and Asia, in some areas of the Middle East and the Mediterranean, and in Papua New Guinea. The geographic distribution of this deficiency is similar to that of sickle cell trait, and is probably also related to the relative resistance it confers against the malaria parasite.

Because the individuals with this deficiency are asymptomatic unless exposed to an "oxidant challenge," the clinical course of the hemolytic anemia is usually self-limited if the causative agent is removed. However, genetic polymorphism accounts for a substantial variability in the severity of the disease. Severely affected patients may have a chronic hemolytic anemia and other sequelae even without known exposure to drugs, infection, and other causative factors. In such patients, neonatal jaundice is also common and can be severe enough to cause death.

BIOCHEMICAL COMMENTS

Before the metabolic toxicity of fructose was appreciated, substitution of fructose for glucose in intravenous solutions, and of fructose for sucrose in enteral tube feeding or diabetic diets, was frequently recommended.

(Enteral tube feeding refers to tubes placed into the gut; parenteral tube feeding refers to tubes placed into the vein, feeding intravenously.) Administration of intravenous fructose to patients with diabetes mellitus or other forms of insulin resistance avoided the hyperglycemia found with intravenous glucose, possibly because fructose metabolism in the liver bypasses the insulin-regulated step at phosphofructokinase-1. However, because of the unregulated flow of fructose through glycolysis, intravenous fructose feeding frequently resulted in lactic acidosis (see Fig. 29.3). In addition, the fructokinase reaction is very rapid, and tissues would become depleted of ATP and phosphate when large quantities of fructose were metabolized over a short period. This would lead to cell death. Fructose is less toxic in the diet or in enteral feeding because of the relatively slow rate of fructose absorption.

Suggested References

Hasler J, Lee S. Acute hemolytic anemia after ingestion of fava beans [letter]. Am J Emerg Med 1993;11:560–561.

Holton JB, Walter JH, Tyfield LA. Galactosemia. In: Scriver CR, Beaudet AL, Valle D, Sly WS, et al., eds. The Metabolic and Molecular Bases of Inherited Disease. 8th Ed. New York: McGraw-Hill, 2001:1553–1587.

Luzatto L, Mehta A, Vuillamy T. Glucose 6-phosphate dehydrogenase deficiency. In: Scriver CR, Beaudet AL, Valle D, Sly WS, et al, eds. The Metabolic and Molecular Bases of Inherited Disease. 8th Ed. New York: McGraw-Hill, 2001:4517–4553.

Sheetz MJ, King GL. Molecular understanding of hyperglycemic adverse effects for diabetic complications. JAMA 2002:2579–2588.

Shibuya A, Hirono A, Ishii S, Fujii, Miwa S. Hemolytic crisis after excessive ingestion of fava beans in a male infant with G6PD Canton. Int J Hematol 1999:233–235.

Steinman B, Gitzelmann R, Van den Berghe G. Disorders of fructose metabolism. In: Scriver CR, Beaudet AL, Valle D, Sly WS, et al, eds. The Metabolic and Molecular Bases of Inherited Disease. 8th Ed. New York: McGraw-Hill, 2001:1489–1520.

 REVIEW QUESTIONS—CHAPTER 29

1. Hereditary fructose intolerance is a rare recessive genetic disease that is most commonly caused by a mutation in exon 5 of the aldolase B gene. The mutation fortuitously creates a new AhaII recognition sequence. To test for the mutation, DNA was extracted from a wife, husband, and their two children, Jack and Jill. The DNA for exon 5 of the aldolase B gene was amplified by polymerase chain reaction (PCR), treated with AhaII, subjected to electrophoresis on an agarose gel, and stained with a dye that binds to DNA.

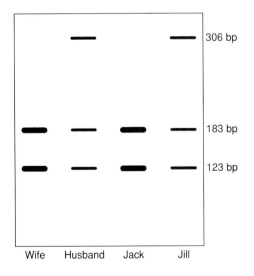

Which of the following conclusions can be made from the data presented?
(A) Both of the children have the disease.
(B) Neither of the children has the disease.
(C) Jill has the disease, Jack does not.
(D) Jack has the disease, Jill does not.
(E) There is not enough information to make a determination

2. On examining the gel himself, the husband became concerned that he might not be the biologic father of one or both of the children. From the pattern on the gel, you can reasonably conclude which of the following?

    (A) He is probably not Jill's father.
    (B) He is probably not Jack's father.
    (C) He could be the father of both children.
    (D) He is probably not the father of either child.
    (E) There is not enough information to make a determination

3. An alcoholic is brought to the Emergency Room for a hypoglycemic coma. Because alcoholics are frequently malnourished, which of the following enzymes can be used to test for a thiamine deficiency?

    (A) Aldolase
    (B) Transaldolase
    (C) Transketolase
    (D) Glucose 6-phosphate dehydrogenase
    (E) UDP-galactose epimerase

4. Intravenous fructose feeding can lead to lactic acidosis caused by which of the following?

    (A) Bypassing the regulated pyruvate kinase step
    (B) Bypassing the regulated PFK-1 step
    (C) Allosterically activating aldolase B
    (D) Allosterically activating lactate dehydrogenase
    (E) Increasing the [ATP]/[ADP] ratio in liver

5. The polyol pathway of sorbitol production and the HMP shunt pathway are linked by which of the following?

    (A) The HMP shunt produces 6-phosphogluconate, an intermediate in the polyol pathway.
    (B) The HMP shunt produces NADPH, which is required for the polyol pathway.
    (C) The HMP shunt produces ribitol, an intermediate of the polyol pathway.
    (D) Both pathways use glucose as the starting material.
    (E) Both pathways use fructose as the starting material.

30 Synthesis of Glycosides, Lactose, Glycoproteins and Glycolipids

*Many of the pathways for interconversion of sugars or the formation of sugar derivatives use activated sugars attached to nucleotides. Both **UDP-glucose** and **UDP-galactose** are used for **glycosyltransferase** reactions in many systems. Lactose, for example, is synthesized from UDP-galactose and glucose in the mammary gland. UDP-glucose also can be oxidized to form UDP-glucuronate, which is used to form **glucuronide derivatives** of bilirubin and xenobiotic compounds. Glucuronide derivatives are generally more readily excreted in urine or bile than the parent compound.*

*In addition to serving as fuel, carbohydrates are often found in **glycoproteins** (carbohydrate chains attached to proteins) and **glycolipids** (carbohydrate chains attached to lipids). **Nucleotide sugars** are used to donate sugar residues for the formation of the glycosidic bonds in both glycoproteins and glycolipids. These carbohydrate groups have many different types of functions.*

*Glycoproteins contain short chains of carbohydrates (oligosaccharides) that are usually branched. These oligosaccharides are generally composed of glucose, galactose, and their amino derivatives. In addition, mannose, L-fucose, and N-acetylneuraminic acid (NANA) are frequently present. The carbohydrate chains grow by the sequential addition of sugars to a **serine** or **threonine** residue of the protein. Nucleotide-sugars are the precursors. Branched carbohydrate chains also may be attached to the amide nitrogen of **asparagine** in the protein. In this case, the chains are synthesized on **dolichol phosphate** and subsequently transferred to the protein. Glycoproteins are found in mucus, in the blood, in compartments within the cell (such as lysosomes), in the extracellular matrix, and embedded in the cell membrane with the carbohydrate portion extending into the extracellular space.*

*Glycolipids belong to the class of **sphingolipids**. They are synthesized from nuceotide-sugars that add monosaccharides sequentially to the hydroxymethyl group of the lipid ceramide (related to sphingosine). They often contain branches of N-acetylneuraminic acid produced from CMP-NANA. They are found in the cell membrane with the carbohydrate portion extruding from the cell surface. These carbohydrates, as well as some of the carbohydrates of glycoproteins, serve as **cell recognition factors**.*

 To help support herself through medical school, **Erna Nemdy** works evenings in a hospital blood bank. She is responsible for assuring that compatible donor blood is available to patients needing blood transfusions.

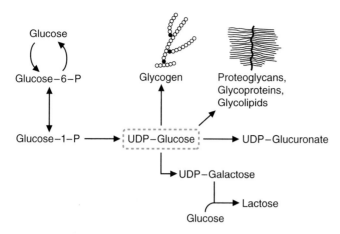

Fig. 30.1. Metabolism of UDP-glucose. The activated glucose moiety of UDP-glucose can be attached by a glycosidic bond to other sugars, as in glycogen or the sugar oligosaccharide and polysaccharide side chains of proteoglycans, glycoproteins, and glycolipids. UDP-glucose also can be oxidized to UDP-glucuronate, or epimerized to UDP-galactose, a precursor of lactose.

As part of her training, Erna has learned that the external surfaces of all blood cells contain large numbers of antigenic determinants. These determinants are often glycoproteins or glycolipids that differ from one individual to another. As a result, all blood transfusions expose the recipient to many foreign immunogens. Most of these, fortunately, do not induce antibodies, or they induce antibodies that elicit little or no immunologic response. For routine blood transfusions, therefore, tests are performed only for the presence of antigens that determine whether the patient's blood type is A, B, AB, or O.

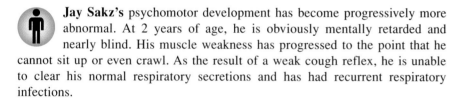

Jay Sakz's psychomotor development has become progressively more abnormal. At 2 years of age, he is obviously mentally retarded and nearly blind. His muscle weakness has progressed to the point that he cannot sit up or even crawl. As the result of a weak cough reflex, he is unable to clear his normal respiratory secretions and has had recurrent respiratory infections.

I. INTERCONVERSIONS INVOLVING NUCLEOTIDE-SUGARS

Activated sugars attached to nucleotides are converted to other sugars, oxidized to sugar acids, and joined to proteins, lipids, or other sugars through glycosidic bonds.

A. Reactions of UDP-Glucose

UDP-glucose is an activated sugar nucleotide that is a precursor of glycogen and lactose, UDP-glucuronate and glucuronides, and the carbohydrate chains in proteoglycans, glycoproteins, and glycolipids (Fig. 30.1). Both proteoglycans and glycosaminoglycans are discussed further in Chapter 49. In the synthesis of many of the carbohydrate portions of these compounds, a sugar is transferred from the nucleotide sugar to an alcohol or other nucleophilic group to form a glycosidic bond (Fig. 30.2). The use of UDP as a leaving group in this reaction provides the energy for formation of the new bond. The enzymes that form glycosidic bonds are sugar transferases (for example, glycogen synthase is a glucosyltransferase). Transferases are also involved in the formation of the glycosidic bonds in bilirubin glucuronides, proteoglycans, and lactose.

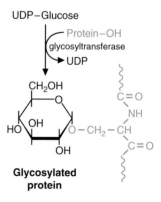

Fig. 30.2. Glycosyltransferases. These enzymes transfer sugars from nucleotide sugars to nucleophilic amino acid residues on proteins, such as the hydroxyl group of serine or the amide group of asparagine. Other transferases transfer specific sugars from a nucleotide sugar to a hydroxyl group of other sugars. The bond formed between the anomeric carbon of the sugar and the nucleophilic group of another compound is a glycosidic bond.

How does glucuronic acid differ from gluconic acid?

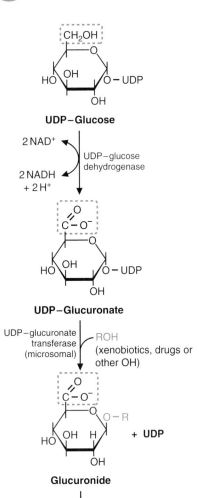

UDP—Glucose

2 NAD⁺

UDP—glucose dehydrogenase

2 NADH + 2 H⁺

UDP—Glucuronate

UDP—glucuronate transferase (microsomal)

ROH (xenobiotics, drugs or other OH)

+ **UDP**

Glucuronide

Bile or urine

Fig. 30.4. Formation of glucuronate and glucuronides. A glycosidic bond is formed between the anomeric hydroxyl of glucuronate and the hydroxyl group of a nonpolar compound. The negatively charged carboxyl group of the glucuronate increases the water solubility and allows otherwise nonpolar compounds to be excreted in the urine or bile.

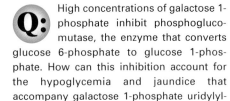 High concentrations of galactose 1-phosphate inhibit phosphoglucomutase, the enzyme that converts glucose 6-phosphate to glucose 1-phosphate. How can this inhibition account for the hypoglycemia and jaundice that accompany galactose 1-phosphate uridylyltransferase deficiency?

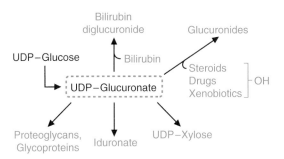

Fig. 30.3. Metabolic routes of UDP-glucuronate. UDP-glucuronate is formed from UDP-glucose (shown in black). Glucuronate from UDP-glucuronate is incorporated into glycosaminoglycans, where certain of the glucuronate residues are converted to iduronate (see Chapter 49). UDP-glucuronate is a precursor of UDP-xylose, another sugar residue incorporated into glycosaminoglycans. Glucuronate is also transferred to the carboxyl groups of bilirubin or the alcohol groups of steroids, drugs, and xenobiotics to form glucuronides. The "ide" in the name glucuronide denotes that these compounds are glycosides. Xenobiotics are pharmacologically, endocrinologically, or toxicologically active substances not endogenously produced and therefore foreign to an organism. Drugs are an example of a xenobiotic.

B. UDP-Glucuronate: A Source of Negative Charges

One of the major routes of UDP-glucose metabolism is the formation of UDP-glucuronate, which serves as a precursor of other sugars and of glucuronides (Fig. 30.3). Glucuronate is formed by the oxidation of the alcohol on C6 of glucose to an acid (through two oxidation states) by an NAD⁺-dependent dehydrogenase (Fig. 30.4). Glucuronate is also present in the diet and can be formed from the degradation of inositol (the sugar alcohol that forms inositol trisphosphate (IP3), an intracellular second messenger for many hormones).

C. Formation of Glucuronides

The function of glucuronate in the excretion of bilirubin, drugs, xenobiotics, and other compounds containing a hydroxyl group is to add negative charges and increase their solubility. Bilirubin is a degradation product of heme that is formed in the reticuloendothelial system and is only slightly soluble in plasma. It is transported to the liver bound to albumin. In the liver, glucuronate residues are transferred from UDP-glucuronate to two carboxyl groups on bilirubin, sequentially forming bilirubin monoglucuronide and bilirubin diglucuronide, the "conjugated" forms of bilirubin (Fig. 30.5). The more soluble bilirubin diglucuronide (as compared with unconjugated bilirubin) is then actively transported into the bile for excretion.

Many xenobiotics, drugs, steroids, and other compounds with hydroxyl groups and a low solubility in water are converted to glucuronides in a similar fashion by glucuronyltransferases present in the endoplasmic reticulum and cytoplasm of the liver and kidney (Table 30.1). This is one of the major conjugation pathways for excretion of these compounds.

 A failure of the liver to transport, store, or conjugate bilirubin results in the accumulation of unconjugated bilirubin in the blood. Jaundice, the yellowish tinge to the skin and the whites of the eyes (sclera) experienced by **Erin Galway**, occurs when plasma becomes supersaturated with bilirubin (>2–2.5 mg/dL), and the excess diffuses into tissues.

When bilirubin levels are measured in the blood, one can measure either indirect bilirubin (this is the nonconjugated form of bilirubin, which is bound to albumin), direct bilirubin (the conjugated, water-soluble form), or total bilirubin (the sum of the direct and indirect levels). If total bilirubin levels are high, then a determination of direct and indirect bilirubin is needed to appropriately determine a cause for the elevation of total bilirubin.

Glucuronate, once formed, can reenter the pathways of glucose metabolism through reactions that eventually convert it to D-xylulose 5-phosphate, an intermediate of the pentose phosphate pathway. In most mammals other than humans, an intermediate of this pathway is the precursor of ascorbic acid (vitamin C). Humans, however, are deficient in this pathway and cannot synthesize vitamin C.

D. Synthesis of UDP-Galactose and Lactose from Glucose

Lactose is synthesized from UDP-galactose and glucose (Fig. 30.6). However, galactose is not required in the diet for lactose synthesis because galactose can be synthesized from glucose.

1. CONVERSION OF GLUCOSE TO GALACTOSE

Galactose and glucose are epimers; they differ only in the stereochemical position of one hydroxyl group. Thus, the formation of UDP-galactose from UDP-glucose is an epimerization (Fig. 30.7). The epimerase does not actually transfer the hydroxyl group; it oxidizes the hydroxyl to a ketone by transferring electrons to NAD^+, and then donates electrons back to re-form the alcohol group on the other side of the carbon.

2. LACTOSE SYNTHESIS

Lactose is unique in that it is synthesized only in the mammary gland of the adult for short periods during lactation. Lactose synthase, an enzyme present in the endoplasmic reticulum of the lactating mammary gland, catalyzes the last step in lactose biosynthesis, the transfer of galactose from UDP-galactose to glucose (see Fig. 30.6). Lactose synthase has two protein subunits, a galactosyltransferase and α-lactalbumin. α-Lactalbumin is a modifier protein synthesized after parturition (childbirth) in response to the hormone prolactin. This enzyme subunit lowers the K_m of the galactosyltransferase for glucose from 1,200 to 1 mM, thereby increasing the rate of lactose synthesis. In the absence of α-lactalbumin, galactosyltransferase transfers galactosyl units to glycoproteins.

Many (60%) full-term newborns develop jaundice, termed neonatal jaundice. This is usually caused by an increased destruction of red blood cells after birth (the fetus has an unusually large number of red blood cells) and an immature bilirubin conjugating system in the liver. This leads to elevated levels of nonconjugated bilirubin, which is deposited in hydrophobic (fat) environments. If bilirubin levels reach a certain threshold at the age of 48 hours, the newborn is a candidate for phototherapy, in which the child is placed under lamps that emit light between the wavelengths of 425 and 475 nm. Bilirubin absorbs this light, undergoes chemical changes, and becomes more water soluble. Usually, within a week of birth, the newborn's liver can handle the load generated from red blood cell turnover.

A: The inhibition of phosphoglucomutase results in hypoglycemia by interfering with both the formation of UDP-glucose (the glycogen precursor) and the degradation of glycogen back to glucose 6-phosphate. Ninety percent of glycogen degradation leads to glucose 1-phosphate, which can only be converted to glucose 6-phosphate by phosphoglucomutase. When phosphoglucomutase activity is inhibited, less glucose-6-P production occurs, and hence, less glucose is available for export. Thus, the stored glycogen is only approximately 10% efficient in raising blood glucose levels, and hypoglycemia results. UDP-glucose levels are reduced because glucose-1-P is required to synthesize UDP-glucose, and in the absence of phosphoglucomutase activity glucose-6-P cannot be converted to glucose-1-P. This prevents the formation of UDP-glucuronate, which is necessary to convert bilirubin to the diglucuronide form for transport into the bile. Bilirubin accumulates in tissues, giving them a yellow color (jaundice).

Table 30.1. Some Compounds Degraded and Excreted as Urinary Glucuronides

Estrogen (female sex hormone)
Progesterone (steroid hormone)
Triiodothyronine (thyroid hormone)
Acetylaminofluorene (xenobiotic carcinogen)
Meprobamate (drug for sleep)
Morphine (painkiller)

A: 6-Phosphogluconate is produced by the first oxidative reaction in the pentose phosphate pathway, in which carbon 1 of glucose is oxidized to a carboxylate. In contrast, glucuronic acid is oxidized at carbon 6 to the carboxylate form.

Q: A pregnant woman who was extremely lactose intolerant asked her physician if she would still be able to breastfeed her infant since she could not drink milk or dairy products. What advice should she be given?

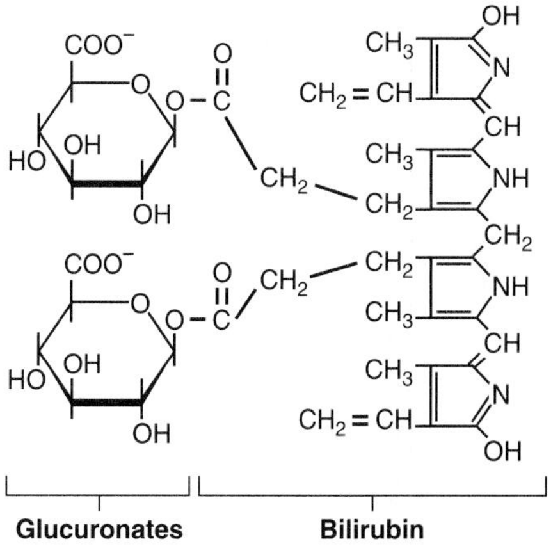

Fig. 30.5. Formation of bilirubin diglucuronide. A glycosidic bond is formed between the anomeric hydroxyl of glucuronate and the carboxylate groups of bilirubin. The addition of the hydrophilic carbohydrate group, and the negatively charged carboxyl group of the glucuronate, increases the water solubility of the conjugated bilirubin and allows the otherwise insoluble bilirubin to be excreted in the urine or bile.

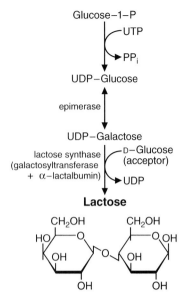

Fig. 30.6. Lactose synthesis. Lactose is a disaccharide composed of galactose and glucose. UDP-galactose for the synthesis of lactose in the mammary gland is usually formed from the epimerization of UDP-glucose. Lactose synthase attaches the anomeric carbon of the galactose to the C4 alcohol group of glucose to form a glycosidic bond. Lactose synthase is composed of a galactosyltransferase and α-lactalbumin, which is a regulatory subunit.

Table 30.2. Some Sugar Nucleotides That Are Precursors for Transferase Reactions

UDP-glucose
UDP-galactose
UDP-glucuronic acid
UDP-xylose
UDP-N-acetylglucosamine
UDP-N-acetylgalactosamine
CMP-N-acetylneuraminic acid
GDP-fucose
GDP-mannose

A: Although the lactose in dairy products is a major source of galactose, the ingestion of lactose is not required for lactation. UDP-galactose in the mammary gland is derived principally from the epimerization of glucose. Dairy products are, however, a major dietary source of Ca^{2+}, so breastfeeding mothers need increased Ca^{2+} from another source.

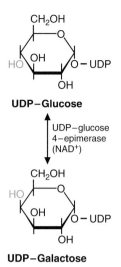

Fig. 30.7. Epimerization of UDP-glucose to UDP-galactose. The epimerization of glucose to galactose occurs on UDP-sugars. The epimerase uses NAD^+ to oxidize the alcohol to a ketone, and then reduce the ketone back to an alcohol. The reaction is reversible; glucose being converted to galactose forms galactose for lactose synthesis, and galactose being converted to glucose is part of the pathway for the metabolism of dietary galactose.

E. Formation of Sugars for Glycolipid and Glycoprotein Synthesis

The transferases that produce the oligosaccharide and polysaccharide side chains of glycolipids and attach sugar residues to proteins are specific for the sugar moiety and for the donating nucleotide (e.g., UDP, CMP, or GDP). Some of the sugar-nucleotides used for glycoprotein, proteoglycan (see Chapter 49) and glycolipid formation are listed in Table 30.2. They include the derivatives of glucose and galactose that we have already discussed, as well as acetylated amino sugars and derivatives of mannose. The reason for the large variety of sugars attached to proteins and lipids is that they have relatively specific and different functions, such as targeting a protein toward a membrane, providing recognition sites on the cell surface for other cells, hormones, or viruses, or acting as lubricants or molecular sieves (see Chapter 42).

The pathways for utilization and formation of many of these sugars are summarized in Figure 30.8. Note that many of the steps are reversible, so that glucose and other dietary sugars enter a common pool from which the diverse sugars can be formed.

The amino sugars are all derived from glucosamine 6-phosphate. To synthesize glucosamine 6-phosphate, an amino group is transferred from the amide of glutamine to fructose 6-phosphate (Fig. 30.9). Amino sugars, such as glucosamine, can then be N-acetylated by an acetyltransferase.

Mannose is found in the diet in small amounts. Like galactose, it is an epimer of glucose, and mannose and glucose are interconverted by epimerization reactions. The interconversion can take place either at the level of fructose 6-phosphate to mannose 6-phosphate, or at the level of the derivatized sugars (see Fig. 30.8).

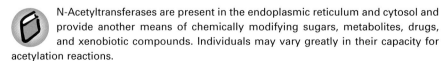

N-Acetyltransferases are present in the endoplasmic reticulum and cytosol and provide another means of chemically modifying sugars, metabolites, drugs, and xenobiotic compounds. Individuals may vary greatly in their capacity for acetylation reactions.

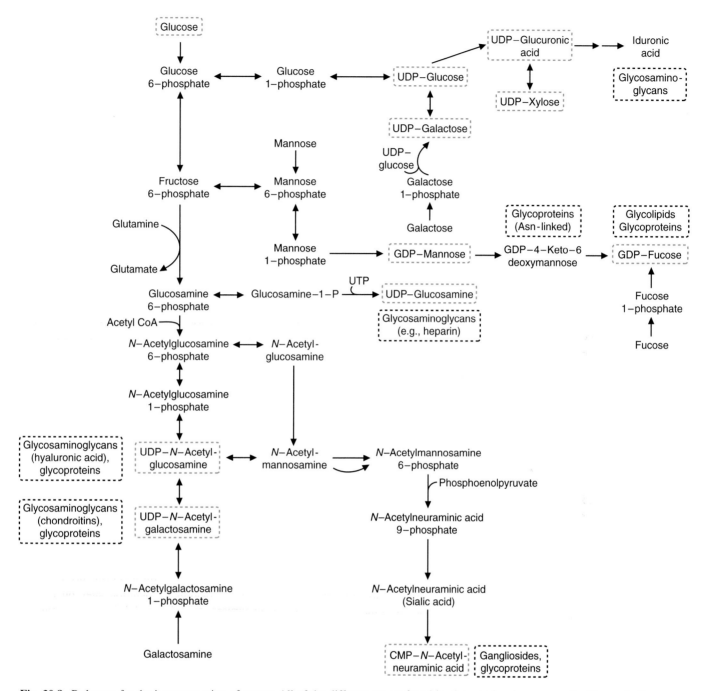

Fig. 30.8. Pathways for the interconversion of sugars. All of the different sugars found in glycosaminoglycans, gangliosides, and other compounds in the body can be synthesized from glucose. Dietary glucose, fructose, galactose, mannose, and other sugars enter a common pool from which other sugars are derived. The activated sugar is transferred from the nucleotide sugar, shown in blue boxes, to form a glycosidic bond with another sugar or amino acid residue. The box next to each nucleotide sugar lists some of the compounds that contain the sugar. Iduronic acid, in the upper right corner of the diagram, is formed only after glucuronic acid is incorporated into a glycosaminoglycan (which is discussed in more detail in Chapter 49).

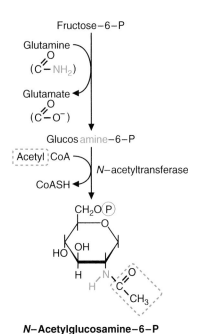

N–Acetylglucosamine–6–P

Fig. 30.9. The formation of *N*-acetylglucosamine 6-phosphate. The amino sugar is formed by a transfer of the amino group from the amide of glutamine to a carbon of the sugar. The amino group is acetylated by the transfer of an acetyl group from acetyl CoA.

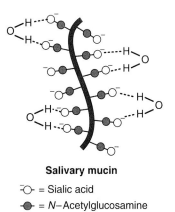

Salivary mucin

⁻◯– = Sialic acid

⁻●– = *N*–Acetylglucosamine

Fig. 30.11. Structure of salivary mucin. The sugars form hydrogen bonds with water. Sialic acid provides a negatively charged carboxylate group. The protein is extremely large, and the negatively charged sialic acids extend the carbohydrate chains so the molecules occupy a large space. All of the salivary glycoproteins are *O*-linked. NANA is a sialic acid.

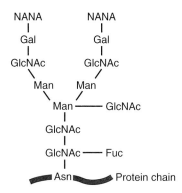

Fig. 30.10. An example of a branched glycoprotein. NANA = *N*-acetylneuraminic acid; Gal= galactose; GlcNAc = *N*-acetylglucosamine; Man = mannose; Fuc = fucose.

N-Acetylmannosamine is the precursor of N-acetylneuraminic acid (NANA, a sialic acid) and GDP-mannose is the precursor of GDP-fucose (see Fig. 30.8). The negative charge on NANA is obtained by the addition of a 3-carbon carboxyl moiety from phosphoenolpyruvate.

II. GLYCOPROTEINS

A. Structure and Function

Glycoproteins contain short carbohydrate chains covalently linked to either serine/threonine or asparagine residues in the protein. These oligosaccharide chains are often branched, and they do not contain repeating disaccharides (Fig. 30.10). Most proteins in the blood are glycoproteins. They serve as hormones, antibodies, enzymes (including those of the blood clotting cascade), and as structural components of the extracellular matrix. Collagen contains galactosyl units and disaccharides composed of galactosyl-glucose attached to hydroxylysine residues (see Chapter 49). The secretions of mucus-producing cells, such as salivary mucin, are glycoproteins (Fig. 30.11).

Although most glycoproteins are secreted from cells, some are segregated in lysosomes, where they serve as the lysosomal enzymes that degrade various types of cellular and extracellular material. Other glycoproteins are produced like secretory proteins, but hydrophobic regions of the protein remain attached to the cell membrane, and the carbohydrate portion extends into the extracellular space (Fig. 30.12)(also see Chapter 15, section I). These glycoproteins serve as receptors for compounds such as hormones, as transport proteins, and as cell attachment and cell–cell recognition sites. Bacteria and viruses also bind to these sites.

B. Synthesis

The protein portion of glycoproteins is synthesized on the endoplasmic reticulum (ER). The carbohydrate chains are attached to the protein in the lumen of the ER and the Golgi complex. In some cases, the initial sugar is added to a serine or a threonine residue in the protein, and the carbohydrate chain is extended by the sequential addition of sugar residues to the nonreducing end. As seen previously in Table 2, UDP-sugars are the precursors for the addition of four of the seven sugars that are usually found in glycoproteins—glucose, galactose, *N*-acetylglucosamine, and *N*-acetylgalactosamine. GDP-sugars are the precursors for the addition of mannose and L-fucose, and CMP-NANA is the precursor for NANA.

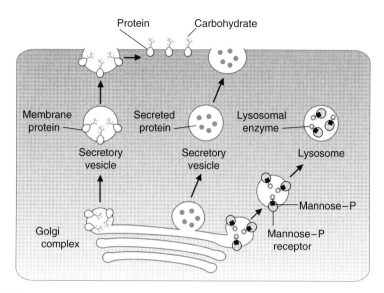

Fig. 30.12. Route from the Golgi complex to the final destination for lysosomal enzymes, cell membrane proteins, and secreted proteins, which include glycoproteins and proteoglycans.

The enzyme that is deficient in I-cell disease is a phosphotransferase located in the Golgi apparatus.

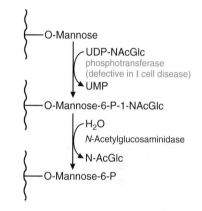

Fig. 30.13. Structure of dolichol phosphate. In humans, the isoprene unit (in brackets) is repeated approximately 17 times (n = ~17).

Dolichol phosphate (Fig. 30.13) (which is synthesized from isoprene units, as discussed in Chapter 34) is involved in transferring branched sugar chains to the amide nitrogen of asparagine residues. Sugars are removed and added as the glycoprotein moves from the ER through the Golgi complex (Fig. 30.14). As discussed in Chapter 10, the carbohydrate chain is used as a targeting marker for lysosomal enzymes.

I-cell (inclusion cell) disease is a rare condition in which lysosomal enzymes lack the mannosephosphate marker that targets them to lysosomes. Consequently, lysosomal enzymes are secreted from the cells. Because lysosomes lack their normal complement of enzymes, undegraded molecules accumulate within membranes inside these cells, forming inclusion bodies.

III. GLYCOLIPIDS

A. Function and Structure

Glycolipids are derivatives of the lipid sphingosine. These sphingolipids include the cerebrosides and the gangliosides (Fig. 30.15; see also Fig. 5.22). They contain ceramide, with carbohydrate moieties attached to its hydroxymethyl group.

Glycolipids are involved in intercellular communication. Oligosaccharides of identical composition are present in both the glycolipids and glycoproteins associated with the cell membrane, where they serve as cell recognition factors. For example, carbohydrate residues in these oligosaccharides are the antigens of the ABO blood group substances (Fig. 30.16).

The phosphotransferase has the unique ability to recognize lysosomal proteins because of their three-dimensional structure, such that they can all be appropriately tagged for transport to the lysosomes.

By identifying the nature of antigenic determinants on the surface of the donor's red blood cells, **Erna Nemdy** is able to classify the donor's blood as belonging to certain specific blood groups. These antigenic determinants are located in the oligosaccharides of the glycoproteins and glycolipids of the cell membranes. The most important blood group in humans is the ABO group, which comprises two antigens, A and B. Individuals with the A antigen on their cells belong to blood group A. Those with B belong to group B, and those with both A and B belong to group AB. The absence of both the A and the B antigen results in blood type O (see Fig. 30.16).

A

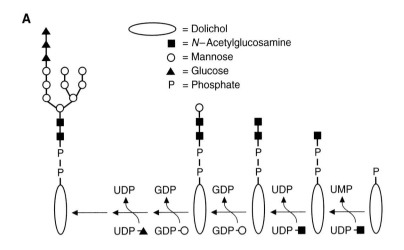

B

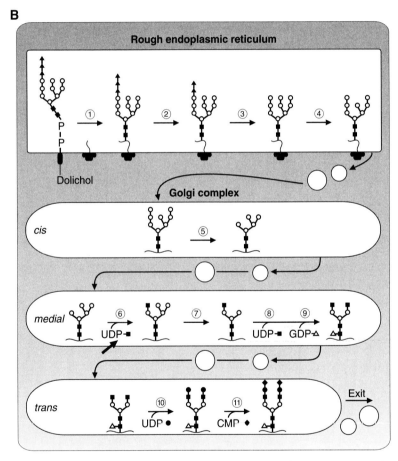

Fig. 30.14. Action of dolichol phosphate in transferring carbohydrate groups to proteins (A) and processing of these carbohydrate groups (B). Transfer of the branched oligosaccharide from dolichol phosphate to a protein in the lumen of the rough endoplasmic reticulum (RER) (step 1) and processing of the oligosaccharide (steps 2–11). Steps 1 through 4 occur in the RER. The glycoprotein is transferred in vesicles to the Golgi complex, where further modifications of the oligosaccharides occur (steps 5–11). B modified with permission from Kornfeld R, Kornfeld S. Annu Rev Biochem 1985;54:640. © 1985 by Annual Reviews, Inc. P = phosphate.

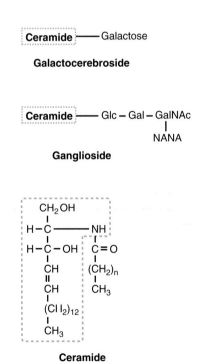

Fig. 30.15. Structures of cerebrosides and gangliosides. In these glycolipids, sugars are attached to ceramide (shown below the glycolipids). The boxed portion of ceramide is sphingosine, from which the name *sphingolipids* is derived.

Blood Type

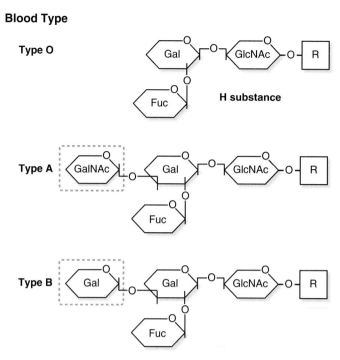

Fig. 30.16. Structures of the blood group substances. Note that these structures are the same except that type A has *N*-acetylgalactosamine (GalNAc) at the nonreducing end, type B has galactose (Gal), and type O has neither. R is either a protein or the lipid ceramide. Each antigenic determinant is boxed. Fuc = fucose; GlcNAc = *N*-acetylglucosamine; Gal = galactose.

The blood group substances are oligosaccharide components of glycolipids and glycoproteins found in most cell membranes. Those located on red blood cells have been studied extensively. A single genetic locus with two alleles determines an individual's blood type. These genes encode glycosyltransferases involved in the synthesis of the oligosaccharides of the blood group substances.

Most individuals can synthesize the H substance, an oligosaccharide that contains a fucose linked to a galactose at the nonreducing end of the blood group substance (see Fig. 30.16). Type A individuals produce an *N*-acetylgalactosamine transferase (encoded by the A gene) that attaches *N*-acetylgalactosamine to the galactose residue of the H substance. Type B individuals produce a galactosyltransferase (encoded by the B gene) that links galactose to the galactose residue of the H substance. Type AB individuals have both alleles and produce both transferases. Thus, some of the oligosaccharides of their blood group substances contain *N*-acetylgalactosamine and some contain galactose. Type O individuals produce a defective transferase, and, therefore, they do not attach either *N*-acetylgalactosamine or galactose to the H substance. Thus, individuals of blood type O have only the H substance.

B. Synthesis

Cerebrosides are synthesized from ceramide and UDP-glucose or UDP-galactose. They contain a single sugar (a monosaccharide). Gangliosides contain oligosaccharides produced from UDP-sugars and CMP-NANA, which is the precursor for the *N*-acetylneuraminic acid residues that branch from the linear chain. The synthesis of the sphingolipids is described in more detail in Chapter 33.

Sphingolipids are produced in the Golgi complex. Their lipid component becomes part of the membrane of the secretory vesicle that buds from the *trans* face of the Golgi. After the vesicle membrane fuses with the cell membrane, the lipid component of the glycolipid remains in the outer layer of the cell membrane, and the carbohydrate component extends into the extracellular space.

Cholera toxin binds to the carbohydrate portion of the GM1 ganglioside to allow its catalytic subunit to enter the cell.

Q: **Erna Nemdy** determined that a patient's blood type was AB. The new surgical resident was eager to give this patient a blood transfusion and, because AB blood is rare and an adequate amount was not available in the blood bank, he requested type A blood. Should Erna give him type A blood for his patient?

Jay Sakz has Tay-Sachs disease, which belongs to a group of gangliosidoses that include Fabry's and Gaucher's diseases. They mainly affect the brain, the skin, and the reticuloendothelial system (e.g., liver and spleen). In these diseases, complex lipids accumulate. Each of these lipids contains a ceramide as part of its structure (Table 30.3). The rate at which the lipid is synthesized is normal. However, the lysosomal enzyme required to degrade it is not very active, either because it is made in deficient quantities because of a mutation in a gene that specifically codes for the enzyme or because a critical protein required to activate the enzyme is deficient. Because the lipid cannot be degraded, it accumulates and causes degeneration of the affected tissues with progressive malfunction, such as the psychomotor deficits that occur as a result of the central nervous system involvement seen in most of these storage diseases.

Table 30.3. Defective Enzymes in the Gangliosidoses

Disease	Enzyme Deficiency	Accumulated Lipid
Fucosidosis	α-Fucosidase	Cer–Glc–Gal–GalNAc–Gal:Fuc H-isoantigen
Generalized gangliosidosis	G_{M1}-β-galactosidase	Cer–Glc–Gal(NeuAc)–GalNAc:Gal G_{M1} ganglioside
Tay-Sachs disease	Hexosaminidase A	Cer–Glc–Gal(NeuAc):GalNAc G_{M2} ganglioside
Tay-Sachs variant or Sandhoff disease	Hexosaminidase A and B	Cer–Glc–Gal–Gal:GalNAc Globoside plus G_{M2} ganglioside
Fabry's disease	α-Galactosidase	Cer–Glc–Gal:Gal Globotriaosylceramide
Ceramide lactoside lipidosis	Ceramide lactosidase (β-galactosidase)	Cer–Glc:Gal Ceramide lactoside
Metachromatic leukodystrophy	Arylsulfatase A	Cer–Gal:OSO_3 3-Sulfogalactosylceramide
Krabbe's disease	β-Galactosidase	Cer:Gal Galactosylceramide
Gaucher's disease	β-Glucosidase	Cer:Glc Glucosylceramide
Niemann-Pick disease	Sphingomyelinase	Cer:P–choline Sphingomyelin
Farber's disease	Ceramidase	Acyl:sphingosine Ceramide

NeuAc, N-acetylneuraminic acid; Cer, ceramide: Glc, glucose; Gal, galactose; Fuc, fucose : site of deficient enzyme reaction.

CLINICAL COMMENTS

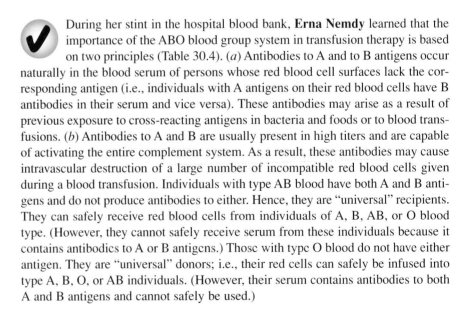

During her stint in the hospital blood bank, **Erna Nemdy** learned that the importance of the ABO blood group system in transfusion therapy is based on two principles (Table 30.4). (*a*) Antibodies to A and to B antigens occur naturally in the blood serum of persons whose red blood cell surfaces lack the corresponding antigen (i.e., individuals with A antigens on their red blood cells have B antibodies in their serum and vice versa). These antibodies may arise as a result of previous exposure to cross-reacting antigens in bacteria and foods or to blood transfusions. (*b*) Antibodies to A and B are usually present in high titers and are capable of activating the entire complement system. As a result, these antibodies may cause intravascular destruction of a large number of incompatible red blood cells given during a blood transfusion. Individuals with type AB blood have both A and B antigens and do not produce antibodies to either. Hence, they are "universal" recipients. They can safely receive red blood cells from individuals of A, B, AB, or O blood type. (However, they cannot safely receive serum from these individuals because it contains antibodies to A or B antigens.) Those with type O blood do not have either antigen. They are "universal" donors; i.e., their red cells can safely be infused into type A, B, O, or AB individuals. (However, their serum contains antibodies to both A and B antigens and cannot safely be used.)

The patient could safely receive type A blood **cells** from another person because he has both A and B antigens on his own cells and does not have antibodies in his serum to either type A or B cells. However, he should not be given type A serum (or type A whole blood) because type A serum contains antibodies to type B antigens, which are present on his cells.

Table 30.4. Characteristics of the ABO Blood Groups

Red cell type	O	A	B	AB
Possible genotypes	OO	AA or AO	BB or BO	AB
Antibodies in serum	Anti-A and B	Anti-B	Anti-A	None
Frequency (in Caucasians)	45%	40%	10%	5%
Can accept blood types	O	A, O	B, O	A, B, AB, O

The second important red blood cell group is the Rh group. It is important because one of its antigenic determinants, the D antigen, is a very potent immunogen, stimulating the production of a large number of antibodies.

The unique carbohydrate composition of the glycoproteins that constitute the antigenic determinants on red blood cells in part contributes to the relative immunogenicity of the A, B, and Rh (D) red blood cell groups in human blood.

Tay-Sachs disease, the problem afflicting **Jay Sakz,** is an autosomal recessive disorder that is rare in the general population (1 in 300,000 births), but its prevalence in Jews of Eastern European extraction (who make up 90% of the Jewish population in the United States) is much higher (1 in 3,600 births). One in 28 Ashkenazi Jews carries this defective gene. Its presence can be discovered by measuring the tissue level of the protein produced by the gene (hexosaminidase A) or by recombinant DNA techniques. Skin fibroblasts of concerned couples planning a family are frequently used for these tests.

Carriers of the affected gene have a reduced but functional level of this enzyme that normally hydrolyzes a specific bond between an N-acetyl-D-galactosamine and a D-galactose residue in the polar head of the ganglioside.

No effective therapy is available. Enzyme replacement has met with little success because of the difficulties in getting the enzyme across the blood-brain barrier.

BIOCHEMICAL COMMENTS

Hexosaminidase A, the enzyme defective in Tay-Sachs disease, is actually composed of two subunits, an α and a β chain. The exact stoichiometry of the active enzyme is unknown, but it may be $\alpha_2\beta_2$. The α subunit is coded for by the HexA gene, whereas the β subunit is coded for by the HexB gene. In Tay-Sachs disease, the α subunit is defective, and hexosaminidase A activity is lost. However, the β subunit can form active tetramers in the absence of the α subunit, and this activity, named hexosaminidase B, which cleaves the glycolipid globoside, retains activity in children with Tay-Sachs disease. Thus, children with Tay-Sachs disease accumulate the ganglioside GM2, but not globoside (Fig. 30.17).

Mutation of the HexB gene, and production of a defective β subunit, leads to inactivation of both hexosaminidase A and B activity. Such a mutation leads to Sandhoff disease. Both activities are lost because both activities require a functional β subunit. The clinical course of this disease is similar to Tay-Sachs but with an accelerated timetable because of the initial accumulation of both GM2 and globoside in the lysosomes.

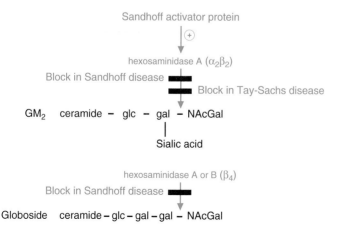

Fig. 30.17. Substrate specificities of hexosaminidase A, B, and the function of the activator protein. Glc = glucose; gal = galactose; NAcGal = N-acetylgalactosamine.

A third type of mutation also can lead to disease symptoms similar to those of Tay-Sachs disease. Children were identified with Tay-Sachs symptoms, but when both hexosaminidase A and B activities were measured in a test tube, they were normal. This disease, ultimately named Sandhoff activator disease, is caused by a mutation in a protein that is needed to activate hexosaminidase A activity. In the absence of the activator, hexosaminidase A activity is minimal, and GM2 initially accumulates in lysosomes. This mutation has no effect on hexosaminidase B activity.

When a glycolipid cannot be degraded because of an enzymatic mutation, it accumulates in residual bodies (vacuoles that contain material that lysosomal enzymes cannot digest). Normal cells contain a small number of residual bodies, but in diseases of lysosomal enzymes, large numbers of residual bodies accumulate within the cell, eventually interfering with normal cell function.

In 70% of the cases of Tay-Sachs disease in persons of Ashkenazai Jewish background, exon 11 of the gene for the α chain of hexosaminidase A contains a mutation. The normal gene sequence encodes a protein with the amino acids arg-ile-ser-tyr-gly-pro-asp in this region, as shown below:

$$\overset{\bullet}{}\quad\overset{10}{}\quad\overset{\bullet}{}\quad\overset{20}{}$$
5'–CGTATATCCTATGGCCCTGAC
arg – ile – ser – tyr – gly – pro – asp

The mutant DNA sequence for this area is shown below:

$$\overset{\bullet}{}\quad\overset{10}{}\quad\overset{\bullet}{}\quad\overset{20}{}$$
5'–CGTATATCT**ATC**CTATGGCCCTGAC
arg – ile – ser – ile – leu – leu – trp – pro –

A four-base insertion (underlined) occurs in the mutated gene, which alters the reading frame of the protein, and also introduces a premature stop codon further down the protein, such that no functional α subunit can be produced.

Suggested References

Gravel RA, Kaback MM, Proia RL, Sandhoff K, et al. The G_{M2} gangliosidoses. In: Scriver CR, Beaudet AL, Valle D, Sly WS, et al eds. The Metabolic and Molecular Bases of Inherited Disease. 8th Ed. New York: McGraw-Hill, 2001:3827–3876.

Kornfeld S, Sly WS. I-cell disease and pseudohurler polydystrophy: disorders of lysosomal enzyme phosphorylation and localization. In: Scriver CR, Beaudet AL, Valle D, Sly WS, et al., eds. The Metabolic and Molecular Bases of Inherited Disease, 8th ed. New York: McGraw-Hill, 2001:3469–3482.

Lloyd KO. The chemistry and immunochemistry of blood group A, B, H and Lewis antigens: past, present and future. Glycoconjugate J 2000:531–541.

 REVIEW QUESTIONS—CHAPTER 30

1. Which of the following best describes a mother with galactosemia caused by a deficiency of galactose 1-phosphate uridylyl transferase?

   (A) She can convert galactose to UDP-galactose for lactose synthesis during lactation.
   (B) She can form galactose 1-phosphate from galactose.
   (C) She can use galactose as a precursor to glucose production.
   (D) She can use galactose to produce glycogen.
   (E) She will have lower than normal levels of serum galactose after drinking milk.

2. The immediate carbohydrate precursors for glycolipid and glycoprotein synthesis are which of the following?

    (A) Sugar phosphates
    (B) Sugar acids
    (C) Sugar alcohols
    (D) Nucleotide sugars
    (E) Acyl-sugars

3. A newborn is diagnosed with neonatal jaundice. In this patient, the bilirubin produced lacks which of the following carbohydrates?

    (A) Glucose
    (B) Gluconate
    (C) Glucuronate
    (D) Galactose
    (E) Galactitol

4. The nitrogen donor for the formation of amino sugars is which of the following?

    (A) Ammonia
    (B) Asparagine
    (C) Glutamine
    (D) Adenine
    (E) Dolichol

5. Which of the following glycolipids would accumulate in a patient with Sandhoff's disease?

    (A) GM1
    (B) Lactosyl-ceramide
    (C) Globoside
    (D) Glucocerebroside
    (E) GM3

31 Gluconeogenesis and Maintenance of Blood Glucose Levels

*During fasting, many of the reactions of glycolysis are reversed as the liver produces glucose to maintain blood glucose levels. This process of **glucose production** is called **gluconeogenesis**.*

*Gluconeogenesis, which occurs primarily in the liver, is the pathway for the synthesis of glucose from compounds other than carbohydrates. In humans, the major precursors of glucose are **lactate**, **glycerol**, and **amino acids**, particularly **alanine**. Except for three key sequences, the reactions of gluconeogenesis are reversals of the steps of glycolysis (Fig. 31.1). The sequences of gluconeogenesis that do not use enzymes of glycolysis involve the irreversible, regulated steps of glycolysis. These three steps are the conversion of (a) pyruvate to phosphoenolpyruvate, (b) fructose 1,6-bisphosphate to fructose 6-phosphate, and (c) glucose 6-phosphate to glucose.*

Some tissues of the body, such as the brain and red blood cells, cannot synthesize glucose on their own, yet depend on glucose for energy. On a long-term basis, most tissues also require glucose for other functions such as the synthesis of the ribose moiety of nucleotides or the carbohydrate portion of glycoproteins and glycolipids. Therefore, to survive, humans must have mechanisms for maintaining blood glucose levels.

*After a meal containing carbohydrates, blood glucose levels rise (Fig. 31.2). Some of the glucose from the diet is stored in the liver as **glycogen**. After 2 or 3 hours of fasting, this glycogen begins to be degraded by the process of **glycogenolysis**, and glucose is released into the blood. As glycogen stores decrease, **adipose triacylglycerols** are also degraded, providing **fatty acids** as an alternative fuel and glycerol for the synthesis of glucose by gluconeogenesis. Amino acids are also released from the muscle to serve as gluconeogenic precursors.*

During an overnight fast, blood glucose levels are maintained by both glycogenolysis and gluconeogenesis. However, after approximately 30 hours of fasting, liver glycogen stores are mostly depleted. Subsequently, gluconeogenesis is the only source of blood glucose.

*Changes in the metabolism of glucose that occur during the switch from the fed to the fasting state are regulated by the hormones **insulin** and **glucagon**. Insulin is elevated in the fed state, and glucagon is elevated during fasting. Insulin stimulates the **transport** of glucose into certain cells such as those in muscle and adipose tissue. Insulin also alters the activity of key enzymes that regulate metabolism, stimulating the storage of fuels. Glucagon counters the effects of insulin, stimulating the release of stored fuels and the conversion of lactate, amino acids, and glycerol to glucose.*

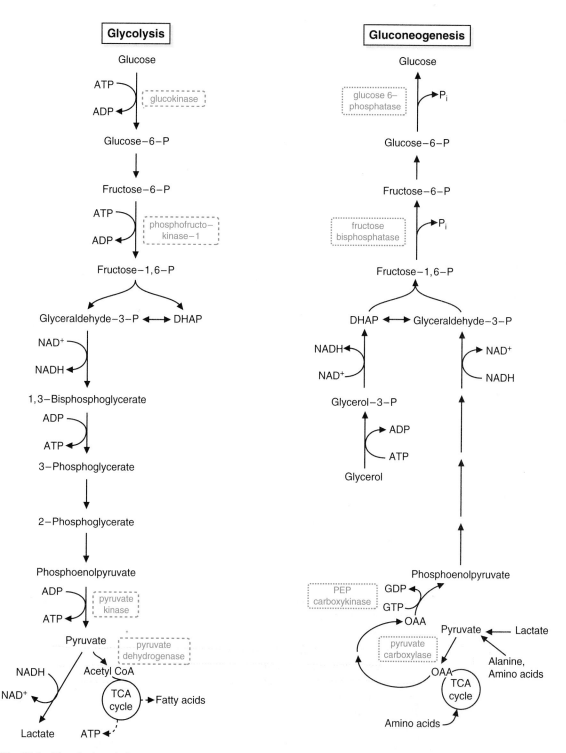

Fig. 31.1. Glycolysis and gluconeogenesis in the liver. The gluconeogenic pathway is almost the reverse of the glycolytic pathway, except for three reaction sequences. At these three steps, the reactions are catalyzed by different enzymes. The energy requirements of these reactions differ, and one pathway can be activated while the other is inhibited.

Fed

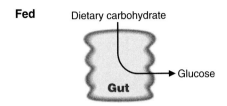

Fasting

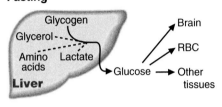

Starved

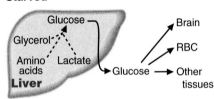

Fig. 31.2. Sources of blood glucose in the fed, fasting, and starved states. RBC = red blood cells.

Q: What clinical signs and symptoms help to distinguish a coma caused by an excess of blood glucose and ketone bodies due to a deficiency of insulin (diabetic ketoacidosis [DKA]) from a coma caused by a sudden lowering of blood glucose (hypoglycemic coma) induced by the inadvertent injection of excessive insulin—the current problem experienced by **Di Abietes?**

Blood glucose levels are maintained not only during fasting, but also during exercise, when muscle cells take up glucose from the blood and oxidize it for energy. During exercise, the liver supplies glucose to the blood by the processes of glycogenolysis and gluconeogenesis.

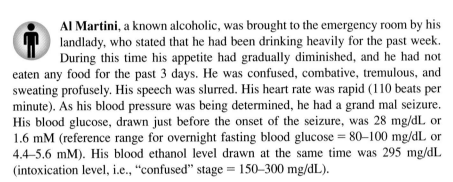

THE WAITING ROOM

Al Martini, a known alcoholic, was brought to the emergency room by his landlady, who stated that he had been drinking heavily for the past week. During this time his appetite had gradually diminished, and he had not eaten any food for the past 3 days. He was confused, combative, tremulous, and sweating profusely. His speech was slurred. His heart rate was rapid (110 beats per minute). As his blood pressure was being determined, he had a grand mal seizure. His blood glucose, drawn just before the onset of the seizure, was 28 mg/dL or 1.6 mM (reference range for overnight fasting blood glucose = 80–100 mg/dL or 4.4–5.6 mM). His blood ethanol level drawn at the same time was 295 mg/dL (intoxication level, i.e., "confused" stage = 150–300 mg/dL).

Emma Wheezer presented to the emergency room 3 days after discharge from the hospital following a 10-day admission for severe refractory bronchial asthma. She required high-dose intravenous dexamethasone (an anti-inflammatory synthetic glucocorticoid) for the first 8 days of her stay. After 2 additional days receiving oral dexamethasone, she was discharged on substantial pharmacologic doses of this steroid and instructed to return to her physician's office in 5 days. She presented now with marked polyuria (increased urination), polydipsia (increased thirst), and muscle weakness. Her blood glucose was 275 mg/dL or 15 mM (reference range = 80–100 mg/dL or 4.4–5.6 mM).

Di Abietes could not remember whether she had taken her 6:00 PM insulin dose, when, in fact, she had done so. Unfortunately, she decided to give herself the evening dose (for the second time). When she did not respond to her alarm clock at 6:00 AM the following morning, her roommate tried unsuccessfully to awaken her. The roommate called an ambulance, and Di was rushed to the hospital emergency room in a coma. Her pulse and blood pressure at admission were normal. Her skin was flushed and slightly moist. Her respirations were slightly slow.

Ann O'Rexia continues to resist efforts on the part of her psychiatrist and family physician to convince her to increase her caloric intake. Her body weight varies between 97 and 99 lb, far below the desirable weight for a woman who is 5 feet 7 inches tall. In spite of her severe diet, her fasting blood glucose levels range from 55 to 70 mg/dL. She denies having any hypoglycemic symptoms.

Otto Shape has complied with his calorie-restricted diet and aerobic exercise program. He has lost another 7 lb and is closing in on his goal of weighing 154 lb. He notes increasing energy during the day, and remains alert during lectures and assimilates the lecture material noticeably better than he did before starting his weight loss and exercise program. He jogs for 45 minutes each morning before breakfast.

Diabetes mellitus (DM) should be suspected if a venous plasma glucose level drawn irrespective of when food was last eaten (a "random" sample of blood glucose) is "unequivocally elevated" (i.e., ≥200 mg/dL), particularly in a patient who manifests the classic signs and symptoms of chronic hyperglycemia (polydipsia, polyuria, blurred vision, headaches, rapid weight loss, sometimes accompanied by nausea and vomiting). To confirm the diagnosis, the patient should fast overnight (10–16 hours), and the blood glucose measurement should be repeated. Values of less than 110 mg/dL are considered normal. Values greater than 140 mg/dL are indicative of DM. Glycosylated hemoglobin should be measured to determine the extent of hyperglycemia over the past 4 to 8 weeks. Values of fasting blood glucose between 111 and 140 mg/dL are designated impaired fasting glucose tolerance (IGT), and further testing should be performed to determine whether these individuals will eventually develop overt diabetes mellitus.

Although the oral glucose tolerance test (OGTT) is contraindicated for patients who clearly have diabetes mellitus, it is used for patients with fasting blood glucose in the IGT range (between 115 and 140 mg/dL). In the OGTT, a nonpregnant patient who has fasted overnight drinks 75 g glucose in an aqueous solution. Blood samples are drawn before the oral glucose load and at 30, 60, 90, and 120 minutes thereafter. If any one of the 30-, 60-, and 90-minute samples and the 120-minute sample are greater than 200 mg/dL, overt DM is indicated.

The diagnosis of IGT and the more severe form of glucose intolerance (DM) is based on blood glucose levels because no more specific characteristic for the disorder exists. The distinction between IGT and DM is clouded by the fact that a patient's blood glucose level may vary significantly with serial testing over time under the same conditions of diet and activity.

The renal tubular transport maximum in the average healthy subject is such that glucose will not appear in the urine until the blood glucose level exceeds 180 mg/dL. As a result, reagent tapes (Tes-Tape or Dextrostix) designed to detect the presence of glucose in the urine are not sensitive enough to establish a diagnosis of early DM.

I. GLUCOSE METABOLISM IN THE LIVER

Glucose serves as a fuel for most tissues of the body. It is the major fuel for certain tissues such as the brain and red blood cells. After a meal, food is the source of blood glucose. The liver oxidizes glucose and stores the excess as glycogen. The liver also uses the pathway of glycolysis to convert glucose to pyruvate, which provides carbon for the synthesis of fatty acids. Glycerol 3-phosphate, produced from glycolytic intermediates, combines with fatty acids to form triacylglycerols, which are secreted into the blood in very-low-density lipoproteins (VLDL; further explained in Chapter 32). During fasting, the liver releases glucose into the blood, so that glucose-dependent tissues do not suffer from a lack of energy. Two mechanisms are involved in this process: glycogenolysis and gluconeogenesis. Hormones, particularly insulin and glucagon, dictate whether glucose flows through glycolysis or whether the reactions are reversed and glucose is produced via gluconeogenesis.

II. GLUCONEOGENESIS

Gluconeogenesis, the process by which glucose is synthesized from noncarbohydrate precursors, occurs mainly in the liver under fasting conditions. Under the more extreme conditions of starvation, the kidney cortex also may produce glucose. For the most part, the glucose produced by the kidney cortex is used by the kidney medulla, but some may enter the bloodstream.

Starting with pyruvate, most of the steps of gluconeogenesis are simply reversals of those of glycolysis (Fig. 31.3). In fact, these pathways differ at only three points. Enzymes involved in catalyzing these steps are regulated so that either glycolysis or gluconeogenesis predominates, depending on physiologic conditions.

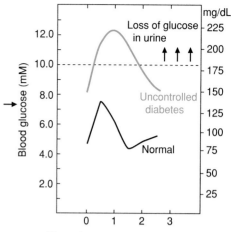

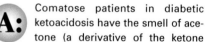
Time after oral glucose load (hours)

 Comatose patients in diabetic ketoacidosis have the smell of acetone (a derivative of the ketone body acetoacetate) on their breath. In addition, DKA patients have deep, relatively rapid respirations typical of acidotic patients (Kussmaul respirations). These respirations result from an acidosis-induced stimulation of the respiratory center in the brain. More CO_2 is exhaled in an attempt to reduce the amount of acid in the body: $H^+ + HCO_3^- \rightarrow H_2CO_3 \rightarrow H_2O + CO_2$ (exhaled).

The severe hyperglycemia of DKA also causes an osmotic diuresis (i.e., glucose entering the urine carries water with it), which, in turn, causes a contraction of blood volume. Volume depletion may be aggravated by vomiting, which is common in patients with DKA. DKA may cause dehydration (dry skin), a low blood pressure, and a rapid heartbeat. These respiratory and hemodynamic alterations are not seen in patients with hypoglycemic coma. The flushed, wet skin of hypoglycemic coma is in contrast to the dry skin observed in DKA.

 Glucocorticoids are naturally occurring steroid hormones. In humans, the major glucocorticoid is cortisol. Glucocorticoids are produced in the adrenal cortex in response to various types of stress (see Chapter 43). One of their actions is to stimulate the degradation of muscle protein. Thus, increased amounts of amino acids become available as substrates for gluconeogenesis. **Emma Wheezer** noted muscle weakness, a result of the muscle-degrading action of the synthetic glucocorticoid dexamethasone, which she was taking for its anti-inflammatory effects.

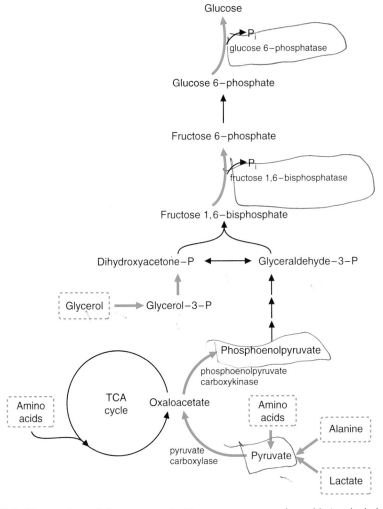

Fig. 31.3. Key reactions of gluconeogenesis. The precursors are amino acids (particularly alanine), lactate, and glycerol. Heavy arrows indicate steps that differ from those of glycolysis.

Because ethanol metabolism only gives rise to acetyl-CoA, the carbons of ethanol cannot be used for gluconeogenesis.

Most of the steps of gluconeogenesis use the same enzymes that catalyze the process of glycolysis. The flow of carbon, of course, is in the reverse direction. Three reaction sequences of gluconeogenesis differ from the corresponding steps of glycolysis. They involve the conversion of pyruvate to phosphoenolpyruvate (PEP) and the reactions that remove phosphate from fructose 1,6-bisphosphate to form fructose 6-phosphate and from glucose 6-phosphate to form glucose (see Fig. 31.3). The conversion of pyruvate to PEP is catalyzed during gluconeogenesis by a series of enzymes instead of the single enzyme used for glycolysis. The reactions that remove phosphate from fructose 1,6-bisphosphate and from glucose 6-phosphate each use single enzymes that differ from the corresponding enzymes of glycolysis. Although phosphate is added during glycolysis by kinases, which use adenosine triphosphate (ATP), it is removed during gluconeogenesis by phosphatases that release P_i via hydrolysis reactions.

A. Precursors for Gluconeogenesis

The three major carbon sources for gluconeogenesis in humans are lactate, glycerol, and amino acids, particularly alanine. Lactate is produced by anaerobic glycolysis in tissues such as exercising muscle or red blood cells, as well as by adipocytes during the fed state. Glycerol is released from adipose stores of triacylglycerol, and amino acids come mainly from amino acid pools in muscle, where they may be obtained by degradation of muscle protein. Alanine, the major gluconeogenic amino acid, is produced in the muscle from other amino acids and from glucose (see Chapter 38).

B. Formation of Gluconeogenic Intermediates from Carbon Sources

The carbon sources for gluconeogenesis form pyruvate, intermediates of the tricarboxylic acid (TCA) cycle, or intermediates common both to glycolysis and gluconeogenesis.

1. LACTATE, AMINO ACIDS, AND GLYCEROL

Pyruvate is produced in the liver from the gluconeogenic precursors lactate and alanine. Lactate dehydrogenase oxidizes lactate to pyruvate, generating NADH (Fig. 31.4A), and alanine aminotransferase converts alanine to pyruvate (see Fig. 31.4B).

Although alanine is the major gluconeogenic amino acid, other amino acids, such as serine, serve as carbon sources for the synthesis of glucose because they also form pyruvate, the substrate for the initial step in the process. Some amino acids form intermediates of the TCA cycle (see Chapter 20), which can enter the gluconeogenic pathway.

The carbons of glycerol are gluconeogenic because they form dihydroxyacetone phosphate (DHAP), a glycolytic intermediate (see Fig. 31.4C)

2. PROPIONATE

Fatty acids with an odd number of carbon atoms, which are obtained mainly from vegetables in the diet, produce propionyl CoA from the three carbons at the ω-end of the chain (see Chapter 23). These carbons are relatively minor precursors of glucose in humans. Propionyl CoA is converted to methylmalonyl CoA, which is rearranged to form succinyl CoA, a 4-carbon intermediate of the TCA cycle that can be used for gluconeogenesis. The remaining carbons of an odd-chain fatty acid form acetyl CoA, from which no net synthesis of glucose occurs.

β-Oxidation of fatty acids produces acetyl CoA. Because the pyruvate dehydrogenase reaction is thermodynamically and kinetically irreversible, acetyl CoA does not form pyruvate for gluconeogenesis. Therefore, if acetyl CoA is to produce glucose, it must enter the TCA cycle and be converted to malate. For every two carbons of acetyl CoA that are converted to malate, two carbons are released as CO_2: one in the reaction catalyzed by isocitrate dehydrogenase and the other in the reaction catalyzed by α-ketoglutarate dehydrogenase. Therefore, there is no *net* synthesis of glucose from acetyl CoA.

In a fatty acid with 19 carbons, how many carbons (and which ones) form glucose?

Excessive ethanol metabolism will block the production of gluconeogenic precursors. Cells have limited amounts of NAD, which exist either as NAD^+ or as NADH. As the levels of NADH rise, those of NAD^+ fall, and the ratio of the concentrations of NADH and NAD^+ ($[NADH]/[NAD^+]$) increases. In the presence of ethanol, which is very rapidly oxidized in the liver, the $[NADH]/[NAD^+]$ ratio is much higher than it is in the normal fasting liver. High levels of NADH drive the lactate dehydrogenase reaction toward lactate. Therefore, lactate cannot enter the gluconeogenic pathway, and pyruvate that is generated from alanine is converted to lactate. Because glycerol is oxidized by NAD^+ during its conversion to DHAP, the conversion of glycerol to glucose is also inhibited when NADH levels are elevated. Consequently, the major precursors lactate, alanine, and glycerol are not used for gluconeogenesis under conditions in which alcohol metabolism is high.

$$CH_3 - CH_2 - OH$$
Ethanol

NAD⁺

NADH + H⁺

$$CH_3 - \overset{\overset{\displaystyle O}{\|}}{CH}$$

Acetaldehyde

NAD⁺

NADH + H⁺

$$CH_3 - \overset{\overset{\displaystyle O}{\|}}{C} - OH$$

Acetate

In some species, propionate is a major source of carbon for gluconeogenesis. Ruminants can produce massive amounts of glucose from propionate. In cows, the cellulose in grass is converted to propionate by bacteria in the rumen. This substrate is then used to generate more than 5 lb glucose each day by the process of gluconeogenesis.

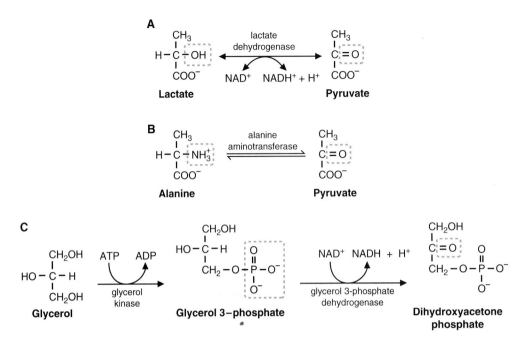

Fig. 31.4. Metabolism of gluconeogenic precursors. A. Conversion of lactate to pyruvate. B. Conversion of alanine to pyruvate. In this reaction, alanine aminotransferase transfers the amino group of alanine to α-ketoglutarate to form glutamate. The coenzyme for this reaction, pyridoxal phosphate, accepts and donates the amino group. C. Conversion of glycerol to dihydroxyacetone phosphate.

Amino acids that form intermediates of the TCA cycle are converted to malate, which enters the cytosol and is converted to oxaloacetate, which proceeds through gluconeogenesis to form glucose. When excessive amounts of ethanol are ingested, elevated NADH levels inhibit the conversion of malate to oxaloacetate in the cytosol. Therefore, carbons from amino acids that form intermediates of the TCA cycle cannot be converted to glucose as readily.

A: Only the three carbons at the ω-end of an odd chain fatty acid that form propionyl CoA are converted to glucose. The remaining 16 carbons of a fatty acid with 19 carbons form acetyl CoA, which does not form any net glucose.

C. Pathway of Gluconeogenesis

Gluconeogenesis occurs by a pathway that reverses many, but not all, of the steps of glycolysis.

1.   CONVERSION OF PYRUVATE TO PHOSPHOENOLPYRUVATE

In glycolysis, PEP is converted to pyruvate by pyruvate kinase. In gluconeogenesis, a series of steps are required to accomplish the reversal of this reaction (Fig. 31.5). Pyruvate is carboxylated by pyruvate carboxylase to form oxaloacetate. This enzyme, which requires biotin, is the catalyst of an anaplerotic (refilling) reaction of the TCA cycle (see Chapter 20). In gluconeogenesis, this reaction replenishes the oxaloacetate that is used for the synthesis of glucose (Fig. 31.6).

The CO_2 that was added to pyruvate to form oxaloacetate is released in the reaction catalyzed by phosphoenolpyruvate carboxykinase (PEPCK), which generates PEP (Fig. 31.7A). For this reaction, GTP provides a source of energy as well as the phosphate group of PEP. Pyruvate carboxylase is found in mitochondria. In various species, PEPCK is located either in the cytosol or in mitochondria, or it is distributed between these two compartments. In humans, the enzyme is distributed about equally in each compartment.

Oxaloacetate, generated from pyruvate by pyruvate carboxylase or from amino acids that form intermediates of the TCA cycle, does not readily cross the mitochondrial membrane. It is either decarboxylated to form PEP by the mitochondrial PEPCK or it is converted to malate or aspartate (see Figs. 31.7B and 31.7C). The conversion of oxaloacetate to malate requires NADH. PEP, malate, and aspartate can be transported into the cytosol.

After malate or aspartate traverse the mitochondrial membrane (acting as carriers of oxaloacetate) and enter the cytosol, they are reconverted to oxaloacetate by reversal of the reactions given above (see Figs. 31.7B and C). The conversion of malate to oxaloacetate generates NADH. Whether oxaloacetate is transported

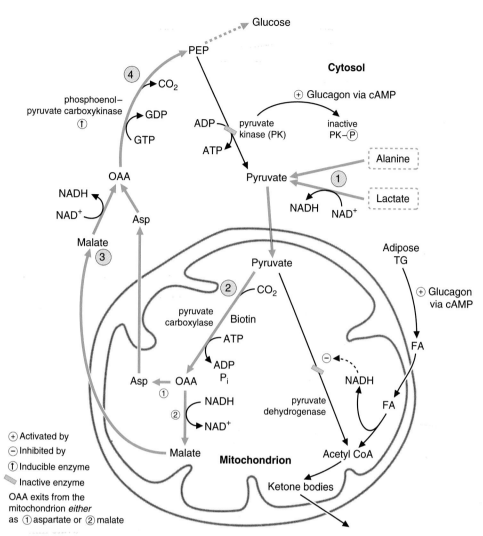

Fig. 31.5. Conversion of pyruvate to phosphoenolpyruvate (PEP). Follow the shaded circled numbers on the diagram, starting with the precursors alanine and lactate. The first step is the conversion of alanine and lactate to pyruvate. Pyruvate then enters the mitochondria and is converted to OAA (circle 2) by pyruvate carboxylase. Pyruvate dehydrogenase has been inactivated by both the NADH and acetyl-CoA generated from fatty acid oxidation, which allows oxaloacetate production for gluconeogenesis. The oxaloacetate formed in the mitochondria is converted to either malate or aspartate to enter the cytoplasm via the malate/aspartate shuttle. Once in the cytoplasm the malate or aspartate is converted back into oxaloacetate (circle 3), and phosphoenolpyruvate carboxykinase will convert it to PEP (circle 4). The white circled numbers are alternate routes for exit of carbon from the mitochondrion using the malate/aspartate shuttle. OAA = oxaloacetate; FA = fatty acid; TG = triacylglycerol.

across the mitochondrial membrane as malate or aspartate depends on the need for reducing equivalents in the cytosol. NADH is required to reduce 1,3-bisphospho-glycerate to glyceraldehyde 3-phosphate during gluconeogenesis.

Oxaloacetate, produced from malate or aspartate in the cytosol, is converted to PEP by the cytosolic PEPCK (see Fig. 31.7A).

2. CONVERSION OF PHOSPHOENOLPYRUVATE TO FRUCTOSE 1,6-BISPHOSPHATE

The remaining steps of gluconeogenesis occur in the cytosol (Fig. 31.8). Starting with PEP as a substrate, the steps of glycolysis are reversed to form glyceraldehyde 3-phosphate. For every two molecules of glyceraldehyde 3-phosphate that are formed, one is converted to dihydroxyacetone phosphate (DHAP). These two triose

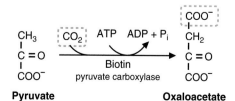

Fig. 31.6. Conversion of pyruvate to oxaloacetate.

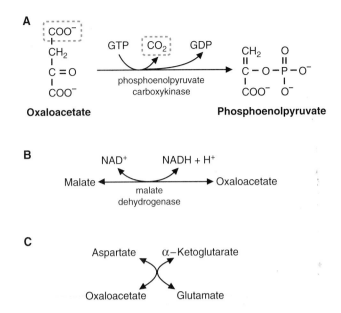

Fig. 31.7. The generation of PEP from gluconeogenic precursors. A. Conversion of oxaloacetate to phosphoenolpyruvate, using PEP carboxykinase. B. Interconversion of oxaloacetate and malate. C. Transamination of aspartate to form oxaloacetate. Note that the cytosolic reaction is the reverse of the mitochondrial reaction as shown in Figure 31.5.

phosphates, DHAP and glyceraldehyde 3-phosphate, condense to form fructose 1,6-bisphosphate by a reversal of the aldolase reaction.

Because glycerol forms DHAP, it enters the gluconeogenic pathway at this level.

3. CONVERSION OF FRUCTOSE 1,6-BISPHOSPHATE TO FRUCTOSE 6-PHOSPHATE

The enzyme fructose 1,6-bisphosphatase releases inorganic phosphate from fructose 1,6-bisphosphate to form fructose 6-phosphate. This is not a reversal of the PFK-1 reaction; ATP is not produced when the phosphate is removed from the 1 position of fructose 1,6-bisphosphate, because that is a low-energy phosphate bond. Rather, inorganic phosphate is released in this hydrolysis reaction. In the next reaction of gluconeogenesis, fructose 6-phosphate is converted to glucose 6-phosphate by the same isomerase used in glycolysis (phosphoglucoisomerase).

4. CONVERSION OF GLUCOSE 6-PHOSPHATE TO GLUCOSE

Glucose 6-phosphatase hydrolyzes P_i from glucose 6-phosphate, and free glucose is released into the blood. As with fructose 1,6-bisphosphatase, this is not a reversal of the glucokinase reaction, because the phosphate bond in glucose 6-phosphate is a low-energy bond, and ATP is not generated at this step.

Glucose 6-phosphatase is located in the membrane of the endoplasmic reticulum. It is used not only in gluconeogenesis, but also to produce blood glucose from the breakdown of liver glycogen.

D. Regulation of Gluconeogenesis

Although gluconeogenesis occurs during fasting, it is also stimulated during prolonged exercise, by a high-protein diet, and under conditions of stress. The factors that promote the overall flow of carbon from pyruvate to glucose include the availability of substrate and changes in the activity or amount of certain key enzymes of glycolysis and gluconeogenesis.

Al Martini had not eaten for 3 days, so he had no dietary source of glucose, and his liver glycogen stores were essentially depleted. He was solely dependent on gluconeogenesis to maintain his blood glucose levels. One of the consequences of ethanol ingestion and the subsequent rise in NADH levels is that the major carbon sources for gluconeogenesis cannot readily be converted to glucose. After his alcoholic binges, Mr. Martini became hypoglycemic. His blood glucose was 28 mg/dL.

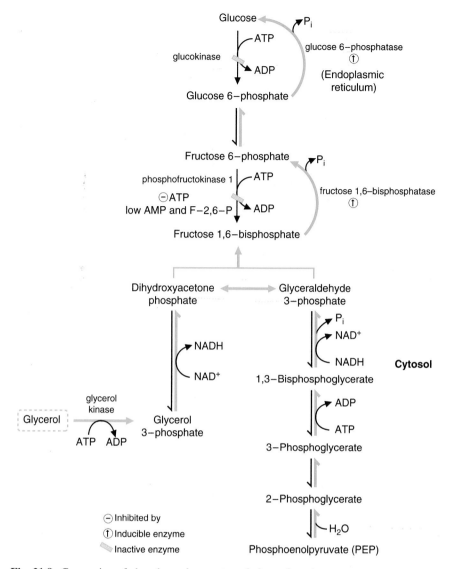

Fig. 31.8. Conversion of phosphoenolpyruvate and glycerol to glucose.

1.   AVAILABILITY OF SUBSTRATE

Gluconeogenesis is stimulated by the flow of its major substrates from peripheral tissues to the liver. Glycerol is released from adipose tissue whenever the levels of insulin are low and the levels of glucagon or the "stress" hormones, epinephrine and cortisol (a glucocorticoid), are elevated in the blood (see Chapter 26). Lactate is produced by muscle during exercise and by red blood cells. Amino acids are released from muscle whenever insulin is low or when cortisol is elevated. Amino acids are also available for gluconeogenesis when the dietary intake of protein is high and intake of carbohydrate is low.

2.   ACTIVITY OR AMOUNT OF KEY ENZYMES

Three sequences in the pathway of gluconeogenesis are regulated:

1. pyruvate → phosphoenolpyruvate
2. fructose 1,6-bisphosphate → fructose 6-phosphate
3. glucose 6-phosphate → glucose.

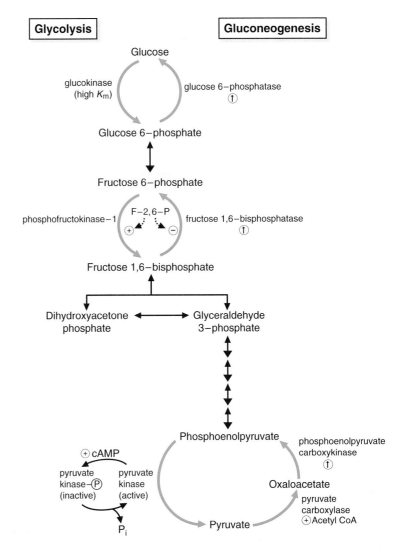

Fig. 31.9. Enzymes involved in regulating the substrate cycles of glycolysis and gluconeogenesis. Heavy arrows indicate the three substrate cycles. F-2,6-P, fructose 2,6-bisphosphate; +, activated by; -, inhibited by; circled ↑, inducible enzyme.

These steps correspond to those in glycolysis that are catalyzed by regulatory enzymes. The enzymes involved in these steps of gluconeogenesis differ from those that catalyze the reverse reactions in glycolysis. The net flow of carbon, whether from glucose to pyruvate (glycolysis) or from pyruvate to glucose (gluconeogenesis), depends on the relative activity or amount of these glycolytic or gluconeogenic enzymes (Fig. 31.9 and Table 31.1).

3.   CONVERSION OF PYRUVATE TO PHOSPHOENOLPYRUVATE

Pyruvate, a key substrate for gluconeogenesis, is derived from lactate and amino acids, particularly alanine. Pyruvate is not converted to acetyl CoA under conditions favoring gluconeogenesis because pyruvate dehydrogenase is relatively inactive. Instead, pyruvate is converted to oxaloacetate by pyruvate carboxylase. Subsequently, oxaloacetate is converted to PEP by PEPCK. Because of the activity state of the enzymes discussed in subsequent sections, PEP reverses the steps of glycolysis, ultimately forming glucose.

Pyruvate dehydrogenase is inactive. Under conditions of fasting, insulin levels are low, and glucagon levels are elevated. Consequently, fatty acids and glycerol are

PEPCK is an example of an inducible enzyme. The gene for the cytosolic form of the enzyme contains regulatory sequences in its 5′-flanking region. cAMP, which is produced as a result of the binding of hormones such as glucagon or epinephrine to receptors on the cell surface, causes one of these sequences to be activated. Glucocorticoids affect a different regulatory sequence. cAMP or glucocorticoids independently cause increased transcription of the PEPCK gene. The mRNA produced during transcription travels to the cytosol combines with ribosomes and is translated, producing increased amounts of the enzyme PEPCK.

Table 31.1. Regulation of Enzymes of Glycolysis and Gluconeogenesis in Liver

A. Glycolytic Enzymes	Mechanism
Pyruvate kinase	Activated by F-1, 6-P
	Inhibited by ATP, alanine
	Inhibited by phosphorylation (glucagon and epinephrine lead to an increase in cAMP levels, which activates protein kinase A)
Phosphofructokinase-1	Activated by F-2,6-P, AMP
	Inhibited by ATP, citrate
Glucokinase	High K_m for glucose
	Induced by insulin

B. Gluconeogenic Enzymes	Mechanism
Pyruvate carboxylase	Activated by acetyl CoA
Phosphoenolpyruvate carboxykinase	Induced by glucagon, epinephrine, glucocorticoids
	Repressed by insulin
Fructose 1,6-bisphosphatase	Inhibited by F-2,6-P, AMP
	Induced during fasting
Glucose 6-phosphatase	Induced during fasting

released from the triacylglycerol stores of adipose tissue. Fatty acids travel to the liver, where they undergo β-oxidation, producing acetyl CoA, NADH, and ATP. As a consequence, the concentration of ADP decreases. These changes result in the phosphorylation of pyruvate dehydrogenase to the inactive form. Therefore, pyruvate is not converted to acetyl CoA.

Pyruvate carboxylase is active. Acetyl CoA, which is produced by oxidation of fatty acids, activates pyruvate carboxylase. Therefore, pyruvate, derived from lactate or alanine, is converted to oxaloacetate.

Phosphoenolpyruvate carboxykinase is induced. Oxaloacetate produces PEP in a reaction catalyzed by PEPCK. Cytosolic PEPCK is an inducible enzyme, which means that the quantity of the enzyme in the cell increases because of increased transcription of its gene and increased translation of its mRNA. The major inducer is cyclic adenosine monophosphate (cAMP), which is increased by hormones that activate adenylate cyclase. Adenylate cyclase produces cAMP from ATP. Glucagon is the hormone that causes cAMP to rise during fasting, whereas epinephrine acts during exercise or stress. cAMP activates protein kinase A, which phosphorylates a set of specific transcription factors (CREB) that stimulate transcription of the PEPCK gene (see Chapter 16 and Fig. 16.18). Increased synthesis of mRNA for PEPCK results in increased synthesis of the enzyme. Cortisol, the major human glucocorticoid, also induces PEPCK.

Pyruvate kinase is inactive. When glucagon is elevated, pyruvate kinase is phosphorylated and inactivated by a mechanism involving cAMP and protein kinase A. Therefore, PEP is not reconverted to pyruvate. Rather, it continues along the pathway of gluconeogenesis. If PEP were reconverted to pyruvate, these substrates would simply cycle, causing a net loss of energy with no net generation of useful products. The inactivation of pyruvate kinase prevents such futile cycling and promotes the net synthesis of glucose.

4. CONVERSION OF FRUCTOSE 1,6-BISPHOSPHATE TO FRUCTOSE 6-PHOSPHATE

The carbons of PEP reverse the steps of glycolysis, forming fructose 1,6-bisphosphate. Fructose 1,6-bisphosphatase acts on this bisphosphate to release inorganic phosphate and produce fructose 6-phosphate. A futile substrate cycle is prevented at

The mechanism of action of steroid hormones on glucose homeostasis differs from that of glucagon or epinephrine (see Chapters 16 and 26). Glucocorticoids are steroid hormones that stimulate gluconeogenesis, in part because they induce the synthesis of PEPCK. **Emma Wheezer** had elevated levels of blood glucose because she was being treated with large pharmacologic doses of dexamethasone, a potent synthetic glucocorticoid.

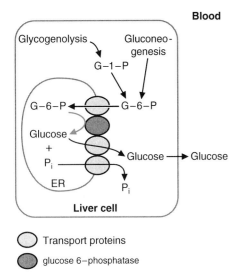

Fig. 31.10. Location and function of glucose 6-phosphatase. Glucose 6-phosphate travels on a transporter (shaded oval) into the endoplasmic reticulum (ER), where it is hydrolyzed by glucose 6-phosphatase (black oval) to glucose and P_i. These products travel back to the cytosol on transporters (shaded ovals).

Glucose 6-phosphatase is used in both glycogenolysis and gluconeogenesis.

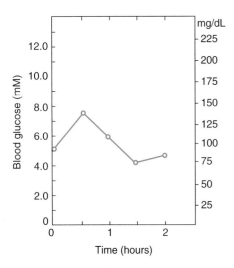

Fig. 31.11. Blood glucose concentrations at various times after a meal.

this step because, under conditions that favor gluconeogenesis, the concentrations of the compounds that activate the glycolytic enzyme PFK-1 are low. These same compounds, fructose 2,6-bisphosphate (whose levels are regulated by insulin and glucagon) and AMP, are allosteric inhibitors of fructose 1,6-bisphosphatase. When the concentrations of these allosteric effectors are low, PFK-1 is less active, fructose 1,6-bisphosphatase is more active, and the net flow of carbon is toward fructose 6-phosphate and, thus, toward glucose. The synthesis of fructose 1,6-bisphosphatase is also induced during fasting.

5. CONVERSION OF GLUCOSE 6-PHOSPHATE TO GLUCOSE

Glucose 6-phosphatase catalyzes the conversion of glucose 6-phosphate to glucose, which is released from the liver cell (Fig. 31.10). The glycolytic enzyme glucokinase, which catalyzes the reverse reaction, is relatively inactive during gluconeogenesis. Glucokinase, which has a high $S_{0.5}$ (K_m) for glucose (see Fig. 9.3), is not very active during fasting because the blood glucose level is lower (approximately 5 mM) than the $S_{0.5}$ of the enzyme.

Glucokinase is also an inducible enzyme. The concentration of the enzyme increases in the fed state, when blood glucose and insulin levels are elevated, and decreases in the fasting state, when glucose and insulin are low.

E. Energy Is Required for the Synthesis of Glucose

During the gluconeogenic reactions, 6 moles of high-energy phosphate bonds are cleaved. Two moles of pyruvate are required for the synthesis of 1 mole of glucose. As 2 moles of pyruvate are carboxylated by pyruvate carboxylase, 2 moles of ATP are hydrolyzed. PEPCK requires 2 moles of GTP (the equivalent of 2 moles of ATP) to convert 2 moles of oxaloacetate to 2 moles of PEP. An additional 2 moles of ATP are used when 2 moles of 3-phosphoglycerate are phosphorylated, forming 2 moles of 1,3-bisphosphoglycerate. Energy in the form of reducing equivalents (NADH) is also required for the conversion of 1,3-bisphosphoglycerate to glyceraldehyde 3-phosphate. Under fasting conditions, the energy required for gluconeogenesis is obtained from β-oxidation of fatty acids.

III. CHANGES IN BLOOD GLUCOSE LEVELS AFTER A MEAL

The metabolic transitions that occur as a person eats a meal and progresses through the various stages of fasting have been described in detail in the previous chapters. This chapter summarizes the concepts presented in these previous chapters. Because a thorough understanding of these concepts is so critical to medicine, a summary is not only warranted but essential.

After a high-carbohydrate meal, blood glucose rises from a fasting level of approximately 80 to 100 mg/dL (~5 mM) to a level of approximately 120 to 140 mg/dL (8 mM) within a period of 30 minutes to 1 hour (Fig. 31.11). The concentration of glucose in the blood then begins to decrease, returning to the fasting range by approximately 2 hours after the meal (see also Chapter 26).

Blood glucose levels increase as dietary glucose is digested and absorbed. The values go no higher than approximately 140 mg/dL in a normal, healthy person because tissues take up glucose from the blood, storing it for subsequent use and oxidizing it for energy. After the meal is digested and absorbed, blood glucose levels decline because cells continue to metabolize glucose.

If blood glucose levels continued to rise after a meal, the high concentration of glucose would cause the release of water from tissues as a result of the osmotic effect of glucose. Tissues would become dehydrated, and their function would be affected. A hyperosmolar coma could result from dehydration of the brain.

Conversely, if blood glucose levels continued to drop after a meal, tissues that depend on glucose would suffer from a lack of energy. If blood glucose levels dropped abruptly, the brain would not be able to produce an adequate amount of ATP. Light-headedness and dizziness would result, followed by drowsiness and, eventually, coma. Red blood cells would not be able to produce enough ATP to maintain the integrity of their membranes. Hemolysis of these cells would decrease the transport of oxygen to the tissues of the body. Eventually, all tissues that rely on oxygen for energy production would fail to perform their normal functions. If the problem were severe enough, death could result.

Devastating consequences of glucose excess or insufficiency are normally avoided because the body is able to regulate its blood glucose levels. As the concentration of blood glucose approaches the normal fasting range of 80 to 100 mg/dL roughly 2 hours after a meal, the process of glycogenolysis is activated in the liver. Liver glycogen is the primary source of blood glucose during the first few hours of fasting. Subsequently, gluconeogenesis begins to play a role as an additional source of blood glucose. The carbon for gluconeogenesis, a process that occurs in the liver, is supplied by other tissues. Exercising muscle and red blood cells provide lactate through glycolysis; muscle also provides amino acids by degradation of protein; and glycerol is released from adipose tissue as triacylglycerol stores are mobilized.

Even during a prolonged fast, blood glucose levels do not decrease dramatically. After 5 to 6 weeks of starvation, blood glucose levels decrease to only approximately 65 mg/dL (Table 31.2).

A. Blood Glucose Levels in the Fed State

The major factors involved in regulating blood glucose levels are the blood glucose concentration itself and hormones, particularly insulin and glucagon.

As blood glucose levels rise after a meal, the increased glucose concentration stimulates the β cells of the pancreas to release insulin (Fig. 31.12). Certain amino acids, particularly arginine and leucine, also stimulate insulin release from the pancreas.

Blood levels of glucagon, which is secreted by the α cells of the pancreas, may increase or decrease, depending on the content of the meal. Glucagon levels decrease in response to a high-carbohydrate meal, but they increase in response to a high-protein meal. After a typical mixed meal containing carbohydrate, protein, and fat, glucagon levels remain relatively constant, whereas insulin levels increase (Fig. 31.13).

Table 31.2. Blood Glucose Levels at Various Stages of Fasting

Glucose (mg/dL)	
Glucose, 700 g/day IV	100
Fasting, 12 hr	80
Starvation, 3 days	70
Starvation, 5–6 weeks	65

Source of data: Ruderman NB, Aoki TT, Cahill GF Jr. Gluconeogenesis and its disorders in man. In: Hanson RW, Mehlman MA, eds. Gluconeogenesis: Its Regulation in Mammalian Species. New York, John Wiley. 1976:517.

When **Di Abietes** inadvertently injected an excessive amount of insulin, she caused an acute reduction in her blood glucose levels 4 to 5 hours later while she was asleep. Had she been awake, she would have first experienced symptoms caused by a hypoglycemia-induced hyperactivity of her sympathetic nervous system (e.g., sweating, tremulousness, palpitations). Eventually, as her hypoglycemia became more profound, she would have experienced symptoms of "neuroglycopenia" (inadequate glucose supply to the brain), such as confusion, speech disturbances, emotional instability, possible seizure activity, and, finally, coma. While sleeping, she had reached this neuroglycopenic stage of hypoglycemia and could not be aroused at 6:00 AM.

Ann O' Rexia, whose intake of glucose and of glucose precursors has been severely restricted, has not developed any of these manifestations. Her lack of hypoglycemic symptoms can be explained by the very gradual reduction of her blood glucose levels as a consequence of near starvation and her ability to maintain blood glucose levels within an acceptable fasting range through hepatic gluconeogenesis. In addition, lipolysis of adipose triacylglycerols produces fatty acids, which are used as fuel and converted to ketone bodies by the liver. The oxidation of fatty acids and ketone bodies by the brain and muscle reduces the need for blood glucose.

In **Di Abiete's** case, the excessive dose of insulin inhibited lipolysis and ketone body synthesis, so these alternative fuels were not available to spare blood glucose. The rapidity with which hypoglycemia was induced could not be compensated for quickly enough by hepatic gluconeogenesis, which was inhibited by the insulin, and hypoglycemia ensued.

A stat finger stick revealed that Di's capillary blood glucose level was less than 20 mg/dL. An intravenous infusion of a 50% solution of glucose was started, and her blood glucose level was determined frequently. When Di regained consciousness, the intravenous solution was eventually changed to 10% glucose. After 6 hours, her blood glucose levels stayed in the upper normal range, and she was able to tolerate oral feedings. She was transferred to the metabolic unit for overnight monitoring. By the next morning, her previous diabetes treatment regimen was reestablished. The reasons that she had developed hypoglycemic coma were explained to Di, and she was discharged to the care of her family doctor.

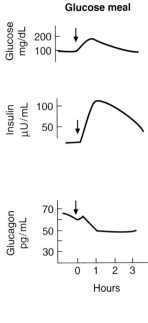

Glucose meal

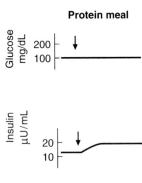

Protein meal

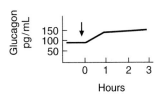

Fig. 31.12. Blood glucose, insulin, and glucagon levels after a high-carbohydrate and a high-protein meal.

1. FATE OF DIETARY GLUCOSE IN THE LIVER

After a meal, the liver oxidizes glucose to meet its immediate energy needs. Any excess glucose is converted to stored fuels. Glycogen is synthesized and stored in the liver, and glucose is converted to fatty acids and to the glycerol moiety that reacts with the fatty acids to produce triacylglycerols. These triacylglycerols are packaged in very-low-density lipoproteins (VLDL) and transported to adipose tissue, where the fatty acids are stored in adipose triacylglycerols.

Regulatory mechanisms control the conversion of glucose to stored fuels. As the concentration of glucose increases in the hepatic portal vein, the concentration of glucose in the liver may increase from the fasting level of 80 to 100 mg/dL (~5 mM) to a concentration of 180 to 360 mg/dL (10–20 mM). Consequently, the velocity of the glucokinase reaction increases because this enzyme has a high $S_{0.5}$ (K_m) for glucose (Fig. 31.14). Glucokinase is also induced by a high-carbohydrate diet; the quantity of the enzyme increases in response to elevated insulin levels.

Insulin promotes the storage of glucose as glycogen by countering the effects of glucagon-stimulated phosphorylation. The response to insulin activates the phosphatases that dephosphorylate glycogen synthase (which leads to glycogen synthase activation) and glycogen phosphorylase (which leads to inhibition of the enzyme) (Fig. 31.15A). Insulin also promotes the synthesis of the triacylglycerols that are released from the liver into the blood as VLDL. The regulatory mechanisms for this process are described in Chapter 33.

2. FATE OF DIETARY GLUCOSE IN PERIPHERAL TISSUES

Almost every cell in the body oxidizes glucose for energy. Certain critical tissues, particularly the brain, other nervous tissue, and red blood cells, especially depend on glucose for their energy supply. The brain requires approximately 150 g glucose per day. In addition, approximately 40 g/day glucose is required by other glucose-dependent tissues. Furthermore, all tissues require glucose for the pentose phosphate pathway, and many tissues use glucose for synthesis of glycoproteins and other carbohydrate-containing compounds.

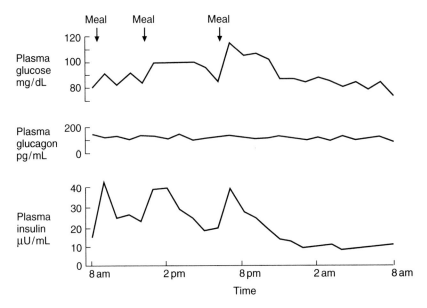

Fig. 31.13. Blood glucose, insulin, and glucagon levels over a 24-hour period in a normal person eating mixed meals. Reprinted with permission from Tasaka Y, Sekine M, Wakatsuki M, et al. Horm Metab Res 1975;7:206. Copyright © Thieme Medical Publishers, Inc.

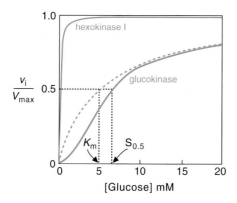

Fig. 31.14. Velocity of the glucokinase reaction.

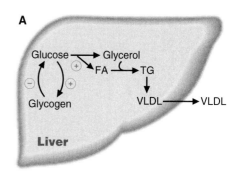

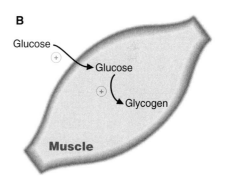

Insulin stimulates the transport of glucose into adipose and muscle cells by promoting the recruitment of glucose transporters to the cell membrane (see Fig. 31.15C). Other tissues, such as the liver, brain, and red blood cells, have a different type of glucose transporter that is not as significantly affected by insulin.

In muscle, glycogen is synthesized after a meal by a mechanism similar to that in the liver (see Fig. 31.15B). Metabolic differences exist between these tissues (see Chapter 28), but, in essence, insulin stimulates glycogen synthesis in resting muscle as it does in the liver. A key difference between muscle and liver is that insulin greatly stimulates the transport of glucose into muscle cells but only slightly stimulates its transport into liver cells.

3. RETURN OF BLOOD GLUCOSE TO FASTING LEVELS

After a meal has been digested and absorbed, blood glucose levels reach a peak and then begin to decline. The uptake of dietary glucose by cells, particularly those in the liver, muscle, and adipose tissue, lowers blood glucose levels. By 2 hours after a meal, blood glucose levels return to the normal fasting level of less than 140 mg/dL.

B. Blood Glucose Levels in the Fasting State

1. CHANGES IN INSULIN AND GLUCAGON LEVELS

During fasting, as blood glucose levels decrease, insulin levels decrease, and glucagon levels rise. These hormonal changes cause the liver to degrade glycogen by the process of glycogenolysis and to produce glucose by the process of gluconeogenesis so that blood glucose levels are maintained.

2. STIMULATION OF GLYCOGENOLYSIS

Within a few hours after a high-carbohydrate meal, glucagon levels begin to rise. Glucagon binds to cell surface receptors and activates adenylate cyclase, causing cAMP levels in liver cells to rise (Fig. 31.16). cAMP activates protein kinase A, which phosphorylates and inactivates glycogen synthase. Therefore, glycogen synthesis decreases.

At the same time, protein kinase A stimulates glycogen degradation by a two-step mechanism. Protein kinase A phosphorylates and activates phosphorylase kinase. This enzyme, in turn, phosphorylates and activates glycogen phosphorylase.

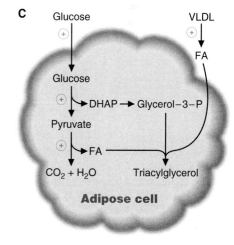

Fig. 31.15. Glucose metabolism in various tissues. A. Effect of insulin on glycogen synthesis and degradation and on VLDL synthesis in the liver. B. Glucose metabolism in resting muscle in the fed state. The transport of glucose into cells and the synthesis of glycogen are stimulated by insulin. C. Glucose metabolism in adipose tissue in the fed state. FA = fatty acids; DHAP = dihydroxyacetone phosphate. FA = fatty acids; TG = triacylglycerols; + = stimulated by insulin; − = inhibited by insulin.

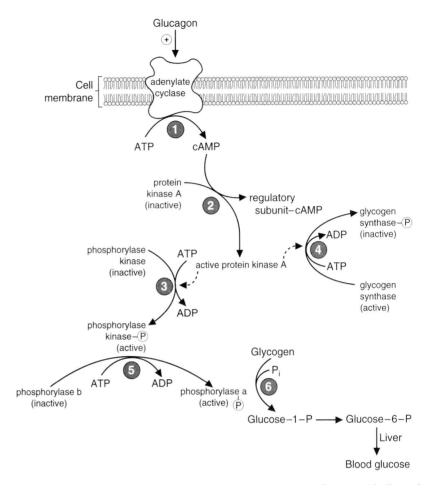

Fig. 31.16. Regulation of glycogenolysis in the liver by glucagon. 1. Glucagon binding to its receptor leads to the activation of adenylate cyclase, which leads to an increase in cAMP levels. 2. cAMP binds to the regulatory subunits of protein kinase A, thereby activating the catalytic subunit. 3. Active protein kinase A phosphorylates and activates phosphorylase kinase, while simultaneously inactivating glycogen synthase (4). 5. Active phosphorylase kinase converts glycogen phosphorylase b to glycogen phosphorylase a. 6. Phosphorylase a degrades glycogen, producing glucose 1-phosphate, which is converted to glucose 6-phosphate, then glucose, for export into the blood.

The pathophysiology leading to an elevation of blood glucose after a meal differs between patients with type 1 diabetes mellitus and those with type 2 diabetes mellitus. **Di Abietes,** who has type 1 disease, cannot secrete insulin adequately in response to a meal because of a defect in the β cells of her pancreas.

Ann Sulin, however, has type 2 disease. In this form of the disorder, the cause of glucose intolerance is more complex, involving at least a delay in the release of relatively appropriate amounts of insulin after a meal combined with a degree of resistance to the actions of insulin in skeletal muscle and adipocytes. Excessive hepatic gluconeogenesis occurs even though blood glucose levels are elevated.

Glycogen phosphorylase catalyzes the phosphorolysis of glycogen, producing glucose 1-phosphate, which is converted to glucose 6-phosphate. Dephosphorylation of glucose 6-phosphate by glucose 6-phosphatase produces free glucose, which then enters the blood.

3. STIMULATION OF GLUCONEOGENESIS

By 4 hours after a meal, the liver is supplying glucose to the blood not only by the process of glycogenolysis but also by the process of gluconeogenesis. Hormonal changes cause peripheral tissues to release precursors that provide carbon for gluconeogenesis, specifically lactate, amino acids, and glycerol.

Regulatory mechanisms promote the conversion of gluconeogenic precursors to glucose (Fig. 31.17). These mechanisms prevent the occurrence of potential futile cycles, which would continuously convert substrates to products while consuming energy but producing no useful result.

These regulatory mechanisms inactivate the glycolytic enzymes pyruvate kinase, phosphofructokinase-1 (PFK-1), and glucokinase during fasting and promote the flow of carbon to glucose via gluconeogenesis. These mechanisms operate at the three steps where glycolysis and gluconeogenesis differ:

1. Pyruvate (derived from lactate and alanine) is converted by the gluconeogenic pathway to phosphoenolpyruvate (PEP). PEP is not reconverted to pyruvate (a potential futile cycle) because glucagon-stimulated phosphorylation inactivates pyruvate kinase. Therefore, PEP reverses the steps of glycolysis and forms fructose 1,6-bisphosphate.

2. Fructose 1,6-bisphosphate is converted to fructose 6-phosphate by a bisphosphatase. Because the glycolytic enzyme PFK-1 is relatively inactive mainly as a result of low fructose 2,6-bisphosphate levels, fructose 6-phosphate is not converted back to fructose 1,6-bisphosphate, and a second potential futile cycle is avoided. The low fructose 2,6-bisphosphate levels are attributable in part to the phosphorylation of phosphofructokinase-2 by protein kinase A, which has been activated in response to glucagon. Fructose 6-phosphate is converted to glucose 6-phosphate.

3. Glucose 6-phosphate is dephosphorylated by glucose 6-phosphatase, forming free glucose. Because glucokinase has a high $S_{0.5}$ (K_m) for glucose, and glucose concentrations are relatively low in liver cells during fasting, glucose is released into the blood. Therefore, the third potential futile cycle does not occur.

Enzymes that participate in gluconeogenesis, but not in glycolysis, are active under fasting conditions. Pyruvate carboxylase is activated by acetyl CoA, derived from oxidation of fatty acids. Phosphoenolpyruvate carboxykinase, fructose 1,6-bisphosphatase, and glucose 6-phosphatase are induced; that is, the quantity of the enzymes increases. Fructose 1,6-bisphosphatase is also active because levels of fructose 2,6-bisphosphate, an inhibitor of the enzyme, are low.

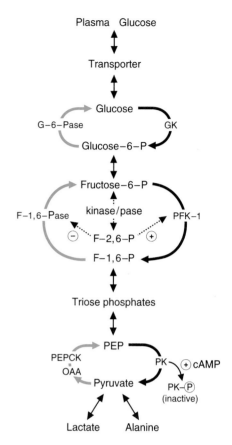

Fig. 31.17. Regulation of gluconeogenesis in the liver. GK = glucokinase; G-6-Pase = glucose 6-phosphatase; PK = pyruvate kinase; OAA = oxaloacetate; PEPCK = phosphoenolpyruvate carboxykinase; F-1,6-Pase = fructose 1,6-bisphosphatase; F-2,6-P = fructose 2,6-bisphosphate; PFK-1 = phosphofructokinase-1.

4. STIMULATION OF LIPOLYSIS

The hormonal changes that occur during fasting stimulate the breakdown of adipose triacylglycerols (see Chapters 3, 33, and 43). Consequently, fatty acids and glycerol are released into the blood (Fig. 31.18). Glycerol serves as a source of carbon for gluconeogenesis. Fatty acids become the major fuel of the body and are oxidized to CO_2 and H_2O by various tissues, which enables these tissues to decrease their utilization of glucose. Fatty acids are also oxidized to acetyl CoA in the liver to provide energy for gluconeogenesis. In a prolonged fast, acetyl CoA is converted to ketone bodies, which enter the blood and serve as an additional fuel source for the muscle and the brain.

C. Blood Glucose Levels during Prolonged Fasting (Starvation)

During prolonged fasting, a number of changes in fuel utilization occur. These changes cause tissues to use less glucose than they use during a brief fast and to use predominantly fuels derived from adipose triacylglycerols (i.e., fatty acids and their derivatives, the ketone bodies). Therefore, blood glucose levels do not decrease drastically. In fact, even after 5 to 6 weeks of starvation, blood glucose levels are still in the range of 65 mg/dL (Fig. 31.19, see Table 31.2).

The major change that occurs in starvation is a dramatic elevation of blood ketone body levels after 3 to 5 days of fasting (see Fig. 31.19). At these levels, the brain and other nervous tissues begin to use ketone bodies and, consequently, they oxidize less glucose, requiring roughly one third as much glucose (approximately 40 g/day) as under normal dietary conditions. As a result of reduced glucose utilization, the rate of gluconeogenesis in the liver decreases, as does the production of urea (see Fig. 31.19). Because in this stage of starvation amino acids, obtained

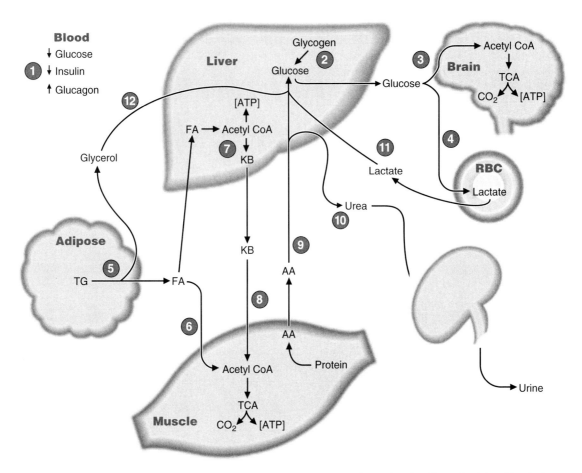

Fig. 31.18. Tissue interrelationships during fasting. 1. Blood glucose levels drop, decreasing insulin and raising blood glucagon levels. 2. Glycogenolysis is induced in the liver to raise blood glucose levels. 3. The brain uses the glucose released by the liver, as do the red blood cells (4). 5. Adipose tissues are induced to release free fatty acids and glycerol from stored triglycerides. 6. The muscle and liver use fatty acids for energy. 7. The liver converts fatty acid derived acetyl-CoA to ketone bodies for export, which the muscles (8) and brain can use for energy. 9. Protein turnover is induced in muscle, and amino acids leave the muscle and travel to the liver for use as gluconeogenic precursors. 10. The high rate of amino acid metabolism in the liver generates urea, which travels to the kidney for excretion. 11. Red blood cells produce lactate, which returns to the liver as a substrate for gluconeogenesis. 12. The glycenol released from adipose tissue is used by the liver set gluconeogenesis. KB = ketone bodies; FA = fatty acids; AA = amino acids; TG = triacylglycerols.

from the degradation of existing proteins, are the major gluconeogenic precursor, reducing glucose requirements in tissues reduces the rate of protein degradation, and, hence, the rate of urea formation. Protein from muscle and other tissues is therefore spared, because there is less need for amino acids for gluconeogenesis.

Body protein, particularly muscle protein, is not primarily a storage form of fuel in the same sense as glycogen or triacylglycerol; proteins have many functions beside fuel storage. For example, proteins function as enzymes, as structural proteins, and in muscle contraction. If tissue protein is degraded to too great an extent, body function can be severely compromised. If starvation continues and no other problems, such as infections, occur, a starving individual usually dies because of severe protein loss that causes malfunction of major organs, such as the heart. Therefore, the increase in ketone body levels that results in the sparing of body protein allows individuals to survive for extended periods without ingesting food.

D. Summary of Sources of Blood Glucose

Immediately after a meal, dietary carbohydrates serve as the major source of blood glucose (Fig. 31.20). As blood glucose levels return to the fasting range

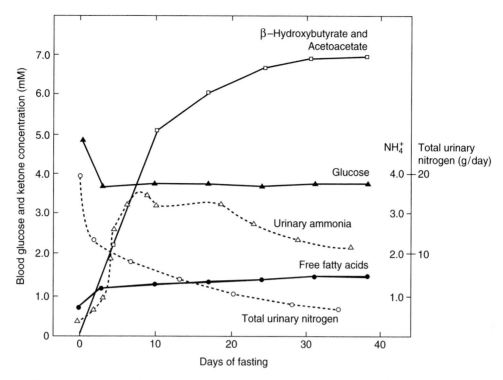

Fig. 31.19. Changes in blood fuels during fasting. The units for fatty acids, glucose, and ketone bodies are millimolar (on left) and for urinary nitrogen and ammonia are grams/day (on right). Modified from Linder MC. Nutritional Biochemistry and Metabolism, 2nd Ed. Stamford, CT: Appleton & Lange, 1991:103. © 1991 Appleton & Lange.

within 2 hours after a meal, glycogenolysis is stimulated and begins to supply glucose to the blood. Subsequently, glucose is also produced by gluconeogenesis.

During a 12-hour fast, glycogenolysis is the major source of blood glucose. Thus, it is the major pathway by which glucose is produced in the basal state (after a 12-hour fast). However, by approximately 16 hours of fasting, glycogenolysis and gluconeogenesis contribute equally to the maintenance of blood glucose.

By 30 hours after a meal, liver glycogen stores are substantially depleted. Subsequently, gluconeogenesis is the primary source of blood glucose.

The mechanisms that cause fats to be used as the major fuel and that allow blood glucose levels to be maintained during periods of food deprivation result in the conservation of body protein and, consequently, permit survival during prolonged fasting for periods often exceeding 1 or more months.

E. Blood Glucose Levels during Exercise

During exercise, mechanisms very similar to those that are used during fasting operate to maintain blood glucose levels. The liver maintains blood glucose levels through both glucagon- and epinephrine-induced glycogenolysis and gluconeogenesis. The use of fuels by muscle during exercise, including the uptake and use of blood glucose, is discussed in Chapter 47.

Otto Shape is able to jog for 45 minutes before eating breakfast without developing symptoms of hypoglycemia in spite of enhanced glucose utilization by skeletal muscle during exercise. He maintains his blood glucose level in an adequate range through hepatic glycogenolysis and gluconeogenesis.

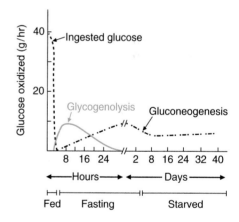

Fig. 31.20. Sources of blood glucose in fed, fasting, and starved states. Note that the scale changes from hours to days. From Ruderman NB, et al. In: Hanson RW, Mehlman MA, eds. Gluconeogenesis: Its Regulation in Mammalian Species. 1976:518. © 1976 John Wiley & Sons.

Remember that muscle glycogen is not used to maintain blood glucose levels; muscle cells lack glucose 6-phosphatase, so glucose cannot be produced from glucose 6-phosphate for export.

Epidemiologic studies have correlated the results of the OGTT with the current and subsequent development of the microvascular complications of DM in the eye (diabetic retinopathy) and in the kidney (diabetic nephropathy). Their development is usually limited to those patients whose fasting blood glucose level exceeds 140 mg/dL (7.8 mM) or whose 2-hour postprandial blood glucose level exceeds 200 mg/dL (11.1 mM).

As a consequence, the success of therapy with diet alone or with diet plus oral hypoglycemic agents is often determined by measuring blood glucose levels during fasting, before breakfast, and 2 hours after a meal. For patients taking an intermediate-acting insulin, blood glucose also may be measured at other times, such as when insulin action is expected to peak after its injection (e.g., around 5:00 PM, when intermediate-acting insulin has been given at 7:00 AM the same day).

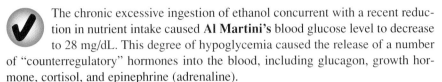

CLINICAL COMMENTS

The chronic excessive ingestion of ethanol concurrent with a recent reduction in nutrient intake caused **Al Martini's** blood glucose level to decrease to 28 mg/dL. This degree of hypoglycemia caused the release of a number of "counterregulatory" hormones into the blood, including glucagon, growth hormone, cortisol, and epinephrine (adrenaline).

Some of the patient's signs and symptoms are primarily the result of an increase in adrenergic nervous system activity after a rapid decrease in blood glucose. The subsequent increase in epinephrine levels in the blood leads to tremulousness, excessive sweating, and rapid heart rate. Other manifestations arise when the brain has insufficient glucose, hence the term "neuroglycopenic symptoms." Mr. Martini was confused, combative, had slurred speech, and eventually had a grand mal seizure. If not treated quickly by intravenous glucose administration, Mr. Martini may have lapsed into a coma. Permanent neurologic deficits and even death may result if severe hypoglycemia is not corrected in 6 to 10 hours.

The elevation in blood glucose that occurred in **Emma Wheezer's** case was primarily a consequence of the large pharmacologic doses of a glucocorticoid that she received in an effort to reduce the intrabronchial inflammatory reaction characteristic of asthmatic bronchospasm. Although the development of hyperglycemia in this case could be classified as a "secondary" form of diabetes mellitus, most patients treated with glucocorticoids do not develop glucose intolerance. Ms. Wheezer, therefore, may have a predisposition to the eventual development of "primary" diabetes mellitus.

In hyperglycemia, increased amounts of glucose enter the urine, causing large amounts of water to be excreted. This "osmotic diuresis" is responsible for the increased volume of urine (polyuria) noted by the patient. Because of increased urinary water loss, the effective circulating blood volume is reduced. Therefore, less blood reaches volume-sensitive receptors in the central nervous system, which then trigger the sensation of thirst, causing increased drinking activity (polydipsia).

A diabetic diet and the tapering of her steroid dose over a period of several weeks gradually returned Ms. Wheezer's blood glucose level into the normal range.

Chronically elevated levels of glucose in the blood may contribute to the development of the microvascular complications of diabetes mellitus, such as diabetic retinal damage, kidney damage, and nerve damage, as well as macrovascular complications such as cerebrovascular, peripheral vascular, and coronary vascular insufficiency. The precise mechanism by which long-term hyperglycemia induces these vascular changes is not fully established.

One postulated mechanism proposes that nonenzymatic glycation (glycosylation) of proteins in vascular tissue alters the structure and functions of these proteins. A protein exposed to chronically increased levels of glucose will covalently bind glucose, a process called glycation or glycosylation. This process is not regulated by enzymes (see Chapter 9). These nonenzymatically glycated proteins slowly form cross-linked protein adducts (often called advanced glycosylation products) within the microvasculature and macrovasculature.

By cross-linking vascular matrix proteins and plasma proteins, chronic hyperglycemia may cause narrowing of the luminal diameter of the microvessels in the retina (causing diabetic retinopathy), the renal glomeruli (causing diabetic nephropathy), and the microvessels supplying peripheral and autonomic nerve fibers (causing diabetic neuropathy). The same process has been postulated to accelerate atherosclerotic change in the macrovasculature, particularly in the brain (causing strokes), the coronary arteries (causing heart attacks), and the peripheral arteries (causing peripheral arterial insufficiency and gangrene). The abnormal lipid metabolism associated with poorly controlled diabetes mellitus also may contribute to the accelerated atherosclerosis associated with this metabolic disorder (see Chapters 33 and 34).

Until recently, it was argued that meticulous control of blood glucose levels in a diabetic patient would not necessarily prevent or even slow these complications of chronic hyperglycemia. The publication of the Diabetes Control and Complications Trial, however, suggests that maintaining long-term euglycemia (normal blood glucose levels) in diabetic patients slows the progress of unregulated glycation of proteins as well as corrects their dyslipidemia. In this way, careful control may favorably affect the course of the microvascular and macrovascular complications of diabetes mellitus in patients such as **Di Abietes** and **Ann Sulin**.

BIOCHEMICAL COMMENTS

Plants are the ultimate source of the earth's supply of glucose. Plants produce glucose from atmospheric CO_2 by the process of photosynthesis (Fig. 31.21A). In contrast to plants, humans cannot synthesize glucose by the fixation of CO_2. Although we have a process called gluconeogenesis, the term may really be a misnomer. Glucose is not generated anew by gluconeogenesis; compounds produced from glucose are simply recycled to glucose. We obtain glucose from the plants, including bacteria, that we eat and, to some extent, from animals in our food supply. We use this glucose both as a fuel and as a source of carbon for the synthesis of fatty acids, amino acids, and other sugars (see Fig. 31.21B). We store glucose as glycogen, which, along with gluconeogenesis, provides glucose when needed for energy (see Fig. 31.21C).

Lactate, one of the carbon sources for gluconeogenesis, is actually produced from glucose by tissues that obtain energy by oxidizing glucose to pyruvate through glycolysis. The pyruvate is then reduced to lactate, released into the bloodstream, and reconverted to glucose by the process of gluconeogenesis in the liver. This process is known as the Cori cycle (Fig. 31.21D).

Carbons of alanine, another carbon source for gluconeogenesis, may be produced from glucose. In muscle, glucose is converted via glycolysis to pyruvate and transaminated to alanine. Alanine from muscle is recycled to glucose in the liver. This process is known as the glucose–alanine cycle (Fig. 31.21E). Glucose also may be used to produce nonessential amino acids other than alanine, which are subsequently reconverted to glucose in the liver by gluconeogenesis. Even the essential amino acids that we obtain from dietary proteins are synthesized in plants and bacteria using glucose as the major source of carbon. Therefore, all amino acids that are converted to glucose in humans, including the essential amino acids, were originally synthesized from glucose.

The production of glucose from glycerol, the third major source of carbon for gluconeogenesis, is also a recycling process. Glycerol is derived from glucose via the dihydroxyacetone phosphate intermediate of glycolysis. Fatty acids are then esterified to the glycerol and stored as triacylglycerol. When these fatty acids are released from the triacylglycerol, the glycerol moiety can travel to the liver and be reconverted to glucose (see Fig. 31.21F).

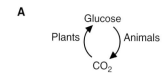

A

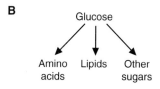

B

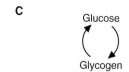

C

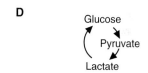

D

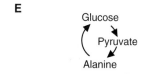

E

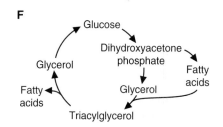

F

Fig. 31.21. Recycling of glucose.

Suggested References

Dimitriadis GD, Raptis SA, Newsholme EA. Integration of some biochemical and physiologic effects of insulin that may play a role in the control of blood glucose concentration. In LeRoith D, Taylor SI,

Olefsky JM, eds. Diabetes Mellitus: A Fundamental and Clinical Text. 2nd Ed. New York: Lippincott, Williams and Wilkins, 2000:161–176.

Granner D, Pilkis S. The genes of hepatic glucose metabolism. J Biol Chem 1990;265:10173–10176.

Gurney AL, Park EA, Liu J, et al. Metabolic regulation of gene transcription. J Nutr 1994;124:15335–15395.

Pilkis S, Granner D. Molecular physiology of the regulation of hepatic gluconeogenesis and glycolysis. Annu Rev Physiol 1992;54:885–909.

The Diabetes Control and Complications Trial Research Group. The effect of intensive treatment of diabetes on the development and progression of long-term complications in insulin-dependent diabetes mellitus. N Engl J Med 1993;329:977–986.

REVIEW QUESTIONS—CHAPTER 31

1. A common intermediate in the conversion of glycerol and lactate to glucose is which of the following?

   (A) Pyruvate
   (B) Oxaloacetate
   (C) Malate
   (D) Glucose 6-phosphate
   (E) Phosphoenolpyruvate

2. A patient presented with a bacterial infection that produced an endotoxin that inhibits phosphoenolpyruvate carboxykinase. In this patient, then, under these conditions, glucose production from which of the following precursors would be inhibited?

   (A) Alanine
   (B) Glycerol
   (C) Even-chain-number fatty acids
   (D) Phosphoenolpyruvate
   (E) Galactose

3. Which of the following statements best describes glucagon?

   (A) It acts as an anabolic hormone.
   (B) It acts on skeletal muscle, liver, and adipose tissue.
   (C) It acts primarily on the liver and adipose tissue.
   (D) Its concentration in the blood increases after a high-carbohydrate meal.
   (E) Its concentration increases in the blood when insulin levels increase.

4. Which of the following is most likely to occur in a normal individual after ingesting a high-carbohydrate meal?

   (A) Only insulin levels decrease.
   (B) Only insulin levels increase.
   (C) Only glucagon levels increase.
   (D) Both insulin and glucagon levels decrease.
   (E) Both insulin and glucagon levels increase.

5. A patient arrives at the hospital in an ambulance. She is currently in a coma. Before lapsing into the coma, her symptoms included vomiting, dehydration, low blood pressure, and a rapid heartbeat. She also had relatively rapid respirations, resulting in more carbon dioxide exhaled. These symptoms are consistent with which of the following conditions?

   (A) The patient lacks a pancreas.
   (B) Ketoalkolosis
   (C) Hypoglycemic coma
   (D) Diabetic ketoacidosis
   (E) Insulin shock in a diabetic patient

Lipid Metabolism

Most of the lipids found in the body fall into the categories of fatty acids and triacylglycerols; glycerophospholipids and sphingolipids; eicosanoids; cholesterol, bile salts, and steroid hormones; and fat-soluble vitamins. These lipids have very diverse chemical structures and functions. However, they are related by a common property: their relative insolublity in water.

Fatty acids, which are stored as triacylglycerols, serve as fuels, providing the body with its major source of energy (Fig. VI.1). Glycerophospholipids and sphingolipids, which contain esterified fatty acids, are found in membranes and in blood lipoproteins at the interfaces between the lipid components of these structures and the surrounding water. These membrane lipids form hydrophobic barriers between subcellular compartments and between cellular constituents and the extracellular milieu. Polyunsaturated fatty acids containing 20 carbons form the eicosanoids, which regulate many cellular processes (Fig. VI.2).

Cholesterol adds stability to the phospholipid bilayer of membranes. It serves as the precursor of the bile salts, detergent-like compounds that function in the process of lipid digestion and absorption (Fig. VI.3). Cholesterol also serves as the precursor of the steroid hormones, which have many actions, including the regulation of metabolism, growth, and reproduction.

The fat-soluble vitamins are lipids that are involved in such varied functions as vision, growth, and differentiation (vitamin A), blood clotting (vitamin K), prevention of oxidative damage to cells (vitamin E), and calcium metabolism (vitamin D).

Triacylglycerols, the major dietary lipids, are digested in the lumen of the intestine (Fig. VI.4). The initial digestive products, free fatty acids and 2-monoacylglycerol, are reconverted to triacylglycerols in intestinal epithelial cells, packaged in lipoproteins known as chylomicrons (so they can safely enter the circulation), and secreted into the lymph. Ultimately, chylomicrons enter the blood, serving as one of the major blood lipoproteins.

Very low density lipoprotein (VLDL) is produced in the liver, mainly from dietary carbohydrate. Lipogenesis is an insulin-stimulated process through which glucose is converted to fatty acids, which are subsequently esterified to glycerol to form the triacylglycerols that are packaged in VLDL and secreted from the liver. Thus, chylomicrons primarily transport dietary lipids, and VLDL transports endogenously synthesized lipids.

The triacylglycerols of chylomicrons and VLDL are digested by lipoprotein lipase (LPL), an enzyme found attached to capillary endothelial cells (see Fig. VI.4). The fatty acids that are released are taken up by muscle and many other tissues and oxidized to CO_2 and water to produce energy (see Chapter 23). After a meal, these fatty acids are taken up by adipose tissue and stored as triacylglycerols.

LPL converts chylomicrons to chylomicron remnants and VLDL to intermediate density lipoprotein (IDL). These products, which have a relatively low triacylglycerol content, are taken up by the liver by the process of endocytosis and degraded by lysosomal action. IDL may also be converted to low density lipoprotein (LDL) by further digestion of triacylglycerol. Endocytosis of LDL occurs in peripheral tissues as well as the liver (Table VI.1), and is the major means of cholesterol transport and delivery to peripheral tissues.

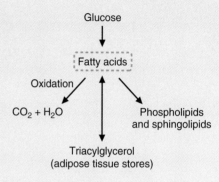

Fig. VI.1. Summary of fatty acid metabolism.

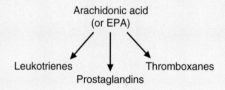

Fig. VI.2. Summary of eicosanoid synthesis. EPA = eicosapentenoic acid.

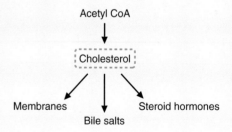

Fig. VI.3. Summary of cholesterol metabolism.

579

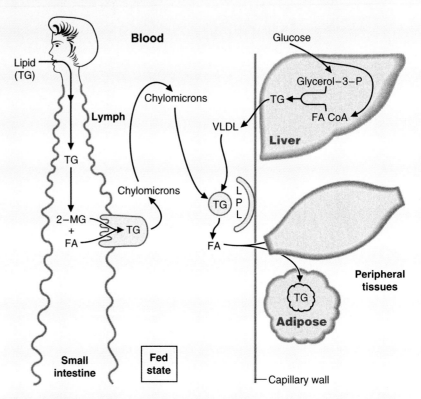

Fig. VI.4. Overview of triacylglycerol metabolism in the fed state. TG = triacylglycerol; 2-MG = 2-monoacylglycerol; FA = fatty acid; circled TG = triacylglycerols of VLDL and chylomicrons; LPL = lipoprotein lipase.

The principal function of high density lipoprotein (HDL) is to transport excess cholesterol obtained from peripheral tissues to the liver and to exchange proteins and lipids with chylomicrons and VLDL. The protein exchange converts "nascent" particles to "mature" particles.

During fasting, fatty acids and glycerol are released from adipose triacylglycerol stores (Fig. VI.5). The glycerol travels to the liver and is used for gluconeogenesis. Only the liver contains glycerol kinase, which is required for glycerol metabolism.

Table VI.1. Blood Lipoproteins

Chylomicrons
- produced in intestinal epithelial cells from dietary fat
- carries triacylglycerol in blood

VLDL (very low density lipoprotein)
- produced in liver mainly from dietary carbohydrate
- carries triacylglycerol in blood

IDL (intermediate density lipoprotein)
- produced in blood (remnant of VLDL after triacylglycerol digestion)
- endocytosed by liver or converted to LDL

LDL (low density lipoprotein)
- produced in blood (remnant of IDL after triacylglycerol digestion; endproduct of VLDL)
- contains high concentration of cholesterol and cholesterol esters
- endocytosed by liver and peripheral tissues

HDL (high density lipoprotein)
- produced in liver and intestine
- exchanges proteins and lipids with other lipoproteins
- functions in the return of cholesterol from peripheral tissues to the liver

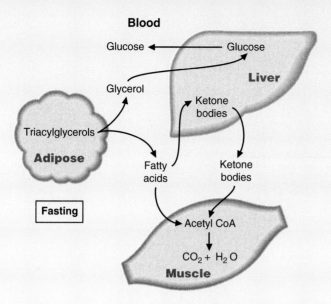

Fig. VI.5. Overview of triacylglycerol metabolism during fasting.

The fatty acids form complexes with albumin in the blood and are taken up by muscle, kidney, and other tissues, where ATP is generated by their oxidation to CO_2 and water. Liver also converts some of the carbon to ketone bodies, which are released into the blood. Ketone bodies are oxidized for energy in muscle, kidney, and other tissues during fasting, and in the brain during prolonged starvation (see Chapter 23).

32 Digestion and Transport of Dietary Lipids

Triacylglycerols are the major fat in the human diet, consisting of three *fatty acids* esterified to a *glycerol* backbone. Limited digestion of these lipids occurs in the mouth (*lingual lipase*) and stomach (*gastric lipase*) because of the low solubility of the substrate. In the intestine, however, the fats are emulsified by *bile salts* that are released from the gallbladder. This increases the available surface area of the lipids for *pancreatic lipase and colipase* to bind and to digest the triglycerides. Degradation products are *free fatty acids* and *2-monoacylglycerol*. When partially digested food enters the intestine, the hormone *cholecystokinin* is secreted by the intestine, which signals the gallbladder to contract and release bile acids, and the pancreas to release digestive enzymes.

In addition to triacylglycerols, phospholipids, cholesterol,, and cholesterol esters (cholesterol esterified to fatty acids) are present in the foods we eat. Phospholipids are hydrolyzed in the intestinal lumen by *phospholipase A2*, and cholesterol esters are hydrolyzed by *cholesterol esterase*. Both of these enzymes are secreted from the pancreas.

The products of enzymatic digestion (free fatty acids, glycerol, *lysophospholipids*, cholesterol) form *micelles* with bile acids in the intestinal lumen. The micelles interact with the enterocyte membrane and allow diffusion of the lipid soluble components across the enterocyte membrane into the cell. The bile acids, however, do not enter the enterocyte at this time. They remain in the intestine, travel further down, and are then reabsorbed and sent back to the liver by the *enterohepatic circulation*. This allows the bile salts to be used multiple times in fat digestion.

The intestinal epithelial cells will resynthesize triacylglycerol from free fatty acids and 2-monoacylglycerol and will package them with a protein, *apolipoprotein B-48*, phospholipids, and cholesterol esters into a soluble lipoprotein particle known as a *chylomicron*. The chylomicrons are secreted into the *lymph* and eventually end up in the circulation, where they can distribute dietary lipids to all tissues of the body.

Once in circulation, the newly released ("nascent") chylomicrons interact with another lipoprotein particle, *HDL* (high-density lipoprotein) and acquire two *apoproteins* from HDL, apoprotein *CII* and *E*. This converts the nascent chylomicron to a "mature" chylomicron. The apoCII on the mature chylomicron activates the enzyme *lipoprotein lipase (LPL)*, which is located on the inner surface of the capillary endothelial cells of muscle and adipose tissue. The LPL digests the triglyceride in the chylomicron, producing free fatty acids and glycerol. The fatty acids enter the adjacent organs either for energy production (muscle) or fat storage (adipocyte). The glycerol that is released is metabolized in the liver.

As the chylomicron loses triglyceride, its density increases and it becomes a *chylomicron remnant*, which is taken up by the liver by receptors that recognize apolipoprotein E. In the liver, the chylomicron remnant is degraded into its component parts for further disposition by the liver.

The lymph system is a network of vessels that surround interstitial cavities in the body. Cells secrete various compounds into the lymph, and the lymph vessels transport these fluids away from the interstitial spaces in the body tissues and into the bloodstream. In the case of the intestinal lymph system, the lymph enters the bloodstream through the thoracic duct. These vessels are designed such that under normal conditions the contents of the blood cannot enter the lymphatic system. The lymph fluid is similar in composition to that of the blood but lacks the cells found in blood.

THE WAITING ROOM

Will Sichel had several episodes of mild back and lower extremity pain over the last year, probably caused by minor sickle cell crises. He then developed severe right upper abdominal pain radiating to his lower right chest and his right flank 36 hours before admission to the emergency room. He states that the pain is not like his usual crisis pain. Intractable vomiting began 12 hours after the onset of these new symptoms. He reports that his urine is the color of iced tea and his stool now has a light clay color.

On physical examination, his body temperature is slightly elevated, and his heart rate is rapid. The whites of his eyes (the sclerae) are obviously jaundiced (a yellow discoloration caused by the accumulation of bilirubin pigment). He is exquisitely tender to pressure over his right upper abdomen.

The emergency room physician suspects that Michael is not in sickle cell crisis but instead has either acute cholecystitis (gallbladder inflammation) or a gallstone lodged in his common bile duct, causing cholestasis (the inability of the bile from the liver to reach his small intestine). His hemoglobin level was low at 7.6 mg/dL (reference range = 12–16) but unchanged from his baseline 3 months earlier. His serum total bilirubin level was 3.2 mg/dL (reference range = 0.2–1.0), and his direct (conjugated) bilirubin level was 0.9 mg/dL (reference range = 0 –0.2).

Intravenous fluids were started, he was not allowed to take anything by mouth, a nasogastric tube was passed and placed on constant suction, and symptomatic therapy was started for pain and nausea. When his condition had stabilized, Michael was sent for an ultrasonographic (ultrasound) study of his upper abdomen.

Al Martini has continued to abuse alcohol and to eat poorly. After a particularly heavy intake of vodka, a steady severe pain began in his upper mid-abdomen. This pain spread to the left upper quadrant and eventually radiated to his mid-back. He began vomiting nonbloody material and was brought to the hospital emergency room with fever, a rapid heart beat, and a mild reduction in blood pressure. On physical examination, he was dehydrated and tender to pressure over the upper abdomen. His vomitus and stool were both negative for occult blood.

Blood samples were sent to the laboratory for a variety of hematologic and chemical tests, including a measurement of serum amylase and lipase, digestive enzymes normally secreted from the exocrine pancreas through the pancreatic ducts into the lumen of the small intestine.

I. DIGESTION OF TRIACYLGLYCEROLS

Triacylglycerols are the major fat in the human diet because they are the major storage lipid in the plants and animals that constitute our food supply. Triacylglycerols contain a glycerol backbone to which three fatty acids are esterified (Fig. 32.1). The main route for digestion of triacylglycerols involves hydrolysis to fatty acids and 2-monoacylglycerols in the lumen of the intestine. However, the route depends to some extent on the chain length of the fatty acids. Lingual and gastric lipases are produced by cells at the back of the tongue and in the stomach, respectively. These lipases preferentially hydrolyze short- and medium-chain fatty acids (containing 12 or fewer carbon atoms) from dietary triacylglycerols. Therefore, they are most active in

Currently, 38% of the calories (kcal) in the typical American diet come from fat. The content of fat in the diet increased from the early 1900s until the 1960s, and then decreased as we became aware of the unhealthy effects of a high-fat diet. According to current recommendations, fat should provide no more than 30% of the total calories of a healthy diet.

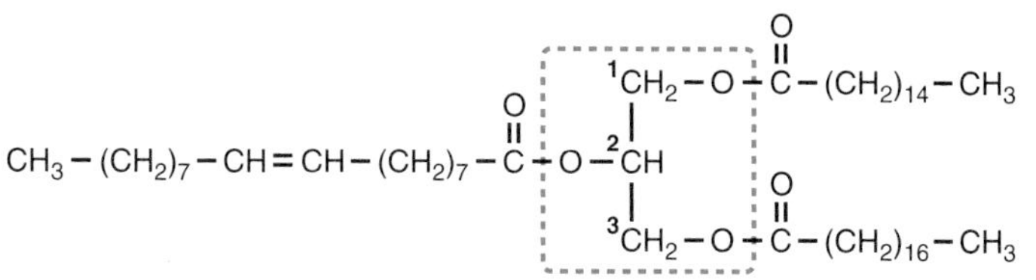

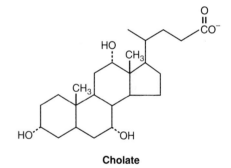

Fig. 32.1. Structure of a triacylglycerol. The glycerol moiety is highlighted, and its carbons are numbered.

infants and young children, who drink relatively large quantities of cow's milk, which contains triacylglycerols with a high percentage of short- and medium-chain fatty acids.

A. Action of Bile Salts

Dietary fat leaves the stomach and enters the small intestine, where it is emulsified (suspended in small particles in the aqueous environment) by bile salts (Fig. 32.2). The bile salts are amphipathic compounds (containing both hydrophobic and hydrophilic components), synthesized in the liver (see Chapter 34 for the pathway) and secreted via the gallbladder into the intestinal lumen. The contraction of the gallbladder and secretion of pancreatic enzymes are stimulated by the gut hormone cholecystokinin, which is secreted by the intestinal cells when stomach contents enter the intestine. Bile salts act as detergents, binding to the globules of dietary fat as they are broken up by the peristaltic action of the intestinal muscle. This emulsified fat, which has an increased surface area as compared with unemulsified fat, is attacked by digestive enzymes from the pancreas (Fig. 32.3).

B. Action of Pancreatic Lipase

The major enzyme that digests dietary triacylglycerols is a lipase produced in the pancreas. Pancreatic lipase is secreted along with another protein, colipase, along with bicarbonate, which neutralizes the acid that enters the intestine with partially digested food from the stomach. Bicarbonate raises the pH of the contents of the intestinal lumen into a range (pH ~ 6) that is optimal for the action of all of the digestive enzymes of the intestine. Bicarbonate secretion from the pancreas is stimulated by the hormone secretin, which is released from the intestine when acid enters the duodenum.

 In patients such as **Will Sichel** who have severe and recurrent episodes of increased red blood cell destruction (hemolytic anemia), greater than normal amounts of the red cell pigment heme must be processed by the liver and spleen. In these organs, heme (derived from hemoglobin) is degraded to bilirubin, which is excreted by the liver in the bile.

If large quantities of bilirubin are presented to the liver as a consequence of acute hemolysis, the capacity of the liver to conjugate it, that is, convert it to the water-soluble bilirubin diglucuronide, can be overwhelmed. As a result, a greater percentage of the bilirubin entering the hepatic biliary ducts in patients with hemolysis is in the less water-soluble forms. In the gallbladder, these relatively insoluble particles tend to precipitate as gallstones rich in calcium bilirubinate. In some patients, one or more stones may leave the gallbladder through the cystic duct and enter the common bile duct. Most pass harmlessly into the small intestine and are later excreted in the stool. Larger stones, however, may become entrapped in the lumen of the common bile duct, where they cause varying degrees of obstruction to bile flow (cholestasis) with associated ductal spasm, producing pain. If adequate amounts of bile salts do not enter the intestinal lumen, dietary fats cannot readily be emulsified and digested.

 The mammary gland produces milk, which is the major source of nutrients for the breastfed human infant. The fatty acid composition of human milk varies, depending on the diet of the mother. However, long-chain fatty acids predominate, particularly palmitic, oleic, and linoleic acids. Although the amount of fat contained in human milk and cow's milk is similar, cow's milk contains more short- and medium-chain fatty acids and does not contain the long-chain, polyunsaturated fatty acids found in human milk that are important in brain development.

Although the concentrations of pancreatic lipase and bile salts are low in the intestinal lumen of the newborn infant, the fat of human milk is still readily absorbed. This is true because lingual and gastric lipases produced by the infant partially compensate for the lower levels of pancreatic lipase. The human mammary gland also produces lipases that enter the milk. One of these lipases, which requires lower levels of bile salts than pancreatic lipase, is not inactivated by stomach acid and functions in the intestine for a number of hours.

Cholate

Fig. 32.2. Structure of a bile salt. The bile salts are derived from cholesterol and retain the cholesterol ring structure. They differ from cholesterol in that the rings in bile salts contain more hydroxyl groups and a polar side chain and lack a 5-6 double bond.

Al Martini's serum levels of pancreatic amylase (which digests dietary starch) and pancreatic lipase were elevated, a finding consistent with a diagnosis of acute and possibly chronic pancreatitis. The elevated levels of these enzymes in the blood are the result of their escape from the inflamed exocrine cells of the pancreas into the surrounding pancreatic veins. The cause of this inflammatory pancreatic process in this case was related to the toxic effect of acute and chronic excessive alcohol ingestion.

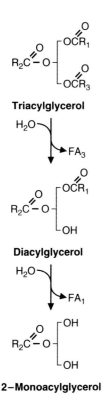

Triacylglycerol

Diacylglycerol

2-Monoacylglycerol

Fig. 32.4. Action of pancreatic lipase. Fatty acids (FA) are cleaved from positions 1 and 3 of the triacylglycerol, and a monoacylglycerol with a fatty acid at position 2 is produced.

Bile salts inhibit pancreatic lipase activity by coating the substrate and not allowing the enzyme access to the substrate. The colipase relieves the bile salt inhibition, and allows the triglyceride to enter the active site of the lipase.

The exocrine pancreas secretes phospholipase A2 in an inactive zymogen form, prophospholipase A2. The enzyme is activated in the intestinal lumen by proteolytic cleavage by trypsin. Pancreatic lipase, however, is secreted in its active form, and only needs to bind colipase and substrate to be active.

Q: When he was finally able to tolerate a full diet, **Al Martini's** stools became bulky, glistening, yellow-brown, and foul smelling. They floated on the surface of the toilet water. What caused this problem?

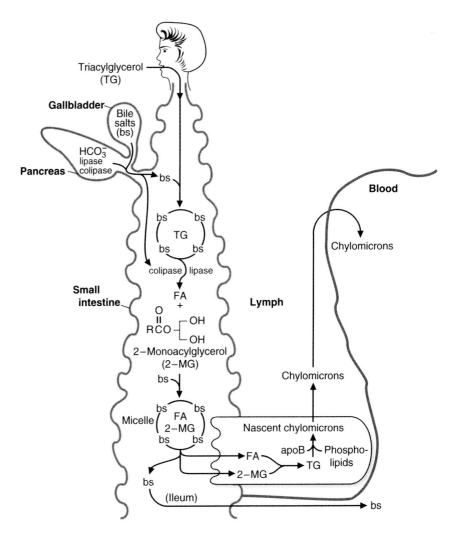

Fig. 32.3. Digestion of triacylglycerols in the intestinal lumen. TG = triacylglycerol; bs = bile salts; FA = fatty acid; 2-MG = 2-monoacylglycerol.

The colipase binds to the dietary fat and to the lipase, thereby increasing lipase activity. Pancreatic lipase hydrolyzes fatty acids of all chain lengths from positions 1 and 3 of the glycerol moiety of the triacylglycerol, producing free fatty acids and 2-monoacylglycerol, i.e., glycerol with a fatty acid esterified at position 2 (Fig. 32.4). The pancreas also produces esterases that remove fatty acids from compounds (such as cholesterol esters) and phospholipase A2 that digests phospholipids to a free fatty acid and a lysophospholipid (Fig. 32.5).

II. ABSORPTION OF DIETARY LIPIDS

The fatty acids and 2-monoacylglycerols produced by digestion are packaged into micelles, tiny microdroplets emulsified by bile salts (see Fig. 32.3). Other dietary lipids, such as cholesterol, lysophospholipids, and fat-soluble vitamins, are also packaged in these micelles. The micelles travel through a layer of water (the unstirred water layer) to the microvilli on the surface of the intestinal epithelial cells, where the fatty acids, 2-monoacylglycerols, and other dietary lipids are absorbed, but the bile salts are left behind in the lumen of the gut.

The bile salts are extensively resorbed when they reach the ileum. Greater than 95% of the bile salts are recirculated, traveling through the enterohepatic circulation

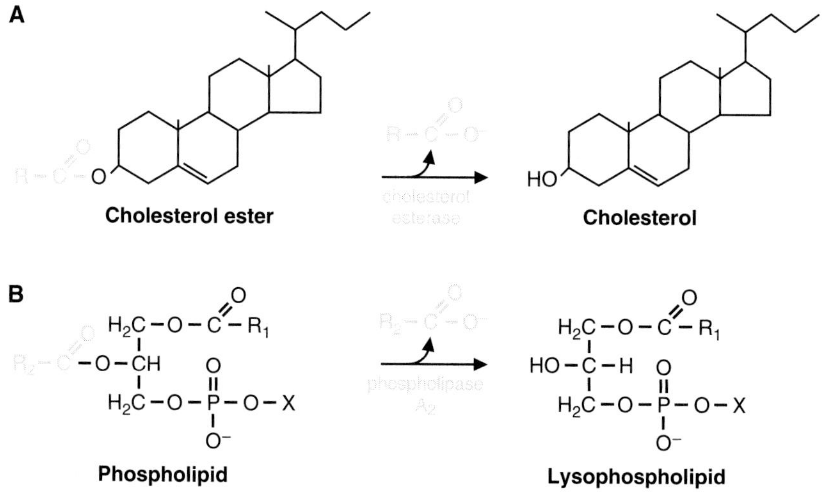

A

Cholesterol ester

Cholesterol

B

$H_2C-O-\overset{\overset{\displaystyle O}{\|}}{C}-R_1$
$-O-CH \quad O$
$H_2C-O-\overset{\overset{\displaystyle \|}{P}}{}-O-X$
$\underset{O^-}{}$

Phospholipid

$H_2C-O-\overset{\overset{\displaystyle O}{\|}}{C}-R_1$
$HO-C-H \quad O$
$H_2C-O-\overset{\overset{\displaystyle \|}{P}}{}-O-X$
$\underset{O^-}{}$

Lysophospholipid

Fig. 32.5. Action of pancreatic esterases (A) and phospholipase A2 (B).

 Al Martini's stool changes are characteristic of steatorrhea (fat-laden stools caused by malabsorption of dietary fats), in this case caused by a lack of pancreatic secretions, particularly pancreatic lipase, which normally digests dietary fat.

Steatorrhea also may be caused by insufficient production or secretion of bile salts. Therefore, **Michael Sichel** might also develop this condition.

to the liver, which secretes them into the bile for storage in the gallbladder and ejection into the intestinal lumen during another digestive cycle (Fig. 32.6).

Short- and medium-chain fatty acids (C4 to C12) do not require bile salts for their absorption. They are absorbed directly into intestinal epithelial cells. Because they do not need to be packaged to increase their solubility, they enter the portal blood (rather than the lymph) and are transported to the liver bound to serum albumin.

For bile salt micelles to form, the concentration of bile salts in the contents of the intestinal lumen must reach 5–15 μmol/mL. This critical concentration of bile salts is therefore required for optimal lipid absorption.

III. SYNTHESIS OF CHYLOMICRONS

Within the intestinal epithelial cells, the fatty acids and 2-monoacylglycerols are condensed by enzymatic reactions in the smooth endoplasmic reticulum to form tri-acylglycerols. The fatty acids are activated to fatty acyl CoA by the same process

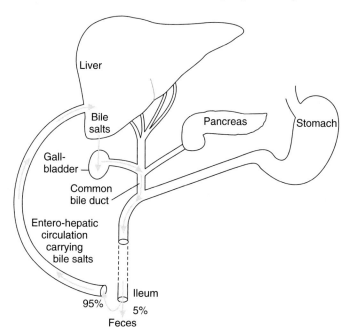

Fig. 32.6. Recycling of bile salts. Bile salts are synthesized in the liver, stored in the gallbladder, secreted into the small intestine, resorbed in the ileum, and returned to the liver via the enterohepatic circulation. Five percent or less of luminal bile acids are excreted in the stool under normal circumstances.

Activation of fatty acids

$$FA \xrightarrow{\text{ATP}} FA-AMP \xrightarrow{\text{CoASH}} FACoA$$
$$\xrightarrow{\quad} AMP$$

Triacylglycerol synthesis

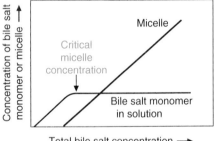

2–Monoacylglycerol   **Diacylglycerol**   **Triacylglycerol**

Fig. 32.7. Resynthesis of triacylglycerols in intestinal epithelial cells. Fatty acids (FA), produced by digestion, are activated in intestinal epithelial cells and then esterified to the 2-monoacylglycerol produced by digestion. The triacylglycerols are packaged in chylomicrons and secreted into the lymph.

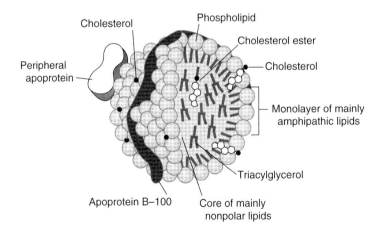

Because the fat-soluble vitamins (A, D, E, and K) are absorbed from micelles along with the long-chain fatty acids and 2-monoacylglycerols, prolonged obstruction of the duct that carries exocrine secretions from the pancreas and the gallbladder into the intestine (via the common duct) could lead to a deficiency of these metabolically important substances. If the obstruction of **Michael Sichel's** common duct continues, he will eventually suffer from a fat soluble vitamin deficiency. (Graph from Devlin T. Textbook of Biochemistry, 3rd Ed. 1992:1084. Copyright © John Wiley & Sons, Inc.)

used for activation of fatty acids before β-oxidation (see Chapter 23). A fatty acyl CoA then reacts with a 2-monoacylglycerol to form a diacylglycerol, which reacts with another fatty acyl CoA to form a triacylglycerol (Fig. 32.7). The reactions for triacylglycerol synthesis in intestinal cells differ from those in liver and adipose cells in that 2-monoacylglycerol is an intermediate in triacylglycerol in intestinal cells, whereas phosphatidic acid is the necessary intermediate in other tissues.

Triacylglycerols are transported in lipoprotein particles because they are insoluble in water. If triacylglycerols directly entered the blood, they would coalesce, impeding blood flow. Intestinal cells package triacylglycerols together with proteins and phospholipids in chylomicrons, which are lipoprotein particles that do not readily coalesce in aqueous solutions (Figs. 32.8 and 32.9). Chylomicrons also contain cholesterol and fat-soluble vitamins. The protein constituents of the lipoproteins are known as apoproteins.

The major apoprotein associated with chylomicrons as they leave the intestinal cells is B-48 (Fig. 32.10). The B-48 apoprotein is structurally and genetically

Fig. 32.8. Example of the structure of a blood lipoprotein. VLDL is depicted. Lipoproteins contain phospholipids and proteins on the surface, with their hydrophilic regions interacting with water. Hydrophobic molecules are in the interior of the lipoprotein. The hydroxyl group of cholesterol is near the surface. In cholesterol esters, the hydroxyl group is esterified to a fatty acid. Cholesterol esters are found in the interior of lipoproteins and are synthesized by reaction of cholesterol with an activated fatty acid (see Chapter 33).

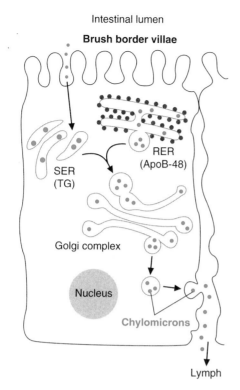

Intestinal lumen

Brush border villae

RER
(ApoB-48)

SER
(TG)

Golgi complex

Nucleus

Chylomicrons

Lymph

Fig. 32.10. Formation and secretion of chylomicrons. The triacylglycerol is produced in the smooth endoplasmic reticulum (SER) of intestinal epithelial cells from the digestive products, fatty acids, and 2-monoacylglycerols. The protein is synthesized in the rough endoplasmic reticulum (RER). The major apoprotein in chylomicrons is B-48. Assembly of the lipoproteins occurs in both the ER and the Golgi complex.

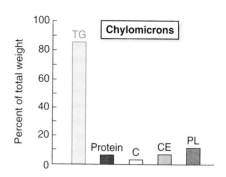

Fig. 32.9. Composition of a typical chylomicron. Although the composition varies to some extent, the major component is triacylglycerol (TG). C = cholesterol; CE = cholesterol ester; PL = phospholipid.

related to the B-100 apoprotein synthesized in the liver that serves as a major protein of another lipid carrier, very-low-density lipoprotein (VLDL). These two apoproteins are encoded by the same gene. In the intestine, the primary transcript of this gene undergoes RNA editing (Fig. 32.11 and see Chapter 15). A stop codon is generated that causes a protein to be produced in the intestine that is 48% of the size of the protein produced in the liver; hence the designations B-48 and B-100.

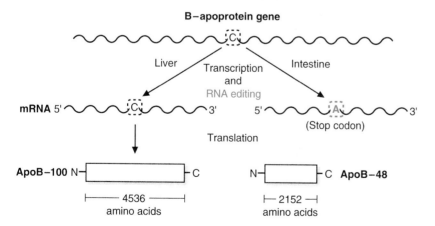

B−apoprotein gene

Liver   Transcription   Intestine
and
RNA editing

mRNA 5'   3'   5'   3'
(Stop codon)

Translation

ApoB−100 N—   —C   N—   —C **ApoB−48**

├— 4536 —┤   ├— 2152 —┤
amino acids   amino acids

Fig. 32.11. B-apoprotein gene. The gene, located on chromosome 2, is transcribed and translated in liver to produce apoB-100, which is 4,536 amino acids in length (one of the longest single-polypeptide chains). In intestinal cells, RNA editing converts a cytosine (C) to an adenine (A), producing a stop codon. Consequently, the B-apoprotein of intestinal cells (apoB-48) contains only 2,152 amino acids. ApoB-48 is 48% of the size of apoB-100.

 Olestra is an artificial fat substitute designed to allow individuals to obtain the taste and food consistency of fat, without the calories from fat. The structure of Olestra is shown below and consists of a sucrose molecule to which fatty acids are esterified to the hydroxyl groups.

Olestra = octa-acyl sucrose
R = fatty acyl group

The fatty acids attached to sucrose are resistant to hydrolysis by pancreatic lipase, so Olestra passes through the intestine intact and is eliminated in the feces. As a result, no useful calories can be obtained through the metabolism of Olestra.

Because of their high triacylglycerol content, chylomicrons are the least dense of the blood lipoproteins. When blood is collected from patients with certain types of hyperlipoproteinemias (high concentrations of lipoproteins in the blood) in which chylomicron levels are elevated, and the blood is allowed to stand in the refrigerator overnight, the chylomicrons float to the top of the liquid and coalesce, forming a creamy layer.

 One manner in which individuals can lose weight is to inhibit the activity of pancreatic lipase. This would result in reduced fat digestion and absorption and a reduced caloric yield from the diet. The drug Orlistat is a chemically synthesized derivative of lipstatin, a natural lipase inhibitor found in certain bacteria. The drug works in the intestinal lumen and forms a covalent bond with the active site serine residue of both gastric and pancreatic lipase, thereby inhibiting their activities. Nondigested triglycerides are not absorbed by the intestine and are eliminated in the feces. Under normal use of the drug, approximately 30% of dietary fat absorption is inhibited. Because excessive nondigested fat in the intestines can lead to gastrointestinal distress related to excessive intestinal gas formation, individuals taking this drug need to follow a reduced daily intake of fat in their diet, which should be evenly distributed amongst the meals of the day.

Blood

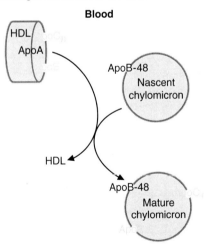

Fig. 32.12. Transfer of proteins from HDL to chylomicrons. Newly synthesized chylomicrons (nascent chylomicrons) mature as they receive apoproteins CII and E from HDL. HDL functions in the transfer of these apoproteins and also in transfer of cholesterol from peripheral tissues to the liver (see Table 1 in the introduction to this section).

The protein component of the lipoproteins is synthesized on the rough endoplasmic reticulum. Lipids, which are synthesized in the smooth endoplasmic reticulum, are complexed with the proteins to form the chylomicrons (see Fig. 32.10).

IV. TRANSPORT OF DIETARY LIPIDS IN THE BLOOD

By the process of exocytosis, chylomicrons are secreted by the intestinal epithelial cells into the chyle of the lymphatic system and enter the blood through the thoracic duct. Chylomicrons begin to enter the blood within 1 to 2 hours after the start of a meal; as the meal is digested and absorbed, they continue to enter the blood for many hours. Initially, the particles are called nascent (newborn) chylomicrons. As they accept proteins from HDL within the lymph and the blood, they become "mature" chylomicrons.

HDL transfers proteins to the nascent chylomicrons, particularly apoprotein E (apoE) and apoprotein CII (apoCII) (Fig. 32.12). ApoE is recognized by membrane receptors, particularly those on the surface of liver cells, allowing ApoE-bearing lipoproteins to enter these cells by endocytosis for subsequent digestion by lysosomes. ApoCII acts as an activator of LPL, the enzyme on capillary endothelial cells, primarily within muscle and adipose tissue, that digests the triacylglycerols of the chylomicrons and VLDL in the blood.

V. FATE OF CHYLOMICRONS

The triacylglycerols of the chylomicrons are digested by LPL attached to the proteoglycans in the basement membranes of endothelial cells that line the capillary walls (Fig. 32.13). LPL is produced by adipose cells, muscle cells (particularly cardiac muscle), and cells of the lactating mammary gland. The isozyme synthesized in adipose cells has a higher K_m than the isozyme synthesized in muscle cells. Therefore, adipose LPL is more active after a meal, when chylomicrons levels are elevated in the blood. Insulin stimulates the synthesis and secretion of adipose LPL, such that after a meal, when triglyceride levels increase in circulation, LPL has been upregulated (through insulin release) to facilitate the hydrolysis of fatty acids from the triglyceride.

The fatty acids released from triacylglycerols by LPL are not very soluble in water. They become soluble in blood by forming complexes with the protein albumin. The major fate of the fatty acids is storage as triacylglycerol in adipose tissue. However, these fatty acids also may be oxidized for energy in muscle and other tissues (see Fig. 32.13). The LPL in the capillaries of muscle cells has a lower K_m than adipose LPL. Thus, muscle cells can obtain fatty acids from blood lipoproteins whenever they are needed for energy, even if the concentration of the lipoproteins is low.

The glycerol released from chylomicron triacylglycerols by LPL may be used for triacylglycerol synthesis in the liver in the fed state.

The portion of a chylomicron that remains in the blood after LPL action is known as a chylomicron remnant. This remnant binds to receptors on hepatocytes (the major cells of the liver), which recognize apoprotein E, and is taken up by the process of endocytosis. Lysosomes fuse with the endocytic vesicles, and the

 Heparin is a complex polysaccharide that is a component of proteoglycans (see Chapter 49). Isolated heparin is frequently used as an anticoagulant, because it binds to antithrombin III (ATIII), and the activated ATIII then binds factors necessary for clotting and inhibits them from working. As LPL is bound to the capillary endothelium through binding to proteoglycans, heparin also can bind to LPL and dislodge it from the capillary wall. This leads to loss of LPL activity and an increase of triglyceride content in the blood.

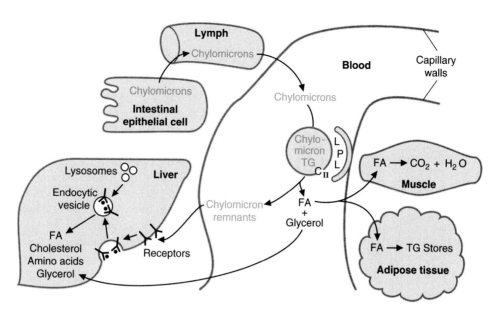

Fig. 32.13. Fate of chylomicrons. Chylomicrons are synthesized in intestinal epithelial cells, secreted into the lymph, pass into the blood, and become mature chylomicrons (see Fig. 32.11). On capillary walls in adipose tissue and muscle, lipoprotein lipase (LPL) activated by ApoC$_{II}$ digests the triacylglycerols (TG) of chylomicrons to fatty acids and glycerol. Fatty acids (FA) are oxidized in muscle or stored in adipose cells as triacylglycerols. The remnants of the chylomicrons are taken up by the liver by receptor-mediated endocytosis. Lysosomal enzymes within the hepatocyte digest the remnants, releasing the products into the cytosol.

chylomicron remnants are degraded by lysosomal enzymes. The products of lysosomal digestion (e.g., fatty acids, amino acids, glycerol, cholesterol, phosphate) can be reused by the cell.

CLINICAL COMMENTS

✔ The upper abdominal ultrasound study showed a large gallstone lodged in **Will Sichel's** common duct with dilation of this duct proximal to the stone. Michael was scheduled for endoscopic retrograde cholangiopancreatography (ERCP). (An ERCP involves cannulation of the common bile duct—and, if necessary, the pancreatic duct—through a tube placed through the mouth and stomach and into the upper small intestine.) With this technique, a stone can be snared in the common duct and removed to relieve an obstruction.

If common duct obstruction is severe enough, bilirubin flows back into the venous blood draining from the liver. As a consequence, serum bilirubin levels, particularly the indirect (unconjugated) fraction, increase. Tissues such as the sclerae of the eye take up this pigment, which causes them to become yellow (jaundiced). **Will Sichel's** condition was severe enough to cause jaundice by this mechanism.

✔ Alcohol excess may produce proteinaceous plugs in the small pancreatic ducts, causing back pressure injury and autodigestion of the pancreatic acini drained by these obstructed channels. This process causes one form of acute pancreatitis. **Al Martini** had an episode of acute alcohol-induced pancreatitis superimposed on a more chronic alcohol-related inflammatory process in the pancreas—in other words, a chronic pancreatitis. As a result of decreased secretion of pancreatic lipase through the pancreatic ducts and into the lumen of the small intestine, dietary fat was not absorbed at a normal rate, and steatorrhea (fat-rich stools) occurred. If abstinence from alcohol does not allow adequate recovery of the enzymatic secretory function of the pancreas, Mr. Martini will have to take a commercial preparation of pancreatic enzymes with meals that contain even minimal amounts of fat.

BIOCHEMICAL COMMENTS

The assembly of chylomicrons within the endoplasmic reticulum of the enterocyte requires the activity of microsomal triglyceride transfer protein (MTP). The protein is a dimer of two nonidentical subunits. The smaller subunit (57 kDa) is protein disulfide isomerase (PDI, see Chapter 7, section IX.A), whereas the larger subunit (97 kDa) contains the triglyceride transfer activity. MTP accelerates the transport of triglycerides, cholesterol esters, and phospholipids across membranes of subcellular organelles. The role of PDI in this complex is not known; the disulfide isomerase activity of this subunit is not needed for triglyceride transport to occur. The lack of triglyceride transfer activity leads to the disease **abetalipoproteinemia**. This disease affects both chylomicron assembly in the intestine and VLDL assembly in the liver. Both particles require a B apoprotein for their assembly (ApoB-48 for chylomicrons, ApoB-100 for VLDL), and MTP binds to the B apoproteins. For both chylomicron and VLDL assembly, a small ApoB–containing particle is first produced within the lumen of the ER. The appropriate apoB is made on the rough endoplasmic reticulum (RER) and is inserted into the ER lumen during its synthesis (see Chapter 15, section IX). As the protein is being translated, lipid (a small amount of triglyceride) begins to associate with the protein, and the lipid association is catalyzed by MTP. This leads to the generation of small ApoB-containing particles; these particles are not formed in patients with abetalipoproteinemia. Thus, it appears as though MTP activity is necessary to transfer triacylglycerol formed within the ER to the ApoB protein. The second stage of particle assembly is the fusion of the initial ApoB particle with triacylglycerol droplets within the ER. MTP also may be required for the transfer of triacylglycerol from the cytoplasm to the lumen of the ER to form this lipid droplet. These steps are depicted in Fig. 32.14.

The symptoms of abetalipoproteinemia include lipid malabsorption (and its accompanying symptoms, such as steatorrhea and vomiting), which can result in caloric deficiencies and weight loss. Because lipid-soluble vitamin distribution occurs through chylomicron circulation, signs and symptoms of deficiencies in the lipid-soluble vitamins may be seen in these patients.

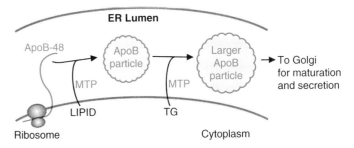

Fig. 32.14. A model of microsomal triglyceride transfer protein (MTP) action. MTP is required to transfer lipid to apoB-48 as it is synthesized, and to transfer lipid from the cytoplasm to the ER lumen.

Suggested References

Berriot-Varoqueaux N, Aggerbeck LP, Samson-Bouma ME, Wetterau JR. The role of the microsomal triglyceride transfer protein in abetalipoproteinemia. Annu Rev Nutr 2000;20:663–697.

Havel RJ, Kane JP. Introduction: structure and metabolism of plasm lipoproteins. In: Scriver CR, Beaudet AL, Valle D, Sly WS, et al., eds. The Metabolic and Molecular Bases of Inherited Disease, vol II, 8th Ed. New York: McGraw-Hill, 2001:2705–2716.

Knopp RH. Drug treatment of lipid disorders. N Engl J Med 1999;341:498–511.

Linder MC, ed. Nutrition and metabolism of fats. In: Nutritional Biochemistry and Metabolism with Clinical Applications. New York: Elsevier, 1991:51–85.

Zlotkin SH. Neonatal nutrition. In: Linder MC, ed. Nutritional Biochemistry and Metabolism with Clinical Applications. New York: Elsevier, 1991:357–360.

 REVIEW QUESTIONS—CHAPTER 32

1. The most abundant component of chylomicrons is which of the following?

   (A) ApoB-48
   (B) Triglyceride
   (C) Phospholipid
   (D) Cholesterol
   (E) Cholesterol ester

2. The conversion of nascent chylomicrons to mature chylomicrons requires which of the following?

   (A) Bile salts
   (B) 2-Monoacylglycerol
   (C) Lipoprotein lipase
   (D) High-density lipoprotein
   (E) Lymphatic system

3. The apoproteins B-48 and B-100 are similar with respect to which of the following?

   (A) They are synthesized from the same gene.
   (B) They are derived by alternative spicing of the same hnRNA.
   (C) ApoB-48 is a proteolytic product of apoB-100.
   (D) Both are found in mature chylomicrons.
   (E) Both are found in very-low-density lipoproteins.

4. Bile salts must reach a particular concentration within the intestinal lumen before they are effective agents for lipid digestion. This is because of which of the following?

   (A) The bile salt concentration must be equal to the triglyceride concentration.
   (B) The bile salt solubility in the lumen is a critical factor.
   (C) The ability of bile salts to bind lipase is concentration dependant.
   (D) The bile salts cannot be reabsorbed in the ileum until they reach a certain concentration.
   (E) The bile salts do not activate lipase until they reach a particular concentration.

5. Type III hyperlipidemia is caused by a deficiency of apoprotein E. Analysis of the serum of patients with this disorder would exhibit which of the following?

   (A) An absence of chylomicrons after eating
   (B) Above-normal levels of VLDL after eating
   (C) Normal triglyceride levels
   (D) Elevated triglyceride levels
   (E) Below-normal triglyceride levels

33 Synthesis of Fatty Acids, Triacylglycerols, and the Major Membrane Lipids

*Fatty acids are synthesized mainly in the liver in humans, with dietary glucose serving as the major source of carbon. Glucose is converted through glycolysis to pyruvate, which enters the mitochondrion and forms both acetyl CoA and oxaloacetate (Fig. 33.1). These two compounds condense, forming citrate. Citrate is transported to the **cytosol**, where it is cleaved to form acetyl CoA, the source of carbon for the reactions that occur on the **fatty acid synthase complex**. The key regulatory enzyme for the process, **acetyl CoA carboxylase**, produces **malonyl CoA** from acetyl CoA.*

*The growing fatty acid chain, attached to the fatty acid synthase complex in the cytosol, is elongated by the sequential addition of 2-carbon units provided by malonyl CoA. **NADPH**, produced by the **pentose phosphate pathway** and **the malic enzyme**, provides **reducing equivalents**. When the growing fatty acid chain is 16 carbons in length, it is released as **palmitate**. After activation to a CoA derivative, palmitate can be elongated and desaturated to produce a series of fatty acids.*

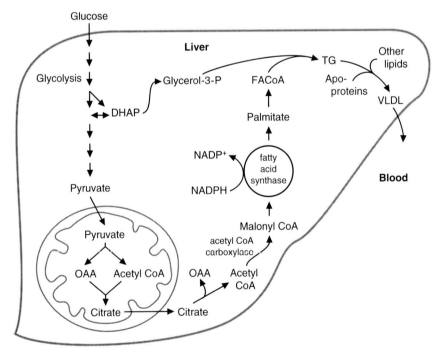

Fig. 33.1. Lipogenesis, the synthesis of triacylglycerols from glucose. In humans, the synthesis of fatty acids from glucose occurs mainly in the liver. Fatty acids (FA) are converted to triacylglycerols (TG), packaged in VLDL, and secreted into the blood. OAA = oxaloacetate.

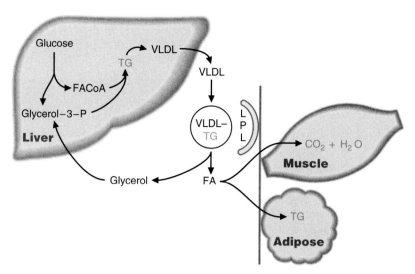

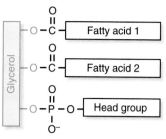

Fig. 33.3. General structure of a glycerophospholipid. The fatty acids are joined by ester bonds to the glycerol moiety. Various combinations of fatty acids may be present. The fatty acid at carbon 2 of the glycerol is usually unsaturated. The head group is the group attached to the phosphate on position 3 of the glycerol moiety. The most common head group is choline, but ethanolamine, serine, inositol, or phosphatidylglycerol also may be present. The phosphate group is negatively charged, and the head group may carry a positive charge (choline and ethanolamine), or both a positive and a negative charge (serine). The inositol may be phosphorylated and, thus, negatively charged.

Fig. 33.2. Fate of VLDL triacylglycerol (TG). The TG of VLDL, produced in the liver, is digested by lipoprotein lipase (LPL) present on the lining cells of the capillaries in adipose and skeletal muscle tissue. Fatty acids are released and either oxidized or stored in tissues as TG. Glycerol is used by the liver and other tissues that contain glycerol kinase. FA = fatty acid (or fatty acyl group).

*Fatty acids, produced in cells or obtained from the diet, are used by various tissues for the synthesis of **triacylglycerols** (the major storage form of fuel) and the **glycerophospholipids** and **sphingolipids** (the major components of cell membranes).*

*In the liver, triacylglycerols are produced from fatty acyl CoA and glycerol 3-phosphate. **Phosphatidic acid** serves as an intermediate in this pathway. The triacylglycerols are not stored in the liver but rather packaged with apoproteins and other lipids in **very-low-density lipoprotein (VLDL)** and secreted into the blood (see Fig. 33.1).*

*In the capillaries of various tissues (particularly adipose tissue, muscle, and the lactating mammary gland), **lipoprotein lipase (LPL)** digests the triacylglycerols of VLDL, forming **fatty acids** and **glycerol** (Fig. 33.2). The glycerol travels to the liver and other tissues where it is used. Some of the fatty acids are oxidized by muscle and other tissues. After a meal, however, most of the fatty acids are converted to triacylglycerols in **adipose cells**, where they are **stored**. These fatty acids are released during fasting and serve as the predominant fuel for the body.*

*Glycerophospholipids are also synthesized from fatty acyl CoA, which forms esters with glycerol 3-phosphate, producing phosphatidic acid. Various head groups are added to carbon 3 of the glycerol 3-phosphate moiety of phosphatidic acid, generating amphipathic compounds such as **phosphatidylcholine, phosphatidylinositol**, and **cardiolipin** (Fig. 33.3). In the formation of **plasmalogens** and **platelet-activating factor (PAF)**, a long-chain fatty alcohol forms an **ether** with carbon 1, replacing the fatty acyl ester (Fig. 33.4). Cleavage of phospholipids is catalyzed by **phospholipases** found in cell membranes, lysosomes, and pancreatic juice.*

*Sphingolipids, which are prevalent in membranes and the myelin sheath of the central nervous system, are built on **serine** rather than glycerol. In the synthesis of sphingolipids, serine and palmityl CoA condense, forming a compound that is related to **sphingosine**. Reduction of this compound, followed by addition of a second fatty acid in amide linkage, produces **ceramide**. Carbohydrate groups attach to ceramide, forming **glycolipids** such as the **cerebrosides, globosides**, and **gangliosides** (Fig. 33.5). The addition of **phosphocholine** to ceramide produces **sphingomyelin**. These sphingolipids are degraded by lysosomal enzymes.*

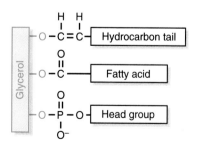

Fig. 33.4. General structure of a plasmalogen. Carbon 1 of glycerol is joined to a long-chain fatty alcohol by an ether linkage. The fatty alcohol group has a double bond between carbons 1 and 2. The head group is usually ethanolamine or choline.

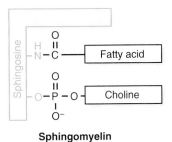

Sphingomyelin

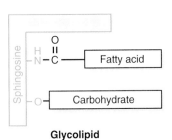

Glycolipid

Fig. 33.5. General structures of the sphingolipids. The "backbone" is sphingosine rather than glycerol. Ceramide is sphingosine with a fatty acid joined to its amino group by an amide linkage. Sphingomyelin contains phosphocholine, whereas glycolipids contain carbohydrate groups.

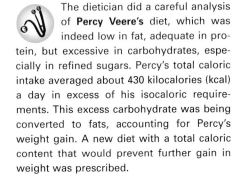

The dietician did a careful analysis of **Percy Veere's** diet, which was indeed low in fat, adequate in protein, but excessive in carbohydrates, especially in refined sugars. Percy's total caloric intake averaged about 430 kilocalories (kcal) a day in excess of his isocaloric requirements. This excess carbohydrate was being converted to fats, accounting for Percy's weight gain. A new diet with a total caloric content that would prevent further gain in weight was prescribed.

THE WAITING ROOM

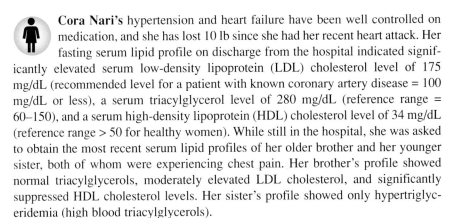

Percy Veere's mental depression slowly responded to antidepressant medication, to the therapy sessions with his psychiatrist, and to frequent visits from an old high school sweetheart whose husband had died several years earlier. While hospitalized for malnutrition, Mr. Veere's appetite returned. By the time of discharge, he had gained back 8 of the 22 lb he had lost and weighed 133 lb.

During the next few months, Mr. Veere developed a craving for "sweet foods" such as the candy he bought and shared with his new friend. After 6 months of this high-carbohydrate courtship, Percy had gained another 22 lb and now weighed 155 lb, just 8 lb more than he weighed when his depression began. He became concerned about the possibility that he would soon be overweight and consulted his dietitian, explaining that he had faithfully followed his low-fat diet but had "gone overboard" with carbohydrates. He asked whether it was possible to become fat without eating fat.

Cora Nari's hypertension and heart failure have been well controlled on medication, and she has lost 10 lb since she had her recent heart attack. Her fasting serum lipid profile on discharge from the hospital indicated significantly elevated serum low-density lipoprotein (LDL) cholesterol level of 175 mg/dL (recommended level for a patient with known coronary artery disease = 100 mg/dL or less), a serum triacylglycerol level of 280 mg/dL (reference range = 60–150), and a serum high-density lipoprotein (HDL) cholesterol level of 34 mg/dL (reference range > 50 for healthy women). While still in the hospital, she was asked to obtain the most recent serum lipid profiles of her older brother and her younger sister, both of whom were experiencing chest pain. Her brother's profile showed normal triacylglycerols, moderately elevated LDL cholesterol, and significantly suppressed HDL cholesterol levels. Her sister's profile showed only hypertriglyceridemia (high blood triacylglycerols).

Colleen Lakker was born 6 weeks prematurely. She appeared normal until about 30 minutes after delivery, when her respirations became rapid at 64 breaths/minute with audible respiratory grunting. The spaces between her ribs (intercostal spaces) retracted inward with each inspiration, and her lips and fingers became cyanotic from a lack of oxygen in her arterial blood. An arterial blood sample indicated a low partial pressure of oxygen (pO_2) and a slightly elevated partial pressure of carbon dioxide (pCO_2). The arterial pH was somewhat suppressed, in part from an accumulation of lactic acid secondary to the hypoxemia (a low level of oxygen in her blood). A chest x-ray showed a fine reticular granularity of the lung tissue, especially in the left lower lobe area. From these clinical data, a diagnosis of respiratory distress syndrome (RDS), also known as hyaline membrane disease, was made.

Colleen was immediately transferred to the neonatal intensive care unit, where, with intensive respiration therapy, she slowly improved.

I. FATTY ACID SYNTHESIS

Fatty acids are synthesized whenever an excess of calories is ingested. The major source of carbon for the synthesis of fatty acids is dietary carbohydrate. An excess of dietary protein also can result in an increase in fatty acid synthesis. In this case, the carbon source is amino acids that can be converted to acetyl CoA or tricarboxylic acid (TCA) cycle intermediates (see Chapter 39). Fatty acid synthesis occurs mainly in the liver in humans, although the process also occurs in adipose tissue.

When an excess of dietary carbohydrate is consumed, glucose is converted to acetyl CoA, which provides the 2-carbon units that condense in a series of reactions on the fatty acid synthase complex, producing palmitate (see Fig. 33.1). Palmitate is then converted to other fatty acids. The fatty acid synthase complex is located in the cytosol, and, therefore, it uses cytosolic acetyl CoA.

A. Conversion of Glucose to Cytosolic Acetyl CoA

The pathway for the synthesis of cytosolic acetyl CoA from glucose begins with glycolysis, which converts glucose to pyruvate in the cytosol (Fig. 33.6). Pyruvate enters mitochondria, where it is converted to acetyl CoA by pyruvate dehydrogenase and to oxaloacetate by pyruvate carboxylase. The pathway pyruvate follows is dictated by the acetyl CoA levels in the mitochondria. When acetyl CoA levels are high, pyruvate dehydrogenase is inhibited, and pyruvate carboxylase activity is stimulated. As oxaloacetate levels increase because of the activity of pyruvate carboxylase, oxaloacetate condenses with acetyl CoA to form citrate. This condensation reduces the acetyl CoA levels, which leads to the activation of pyruvate dehydrogenase and inhibition of pyruvate carboxylase. Through such reciprocal regulation, citrate can be continuously synthesized and transported across the inner mitochondrial membrane. In the cytosol, citrate is cleaved by citrate lyase to re-form acetyl CoA and oxaloacetate. This circuitous route is required because pyruvate dehydrogenase, the enzyme that converts pyruvate to acetyl CoA, is found only in mitochondria and because acetyl CoA cannot directly cross the mitochondrial membrane.

The NADPH required for fatty acid synthesis is generated by the pentose phosphate pathway (see Chapter 29) and from recycling of the oxaloacetate produced by citrate lyase (Fig. 33.7). Oxaloacetate is converted back to pyruvate in two steps: the reduction of oxaloacetate to malate by NAD^+-dependent malate dehydrogenase and the oxidative decarboxylation of malate to pyruvate by an $NADP^+$-dependent malate dehydrogenase (malic enzyme) (Fig. 33.8). The pyruvate formed by malic enzyme is reconverted to citrate. The NADPH that is generated by malic enzyme, along with the NADPH generated by glucose 6-phosphate and gluconate 6-phosphate dehydrogenases in the pentose phosphate pathway, is used for the reduction reactions that occur on the fatty acid synthase complex (Fig. 33.9).

The generation of cytosolic acetyl CoA from pyruvate is stimulated by elevation of the insulin/glucagon ratio after a carbohydrate meal. Insulin activates pyruvate dehydrogenase by stimulating the phosphatase that dephosphorylates the enzyme to

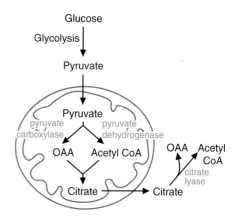

Fig. 33.6. Conversion of glucose to cytosolic acetyl CoA. OAA = oxaloacetate.

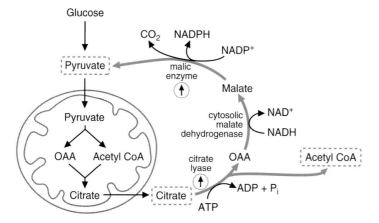

Fig. 33.7. Fate of citrate in the cytosol. Citrate lyase is also called citrate cleavage enzyme. OAA = oxaloacetate; circled ↑ = inducible enzyme.

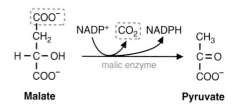

Fig. 33.8. Reaction catalyzed by malic enzyme. This enzyme is also called the decarboxylating or NADP-dependent malate dehydrogenase.

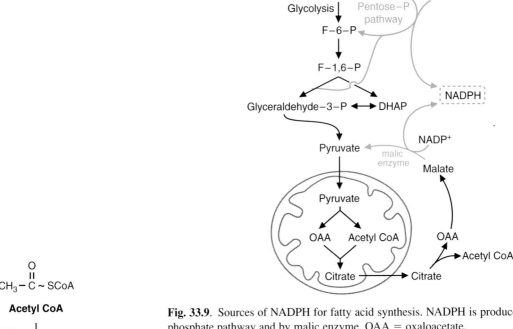

Fig. 33.9. Sources of NADPH for fatty acid synthesis. NADPH is produced by the pentose phosphate pathway and by malic enzyme. OAA = oxaloacetate.

an active form (see Chapter 20). The synthesis of malic enzyme, glucose 6-phosphate dehydrogenase, and citrate lyase is induced by the high insulin/glucagon ratio. The ability of citrate to accumulate, and leave the mitochondrial matrix for the synthesis of fatty acids, is attributable to the allosteric inhibition of isocitrate dehydrogenase by high energy levels within the matrix under these conditions. The concerted regulation of glycolysis and fatty acid synthesis is described in Chapter 36.

B. Conversion of Acetyl CoA to Malonyl CoA

Cytosolic acetyl CoA is converted to malonyl CoA, which serves as the immediate donor of the 2-carbon units that are added to the growing fatty acid chain on the fatty acid synthase complex. To synthesize malonyl CoA, acetyl CoA carboxylase adds a carboxyl group to acetyl CoA in a reaction requiring biotin and adenosine triphosphate (ATP) (Fig. 33.10).

Acetyl CoA carboxylase is the rate-limiting enzyme of fatty acid synthesis. Its activity is regulated by phosphorylation, allosteric modification, and induction/repression of its synthesis (Fig. 33.11). Citrate allosterically activates acetyl CoA carboxylase by causing the individual enzyme molecules (each composed of 4 subunits) to polymerize. Palmityl CoA, produced from palmitate (the endproduct of fatty acid synthase activity), inhibits acetyl CoA carboxylase. Phosphorylation by an AMP-dependent protein kinase inhibits the enzyme in the fasting state when energy levels are low. The enzyme is activated by dephosphorylation in the fed state when energy and insulin levels are high. A high insulin/glucagon ratio also results in induction of the synthesis of both acetyl CoA carboxylase and the next enzyme in the pathway, fatty acid synthase.

C. Fatty Acid Synthase Complex

As an overview, fatty acid synthase sequentially adds 2-carbon units from malonyl CoA to the growing fatty acyl chain to form palmitate. After the addition of each 2-carbon unit, the growing chain undergoes two reduction reactions that require NADPH.

$$O$$
$$||$$
$$CH_3 - C \sim SCoA$$

Acetyl CoA

CO_2

Biotin

acetyl CoA carboxylase

ATP

ADP + P_i

$$O \qquad O$$
$$|| \qquad ||$$
$$^-O - C - CH_2 - C \sim SCoA$$

Malonyl CoA

Fig. 33.10. Reaction catalyzed by acetyl CoA carboxylase. CO_2 is covalently attached to biotin, which is linked by an amide bond to the ε-amino group of a lysine residue of the enzyme. Hydrolysis of ATP is required for the attachment of CO_2 to biotin.

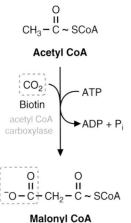 AMP is a much more sensitive indicator of low energy levels because of the adenylate kinase reaction. The [AMP] to [ATP] ratio is proportional to the square of the [ADP] to [ATP] ratio, so a fivefold change in ADP levels corresponds to a 25-fold change in AMP levels.

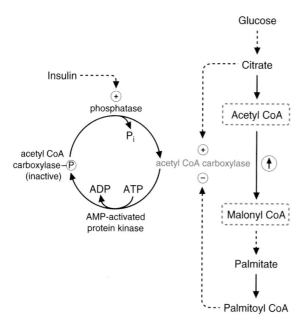

Fig. 33.11. Regulation of acetyl CoA carboxylase. This enzyme is regulated allosterically, both positively and negatively, by phosphorylation (circled P) and dephosphorylation, and by diet-induced induction (circled ↑). It is active in the dephosphorylated state when citrate causes it to polymerize. Dephosphorylation is catalyzed by an insulin-stimulated phosphatase. Low energy levels, via activation of an AMP-dependent protein kinase, cause the enzyme to be phosphorylated and inactivated. The ultimate product of fatty acid synthesis, palmitate, is converted to its CoA derivative palmityl CoA, which inhibits the enzyme. A high-calorie diet increases the rate of transcription of the gene for acetyl CoA carboxylase, whereas a low-calorie diet reduces transcription of this gene.

Fatty acid synthase is a large enzyme composed of two identical dimers, which each have seven catalytic activities and an acyl carrier protein (ACP) segment in a continuous polypeptide chain. The ACP segment contains a phosphopantetheine residue that is derived from the cleavage of coenzyme A (Fig. 33.12). The two dimers associate in a head-to-tail arrangement, so that the phosphopantetheinyl sulfhydryl group on one subunit and a cysteinyl sulfhydryl group on another subunit are closely aligned.

In the initial step of fatty acid synthesis, an acetyl moiety is transferred from acetyl CoA to the ACP phosphopantetheinyl sulfhydryl group of one subunit, and then to the cysteinyl sulfhydryl group of the other subunit. The malonyl moiety from malonyl CoA then attaches to the ACP phosphopantetheinyl sulfhydryl group of the first subunit. The acetyl and malonyl moieties condense, with the release of the malonyl carboxyl group as CO_2. A 4-carbon α-keto acyl chain is now attached to the ACP phosphopantetheinyl sulfhydryl group (Fig. 33.13).

A series of three reactions reduces the 4-carbon keto group to an alcohol, removes water to form a double bond, and reduces the double bond (Fig. 33.14). NADPH provides the reducing equivalents for these reactions. The net result is that the original acetyl group is elongated by two carbons.

The 4-carbon fatty acyl chain is then transferred to the cysteinyl sulfhydryl group and subsequently condenses with a malonyl group. This sequence of reactions is repeated until the chain is 16 carbons in length. At this point, hydrolysis occurs, and palmitate is released (Fig. 33.15).

Palmitate is elongated and desaturated to produce a series of fatty acids. In the liver, palmitate and other newly synthesized fatty acids are converted to triacylglycerols that are packaged into VLDL for secretion.

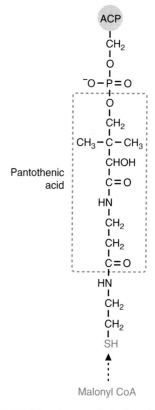

Fig. 33.12. Phosphopantetheinyl residue of the fatty acid synthase complex. The portion derived from the vitamin, pantothenic acid, is indicated. Phosphopantetheine is covalently linked to a serine residue of the acyl carrier protein (ACP) segment of the enzyme. The sulfhydryl group reacts with malonyl CoA to form a thioester.

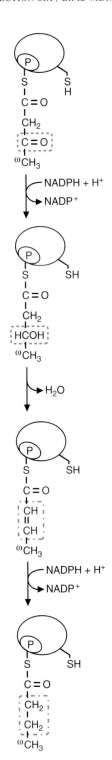

Fig. 33.14. Reduction of a β-ketoacyl group on the fatty acid synthase complex. NADPH is the reducing agent.

Q: Where does the methyl group of the first acetyl CoA that binds to fatty acid synthase appear in palmitate, the final product?

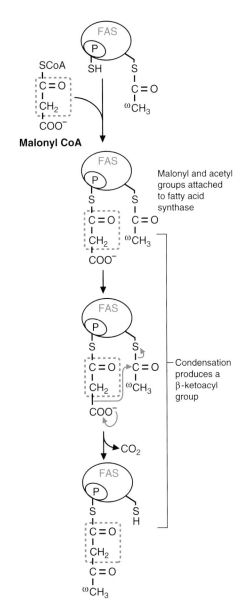

Fig. 33.13. Addition of a 2-carbon unit to an acetyl group on fatty acid synthase. The malonyl group attaches to the phosphopantetheinyl residue (P) of the ACP of the fatty acid synthase. The acetyl group, which is attached to a cysteinyl sulfhydryl group, condenses with the malonyl group. CO_2 is released, and a 3-ketoacyl group is formed. The carbon that eventually forms the ω-methyl group of palmitate is labeled ω.

In the liver, the oxidation of newly synthesized fatty acids back to acetyl CoA via the mitochondrial β-oxidation pathway is prevented by malonyl CoA. Carnitine:palmitoyltransferase I, the enzyme involved in the transport of long-chain fatty acids into mitochondria (see Chapter 23), is inhibited by malonyl CoA (Fig. 33.16). Malonyl CoA levels are elevated when acetyl CoA carboxylase is activated, and, thus, fatty acid oxidation is inhibited while fatty acid synthesis is proceeding. This inhibition prevents the occurrence of a futile cycle.

D. Elongation of Fatty Acids

After synthesis on the fatty acid synthase complex, palmitate is activated, forming palmityl CoA. Palmityl CoA and other activated long-chain fatty acids can be

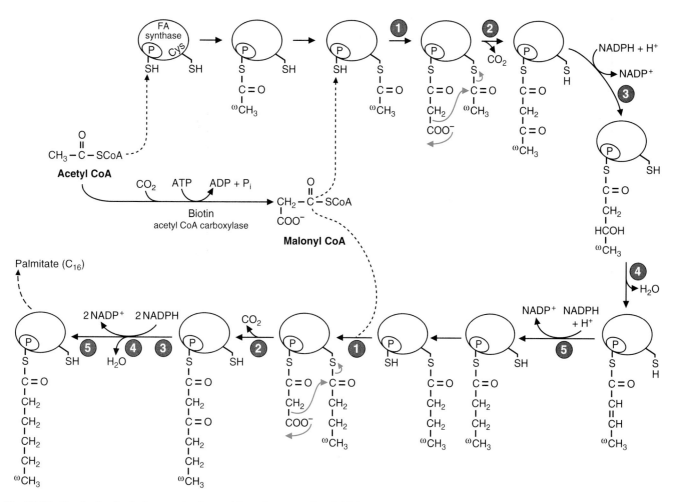

Fig. 33.15. Synthesis of palmitate on the fatty acid synthase complex. Initially, acetyl CoA adds to the synthase. It provides the ω-methyl group of palmitate. Malonyl CoA provides the 2-carbon units that are added to the growing fatty acyl chain. The addition and reduction steps are repeated until palmitate is produced. 1. Transfer of the malonyl group to the phosphopantetheinyl residue. 2. Condensation of the malonyl and fatty acyl groups. 3. Reduction of the β-ketoacyl group. 4. Dehydration. 5. Reduction of the double bond. P = a phosphopantetheinyl group attached to the fatty acid synthase complex; Cys-SH = a cysteinyl residue.

elongated, two carbons at a time, by a series of reactions that occur in the endoplasmic reticulum (Fig. 33.17). Malonyl CoA serves as the donor of the 2-carbon units, and NADPH provides the reducing equivalents. The series of elongation reactions resemble those of fatty acid synthesis except that the fatty acyl chain is attached to coenzyme A rather than to the phosphopantetheinyl residue of an ACP. The major elongation reaction that occurs in the body involves the conversion of palmityl CoA (C16) to stearyl CoA (C18). Very-long-chain fatty acids (C22 to C24) are also produced, particularly in the brain.

E. Desaturation of Fatty Acids

Desaturation of fatty acids involves a process that requires molecular oxygen (O_2), NADH, and cytochrome b_5. The reaction, which occurs in the endoplasmic reticulum, results in the oxidation of both the fatty acid and NADH (Fig. 33.18). The most common desaturation reactions involve the placement of a double bond between carbons 9 and 10 in the conversion of palmitic acid to palmitoleic acid (16:1, Δ^9) and the conversion of stearic acid to oleic acid (18:1, Δ^9). Other positions that can be desaturated in humans include carbons 4, 5, and 6.

A: The methyl group of acetyl CoA becomes the ω-carbon (the terminal methyl group) of palmitate. Each new 2-carbon unit is added to the carboxyl end of the growing fatty acyl chain (see Fig. 33.13).

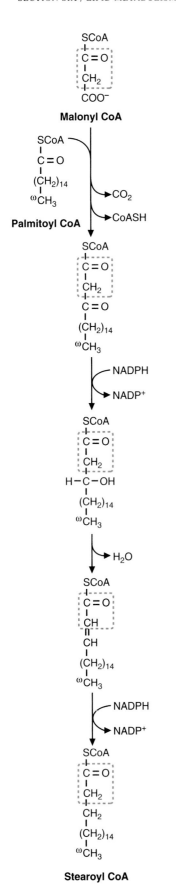

Fig. 33.17. Elongation of long-chain fatty acids in the endoplasmic reticulum.

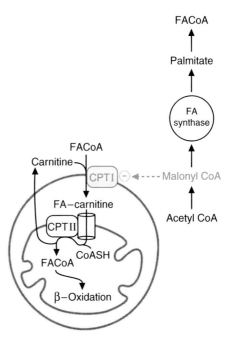

Fig. 33.16. Inhibition of carnitine:palmitoyltransferase (CPTI, also called carnitine:acyl-transferase I) by malonyl CoA. During fatty acid synthesis, malonyl CoA levels are high. This compound inhibits CPTI, which is involved in the transport of long-chain fatty acids into mitochondria for β-oxidation. This mechanism prevents newly synthesized fatty acids from undergoing immediate oxidation.

Polyunsaturated fatty acids with double bonds three carbons from the methyl end (ω3 fatty acids) and six carbons from the methyl end (ω6 fatty acids) are required for the synthesis of eicosanoids (see Chapter 35). Because humans cannot synthesize these fatty acids de novo (i.e., from glucose via palmitate), they must be present in the diet or the diet must contain other fatty acids that can be converted to these fatty acids. We obtain ω6 and ω3 polyunsaturated fatty acids mainly from dietary plant oils that contain the ω6 fatty acid linoleic acid (18:2, $\Delta^{9,12}$) and the ω3 fatty acid α-linolenic acid (18:3, $\Delta^{9,12,15}$). In the body, linoleic acid can be converted by elongation and desaturation reactions to arachidonic acid (20:4, $\Delta^{5,8,11,14}$), which is used for the synthesis of the major class of human prostaglandins and other eicosanoids (Fig. 33.19). Elongation and desaturation of α-linolenic acid produces eicosapentaenoic acid (EPA; 20:5, $\Delta^{5,8,11,14,17}$), which is the precursor of a different class of eicosanoids (see Chapter 35).

Plants are able to introduce double bonds into fatty acids in the region between C10 and the ω-end and therefore can synthesize ω3 and ω6 polyunsaturated fatty acids. Fish oils also contain ω3 and ω6 fatty acids, particularly eicosapentaenoic acid (EPA; ω3, 20:5, Δ5, 8, 11, 14, 17) and docosahexaenoic acid (DHA; ω3,22:6, Δ4,7,10,13,16,19). The fish obtain these fatty acids by eating phytoplankton (plants that float in water).

Arachidonic acid is listed in some textbooks as an essential fatty acid. Although it is an ω6 fatty acid, it is not essential in the diet if linoleic acid is present because arachidonic acid can be synthesized from dietary linoleic acid (see Fig. 33.19).

The essential fatty acid linoleic acid is required in the diet for at least three reasons: (a) It serves as a precursor of arachidonic acid from which eicosanoids are produced. (b) It covalently binds another fatty acid attached to cerebrosides in the skin, forming an unusual lipid (acylglucosylceramide) that helps to make the skin impermeable to water. This function of linoleic acid may help to explain the red, scaly dermatitis and other skin problems associated with a dietary deficiency of essential fatty acids. (c) It is the precursor of C22:6ω3, an important neuronal fatty acid.

The other essential fatty acid, α-linolenic acid (18:3, Δ9, 12, 15), also forms eicosanoids.

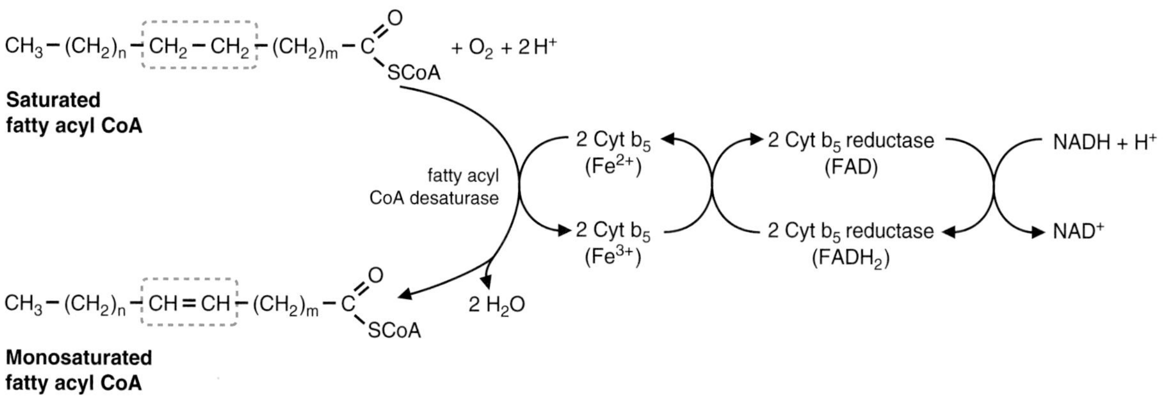

Fig. 33.18. Desaturation of fatty acids. The process occurs in the endoplasmic reticulum and uses molecular oxygen. Both the fatty acid and NADH are oxidized. Human desaturases cannot introduce double bonds between carbon 9 and the methyl end. Therefore, m is equal to or less than 7.

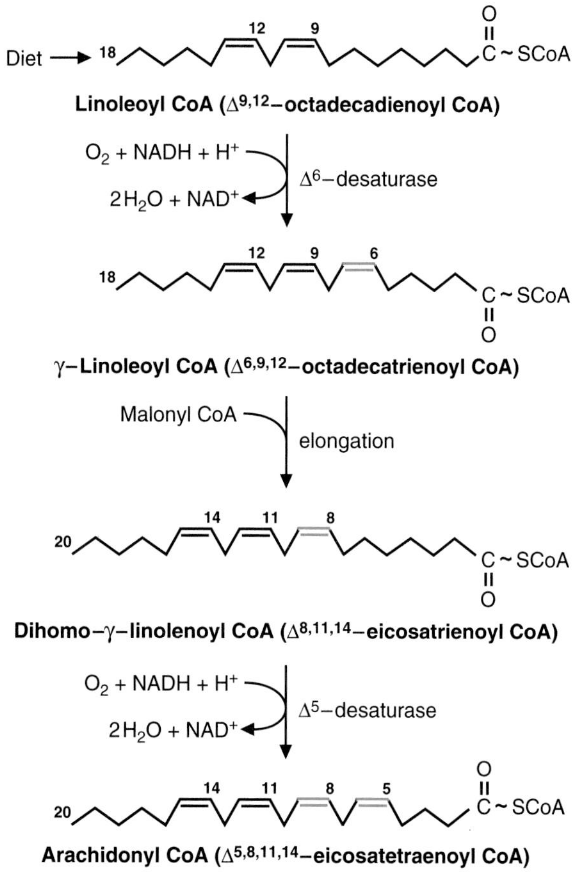

Fig. 33.19. Conversion of linoleic acid to arachidonic acid. Dietary linoleic acid (as linoleoyl CoA) is desaturated at carbon 6, elongated by 2 carbons, and then desaturated at carbon 5 to produce arachidonyl CoA.

II. SYNTHESIS OF TRIACYLGLYCEROLS AND VLDL PARTICLES

In liver and adipose tissue, triacylglycerols are produced by a pathway containing a phosphatidic acid intermediate (Fig. 33.20). Phosphatidic acid is also the precursor of the glycerolipids found in cell membranes and the blood lipoproteins.

The sources of glycerol 3-phosphate, which provides the glycerol moiety for triacylglycerol synthesis, differ in liver and adipose tissue. In liver, glycerol 3-phosphate

Recent experiments have shown functional glycerol kinase activity in muscle cells. The significance of this finding is under investigation, but it may indicate that muscle has a greater capacity for fatty acid synthesis than previously believed.

is produced from the phosphorylation of glycerol by glycerol kinase or from the reduction of dihydroxyacetone phosphate derived from glycolysis. Adipose tissue lacks glycerol kinase and can produce glycerol 3-phosphate only from glucose via dihydroxyacetone phosphate. Thus, adipose tissue can store fatty acids only when glycolysis is activated, i.e., in the fed state.

In both adipose tissue and liver, triacylglycerols are produced by a pathway in which glycerol 3-phosphate reacts with fatty acyl CoA to form phosphatidic acid. Dephosphorylation of phosphatidic acid produces diacylglycerol. Another fatty acyl CoA reacts with the diacylglycerol to form a triacylglycerol (see Fig. 33.20).

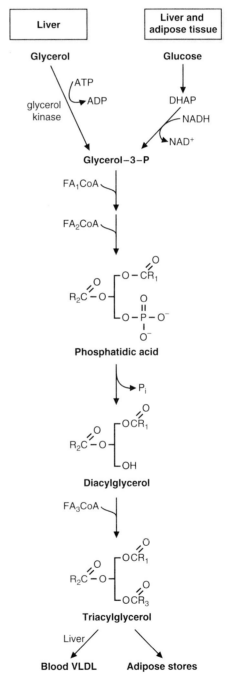

Fig. 33.20. Synthesis of triacylglycerol in liver and adipose tissue. Glycerol 3-phosphate is produced from glucose in both tissues. It is also produced from glycerol in liver, but not in adipose tissue, which lacks glycerol kinase. The steps from glycerol 3-phosphate are the same in the two tissues. FA = fatty acyl group.

Adipose tissue also undergoes glyceroneogenesis, the process of synthesizing glycerol from gluconeogenic precursors in the blood, such as alanine, aspartate, and malate. Glyceroneogenesis occurs primarily in the fasting state and is dependent on the induction of cytoplasmic PEPCK in the adipocyte. The re-synthesis of triglycerides by adipose tissue during fasting modulates the release of fatty acids in the circulation. Mice that have been engineered to not express PEPCK in adipose tissue display reduced levels of triglyceride in their adipocytes; mice that overproduce adipocyte PEPCK were obese. Thus, although activation of hormone-sensitive lipase during fasting results in the release of fatty acids from adipocytes, the release is carefully modulated through glyceroneogenesis and re-synthesis of triglycerides.

Adipocyte; fasting conditions

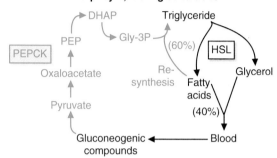

The triacylglycerol, which is produced in the smooth endoplasmic reticulum of the liver, is packaged with cholesterol, phospholipids, and proteins (synthesized in the rough endoplasmic reticulum) to form VLDL (Fig. 33.21). The microsomal triglyceride transfer protein (MTP), which is required for chylomicron assembly, is also required for VLDL assembly. The major protein of VLDL is apoB-100. There is one long apoB-100 molecule wound through the surface of each VLDL particle. ApoB-100 is encoded by the same gene as the apoB-48 of chylomicrons, but is a longer protein (see Fig. 32.11). In intestinal cells, RNA editing produces a smaller mRNA and, thus, a shorter protein, apoB-48.

VLDL is processed in the Golgi complex and secreted into the blood by the liver (Figs. 33.22 and 33.23). The fatty acid residues of the triacylglycerols ultimately are stored in the triacylglycerols of adipose cells. Note that, in comparison to chylomicrons (see Chapter 32), VLDL particles are more dense, as they contain a lower percentage of triglyceride than do the chylomicrons. Similar to chylomicrons, VLDL particles are first synthesized in a nascent form, and on entering the circulation they acquire apoproteins CII and E from HDL particles to become mature VLDL particles.

Abetalipoproteinemia, which is due to a lack of MTP (microsomal triglyceride transfer protein; see Chapter 32) activity, results in an inability to assemble both chylomicrons in the intestine and VLDL particles in the liver.

Q: Why do some alcoholics have high VLDL levels?

The fact that a number of different abnormal lipoprotein profiles were found in **Cora Nari** and her siblings, and that each had evidence of coronary artery disease, suggests that Cora has familial combined hyperlipidemia (FCH). This diagnostic impression is further supported by the finding that Cora's profile of lipid abnormalities appeared to change somewhat from one determination to the next, a characteristic of FCH. This hereditary disorder of lipid metabolism is believed to be quite common, with an estimated prevalence of about 1 per 100 population.

The mechanisms for FCH are incompletely understood but may involve a genetically determined increase in the production of apoprotein B-100. As a result, packaging of VLDL is increased, and blood VLDL levels may be elevated. Depending on the efficiency of lipolysis of VLDL by LPL, VLDL levels may be normal and LDL levels may be elevated, or both VLDL and LDL levels may be high. In addition, the phenotypic expression of FCH in any given family member may be determined by the degree of associated obesity, the diet, the use of specific drugs, or other factors that change over time.

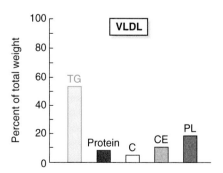

Fig. 33.21. Composition of a typical VLDL particle. The major component is triacylglycerol (TG). C = cholesterol; CE = cholesterol ester; PL = phospholipid.

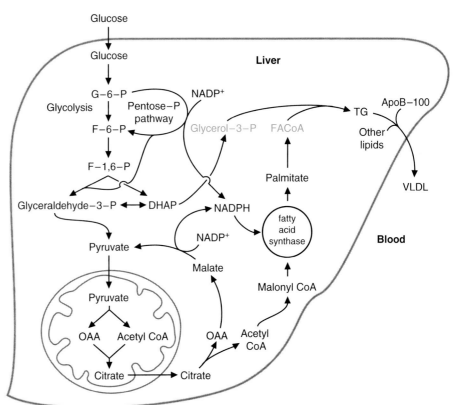

Fig. 33.22. Synthesis of VLDL from glucose in the liver. G-6-P = glucose 6-phosphate; F-6-P = fructose 6-phosphate; F-1,6-BP = fructose 1,6-bisphosphate; FA = fatty acyl group; TG = triacylglycerol.

III. FATE OF VLDL TRIACYLGLYCEROL

Lipoprotein lipase (LPL), which is attached to the basement membrane proteoglycans of capillary endothelial cells, cleaves the triacylglycerols in both VLDL and chylomicrons, forming fatty acids and glycerol. The C-II apoprotein, which these lipoproteins obtain from HDL, activates LPL. The low K_m of the muscle LPL isozyme permits muscle to use the fatty acids of chylomicrons and VLDL as a source of fuel even when the blood concentration of these lipoproteins is very low. The isozyme in adipose tissue has a high K_m and is most active after a meal, when blood levels of chylomicrons and VLDL are elevated. The fate of the VLDL particle after triglyceride has been removed by LPL is the generation of an IDL particle (intermediate-density lipoprotein), which can further lose triglyceride to become an LDL particle (low-density lipoprotein). The fate of the IDL and LDL particles is discussed in Chapter 34.

Fatty acids for VLDL synthesis in the liver may be obtained from the blood or they may be synthesized from glucose. In a healthy individual, the major source of the fatty acids of VLDL triacylglycerol is excess dietary glucose. In individuals with diabetes mellitus, fatty acids mobilized from adipose triacylglycerols in excess of the oxidative capacity of tissues are a major source of the fatty acids re-esterified in liver to VLDL triacylglycerol. These individuals frequently have elevated levels of blood triacylglycerols.

A: In alcoholism, NADH levels in the liver are elevated (see Chapter 25). High levels of NADH inhibit the oxidation of fatty acids. Therefore, fatty acids, mobilized from adipose tissue, are re-esterified to glycerol in the liver, forming triacylglycerols, which are packaged into VLDL and secreted into the blood. Elevated VLDL is frequently associated with chronic alcoholism. As alcohol-induced liver disease progresses, the ability to secrete the triacylglycerols is diminished, resulting in a fatty liver.

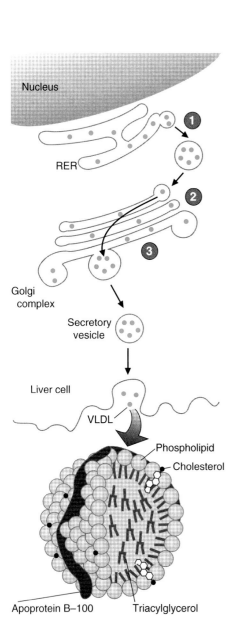

Fig. 33.23. Synthesis, processing, and secretion of VLDL. Proteins synthesized on the rough endoplasmic reticulum (RER) are packaged with triacylglycerols in the ER and Golgi complex to form VLDL. VLDL are transported to the cell membrane in secretory vesicles and secreted by endocytosis. Blue dots represent VLDL particles. An enlarged VLDL particle is depicted at the bottom of the figure.

IV. STORAGE OF TRIACYLGLYCEROLS IN ADIPOSE TISSUE

After a meal, the triacylglycerol stores of adipose tissue increase (Fig. 33.24). Adipose cells synthesize LPL and secrete it into the capillaries of adipose tissue when the insulin/glucagon ratio is elevated. This enzyme digests the triacylglycerols of both chylomicrons and VLDL. The fatty acids enter adipose cells and are activated, forming fatty acyl CoA, which reacts with glycerol 3-phosphate to form triacylglycerol by the same pathway used in the liver (see Fig. 33.20). Because adipose tissue lacks glycerol kinase and cannot use the glycerol produced by LPL, the glycerol travels through the blood to the liver, which uses it for the synthesis of triacylglycerol. In adipose cells, glycerol 3-phosphate is derived from glucose.

In addition to stimulating the synthesis and release of LPL, insulin stimulates glucose metabolism in adipose cells. Insulin leads to the activation of the glycolytic enzyme phosphofructokinase-1 by an activation of PFK-2, which increases fructose 2,6-bisphosphate levels. Insulin also stimulates the dephosphorylation of pyruvate dehydrogenase, so that the pyruvate produced by glycolysis can be oxidized in the TCA cycle. Furthermore, insulin stimulates the conversion of glucose to fatty acids in adipose cells, although the liver is the major site of fatty acid synthesis in humans.

V. RELEASE OF FATTY ACIDS FROM ADIPOSE TRIACYLGLYCEROLS

During fasting, the decrease of insulin and the increase of glucagon cause cAMP levels to rise in adipose cells, stimulating lipolysis (Fig. 33.25). Protein kinase A phosphorylates hormone-sensitive lipase to produce a more active form of the enzyme. Hormone-sensitive lipase, also known as adipose triacylglycerol lipase, cleaves a fatty acid from a triacylglycerol. Subsequently, other lipases complete the process of lipolysis, and fatty acids and glycerol are released into the blood. Simultaneously, to regulate the amount of fatty acids released into circulation, triglyceride synthesis occurs along with glyceroneogenesis.

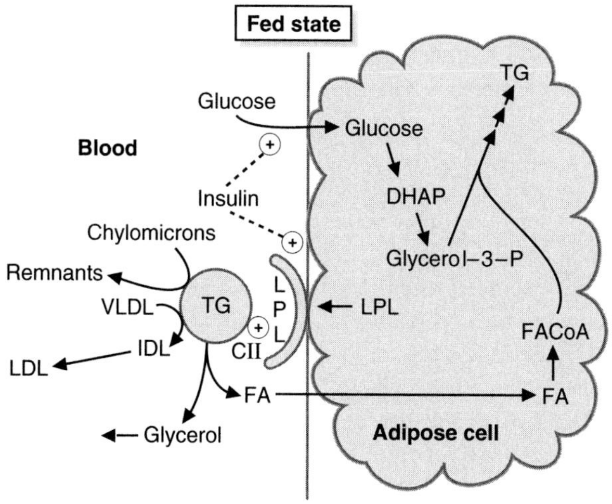

Q: In some cases of hyperlipidemia, LPL is defective. If a blood lipid profile is performed on patients with an LPL deficiency, which lipids would be elevated?

Because the fatty acids of adipose triacylglycerols come both from chylomicrons and VLDL, we produce our major fat stores both from dietary fat (which produces chylomicrons) and dietary sugar (which produces VLDL). An excess of dietary protein also can be used to produce the fatty acids for VLDL synthesis.

The dietician carefully explained to **Percy Veere** that we can become fat from eating excess fat, excess sugar, or excess protein.

Fig. 33.24. Conversion of the fatty acid (FA) from the triacylglycerols (TG) of chylomicrons and VLDL to the TG stored in adipose cells. Note that insulin stimulates both the transport of glucose into adipose cells and the secretion of LPL from the cells. Glucose provides the glycerol 3-phosphate for TG synthesis. Insulin also stimulates the synthesis and secretion of lipoprotein lipase (LPL). Apoprotein C-II activates LPL.

A: Individuals with a defective LPL have high blood triacylglycerol levels. Their levels of chylomicrons and VLDL (which contain large amounts of triacylglycerols) are elevated because they are not digested at the normal rate by LPL.

LPL can be dissociated from capillary walls by treatment with heparin (a glycosaminoglycan). Measurements can be made on blood after heparin treatment to determine whether LPL levels are abnormal.

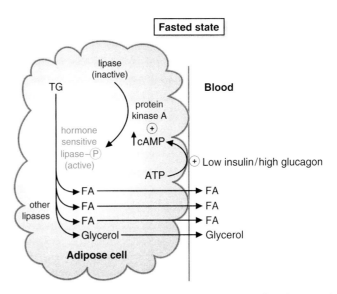

Fig. 33.25. Mobilization of adipose triacylglycerol (TG). In the fasted state, when insulin levels are low and glucagon is elevated, intracellular cAMP increases and activates protein kinase A, which phosphorylates hormone-sensitive lipase (HSL). Phosphorylated HSL is active and initiates the breakdown of adipose TG. Recall, however, that re-esterification of fatty acids does occur, along with glyceroneogenesis, in the fasted state. HSL is also called triacylglycerol lipase. FA = fatty acid.

The fatty acids, which travel in the blood complexed with albumin, enter cells of muscle and other tissues, where they are oxidized to CO_2 and water to produce energy. During prolonged fasting, acetyl CoA produced by β-oxidation of fatty acids in the liver is converted to ketone bodies, which are released into the blood. The glycerol derived from lipolysis in adipose cells is used by the liver during fasting as a source of carbon for gluconeogenesis.

VI. METABOLISM OF GLYCEROPHOSPHOLIPIDS AND SPHINGOLIPIDS

Fatty acids, obtained from the diet or synthesized from glucose, are the precursors of glycerophospholipids and of sphingolipids (Fig. 33.26). These lipids are major components of cellular membranes. Glycerophospholipids are also components of blood lipoproteins, bile, and lung surfactant. They are the source of the polyunsaturated fatty acids, particularly arachidonic acid, that serve as precursors of the eicosanoids (e.g., prostaglandins, thromboxanes, leukotrienes; see Chapter 35). Ether glycerophospholipids differ from other glycerophospholipids in that the alkyl or alkenyl chain (an alkyl chain with a double bond) is joined to carbon 1 of the glycerol moiety by an ether rather than an ester bond. Examples of ether lipids are the plasmalogens and platelet activating factor. Sphingolipids are particularly important in forming the myelin sheath surrounding nerves in the central nervous system, and in signal transduction.

In glycerolipids and ether glycerolipids, glycerol serves as the backbone to which fatty acids and other substituents are attached. Sphingosine, derived from serine, provides the backbone for sphingolipids.

A. Synthesis of Phospholipids Containing Glycerol

1. GLYCEROPHOSPHOLIPIDS

The initial steps in the synthesis of glycerophospholipids are similar to those of triacylglycerol synthesis. Glycerol 3-phosphate reacts with fatty acyl CoA to form

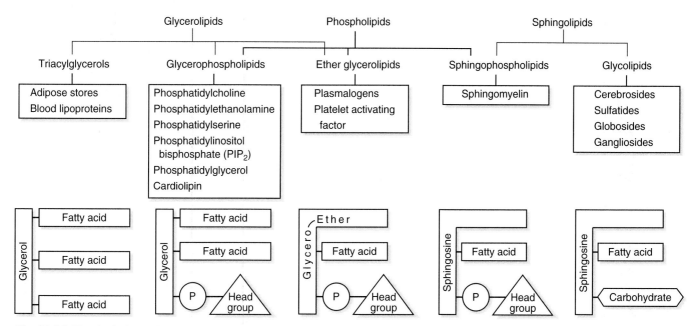

Fig. 33.26. Types of glycerolipids and sphingolipids. Glycerolipids contain glycerol, and sphingolipids contain sphingosine. The category of phospholipids overlaps both glycerolipids and sphingolipids. The head groups include choline, ethanolamine, serine, inositol, glycerol, and phosphatidylglycerol. The carbohydrates are monosaccharides (which may be sulfated), oligosaccharides, and oligosaccharides with branches of *N*-acetylneuraminic acid. P = phosphate.

phosphatidic acid. Two different mechanisms are then used to add a head group to the molecule (Fig. 33.27). A head group is a chemical group, such as choline or serine, attached to carbon 3 of a glycerol moiety that contains hydrophobic groups, usually fatty acids, at positions 1 and 2. Head groups are hydrophilic, either charged or polar.

In the first mechanism, phosphatidic acid is cleaved by a phosphatase to form diacylglycerol (DAG). DAG then reacts with an activated head group. In the synthesis of phosphatidylcholine, the head group choline is activated by combining with CTP to form CDP-choline (Fig. 33.28). Phosphocholine is then transferred to carbon 3 of DAG, and CMP is released. Phosphatidylethanolamine is produced by a similar reaction involving CDP-ethanolamine.

Various types of interconversions occur among these phospholipids (see Fig. 33.28). Phosphatidylserine is produced by a reaction in which the ethanolamine moiety of

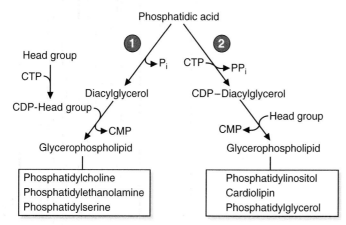

Fig. 33.27. Strategies for addition of the head group to form glycerophospholipids. In both cases, CTP is used to drive the reaction.

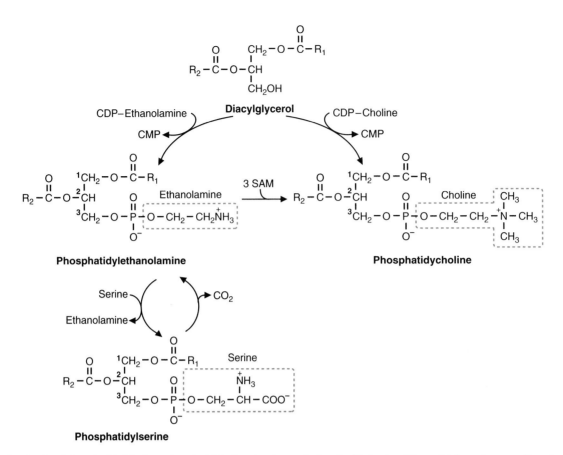

Fig. 33.28. Synthesis of phosphatidylcholine, phosphatidylethanolamine, and phosphatidylserine. The multiple pathways reflect the importance of phospholipids in membrane structure. For example, phosphatidylcholine (PC) can be synthesized from dietary choline when it is available. If choline is not available, PC can be made from dietary carbohydrate, although the amount synthesized is inadequate to prevent choline deficiency. SAM is S-adenosylmethionine, a methyl group donor for many biochemical reactions (see Chapter 40).

Phosphatidylcholine (lecithin) is not required in the diet because it can be synthesized in the body. The components of phosphatidylcholine (including choline) all can be produced, as shown in Figure 33.28. A pathway for de novo choline synthesis from glucose exists, but the rate of synthesis is inadequate to provide for the necessary amounts of choline. Thus, choline has been classified as an essential nutrient, with an AI (adequate intake) of 425 mg/day in females and 550 mg/day in males.

Because choline is widely distributed in the food supply, primarily in phosphatidylcholine (lecithin), deficiencies have not been observed in humans on a normal diet. Deficiencies may occur, however, in patients on total parenteral nutrition (TPN), i.e., supported solely by intravenous feeding. The fatty livers that have been observed in these patients probably result from a decreased ability to synthesize phospholipids for VLDL formation.

phosphatidylethanolamine is exchanged for serine. Phosphatidylserine can be converted back to phosphatidylethanolamine by a decarboxylation reaction. Phosphatidylethanolamine can be methylated to form phosphatidylcholine (see Chapter 40).

In the second mechanism for the synthesis of glycerolipids, phosphatidic acid reacts with CTP to form CDP-diacylglycerol (Fig. 33.29). This compound can react with phosphatidylglycerol (which itself is formed from the condensation of CDP-diacylglycerol and glycerol 3-phosphate) to produce cardiolipin or with inositol to produce phosphatidylinositol. Cardiolipin is a component of the inner mitochondrial membrane. Phosphatidylinositol can be phosphorylated to form phosphatidylinositol 4,5-bisphosphate (PIP_2), which is a component of cell membranes. In response to signals such as the binding of hormones to membrane receptors, PIP_2 can be cleaved to form the second messengers diacylglycerol and inositol triphosphate (see Chapter 11).

2. ETHER GLYCEROLIPIDS

The ether glycerolipids are synthesized from the glycolytic intermediate dihydroxyacetone phosphate (DHAP). A fatty acyl CoA reacts with carbon 1 of DHAP, forming an ester (Fig. 33.30). This fatty acyl group is exchanged for a fatty alcohol, produced by reduction of a fatty acid. Thus, the ether linkage is formed. Then the keto group on carbon 2 of the DHAP moiety is reduced and esterified to a fatty acid. Addition of the head group proceeds by a series of reactions analogous to those for synthesis of phosphatidylcholine. Formation of a double bond between carbons 1 and 2 of the alkyl group produces a plasmalogen. Ethanolamine plasmalogen is found in

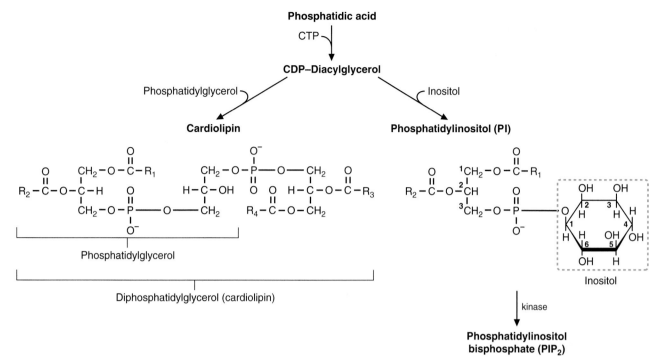

Fig. 33.29. Synthesis of cardiolipin and phosphatidylinositol.

The respiratory distress syndrome (RDS) of a premature infant such as **Colleen Lakker** is, in part, related to a deficiency in the synthesis of a substance known as lung surfactant. The major constituents of surfactant are dipalmitoylphosphatidyl-choline, phosphatidylglycerol, apoproteins (surfactant proteins: Sp-A,B,C), and cholesterol.

**Dipalmitoylphosphatidycholine,
the major component of
lung surfactant**

These components of lung surfactant normally contribute to a reduction in the surface tension within the air spaces (alveoli) of the lung, preventing their collapse. The premature infant has not yet begun to produce adequate amounts of lung surfactant.

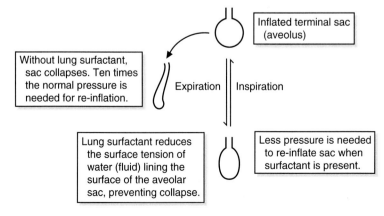

The effect of lung surfactant

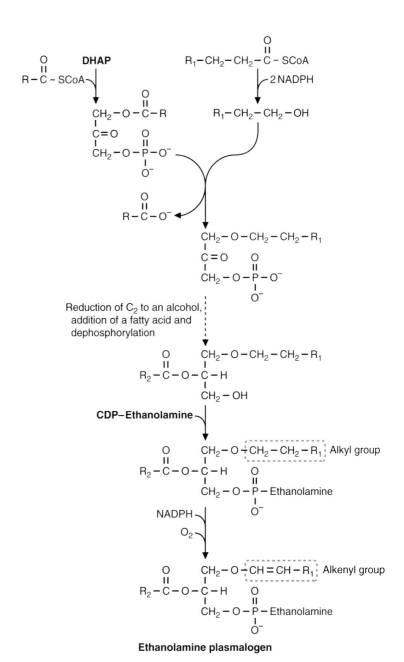

Fig. 33.30. Synthesis of a plasmalogen.

myelin and choline plasmalogen in heart muscle. Platelet-activating factor (PAF) is similar to choline plasmalogen except that an acetyl group replaces the fatty acyl group at carbon 2 of the glycerol moiety, and the alkyl group on carbon 1 is saturated. PAF is released from phagocytic blood cells in response to various stimuli. It causes platelet aggregation, edema, and hypotension, and it is involved in the allergic response. Plasmalogen synthesis occurs within peroxisomes, and, in individuals with Zellweger's syndrome (a defect in peroxisome biogenesis), plasmalogen synthesis is compromised. If severe enough, this syndrome leads to death at an early age.

B. Degradation of Glycerophospholipids

Phospholipases located in cell membranes or in lysosomes degrade glycerophospholipids. Phospholipase A1 removes the fatty acyl group on carbon 1 of the glycerol moiety, and phospholipase A2 removes the fatty acid on carbon 2 (Fig. 33.31). The C2 fatty acid in cell membrane phospholipids is usually an unsaturated fatty acid,

Phospholipase A2 provides the major repair mechanism for membrane lipids damaged by oxidative free radical reactions. Arachidonic acid, which is a polyunsaturated fatty acid, can be peroxidatively cleaved in free radical reactions to malondialdehyde and other products. Phospholipase A2 recognizes the distortion of membrane structure caused by the partially degraded fatty acid and removes it. Acyltransferases then add back a new arachidonic acid molecule.

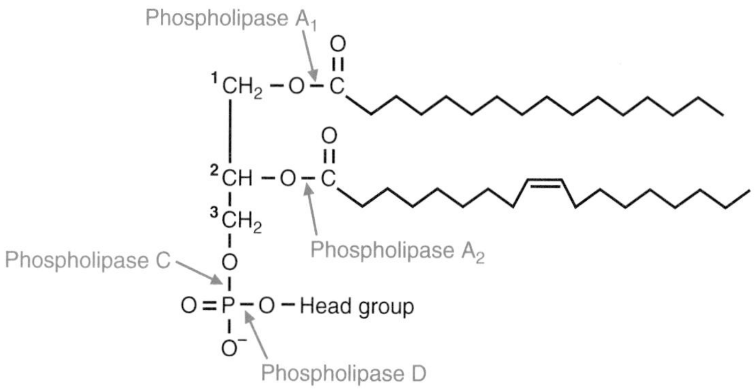

Fig. 33.31. Bonds cleaved by phospholipases.

which is frequently arachidonic acid. It is removed in response to signals for the synthesis of eicosanoids. The bond joining carbon 3 of the glycerol moiety to phosphate is cleaved by phospholipase C. Hormonal stimuli activate phospholipase C, which hydrolyzes PIP_2 to produce the second messengers DAG and inositol triphosphate (IP_3). The bond between the phosphate and the head group is cleaved by phospholipase D, producing phosphatidic acid and the free alcohol of the head group.

C. Sphingolipids

Sphingolipids serve in intercellular communication and as the antigenic determinants of the ABO blood group. Some are used as receptors by viruses and bacterial toxins, although it is unlikely that this was the purpose for which they originally evolved. Before the functions of the sphingolipids were elucidated, these compounds appeared to be inscrutable riddles. They were, therefore, named for the Sphinx of Thebes, who killed passersby that could not solve her riddle.

The synthesis of sphingolipids begins with the formation of ceramide (Fig. 33.32). Serine and palmityl CoA condense to form a product that is reduced. A very-long-chain fatty acid (usually containing 22 carbons) forms an amide with the amino group, a double bond is generated, and ceramide is formed.

Ceramide reacts with phosphatidylcholine to form sphingomyelin, a component of the myelin sheath (Fig. 33.33). Ceramide also reacts with UDP-sugars to form cerebrosides (which contain a single monosaccharide, usually galactose or glucose). Galactocerebroside may react with 3'-phosphoadenosine 5'-phosphosulfate (PAPS, an active sulfate donor; Figure 33.34) to form sulfatides, the major sulfolipids of the brain.

Additional sugars may be added to ceramide to form globosides, and gangliosides are produced by the addition of N-acetylneuraminic acid (NANA) as branches from the oligosaccharide chains (see Fig. 33.33 and Chapter 30).

Sphingolipids are degraded by lysosomal enzymes (see Chapter 30). Deficiencies of these enzymes result in a group of lysosomal storage diseases known as the sphingolipidoses.

CLINICAL COMMENTS

If **Percy Veere** had continued to eat a hypercaloric diet rich in carbohydrates, he would have become obese. In an effort to define obesity, it has been agreed internationally that the ratio of the patient's body weight in kilograms and their height in meters squared (W/H^2) is the most useful and reproducible measure. This ratio is referred to as the body mass index or BMI. Normal men and women fall into the range of 20 to 25. Percy's current value is 21.3 and rising.

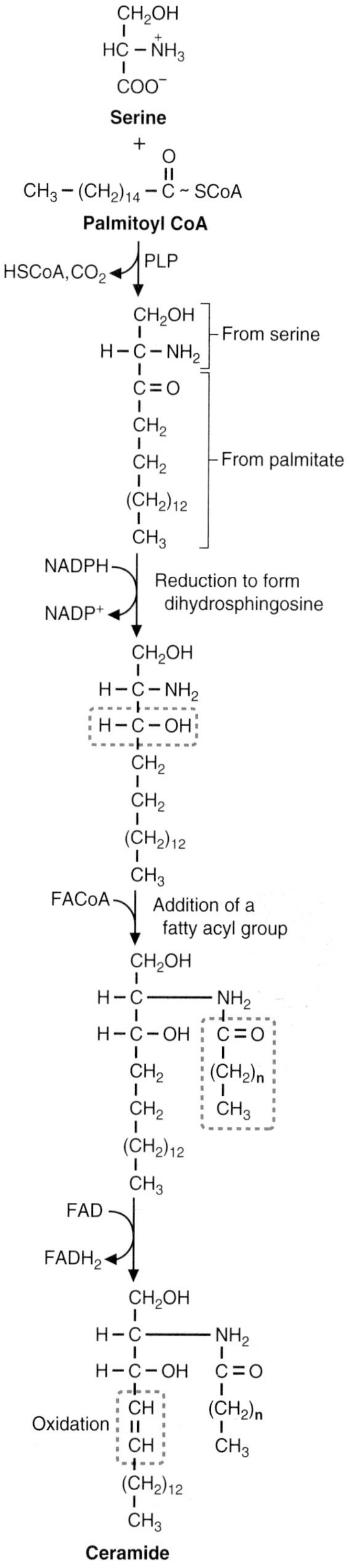

Fig. 33.32. Synthesis of ceramide. The changes that occur in each reaction are highlighted. PLP = pyridoxal phosphate.

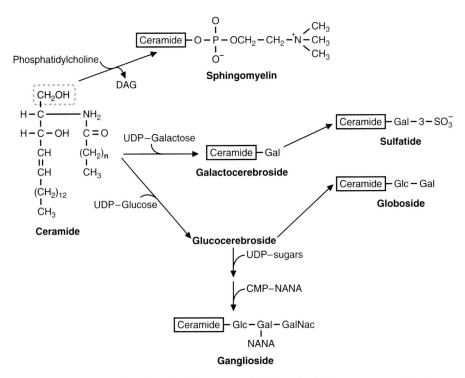

Fig. 33.33. Synthesis of sphingolipids from ceramide. Phosphocholine or sugars add to the hydroxymethyl group of ceramide (in blue) to form sphingomyelins, cerebrosides, sulfatides, globosides, and gangliosides. Gal = galactose; Glc = gucose; GalNAc = *N*-acetylgalactosamine; NANA = *N*-acetylneuraminic acid.

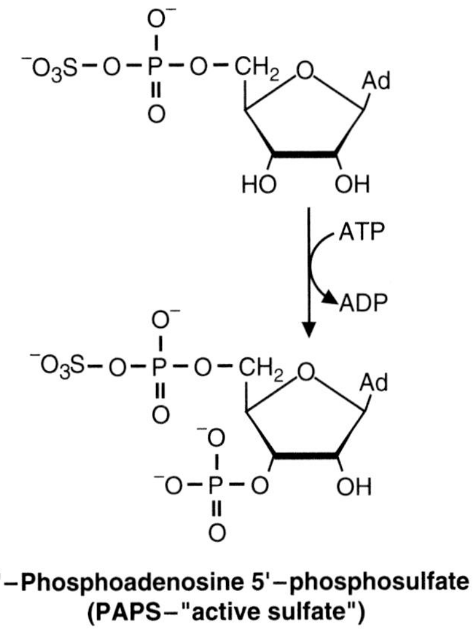

Fig. 33.34. The synthesis of 3'-phosphoadenosine 5'-phosphosulfate (PAPS), an active sulfate donor. PAPS donates sulfate groups to cerebrosides to form sulfatides and is also involved in glycosaminoglycan biosynthesis (see Chapter 49). Ad = adenosine.

Approximately 36 million people in the United States have a BMI greater than 27.8 (for men) or 27.3 (for women). At this level of obesity, which is quite close to a 20% weight increase above the "ideal" or desirable weight, an attempt at weight loss should be strongly advised. The idea that obesity is a benign condition unless accompanied by other risk factors for cardiovascular disease is disputed by several long-term, properly controlled prospective studies. These studies show that obesity is an independent risk factor not only for heart attacks and strokes, but for the development of insulin resistance, type 2 diabetes mellitus, hypertension, and gallbladder disease.

Percy did not want to become overweight and decided to follow his new diet faithfully.

Because **Cora Nari's** lipid profile indicated an elevation in both serum triacylglycerols and LDL cholesterol, she was classified as having a combined hyperlipidemia. The dissimilarities in the lipid profiles of Cora and her two siblings, both of whom were experiencing anginal chest pain, is characteristic of the multigenic syndrome referred to as familial combined hyperlipidemia (FCH).

Approximately 1% of the North American population has FCH. It is the most common cause of coronary artery disease in the United States. In contrast to patients with familial hypercholesterolemia (FH), patients with FCH do not have fatty deposits within the skin or tendons (xanthomas) (see Chapter 34). In FCH, coronary artery disease usually appears by the fifth decade of life.

Treatment of FCH includes restriction of dietary fat. Patients who do not respond adequately to dietary therapy are treated with antilipidemic drugs. Selection of the appropriate antilipidemic drugs depends on the specific phenotypic expression of the patient's multigenic disease as manifest by their particular serum lipid profile. In Cora's case, a decrease in both serum triacylglycerols and LDL cholesterol must be achieved. If possible, her serum HDL cholesterol level should also be raised to a level above 40 mg/dL.

To accomplish these therapeutic goals, her physician initially prescribed fast-release nicotinic acid (niacin), because this agent has the potential to lower serum triacylglycerol levels and cause a reciprocal rise in serum HDL cholesterol levels, as well as to lower serum total and LDL cholesterol levels. The mechanisms suggested for niacin's triacylglycerol-lowering action include enhancement of the action of LPL, inhibition of lipolysis in adipose tissue, and a decrease in esterification of triacylglycerols in the liver (see Table 34.5). The mechanism by which niacin lowers the serum total and LDL cholesterol levels is related to the decrease in hepatic production of VLDL. When the level of VLDL in the circulation decreases, the production of its daughter particles, IDL and LDL, also decreases. Cora found niacin's side effects of flushing and itching to be intolerable, and the drug was discontinued.

Pravastatin was given instead. Pravastatin inhibits cholesterol synthesis by inhibiting hydroxymethylglutaryl CoA (HMG-CoA) reductase, the rate-limiting enzyme in the pathway (see Chapter 34). After 3 months of therapy, pravastatin decreased Cora's LDL cholesterol from a pretreatment level of 175 to 122 mg/dL (still higher than the recommended treatment goal of 100 mg/dL or less in a patient with established coronary artery disease). Her fasting serum triacylglycerol concentration was decreased from a pretreatment level of 280 to 178 mg/dL (a treatment goal for serum triacylglycerol when the pretreatment level is less than 500 mg/dL has not been established).

Colleen Lakker suffered from respiratory distress syndrome (RDS), which is a major cause of death in the newborn. RDS is preventable if prematurity can be avoided by appropriate management of high-risk pregnancy and labor. Before delivery, the obstetrician must attempt to predict and possibly treat pulmonary prematurity in utero. For example, estimation of fetal head circumference by ultrasonography, monitoring for fetal arterial oxygen saturation, and determination of the ratio of the concentrations of phosphatidylcholine (lecithin) and that of sphingomyelin in the amniotic fluid may help to identify premature infants who are predisposed to RDS (Fig. 33.35).

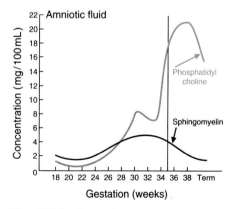

Fig. 33.35. Comparison of phosphatidylcholine and sphingomyelin in amniotic fluid. Phosphatidylcholine is the major lipid in lung surfactant. The concentration of phosphatidylcholine relative to sphingomyelin rises at 35 weeks of gestation, indicating pulmonary maturity.

The administration of synthetic corticosteroids 48 to 72 hours before delivery of a fetus of less than 33 weeks of gestation in women who have toxemia of pregnancy, diabetes mellitus, or chronic renal disease may reduce the incidence or mortality of RDS by stimulating fetal synthesis of lung surfactant.

The administration of one dose of surfactant into the trachea of the premature infant immediately after birth may transiently improve respiratory function but does not improve overall mortality. In Colleen's case, intensive therapy allowed her to survive this acute respiratory complication of prematurity.

BIOCHEMICAL COMMENTS

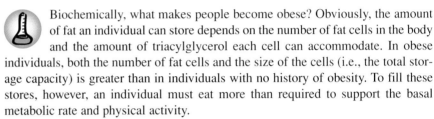

Biochemically, what makes people become obese? Obviously, the amount of fat an individual can store depends on the number of fat cells in the body and the amount of triacylglycerol each cell can accommodate. In obese individuals, both the number of fat cells and the size of the cells (i.e., the total storage capacity) is greater than in individuals with no history of obesity. To fill these stores, however, an individual must eat more than required to support the basal metabolic rate and physical activity.

Fat cells begin to proliferate early in life, starting in the third trimester of gestation. Proliferation essentially ceases before puberty, and thereafter fat cells change mainly in size. However, some increase in the number of fat cells can occur in adulthood if preadipocytes are induced to proliferate by growth factors and changes in the nutritional state. Weight reduction results in a decrease in the size of fat cells rather than a decrease in number. After weight loss, the amount of LPL, an enzyme involved in the transfer of fatty acids from blood triacylglycerols to the triacylglycerol stores of adipocytes, increases. In addition, the amount of mRNA for LPL also increases. All of these factors suggest that individuals who become obese, particularly those who do so early in life, will have difficulty losing weight and maintaining a lower body adipose mass.

Signals that initiate or inhibit feeding are extremely complex and include psychological and hormonal factors as well as neurotransmitter activity. These signals are integrated and relayed through the hypothalamus. Destruction of specific regions of the hypothalamus can lead to overeating and obesity or to anorexia and weight loss. Overeating and obesity are associated with damage to the ventromedial or the paraventricular nucleus, whereas weight loss and anorexia are related to damage to more lateral hypothalamic regions. Compounds that act as satiety signals have been identified in brain tissue and include leptin and glucagon-like peptide-1 (GLP-1). Appetite suppressors developed from compounds such as these may be used in the future for the treatment of obesity.

Recently it has become apparent that the adipocyte, in addition to storing triacylglycerol, secretes hormones that regulate both glucose and fat metabolism. The hormones leptin, resistin (resists insulin action), and adiponectin (also known as Acrp30) are all secreted from adipocytes under different conditions. The role of these hormones has been best understood in mouse models; unfortunately, extrapolation to the human condition has been difficult. In mice, leptin is released from adipocytes as triglyceride levels increase and signals the hypothalamus to reduce eating and to increase physical activity. Mice lacking the ability to secrete leptin (the ob mouse), or respond to leptin (the db mouse) are obese. Injecting leptin into ob mice allows them to lose weight.

The adipocytes in mice have been shown to release a hormone known as resistin. This hormone may contribute to insulin resistance in these animals. The mechanism by which resistin causes an insensitivity of cells to the actions of insulin is unknown. It is of great interest, however, that the class of drugs known as thiazolidinediones, which are given to individuals with type 2 diabetes, suppress resistin transcription, reduce resistin levels, and increase sensitivity to insulin in these patients. Additionally, thiazolidinediones may upregulate adipose PEPCK, resulting in a reduced fatty acid output from the adipocyte because of increased glyceroneogenesis.

In humans, adiponectin is secreted from adipocytes in inverse proportion to their adipose mass, lean individuals secreting more adiponectin than obese individuals. This is the exact opposite of leptin secretion. The effects of adiponectin, and how it interacts with resistin and leptin, are active areas of current research.

Further complicating the issue of glucose and lipid homeostasis is the effect of nuclear receptors known as peroxisome proliferator activated receptors (PPAR). These nuclear receptors (see Chapter 10) exist in three forms; α, β/δ, and γ. PPARγ is found in highest levels in adipocytes, and activation of the receptor leads to gene transcription, which is necessary for adipocyte differentiation and regulation of lipid metabolism. The thiazolidinediones activate PPARγ, which leads to a decrease in circulating resistin levels. Understanding more about the physiologic regulators of PPARγ is also an active area of research. The role of PPAR in liver is discussed in Chapter 46.

Although an increase in food intake beyond the daily requirements results in an increase in body weight and in fat stores, there is a large variation among individuals in the amount of weight gained for a given number of excess calories consumed. Both genetic and environmental factors influence the development of obesity. Studies of identical twins who were purposely overfed showed that the amount of weight gained was more similar within sets than between sets. Other studies of identical and fraternal twins, in which the members of a set were reared apart, support the conclusion that heredity plays a major role in determining body weight.

Suggested Readings

Beale EG, Hammer RE, Antoine B, Forest C. Glyceroneogenesis comes of age. FASEB J. 2002;16:1695–1696.

Berg AH, Combs TP, Scherer PE. ACRP30/adiponectin: an adipokine regulating glucose and lipid metabolism. Trends in Endocrinology and Metabolism 2002;13:84–89.

Bouchard C, Tremblay A, Despres J-P, et al. The response to long-term overfeeding in identical twins. N Engl J Med 1990;322:1477–1482.

Girard J, Perderbeau D, Foufelle F, Prip-Buus C, Ferre P. Regulation of lipogenic enzyme gene expression by nutrients and hormones. FASEB J 1994;8:36–42.

Kern PA, Ong JM, Bahman S, Carty J. The effects of weight loss on the activity and expression of adipose-tissue lipoprotein lipase in very obese humans. N Engl J Med 1990;322:1053–1059.

Picard F, Auwerx, J. PPARγand glucose homeostasis. Annu Rev Nutr 2002;22:167–197.

Steppen CM et al. The hormone resistin links obesity to diabetes. Nature 2001;409:307–312.

Stunkard A, Harris J, Pedersen N, McClearn G. The body-mass index of twins who have been reared apart. N Engl J Med 1990;322:1483–1487.

Sweeney G. Leptin signaling. Cellular Signalling 2002;14:655–663.

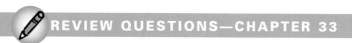 **REVIEW QUESTIONS—CHAPTER 33**

1. Which of the following is involved in the synthesis of triacylglycerols in adipose tissue?

    (A) Fatty acids obtained from chylomicrons and VLDL
    (B) Glycerol 3-phosphate derived from blood glycerol
    (C) 2-Monoacylglycerol as an obligatory intermediate
    (D) Lipoprotein lipase to catalyze the formation of ester bonds
    (E) Acetoacetyl CoA as an obligatory intermediate

2. A molecule of palmitic acid, attached to carbon 1 of the glycerol moiety of a triacylglycerol, is ingested and digested. It passes into the blood, is stored in a fat cell, and ultimately is oxidized to carbon dioxide and water in a muscle cell. Choose the molecular complex in the blood in which the palmitate residue is carried from the lumen of the gut to the surface of the gut epithelial cell.

   (A) VLDL
   (B) Chylomicron
   (C) Fatty acid-albumin complex
   (D) Bile salt micelle
   (E) LDL

3. A patient with hyperlipoproteinemia would be most likely to benefit from a low-carbohydrate diet if the lipoproteins that are elevated in blood are which of the following?

   (A) Chylomicrons
   (B) VLDL
   (C) HDL
   (D) LDL
   (E) IDL

4. Which of the following is a characteristic of sphingosine?

   (A) It is converted to ceramide by reacting with a UDP-sugar.
   (B) It contains a glycerol moiety.
   (C) It is synthesized from palmitoyl CoA and serine.
   (D) It is a precursor of cardiolipin.
   (E) It is only synthesized in neuronal cells.

5. Newly synthesized fatty acids are not immediately degraded because of which of the following?

   (A) Tissues that synthesize fatty acids do not contain the enzymes that degrade fatty acids.
   (B) High NADPH levels inhibit β-oxidation.
   (C) In the presence of insulin, the key fatty acid degrading enzyme is not induced.
   (D) Newly synthesized fatty acids cannot be converted to their CoA derivatives.
   (E) Transport of fatty acids into mitochondria is inhibited under conditions in which fatty acids are being synthesized.

34 Cholesterol Absorption, Synthesis, Metabolism, and Fate

*Cholesterol is one of the most highly recognized molecules in human biology, in part because of a direct relationship between its concentrations in blood and tissues and the development of **atherosclerotic vascular disease**. Cholesterol, which is transported in the blood in **lipoproteins** because of its absolute insolubility in water, serves as a **stabilizing component of cell membranes** and as a precursor of the **bile salts** and **steroid hormones**. Precursors of cholesterol are converted to **ubiquinone, dolichol**, and, in the skin, to **cholecalciferol, the active form of vitamin D**. As a **major component of blood lipoproteins,** cholesterol can appear in its free, unesterified form in the outer shell of these macromolecules and as cholesterol esters in the lipoprotein core.*

*Cholesterol is obtained from the diet or synthesized by a pathway that occurs in most cells of the body, but to a greater extent in cells of the liver and intestine. The precursor for cholesterol synthesis is **acetyl CoA**, which can be produced from glucose, fatty acids, or amino acids. Two molecules of acetyl CoA form **acetoacetyl CoA**, which condenses with another molecule of acetyl CoA to form **hydroxymethylglutaryl CoA (HMG-CoA)**. Reduction of HMG-CoA produces **mevalonate**. This reaction, catalyzed by **HMG-CoA reductase**, is the major rate-limiting step of cholesterol synthesis. Mevalonate produces isoprene units that condense, eventually forming **squalene**. Cyclization of squalene produces the steroid ring system, and a number of subsequent reactions generate cholesterol. The adrenal cortex and the gonads also synthesize cholesterol in significant amounts and use it as a precursor for steroid hormone synthesis.*

*Cholesterol is packaged in **chylomicrons** in the intestine and in **very-low-density lipoprotein (VLDL)** in the liver. It is transported in the blood in these lipoprotein particles, which also transport triacylglycerols. As the triacylglycerols of the blood lipoproteins are digested by lipoprotein lipase, chylomicrons are converted to **chylomicron remnants,** and VLDL is converted to **intermediate-density lipoprotein (IDL)** and subsequently to **low-density lipoprotein (LDL)**. These products return to the liver, where they bind to receptors in cell membranes and are taken up by endocytosis and digested by lysosomal enzymes. LDL is also endocytosed by nonhepatic (peripheral) tissues. Cholesterol and other products of lysosomal digestion are released into the cellular pools. The liver uses this recycled cholesterol, and the cholesterol that is synthesized from acetyl CoA, to produce VLDL and to synthesize bile salts.*

*Intracellular cholesterol obtained from blood lipoproteins decreases the synthesis of cholesterol within cells, stimulates the storage of cholesterol as cholesterol esters, and decreases the synthesis of **LDL receptors**. LDL receptors are found on the surface of the cells and bind various classes of lipoproteins prior to endocytosis.*

*Although high-density lipoprotein (HDL) contains triacylglycerols and cholesterol, its function is very different from that of the chylomicrons and VLDL, which transport triacylglycerols. HDL exchanges proteins and lipids with the other lipoproteins in the blood. HDL transfers **apolipoprotein E (apoE) and apoC$_{II}$** to chylomicrons and VLDL. After digestion of the VLDL triacylglycerols, apoE and apoC$_{II}$ are transferred back to HDL. In addition, HDL obtains cholesterol from*

619

*other lipoproteins and from cell membranes and converts it to **cholesterol esters** by the **lecithin:cholesterol acyltransferase (LCAT)** reaction. Then HDL either directly transports cholesterol and cholesterol esters to the liver or transfers cholesterol esters to other lipoproteins via the **cholesterol ester transfer protein (CETP)**. Ultimately, lipoprotein particles carry the cholesterol and cholesterol esters to the liver, where endocytosis and lysosomal digestion occur. Thus, **"reverse cholesterol transport"** (i.e., the return of cholesterol to the liver) is a major function of HDL.*

*Elevated levels of cholesterol in the blood are associated with the formation of **atherosclerotic plaques** that can occlude blood vessels, causing heart attacks and strokes. Although high levels of LDL cholesterol are especially atherogenic, high levels of HDL cholesterol are protective because HDL particles are involved in the process of removing cholesterol from tissues, such as the lining cells of vessels, and returning it to the liver.*

Bile salts, which are produced in the liver from cholesterol obtained from the blood lipoproteins or synthesized from acetyl CoA, are secreted into the bile. They are stored in the gallbladder and released into the intestine during a meal. The bile salts emulsify dietary triacylglycerols, thus aiding in digestion. The digestive products are absorbed by intestinal epithelial cells from bile salt micelles, tiny microdroplets that contain bile salts at their water interface. After the contents of the micelles are absorbed, most of the bile salts travel to the ileum, where they are resorbed and recycled by the liver. Less than 5% of the bile salts that enter the lumen of the small intestine are eventually excreted in the feces.

Although the fecal excretion of bile salts is relatively low, it is a major means by which the body disposes of the steroid nucleus of cholesterol. Because the ring structure of cholesterol cannot be degraded in the body, it is excreted mainly in the bile as free cholesterol and bile salts.

The steroid hormones, derived from cholesterol, include the adrenal cortical hormones (e.g., cortisol, aldosterone, and the adrenal sex steroids dehydroepiandrosterone [DHEA] and androstenedione) and the gonadal hormones (e.g., the ovarian and testicular sex steroids, such as testosterone and estrogen).

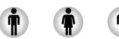

THE WAITING ROOM

At his current office visit, **Ivan Applebod's** case was reviewed by his physician. Mr. Applebod has several of the major risk factors for coronary heart disease (CHD). These include a sedentary lifestyle, marked obesity, hypertension, hyperlipidemia, and early non–insulin-dependent diabetes mellitus (NIDDM). Unfortunately, he has not followed his doctor's advice with regard to a diabetic diet designed to affect a significant loss of weight, nor has he followed an aerobic exercise program. As a consequence, his weight has gone from 270 to 281 lb. After a 14-hour fast, his serum glucose is now 214 mg/dL (normal, <110), and his serum total cholesterol level is 314 mg/dL (desired level is 200 or less). His serum triacylglycerol level is 295 mg/dL (desired level is 150 or less), and his serum HDL cholesterol is 24 mg/dL (desired level is ≥40 for a male). His calculated serum LDL cholesterol level is 231 mg/dL (desired level for a person with two or more risk factors for CHD is 130 mg/dL or less, unless one of the risk factors is diabetes mellitus, in which case, the LDL cholesterol level should be < 100 mg/dL).

Ann Jeina was carefully followed by her physician after she survived her heart attack. Before discharge from the hospital, after a 14-hour fast, her serum triacylglycerol level was 158 mg/dL (slightly above the upper range of normal), and her HDL cholesterol level was low at 32 mg/dL (normal for women is ≥50). Her serum total cholesterol level was elevated at 420 mg/dL (reference range, ≤200 for a female with known CHD). From these values, her LDL cholesterol level was calculated to be 356 mg/dL (desirable level for a person with established heart disease is <100).

Both of Ms. Jeina's younger brothers had "very high" serum cholesterol levels, and both had suffered heart attacks in their mid-forties. With this information, a tentative diagnosis of familial hypercholesterolemia, type IIA was made, and the patient was started on a step I diet as recommended by the National Cholesterol Education Program (NCEP) Adult Treatment Panel III. This panel recommends that decisions with regard to when dietary and drug therapy are initiated based on the serum LDL cholesterol level, as depicted in Table 34.1.

Because a Step I diet (Table 34.2) usually lowers serum total and LDL cholesterol levels by no more than 15%, it is likely that Ms. Jeina's diet will eventually have to be further restricted in cholesterol and fat and that one or more lipid-lowering drugs will have to be added to her treatment plan.

Vera Leizd is a 34-year-old woman in whom pubertal changes began at age 12, leading to the development of normal secondary sexual characteristics and the onset of menses at age 13. Her menstrual periods occurred on a monthly basis over the next 7 years, but the flow was scant. At age 20, she noted a gradual increase in the intermenstrual interval from her normal of 28 days to 32 to 38 days. The volume of her menstrual flow also gradually diminished. After 7 months, her menstrual periods ceased. She complained of increasing oiliness of her skin, the appearance of acnelike lesions on her face and upper back, and the appearance of short dark terminal hairs on the mustache and sideburn areas of her face. The amount of extremity hair also increased, and she noticed a disturbing loss of hair from her scalp.

Until recently, the concentration of LDL cholesterol could only be directly determined by sophisticated laboratory techniques not available for routine clinical use. As a consequence, the LDL cholesterol concentration in the blood was derived indirectly by using the Friedewald formula: the sum of the HDL cholesterol level and the triacylglycerol (TG) level divided by 5 (which gives an estimate of the VLDL cholesterol level) subtracted from the total cholesterol level.

LDL cholesterol =
Total cholesterol − [HDL cholesterol + (TG/5)]

This equation yields inaccurate LDL cholesterol levels 15 to 20% of the time and fails completely when serum triacylglycerol levels exceed 400 mg/dL.

A recently developed test called "LDL direct" isolates LDL cholesterol by using a special immunoseparation reagent. Not only is this direct assay for LDL cholesterol more accurate than the indirect Friedewald calculation, it also is not affected by mildly to moderately elevated serum triacylglycerol levels and can be used for a patient who has not fasted. It does not require the expense of determining serum total cholesterol, HDL cholesterol, and triacylglycerol levels.

I. INTESTINAL ABSORPTION OF CHOLESTEROL

Cholesterol absorption by intestinal cells is a key regulatory point in human sterol metabolism because it ultimately determines what percentage of the 1,000 mg of biliary cholesterol produced by the liver each day and what percentage of the

Table 34.1. ATP III: LDL-C Goals and Cut Points for Therapy in Different Risk Categories

Risk Category	LDL Goal (mg/dL)	LDL level at which to initiate therapeutic lifestyle changes (mg/dL)	LDL level at which to consider drug therapy (mg/dL)
CHD or CHD risk equivalents (10-year risk >20%)	<100	≥100	≥130 (100-129: drug optional)
2+ Risk factors (10-year risk ≤20%)	<130	≥130	10-Year risk 10%-20%: ≥130 10-year risk <10%: ≥160
0–1 risk factor	<160	≥160	≥190 (160–189: LDL-lowering drug optional)

LDL-C = low-density lipoprotein cholesterol; CHD = coronary heart disease.
Source: Executive summary of the third report of the National Cholesterol Education Programs (NCEP) Expert panel on detection, evaluation, and treatment of high blood cholesterol in Adults (Adult Treatment Panel III). Final Report, Circulation 2002;106:3145–3457.

Table 34.2: Dietary Therapy of Elevated Blood Cholesterol

Nutrient	Step I Diet	Step II Diet[a]
Cholesterol[b]	<300 mg/day	<200 mg/day
Total fat	≤30%[b]	30%
Saturated fat	8–10%	<7%
Polyunsaturated fat	≤10%	≤10%
Monounsaturated fat	≤15%	≤15%
Carbohydrates	≥55%	≥55%
Protein	~15%	~15%
Calories	To achieve and maintain desirable body weight	

Based on: NCEP. Second Report of the Adult Treatment Panel, JAMA, 1993;269(23):3015–3023.
[a]The Step II diet is applied if 3 months on the Step I diet has failed to reduce blood cholesterol to the desired level (see Table 34.1).
[b]Except for the values given in mg/day, all the values are percentage of total calories eaten daily.

300 mg of dietary cholesterol entering the gut per day is eventually absorbed into the blood. In normal subjects, approximately 55% of this intestinal pool enters the blood through the enterocyte each day. The details of cholesterol absorption from dietary sources was outlined in Chapter 32.

Although the absorption of cholesterol from the intestinal lumen is a diffusion-controlled process, there is also a mechanism to remove unwanted or excessive cholesterol and plant sterols from the enterocyte. The transport of sterols out of the enterocyte, and into the lumen, is related to the products of genes that code for the adenosine triphosphate (ATP)-binding cassette (ABC) protein family, ABC1, ABCG5, and ABCG8. These proteins couple ATP hydrolysis to the transport of unwanted or excessive cholesterol and plant sterols (phytosterols) from the enterocyte back into the gut lumen. Cholesterol cannot be metabolized to CO_2 and water and is, therefore, principally eliminated from the body in the feces as unreabsorbed sterols and bile acids. ABC protein expression increases the amount of sterols present in the gut lumen, with the potential to increase elimination of the sterols into the feces. Patients with a condition known as phytosterolemia (a rare autosomal recessive disease, also known as sitosterolemia) have a defect in the function of either ABCG5 or ABCG8 in the enterocytes, thereby leading to the accumulation of cholesterol and phytosterols within these cells. These eventually reach the bloodstream, markedly elevating the level of cholesterol and phytosterol in the blood. This accounts for the increased cardiovascular morbidity in individuals with this disorder. From these experiments of nature, it is clear that agents that either amplify the expression of the ABC proteins within enterocytes, or block cholesterol absorption from the lumen, have therapeutic potential in the treatment of patients with hypercholesterolemia. Ezetimibe, now available for clinical use, is a compound that is structurally different from the sterols. Its primary action in lowering serum cholesterol levels is to block cholesterol absorption through a specific but as yet poorly characterized cholesterol absorption mechanism in the brush border of enterocytes. It also may induce ABC protein expression, but this action is relatively unimportant in reducing net cholesterol absorption. The reduction of cholesterol absorption from the intestinal lumen has been shown to reduce blood levels of LDL cholesterol.

II. CHOLESTEROL SYNTHESIS

Cholesterol is an alicyclic compound whose basic structure includes the perhydrocyclopentanophenanthrene nucleus containing four fused rings (Figure 34.1). In its "free" form, the cholesterol molecule contains 27 carbon atoms, a simple hydroxyl group at C3, a double bond between C5 and C6, an eight-membered hydrocarbon chain attached to carbon 17 in the D ring, a methyl group (carbon 19) attached to carbon 10, and a second methyl group (carbon 18) attached to carbon 13 (Figure 34.2).

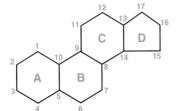

Fig. 34.1. The basic ring structure of sterols; the perhydrocyclopentanophenanthrene nucleus. Each ring is labeled either A, B, C, or D.

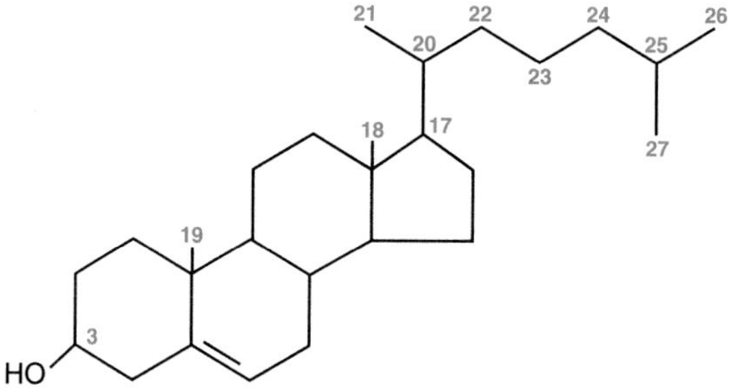

Fig. 34.2. The structure of cholesterol.

Approximately one third of plasma cholesterol exists in the free (or unesterified) form. The remaining two thirds exists as cholesterol esters in which a long-chain fatty acid (usually linoleic acid) is attached by ester linkage to the hydroxyl group at C-3 of the A ring. The proportions of free and esterified cholesterol in the blood can be measured using methods such as high-performance liquid chromatography (HPLC).

The structure of cholesterol suggests that its synthesis involves multimolecular interactions; yet all of the 27 carbons are derived from one precursor, acetyl CoA. Acetyl CoA can be obtained from several sources, including the beta oxidation of fatty acids, the oxidation of ketogenic amino acids, such as leucine and lysine, and the pyruvate dehydrogenase reaction. Carbons 1, 2, 5, 7, 9, 13, 15, 18, 19, 20, 22, 24, 26, and 27 of cholesterol are derived from the methyl group of acetyl CoA and the remaining 12 carbons of cholesterol from the carboxylate atom of acetyl CoA.

The synthesis of cholesterol requires significant reducing power, which is supplied in the form of NADPH. The latter is provided by glucose-6-phosphate dehydrogenase and 6-phosphogluconate dehydrogenase of the hexose monophosphate shunt pathway (see Chapter 29). Cholesterol synthesis occurs in the cytosol, requiring hydrolysis of high-energy thioester bonds of acetyl CoA and phosphoanhydride bonds of ATP. Its synthesis occurs in four stages.

A. Stage 1: Synthesis of Mevalonate from Acetyl CoA

The first stage of cholesterol synthesis leads to the production of the intermediate mevalonate (Fig. 34.3). *The synthesis of mevalonate is the committed, rate-limiting step in cholesterol formation.* In this cytoplasmic pathway, two molecules of acetyl CoA condense, forming acetoacetyl CoA, which then condenses with a third molecule of acetyl CoA to yield the 6-carbon compound β-hydroxy- β-methylglutaryl-CoA (HMG-CoA). The HMG-CoA synthase in this reaction is present in the cytosol and is distinct from the mitochondrial HMG-CoA synthase that catalyses HMG-CoA synthesis involved in ketone body production. *The committed step and major point of regulation of cholesterol synthesis in stage 1 involves reduction of HMG-CoA to mevalonate, a reaction catalyzed by HMG-CoA reductase, an enzyme embedded in the membrane of the endoplasmic reticulum.* HMG-CoA reductase contains eight membrane-spanning domains, and the amino terminal domain, which faces the cytoplasm, contains the enzymatic activity. The reducing equivalents for this reaction are donated by two molecules of NADPH. The regulation of the activity of HMG-CoA reductase is controlled in multiple ways.

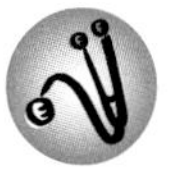

1. TRANSCRIPTIONAL CONTROL

The rate of synthesis of HMG-CoA reductase messenger RNA (mRNA) is controlled by one of the family of sterol regulatory element binding proteins (SREBPs)(Fig. 34.4A). These transcription factors belong to the helix-loop-helix-

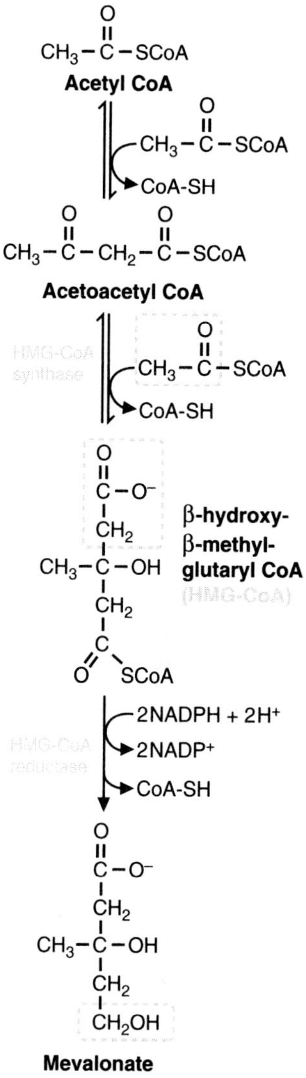

Fig. 34.3. The conversion of three molecules of acetyl-CoA to mevalonic acid.

Ann Jeina's serum total and LDL cholesterol levels improved only modestly after 3 months on a Step I diet. Three additional months on a more severe low-fat diet (Step II diet) brought little further improvement. The next therapeutic step would be to initiate lipid-lowering drug therapy (see Table 34.5).

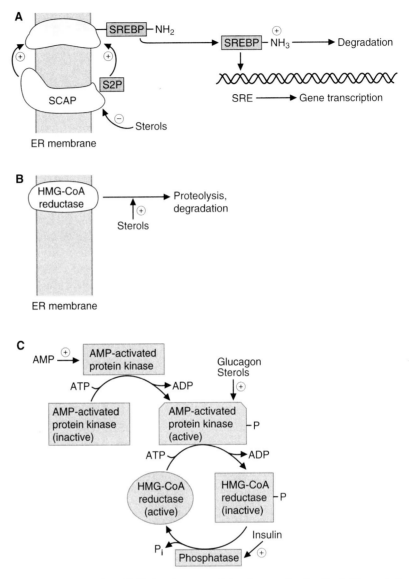

Fig. 34.4. Regulation of HMG-CoA reductase activity. See text for details. A. Transcriptional control. B. Regulation by proteolysis. C. Regulation by phosphorylation.

leucine zipper (bHlH-Zip) family of transcription factors that directly activate the expression of more than 30 genes dedicated to the synthesis and uptake of cholesterol, fatty acids, triacylglycerols, and phospholipids as well as the production of the NADPH cofactors required to synthesize these molecules.

SREBP1-a specifically enhances transcription of genes required for HMG-CoA reductase expression by binding to the sterol regulatory element (SRE) upstream of the reductase gene. When bound, the rate of transcription is increased. SREBPs, after synthesis, are integral ER proteins, and the active component of the protein is released by two proteases, SCAP (**S**REBP **c**leavage-**a**ctivating **p**rotein) and S2P (site 2 protease). Once released, the active amino terminal component travels to the nucleus to bind to SREs. The soluble SREBPs are rapidly turned over and need to be continuously produced to effectively stimulate reductase mRNA transcription. When cytoplasmic sterol levels rise, the sterols bind to SCAP and inactivate it, thereby leading to a decrease in transcription of the reductase gene, and less reductase protein being produced.

2. PROTEOLYTIC DEGRADATION OF HMG-CoA REDUCTASE

Rising levels of cholesterol and bile salts in cells that synthesize these molecules also may cause a change in the oligomerization state of the membrane domain of HMG-CoA reductase, rendering the enzyme more susceptible to proteolysis (see Fig. 34.4B). This, in turn, decreases its activity. The membrane domains of HMG-CoA reductase contain sterol-sensing regions, which are similar to those in SCAP.

3. REGULATION BY COVALENT MODIFICATION

In addition to the inductive and repressive influences cited above, the activity of the reductase is also regulated by phosphorylation and dephosphorylation (see Fig. 34.4C). Elevated glucagon levels increase phosphorylation of the enzyme, thereby inactivating it, whereas hyperinsulinemia increases the activity of the reductase by activating phosphatases, which dephosphorylate the reductase. Increased levels of intracellular sterols also may increase phosphorylation of HMG-CoA reductase, thereby reducing its activity as well (feedback suppression). Thyroid hormone also increases enzyme activity, whereas glucocorticoids decrease its activity. The enzyme that phosphorylates HMG-CoA reductase is the adenosine monophosphate (AMP)-activated protein kinase, which itself is regulated by phosphorylation by the AMP-activated protein kinase kinase. Thus, cholesterol synthesis decreases when ATP levels are low and increases when ATP levels are high. This will become very clear once the further reactions of the biosynthetic pathway of cholesterol are discussed.

B. Stage 2: Conversion of Mevalonate to Two Activated Isoprenes

In the second stage of cholesterol synthesis, three phosphate groups are transferred from three molecules of ATP to mevalonate (Fig. 34.5). The purpose of these phosphate transfers is to activate both carbon 5 and the hydroxyl group on carbon 3 for further reactions in which these groups will leave the molecule. The phosphate group attached to the C-3 hydroxyl group of mevalonate in the 3-phospho-5-pyrophosphomevalonate intermediate is removed along with the carboxyl group on C-1. This produces a double bond in the 5-carbon product, Δ^3-isopentenyl pyrophosphate, the first of two activated isoprenes necessary for the synthesis of cholesterol. The second activated isoprene is formed when Δ^3-isopentenyl pyrophosphate is isomerized to dimethylallyl pyrophosphate (see Fig. 34.5).

C. Stage 3: Condensation of Six Activated 5-Carbon Isoprenes to Form the 30-Carbon Squalene

The next stage in the biosynthesis of cholesterol involves the head-to-tail condensation of isopentenylpyrophosphate and dimethylallyl pyrophosphate. In this reaction, one pyrophosphate group is displaced, and a 10-carbon chain, known as geranyl pyrophosphate, is generated (Fig. 34.6). (The "head" refers to the end to which pyrophosphate is joined.) Geranyl pyrophosphate then undergoes another head-to-tail condensation with isopentenyl pyrophosphate, resulting in the formation of the 15-carbon intermediate, farnesyl pyrophosphate. After this, two molecules of farnesyl pyrophosphate undergo a head-to-head fusion, and both pyrophosphate groups are removed to form squalene, a compound first isolated from the liver of sharks (genus Squalus). Squalene contains 30 carbons (24 in the main chain and 6 in the methyl group branches; see Fig. 34.6).

Farnesyl and geranyl groups can form covalent bonds with proteins, particularly the G proteins and certain protooncogene products involved in signal transduction. These hydrophobic groups anchor the proteins in the cell membrane.

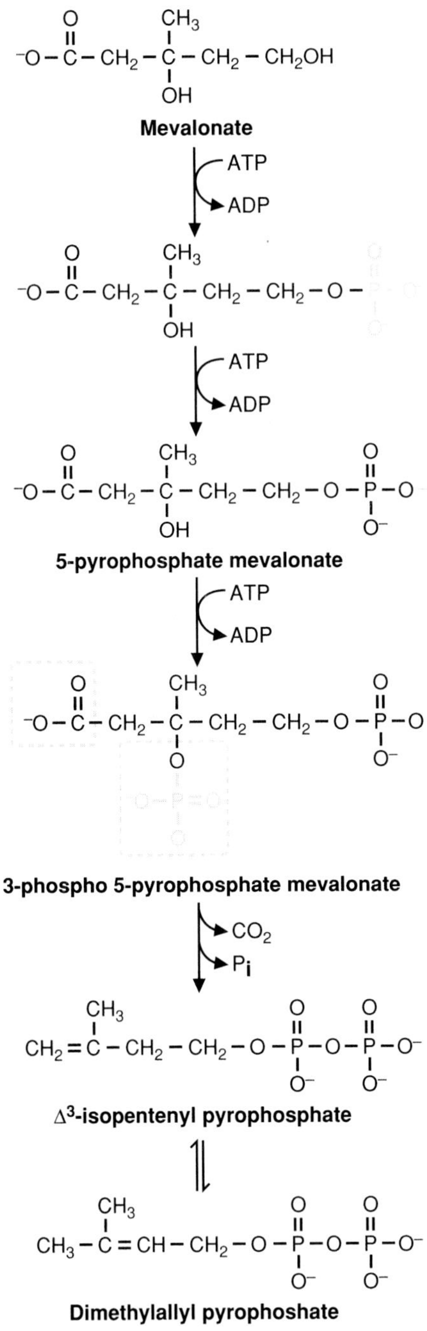

Fig. 34.5. The formation of activated isoprene units (Δ^3-isopentenyl pyrophosphate and dimethylallyl pyrophosphate) from mevalonic acid. Note the large ATP requirement for these steps.

D. Stage 4: Conversion of Squalene to the Four-Ring Steroid Nucleus

The enzyme squalene monooxygenase adds a single oxygen atom from O_2 to the end of the squalene molecule, forming an epoxide. NADPH then reduces the other oxygen atom of O_2 to H_2O. The unsaturated carbons of the squalene 2, 3- epoxide are aligned in a way that allows conversion of the linear squalene epoxide into a cyclic structure. The cyclization leads to the formation of lanosterol, a sterol with the four-ring structure characteristic of the steroid nucleus. A series of complex

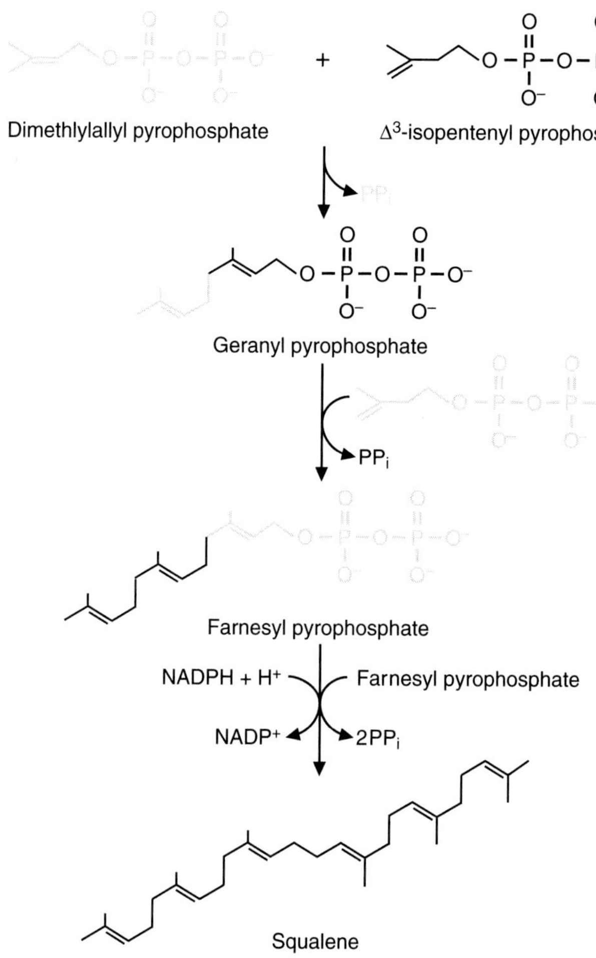

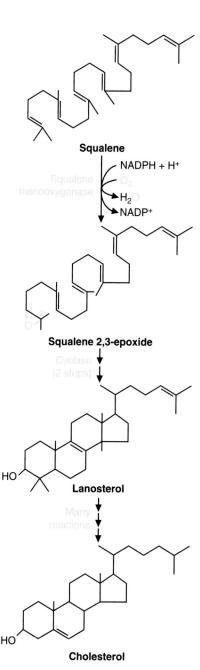

Fig. 34.6. The formation of squalene from six isoprene units. The activation of the isoprene units drives their condensation to form geranyl pyrophosphate, farnesyl pyrophosphate, and squalene.

reactions, containing many steps and elucidated in the late 1950s, leads to the formation of cholesterol (Fig. 34.7).

III. SEVERAL FATES OF CHOLESTEROL

Almost all mammalian cells are capable of producing cholesterol. Most of the biosynthesis of cholesterol, however, occurs within liver cells, although the gut, the adrenal cortex, and the gonads (as well as the placenta in pregnant women) also produce significant quantities of the sterol. Although a fraction of hepatic cholesterol is used for the synthesis of hepatic membranes, the bulk of synthesized cholesterol is secreted from the hepatocyte as one of three moieties: cholesterol esters, biliary cholesterol, or bile acids. Cholesterol ester production in the liver is catalyzed by acyl-CoA-cholesterol acyl transferase (ACAT). ACAT catalyzes the transfer of a fatty acid from coenzyme A to the hydroxyl group on carbon 3 of cholesterol (Fig. 34.8). Cholesterol esters are more hydrophobic than is free cholesterol. The liver packages some of the esterified cholesterol into the hollow core of lipoproteins, primarily VLDL. VLDL is secreted from the hepatocyte into the blood and transports the cholesterol esters (and triacylglycerols, phospholipids, apoproteins, etc.) to the tissues that require greater amounts of cholesterol than they can synthesize de novo. These tissues then use the cholesterol for the synthesis of membranes,

Fig. 34.7. The conversion of squalene to cholesterol. Squalene is shown in a different conformation than that of Fig. 34.6 to better indicate how the cyclization reaction occurs.

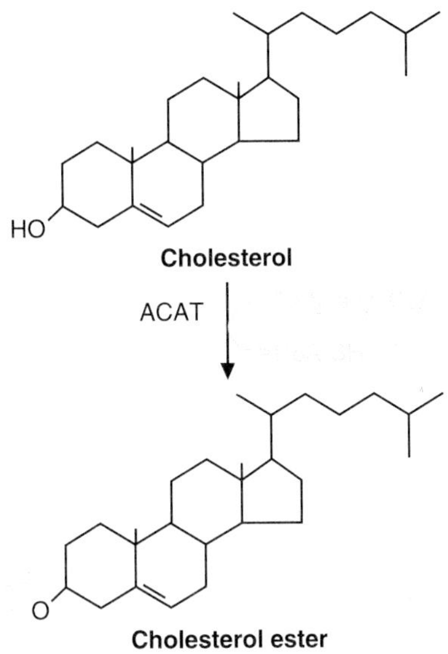

Cholesterol

ACAT

Cholesterol ester

Fig. 34.8. The ACAT reaction, producing cholesterol esters. ACAT = acyl-CoA:cholesterol acyl transferase.

for the formation of steroid hormones, and for the biosynthesis of vitamin D. The residual cholesterol esters not used in these ways are stored in the liver for later use. The hepatic cholesterol pool also serves as a source of cholesterol for the synthesis of the relatively hydrophilic bile acids and their salts. These derivatives of cholesterol are highly effective detergents because they contain both polar and nonpolar regions. They are introduced in the biliary ducts of the liver. They are stored and concentrated in the gallbladder and later discharged into the gut in response to the ingestion of food. They aid in the digestion of intraluminal lipids by forming micelles with them, which increases the surface area of lipids exposed to the digestive action of intraluminal lipases. Free cholesterol also enters the gut lumen via the biliary tract (approximately 1,000 mg daily, which mixes with 300 mg dietary cholesterol to form an intestinal pool, roughly 55% of which is resorbed by the enterocytes and enters the bloodstream daily). On a low-cholesterol diet, the liver will synthesize approximately 800 mg cholesterol per day to replace bile salts and cholesterol lost from the enterohepatic circulation into the feces. Conversely, a greater intake of dietary cholesterol suppresses the rate of hepatic cholesterol synthesis (feedback repression).

IV. SYNTHESIS OF BILE SALTS

A. Conversion of Cholesterol to Cholic Acid and Chenocholic Acid

Bile salts are synthesized in the liver from cholesterol by reactions that hydroxylate the steroid nucleus and cleave the side chain. In the first reaction, an α-hydroxyl group is added to carbon 7 (on the α side of the B ring). The activity of the 7 α-hydroxylase that catalyzes this rate-limiting step is decreased by bile salts (Fig. 34.9).

In subsequent steps, the double bond in the B ring is reduced, and an additional hydroxylation may occur. Two different sets of compounds are produced. One set has α-hydroxyl groups at positions 3, 7, and 12, and produces the cholic acid series

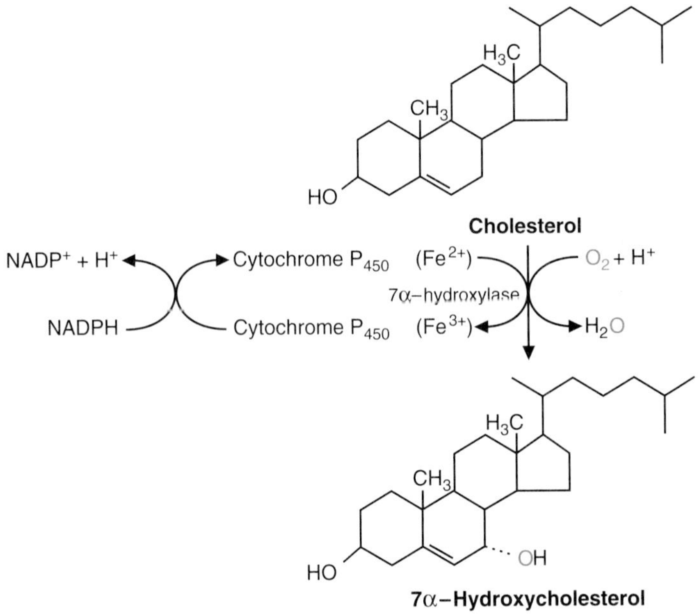

Cholesterol

NADP$^+$ + H$^+$ Cytochrome P$_{450}$ (Fe^{2+})   O$_2$ + H$^+$

7α–hydroxylase

NADPH   Cytochrome P$_{450}$ (Fe^{3+})   H$_2$O

7α–Hydroxycholesterol

Fig. 34.9. The reaction catalyzed by 7α-hydroxylase. An α-hydroxyl group is formed at position 7 of cholesterol. This reaction, which is inhibited by bile salts, is the rate-limiting step in bile salt synthesis.

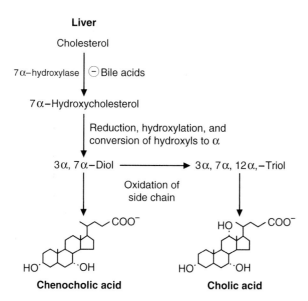

Fig. 34.10. Synthesis of bile salts. Two sets of bile salts are generated; one with α-hydroxyl groups at positions 3 and 7 (the chenocholate series), and the other with α-hydroxyls at positions 3, 7 and 12 (the cholate series).

of bile salts. The other set has α-hydroxyl groups only at positions 3 and 7 and produces the chenocholic acid series (Fig. 34.10). Three carbons are removed from the side chain by an oxidation reaction. The remaining 5-carbon fragment attached to the ring structure contains a carboxyl group (see Fig. 34.10).

The pK of the bile acids is approximately 6. Therefore, in the contents of the intestinal lumen, which normally have a pH of 6, approximately 50% of the molecules are present in the protonated form, and 50% are ionized, which forms bile salts. (The terms *bile acids* and *bile salts* are often used interchangeably, but *bile salts* actually refer to the ionized form of the molecule.)

B. Conjugation of Bile Salts

The carboxyl group at the end of the side chain of the bile salts is activated by a reaction that requires ATP and coenzyme A (CoA). The CoA derivatives can react with either glycine or taurine (which is derived from cysteine), forming amides that are known as the conjugated bile salts. In glycocholic acid and glycochenocholic acid, the bile acids are conjugated with glycine. These compounds have a pK of approximately 4, so compared to their unconjugated forms, a higher percentage of the molecules is present in the ionized form at the pH of the intestine. The taurine conjugates, taurocholic and taurochenocholic acid, have a pK of approximately 2. Therefore, compared with the glycoconjugates, an even greater percentage of the molecules of these conjugates are ionized in the lumen of the gut (Fig. 34.11).

V. FATE OF THE BILE SALTS

The bile salts are produced in the liver and secreted into the bile (Fig. 34.12), They are stored in the gallbladder and released into the intestine during a meal, where they serve as detergents that aid in the digestion of dietary lipids (see Chapter 32).

Intestinal bacteria deconjugate and dehydroxylate the bile salts, removing the glycine and taurine residues and the hydroxyl group at position 7. The bile salts that lack a hydroxyl group at position 7 are called secondary bile salts. The deconjugated and dehydroxylated bile salts are less soluble and, therefore, less readily resorbed from the intestinal lumen than the bile salts that have not been subjected to bacterial

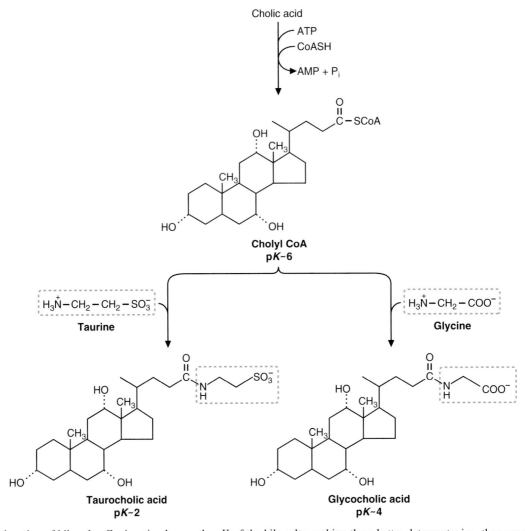

Fig. 34.11. Conjugation of bile salts. Conjugation lowers the pK of the bile salts, making them better detergents; i.e., they are more ionized in the contents of the intestinal lumen (pH ≈ 6) than are the unconjugated bile salts (pK ≈ 6). The reactions are the same for the chenocholic acid series of bile salts.

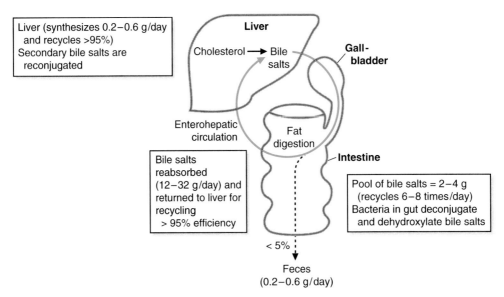

Fig. 34.12. Overview of bile salt metabolism.

action (Fig. 34.13). Lithocholic acid, a secondary bile salt that has a hydroxyl group only at position 3, is the least soluble bile salt. Its major fate is excretion.

Greater than 95% of the bile salts are resorbed in the ileum and return to the liver via the enterohepatic circulation (via the portal vein; see Fig. 34.12). The secondary bile salts may be reconjugated in the liver, but they are not rehydroxylated. The bile salts are recycled by the liver, which secretes them into the bile. This enterohepatic recirculation of bile salts is extremely efficient. Less than 5% of the bile salts entering the gut are excreted in the feces each day. Because the steroid nucleus cannot be degraded in the body, the excretion of bile salts serves as a major route for removal of the steroid nucleus and, thus, of cholesterol from the body.

VI. TRANSPORT OF CHOLESTEROL BY THE BLOOD LIPOPROTEINS

Because they are hydrophobic and essentially insoluble in the water of the blood, cholesterol and cholesterol esters, like triacylglycerols and phospholipids, must be transported through the bloodstream packaged as lipoproteins. These macromolecules are water-soluble. Each lipoprotein particle is composed of a core of hydrophobic lipids such as cholesterol esters and triacylglycerols surrounded by a shell of polar lipids (the phospholipids), which allows a hydration shell to form around the lipoprotein (see Fig. 32.9). This occurs when the positive charge of the nitrogen atom of the phospholipid (phosphatidylcholine, phosphatidylethanolamine, or phosphatidylserine) forms an ionic bond with the negatively charged hydroxyl ion of the environment. In addition, the shell contains a variety of apoproteins that also increase the water solubility of the lipoprotein. Free cholesterol molecules are dispersed throughout the lipoprotein shell to stabilize it in a way that allows it to maintain its spherical shape. The major carriers of lipids are chylomicrons (see Chapter 32), VLDL, and HDL. Metabolism of VLDL will lead to IDL and LDL. Metabolism of chylomicrons leads to chylomicron remnant formation.

Through this carrier mechanism, lipids leave their tissue of origin, enter the bloodstream, and are transported to the tissues, where their components will be either used in synthetic or oxidative process or stored for later use. The apoproteins ("apo" describes the protein within the shell of the particle in its lipid-free form) not only add to the hydrophilicity and structural stability of the particle but have other functions as well: (1) they activate certain enzymes required for normal lipoprotein metabolism and (2) they act as ligands on the surface of the lipoprotein that target specific receptors on peripheral tissues that require lipoprotein delivery for their innate cellular function.

Ten principal apoproteins have been characterized. Their tissue source, molecular mass, distribution within lipoproteins, and metabolic functions are shown in Table 34.3.

The lipoproteins themselves are distributed among eight major classes. Some of their characteristics are shown in Table 34.4. Each class of lipoprotein has a specific function determined by its apolipoprotein content, its tissue of origin, and the proportion of the macromolecule made up of triacylglycerols, cholesterol esters, free cholesterol, and phospholipids (see Tables 34.3 and 34.4).

A. The Chylomicrons

Chylomicrons are the largest of the lipoproteins and the least dense because of their rich triacylglycerol content. They are synthesized from dietary lipids (the "exogenous" lipoprotein pathway) within the epithelial cells of the small intestine and then secreted into the lymphatic vessels draining the gut (see Fig. 32.13). They enter the bloodstream via the left subclavian vein. The major apoproteins of chylomicrons are apoB-48, apoC$_{II}$, and apoE (see Table 34.3). The apoC$_{II}$ activates lipoprotein lipase

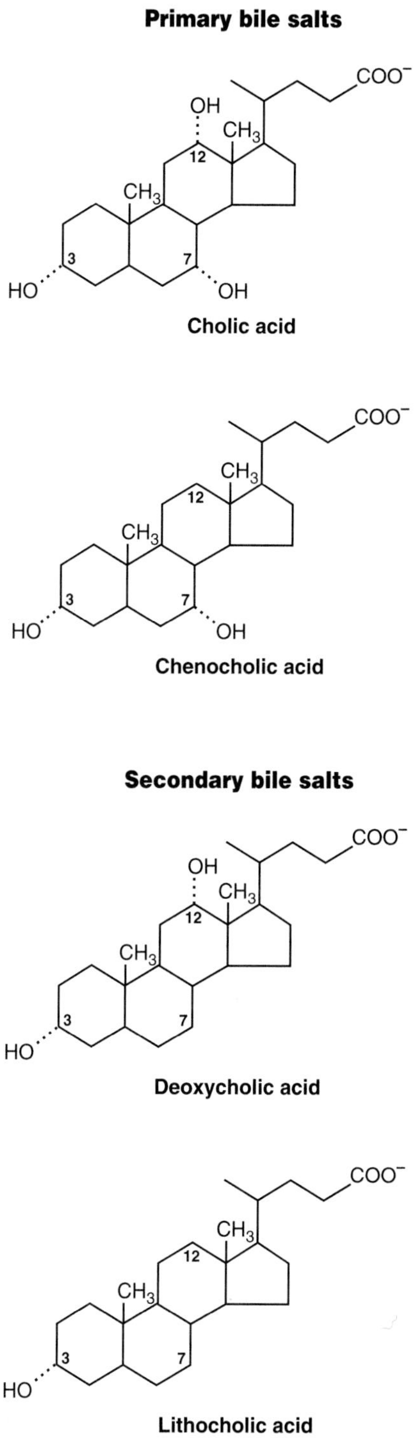

Primary bile salts

Cholic acid

Chenocholic acid

Secondary bile salts

Deoxycholic acid

Lithocholic acid

Fig. 34.13. Structures of the primary and secondary bile salts. Primary bile salts form conjugates with taurine or glycine in the liver. After secretion into the intestine, they may be deconjugated and dehydroxylated by the bacterial flora, forming secondary bile salts. Note that dehydroxylation occurs at position 7, forming the deoxy family of bile salts.

Table 34.3. CHARACTERISTICS OF THE MAJOR APOPROTEINS

Apoprotein	Primary Tissue Source	Molecular Mass (Daltons)	Lipoprotein Distribution	Metabolic Function
ApoA-1	Intestine, liver	28,016	HDL (chylomicrons)	Activates LCAT; structural component of HDL
ApoA-II	Liver	17,414	HDL (chylomicrons)	Unknown
ApoA-IV	Intestine	46,465	HDL (chylomicrons)	Unknown (may facilitate transport of other apoproteins between HDL and chylomicrons)
ApoB-48	Intestine	264,000	Chylomicrons	Assembly and secretion of chylomicrons from small bowel
ApoB-100	Liver	540,000	VLDL, IDL, LDL	VLDL assembly and secretion structured protein of VLDL, IDL, and LDL ligand for LDL receptor
ApoC-1	Liver	6,630	Chylomicrons, VLDL, IDL, HDL	Unknown; may inhibit hepatic uptake of chylomicron and VLDL remnants
ApoC-II	Liver	8,900	Chylomicrons, VLDL, IDL, HDL	Cofactor activator of lipoprotein lipase (LPL)
ApoC-III	Liver	8,800	Chylomicrons, VLDL, IDL, HDL	Inhibitor of LPL; may inhibit hepatic uptake of chylomicrons and VLDL remnants
ApoE	Liver	34,145	Chylomicron remnants, VLDL, IDL, HDL	Ligand for binding of several lipoproteins to the LDL receptor, to the LDL receptor-related protein (LRP) and possibly to a separate apo-E receptor.
Apo(a)	Liver		Lipoprotein "little" a (Lp(a))	Unknown

(LPL), an enzyme that projects into the lumen of capillaries in adipose tissue, cardiac muscle, skeletal muscle, and the acinar cells of mammary tissue. This activation allows LPL to hydrolyze the chylomicrons, leading to the release of free fatty acids derived from core triacylglycerides of the lipoprotein into these target cells. The muscle cells then oxidize the fatty acids as fuel while the adipocytes and mammary cells store them as triacylglycerols (fat) or, in the case of the lactating breast, use them for milk formation. The partially hydrolyzed chylomicrons remaining in the bloodstream (the **chylomicron remnants**), now partly depleted of their core triacylglycerols, retain their apoE and apoB48 proteins. Receptors in the plasma membranes of the liver cells bind to apoE on the surface of these remnants, allowing them to be taken up by the liver through a process of receptor-mediated endocytosis (see below).

B. Very-Low-Density Lipoproteins (VLDL)

If dietary intake of fatty acids exceeds the immediate fuel requirements of the liver, the excess fatty acids are converted to triacylglycerols, which, along with free and esterified cholesterol, phospholipids, and a variety of apoproteins (see Table 34.3),

Table 34.4. CHARACTERISTICS OF THE MAJOR LIPOPROTEINS

Lipoprotein	Density Range (g/mL)	Particle Diameter (MM) range	Electrophoretic Mobility	Lipid (%)* TG	Chol	PL	Function
Chylomicrons	0.930	75–1200	Origin	80–95	2–7	3–9	Deliver dietary lipids
Chylomicron remnants	0.930–1.006	30–80	Slow pre β				Return dietary lipids to the liver
VLDL	0.930–1.006	30–80	Pre β	55–80	5–15	10–20	Deliver endogenous lipids
IDL	1.006–1.019	25–35	Slow pre β	20–50	20–40	15–25	Return endogenous lipids to the liver; precursor of LDL
LDL	1.019–1.063	18–25	β	5–15	40–50	20–25	Deliver cholesterol to cells
HDL₂	1.063–1.125	9–12	α	5–10	15–25	20–30	Reverse cholesterol transport
HDL₃	1.125–1.210	5–9	α				Reverse cholesterol transport
Lip(a)	1.050–1.120	25	Pre β				

*The remaining percent composition is composed of apoproteins.
Abbreviations: TG, Triacylglycerols; Chol, the sum of free and esterified cholesterol; PL, phospholipid; VLDL = very-low-density lipoproteins; IDL, intermediate-density lipoproteins; LDL, low-density lipoproteins; HDL, high-density lipoproteins.

including apoB-100, apoC$_{II}$, and apoE, are packaged to form VLDL. These particles are then secreted from the liver (the "endogenous" pathway of lipoprotein metabolism) into the bloodstream (Fig. 34.14). The density, particle size, and lipid content of VLDL particles are given in Table 34.3. These particles are then transported from the hepatic veins to capillaries in skeletal and cardiac muscle and adipose tissue, as well as lactating mammary tissues, where lipoprotein lipase is activated by apoC$_{II}$ in the VLDL particles. The activated enzyme facilitates the hydrolysis of the triacylglycerol in VLDL, causing the release of fatty acids and glycerol from a portion of core triacylglycerols. These fatty acids are oxidized as fuel by muscle cells, used in the resynthesis of triacylglycerols in fat cells, and used for milk production in the lactating breast. The residual particles remaining in the bloodstream are called **VLDL remnants**. Approximately 50% of these remnants are taken up from the blood by liver cells through the binding of VLDL apoE to the hepatocyte plasma membrane apoE receptor followed by endocytic internalization of the VLDL remnant.

C. Intermediate-Density Lipoprotein (IDL) and Low-Density Lipoproteins (LDL)

Approximately half of the VLDL remnants are not taken up by the liver but, instead, have additional core triacylglycerols removed to form IDL, a specialized class of VLDL remnants. With the removal of additional triacylglycerols from IDL through the action of hepatic triglyceride lipase within hepatic sinusoids, LDL is generated from IDL. As seen in Table 34.4, the LDL particles are rich in cholesterol and cholesterol esters. Approximately 60% of the LDL is transported back to the liver, where its apoB-100 binds to specific apoB-100 receptors in the liver cell plasma membranes, allowing particles to be endocytosed into the hepatocyte. The remaining 40% of LDL particles are carried to extrahepatic tissues such as adrenocortical

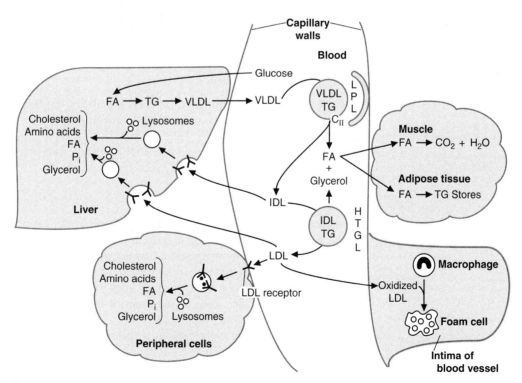

Fig. 34.14. Fate of VLDL. VLDL triacylglycerol (TG) is degraded by LPL, forming IDL. IDL can either be endocytosed by the liver through a receptor-mediated process or further digested, mainly by hepatic triacylglycerol lipase (HTGL), to form LDL. LDL may be endocytosed by receptor-mediated processes in the liver or in peripheral cells. LDL also may be oxidized and taken up by "scavenger" receptors on macrophages. The scavenger pathway plays a role in atherosclerosis. FA = fatty acids; Pi = inorganic phosphate.

and gonadal cells that also contain apoB-100 receptors, allowing them to internalize the LDL particles and use their cholesterol for the synthesis of steroid hormones. Some of the cholesterol of the internalized LDL is used for membrane synthesis and vitamin D synthesis as well. If an excess of LDL particles is present in the blood, this specific receptor-mediated uptake of LDL by hepatic and nonhepatic tissue becomes saturated. The "excess" LDL particles are now more readily available for nonspecific uptake of LDL by macrophages (scavenger cells) present near the endothelial cells of arteries. This exposure of vascular endothelial cells to high levels of LDL is believed to induce an inflammatory response by these cells, a process suggested to initiate the complex cascade of atherosclerosis discussed below.

D. High-Density Lipoprotein (HDL)

The fourth class of lipoproteins is HDL, which plays several roles in whole body lipid metabolism.

1. SYNTHESIS OF HDL

HDL particles can be created by a number of mechanisms. The first is synthesis of nascent HDL by the liver and intestine as a relatively small molecule whose shell, like that of other lipoproteins, contains phospholipids, free cholesterol, and a variety of apoproteins, predominant among which are apoA1, apoAII, apoC$_I$, and apoC$_{II}$ (see Table 34.3). Very low levels of triacylglycerols or cholesterol esters are found in the hollow core of this early, or nascent, version of HDL.

A second method for HDL generation is the budding of apoproteins from chylomicrons and VLDL particles as they are digested by lipoprotein lipase. The apoproteins (particularly AI) and shells can then accumulate more lipid, as described below.

A third method for HDL generation is free apoprotein AI, which may be shed from other circulating lipoproteins. AI will acquire cholesterol and phospholipids from other lipoproteins and cell membranes, to form a nascent-like HDL particle within the circulation.

2. MATURATION OF NASCENT HDL

In the process of maturation, the nascent HDL particles accumulate phospholipids and cholesterol from cells lining the blood vessels. As the central hollow core of nascent HDL progressively fills with cholesterol esters, HDL takes on a more globular shape to eventually form the mature HDL particle. The transfer of lipids to nascent HDL does not require enzymatic activity.

3. REVERSE CHOLESTEROL TRANSPORT

A major benefit of HDL particles derives from their ability to remove cholesterol from cholesterol-laden cells and to return the cholesterol to the liver, a process known as reverse cholesterol transport. This is particularly beneficial in vascular tissue; by reducing cellular cholesterol levels in the subintimal space, the likelihood that foam cells (lipid-laden macrophages that engulf oxidized LDL-cholesterol and represent an early stage in the development of atherosclerotic plaque) will form within the blood vessel wall is reduced.

Reverse cholesterol transport requires a directional movement of cholesterol from the cell to the lipoprotein particle. Cells contain the protein ABC1 (ATP-binding cassette protein 1) which uses ATP hydrolysis to move cholesterol from the inner leaflet of the membrane to the outer leaflet. Once the cholesterol has reached the outer membrane leaflet, the HDL particle can accept it, but if the cholesterol is not modified within the HDL particle, the cholesterol can leave the particle by the same route that it entered. To trap the cholesterol within the HDL core, the HDL particle acquires the enzyme LCAT from the circulation (LCAT is synthesized and secreted by the liver). LCAT catalyzes the transfer of a fatty acid from the 2-position of lecithin (phosphatidylcholine) in the phospholipid shell of the particle to the 3-hydroxyl group of cholesterol, forming a cholesterol ester (Fig. 34.15). The cholesterol ester migrates to the core of the HDL particle and is no longer free to return to the cell.

Elevated levels of lipoprotein-associated cholesterol in the blood, particularly that associated with LDL but also that in the more triacylglycerol-rich lipoproteins, are associated with the formation of cholesterol-rich atheromatous plaque in the vessel wall, eventually leading to diffuse atherosclerotic vascular disease resulting in acute cardiovascular events, such as a myocardial infarction, a stroke, or symptomatic peripheral vascular insufficiency. High levels of HDL in the blood, therefore, are believed to be vasculoprotective, because these high levels increase the rate of reverse cholesterol transport "away" from the blood vessels and "toward" the liver ("out of harm's way").

4. FATE OF HDL CHOLESTEROL

Mature HDL particles can bind to specific receptors on hepatocytes (such as the apoE receptor), but the primary means of clearance of HDL from the blood is through its uptake by the scavenger receptor SR-B1. This receptor is present on many cell types. It does not carry out endocytosis per se, but once the HDL particle

 Two genetically determined disorders, familial HDL deficiency and Tangier disease, result from mutations in the ATP-binding cassette 1 (ABC 1) protein. Cholesterol-depleted HDL cannot transport free cholesterol from cells that lack the ability to express this protein. As a consequence, HDL is rapidly degraded. These disorders have established a role for ABC 1 protein in the regulation of HDL levels in the blood.

 Because **Ann Jeina** continued to experience intermittent chest pain, in spite of good control of her hypertension and a 20-lb weight loss, her physician decided that a 2-drug regimen to lower her blood LDL cholesterol level must be added to the dietary measures already in place. Consequently, treatment with cholestyramine, a resin that binds some of the bile salts in the intestinal lumen, and the HMG-CoA reductase inhibitor pravastatin was initiated.

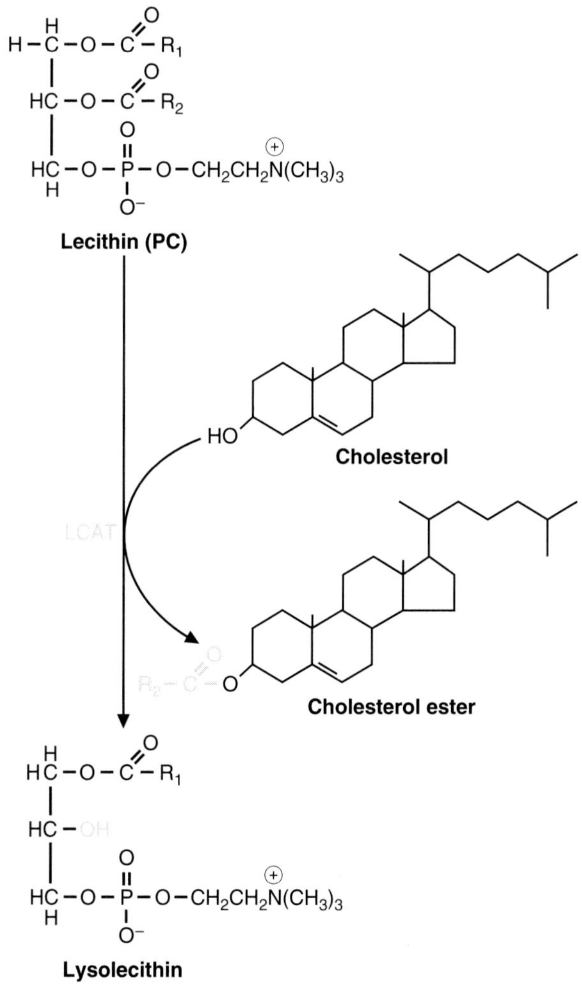

Fig. 34.15. The reaction catalyzed by LCAT. R1 = saturated fatty acid. R2 = unsaturated fatty acid.

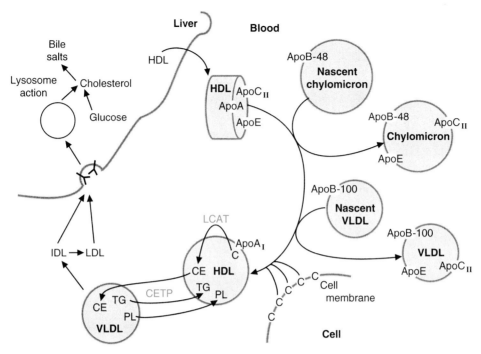

Fig. 34.16. Functions and fate of HDL. Nascent HDL is synthesized in liver and intestinal cells. It exchanges proteins with chylomicrons and VLDL. HDL picks up cholesterol (C) from cell membranes. This cholesterol is converted to cholesterol ester (CE) by the LCAT reaction. HDL transfers CE to VLDL in exchange for triacylglycerol (TG). The cholesterol ester transfer protein (CETP) mediates this exchange. PL = phospholipids.

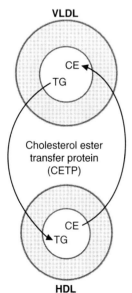

Fig. 34.17. Function of cholesterol ester transfer protein (CETP). CETP transfers cholesterol esters (CE) from HDL to VLDL in exchange for triacylglycerol (TG).

is bound to the receptor, its cholesterol and cholesterol esters are transferred into the cells. When depleted of cholesterol and its esters, the HDL particle dissociates from the SR-B1 receptor and re-enters the circulation. SR-B1 receptors can be upregulated in certain cell types that require cholesterol for biosynthetic purposes, such as the cells that produce the steroid hormones. The SR-B1 receptors are not downregulated when cholesterol levels are high.

5.   HDL INTERACTIONS WITH OTHER PARTICLES

In addition to its ability to pick up cholesterol from cell membranes, HDL also exchanges apoproteins and lipids with other lipoproteins in the blood. For example, HDL transfers apolipoprotein E (apoE) and apolipoprotein CII (apoC$_{II}$) to chylomicrons and to VLDL. The apoC$_{II}$ stimulates the degradation of the triacylglycerols of chylomicrons and VLDL by activating LPL (Fig. 34.16). After digestion of the chylomicrons and the VLDL triacylglycerols, apoE and apoCII are transferred back to HDL. When HDL obtains free cholesterol from cell membranes, the free cholesterol is esterified at the third carbon of the A ring via the LCAT reaction (see Fig. 34.14). From this point, HDL either transports the free cholesterol and cholesterol esters directly to the liver, as described above, or by CETP to circulating triacylglycerol-rich lipoproteins such as VLDL and VLDL remnants (see Fig. 34.16). In exchange, triacylglycerols from the latter lipoproteins are transferred to HDL (Fig. 34.17). The greater the concentration of triacylglycerol-rich lipoproteins in the blood, the greater the rate of these exchanges. Thus, the CETP exchange pathway may explain the observation that whenever triacylglycerol-rich lipoproteins are present in the blood in high concentrations, the amount of cholesterol reaching the liver via cholesterol-enriched VLDL and VLDL remnants increases, and a proportional reduction in the total amount of cholesterol and cholesterol esters that are directly transferred to the liver via HDL occurs. Mature

HDL particles are designated as HDL$_3$; after the CETP reaction and loss of cholesterol and gain of triacylglycerol, the particles become larger and are designated as HDL$_2$ particles (see Table 34.4).

VII. LIPOPROTEINS ENTER CELLS BY RECEPTOR-MEDIATED ENDOCYTOSIS

As stated earlier, each lipoprotein particle contains specific apoproteins on its surface that act as ligands for specific plasma membrane receptors on target tissues such as the liver, the adrenal cortex, the gonads, and other cells that require one or more of the components of the lipoproteins. With the exception of the scavenger receptor SR-B1, the interaction of ligand and receptor initiates the process of endocytosis depicted for LDL in Figure 34.18. The receptors for LDL, for example, are found in specific areas of the plasma membrane of the target cell for circulating lipoproteins. These are known as coated pits, and they contain a unique protein called clathrin. The plasma membrane in the vicinity of the receptor–LDL complex invaginates and fuses to form an endocytic vesicle. These vesicles then fuse with lysosomes, acidic subcellular vesicles that contain a number of degradative enzymes. The cholesterol esters of LDL are hydrolyzed to form free cholesterol, which is rapidly reesterified through the action of ACAT. This rapid reesterification is necessary to avoid the damaging effect of high levels of free cholesterol on cellular membranes. The newly esterified cholesterol contains primarily oleate or palmitoleate (monounsaturated fatty acids), unlike those of the cholesterol esters in LDL, which are rich in linoleate, a polyunsaturated fatty acid.

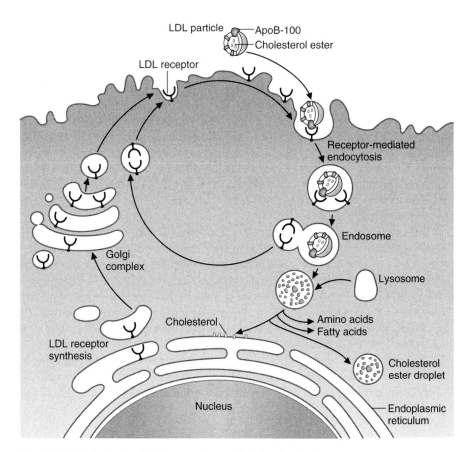

Fig. 34.18. Cholesterol uptake by receptor-mediated endocytosis.

As is true for the synthesis and activity of HMG CoA reductase, the synthesis of the LDL receptor itself is subject to feedback inhibition by increasing levels of cholesterol within the cell. One probable mechanism for this feedback regulation involves one or more of the SREBP described earlier. These proteins or the cofactors that are required for the full expression of genes that code for the LDL receptor are also capable of sensing the concentration of sterols within the cell. When sterol levels are high, the process that leads to the binding of the SREBP to the sterol regulatory element of these genes is suppressed (see Fig. 34.4). The rate of synthesis from mRNA for the LDL receptor is diminished under these circumstances. This, in turn, appropriately reduces the amount of cholesterol that can enter these cholesterol-rich cells by receptor-mediated endocytosis (downregulation of receptor synthesis). When the intracellular levels of cholesterol decrease, these processes are reversed, and cells act to increase their cholesterol levels. Both synthesis of cholesterol from acetyl CoA and synthesis of LDL receptors are stimulated. An increased number of receptors (upregulation of receptor synthesis) results in an increased uptake of LDL cholesterol from the blood, with a subsequent reduction of LDL-cholesterol levels. At the same time, the cellular cholesterol pool is replenished.

VIII.   LIPOPROTEIN RECEPTORS

The best-characterized lipoprotein receptor, the LDL receptor, specifically recognizes apoB-100 and apo E. Therefore, this receptor binds VLDL, IDL, and chylomicron remnants in addition to LDL. The binding reaction is characterized by its saturability and occurs with high affinity and a narrow range of specificity. Other receptors, such as the LDL receptor-related proteins (LRP) and the macrophage scavenger receptor (notably types SR-A1 and SR-A2, which are located primarily near the endothelial surface of vascular endothelial cells), have broad specificity and bind many other ligands in addition to the blood lipoproteins.

A. The LDL Receptor

The LDL receptor has a mosaic structure encoded by a gene that was assembled by a process known as exon shuffling. It is composed of six different regions (Fig. 34.19). The first region, at the amino terminus, contains the LDL-binding region, a cysteine-rich sequence of 40 residues. Acidic side chains in this region bind ionic calcium. When these side chains are protonated, calcium is released from its binding sites. This release leads to conformational changes that allow the LDL to disconnect from its receptor docking site. Disulfide bonds, formed from the cysteine residues, have a stabilizing influence on the structural integrity of this portion of the receptor.

The second region of the receptor contains domains that are homologous with epidermal growth factor (EGF) as well as a complex consisting of six repeats that resemble the blades of the transducin beta subunit forming a propeller like moiety.

The third region of the LDL receptor contains a chain of N-linked oligosaccharides, whereas the fourth region contains a domain that is rich in serine and threonine and contains O-linked sugars. This region may have a role in physically extending the receptor away from the membrane so that the LDL-binding region is accessible to the LDL molecule.

The fifth region contains 22 hydrophobic residues constituting the membrane-spanning unit of the receptor, whereas the sixth region extends into the cytosol, where it regulates the interaction between the C-terminal domain of the LDL receptor and the clathrin-containing coated pit where the process of receptor-mediated endocytosis is initiated.

The number of LDL receptors, the binding of LDL to its receptors, and the postreceptor binding process can be diminished for a variety of reasons, all of which

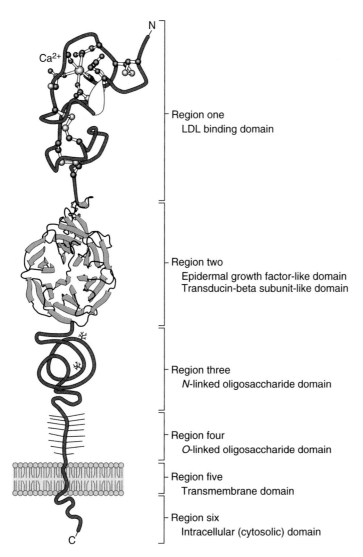

Fig. 34.19. Structure of the LDL receptor. The protein has six major regions.

may lead to an accumulation of LDL cholesterol in the blood and premature atherosclerosis. These abnormalities can result from mutations in one (heterozygous—
seen in approximately 1 in 500 people) or both (homozygous—seen in about 1 in 1
million people) alleles for the LDL receptor (familial hypercholesterolemia). Heterozygotes produce approximately half of the normal complement of LDL receptors, whereas the homozygotes produce almost no LDL receptor protein (receptor
negative familial hypercholesterolemia). The latter have serum total cholesterol levels in the range of 500 to 800 mg/dL. In a subset of patients with familial hypercholesterolemia, the LDL receptor is normally synthesized and transported to the cell
surface, but an amino acid substitution or deletion leads to changes in the protein's
structure such that LDL-binding is impaired. As a result, cholesterol does not enter
the target cell from the bloodstream and, therefore, cannot feedback negatively on
cholesterol biosynthesis in the cell. As a result, the serum cholesterol level rises. A
third form of familial hypercholesterolemia involves a genetic defect in the transport or migration mechanism that normally delivers the LDL receptor from its point
of synthesis within the cell to its proper location in that cell's plasma membrane.
Genetic mutations can lead to yet another form of familial hypercholesterolemia in
which a structural change occurs in the carboxy terminus of the LDL receptor.

 Ann Jeina's blood lipid levels (in
mg/dL) were:

Triacylglycerol	158
Total cholesterol	420
HDL cholesterol	32
LDL cholesterol	356

She was diagnosed as having familial
hypercholesterolemia (FH) type IIA, which is
caused by genetic defects in the gene that
encodes the LDL receptor (see Biochemical
Comments). As a result of the receptor defect,
LDL cannot readily be taken up by cells, and
its concentration in the blood is elevated.

LDL particles contain a high percentage,
by weight, of cholesterol and cholesterol
esters, more than other blood lipoproteins.
However, LDL triacylglycerol levels are low
because LDL is produced by digestion of the
triacylglycerols of VLDL and IDL. Therefore,
individuals with a type IIA hyperlipoproteinemia have very high blood cholesterol levels,
but their levels of triacylglycerols may be in or
near the normal range (see Table 34.4).

Ivan Applebod's blood lipid levels were:

Triacylglycerol	295
Total cholesterol	314
HDL cholesterol	24
LDL cholesterol	231

The elevated serum levels of LDL cholesterol found in patients such as **Ivan Applebod** who have type 2 diabetes mellitus is multifactorial. One of the mechanisms responsible for this increase involves the presence of chronically elevated levels of glucose in the blood of poorly controlled diabetics. This prolonged hyperglycemia increases the rate of nonenzymatic attachment of glucose to various proteins in the body, a process referred to as glycation or glycosylation of proteins.

Glycation may adversely affect the structure or the function of the protein involved. For example, glycation of the LDL receptor and of proteins in the LDL particle may interfere with the normal "fit" of LDL particles with their specific receptors. As a result, less circulating LDL is internalized into cells by receptor-mediated endocytosis, and the serum LDL cholesterol level rises.

Although such patients are able to place structurally normal LDL receptors in the plasma membrane of the cell, they are unable to internalize the LDL–LDL receptor complex because they cannot properly translocate the complex into the clathrin-containing coated pits. The spectrum of mutations of the LDL receptor gene is shown in Figure 34.20.

B. LDL Receptor-Related Protein (LRP)

LRP is structurally related to the LDL receptor but recognizes a broader spectrum of ligands. In addition to lipoproteins, it binds the blood proteins α_2-macroglobulin (a protein that inhibits blood proteases) and tissue plasminogen activator (TPA) and its inhibitors. The LRP receptor recognizes the apoE of lipoproteins and binds remnants produced by the digestion of the triacylglycerols of chylomicrons and VLDL by LPL. Thus, one of its functions is believed to be the clearance of these remnants from the blood. The LRP receptor is abundant in the cell membranes of the liver, brain, and placenta. In contrast to the LDL receptor, synthesis of the LRP receptor is not significantly affected by an increase in the intracellular concentration of cholesterol. However, insulin causes the number of these receptors on the cell surface to increase, consistent with the need for removal of chylomicron remnants that otherwise would accumulate after eating a meal.

C. Macrophage Scavenger Receptor

Some cells, particularly the phagocytic macrophages, have nonspecific receptors known as "scavenger" receptors that bind various types of molecules, including oxidatively modified LDL particles. There are a number of different types of scavenger receptors. SR-B1 is used primarily for HDL binding, whereas the scavenger receptors expressed on macrophages are SR-A1 and SR-A2. Modification of LDL frequently involves oxidative damage, particularly of polyunsaturated fatty acyl groups (see Chapter 24). In contrast to the LDL receptors, the scavenger receptors

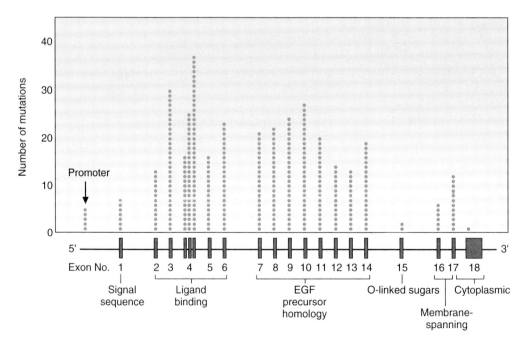

Fig. 34.20. Location of 353 point mutations and small deletions/insertions (<25 bp) in the LDL receptor gene in individuals with familial hypercholesterolemia (FH). Exons are shown as vertical boxes and introns as the lines connecting them. The figure was obtained from Goldstein JL Hobbs HH, Brown MS. Familial hypercholesterolemia. In: Scriver CR, Beaudet AL, Sly WS, Valle D, et al., eds. The Metabolic and Molecular Bases of Inherited Disease. 8th Ed., vol III. New York: McGraw-Hill, 2001:2863–2913.

are not subject to downregulation. The continued presence of scavenger receptors in the cell membrane allows the cells to take up oxidatively modified LDL long after intracellular cholesterol levels are elevated. When the macrophages become engorged with lipid, they are called foam cells. An accumulation of these foam cells in the subendothelial space of blood vessels form the earliest gross evidence of a developing atherosclerotic plaque known as a fatty streak.

The processes that cause oxidation of LDL involve superoxide radicals, nitric oxide, hydrogen peroxide, and other oxidants (see Chapter 24). Antioxidants, such as vitamin E, ascorbic acid (vitamin C), and carotenoids, may be involved in protecting LDL from oxidation.

IX. ANATOMIC AND BIOCHEMICAL ASPECTS OF ATHEROSCLEROSIS

The normal artery is composed of three distinct layers (Fig. 34.21). That which is closest to the lumen of the vessel, the intima, is lined by a monolayer of endothelial cells that are bathed by the circulating blood. Just beneath these specialized cells lies the subintimal extracellular matrix, in which some vascular smooth muscle cells are embedded (the subintimal space). The middle layer, known as the tunica media, is separated from the intima by the internal elastic lamina. The tunica media contains lamellae of smooth muscle cells surrounded by an elastin- and collagen-rich matrix. The external elastic lamina forms the border between the tunica media and the outermost layer, the adventitia. This layer contains nerve fibers and mast cells. It is the origin of the vasa vasorum, which supply blood to the outer two thirds of the tunica media.

The initial step in the development of an atherosclerotic lesion within the wall of an artery is the formation of a fatty streak. The latter represents an accumulation of lipid-ladened macrophages or foam cells in the subintimal space. These fatty streaks are visible as a yellow-white linear streak that bulges slightly into the lumen of the vessel. These streaks are initiated when one or more known "vascular risk factors for atherosclerosis," all of which have the potential to injure the vascular endothelial cells, reach a critical threshold at the site of future lesions. Examples of such risk factors include elevated intra-arterial pressure (arterial hypertension), elevated circulating levels of various lipids such as LDL, chylomicron remnants, and VLDL remnants, or low levels of circulating HDL, cigarette smoking, chronic elevations in blood glucose levels, high circulating levels of the vasoconstricting octapeptide angiotensin II, and others. The resulting insult to

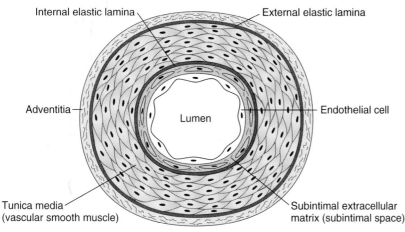

Fig. 34.21. The different layers of the arterial wall.

In addition to dietary therapy, aimed at reducing her blood cholesterol levels, **Ann Jeina** was treated with pravastatin, an HMG-CoA reductase inhibitor. The HMG-CoA reductase inhibitors decrease the rate of synthesis of cholesterol in cells. As cellular cholesterol levels decrease, the synthesis of LDL receptors increases. As the number of receptors rises on the cell surface, the uptake of LDL is increased. Consequently, the blood level of LDL cholesterol decreases.

 HDL is considered to be the "good cholesterol," because it accepts free cholesterol from peripheral tissues, such as cells in the walls of blood vessels. This cholesterol is converted to cholesterol ester, part of which is transferred to VLDL by CETP, and returned to the liver by IDL and LDL. The remainder of the cholesterol is transferred directly as part of the HDL molecule to the liver. The liver reutilizes the cholesterol in the synthesis of VLDL, converts it to bile salts, or excretes it directly into the bile. HDL therefore tends to lower blood cholesterol levels. Lower blood cholesterol levels correlate with a lower rates of death of atherosclerosis.

 In patients such as **Ann Jeina** and **Ivan Applebod**, who have elevated levels of VLDL or LDL, HDL levels are often low. These patients are predisposed to atherosclerosis and suffer from a high incidence of heart attacks and strokes.

Exercise and estrogen administration both increase HDL levels. This is one of the reasons exercise is often recommended to aid in the prevention or treatment of heart disease, and estrogen replacement therapy (ERT) is often prescribed for postmenopausal women. Before menopause, the incidence of heart attacks is relatively low in women, but it rises after menopause and increases to the level found in men by the age of 65 or 70 years. Moderate consumption of ethanol (alcohol) has also been correlated with increased HDL levels. Recent studies suggest that the beneficial amount of ethanol may be quite low, about two small glasses of wine a day, and that beneficial effects ascribed to ethanol may result from other components of wine and alcoholic beverages. In spite of the evidence that postmenopausal estrogen replacement therapy decreases circulating levels of LDL and increases HDL levels, recent data suggest that ERT may actually increase the rate of atherosclerotic vascular disease in these women. As a result, the accepted indications for ERT are now limited to intolerable "hot flashes" or vaginal dryness.

endothelial cells may trigger these cells to secrete adhesion molecules that bind to circulating monocytes and markedly slow their rate of movement past the endothelium. When sufficiently slowed, these monocytic cells accumulate and have access to the physical spaces that exist between endothelial cells. This accumulation of monocytic cells resembles the classical inflammatory response to injury. These changes have led to the suggestion that atherosclerosis is, in fact, an inflammatory disorder and, therefore, is one that might be prevented or attenuated through the use of anti-inflammatory agents such as acetylsalicylic acid (e.g., aspirin) and HMG CoA reductase inhibitors (statins), which have been shown to suppress the inflammatory cascade as well as to inhibit the action of HMG CoA reductase.

The monocytic cells are transformed into macrophages that migrate through the spaces between endothelial cells. They enter the subintimal space under the influence of chemoattractant cytokines (e.g., chemokine macrophage chemoattractant protein I) secreted by vascular cells in response to exposure to oxidatively modified fatty acids within the lipoproteins.

The macrophages can replicate and exhibit augmented expression of receptors that recognize oxidatively modified lipoproteins. Unlike the classic LDL receptors on liver and many nonhepatic cells, these macrophage-bound receptors are high-capacity, low-specificity receptors (scavenger receptors). They bind to and internalize oxidatively modified fatty acids within LDLs to become subintimal foam cells as described previously. As these foam cells accumulate, they deform the overlying endothelium, causing microscopic separations between endothelial cells, exposing these foam cells and underlying extracellular matrix to the blood. These exposed areas serve as sites for platelet adhesion and aggregation. Activated platelets secrete cytokines that perpetuate this process and increase the potential for thrombus (clot) formation locally. As the evolving plaque matures, a fibrous cap forms over its expanding "roof," which now bulges into the vascular lumen, thereby partially occluding it. Vascular smooth muscle cells now migrate from the tunica media to the subintimal space and secrete additional plaque matrix material. The smooth muscle cells also secrete metalloproteinases that thin the fibrous cap near its "elbow" at the periphery of the plaque. This thinning progresses until the fibrous cap ruptures, allowing the plaque contents to physically contact the procoagulant elements present within the circulation. This leads to acute thrombus formation. If this thrombus completely occludes the remaining lumen of the vessel, an infarction of tissues distal to the occlusion (i.e., an acute myocardial infarction) may occur (Fig. 34.22). Most plaques that rupture also contain focal areas of calcification, which appears to result from the induction of the same cluster of genes as those that promote the formation of bone. The inducers for this process include oxidized sterols as well as transforming growth factor beta (TGF-β) derived from certain vascular cells.

Finally, high intraluminal shear forces develop in these thinning or eroded areas of the plaque's fibrous cap, inducing macrophages to secrete additional metalloproteinases that further degrade the arterial-fibrous cap matrix. This contributes further to plaque rupture and thrombus formation (see Fig. 34.22). The consequence is a macrovascular ischemic event such as an acute myocardial infarction (AMI) or an acute cerebrovascular accident (CVA).

 Lipoprotein(a) is essentially an LDL particle that is covalently bound to apoprotein(a). It is called "lipoprotein little a" to avoid confusion with the apoprotein A found in HDL. The structure of apoprotein(a) is very similar to that of plasminogen, a precursor of the protease plasmin that degrades fibrin, a major component of blood clots. Lipoprotein(a), however, cannot be converted to active plasmin. There are reports that high concentrations of lipoprotein(a) correlate with an increased risk of coronary artery disease, even in patients in whom the lipid profile is otherwise normal.

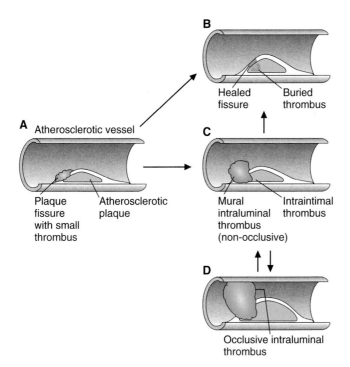

Fig. 34.22. Evolution of an atherosclerotic plaque. Plaque capsule eroded near the "elbow" of plaque creating an early plaque fissure (A), which may heal as plaque increases in size (B) or may grow as thrombus expands, having an intraluminal portion and an intraintimal portion (C). If the fissure is not properly sealed, the thrombus may grow and completely occlude the vessel lumen (D), causing an acute infarction of tissues downstream of the vessel occlusion.

X. STEROID HORMONES

Cholesterol is the precursor of all five classes of steroid hormones: glucocorticoids, mineralcorticoids, androgens, estrogens, and progestins. These hormones are synthesized in the adrenal cortex, ovaries, testes, and ovarian corpus luteum. Steroid hormones are transported through the blood from their sites of synthesis to their target organs, where, because of their hydrophobicity, they cross the cell membrane and bind to specific receptors in either the cytoplasm or nucleus. The bound receptors then bind to DNA to regulate gene transcription (see Chapter 16, section III.C.2, and Fig. 16.13). Because of their hydrophobicity, steroid hormones must be complexed with a serum protein. Serum albumin can act as a nonspecific carrier for the steroid hormones, but there are specific carriers as well. The cholesterol used for steroid hormone synthesis is either synthesized in the tissues from acetyl CoA, extracted from intracellular cholesterol ester pools, or taken up by the cell in the form of cholesterol-containing lipoproteins (either internalized by the LDL-receptor, or absorbed by the SR-B1 receptor). In general, glucocorticoids and progestins contain 21 carbons, androgens contain 19 carbons, and estrogens contain 18 carbons. The specific complement of enzymes present in the cells of an organ determines which hormones the organ can synthesize.

The oxidative reactions that lead to the synthesis and secretion of glucocorticoids such as cortisol are stimulated by adrenal corticotrophic hormone (ACTH). The role of cortisol as a stress-released hormone is discussed in Chapter 43.

Mineralocorticoids such as aldosterone are also synthesized in the adrenal cortex and are secreted in response to angiotensin II or III, rising potassium levels in the blood, or hyponatremia (low levels of sodium ions in the blood). Aldosterone stimulates sodium reuptake in the kidney, sweat glands, salivary glands, and other

Vera Leizd consulted her gynecologist, who confirmed that her problems were probably the result of an excess production of androgens (virilization) and ordered blood and urine studies to determine whether Vera's adrenal cortices or her ovaries were causing her virilizing syndrome.

Cytochrome P450$_{C11}$, another enzyme located in the mitochondrial membrane, catalyzes β-hydroxylation at C11. Hydroxylations at C17 and C21 are catalyzed by two enzymes located in the membranes of the endoplasmic reticulum (P450$_{C17}$ for 17α-hydroxylation and P450$_{C21}$ for 21-hydroxylation).

tissues, with a resultant increase in extracellular fluid volume and eventually in blood pressure. The angiotensins are produced in response to a reduction in extracellular fluid volume, which may occur as a result of such things as excessive sweating, persistent vomiting without sufficient rehydration, or bleeding without adequate replacement of blood.

Androgens such as testosterone are synthesized in the Leydig cells of the testes and to a lesser extent in the ovary and are secreted in response to luteinizing hormone (LH). In males, testosterone is commonly converted to dihydrotestosterone, a higher-affinity form of the hormone, within specific target tissues. This active form of the hormone stimulates the production of sperm proteins in Sertoli cells and the development of secondary sex characteristics.

Estrogens such as 17-β-estradiol are synthesized in the ovarian follicle and the corpus luteum, from which their secretion is stimulated by follicle-stimulating hormone (FSH). In the female, 17 β-estradiol feeds back negatively on the synthesis and secretion of the pituitary gonadotropins, such as FSH. Estrogen and progesterone prepare the uterine endometrium for implantation of the fertilized ovum, and among other actions promotes differentiation of the mammary gland.

Progestogens such as progesterone are synthesized in the corpus luteum, and their secretion is stimulated by LH. As mentioned, in concert with estradiol, progesterone prepares the uterine endometrium for implantation of the fertilized ovum and acts as a differentiation factor in mammary gland development.

The biosynthesis of glucocorticoids and mineralocorticoids (in the adrenal cortex), and that of sex steroids (in the adrenal cortex and gonads), requires four cytochrome P450 enzymes (see Chapter 24). These monooxygenases are involved in the transfer of electrons from NADPH through electron transfer protein intermediates to molecular oxygen, which then oxidizes a variety of the ring carbons of cholesterol.

Cholesterol is converted to progesterone in the first two steps of synthesis of all steroid hormones. Cytochrome P450$_{SCC}$ side-chain cleavage enzyme (previously referred to as cholesterol desmolase) is located in the mitochondrial inner membrane and removes six carbons from the side chain of cholesterol, forming pregnenolone, which has 21 carbons (Fig. 34.23). The next step, the conversion of pregnenolone to progesterone, is catalyzed by 3 β-hydroxysteroid dehydrogenase, an enzyme that is not a member of the cytochrome P450 family. Other steroid hormones are produced from progesterone by reactions that involve members of the P450 family. As the synthesis of the steroid hormones is discussed, notice how certain enzymes are used in more than one pathway. Defects in such enzymes will lead to multiple abnormalities in steroid synthesis, which, in turn, results in a variety of abnormal phenotypes.

A. Synthesis of Cortisol

The adrenocortical biosynthetic pathway that leads to cortisol synthesis occurs in the middle layer of the adrenal cortex known as the zona fasciculata. Free cholesterol is transported by an intracellular carrier protein to the inner mitochondrial membrane of cells (Fig. 34.24), where the side chain is cleaved to form pregnenolone. Pregnenolone returns to the cytosol, where it forms progesterone.

In the membranes of the endoplasmic reticulum, the enzyme P450$_{C17}$ catalyzes the hydroxylation of C17 of progesterone or pregnenolone and can also catalyze the cleavage of the 2-carbon side chain of these compounds at C17 (a C17-C20 lyase activity). These two separate functions of the same enzyme allow further steroid synthesis to proceed along two separate pathways: the 17-hydroxylated steroids that retain their side chains are precursors of cortisol (C21), whereas those from which the side chain was cleaved (C19 steroids) are precursors of androgens (male sex hormones) and estrogens (female sex hormones).

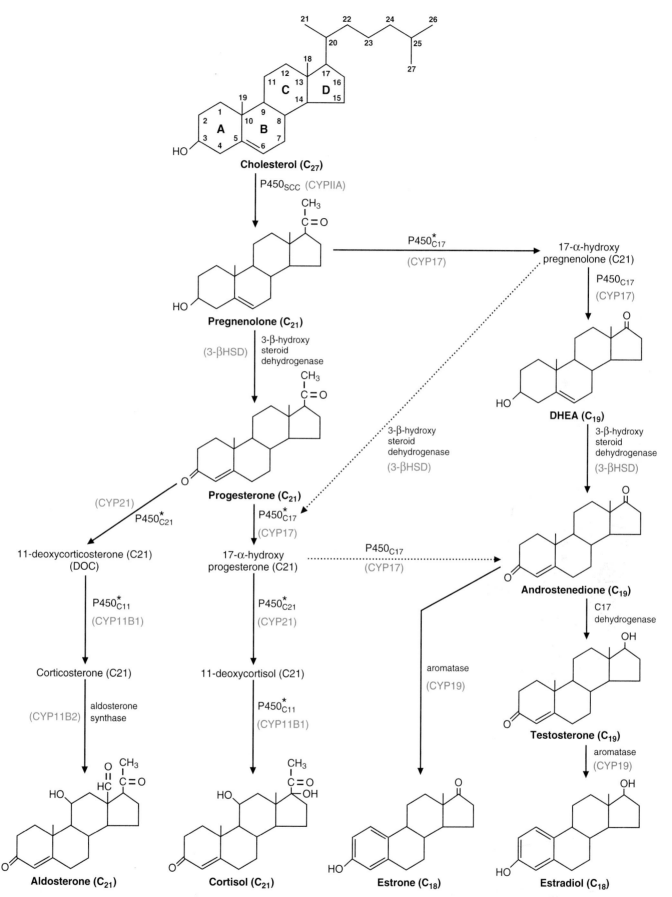

Fig. 34.23. Synthesis of the steroid hormones. The rings of the precursor, cholesterol, are lettered. Dihydrotestosterone is produced from testosterone by reduction of the carbon–carbon double bond in ring A. Structural changes between the precursor and final hormone are noted in blue. DHEA = dehydroepiandrosterone. The dashed lines indicate alternative pathways to the major pathways indicated. The starred enzymes are those that may be defective in the condition congenital adrenal hyperplasia.

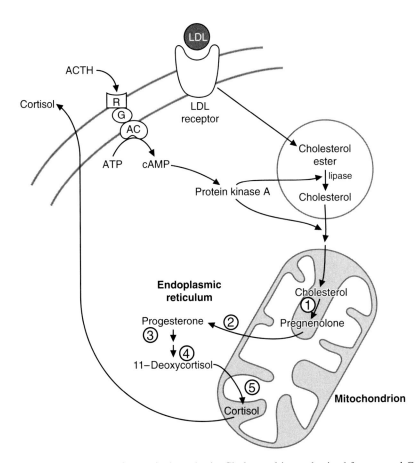

Fig. 34.24. Cellular route for cortisol synthesis. Cholesterol is synthesized from acetyl CoA or derived from low-density lipoprotein (LDL), which is endocytosed and digested by lysosomal enzymes. Cholesterol is stored in cells of the adrenal cortex as cholesterol esters. ACTH signals the cell to convert cholesterol to cortisol. 1 = cholesterol desmolase (involved in side chain cleavage); 2 = 3β-hydroxysteroid dehydrogenase; 3 = 17α-hydroxylase; 4 = 21-hydroxylase; 5 = 11β-hydroxylase.

In the pathway of cortisol synthesis, the 17-hydroxylation of progesterone yields 17-α-hydroxyprogesterone, which, along with progesterone, is transported to the smooth endoplasmic reticulum. There the membrane-bound $P450_{C21}$ (21-α-hydroxylase) enzyme catalyzes the hydroxylation of C21 of 17-α-hydroxyprogesterone to form 11-deoxycortisol (and of progesterone to form deoxycorticosterone [DOC], a precursor of the mineralocorticoid, aldosterone; see Fig. 34.23).

The final step in cortisol synthesis requires transport of 11-deoxycortisol back to the inner membrane of the mitochondria, where $P450_{C11}$ (11-β-hydroxylase) receives electrons from electron transport protein intermediates (adrenodoxin, which when oxidized is reduced by adrenodoxin reductase). The enzyme then transfers these reducing equivalents by way of oxygen to 11-deoxycortisol for hydroxylation at C11 to form cortisol. The rate of biosynthesis of cortisol and other adrenal steroids is dependent on stimulation of the adrenal cortical cells by adrenocorticotropic hormone (ACTH).

B. Synthesis of Aldosterone

The synthesis of the potent mineralocorticoid aldosterone in the zona glomerulosa of the adrenal cortex also begins with the conversion of cholesterol to progesterone (see Figs. 34.23 and 34.24). Progesterone is then hydroxylated at C21, a reaction catalyzed by $P450_{C21}$, to yield DOC. The $P450_{C11}$ enzyme system then catalyzes the reactions that convert DOC to corticosterone. The terminal steps in aldosterone synthesis, catalyzed by the P450 aldosterone system, involve the oxidation of corticosterone to 18-hydroxycorticosterone, which is oxidized to aldosterone.

The primary stimulus for aldosterone production is the octapeptide angiotensin II, although hyperkalemia (greater than normal levels of potassium in the blood) or hyponatremia (less than normal levels of sodium in the blood) may directly stimulate aldosterone synthesis as well. ACTH has a permissive action in aldosterone production. It allows cells to respond optimally to their primary stimulus, angiotensin II.

C. Synthesis of the Adrenal Androgens

Adrenal androgen biosynthesis proceeds from cleavage of the 2-carbon side chain of 17-hydroxypregnenolone at C17 to form the 19-carbon adrenal androgen dehydroepiandrosterone (DHEA) and its sulfate derivative (DHEAS) in the zona reticulosum of the adrenal cortex (see Fig. 34.23). These compounds, which are weak androgens, represent a significant percentage of the total steroid production by the normal adrenal cortex, and are the major androgens synthesized in the adrenal gland.

Androstenedione, another weak adrenal androgen, is produced when the 2-carbon side chain is cleaved from 17α-hydroxyprogesterone by the C17-C20 lyase activity of $P450_{C17}$. This androgen is converted to testosterone primarily in extraadrenal tissues. Although the adrenal cortex makes very little estrogen, the weak adrenal androgens may be converted to estrogens in the peripheral tissues, particularly in adipose tissue (Fig. 34.25).

D. Synthesis of Testosterone

Luteinizing hormone (LH) from the anterior pituitary stimulates the synthesis of testosterone and other androgens by the Leydig cells of the human testicle. In many ways, the pathways leading to androgen synthesis in the testicle are similar to those described for the adrenal cortex. In the human testicle, the predominant pathway leading to testosterone synthesis is through pregnenolone to 17-α-hydroxypregnenolone to DHEA (the Δ^5 pathway), and then from DHEA to androstenedione, and from androstenedione to testosterone (see Fig. 34.23). As for all steroids, the rate-limiting step in testosterone production is the conversion of cholesterol to pregnenolone. LH controls the rate of side-chain cleavage from cholesterol at carbon 21 to form pregnenolone, and thus regulates the rate of

Congenital adrenal hyperplasia (CAH) is a group of diseases caused by a genetically determined deficiency in a variety of enzymes required for cortisol synthesis. The most common deficiency is that of 21-α hydroxylase, the activity of which is necessary to convert progesterone to 11-deoxycorticosterone and 17-α hydroxy progesterone to 11-deoxycortisol. Thus, this deficiency reduces both aldosterone and cortisol production, without affecting androgen production. If the enzyme deficiency is severe, the precursors for aldosterone and cortisol production are shunted to androgen synthesis, producing an overabundance of androgens, which leads to prenatal masculinization in females and postnatal virilization of males. Another enzyme deficiency in this group of diseases is that of 11-β hydroxylase, which results in the accumulation of 11-deoxycorticosterone. An excess of this mineralocorticoid leads to hypertension (through binding of 11-deoxycorticosterone to the aldosterone receptor). In this form of CAH, 11-deoxycortisol also accumulates, but its biologic activity is minimal, and no specific clinical signs and symptoms result. The androgen pathway is unaffected, and the increased ACTH levels may increase the levels of adrenal androgens in the blood. A third possible enzyme deficiency is that of 17-α hydroxylase. A defect in 17-α hydroxylase leads to aldosterone excess and hypertension; however, because adrenal androgen synthesis requires this enzyme, no virilization occurs in these patients.

Hyperplasia or tumors of the adrenal cortex that produce excess aldosterone result in a condition known as primary aldosteronism, which is characterized by enhanced sodium and water retention, resulting in hypertension.

Although aldosterone is the major mineralocorticoid in humans, excessive production of a weaker mineralocorticoid, DOC, which occurs in patients with a deficiency of the 11-hydroxylase (the $P450_{C11}$ enzyme), may lead to clinical signs and symptoms of mineralocorticoid excess even though aldosterone secretion is suppressed in these patients.

Androstenedione can be purchased at health food stores under the name Andros. It is touted to improve athletic performance through its ability to be converted to testosterone. Its use has been banned by most major sports, although in 1998 it was a legal supplement in baseball. During that year, the drug received a lot of publicity, as the supplement had been used by a player who broke the major league home run record.

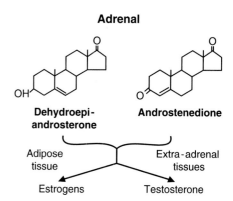

Adrenal

Dehydroepi-androsterone

Androstenedione

Adipose tissue

Extra-adrenal tissues

Estrogens

Testosterone

Fig. 34.25. Adrenal androgens. These weak androgens are converted to testosterone or estrogens in other tissues.

Biologically, the most potent circulating androgen is testosterone. Approximately 50% of the testosterone in the blood in a normal woman is produced equally in the ovaries and in the adrenal cortices. The remaining half is derived from ovarian and adrenal androstenedione, which, after secretion into the blood, is converted to testosterone in adipose tissue, muscle, liver, and skin. The adrenal cortex, however, is the major source of the relatively weak androgen dehydroepiandrosterone (DHEA). The serum concentration of its stable metabolite, DHEAS, is used as a measure of adrenal androgen production in hyperandrogenic patients with diffuse excessive growth of secondary sexual hair, e.g., facial hair as well as that in the axillae, the suprapubic area, the chest, and the upper extremities.

Q: The results of the blood tests on **Vera Leizd** showed that her level of testosterone was normal but that her serum dehydroepiandrosterone sulfate (DHEAS) level was significantly elevated. Which tissue was the most likely source of the androgens that caused Vera's hirsutism (a male pattern of secondary sexual hair growth)?

Ergosterol is the provitamin of vitamin D_2, which differs from 7-dehydrocholesterol and vitamin D_3, respectively, only by having a double bond between C22 and C23 and a methyl group at C24. Vitamin D_2 is the constituent in many commercial vitamin preparations and in irradiated milk and bread. The antirachitic potencies of D_2 and D_3 in humans are equal, but both must be converted to 25-(OH)-cholecalciferol and eventually to the active form calcitriol (1,25-$(OH)_2D_3$) for biologic activity.

Rickets is a disorder of young children caused by a deficiency of vitamin D. Low levels of calcium and phosphorus in the blood are associated with skeletal deformities in these patients.

testosterone synthesis. In its target cells, the double bond in ring A of testosterone is reduced through the action of 5-α reductase, forming the active hormone dihydrotestosterone (DHT).

E. Synthesis of Estrogens and Progesterone

Ovarian production of estrogens, progestins (compounds related to progesterone), and androgens requires the activity of the cytochrome P450 family of oxidative enzymes used for the synthesis of other steroid hormones. Ovarian estrogens are C18 steroids with a phenolic hydroxyl group at C3 and either a hydroxyl group (estradiol) or a ketone group (estrone) at C17. Although the major steroid-producing compartments of the ovary (the granulosa cell, the theca cell, the stromal cell, and the cells of the corpus luteum) have all of the enzyme systems required for the synthesis of multiple steroids, the granulosa cells secrete primarily estrogens, the thecal and stromal cells secrete primarily androgens, and the cells of the corpus luteum secrete primarily progesterone.

The ovarian granulosa cell, in response to stimulation by follicle-stimulating hormone (FSH) from the anterior pituitary gland and through the catalytic activity of P450 aromatase, converts testosterone to estradiol, the predominant and most potent of the ovarian estrogens (see Fig. 34.23). Similarly, androstenedione is converted to estrone in the ovary, although the major site of estrone production from androstenedione occurs in extraovarian tissues, principally skeletal muscle and adipose tissue.

XI. VITAMIN D SYNTHESIS

Vitamin D is unique in that it can be either obtained from the diet (as vitamin D_2 or D_3) or synthesized from a cholesterol precursor, a process that requires reactions in the skin, liver, and intestine. The calciferols, including several forms of vitamin D, are a family of steroids that affect calcium homeostasis (Fig. 34.26). Cholecalciferol (vitamin D_3) requires ultraviolet light for its production from 7-dehydrocholesterol present in cutaneous tissues (skin) in animals and from ergosterol in plants. This irradiation cleaves the carbon–carbon bond at C9–C10 to open the B ring to form cholecalciferol, an inactive precursor of 1,25-$(OH)_2$-cholecalciferol (calcitriol). Calcitriol is the most potent biologically active form of vitamin D (see Fig. 34.26).

The formation of calcitriol from cholecalciferol begins in the liver and ends in the kidney, where the pathway is regulated. In this activation process, carbon 25 of vitamin D_2 or D_3 is hydroxylated in the microsomes of the liver to form 25-hydroxycholecalciferol (calcidiol). Calcidiol circulates to the kidney bound to vitamin D–binding globulin (transcalciferin). In the proximal convoluted tubule of the kidney, a mixed function oxidase, which requires molecular O_2 and NADPH as cofactors, hydroxylates carbon 1 on the A ring to form calcitriol. This step is tightly regulated and is the rate-limiting step in the production of the active hormone.

1,25-$(OH)_2D_3$ (calcitriol) is approximately 100 times more potent than 25-$(OH)D_3$ in its actions, yet 25-$(OH)D_3$ is present in the blood in a concentration that may be 100 times greater, which suggests that it may play some role in calcium and phosphorus homeostasis.

The biologically active forms of vitamin D are sterol hormones and, like other steroids, diffuse passively through the plasma membrane. In the intestine, bone, and kidney, the sterol then moves into the nucleus and binds to specific vitamin D_3 receptors. This complex activates genes that encode proteins mediating the action of active vitamin D_3. In the intestinal mucosal cell, for example, transcription of genes encoding calcium-transporting proteins is activated. These proteins are capable of carrying Ca^{2+} (and phosphorus) absorbed from the gut lumen across the cell, making it available for eventual passage into the circulation.

CLINICAL COMMENTS

Ann Jeina is typical of patients with essentially normal serum triacylglycerol levels and elevated serum total cholesterol levels that are repeatedly in the upper 1% of the general population (e.g., 325–500 mg/dL). When similar lipid abnormalities are present in other family members in a pattern of autosomal dominant inheritance and no secondary causes for these lipid alterations (e.g., hypothyroidism) are present, the entity referred to as "familial hypercholesterolemia (FH), type IIA" is the most likely cause of this hereditary dyslipidemia.

FH is a genetic disorder caused by an abnormality in one or more alleles responsible for the formation or the functional integrity of high-affinity LDL receptors on the plasma membrane of cells that normally initiate the internalization of circulating LDL and other blood lipoproteins. Heterozygotes for FH (1 in 500 of the population) have roughly one half of the normal complement or functional capacity of such receptors, whereas homozygotes (1 in 1 million of the population) have essentially no functional LDL receptors. The rare patient with the homozygous form of FH has a more extreme elevation of serum total and LDL cholesterol than does the heterozygote and, as a result, has a more profound predisposition to premature coronary artery disease.

Chronic hypercholesterolemia not only may cause the deposition of lipid within vascular tissues leading to atherosclerosis but also may cause the deposition of lipid within the skin and eye. When this occurs in the medial aspect of the upper and lower eyelids, it is referred to as xanthelasma. Similar deposits known as xanthomas may occur in the iris of the eye (arcus lipidalis) as well as the tendons of the hands ("knucklepads") and Achilles tendons.

Although therapy aimed at inserting competent LDL receptor genes into the cells of patients with homozygous FH is undergoing clinical trials, the current approach in the heterozygote is to attempt to increase the rate of synthesis of LDL receptors in cells pharmacologically.

Ann Jeina was treated with cholestyramine, a resin that binds some of the bile salts in the intestine, causing these resin-bound salts to be carried into the feces rather than recycled to the liver. The liver must now synthesize more bile salts, which lowers the intrahepatic free cholesterol pool. As a result, hepatic LDL receptor synthesis is induced, and more circulating LDL is taken up by the liver.

HMG-CoA reductase inhibitors, such as pravastatin, also stimulate the synthesis of additional LDL receptors but do so by inhibiting HMG-CoA reductase, the rate-limiting enzyme for cholesterol synthesis. The subsequent decline in the intracellular free cholesterol pool also stimulates the synthesis of additional LDL receptors. These additional receptors reduce circulating LDL-cholesterol levels by increasing receptor-mediated endocytosis of LDL particles.

A combination of strict dietary and dual pharmacologic therapy, aimed at decreasing the cholesterol levels of the body, is usually quite effective in cor-

Ann Jeina was treated with a statin (pravastatin) and cholestyramine, a bile acid sequestrant. With the introduction of the cholesterol absorption blocker ezetimibe, the use of cholestyramine with its high level of gastrointestinal side effects may decline. Ezetimibe reduces the percentage of absorption of free cholesterol present in the lumen of the gut and hence the amount of cholesterol available to the enterocyte to package into chylomicrons. This, in turn, reduces the amount of cholesterol returning to the liver in chylomicron remnants. The net result is a reduction in the cholesterol pool in hepatocytes. The latter induces the synthesis of an increased number of LDL receptors by the liver cells. As a consequence, the capacity of the liver to increase hepatic uptake of LDL from the circulation leads to a decrease in serum LDL levels.

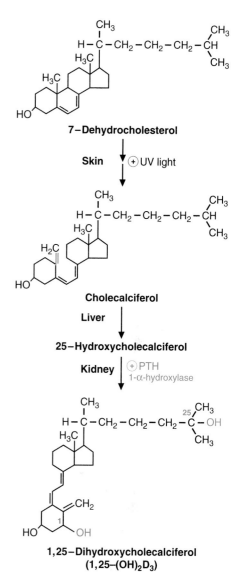

Fig. 34.26. Synthesis of active vitamin D. (1, 25-di (OH)$_2$D$_3$) is produced from 7-dehydrocholesterol, a precursor of cholesterol. In the skin, ultraviolet (UV) light produces cholecalciferol, which is hydroxylated at the 25-position in the liver and the 1-position in the kidney to form the active hormone.

Vera Leizd's hirsutism was most likely the result of a problem in her adrenal cortex that caused excessive production of DHEA.

recting the lipid abnormality and, hopefully, the associated risk of atherosclerotic cardiovascular disease in patients with heterozygous familial hypercholesterolemia.

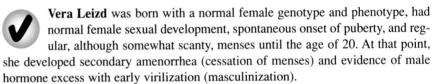 Low-density lipoprotein cholesterol is the primary target of cholesterol-lowering therapy because both epidemiologic and experimental evidence strongly suggest a benefit of lowering serum LDL cholesterol in the prevention of atherosclerotic cardiovascular disease. Similar evidence for raising subnormal levels of serum HDL cholesterol is less conclusive but adequate to support such efforts, particularly in high-risk patients, such as **Ivan Applebod**, who have multiple cardiovascular risk factors. The first-line therapy in this attempt is non-pharmacologic and includes such measures as increasing aerobic exercise, weight loss in overweight patients, avoidance of excessive alcohol intake, reducing the intake of refined sugars, and cessation of smoking. If these efforts fail, drug therapy to raise serum HDL cholesterol levels must be considered.

So far, Mr. Applebod has failed in his attempts to diet and exercise. His LDL cholesterol level is 231 mg/dL. According to Table 34.1, he is a candidate for more stringent dietary therapy and for drug treatment. He could be given an HMG CoA reductase inhibitor such as pravastatin and, perhaps, a bile salt–binding resin such as cholestyramine. Other lipid-lowering drugs such as the fibric acid derivatives and ezetimibe, which also decrease triacylglycerol levels and potentially increase HDL levels, should be considered (Table 34.5).

Vera Leizd was born with a normal female genotype and phenotype, had normal female sexual development, spontaneous onset of puberty, and regular, although somewhat scanty, menses until the age of 20. At that point, she developed secondary amenorrhea (cessation of menses) and evidence of male hormone excess with early virilization (masculinization).

The differential diagnosis included an ovarian versus an adrenocortical source of the excess androgenic steroids. A screening test to determine whether

Table 34.5. Mechanism(s) of Action and Efficacy of Lipid-Lowering Agents

Agent	Mechanism of Action	Percentage change in serum lipid level (monotherapy)			
		Total cholesterol	LDL-cholesterol	HDL cholesterol	Triacylglycerols
Statins	Inhibits HMG-CoA reductase activity	↓15–60%	↓ 20–60%	↑ 5–15%	↓10–40%
Bile acid resins	Increase fecal excretion of bile salts	↓15–20%	↓10–25%	↑ 3–5%	Variable, depending on pretreatment level of triacylglycerols (may increase)
Niacin	Activates LPL; reduces hepatic production of VLDL; reduces catabolism of HDL	↓ 22–25%	↓10–25%	↑ 15–35%	↓ 20–50%
Fibrates	Antagonizes PPAR-α causing an increase in LPL activity, a decrease in apoprotein C-III production, and an increase in apoprotein A-I production.	↓12–15%	Variable, depending on pretreatment levels of other lipids	↑ 5–15%	↓ 20–50%
Ezetimibe	Reduces intestinal absorption of free cholesterol from the gut lumen	↓10–15%	↓ 15–20%	↑ 1–3%	↓ 5–8% if triacylglycerols are high pretreatment

Abbreviations: LPL, lipoprotein lipase; LDL, low-density lipoprotein; HDL, high-density lipoprotein; triacylglycerols, triglycerides; PPAR, peroxisome proliferators-activated receptor (the Table is adapted from Circulation 2002; 106:3145–3457).

the adrenal cortex or the ovary is the source of excess male hormone involves the measurement of the concentration of dehydroepiandrosterone sulfate (DHEAS) in the patient's plasma, because the adrenal cortex makes most of the DHEA, and the ovary makes little or none. Vera's plasma DHEAS level was moderately elevated, identifying her adrenal cortices as the likely source of her virilizing syndrome.

If the excess production of androgens is not the result of an adrenal tumor, but the result of a defect in the pathway for cortisol production, the simple treatment is to administer glucocorticoids by mouth. The rationale for such treatment can be better understood by reviewing Fig. 34.23. If **Vera Leizd** has a genetically determined partial deficiency in the $P450_{C11}$ enzyme system needed to convert 11-deoxycortisol to cortisol, her blood cortisol levels would fall. By virtue of the normal positive feedback mechanism, a subnormal level of cortisol in the blood would induce the anterior pituitary to make more ACTH. The latter would not only stimulate the cortisol pathway to increase cortisol synthesis to normal but, in the process, would also induce increased production of adrenal androgens such as DHEA and DHEAS. The increased levels of the adrenal androgens (although relatively weak androgens) would cause varying degrees of virilization, depending on the severity of the enzyme deficiency. The administration of a glucocorticoid by mouth would suppress the high level of secretion of ACTH from the anterior pituitary gland that occurs in response to the reduced levels of cortisol secreted from the adrenal cortex. Treatment with prednisone (a synthetic glucocorticoid), therefore, will prevent the ACTH-induced overproduction of adrenal androgens. However, when ACTH secretion returns to normal, endogenous cortisol synthesis falls below normal. The administered prednisone brings the net glucocorticoid activity in the blood back to physiologic levels. Vera's adrenal androgen levels in the blood returned to normal after several weeks of therapy with prednisone (a synthetic glucocorticoid). As a result, her menses eventually resumed, and her virilizing features slowly resolved.

Because Vera's symptoms began in adult life, her genetically determined adrenal hyperplasia is referred to as a "nonclassic" or "atypical" form of the disorder. A more severe enzyme deficiency leads to the "classic" disease, which is associated with excessive fetal adrenal androgen production in utero and, therefore, manifests itself at birth, often with ambiguous external genitalia and virilizing features in the female neonate.

BIOCHEMICAL COMMENTS

Defects in the LDL receptor gene are responsible for the elevated blood levels of LDL, and thus of cholesterol, in FH. Over 300 mutations have been found in the LDL receptor gene, affecting all stages in the production and functioning of the receptor.

The LDL receptor gene, which contains 18 exons and is 45 kilobases (kb) in length, is located on the short arm of chromosome 19. The exons share sequences for the C9 component of complement (a blood protein involved in the immune response), and the *N*-linked oligosaccharide domain is homologous to the genes for the precursor of EGF and also for three proteases of the blood clotting system, Factors IX and X and protein C (see Chapter 45). The LDL receptor gene encodes a glycoprotein that contains 839 amino acids.

Heterozygotes for FH have one normal and one mutant allele. Their cells produce approximately half the normal amount of receptor and take up LDL at about half the normal rate. Homozygotes have two mutant alleles, which may either be identical or differ. They produce very little functional receptor.

The genetic mutations are mainly deletions, but insertions or duplications also occur, as well as missense and nonsense point mutations (see Fig. 34.20). Four classes of mutations have been identified. The first class involves "null" alleles that either direct the synthesis of no protein at all or a protein that cannot be precipitated by antibodies to the LDL receptor. In the second class, the alleles encode proteins, but they cannot be transported to the cell surface. The third class of mutant alleles encodes proteins that reach the cell surface but cannot bind LDL normally. Finally, the fourth class encodes proteins that reach the surface and bind LDL but fail to cluster and internalize the LDL particles. The result of each of these mutations is that blood levels of LDL are elevated because cells cannot take up these particles at a normal rate.

Suggested References

Goldstein JL, Hobbs HH, Brown MS. Familial hypercholesterolemia. In: Scriver CR, Beaudet AL, Sly WS, Valle D, et al., eds. The Metabolic and Molecular Bases of Inherited Disease. 8th Ed., vol III. New York: McGraw-Hill, 2001:2863–2913.

Jeon H, Meng W, Takagi J, Eck MG, Springer TA, Blacklow SC. Implications for familial hypercholesterolemia from the structure of the LDL receptor YWTD-EGF domain pair. Nature Struct Biol 2001;8:499–504.

Nimpf J, Schneider WJ. From cholesterol transport to signal transduction: Low density lipoprotein receptor, very low density lipoprotein receptor, and apolipoprotein E receptor-2. Biochim Biophys Acta 2000;1529:287–298.

Yokoyama S.. Release of cellular cholesterol molecular mechanism for cholesterol homeostasis in cells and in the body. Biochim Biophys Acta 2000;1529:231–244.

 REVIEW QUESTIONS—CHAPTER 34

1. Which of the following steps in the biosynthesis of cholesterol is the committed rate-limiting step?

    (A) The condensation of acetoacetyl-CoA with a molecule of acetyl-CoA to yield β-hydroxy-β methylglutaryl-CoA (HMG-CoA)
    (B) The reduction of HMG-CoA to mevalonate
    (C) The conversion of mevalonate to two activated isoprenes
    (D) The formation of farnesyl pyrophosphate
    (E) Condensation of six activated isoprene units to form squalene

2. Considering the final steps in cholesterol biosynthesis, when squalene is eventually converted to lanosterol, which of the following statements is correct?

    (A) All of the sterols have three fused rings (the steroid nucleus) and are alcohols with a hydroxyl group at C-3.
    (B) The action of squalene monooxygenase oxidizes carbon 14 of the squalene chain, forming an epoxide.
    (C) Squalene monooxygenase is considered a mixed function oxidase because it catalyzes a reaction in which only one of the oxygen atoms of O_2 is incorporated into the organic substrate.
    (D) Squalene monooxygenase uses reduced flavin nucleotides (e.g., FAD(2H)) as the cosubstrate in the reaction.
    (E) Squalene is joined at carbons 1 and 30 to form the fused ring structure of sterols.

3. Of the major risk factors for the development of atherosclerotic cardiovascular disease (ASCVD) such as sedentary lifestyle, obesity, cigarette smoking, diabetes mellitus, hypertension, and hyperlipidemia, which one, if present, is the only risk factor in a given patient without a history of having had a myocardial infarction that requires that the therapeutic goal for the serum LDL cholesterol level be < 100mg/dL?

    (A) Obesity
    (B) Cigarette smoking
    (C) Diabetes mellitus
    (D) Hypertension
    (E) Sedentary lifestyle

4. Which one of the following apoproteins acts as a cofactor activator of the enzyme lipoprotein lipase (LPL)?

    (A) ApoC-III
    (B) ApoC-II
    (C) ApoB-100
    (D) ApoB-48
    (E) ApoE

5. Which one of the following sequences places the lipoproteins in the order of most dense to least dense?

    (A) HDL/VLDL/chylomicrons/LDL
    (B) HDL/LDL/VLDL/chylomicrons
    (C) LDL/chylomicrons/HDL/VLDL
    (D) VLDL/chylomicrons/LDL/HDL
    (E) LDL/chylomicrons/VLDL/HDL

35 Metabolism of the Eicosanoids

*The **eicosanoids**, which include the **prostaglandins** (PG), **thromboxanes** (TX), and **leukotrienes** (LT), are among the most potent regulators of cellular function in nature and are produced by almost every cell in the body. They act mainly as "local" hormones, affecting the cells that produce them or neighboring cells of a different type.*

*Eicosanoids participate in many processes in the body, particularly the **inflammatory response** that occurs after **infection** or **injury**. The inflammatory response is the sum of the body's efforts to destroy invading organisms and to repair damage. It includes the control of bleeding through the formation of blood clots. In the process of protecting the body from a variety of insults, the inflammatory response can produce **symptoms** such as **pain**, **swelling**, and **fever**. An exaggerated or inappropriate expression of the normal inflammatory response may occur in individuals who have **allergic** or **hypersensitivity** reactions.*

*In addition to participating in the inflammatory response, eicosanoids also regulate **smooth muscle contraction** (particularly in the intestine and uterus). They increase **water** and **sodium excretion** by the kidney and are involved in **regulating blood pressure**. They frequently serve as modulators; some eicosanoids stimulate and others inhibit the same process. For example, some serve as constrictors and others as dilators of blood vessels. They are also involved in regulating **bronchoconstriction** and **bronchodilation**.*

Eicosanoids are derived from polyunsaturated fatty acids containing 20 carbon atoms, which are found in cell membranes esterified to membrane phospholipids. Arachidonic acid, derived from the diet or synthesized from linoleate, is the compound from which most of the eicosanoids are produced in the body. Compounds that serve as signals for eicosanoid production bind to cell membrane receptors and activate phospholipases that cleave the polyunsaturated fatty acids from cell membrane phospholipids (Fig. 35.1).

*Arachidonic acid is enzymatically metabolized by three major pathways. The two pathways that have been most thoroughly studied are the **cyclooxygenase** pathway (which produces prostaglandins and thromboxanes) and the **lipoxygenase** pathway (which produces leukotrienes). The **cytochrome P450** pathway generates eicosanoids with less well-defined physiologic functions. **Isoprostanes** are a relatively new class of eicosanoids derived from nonenzymatic free radical–catalyzed reactions. The isoprostanes are similar to prostaglandins in structure and may play a role in inflammatory responses and free radical–mediated tissue injury. In brain tissue, arachidonic acid can be coupled to ethanolamine to generate **anandamide**. This compound can bind and activate cannabinoid receptors with actions similar to those of Δ^9-tetrahydrocannabinol (THC).*

*Many eicosanoids have very **short half-lives**, in the range of a few minutes or less. They are rapidly inactivated and excreted.*

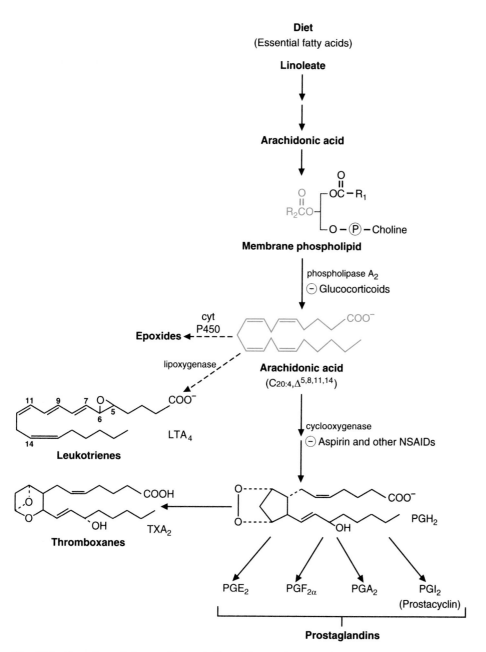

Fig. 35.1. Overview of eicosanoid metabolism. Eicosanoids are produced from fatty acids released from membrane phospholipids. In humans, arachidonic acid is the major precursor of the eicosanoids, which include the prostaglandins, leukotrienes, and thromboxanes. The circled minus sign = inhibits; cyt = cytochrome.

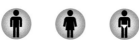

THE WAITING ROOM

Since her admission to the hospital for an acute myocardial infarction, **Ann Jeina** has been taking the bile salt sequestrant cholestyramine and the HMG-CoA reductase inhibitor pravastatin to lower her blood cholesterol levels (see Chapter 34). She also takes 160 mg acetylsalicylic acid (ASA; aspirin) each day. At her most recent visit to her cardiologist, she asked whether she should

"Eicosa" is the Greek word for the number 20. Eicosanoids are synthesized from polyunsaturated fatty acids with 20 carbon atoms.

The composition of the diet affects the fatty acid content of membrane phospholipids. Individuals with a high content of saturated fatty acids in their diets have a high content of saturated fatty acids in their membrane lipids. Likewise, individuals with a high content of polyunsaturated fatty acids in their diets have a high content of polyunsaturated fatty acids in their membrane lipids.

Dietary deficiencies of essential fatty acids are rare. However, some cases have been reported in patients receiving total parenteral nutrition (TPN). Although the most obvious symptom is a red scaly dermatitis, deficiencies of essential fatty acids also result in a decreased availability of precursors for eicosanoid synthesis.

continue to take aspirin because she no longer has any chest pain. She was told that the use of aspirin in her case was not to alleviate pain but to reduce the risk of a second heart attack and that she should continue to take this drug for the remainder of her life unless a complication, such as gastrointestinal bleeding, occurred as a result of its use.

Emma Wheezer has done well with regard to her respiratory function since her earlier hospitalization for an acute asthmatic attack. She has been maintained on two puffs of triamcinolone acetonide, a potent inhaled corticosteroid, three times per day, and has not required systemic steroids for months. The glucose intolerance precipitated by high intravenous and oral doses of the synthetic glucocorticoid dexamethasone during her earlier hospitalization resolved after this drug was discontinued. She has come to her doctor now because she is concerned that the low-grade fever and cough she has developed over the last 36 hours may trigger another acute asthma attack.

I. SOURCE OF THE EICOSANOIDS

The most abundant and therefore the most common precursor of the eicosanoids is arachidonic acid (eicosatetraenoic acid, $\omega 6,20:4,\Delta 5,8,11,14$), a polyunsaturated fatty acid with 20 carbons and 4 double bonds (see Fig. 35.1). It is esterified to phospholipids located in the lipid bilayer that constitutes the plasma membrane of the cell. Because arachidonic acid cannot be synthesized de novo in the body, the diet must contain arachidonic acid or other fatty acids from which arachidonic acid can be produced. The major dietary precursor for arachidonic acid synthesis is the essential fatty acid linoleate, which is present in plant oils (see Chapter 33).

The arachidonic acid present in membrane phospholipids is released from the lipid bilayer as a consequence of the activation of membrane-bound phospholipase A2 or C (see Fig. 33.31 and Fig. 35.2). This activation occurs when a variety of stimuli (agonists), such as histamine and the cytokines, interact with a specific plasma membrane receptor on the target cell surface. Phospholipase A2 is specific for the sn-2 position of phosphoacylglycerols, the site of attachment of arachidonic acid to the glycerol moiety. Phospholipase C hydrolyzes phosphorylated inositol

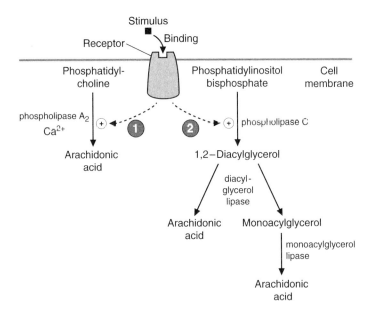

Fig. 35.2. Release of arachidonic acid from membrane lipids. The binding of a stimulus to its receptor activates pathway 1 or 2.

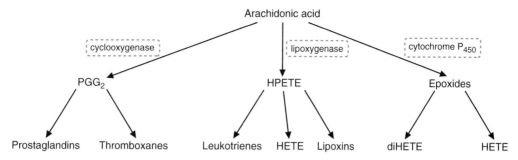

Fig. 35.3. Pathways for the metabolism of arachidonic acid.

from the inositol glycerophospholipids, generating a diacylglycerol containing arachidonic acid. This arachidonic acid is subsequently released by the action of other lipases.

II. PATHWAYS FOR EICOSANOID SYNTHESIS

After arachidonic acid is released into the cytosol, it is converted to eicosanoids by a variety of enzymes with activities that vary among tissues. This variation explains why some cells, such as those in the vascular endothelium, synthesize prostaglandins E_2 and I_2 (PGE_2 and PGI_2) whereas cells, such as platelets, synthesize primarily thromboxane A_2 (TXA_2) and 12-hydroxyeicosatetraenoic acid (12-HETE).

Three major pathways for the metabolism of arachidonic acid occur in various tissues (Fig. 35.3). The first of these, the cyclooxygenase pathway, leads to the synthesis of prostaglandins and thromboxanes. The second, the lipoxygenase pathway, yields the leukotrienes, HETEs, and lipoxins. The third pathway, catalyzed by the cytochrome P450 system, is responsible for the synthesis of the epoxides, HETEs, and diHETEs.

A. Cyclooxygenase Pathway: Synthesis of the Prostaglandins and Thromboxanes

1. STRUCTURES OF THE PROSTAGLANDINS

Prostaglandins are fatty acids containing 20 carbon atoms, including an internal 5-carbon ring. In addition to this ring, each of the biologically active prostaglandins has a hydroxyl group at carbon 15, a double bond between carbons 13 and 14, and various substituents on the ring (Fig. 35.4)

The nomenclature for the prostaglandins (PGs) involves the assignment of a capital letter (PGE), an Arabic numeral subscript (PGE_1), and, for the PGF family, a Greek letter subscript (e.g., $PGF_{2\alpha}$). The capital letter, in this case "F," refers to the ring substituents shown in figure 35.5.

The subscript that follows the capital letter (PGF_1) refers to the PG series 1, 2, or 3, determined by the number of unsaturated bonds present in the linear portion of the hydrocarbon chain (Fig. 35.6). It does not include double bonds in the internal ring. Prostaglandins of the 1-series have one double bond (between carbons 13 and 14). The 2-series has two double bonds (between carbons 13 and 14, and 5 and 6), and the 3-series has three double bonds (between carbons 13 and 14, 5 and 6, and 17 and 18). The double bonds between carbons 13 and 14 are *trans*; the others are *cis*.

The Greek letter subscript, found only in the F series, refers to the position of the hydroxyl group at carbon 9. This hydroxyl group primarily exists in the α position, where it lies below the plane of the ring, as does the hydroxyl group at carbon 11 (see Figs. 35.4 and 35.5).

Inflammation involving the mucosal and smooth muscle layers of the respiratory tract plays a major role in the development of acute asthmatic bronchospasm in patients such as **Emma Wheezer**. Dexamethasone and other potent glucocorticoids are capable of preventing or suppressing this inflammation.

In part, the glucocorticoids act by inhibiting the recruitment of leukocytes and monocytes–macrophages into affected areas. They also limit the ability of these cells to elaborate a variety of chemotactic factors and other substances, such as certain eicosanoids, which enhance the inflammatory process. Glucocorticoids, for example, suppress the transcription and translation of the inducible form of the cyclooxygenase enzyme, COX-2. Glucocorticoids also induce the synthesis of a protein or family of proteins (lipocortins or macrocortins) that inhibit the activity of phospholipase A_2. As a result, the synthesis of prostaglandins and leukotrienes is decreased, and the inflammatory response in bronchial tissues is reduced (see Figs. 35.1 and 35.2).

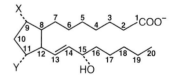

Fig. 35.4. Structural features common to the biologically active prostaglandins. These compounds have 20 carbons, with a carboxyl group at carbon 1. Carbons 8 through 12 form a five-membered ring with substituents (usually a hydroxyl or keto group) at carbons 9 (X) and 11 (Y). Carbon 15 contains a hydroxyl group, and a *trans* double bond connects carbons 13 and 14. Double bonds also may be present between carbons 5 and 6 and between carbons 17 and 18 (see Fig. 35.6).

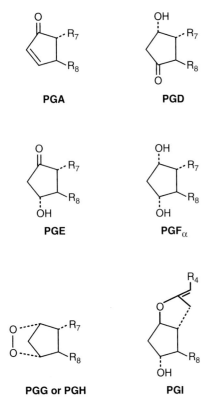

PGA

PGD

PGE

PGF$_\alpha$

PGG or PGH

PGI

Fig. 35.5. Ring substituents of the prostaglandins (PG). The letter after PG denotes the configuration of the ring and its substituents. R_4, R_7, and R_8 represent the non-ring portions of the molecule. R_4 contains four carbons (including the carboxyl group). R_7 and R_8 contain seven and eight carbons, respectively, and correspond to the 1-, 2-, or 3-series shown in Figure 35.6. Note that the prostacyclins (PGI) contain two rings.

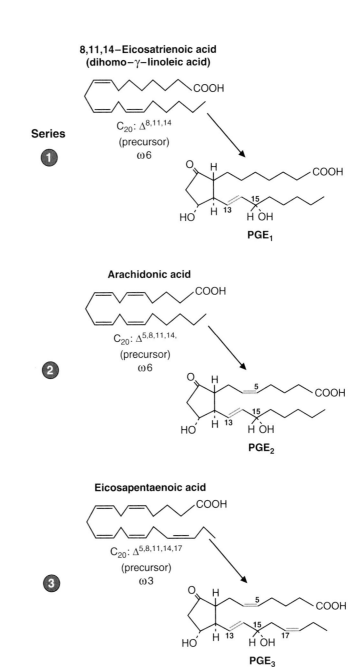

Fig. 35.6. Prostaglandins of the 1-, 2-, and 3-series and their precursors. The numeral (as a subscript in the name of the compound) refers to the number of double bonds in the non-ring portion of the prostaglandin. *Trans* double bonds are at position 13, and *cis* double bonds at positions 5 and 17. The hydroxyl group at carbon 15 is required for biologic activity.

2. STRUCTURE OF THE THROMBOXANES

The thromboxanes, derived from arachidonic acid via the cyclooxygenase pathway, closely resemble the prostaglandins in structure except that they contain a 6-membered ring that includes an oxygen atom (Fig. 35.7). The most common thromboxane, TXA_2, contains an additional oxygen atom attached both to carbon 9 and carbon 11 of the ring.

The thromboxanes were named for their action in producing blood clots (thrombi).

3. BIOSYNTHESIS OF THE PROSTAGLANDINS AND THROMBOXANES

Only the biosynthesis of those prostaglandins derived from arachidonic acid (e.g., the 2-series, such as PGE_2, PGI_2, TXA_2) are described, because those derived from eicosatrienoic acid (the 1-series) or from eicosapentaenoic acid (the 3-series) are present in very small amounts in humans on a normal diet (see Fig. 35.6).

The biochemical reactions that lead to the synthesis of prostaglandins and thromboxanes are illustrated in figure 35.8. The initial step, which is catalyzed by a cyclooxygenase, forms the five-membered ring and adds four atoms of oxygen (two between carbons 9 and 11, and two at carbon 15) to form the unstable endoperoxide, PGG_2. The hydroperoxy group at carbon 15 is quickly reduced to a hydroxyl group by a peroxidase to form another endoperoxide, PGH_2.

The next step is tissue specific (see Fig. 35.8). Depending on the type of cell involved, PGH_2 may be reduced to PGE_2 or PGD_2 by specific isomerases (PGE synthase and PGD synthase). PGE_2 may be further reduced by PGE 9-ketoreductase to form $PGF_{2\alpha}$. $PGF_{2\alpha}$ also may be formed directly from PGH_2 by the action of an endoperoxide reductase. Some of the major functions of the prostaglandins are listed in Table 35.1.

PGH_2 may be converted to the thromboxane TXA_2, a reaction catalyzed by TXA synthase (see Fig. 35.8). This enzyme is present in high concentration in platelets. In the vascular endothelium, however, PGH_2 is converted to the prostaglandin PGI_2

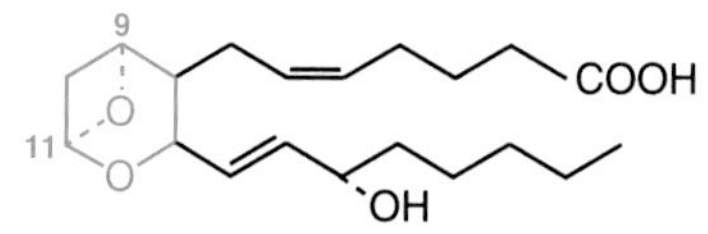

Thromboxane A₂
(TXA₂)

Fig. 35.7. The thromboxane ring. In contrast to the prostaglandins, which have a five-membered carbon ring, thromboxanes have a six-membered ring (shown in blue) containing an oxygen atom. Substituents are attached to the ring at carbons 9 and 11. In the case of TXA_2 (shown above), an oxygen atom connects carbons 9 and 11.

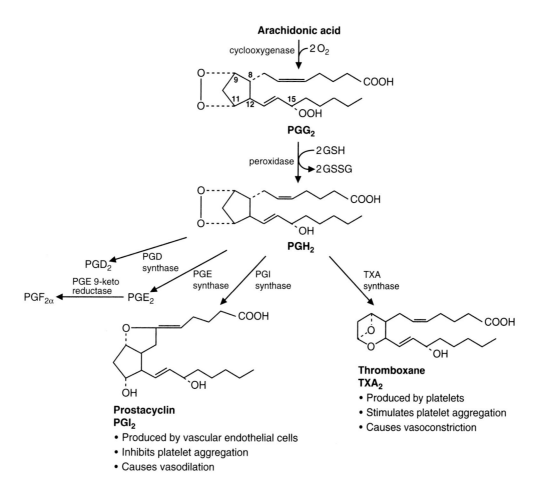

Fig. 35.8. Formation of prostaglandins (including the prostacyclin PGI_2) and thromboxane TXA_2 from arachidonic acid. The conversion of arachidonic acid to PGH_2 is catalyzed by a membrane-bound enzyme, prostaglandin endoperoxide synthase, which has cyclooxygenase and peroxidase activities. The reducing agent is glutathione (GSH), which is oxidized to GSSG.

The predominant eicosanoid in platelets is TXA$_2$, a potent vasoconstrictor and a stimulator of platelet aggregation. The latter action initiates thrombus formation at sites of vascular injury as well as in the vicinity of a ruptured atherosclerotic plaque in the lumen of vessels such as the coronary arteries. Such thrombi may cause sudden total occlusion of the vascular lumen, causing acute ischemic damage to tissues distal to the block (i.e., acute myocardial infarction).

Aspirin, by covalently acetylating the active site of cyclooxygenase, blocks the production of TXA$_2$ from its major precursor, arachidonic acid. By causing this mild hemostatic defect, low-dose aspirin has been shown to be effective in prevention of acute myocardial infarction (see Clinical Comments). For **Ivan Applebod** (who has symptoms of coronary heart disease), aspirin is used to prevent a first heart attack (primary prevention). For **Ann Jeina** and **Cora Nari** (who already have had heart attacks), aspirin is used to prevent a second heart attack (secondary prevention).

Diets that include cold water fish (e.g., salmon, mackerel, brook trout, herring), with a high content of polyunsaturated fatty acids, eicosapentaenoic acid (EPA), and docosahexaenoic acid (DHA) (see Chapter 33), result in a high content of these fatty acids in membrane phospholipids. It has been suggested that such diets are effective in preventing heart disease, in part because they lead to formation of more TXA$_3$ relative to TXA$_2$. TXA$_3$ is less effective in stimulating platelet aggregation than its counterpart in the 2-series, TXA$_2$.

Table 35.1. Some Functions of the Prostaglandins

PGI$_2$, PGE$_2$, PGD$_2$
   Increase
      Vasodilation
      cAMP
   Decrease
      Platelet aggregation
      Leukocyte aggregation
      IL-1[a] and IL-2
      T-cell proliferation
      Lymphocyte migration
PGF$_{2\alpha}$
   Increases
      Vasoconstriction
      Bronchoconstriction
      Smooth muscle contraction

[a] IL = interleukin, a cytokine that augments the activity of many cells in the immune system.

Table 35.2. Some Functions of Thromboxane A$_2$

Increases
   Vasoconstriction
   Platelet aggregation
   Lymphocyte proliferation
   Bronchoconstriction

(prostacyclin) by PGI synthase (see Fig. 35.8). TXA$_2$ and PGI$_2$ have important antagonistic biologic effects on vasomotor and smooth muscle tone and on platelet aggregation. Some of the known functions of the thromboxanes are listed in Table 35.2.

In the 1990s, the cyclooxygenase enzyme was found to exist as two distinct isoforms, designated COX-1 and COX-2. COX-1 is regarded as a constitutive form of the enzyme, widely expressed in almost all tissues, and involved in the production of prostaglandins and thromboxanes for "normal" physiologic functions. COX-2 is an inducible form of the enzyme regulated by a variety of cytokines and growth factors. COX-2 mRNA and protein levels are usually low in most healthy tissue, but are expressed at high levels in inflamed tissue.

Because of the importance of prostaglandins in mediating the inflammatory response, drugs that block prostaglandin production should provide relief from pain. The cyclooxygenase enzyme is inhibited by all nonsteroidal anti-inflammatory drugs (NSAIDs) such as aspirin (acetylsalicylic acid). Aspirin transfers an acetyl group to the enzyme, irreversibly inactivating it (Fig. 35.9). Other NSAIDs (e.g., acetaminophen, ibuprofen) act as reversible inhibitors of cyclooxygenase. Acetaminophen is the major ingredient in Tylenol, and ibuprofen is the major ingredient in other NSAIDs such as Motrin, Nuprin, and Advil (see Fig. 35.9). Although having some relative selectivity for inhibiting either COX-1 or COX-2,

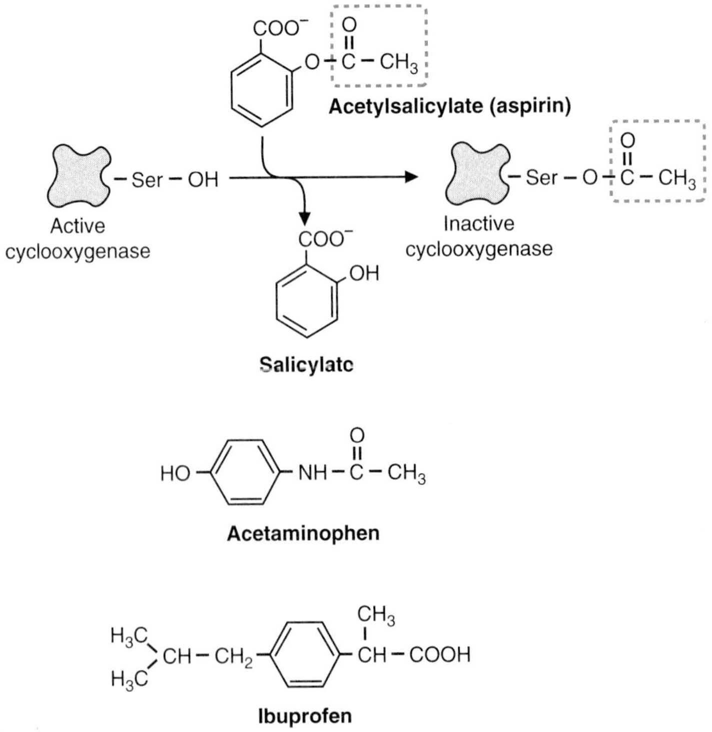

Fig. 35.9. Action of aspirin and other nonsteroidal anti-inflammatory drugs.

NSAIDs block the activity of both isoforms. These findings have provided the impetus for the development of selective COX-2 inhibitors, which are proposed to act as potent anti-inflammatory agents by inhibiting COX-2 activity, without the gastrointestinal and anti-platelet side effects commonly associated with NSAID use. These NSAID adverse effects are thought to be a result of COX-1 inhibition. Examples of these newer selective COX-2 inhibitors are celecoxib (Celebrex) and rofecoxib (Vioxx).

4. INACTIVATION OF THE PROSTAGLANDINS AND THROMBOXANES

Prostaglandins and thromboxanes are rapidly inactivated. Their half-lives ($t_{1/2}$) range from seconds to minutes. The prostaglandins are inactivated by oxidation of the 15-hydroxy group, critical for their activity, to a ketone. The double bond at carbon 13 is reduced. Subsequently, both β- and ω-oxidation of the non-ring portions occur, producing dicarboxylic acids that are excreted in the urine. Active TXA_2 is rapidly metabolized to TXB_2 by cleavage of the oxygen bridge between carbons 9 and 11 to form two hydroxyl groups. TXB_2 has no biologic activity.

B. Lipoxygenase Pathway: Synthesis of the Leukotrienes, HETE, and Lipoxins

In addition to serving as a substrate for the cyclooxygenase pathway, arachidonic acid also acts as a substrate for the lipoxygenase pathway. The lipoxygenase enzymes catalyze the incorporation of an oxygen molecule onto a carbon of one of several double bonds of arachidonic acid, forming a hydroperoxy (–OOH) group at these positions. With this oxygenation, the double bond isomerizes to a position one carbon removed from the hydroperoxy group and is transformed from the *cis* to the *trans* configuration (Fig. 35.10). The unstable hydroperoxy group is then converted to the more stable hydroxy group.

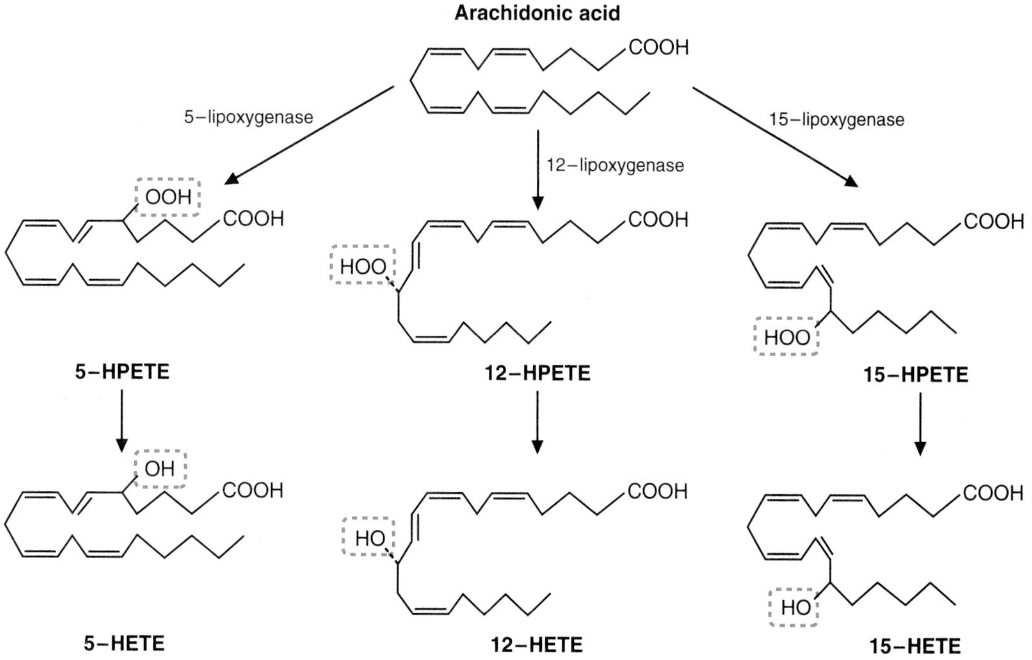

Fig. 35.10. Action of lipoxygenases in the formation of HPETEs and HETEs. Lipoxygenases add hydroperoxy groups at position 5, 12, or 15 with rearrangement of the double bond. HPETEs are unstable and are rapidly reduced to form HETEs or converted to leukotrienes and lipoxins (see Figs. 35.11 and 35.12).

Leukotrienes were so named because they are synthesized in leukocytes and contain the typical triene structure, i.e., three double bonds in series (in this case, at positions 7, 9, and 11) (see Fig. 35.11).

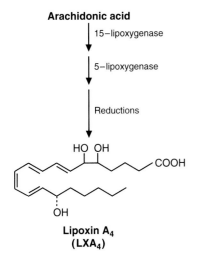

Arachidonic acid

15–lipoxygenase

5–lipoxygenase

Reductions

Lipoxin A$_4$
(LXA$_4$)

Fig. 35.12. Formation of the lipoxins. These compounds contain three hydroxyl groups.

Lipoxygenases may act at carbons 5, 12, or 15. The type of lipoxygenase varies from tissue to tissue. For example, polymorphonuclear leukocytes contain primarily 5-lipoxygenase, platelets are rich in 12-lipoxygenase, and eosinophilic leukocytes contain primarily 15-lipoxygenase.

1. LEUKOTRIENE SYNTHESIS

As shown in figure 35.11, the synthesis of the leukotrienes begins with the formation of hydroperoxyeicosatetraenoic acids (HPETEs). This product is either reduced to the corresponding hydroxy metabolites, HETEs (see Fig. 35.10), or it is metabolized to form leukotrienes or lipoxins (see Figs. 35.11 and 35.12). The major leukotrienes are produced by 5-lipoxygenase.

In leukocytes and mast cells, 5-HPETE is converted to an epoxide, leukotriene A$_4$ (LTA$_4$). The subscript number 4 refers to the presence of four double bonds in the leukotriene. Three of the double bonds (7, 9, 11) are conjugated, that is, they form a triene.

Other functional leukotrienes are formed from LTA$_4$ by one of two pathways. In the first, LTA$_4$ is converted to LTB$_4$, a 5,12-dihydroxy derivative. The second metabolic pathway involves the addition of reduced glutathione to carbon 6 to form LTC$_4$, a reaction catalyzed by glutathione S-transferase. Glutamate is removed from the glutathione moiety of LTC$_4$ through the action of γ-glutamyl transpeptidase to form LTD$_4$. A dipeptidase then cleaves the glycine residue from LTD$_4$ to form LTE$_4$ (see Fig. 35.11). The major functions of some of the leukotrienes are listed in Table 35.3.

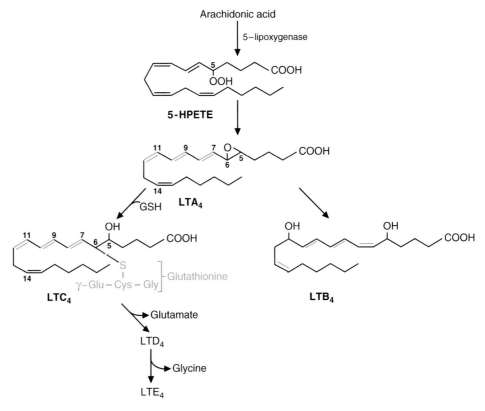

Fig. 35.11. Formation of leukotrienes and their glutathione (GSH) derivatives. HPETE = hydroperoxyeicosatetraenoic acids; LT = leukotriene (thus, LTA$_4$ is leukotriene A$_4$).

2. LIPOXIN SYNTHESIS AND ACTIONS

The lipoxins are formed through the action of 15-lipoxygenase followed by the action of 5-lipoxygenase on arachidonic acid. A series of reductions of the resultant hydroperoxy groups leads to the formation of trihydroxy derivatives of arachidonic acid known as the lipoxins (see Fig. 35.12). Lipoxins induce chemotaxis and stimulate superoxide anion production in leukocytes.

C. Cytochrome P450 Pathway: Synthesis and Actions of Epoxides, HETEs, and diHETES

A third mechanism for the oxygenation of arachidonic acid involves the cytochrome P450 pathway. The activity of the monooxygenases in this microsomal system yields epoxides, certain forms of HETEs (e.g., ω-hydroxy derivatives), and diol forms (diHETEs) (Fig. 35.13). The biologic activities of these compounds include actions in ocular, vascular, endocrine, and renal systems. Some of these actions are attributed to inhibition of Na^+, K^+-ATPase. The physiologic role of these compounds remains to be fully characterized.

D. Isoprostane Synthesis

Isoprostanes are derived from arachidonic acid by lipid peroxidation, initiated by free radicals. There is no enzymatic mechanism for their production. Arachidonic acid, while still a component of a phospholipid, undergoes free radical damage, and then phospholipase A2 removes the altered eicosanoid from the phospholipid and releases it into circulation (Fig. 35.14). The level of isoprostanes in the urine can be used as a measure of the oxidative stress of a patient and is a useful biologic marker for patients undergoing oxidative stress caused by a variety of disorders. Surprisingly, these altered arachidonic acid molecules also have biologic activity when measured on cultured cells; it is not known whether intracellular levels reach high enough concentrations to elicit these biologic effects. The best studied isoprostane is similar to $PGF_{2\alpha}$, and this molecule has similar effects on cultured cells as does $PGF_{2\alpha}$ (see Table 35.1).

E. Endocannabinoid Synthesis

Endocannabinoids are endogenous ligands for the cannabinoid receptor, with effects primarily in the nervous system. Anandamide was the first such ligand isolated and identified. Anandamide is synthesized in neurons from phosphatidylethanolamine, as outlined in figure 35.15. The biosynthetic pathway is unique in transferring an arachidonic acid group from the 2-position to the free amino group on ethanolamine, and then using a unique phospholipase D to cleave the modified ethanolamine from the phospholipid. The synthesis of anandamide is regulated, in part, by agonists that cause calcium influx into nerve cells. Once anandamide is released, it acts as a retrograde messenger, binding to receptors on the presynaptic membrane that alter ion fluxes such that neurotransmitter release from the presynaptic neuron can be increased and an analgesic effect obtained. Anandamide is degraded by the enzyme fatty acid amide hydrolase, which splits anandamide to arachidonic acid and ethanolamine. The hydrolase enzyme is the target of drug research, because inhibiting the action of this enzyme will prolong the analgesic effects induced by anandamide.

III. MECHANISM OF ACTION OF THE EICOSANOIDS

The eicosanoids have a wide variety of physiologic effects, which are generally initiated through an interaction of the eicosanoid with a specific receptor on the plasma membrane of a target cell (Table 35.4). This eicosanoid-receptor binding either activates the adenylate cyclase-cAMP-protein kinase A system (PGE, PGD,

Table 35.3. Some Functions of Leukotrienes

LTB$_4$
Increases
Vascular permeability
T-cell proliferation
Leukocyte aggregation
INF-γ
IL-1
IL-2
LTC$_4$ and LTD$_4$
Increase
Bronchoconstriction
Vascular permeability
INF-γ

Abbreviations: INF = interferon; IL = interleukin.

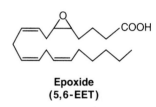

**Epoxide
(5,6-EET)**

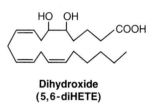

**Dihydroxide
(5,6-diHETE)**

Fig. 35.13. Examples of compounds produced from arachidonic acid by the cytochrome P450 pathway.

 Recall that oxidative stress results from reactive oxygen or nitrogen species that are not fully neutralized by anti-oxidants (see Chapter 24). The increase in reactive oxygen and nitrogen species results in protein, lipid, and nucleic acid modifications. Many neurodegenerative diseases, such as Alzheimer disease, Parkinson disease, and Lou Gehrig disease, have in common increased oxidative stress.

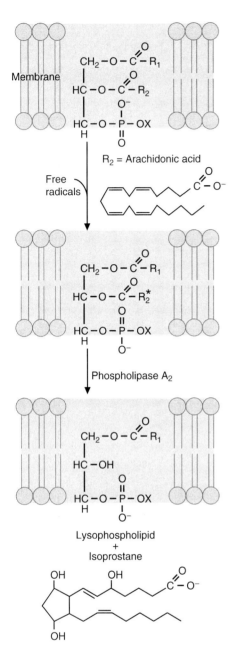

Fig. 35.14. Generation of an isoprostane. Radical damage to a phospholipid on the arachidonic acid residue at position 2 generates an isoprostane, which is then removed from the damaged phospholipid by phospholipase A2. The example of an isoprostane shown in this figure is just one of many that can be produced.

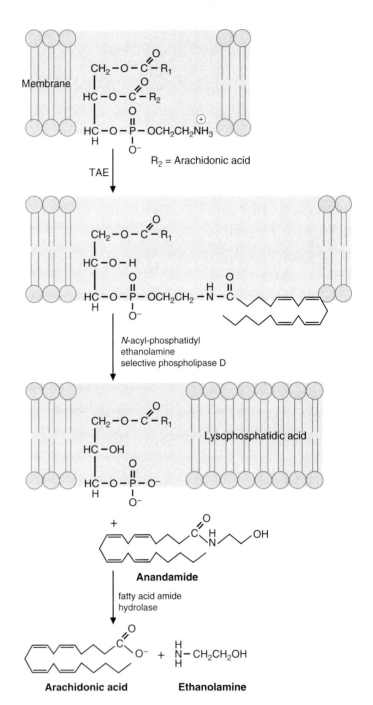

Fig. 35.15. Anandamide synthesis and degradation. TAE = transacylase.

Table 35.4. Prostaglandin and Thromboxane Receptors

Receptor	Type Ligand	G-protein coupled	cAMP response	Calcium response
DP	PGD series	Yes	Increase	None
EP1	PGE series	Yes	None	Increase
EP2	PGE series	Yes	Increase	None
EP3	PGE series	Yes	Decrease	None
EP4	PGE series	Yes	Increase	None
FP	PGF series	Yes	None	Increase
IP	PGI series	Yes	Increase	None
TP	Thromboxane A	Yes	None	Increase

and PGI series) or causes an increase in the level of calcium in the cytosol of target cells ($PGF_{2\alpha}$, TXA_2, the endoperoxides, and the leukotrienes).

In some systems, the eicosanoids appear to modulate the degree of activation of adenylate cyclase in response to other stimuli. In these instances, the eicosanoid may bind to a regulatory subunit of the GTP-binding proteins (G proteins) within the plasma membrane of the target cell (see Chapter 11). If the eicosanoid binds to the stimulatory subunit, the effect of the stimulus is amplified. Conversely, if the eicosanoid binds to the inhibitory subunit, the cellular response to the stimulus is reduced. Through these influences on the activation of adenylate cyclase, eicosanoids contribute to the regulation of cell function.

Some of the biologic effects of certain eicosanoids occur as a result of a paracrine or autocrine action. One paracrine action is the contraction of vascular smooth muscle cells caused by TXA_2 released from circulating platelets (vasoconstriction). An autocrine action of eicosanoids is exemplified by platelet aggregation induced by TXA_2 produced by the platelets themselves.

The eicosanoids influence the cellular function of almost every tissue of the body. Certain organ systems are affected to a greater degree than others.

CLINICAL COMMENTS

 In the presence of aspirin, cyclooxygenase is irreversibly inactivated by acetylation. New cyclooxygenase molecules are not produced in platelets, because these cells have no nuclei and, therefore, cannot synthesize new mRNA. Thus, the inhibition of cyclooxygenase by aspirin persists for the lifespan of the platelet (7–10 days). When aspirin is taken daily at doses between 81 and 325 mg, new platelets are affected as they are generated. Higher doses do not improve efficacy but do increase side effects, such as gastrointestinal bleeding and easy bruisability.

Patients with established or suspected atherosclerotic coronary disease, such as **Ann Jeina, Cora Nari,** and **Ivan Applebod,** benefit from the action of low-dose aspirin (approximately 162 mg/day), which produces a mild defect in hemostasis. This action of aspirin helps to prevent thrombus formation in the area of an atherosclerotic plaque at critical sites in the vascular tree.

Corticosteroids reduce inflammation, in part, through their inhibitory effect on phospholipase A2. In addition, suppression of COX-2 induction is now thought to be a primary anti-inflammatory mechanism of action for glucocorticoids. Despite the unquestionable value of glucocorticoid therapy in a variety of diseases associated with acute inflammation of tissues, the suppression of the inflammatory response with pharmacologic doses of corticosteroids is potentially hazardous. The sudden appearance of temporary glucose intolerance when **Emma Wheezer** was treated with large doses of dexamethasone, a gluconeogenic steroid (glucocorticoid), is just one of the many potential adverse effects of this class of drugs when given systemically in pharmacologic doses over an extended period. The inhaled steroids, conversely, have far fewer systemic side effects because their absorption across the bronchial mucosa into the circulation is very limited. This property allows them to be used over prolonged periods in the treatment of asthma. The fact that inhalation allows direct delivery of the agent to the primary site of inflammation adds to their effectiveness in the treatment of these patients.

Although our knowledge of the spectrum of biologic actions of the endogenous eicosanoids is incomplete, several actions are well-enough established to allow their application in a variety of clinical situations or diseases. For example, drugs that are analogs of PGE_1 and PGE_2 suppress gastric ulceration, in part by inhibiting secretion of hydrochloric acid in the mucosal cells of the stomach. Analogs of PGE_1 are used in the treatment of sexual impotence. Men with certain forms of sexual impotence can self-inject this agent into the corpus cavernosum of the penis to induce immediate but temporary penile tumescence. The erection lasts for 1 to 3 hours. The stimulatory action of PGE_2 and $PGF_{2\alpha}$ on uterine muscle contraction has led to the use of these prostaglandins to induce labor and to control postpartum bleeding. PGE_1 is also used as palliative therapy in neonates with congenital heart defects to maintain patency of the ductus arteriosus until surgery can be performed. Analogs of PGI_2 have been shown to be effective in the treatment of primary pulmonary hypertension.

BIOCHEMICAL COMMENTS

 Inflammation is the response of the body to infection or injury, directed at destroying the infectious agents and repairing the damaged areas. It involves an increase of the blood supply to the affected region by means of

Although uncomfortable, the pain, swelling, and fever that are part of the inflammatory response serve as an important warning sign that the host is threatened and that some specific counteractions must be taken against the offending agent or process. Although the use of anti-inflammatory drugs may bring welcome symptomatic relief, their use may, in part, diminish the effectiveness of the host's response to the inciting agent.

vasodilation. The capillaries become more permeable so that fluid, large molecules, and white blood cells can cross, leaving the blood and entering the tissue. White blood cells (particularly neutrophils and monocytes) move by chemotaxis to the injured site. Redness (rubor), heat (calor), swelling (tumor), and pain (dolor) are associated with the inflammatory process. Redness and heat are caused by the increased blood flow. Swelling is the result of the increased movement of fluid and white blood cells into the area of inflammation. Pain is caused by the release of chemical compounds and the compression of nerves in the vicinity of the inflammatory process.

The chemical mediators of inflammation usually are produced by activation of complement (a family of blood proteins that are cleaved to form active fragments) or of the blood clotting cascade (see Chapter 45). These processes cause the release of histamine from mast cells, and the production of kinins by cleavage of kininogens. Among their other effects, both histamine and kinins increase vascular permeability. They stimulate the synthesis of eicosanoids that act on the motility and metabolism of white blood cells and cause the aggregation of platelets to arrest bleeding. Some of the prostaglandins act on thermoregulatory centers of the brain, producing fever. Cytokines are also released that stimulate the proliferation of cells involved in the immune response.

Suggested References

Brash AR. Lipoxygenases: occurrence, functions, catalysis, and acquisition of substrate. J Biol Chem 1999;274:23679–23682.

Dimarzo V, Bisogno T, and DePetrocellis L. Anandamide: some like it hot. Trends Pharm Sci 2001;22:346–349.

Halushka PV. Prostaglandins and related compounds. In: Goldman L and Bennett JC, eds. Cecil Textbook of Medicine. Philadelphia: WB Saunders, 2000:1189–1194.

Marnett LJ, Rowlinson SW, Goodwin DC, Kalgutkar AS, Lanzo CA. Arachidonic acid oxygenation by COX-1 and COX-2: Mechanisms of catalysis and inhibition. J Biol Chem 1999;274:22903–22906.

Morrow JD, Roberts LJ II. Lipid-derived autacoids. In: Hardman JG, Limbird LE, eds. Goodman and Gilman's The Pharmacological Basis of Therapeutics. New York: McGraw-Hill, 2001:669–680.

 REVIEW QUESTIONS—CHAPTER 35

1. In humans, prostaglandins are primarily derived from which of the following?

   (A) Glucose
   (B) Acetyl CoA
   (C) Arachidonic acid
   (D) Oleic acid
   (E) Leukotrienes

2. Aspirin will inhibit which of the following reaction pathways?

   (A) Arachidonic acid → thromboxanes
   (B) Arachidonic acid → leukotrienes
   (C) Arachidonic acid → phospholipids
   (D) Linoleic acid → arachidonic acid
   (E) Acetyl CoA → linoleic acid

3. Which of the following drugs leads to the covalent modification, and inactivation, of both the COX-1 and COX-2 enzymes?

    (A) Aspirin
    (B) Tylenol
    (C) Celebrex
    (D) Vioxx
    (E) Advil

4. Thromboxane A2, which is found in high levels in platelets, aids in wound repair through induction of which of the following activities?

    (A) Inhibits COX-2 gene expression
    (B) Inhibits COX-1 gene expression
    (C) Vasoconstriction
    (D) Vasodilation
    (E) Bronchodilation

5. Certain prostaglandins, when binding to their receptor, induce an increase in intracellular calcium levels. The signal that leads to the elevation of intracellular calcium is initiated by which of the following enzymes?

    (A) Protein kinase A
    (B) Phospholipase C
    (C) Phospholipase A2
    (D) Protein kinase C
    (E) Cyclooxygenase

36 Integration of Carbohydrate and Lipid Metabolism

The purpose of this chapter is to summarize and integrate the major pathways for the utilization of carbohydrates and fats as fuels. We will concentrate on reviewing the regulatory mechanisms that determine the flux of metabolites in the fed and fasting states, integrating the pathways that were described separately under carbohydrate and lipid metabolism. The next section of the book covers the mechanisms by which the pathways of nitrogen metabolism are coordinated with fat and carbohydrate metabolism.

*For the species to survive, it is necessary for us to store excess food when we eat and to use these stores when we are fasting. Regulatory mechanisms direct compounds through the pathways of metabolism involved in the storage and utilization of fuels. These mechanisms are controlled by **hormones**, by the **concentration of available fuels**, and by the **energy needs** of the body.*

*Changes in hormone levels, in the concentration of fuels, and in energy requirements affect the activity of key enzymes in the major pathways of metabolism. Intracellular **enzymes** are generally regulated by **activation and inhibition**, by **phosphorylation and dephosphorylation** (or other covalent modifications), by **induction and repression** of synthesis, and by **degradation**. Activation and inhibition of enzymes cause immediate changes in metabolism. Phosphorylation and dephosphorylation of enzymes affect metabolism slightly less rapidly. Induction and repression of enzyme synthesis are much slower processes, usually affecting metabolic flux over a period of hours. Degradation of enzymes decreases the amount available to catalyze reactions.*

*The pathways of metabolism have **multiple control points** and **multiple regulators** at each control point. The function of these complex mechanisms is to produce a graded response to a stimulus and to provide sensitivity to multiple stimuli so that an exact balance is maintained between flux through a given step (or series of steps) and the need or use for the product. Pyruvate dehydrogenase is an example of an enzyme that has multiple regulatory mechanisms. Regardless of insulin levels, the enzyme cannot become fully activated in the presence of products and absence of substrates.*

*The major hormones that regulate the pathways of fuel metabolism are **insulin** and **glucagon**. In liver, all effects of glucagon are reversed by insulin, and some of the pathways that insulin activates are inhibited by glucagon. Thus, the pathways of carbohydrate and lipid metabolism are generally regulated by changes in the **insulin/glucagon ratio**.*

*Although **glycogen** is a critical storage form of fuel because blood glucose levels must be carefully maintained, adipose **triacylglycerols** are quantitatively the major fuel store in the human. After a meal, both dietary glucose and fat are stored in adipose tissue as triacylglycerol. This fuel is released during fasting, when it provides the main source of energy for the tissues of the body. The length of time we can survive without food depends mainly on the size of our bodies' fat stores.*

THE WAITING ROOM

Within 2 months of her surgery to remove a benign insulin-secreting β cell tumor of the pancreas, **Bea Selmass** was again jogging lightly. She had lost the 8 lb that she had gained in the 6 weeks before her surgery. Because her hypoglycemic episodes were no longer occurring, she had no need to eat frequent carbohydrate snacks to prevent the adrenergic and neuroglycopenic symptoms that she had experienced when her tumor was secreting excessive amounts of insulin.

A few months after her last hospitalization, **Di Abietes** was once again brought to the hospital emergency room in diabetic ketoacidosis (DKA). Blood samples for glucose and electrolytes were drawn repeatedly during the first 24 hours. The hospital laboratory reported that the serum in each of these specimens appeared opalescent rather than having its normal clear or transparent appearance. This opalescence results from light scattering caused by the presence of elevated levels of triacylglycerol-rich lipoproteins in the blood

When **Ann Sulin** initially presented with type 2 diabetes mellitus at age 39, she was approximately 30 lb above her ideal weight. Her high serum glucose levels were accompanied by abnormalities in her 14-hour fasting lipid profile. Her serum total cholesterol, low-density lipoprotein (LDL) cholesterol, and triacylglycerol levels were elevated, and her serum high-density lipoprotein (HDL) cholesterol level was below the normal range.

I. REGULATION OF CARBOHYDRATE AND LIPID METABOLISM IN THE FED STATE

A. Mechanisms That Affect Glycogen and Triacylglycerol Synthesis in Liver

After a meal, the liver synthesizes glycogen and triacylglycerol. The level of glycogen stored in the liver can increase from approximately 80 g after an overnight fast to a limit of approximately 200–300 g. Although the liver synthesizes triacylglycerol, it does not store this fuel but rather packages it in very-low-density lipoprotein (VLDL) and secretes it into the blood. The fatty acids of the VLDL triacylglycerols secreted from the liver are stored as adipose triacylglycerols. Adipose tissue has an almost infinite capacity to store fat, limited mainly by the ability of the heart to pump blood through the capillaries of the expanding adipose mass. Although we store fat throughout our bodies, it tends to accumulate in places where it does not interfere too much with our mobility: in the abdomen, hips, thighs, and buttocks.

Both the synthesis of liver glycogen and the conversion by the liver of dietary glucose to triacylglycerol (lipogenesis) are regulated by mechanisms involving key enzymes in these pathways.

1. GLUCOKINASE

After a meal, glucose can be converted to glycogen or to triacylglycerol in the liver. For both processes, glucose is first converted to glucose 6-phosphate by glucokinase, a liver enzyme that has a high K_m for glucose (Fig. 36.1). Because of the enzyme's low affinity for glucose, this enzyme is most active in the fed state, when the concentration of glucose is particularly high because the hepatic portal vein

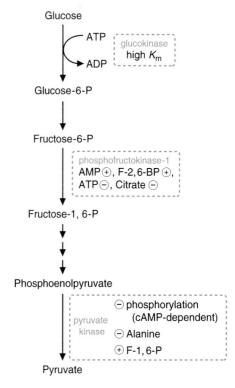

Fig. 36.1. Regulation of glucokinase, PFK-1, and pyruvate kinase in the liver.

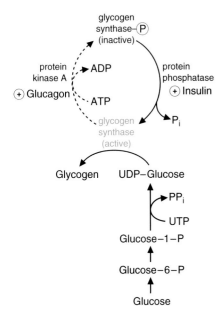

Fig. 36.2. Regulation of glycogen synthase. This enzyme is phosphorylated by a series of kinases, which are initiated by the cAMP-dependent protein kinase, under fasting conditions. It is dephosphorylated and active after a meal, and glycogen is stored. Circled P = phosphate; a circled + sign = activated by; a circled − sign = inhibited by.

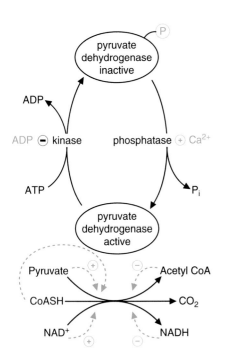

Fig. 36.3. Regulation of pyruvate dehydrogenase (PDH). A kinase associated with the PDH complex phosphorylates and inactivates the enzyme.

carries digestive products directly from the intestine to the liver. Synthesis of glucokinase is also induced by insulin (which is elevated after a meal) and repressed by glucagon (which is elevated during fasting). In keeping with the liver's function in maintaining blood glucose levels, this system is set up such that the liver can only metabolize glucose when sugar levels are high, and not when sugar levels are low.

2. GLYCOGEN SYNTHASE

In the conversion of glucose 6-phosphate to glycogen, the key regulatory enzyme is glycogen synthase. This enzyme is activated by the dephosphorylation that occurs when insulin is elevated and glucagon is decreased (Fig. 36.2) and by the increased level of glucose.

3. PHOSPHOFRUCTOKINASE-1 AND PYRUVATE KINASE

For lipogenesis, glucose 6-phosphate is converted through glycolysis to pyruvate. Key enzymes that regulate this pathway in the liver are phosphofructokinase-1 (PFK-1) and pyruvate kinase. PFK-1 is allosterically activated in the fed state by fructose 2,6-bisphosphate and adenosine monophosphate (AMP) (see Fig. 36.1). Phosphofructokinase-2, the enzyme that produces the activator fructose 2,6-bisphosphate, is dephosphorylated and active after a meal (see Chapter 22). Pyruvate kinase is also activated by dephosphorylation, which is stimulated by the increase of the insulin/glucagon ratio in the fed state (see Fig. 36.1).

4. PYRUVATE DEHYDROGENASE AND PYRUVATE CARBOXYLASE

The conversion of pyruvate to fatty acids requires a source of acetyl CoA in the cytosol. Pyruvate can only be converted to acetyl CoA in mitochondria, so it enters mitochondria and forms acetyl CoA through the pyruvate dehydrogenase (PDH) reaction. This enzyme is dephosphorylated and most active when its supply of substrates and adenosine diphosphate (ADP) is high, its products are used, and insulin is present (Fig. 36.3).

Pyruvate is also converted to oxaloacetate. The enzyme that catalyzes this reaction, pyruvate carboxylase, is activated by acetyl CoA. Because acetyl CoA cannot directly cross the mitochondrial membrane to form fatty acids in the cytosol, it condenses with oxaloacetate, producing citrate. The citrate that is not required for tricarboxylic acid (TCA) cycle activity crosses the membrane and enters the cytosol.

As fatty acids are produced under conditions of high energy, the high NADH/NAD$^+$ ratio in the mitochondria inhibits isocitrate dehydrogenase, which leads to citrate accumulation within the mitochondrial matrix. As the citrate accumulates, it is transported out into the cytosol to donate carbons for fatty acid synthesis.

5. CITRATE LYASE, MALIC ENZYME, AND GLUCOSE 6-PHOSPHATE DEHYDROGENASE

In the cytosol, citrate is cleaved by citrate lyase, an inducible enzyme, to form oxaloacetate and acetyl CoA (Fig. 36.4). The acetyl CoA is used for fatty acid biosynthesis and for cholesterol synthesis, pathways that are activated by insulin. Oxaloacetate is recycled to pyruvate via cytosolic malate dehydrogenase and malic enzyme, which is inducible. Malic enzyme generates NADPH for the reactions of the fatty acid synthase complex. NADPH is also produced by the two enzymes of the pentose phosphate pathway (see Chapter 29), glucose 6-phosphate dehydrogenase and 6-phosphogluconate dehydrogenase. Glucose 6-phosphate dehydrogenase is also induced by insulin.

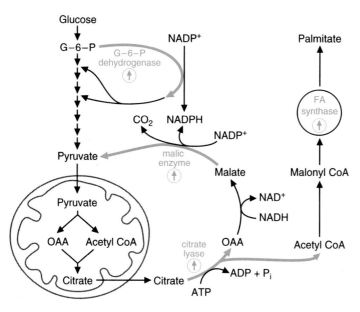

Fig. 36.4. Regulation of citrate lyase, malic enzyme, glucose 6-phosphate dehydrogenase, and fatty acid synthase. Citrate lyase, which provides acetyl CoA for fatty acid biosynthesis, the enzymes that provide NADPH (malic enzyme, glucose 6-phosphate dehydrogenase), as well as fatty acid synthase, are inducible (circled ↑).

6. ACETYL CoA CARBOXYLASE

Acetyl CoA is converted to malonyl CoA, which provides the 2-carbon units for elongation of the growing fatty acyl chain on the fatty acid synthase complex. Acetyl CoA carboxylase, the enzyme that catalyzes the conversion of acetyl CoA to malonyl CoA, is controlled by three of the major mechanisms that regulate enzyme activity (Fig. 36.5). It is activated by citrate, which causes the enzyme to

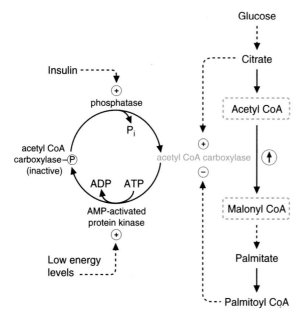

Fig. 36.5. Regulation of acetyl CoA carboxylase (AcC). AcC is regulated by activation and inhibition, by phosphorylation (mediated by the AMP-activated protein kinase) and dephosphorylation (via an insulin-stimulated phosphatase), and by induction and repression. It is active in the fed state.

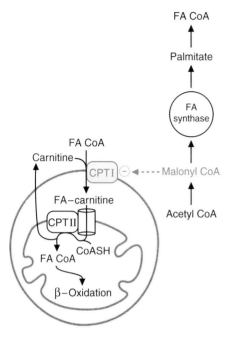

FA CoA

↑

Palmitate

↑

Fig. 36.6. Inhibition of transport of fatty acids (FA) into mitochondria by malonyl CoA. In the fed state, malonyl CoA (the substrate for fatty acid synthesis produced by acetyl CoA carboxylase) is elevated. It inhibits CPTI, preventing the transport of long-chain fatty acids into mitochondria. Therefore, substrate is not available for β-oxidation and ketone body synthesis.

 Why does **Ann Sulin** have a hypertriglyceridemia?

 Di Abietes has insulin-dependent diabetes mellitus (type 1), a disease associated with a severe deficiency or absence of insulin production by the β cells of the pancreas. One of the effects of insulin is to stimulate production of LPL. Because of low insulin levels, **Di Abietes** tends to have low levels of this enzyme. Hydrolysis of the triacylglycerols in chylomicrons and in VLDL is decreased, and hypertriglyceridemia results.

polymerize, and inhibited by long-chain fatty acyl CoA. A phosphatase stimulated by insulin activates the enzyme by dephosphorylation. The third means by which this enzyme is regulated is induction: the quantity of the enzyme increases in the fed state.

Malonyl CoA, the product of the acetyl CoA carboxylase reaction, provides the carbons for the synthesis of palmitate on the fatty acid synthase complex. Malonyl CoA also inhibits carnitine:palmitoyltransferase I (CPTI, also known as carnitine:acyltransferase I), the enzyme that prepares long-chain fatty acyl CoA for transport into mitochondria (Fig. 36.6). In the fed state, when acetyl CoA carboxylase is active and malonyl CoA levels are elevated, newly synthesized fatty acids are converted to triacylglycerols for storage, rather than being transported into mitochondria for oxidation and ketone body formation.

7. FATTY ACID SYNTHASE COMPLEX

In a well-fed individual, the quantity of the fatty acid synthase complex is increased (see Fig. 36.4). The genes that produce this enzyme complex are induced by increases in the insulin/glucagon ratio. The amount of the complex increases slowly after a few days of a high-carbohydrate diet.

Glucose 6-phosphate dehydrogenase, which generates NADPH in the pentose phosphate pathway, and malic enzyme, which produces NADPH, are also induced by the increase of insulin.

The palmitate produced by the synthase complex is converted to palmityl CoA and elongated and desaturated to form other fatty acyl CoA molecules, which are converted to triacylglycerols. These triacylglycerols are packaged and secreted into the blood as VLDL.

B. Mechanisms That Affect the Fate of Chylomicrons and VLDL

The lipoprotein triacylglycerols in chylomicrons and VLDL are hydrolyzed to fatty acids and glycerol by lipoprotein lipase (LPL), an enzyme attached to endothelial cells of capillaries in muscle and adipose tissue. The enzyme found in muscle, particularly heart muscle, has a low K_m for these blood lipoproteins. Therefore, it acts even when these lipoproteins are present at very low concentrations in the blood. The fatty acids enter muscle cells and are oxidized for energy. The enzyme found in adipose tissue has a higher K_m and is most active after a meal when blood lipoprotein levels are elevated.

C. Mechanisms That Affect Triacylglycerol Storage in Adipose Tissue

Insulin stimulates adipose cells to synthesize and secrete LPL, which hydrolyzes the chylomicron and VLDL triacylglycerols. The C_{II} apoprotein, donated to chylomicrons and VLDL by HDL, activates LPL (Fig. 36.7).

Fatty acids released from chylomicrons and VLDL by LPL are stored as triacylglycerols in adipose cells. The glycerol released by LPL is not used by adipose cells because they lack glycerol kinase. Glycerol can be used by liver cells, however, because these cells do contain glycerol kinase. In the fed state, liver cells convert glycerol to the glycerol moiety of the triacylglycerols of VLDL, which is secreted from the liver to distribute the newly synthesized triglycerides to the tissues.

Insulin causes the number of glucose transporters in adipose cell membranes to increase. Glucose enters these cells, and is oxidized, producing energy and providing the glycerol 3-phosphate moiety for triacylglycerol synthesis (via the dihydroxyacetone phosphate intermediate of glycolysis).

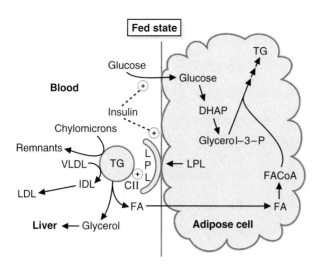

Fig. 36.7. Regulation of the storage of triacylglycerols (TG) in adipose tissue. Insulin stimulates the secretion of LPL from adipose cells and the transport of glucose into these cells. ApoC$_{II}$ activates LPL. FA = fatty acids.

II. REGULATION OF CARBOHYDRATE AND LIPID METABOLISM DURING FASTING

A. Mechanisms in Liver That Serve to Maintain Blood Glucose Levels

During fasting, the insulin/glucagon ratio decreases. Liver glycogen is degraded to produce blood glucose because enzymes of glycogen degradation are activated by cAMP-directed phosphorylation (Fig. 36.8). Glucagon stimulates adenylate cyclase to produce cAMP, which activates protein kinase A. Protein kinase A phosphorylates phosphorylase kinase, which then phosphorylates and activates glycogen phosphorylase. Protein kinase A also phosphorylates but, in this case, **in**activates glycogen synthase.

Gluconeogenesis is stimulated because the synthesis of phosphoenolpyruvate carboxykinase, fructose 1,6-bisphosphatase, and glucose 6-phosphatase is induced and because there is an increased availability of precursors. Fructose 1,6-bisphosphatase is also activated because the levels of its inhibitor, fructose 2,6-bisphosphate, are low (Fig. 36.9). During fasting, the activity of the corresponding enzymes of glycolysis is decreased.

B. Mechanisms That Affect Lipolysis in Adipose Tissue

During fasting, as blood insulin levels fall and glucagon levels rise, the level of cAMP rises in adipose cells. Consequently, protein kinase A is activated and causes phosphorylation of hormone-sensitive lipase (HSL). The phosphorylated form of this enzyme is active and cleaves fatty acids from triacylglycerols (Fig. 36.10). Other hormones (e.g., epinephrine, adrenocorticotropic hormone [ACTH], growth hormone) also activate this enzyme (see Chapter 43). Glyceroneogenesis and resynthesis of triglyceride by the adipocyte regulates the rate of release of fatty acids during fasting.

C. Mechanisms That Affect Ketone Body Production by the Liver

As fatty acids are released from adipose tissue during fasting, they travel in the blood complexed with albumin. These fatty acids are oxidized by various tissues, particularly muscle. In the liver, fatty acids are transported into mitochondria

Ann Sulin has type 2 diabetes mellitus. She produces insulin, but her adipose tissue is resistant to its actions. Therefore, her adipose tissue does not produce as much LPL as a normal person, which is one of the reasons why VLDL and chylomicrons remain elevated in her blood.

Twenty to thirty percent of patients with an insulinoma gain weight as part of their syndrome. **Bea Selmass** gained 8 lb in the 6 weeks before her surgery. Although she was primed by her high insulin levels both to store and to use fuel more efficiently, she would not have gained weight if she had not consumed more calories than she required for her daily energy expenditure during her illness (see Chapter 1). Bea consumed extra carbohydrate calories, mostly as hard candies and table sugar, to avoid the symptoms of hypoglycemia.

Induction of enzyme synthesis requires activation of transcription factors. One of the factors that is activated is CREB, which stands for cAMP response element binding protein. CREB is phosphorylated and activated by the cAMP-dependent protein kinase, which itself is activated on glucagon or epinephrine stimulation. A second set of transcription factors activated are the C/EPBs (CCAAT/ enhancer binding proteins), although the regulation of their activity is still under investigation.

Di Abietes suffers from hyperglycemia because her insulin levels tend to be low and her glucagon levels tend to be high. Her muscle and adipose cells do not take glucose up at a normal rate, and she produces glucose by glycogenolysis and gluconeogenesis. As a result, her blood glucose levels are elevated.

Ann Sulin is in a similar metabolic state. However, in this case, she produces insulin, but her tissues are resistant to its actions.

Would **Ann Sulin's** serum triacylglycerol level be elevated?

A: Because the adipose tissue of individuals with type 2 diabetes mellitus is relatively resistant to insulin's inhibition of HSL and its stimulation of LPL, **Ann Sulin's** serum triacylglycerol level would be elevated for the same reasons as those that caused the hypertriglyceridemia in **Di Abietes**.

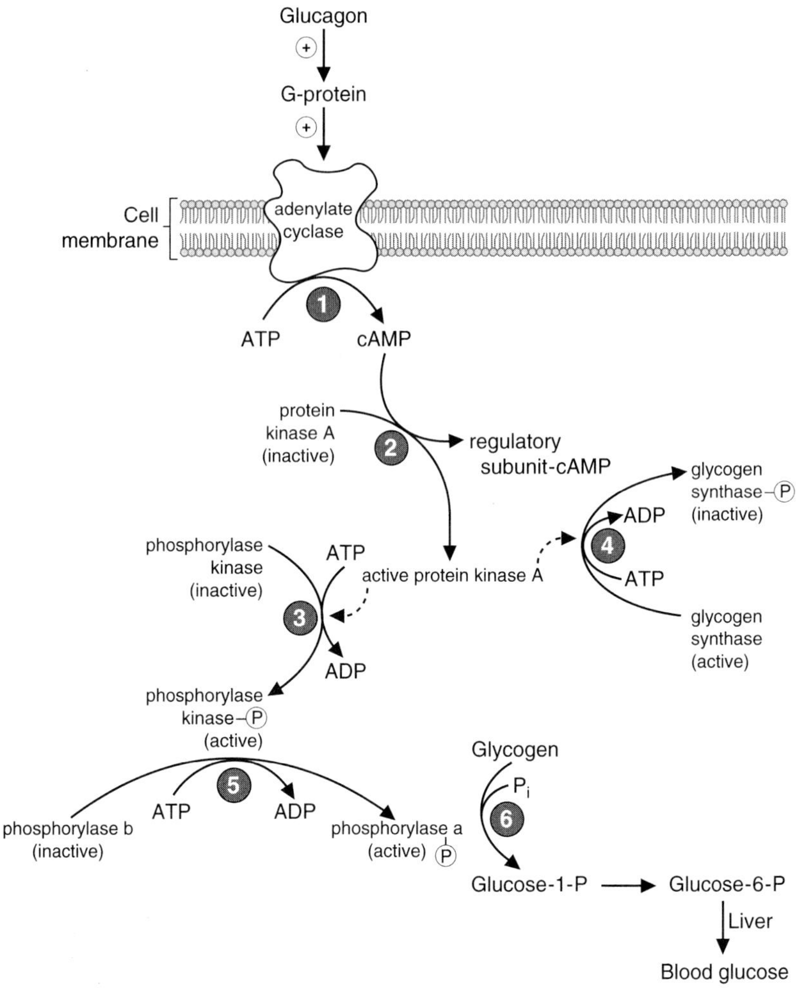

Glucagon

⊕

G-protein

⊕

Cell membrane

adenylate cyclase

①

ATP → cAMP

protein kinase A (inactive)

②

regulatory subunit-cAMP

active protein kinase A

phosphorylase kinase (inactive)

ATP

③

ADP

phosphorylase kinase-Ⓟ (active)

④

ADP

glycogen synthase-Ⓟ (inactive)

ATP

glycogen synthase (active)

phosphorylase b (inactive)

ATP

⑤

ADP

phosphorylase a (active) Ⓟ

Glycogen

Pi

⑥

Glucose-1-P ⟶ Glucose-6-P

Liver

Blood glucose

Fig. 36.8. Regulation of the enzymes of glycogen degradation in the liver. 1. Glucagon (or epinephrine) binds to its cell membrane receptor, initially activating a G protein, which activates adenylate cyclase. 2. As cAMP levels rise, inhibitory subunits are removed from protein kinase A, which now phosphorylates phosphorylase kinase (step 3). 4. The cAMP-dependent protein kinase also phosphorylates glycogen synthase, inactivating the enzyme. 5. Phosphorylated phosphorylase kinase phosphorylates glycogen phosphorylase. 6. Phosphorylated glycogen phosphorylase catalyzes the phosphorolysis of glycogen, producing glucose 1-phosphate. These events occur during fasting and produce glucose to maintain a relatively constant level of blood glucose.

Insulin normally inhibits lipolysis by decreasing the lipolytic activity of HSL in the adipocyte. Individuals such as **Di Abietes**, who have a deficiency of insulin, have an increase in lipolysis and a subsequent increase in the concentration of free fatty acids in the blood. The liver, in turn, uses some of these fatty acids to synthesize triacylglycerols, which then are used in the hepatic production of VLDL. VLDL is not stored in the liver but is secreted into the blood, raising its serum concentration. Di also has low levels of LPL because of decreased insulin levels. Her hypertriglyceridemia is the result, therefore, of both overproduction of VLDL by the liver and decreased breakdown of VLDL triacylglycerol for storage in adipose cells.

The serum begins to appear cloudy when the triacylglycerol level reaches 200 mg/dL. As the triacylglycerol level increases still further, the degree of serum opalescence increases proportionately.

because acetyl CoA carboxylase is inactive, malonyl CoA levels are low, and CPTI (carnitine:acyltransferase I) is active (see Fig. 36.6). Acetyl CoA, produced by β-oxidation, is converted to ketone bodies. Ketone bodies are used as an energy source by many tissues (Table 36.1) to spare the use of glucose and the necessity of degrading muscle protein to provide the precursors for gluconeogenesis. The high levels of acetyl CoA in the liver (derived from fat oxidation) inhibit pyruvate dehydrogenase (which prevents pyruvate from being converted to acetyl CoA) and activate pyruvate carboxylase, which produces oxaloacetate for gluconeogenesis. The oxaloacetate does not condense with acetyl CoA to form citrate for two reasons. The first is that under these conditions (a high rate of fat oxidation in the liver mitochondria), energy levels in the mitochondrial matrix are high; that is, there are high levels of NADH and ATP present. The high NADH level inhibits isocitrate dehydrogenase. As a result, citrate accumulates and inhibits citrate synthase from producing more citrate. The second reason that citrate synthesis is depressed is that the

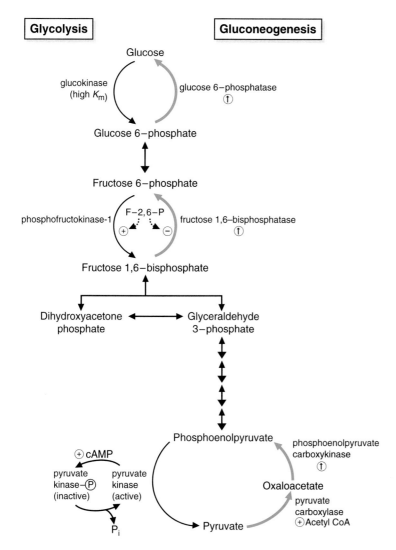

Fig. 36.9. Regulation of gluconeogenesis and glycolysis during fasting. The gluconeogenic enzymes phosphoenolpyruvate carboxykinase, fructose 1,6-bisphosphatase, and glucose 6-phosphatase are induced. Fructose 1,6-bisphosphatase is also active because, during fasting, the level of its inhibitor, fructose 2,6-bisphosphate, is low. The corresponding enzymes of glycolysis are not very active during fasting. The rate of glucokinase is low because it has a high K_m for glucose and the glucose concentration is low. Phosphofructokinase-1 is not very active because the concentration of its activator fructose 2,6-bisphosphate is low. Pyruvate kinase is inactivated by cAMP-mediated phosphorylation.

Table 36.1. Fuel Utilization by Various Tissues during Starvation (Fasting)

Tissue	Glucose	Fatty Acids	Ketone Bodies
Nervous system	++	−	++
Skeletal muscle	−	++	++
Heart muscle	−	++	++
Liver	−	++	−
Intestinal epithelial cells	−	−	++
Kidney	−	+	+

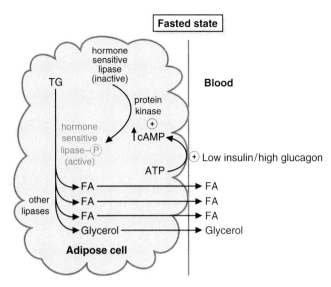

Fasted state

hormone
sensitive
lipase
(inactive)

TG

protein
kinase

$\uparrow$cAMP

hormone
sensitive
lipase–Ⓟ
(active)

ATP

Ⓐ Low insulin/high glucagon

Blood

other
lipases

FA ——— FA
FA ——— FA
FA ——— FA
Glycerol ——— Glycerol

Adipose cell

Fig. 36.10. Regulation of hormone-sensitive lipase (HSL) in adipose tissue. During fasting, the glucagon/insulin ratio rises, causing cAMP levels to be elevated. Protein kinase A is activated and phosphorylates HSL, activating this enzyme. HSL-P initiates the mobilization of adipose triacylglycerol by removing a fatty acid (FA). Other lipases then act, producing fatty acids and glycerol. Insulin stimulates the phosphatase that inactivates HSL in the fed state.

high $NADH/NAD^+$ ratio also diverts oxaloacetate into malate, such that the malate can exit the mitochondria (via the malate/aspartate shuttle) for use in gluconeogenesis.

D. Regulation of the Use of Glucose and Fatty Acids by Muscle

During exercise, the fuel that is used initially by muscle cells is muscle glycogen. As exercise continues and the blood supply to the tissue increases, glucose is taken up from the blood and oxidized. Liver glycogenolysis and gluconeogenesis replenish the blood glucose supply. However, as insulin levels drop, the concentration of GLUT4 transporters in the membrane is reduced, thereby reducing glucose entry from the circulation into the muscle.

Thus, as fatty acids become available because of increased lipolysis of adipose triacylglycerols, the exercising muscle begins to oxidize fatty acids. β-Oxidation produces NADH and acetyl CoA, which slow the flow of carbon from glucose through the reaction catalyzed by pyruvate dehydrogenase (see Fig. 36.3). Thus, the oxidation of fatty acids provides a major portion of the increased demand for ATP generation and spares blood glucose.

III. THE IMPORTANCE OF AMP AND FRUCTOSE 2,6-BISPHOSPHATE

The switch between catabolic and anabolic pathways is often regulated by the levels of AMP and fructose 2,6-bisphosphate in cells, particularly the liver. It is logical for AMP to be a critical regulator. As a cell uses ATP in energy-requiring pathways, the levels of AMP accumulate more rapidly than that of ADP because of the adenylate kinase reaction (2 ADP → ATP and AMP). The rise in AMP levels then signals that more energy is required (usually through allosteric binding sites on enzymes and the activation of the AMP-activated protein kinase), and the cell will switch to the activation of catabolic pathways. As AMP levels drop, and ATP levels rise, the anabolic pathways are now activated to store the excess energy.

Muscle GLUT4 transporters also can be induced by AMP levels (see Chapter 47), through the actions of the AMP-activated protein kinase. Thus, if energy levels are very low, and AMP levels increase, glucose can still be transported from the circulation into the muscle to provide energy. This most often occurs during exercise.

The levels of fructose 2,6-bisphosphate are also critical in regulating glycolysis versus gluconeogenesis in the liver. Under conditions of high blood glucose, and insulin release, fructose 2,6 bisphosphate levels will be high because PFK-2 will be in its activated state. The fructose 2,6 bisphosphate activates PFK-1, and inhibits fructose 2,6 bisphosphatase, thereby allowing glycolysis to proceed. When blood glucose levels are low, and glucagon is released, PFK-2 is phosphorylated by the cAMP-dependent protein kinase and is inhibited, thereby lowering fructose 2,6-bisphosphate levels and inhibiting glycolysis, while favoring gluconeogenesis.

CLINICAL COMMENTS

Bea Selmass's younger sister was very concerned that Bea's pancreatic tumor might be genetically determined or potentially malignant, so she accompanied Bea to her second postoperative visit to the endocrinologist. The doctor explained that insulinomas may be familial in up to 20% of cases and that in 10% of patients with insulinomas, additional secretory neoplasms may occur in the anterior pituitary or the parathyroid glands (a genetically determined syndrome known as multiple endocrine neoplasia, type I or, simply, MEN I). Bea's tumor showed no evidence of malignancy, and the histologic slides, although not always definitive, showed a benign-appearing process. The doctor was careful to explain, however, that close observation for recurrent hypoglycemia and for the signs and symptoms suggestive of other facets of MEN I would be necessary for the remainder of Bea's and her immediate family's life.

Diabetes mellitus is a well-accepted risk factor for the development of coronary artery disease; the risk is three to four times higher in the diabetic than in the nondiabetic population. Although chronically elevated serum levels of chylomicrons and VLDL may contribute to this atherogenic predisposition, the premature vascular disease seen in **Di Abietes** and other patients with type 1 diabetes mellitus, as well as **Ann Sulin** and other patients with type 2 diabetes mellitus, is also related to other abnormalities in lipid metabolism. Among these are the increase in glycation (nonenzymatic attachment of glucose molecules to proteins) of LDL apoproteins as well as glycation of the proteins of the LDL receptor, which occurs when serum glucose levels are chronically elevated. These glycations interfere with the normal interaction or "fit" of the circulating LDL particles with their specific receptors on cell membranes. As a consequence, the rate of uptake of circulating LDL by the normal target cells is diminished. The LDL particles, therefore, remain in the circulation and eventually bind nonspecifically to "scavenger" receptors located on macrophages adjacent to the endothelial surfaces of blood vessels, one of the early steps in the process of atherogenesis.

BIOCHEMICAL COMMENTS

All of the material in this chapter was presented previously. However, because this information is so critical for understanding biochemistry in a way that will allow it to be used in interpreting clinical situations, it was summarized in this chapter. In addition, the information previously presented under carbohydrate metabolism was integrated with lipid metabolism. We have, for the most part, left out the role of allosteric modifiers and other regulatory mechanisms that finely coordinate these processes to an exquisite level. Because such details may be important for specific clinical situations, we hope this summary will serve as a framework to which the details can be fitted as students advance in their clinical studies.

Because **Di Abietes** produces very little insulin, she is prone to developing ketoacidosis. When insulin levels are low, HSL of adipose tissue is very active, resulting in increased lipolysis. The fatty acids that are released travel to the liver, where they are converted to the triacylglycerols of VLDL. They also undergo β-oxidation and conversion to ketone bodies. If Di does not take exogenous insulin or if her insulin levels decrease abruptly for some physiologic reason, she may develop a ketoacidosis (DKA). In fact, she has had repeated bouts of DKA.

For reasons that are not as well understood, individuals with type 2 diabetes mellitus, such as **Ann Sulin**, do not tend to develop ketoacidosis. One possible explanation is that the insulin resistance is tissue-specific; the insulin sensitivity of adipocytes may be greater than that of muscle and liver. Such a tissue-specific sensitivity would lead to less fatty acids being released from adipocytes in type 2 diabetes than in type 1 diabetes, although in both cases the release of fatty acids would be greater than that of an individual without the disease.

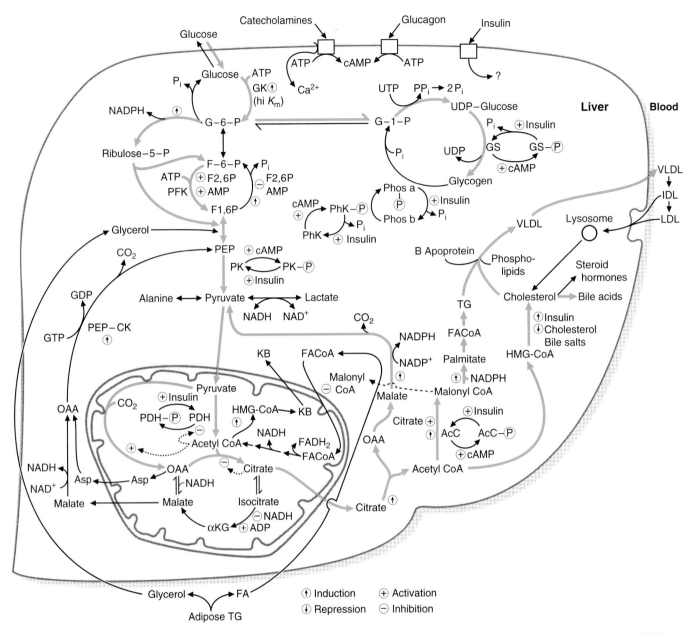

Fig. 36.11. Regulation of carbohydrate and lipid metabolism in the liver. Solid blue arrows indicate the flow of metabolites in the fed state. Solid black arrows indicate the flow during fasting. G = glucose; GK = glucokinase; F = fructose; PFK = phosphofructokinase-1; PEP = phosphoenolpyruvate; PK = pyruvate kinase; OAA = oxaloacetate; αKG = α-ketoglutarate; GS = glycogen synthase; Phos = glycogen phosphorylase; PhK = phosphorylase kinase; AcC = acetyl CoA carboxylase; FA = fatty acid or fatty acyl group; TG = triacylglycerol; circled P = phosphate group.

Figure 36.11 is a comprehensive figure, and Tables 36.2 and 36.3 provide a list of the major regulatory enzymes of carbohydrate and lipid metabolism in the liver, an order to the events that occur, and the mechanisms by which they are controlled. This figure and tables should help students to integrate this mass of material.

Now that many of the details of the pathways have been presented, it would be worthwhile to re-read the first three chapters of this book. A student who understands biochemistry within the context of fuel metabolism is in a very good position to solve clinical problems that involve metabolic derangements.

Table 36.2. Flowchart of Changes in Liver Metabolism

When blood sugar increases:
Insulin is released, which leads
  to the *dephosphorylation* of:

- PFK-2 (now active)
- Pyruvate kinase (now active)
- Glycogen synthase (now active)

- Phosphorylase kinase (now inactive)

- Glycogen phosphorylase (now inactive)

- Pyruvate dehydrogenase (now active)

- Acetyl CoA Carboxylase (now active)

Which leads to *active*
- Glycolysis
- Fatty acid synthesis
- Glycogen synthesis

When blood sugar decreases:
Glucagon is released, which
  leads to the *phosphorylation*
  of:
- PFK-2 (now inactive)
- Pyruvate kinase (now inactive)
- Glycogen synthase (now inactive)

- Phosphorylase kinase (now active)

- Glycogen phosphorylase (now active)

- Pyruvate dehydrogenase (now inactive)

- Acetyl CoA Carboxylase (now inactive)

Which leads to *active*
- Glycogenolysis
- Fatty acid oxidation
- Gluconeogenesis

Table 36.3. Regulation of Liver Enzymes Involved in Glycogen, Blood Glucose, and Triacylglycerol Synthesis and Degradation

LIVER ENZYMES REGULATED BY ACTIVATION/INHIBITION		
Enzyme	**Activated By**	**State in Which Active**
Phosphofructokinase-1	Fructose-2,6-bisP, AMP	Fed
Pyruvate carboxylase	Acetyl CoA	Fed and fasting
Acetyl CoA carboxylase	Citrate	Fed
Carnitine: palmitoyltransferase I	Loss of inhibitor (malonyl CoA)	Fasting

LIVER ENZYMES REGULATED BY PHOSPHORYLATION/DEPHOSPHORYLATION		
Enzyme	**Active Form**	**State in Which Active**
Glycogen synthase	Dephosphorylated	Fed
Phosphorylase kinase	Phosphorylated	Fasting
Glycogen phosphorylase	Phosphorylated	Fasting
Phosphofructokinase-2/F-2, 6-bisphosphatase (acts as a kinase, increasing fructose- 2,6-bisP levels)	Dephosphorylated	Fed
Phosphofructokinase-2/F-2, 6-bisphosphatase (acts as a phosphatase, decreasing fructose- 2,6-bisP levels)	Phosphorylated	Fasting
Pyruvate kinase	Dephosphorylated	Fed
Pyruvate dehydrogenase	Dephosphorylated	Fed
Acetyl CoA carboxylase	Dephosphorylated	Fed

LIVER ENZYMES REGULATED BY INDUCTION/REPRESSION		
Enzyme	**State in Which Induced**	**Process Affected**
Glucokinase	Fed	Glucose → TG
Citrate lyase	Fed	Glucose → TG
Acetyl CoA carboxylase	Fed	Glucose → TG
Fatty acid synthase	Fed	Glucose → TG
Malic enzyme	Fed	Production of NADPH
Glucose-6-P dehydrogenase	Fed	Production of NADPH
Glucose 6-phosphatase	Fasted	Production of blood glucose
Fructose 1, 6-bisphosphatase	Fasted	Production of blood glucose
Phosphoenolpyruvate carboxykinase	Fasted	Production of blood glucose

Suggested References

Iritani N. Nutritional and hormonal regulation of lipogenic-enzyme gene expression in rat liver. Eur J Biochem 1992:205:433–442.

Jump DB, Clarke SD. Regulation of gene expression by dietary fat. Annu Rev Nutr 1999; 19:63–90.

Klip A, Tsakiridis T, Marette A, Ortiz PA. Regulation of expression of glucose transporters by glucose: a review of studies in vivo and in cell cultures. FASEB J 1994;8:43–53.

Pilkis SJ, Granner DK. Molecular physiology of the regulation of hepatic gluconeogenesis and glycolysis. Annu Rev Physiol 1992;54:885–909.

Roesler WJ. What is a cAMP response unit? Mol Cell Endocrinol 2000;162:1–7.

Sugden MC, Holness MJ. Interactive regulation of the pyruvate dehydrogenase complex and the carnitine palmitoyltransferase system. FASEB J 1994;8:54–61.

Vaulont S, Kahn A. Transcriptional control of metabolic regulation genes by carbohydrates. FASEB J 1994:8:28–35.

 REVIEW QUESTIONS—CHAPTER 36

1. A 20-year-old woman with diabetes mellitus was admitted to the hospital in a semiconscious state with fever, nausea, and vomiting. Her breath smelled of acetone. A urine sample was strongly positive for ketone bodies. Which of the following statements is correct concerning this woman?

    (A) A blood glucose test would probably show that her blood glucose level was well below 80 mg/dL.
    (B) An insulin injection would decrease her ketone body production.
    (C) She should be given a glucose infusion to regain consciousness.
    (D) Glucagon should be administered to stimulate glycogenolysis and gluconeogenesis in the liver.
    (E) The acetone was produced by decarboxylation of the ketone body β-hydroxybutyrate.

2. A woman was told by her physician to go on a low-fat diet. She decided to continue to consume the same number of calories by increasing her carbohydrate intake while decreasing her fat intake. Which of the following blood lipoprotein levels would be decreased as a consequence of her diet?

    (A) VLDL
    (B) IDL
    (C) HDL
    (D) Chylomicrons
    (E) HDL

3. Assume that an individual has been eating excess calories daily such that they will gain weight. Under which of the following conditions would the person gain weight most rapidly?

    (A) If all the excess calories were due to carbohydrate
    (B) If all the excess calories were due to triacylglycerol
    (C) If all the excess calories were split 50%–50% between carbohydrate and triacylglycerol
    (D) If all the excess calories were split 25%–75% between carbohydrate and triacylglycerol
    (E) It makes no difference what form the excess calories are in

4. A chronic alcoholic has been admitted to the hospital because of a severe hypoglycemic episode brought about by excessive alcohol consumption for the past 5 days. A blood lipid analysis indicates much higher than expected VLDL levels. The elevated VLDL is attributable to which of the following underlying causes?

    (A) Alcohol-induced inhibition of lipoprotein lipase
    (B) Elevated NADH levels in the liver
    (C) Alcohol-induced transcription of the apoB-100 gene
    (D) NADH activation of phosphoenolpyruvate carboxykinase
    (E) Acetaldehyde induction of enzymes on the endoplasmic reticulum

5. Certain patients with abetalipoproteinemia frequently have difficulties in maintaining blood volume; their blood has trouble clotting. This symptom is attributable to which of the following?

    (A) Inability to produce chylomicrons
    (B) Inability to produce VLDL
    (C) Inability to synthesize clotting factors
    (D) Inability to synthesize fatty acids
    (E) Inability to absorb short-chain fatty acids

Nitrogen Metabolism

Dietary proteins are the primary source of the nitrogen that is metabolized by the body (Fig. 1). Amino acids, produced by digestion of dietary proteins, are absorbed through intestinal epithelial cells and enter the blood. Various cells take up these amino acids, which enter the cellular pools. They are used for the synthesis of proteins and other nitrogen-containing compounds or they are oxidized for energy.

Protein synthesis, the translation of mRNA on ribosomes (see Chapter 15), is a dynamic process. Within the body, proteins are constantly being synthesized and degraded, partially draining and then refilling the cellular amino acid pools.

Compounds derived from amino acids include cellular proteins, hormones, neurotransmitters, creatine phosphate, the heme of hemoglobin and the cytochromes, the skin pigment melanin, and the purine and pyrimidine bases of nucleotides and nucleic acids. In fact, all of the nitrogen-containing compounds of the body are synthesized from amino acids. Many of these pathways are outlined in the following chapters of the book.

In addition to serving as the precursors for the nitrogen-containing compounds of the body and as the building blocks for protein synthesis, amino acids are also a source of energy. Amino acids are directly oxidized or they are converted to glucose and then oxidized or stored as glycogen. They also may be converted to fatty acids and stored as adipose triacylglycerols. Glycogen and triacylglycerols are oxidized during periods of fasting. The liver is the major site of amino acid oxidation. However, most tissues can oxidize the branched-chain amino acids (leucine, isoleucine, and valine).

Before the carbon skeletons of amino acids are oxidized, the nitrogen must be removed. Amino acid nitrogen forms ammonia, which is toxic to the body. In the liver, ammonia and the amino groups from amino acids are converted to urea, which is nontoxic, water-soluble, and readily excreted in the urine. The process by which urea is produced is known as the urea cycle. The liver is the organ responsible for producing urea. Branched-chain amino acids can be oxidized in many tissues, but the nitrogen must always travel to the liver for disposal.

Although urea is the major nitrogenous excretory product of the body, nitrogen is also excreted in other compounds (Table 1). Uric acid is the degradation product

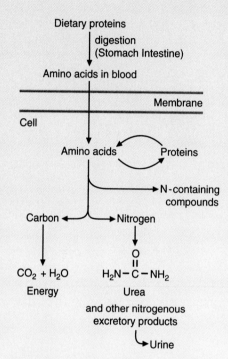

Fig. 1. Summary of amino acid metabolism. Dietary proteins are digested to amino acids in the stomach and intestine, which are absorbed by the intestinal epithelium, transferred to the circulation, and taken up by cells. Amino acids are used to synthesize proteins and other nitrogen-containing compounds. The carbon skeletons of amino acids are also oxidized for energy, and the nitrogen is converted to urea and other nitrogenous excretory products.

Table 1. Major Nitrogenous Urinary Excretory Products

Amount excreted in urine/day[a]		
Urea[b]	12–20 g urea nitrogen (12,000–20,000 mg)	
NH_4^+	140–1,500 mg ammonia nitrogen	
Creatinine	Males:	14–26 mg/kg
	Females:	11–20 mg/kg
Uric acid	250–750 mg	

[a]The amounts are expressed in units generally reported by clinical laboratories. Note that the amounts for creatinine and uric acid are for the whole compound, whereas those for urea and ammonia are for the nitrogen content.

[b]Under normal circumstances, approximately 90% of the nitrogen excreted in the urine is in the form of urea. The exact amounts of each component vary, however, depending on dietary protein intake and physiologic state. For instance, NH_4^+ excretion increases during an acidosis because the kidney secretes ammonia to bind protons in the urine.

The healthy human adult is in nitrogen balance; in other words, the amount of nitrogen excreted each day (mainly in the urine) equals the amount consumed (mainly as dietary protein). Negative nitrogen balance occurs when the amount of nitrogen excreted is greater than the amount consumed, and positive nitrogen balance occurs when the amount excreted is less than that consumed (see Chapter 1).

Table 2. Amino Acids Synthesized in the Body[a]

From Glucose	From an Essential Amino Acid
Serine	Tyrosine (from phenylalanine)
Glycine	
Cysteine[b]	
Alanine	
Aspartate	
Asparagine	
Glutamate	
Glutamine	
Proline	
Arginine	

[a]These amino acids are called "nonessential" or "dispensable," terms that refer to dietary requirements. Of course, within the body, they are necessary. We cannot survive without them.
[b]Although the carbons of cysteine can be derived from glucose, its sulfur is obtained from the essential amino acid methionine.

of the purine bases, creatinine is produced from creatine phosphate, and ammonia is released from glutamine, particularly by the kidney, where it helps to buffer the urine by reacting with protons to form ammonium ions (NH_4^+). These compounds are excreted mainly in the urine, but substantial amounts are also lost in the feces and through the skin. Small amounts of nitrogen-containing metabolites are formed from the degradation of neurotransmitters, hormones, and other specialized amino acid products and excreted in the urine. Some of these degradation products, such as bilirubin (formed from the degradation of heme), are excreted mainly in the feces.

Eleven of the 20 amino acids used to form proteins are synthesized in the body if an adequate amount is not present in the diet (Table 2). Ten of these amino acids can be produced from glucose; the 11th, tyrosine, is synthesized from the essential amino acid phenylalanine. It should be noted that cysteine, one of the 10 amino acids produced from glucose, obtains its sulfur atom from the essential amino acid methionine.

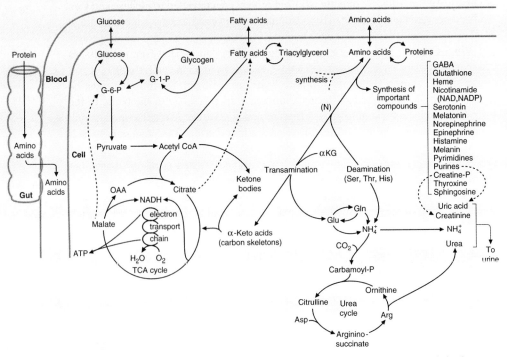

Fig. 2. Overview of nitrogen metabolism. The metabolism of nitrogen-containing compounds is shown on the right and that of glucose and fatty acids is shown on the left. This figure shows a hypothetical, composite cell. No single cell type has all of these pathways. Many of the pathways shown are described in the next few chapters. αKG = α-ketoglutarate; OAA = oxaloacetate; G-6-P = glucose 6-phosphate; G-1-P = glucose 1-phosphate.

Nine amino acids are essential in the human. "Essential" means that the carbon skeleton cannot be synthesized and, therefore, these amino acids are required in the diet (Table 3). The essential amino acids are also called the indispensable amino acids. Arginine is essential during periods of growth; in adults it is no longer considered essential.

After nitrogen is removed from amino acids, the carbon skeletons are oxidized (Fig. 2). Most of the carbons are converted to pyruvate, intermediates of the tricarboxylic acid (TCA) cycle, or to acetyl CoA. In the liver, particularly during fasting, these carbons may be converted to glucose or to ketone bodies and released into the blood. Other tissues then oxidize the glucose and ketone bodies. Ultimately, the carbons of the amino acids are converted to CO_2 and H_2O.

Table 3. Amino Acids Essential in the Diet

Lysine
Isoleucine
Leucine
Threonine
Valine
Tryptophan
Phenylalanine
Methionine
Histidine
Arginine (not required by the adult, but required for growth)

37 Protein Digestion and Amino Acid Absorption

*Proteolytic enzymes (also called **proteases**) break down dietary proteins into their constituent amino acids in the **stomach** and the **intestine**. Many of these digestive proteases are synthesized as larger, inactive forms known as **zymogens**. After zymogens are secreted into the digestive tract, they are cleaved to produce the active proteases.*

*In the stomach, **pepsin** begins the digestion of proteins by hydrolyzing them to smaller polypeptides. The contents of the stomach pass into the small intestine, where enzymes produced by the exocrine pancreas act. The pancreatic proteases (**trypsin, chymotrypsin, elastase,** and the **carboxypeptidases**) cleave the polypeptides into oligopeptides and amino acids.*

*Further cleavage of the oligopeptides to amino acids is accomplished by enzymes produced by the intestinal epithelial cells. These enzymes include **aminopeptidases** located on the brush border and other peptidases located within the cells. Ultimately, the amino acids produced by protein digestion are absorbed through the **intestinal epithelial cells** and enter the **blood**.*

*A large number of overlapping transport systems exist for amino acids in cells. Some systems contain **facilitative transporters**, whereas others express **sodium-linked tranporters**, which allow the **active transport** of amino acids into cells. Defects in amino acid transport can lead to disease.*

*Proteins are also continually synthesized and degraded (**turnover**) in cells. A wide variety of proteases exist in cells to carry out this activity. **Lysosomal proteases (cathepsins)** degrade proteins that enter lysosomes. Cytoplasmic proteins targeted for turnover are covalently linked to the small protein **ubiquitin**, which then interacts with a large protein complex, the **proteasome,** to degrade the protein in an adenosine triphosphate (ATP)-dependent process. The amino acids released from proteins during turnover can then be used for the synthesis of new proteins or for energy generation.*

THE WAITING ROOM

Sissy Fibrosa, a young child with cystic fibrosis, has had repeated bouts of bronchitis caused by *Pseudomonas aeruginosa*. With each of these infections, her response to aerosolized antibiotics has been good. However, her malabsorption of food continues, resulting in foul-smelling, glistening, bulky stools. Her growth records show a slow decline. She is now in the 24th percentile for height and the 20th percentile for weight. She is often listless and irritable, and she tires easily. When her pediatrician discovered that her levels of the serum proteins

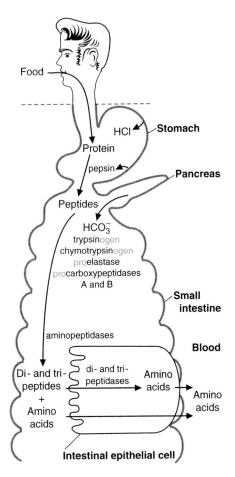

Fig. 37.1. Digestion of proteins. The proteolytic enzymes, pepsin, trypsin, chymotrypsin, elastase, and the carboxypeptidases, are produced as zymogens (the [pro] and [ogen] accompanying the enzyme name) that are activated by cleavage after they enter the gastrointestinal lumen (see Fig. 37.2).

Kwashiorkor, a common problem of children in Third World countries, is caused by a deficiency of protein in a diet that is adequate in calories. Children with kwashiorkor suffer from muscle wasting and a decreased concentration of plasma proteins, particularly albumin. The result is an increase in interstitial fluid that causes edema and a distended abdomen that make the children appear "plump" (see Chapter 44). The muscle wasting is caused by the lack of essential amino acids in the diet; existing proteins must be broken down to produce these amino acids for new protein synthesis.

These problems may be compounded by a decreased ability to produce digestive enzymes and new intestinal epithelial cells because of a decreased availability of amino acids for the synthesis of new proteins.

albumin, transferrin, and thyroid hormone binding prealbumin (transthyretin) were low to low-normal (indicating protein malnutrition), Sissy was given enteric-coated microspheres of pancreatic enzymes. Almost immediately, the character of Sissy's stools became more normal and she began gaining weight. In the next 6 months, her growth curves showed improvement, and she seemed brighter, more active, and less irritable.

For the first few months after a painful episode of renal colic, during which he passed a kidney stone (see Chapter 6), **Cal Kulis** had faithfully maintained a high daily fluid intake and had taken the medication required to increase the pH of his urine. Because he has cystinuria, these measures were necessary to increase the solubility of the large amounts of cystine present in his urine and, thereby, to prevent further formation of kidney stones (calculi). With time, however, he became increasingly complacent about his preventive program. After failing to take his medication for a month, he experienced another severe episode of renal colic with grossly bloody urine. Fortunately, he passed the stone spontaneously, after which he vowed to faithfully comply with therapy.

His mother heard that some dietary amino acids were not absorbed in patients with cystinuria and asked whether any dietary changes would reduce Cal's chances of developing additional renal stones.

I. PROTEIN DIGESTION

The digestion of proteins begins in the stomach and is completed in the intestine (Fig. 37.1). The enzymes that digest proteins are produced as inactive precursors (zymogens) that are larger than the active enzymes. The inactive zymogens are secreted from the cells in which they are synthesized and enter the lumen of the digestive tract, where they are cleaved to smaller forms that have proteolytic activity (Fig. 37.2). These active enzymes have different specificities; no single enzyme can completely digest a protein. However, by acting in concert, they can digest dietary proteins to amino acids and small peptides, which are cleaved by peptidases associated with intestinal epithelial cells

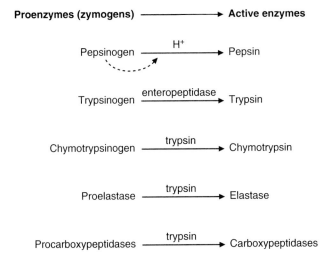

Fig. 37.2. Activation of the gastric and pancreatic zymogens. Pepsinogen catalyzes its own cleavage as the pH of the stomach drops. Trypsinogen is cleaved by enteropeptidase in the intestine to form the active protease trypsin. Trypsin then plays a key role by catalyzing the cleavage and activation of the other pancreatic zymogens.

A. Digestion of Proteins in the Stomach

Pepsinogen is secreted by the chief cells of the stomach. The gastric parietal cells secrete HCl. The acid in the stomach lumen alters the conformation of pepsinogen so that it can cleave itself, producing the active protease pepsin. Thus, the activation of pepsinogen is autocatalytic.

Dietary proteins are denatured by the acid in the stomach. This serves to inactivate the proteins and partially unfolds them such that they are better substrates for proteases. However, at the low pH of the stomach, pepsin is not denatured and acts as an endopeptidase, cleaving peptide bonds at various points within the protein chain. Although pepsin has a fairly broad specificity, it tends to cleave peptide bonds in which the carboxyl group is provided by an aromatic or acidic amino acid (Fig. 37.3). Smaller peptides and some free amino acids are produced.

B. Digestion of Proteins by Enzymes from the Pancreas

As the gastric contents empty into the intestine, they encounter the secretions from the exocrine pancreas. One of these secretions is bicarbonate, which, in addition to neutralizing the stomach acid, raises the pH such that the pancreatic proteases, which are also present in pancreatic secretions, can be active. As secreted, these pancreatic proteases are in the inactive proenzyme form (zymogens). Because the active forms of these enzymes can digest each other, it is important for their zymogen forms all to be activated within a short span of time. This feat is accomplished by the cleavage of trypsinogen to the active enzyme trypsin, which then cleaves the other pancreatic zymogens, producing their active forms (see Fig. 37.2).

The zymogen trypsinogen is cleaved to form trypsin by enteropeptidase (a protease, formerly called enterokinase) secreted by the brush-border cells of the small intestine. Trypsin catalyzes the cleavages that convert chymotrypsinogen to the active enzyme chymotrypsin, proelastase to elastase, and the procarboxypeptidases to the carboxypeptidases. Thus, trypsin plays a central role in digestion because it both cleaves dietary proteins and activates other digestive proteases produced by the pancreas.

Trypsin, chymotrypsin, and elastase are serine proteases (see Chapter 9) that act as endopeptidases. Trypsin is the most specific of these enzymes, cleaving peptide bonds in which the carboxyl (carbonyl) group is provided by lysine or arginine (see Fig. 37.3). Chymotrypsin is less specific but favors residues that contain hydrophobic or acidic amino acids. Elastase cleaves not only elastin (for which it was named) but also other proteins at bonds in which the carboxyl group is contributed by amino acid residues with small side chains (alanine, glycine, or serine). The actions of these pancreatic endopeptidases continue the digestion of dietary proteins begun by pepsin in the stomach.

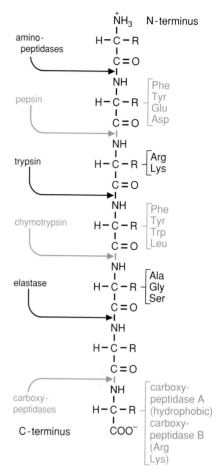

Fig. 37.3. Action of the digestive proteases. Pepsin, trypsin, chymotrypsin, and elastase are endopeptidases; they hydrolyze peptide bonds within chains. The others are exopeptidases; aminopeptidases remove the amino acid at the N-terminus and the carboxypeptidases remove the amino acid at the C terminus. For each proteolytic enzyme, the amino acid residues involved in the peptide bond that is cleaved are listed beside the R group to the right of the enzyme name.

Recall that the exocrine pancreas, in addition to secreting proteolytic zymogens, also secretes amylase for starch digestion and lipase and co-lipase for dietary triacylglycerol digestion.

Elastase is also found in neutrophils, white blood cells that have the job of engulfing and destroying invading bacteria. Neutrophils frequently act in the lung, and elastase is sometimes released into the lung as the neutrophils work. In normal individuals, the released elastase is blocked from destroying lung cells by the action of circulating α-1-antitrypsin, a protease inhibitor synthesized and secreted by the liver. Certain individuals have a genetic mutation that leads to the production of an inactive α-1-antitrypsin protein (α-1-antitrypsin deficiency). The lack of this enzyme activity leads to the development of emphysema caused by proteolytic destruction of lung cells, which results in a reduction in the expansion/contraction capability of the lungs.

Patients with cystic fibrosis, such as **Sissy Fibrosa**, have a genetically determined defect in the function of the chloride channels. In the pancreatic secretory ducts, which carry pancreatic enzymes into the lumen of the small intestines, this defect causes inspissation (drying and thickening) of pancreatic exocrine secretions, eventually leading to obstruction of these ducts. One result of this problem is the inability of pancreatic enzymes to enter the intestinal lumen to digest dietary proteins.

The pancreas synthesizes and stores the zymogens in secretory granules. The pancreas also synthesizes a secretory trypsin inhibitor. The need for the inhibitor is to block any trypsin activity that may occur from accidental trypsinogen activation. If the inhibitor were not present, trypsinogen activation would lead to the activation of all of the zymogens in the pancreas, which would lead to the digestion of intracellular pancreatic proteins. Such episodes can lead to pancreatitis.

Q: Why do patients with cystinuria and Hartnup disease have a hyperaminoaciduria without an associated hyperaminoacidemia?

Hartnup disease is another genetically determined and relatively rare autosomal recessive disorder. It is caused by a defect in the transport of neutral amino acids across both intestinal and renal epithelial cells. The signs and symptoms are, in part, caused by a deficiency of essential amino acids (see Clinical Comments). Cystinuria and Hartnup disease involve defects in two different transport proteins. In each case, the defect is present both in intestinal cells, causing malabsorption of the amino acids from the digestive products in the intestinal lumen and in kidney tubular cells, causing a decreased resorption of these amino acids from the glomerular filtrate.

Trace amounts of polypeptides pass into the blood. They may be transported through intestinal epithelial cells, probably by pinocytosis, or they may slip between the cells that line the gut wall. This process is particularly troublesome for premature infants, because it can lead to allergies caused by proteins in their food.

The smaller peptides formed by the action of trypsin, chymotrypsin, and elastase are attacked by exopeptidases, which are proteases that cleave one amino acid at a time from the end of the chain. Procarboxypeptidases, zymogens produced by the pancreas, are converted by trypsin to the active carboxypeptidases. These exopeptidases remove amino acids from the carboxyl ends of peptide chains. Carboxypeptidase A preferentially releases hydrophobic amino acids, whereas carboxypeptidase B releases basic amino acids (arginine and lysine).

C. Digestion of Proteins by Enzymes from Intestinal Cells

Exopeptidases produced by intestinal epithelial cells act within the brush border and also within the cell. Aminopeptidases, located on the brush border, cleave one amino acid at a time from the amino end of peptides. Intracellular peptidases act on small peptides that are absorbed by the cells.

The concerted action of the proteolytic enzymes produced by cells of the stomach, pancreas, and intestine cleaves dietary proteins to amino acids. The digestive enzymes digest themselves as well as dietary protein. They also digest the intestinal cells that are regularly sloughed off into the lumen. These cells are replaced by cells that mature from precursor cells in the duodenal crypts. The amount of protein that is digested and absorbed each day from digestive juices and cells released into the intestinal lumen may be equal to, or greater than, the amount of protein consumed in the diet (50–100 g).

II. ABSORPTION OF AMINO ACIDS

Amino acids are absorbed from the intestinal lumen through secondary active Na^+-dependent transport systems and through facilitated diffusion.

A. Cotransport of Na^+ and Amino Acids

Amino acids are absorbed from the lumen of the small intestine principally by semispecific Na^+-dependent transport proteins in the luminal membrane of the intestinal cell brush border, similar to that already seen for carbohydrate transport (Fig 37.4). The cotransport of Na^+ and the amino acid from the outside of the apical membrane to the inside of the cell is driven by the low intracellular Na^+ concentration. Low intracellular Na^+ results from the pumping of Na^+ out of the cell by a Na^+,K^+-ATPase on the serosal membrane. Thus, the primary transport mechanism is the creation of a sodium gradient; the secondary transport process is the coupling of amino acids to the influx of sodium. This mechanism allows the cells to concentrate amino acids from the intestinal lumen. The amino acids are then transported out of the cell into the interstitial fluid principally by facilitated transporters in the serosal membrane (see Fig. 37.4).

At least six different Na^+-dependent amino acid carriers are located in the apical brush border membrane of the epithelial cells. These carriers have an overlapping specificity for different amino acids. One carrier preferentially transports neutral amino acids, another transports proline and hydroxyproline, a third preferentially transports acidic amino acids, and a fourth transports basic amino acids (lysine, arginine, the urea cycle intermediate ornithine) and cystine (two cysteine residues linked by a disulfide bond). In addition to these Na^+-dependent carriers, some amino acids are transported across the luminal membrane by facilitated transport carriers. Most amino acids are transported by more than one transport system.

As with glucose transport, the Na^+-dependent carriers of the apical membrane of the intestinal epithelial cells are also present in the renal epithelium. However, different isozymes are present in the cell membranes of other tissues. Conversely, the facilitated transport carriers in the serosal membrane of the intestinal epithelia are similar to those found in other cell types in the body. During starvation, the intestinal epithelia, like these other cells, take up amino acids from the blood to use as an energy source. Thus, amino acid transport across the serosal membrane is bidirectional.

Table 37.1. A Partial Listing of Amino Acid Transport Systems[a]

System Name	Sodium-dependent?	Specificity	Tissues Expressed
A	Yes	Small amino acids (ala, ser, gln)	Many
ASC	Yes	Small amino acids (ala, ser, cys)	Many
N	Yes	Gln, asn, his	Liver
L	No	Branched and aromatic amino acids	Many
$B^{0,+}$	Yes	Basic amino acids	Intestine (brush border)[b]
ATB^0	Yes	Zwitterionic amino acids (monoamino, monocarboxylic acid amino acids)	Intestine and kidney[c]
X_{AG}^-	Yes	Anionic amino acids	Intestine (brush border)
Imino	Yes	Pro, hypro, gly	Intestine (brush border)

[a] Not all transport systems are listed.
[b] This system is most likely defective in cystinuria.
[c] This system is most likely defective in Hartnup disease.

B. Transport of Amino Acids into Cells

Amino acids that enter the blood are transported across cell membranes of the various tissues principally by Na^+-dependent cotransporters and, to a lesser extent, by facilitated transporters (Table 37.1). In this respect, amino acid transport differs from glucose transport, which is Na^+-dependent transport in the intestinal and renal epithelium but facilitated transport in other cell types. The Na^+ dependence of amino acid transport in liver, muscle, and other tissues allows these cells to concentrate amino acids from the blood. These transport proteins have a different genetic basis, amino acid composition, and somewhat different specificity than those in the luminal membrane of intestinal epithelia. They also differ somewhat between tissues. For instance, the N system for glutamine uptake is present in the liver but either not present in other tissues or present as an isoform with different properties. There is also some overlap in specificity of the transport proteins, with most amino acids being transported by more than one carrier.

III. PROTEIN TURNOVER AND REPLENISHMENT OF THE INTRACELLULAR AMINO ACID POOL

The amino acid pool within cells is generated both from dietary amino acids and from the degradation of existing proteins within the cell. All proteins within cells have a half-life ($t_{1/2}$), a time at which 50% of the protein that was synthesized at a particular time will have been degraded. Some proteins are inherently short-lived, with half-lives of 5 to 20 minutes. Other proteins are present for extended periods, with half-lives of many hours, or even days. Thus, proteins are continuously being

Cal Kulis and other patients with cystinuria have a genetically determined defect in the transport of cystine and the basic amino acids, lysine, arginine, and ornithine, across the brush-border membranes of cells in both their small intestine and renal tubules. However, they do not appear to have any symptoms of amino acid deficiency, in part because the amino acids cysteine (which is oxidized in blood and urine to form the disulfide cystine) and arginine can be synthesized in the body (i.e., they are "nonessential" amino acids). Ornithine (an amino acid that is not found in proteins but serves as an intermediate of the urea cycle) can also be synthesized. The most serious problem for these patients is the insolubility of cystine, which can form kidney stones that may lodge in the ureter, causing bleeding and severe pain.

A: Patients with cystinuria and Hartnup disease have defective transport proteins in both the intestine and the kidney. These patients do not absorb the affected amino acids at a normal rate from the digestive products in the intestinal lumen. They also do not readily resorb these amino acids from the glomerular filtrate into the blood. Therefore, they do not have a hyperaminoacidemia (a high concentration in the blood). Normally, only a few percent of the amino acids that enter the glomerular filtrate are excreted in the urine; most are resorbed. In these diseases, much larger amounts of the affected amino acids are excreted in the urine, resulting in a hyperaminoaciduria.

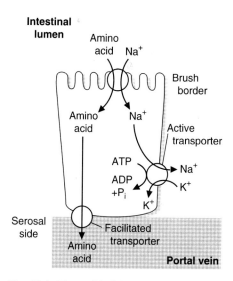

Fig. 37.4. Transepithelial amino acid transport. Na^+-dependent carriers transport both Na^+ and an amino acid into the intestinal epithelial cell from the intestinal lumen. Na^+ is pumped out on the serosal side (across the basolateral membrane) in exchange for K^+ by the Na^+,K^+-ATPase. On the serosal side, the amino acid is carried by a facilitated transporter down its concentration gradient into the blood. This process is an example of secondary active transport.

Protein turnover is quite extensive. For example, red blood cells have a lifespan of 120 days. Every day 3×10^{11} (300,000 million) red blood cells die and are phagocytosed. The hemoglobin in these cells is degraded to amino acids by lysosomal proteases, and these amino acids are reutilized. Approximately 6 lb hemoglobin is recycled in this way every year. As the aged cells are dying, newly generated reticulocytes are synthesizing hemoglobin in preparation for their conversion into new red blood cells, which replace the dying cells.

Adults cannot increase the amount of muscle or other body proteins by eating an excess amount of protein. If dietary protein is consumed in excess of our needs, it is converted to glycogen and triacylglycerols, which are then stored.

synthesized and degraded in the body, using a variety of enzyme systems to do so (Table 37.2). Examples of proteins that undergo extensive synthesis and degradation are hemoglobin, muscle proteins, digestive enzymes, and the proteins of cells sloughed off from the gastrointestinal tract. Hemoglobin is produced in reticulocytes and reconverted to amino acids by the phagocytic cells that remove mature red blood cells from the circulation on a daily basis. Muscle protein is degraded during periods of fasting, and the amino acids are used for gluconeogenesis. After ingestion of protein in the diet, muscle protein is resynthesized.

A large amount of protein is recycled daily in the form of digestive enzymes, which are themselves degraded by digestive proteases. In addition, approximately one fourth of the cells lining the walls of the gastrointestinal tract are lost each day and replaced by newly synthesized cells. As cells leave the gastrointestinal wall, their proteins and other components are digested by enzymes in the lumen of the gut, and the products are absorbed. Only approximately 6% (roughly 10 g) of the protein that enters the digestive tract (including dietary proteins, digestive enzymes, and the proteins in sloughed-off cells) is excreted in the feces each day. The remainder is recycled.

Proteins are also recycled within cells. The differences in amino acid composition of the various proteins of the body, the vast range in turnover times ($t_{1/2}$), and the recycling of amino acids are all important factors that help to determine the requirements for specific amino acids and total protein in the diet. The synthesis of many enzymes is induced in response to physiologic demand (such as fasting or feeding). These enzymes are continuously being degraded. Intracellular proteins are also damaged by oxidation and other modifications that limit their function. Mechanisms for intracellular degradation of unnecessary or damaged proteins involve lysosomes and the ubiquitin/proteasome system.

A. Lysosomal Protein Turnover

Lysosomes participate in the process of autophagy, in which intracellular components are surrounded by membranes that fuse with lysosomes, and endocytosis (see Chapter 10). Autophagy is a complex regulated process in which cytoplasm is sequestered into vesicles and delivered to the lysosomes. Within the lysosomes, the cathepsin family of proteases degrades the ingested proteins to individual amino acids. The recycled amino acids can then leave the lysosome and rejoin the intracellular amino acid pool. Although the details of how autophagy is induced are still not known, starvation of a cell is a trigger to induce this process. This will allow old proteins to be recycled and the newly released amino acids used for new protein synthesis, to enable the cell to survive starvation conditions.

Table 37.2. Proteases Involved in Protein Turnover/Degradation

Classification	Mechanism	Role
Cathepsins	Cysteine proteases	Lysosomal enzymes
Caspases	Cysteine proteases, which cleave after aspartate	Apoptosis; activated from pro-caspases (see Chapter 18)
Matrix metalloproteinases	Require zinc for catalysis	Model extracellular matrix components; regulated by TIMPs (tissue inhibitors of matrix metalloproteinases)
Proteasome	Large complex that degrades ubiquitin-tagged proteins	Protein turnover
Serine proteases	Active site serine in a catalytic triad with histidine and aspartic acid	Digestion and blood clotting; activated usually from zymogens (see Chapter 45)
Calpains	Calcium-dependent cysteine proteases	Many different cellular roles

B. The Ubiquitin-Proteasome Pathway

Ubiquitin is a small protein (76 amino acids) that is highly conserved. Its amino acid sequence in yeast and humans differs by only three residues. Ubiquitin targets intracellular proteins for degradation by covalently binding to the ϵ-amino group of lysine residues. This is accomplished by a three-enzyme system that adds ubiquitin to proteins targeted for degradation. Oftentimes, the target protein is polyubiquitinylated, in which additional ubiquitin molecules are added to previous ubiquitin molecules, forming a long ubiquitin tail on the target protein. After polyubiquitinylation is complete, the targeted protein is released from the three-enzyme complex.

A protease complex, known as the proteasome, then degrades the targeted protein, releasing intact ubiquitin that can again mark other proteins for degradation (Figure 37.5). The basic proteasome is a cylindrical 20S protein complex with multiple internal proteolytic sites. ATP hydrolysis is used both to unfold the tagged protein and to push the protein into the core of the cylinder. The complex is regulated by cap protein complexes, which bind the ubiquinylated protein (a step that requires ATP) and deliver them to the complex. After the target protein is degraded, the ubiquitin is released intact and recycled. The resultant amino acids join the intracellular pool of free amino acids. Different cap complexes alter the specificity of the proteasome. For example, the PA700 cap is required for ubiquinylated proteins, whereas the PA28 cap targets only short peptides to the complex.

Another protein modification, which occurs through a three-enzyme complex similar to that required for ubiquitin addition, is SUMOylation. SUMO stands for small ubiquitin-like modifier, and when proteins are tagged with SUMO their activites are altered (either positively or negatively, depending on the protein). SUMOylation presents yet another means of fine-tuning existing regulatory systems.

Many proteins that contain regions rich in the amino acids proline (P), glutamate (E), serine (S), and threonine (T) have short half-lives. These regions are known as PEST sequences, based on the one-letter abbreviations used for these amino acids. Most of the amino acids that contain PEST sequences are hydrolyzed by the ubiquitin-proteasome system.

CLINICAL COMMENTS

Sissy Fibrosa's growth and weight curves were both subnormal until her pediatrician added pancreatic enzyme supplements to her treatment plan. These supplements digest dietary protein, releasing essential and other amino acids from the dietary protein that are then absorbed by the endothelial cells of Sissy's small intestine, through which they are transported into the blood. A discernable improvement in Sissy's body weight and growth curves was noted within months of the start of this therapy.

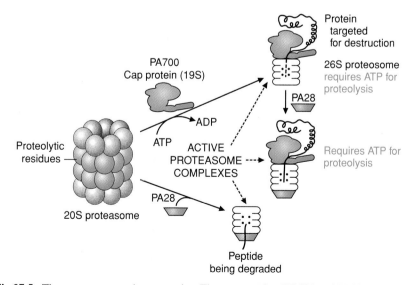

Fig 37.5. The proteasome and cap proteins. The cap proteins (PA700 and PA28) regulate the activity of this proteolytic complex by recruiting to the complex the substrates for proteolysis. The ATP requirement is to unfold and denature the proteins targeted for destruction, although the PA28 protease complex does not require ATP.

Apart from the proportions of essential amino acids present in various foods, the quality of a dietary protein is also determined by the rate at which it is digested and, in a more general way, by its capacity to contribute to the growth of the infant. In this regard, the proteins in foods of animal origin are more digestible than are those derived from plants. For example, the digestibility of proteins in eggs is approximately 97%; that for meats, poultry, and fish is 85 to 100%, and that from wheat, soybeans, and other legumes ranges from 75 to 90%.

The official daily dietary "protein requirement" accepted by the U.S. and Canadian governments is 0.8 g of protein per kilogram of desirable body weight for adults (approximately 56 g for an adult male and 44 g for an adult female). On an average weight basis, the requirement per kilogram is much greater for infants and children. This fact underscores the importance of improving **Sissy Fibrosa's** protein digestion to optimize her potential for normal growth and development.

In patients with cystinuria, such as **Cal Kulis**, the inability to normally absorb cystine and basic amino acids from the gut and the increased loss of these amino acids in the urine would be expected to cause a deficiency of these compounds in the blood. However, because three of these amino acids can be synthesized in the body (i.e., they are nonessential amino acids), their concentrations in the plasma remain normal, and clinical manifestations of a deficiency state do not develop. It is not clear why symptoms related to a lysine deficiency have not been observed.

In the disorder that was first observed in the Hartnup family and bears their name, the intestinal and renal transport defect involves the neutral amino acids (monoamine, monocarboxylic acids), including a number of the essential amino acids (isoleucine, leucine, phenylalanine, threonine, tryptophan, and valine) as well as certain nonessential amino acids (alanine, serine, and tyrosine). A reduction in the availability of these essential amino acids would be expected to cause a variety of clinical disorders. Yet children with the Hartnup disorder identified by routine newborn urine screening almost always remain clinically normal.

However, some patients with the Hartnup biochemical phenotype eventually develop pellagra-like manifestations, which usually include a photosensitivity rash, ataxia, and neuropsychiatric symptoms. Pellagra results from a dietary deficiency of the vitamin niacin or the essential amino acid tryptophan, which are both precursors for the nicotinamide moiety of NAD and NADP. In asymptomatic patients, the transport abnormality may be incomplete and so subtle as to allow no phenotypic expression of Hartnup disease. These patients also may be capable of absorbing some small peptides that contain the neutral amino acids.

The only rational treatment of patients having pellagra-like symptoms is the administration of niacin (nicotinic acid) in oral doses up to 300 mg/day. Although the rash, ataxia, and neuropsychiatric manifestations of niacin deficiency may disappear, the hyperaminoaciduria and intestinal transport defect do not respond to this therapy. In addition to niacin, a high-protein diet may benefit some patients.

BIOCHEMICAL COMMENTS

The γ-glutamyl cycle is necessary for the synthesis of glutathione, a compound that protects cells from oxidative damage (see Chapter 24). When originally discovered, the cycle was thought to be important in amino acid transport, but its involvement in such transport is now thought to be limited to salvage of cysteine. The enzymes of the cycle are present in many tissues, although certain tissues lack one or more of the enzymes of the cycle.

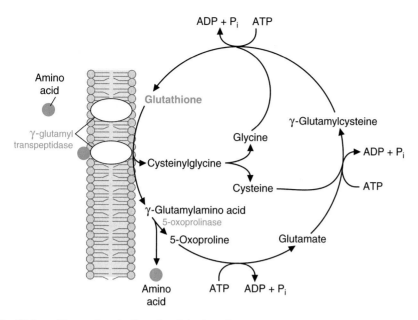

Fig. 37.6. γ-Glutamyl cycle. In cells of the intestine and kidney, amino acids can be transported across the cell membrane by reacting with glutathione (γ-glutamyl-cysteinyl-glycine) to form a γ-glutamyl amino acid. The amino acid is released into the cell, and glutathione is resynthesized. However, the major role of this cycle is glutathione synthesis, and many tissues lack the transpeptidase and 5-oxo-prolinase activities.

The entire cycle is presented in Figure 37.6. In this case, the extracellular amino acid reacts with glutathione (γ-glutamyl-cysteinyl-glycine) in a reaction catalyzed by a transpeptidase present in the cell membrane. A γ-glutamyl amino acid is formed, which travels across the cell membrane and releases the amino acid into the cell. The other products of these two reactions are reconverted to glutathione.

The reactions converting glutamate to glutathione in the γ-glutamyl cycle are the same reactions required for the synthesis of glutathione. The enzymes for glutathione synthesis, but not the transpeptidase, are found in most tissues. The oxoprolinase is also missing from many tissues, such that the major role of this pathway is one of glutathione synthesis from glutamate, cysteine, and glycine. The transpeptidase is the only protease in the cell that can break the γ-glutamyl linkage in glutathione. Glutathione is also involved in reducing compounds such as hydrogen peroxide (see Chapter 21). It also protects cells, in particular erythrocytes, from oxidative damage, through formation of oxidized glutathione, two glutathione residues connected by a disulfide bond.

Suggested References

Argiles JF, Lopez-Soriano FJ. Intestinal amino acid transport: an overview. Int J Biochem 1990;22:931–939.

Christensen HN. Role of amino acid transport and countertransport in nutrition and metabolism. Physiol Rev 1990;70:43–77.

Demartino GN, Slaughter CA. The proteasome, a novel protease regulated by multiple mechanisms. J Biol Chem 1999;274:22123–22126.

Larrson A, Anderson ME. Glutathione synthetase deficiency and other disorders of the γ-glutamyl cycle. In: Scriver CR, Beaudet AL, Valle D, Sly WS, et al., eds. The Metabolic and Molecular Bases of Inherited Disease, vol II, 8th Ed. New York: McGraw-Hill, 2001:2205–2216.

Palacin M, Estevez R, Bertran J, Zorzano A. Molecular biology of mammalian plasma membrane amino acid transporters. Physiol Rev 1998;78:969–1054.

REVIEW QUESTIONS—CHAPTER 37

1. An individual with a deficiency in the conversion of trypsinogen to trypsin would be expected to experience a more detrimental effect on protein digestion than an individual who was defective in any of the other digestive proteases. This is due to which of the following?

    (A) Trypsin has a greater and wider range of substrates to act on.
    (B) Trypsin activates pepsinogen, so digestion can begin in the stomach.
    (C) Trypsin activates the other zymogens that are secreted by the pancreas.
    (D) Trypsin activates enteropeptidase, which is needed to activate the other pancreatic zymogens.
    (E) Trypsin inhibits intestinal motility, so the substrates can be hydrolyzed for longer periods.

2. An individual has been shown to have a deficiency in an intestinal epithelial cell amino acid transport system for leucine. However, the individual shows no symptoms of amino acid deficiency. This could be due to which of the following?

    (A) The body synthesizes leucine to compensate for the transport defect.
    (B) The kidney reabsorbs leucine and sends it to other tissues.
    (C) There are multiple transport systems for leucine.
    (D) Isoleucine takes the place of leucine in proteins.
    (E) Leucine is not necessary for bulk protein synthesis.

3. Kwashiorkor can result from which of the following?

    (A) Consuming a calorie-deficient diet that is also deficient in protein
    (B) Consuming a calorie-adequate diet that is deficient in carbohydrates
    (C) Consuming a calorie-adequate diet that is deficient in fatty acids
    (D) Consuming a calorie-adequate diet that is deficient in proteins
    (E) Consuming a calorie-deficient diet that is primarily proteins

4. Which of the following enzymes is activated through an autocatalytic process?

    (A) Enteropeptidase
    (B) Trypsinogen
    (C) Pepsinogen
    (D) Aminopeptidase
    (E) Proelastase

5. Children with kwashiorkor usually have a fatty liver. This is due to which of the following?

    (A) The high fat content of their diet
    (B) The high carbohydrate content of their diet
    (C) The high protein content of their diet
    (D) The lack of substrates for gluconeogenesis in the liver
    (E) The lack of substrates for protein synthesis in the liver
    (F) The lack of substrates for glycogen synthesis in the liver

38 Fate of Amino Acid Nitrogen: Urea Cycle

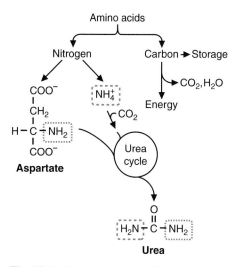

Fig 38.1. Fate of amino acid carbons and nitrogen. Amino acid carbon can be used either for energy storage (glycogen, fatty acids) or for energy. Amino acid nitrogen is used for urea synthesis. One nitrogen of urea comes from NH_4^+, the other from aspartate.

*In comparison with carbohydrate and lipid metabolism, the metabolism of amino acids is complex. We must be concerned not only with the fate of the carbon atoms of the amino acids but also with the fate of the **nitrogen**. During their metabolism, amino acids travel in the blood from one tissue to another. Ultimately, most of the nitrogen is converted to **urea** in the **liver** and the carbons are oxidized to CO_2 and H_2O by a number of tissues (Fig. 38.1).*

After a meal that contains protein, amino acids released by digestion (see Chapter 37) pass from the gut through the hepatic portal vein to the liver (see Fig. 38.2A). In a normal diet containing 60 to 100 g protein, most of the amino acids are used for the synthesis of proteins in the liver and in other tissues. Excess amino acids may be converted to glucose or triacylglycerol.

*During fasting, muscle protein is cleaved to amino acids. Some of the amino acids are partially oxidized to produce energy (see Fig. 38.2B). Portions of these amino acids are converted to **alanine** and **glutamine**, which, along with other amino acids, are released into the blood. Glutamine is oxidized by various tissues, including the **lymphocytes**, **gut**, and **kidney**, which convert some of the carbons and nitrogen to alanine. Alanine and other amino acids travel to the liver, where the carbons are converted to glucose and ketone bodies and the nitrogen is converted to urea, which is excreted by the kidneys. Glucose, produced by gluconeogenesis, is subsequently oxidized to CO_2 and H_2O by many tissues, and ketone bodies are oxidized by tissues such as muscle and kidney.*

*Several enzymes are important in the process of interconverting amino acids and in removing nitrogen so that the carbon skeletons can be oxidized. These include **dehydratases**, **transaminases**, **glutamate dehydrogenase**, **glutaminase**, and **deaminases**.*

*The conversion of amino acid nitrogen to urea occurs mainly in the liver. Urea is formed in the urea cycle from NH_4^+, bicarbonate, and the nitrogen of **aspartate** (see Fig. 38.1). Initially, NH_4^+, bicarbonate, and ATP react to produce **carbamoyl phosphate**, which reacts with **ornithine** to form **citrulline**. Aspartate then reacts with citrulline to form **argininosuccinate**, which releases **fumarate**, forming **arginine**. Finally, **arginase** cleaves arginine to release urea and regenerate ornithine. The cycle is regulated in a **feed-forward** manner, such that when amino acid degradation is occurring, the rate of the cycle is increased.*

THE WAITING ROOM

Percy Veere and his high school friend decided to take a Caribbean cruise, during which they sampled the cuisine of many of the islands on their itinerary. One month after their return to the United States, Percy complained of

697

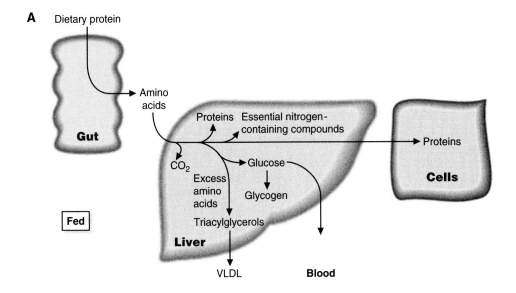

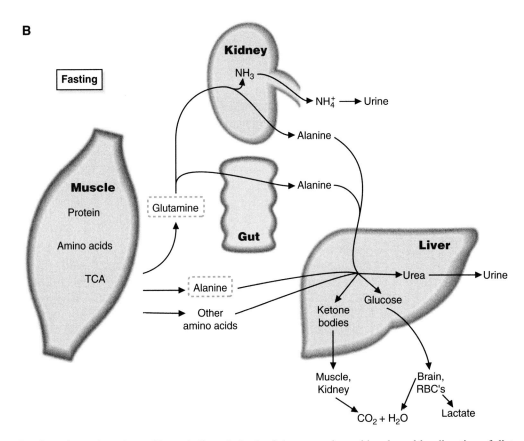

Fig 38.2. Roles of various tissues in amino acid metabolism. A. In the fed state, amino acids released by digestion of dietary proteins travel through the hepatic portal vein to the liver, where they are used for the synthesis of proteins, particularly the blood proteins, such as serum albumin. Excess amino acids are converted to glucose or to triacylglycerols. The latter are then packaged and secreted in VLDL. The glucose produced from amino acids in the fed state is stored as glycogen or released into the blood if blood glucose levels are low. Amino acids that pass through the liver are converted to proteins in cells of other tissues. B. During fasting, amino acids are released from muscle protein. Some enter the blood directly. Others are partially oxidized and the nitrogen stored in the form of alanine and glutamine, which enter the blood. In the kidney, glutamine releases ammonia into the urine and is converted to alanine and serine. In the cells of the gut, glutamine is converted to alanine. Alanine (the major gluconeogenic amino acid) and other amino acids enter the liver, where their nitrogen is converted to urea, which is excreted in the urine, and their carbons to glucose and ketone bodies, which are oxidized by various tissues for energy.

severe malaise, loss of appetite, nausea, vomiting, and arthralgias (joint pains). He had a low-grade fever and noted a persistent and increasing pain in the area of his liver. His friend noted a yellow discoloration of the whites of Percy's eyes and skin. Percy's urine turned the color of iced tea, and his stool became a light-clay color. His doctor found his liver to be enlarged and tender. Liver function tests were ordered.

Serologic testing for viral hepatitis type B, C, and D were nonreactive, but fecal studies showed "shedding" of hepatitis virus type A. Tests for antibodies to antigens of the hepatitis A virus (anti-HAV) in the serum were positive for the immunoglobulin M type.

A diagnosis of acute viral hepatitis type A was made, probably contracted from virus-contaminated food Percy had eaten while on his cruise. His physician explained that there was no specific treatment for type A viral hepatitis but recommended symptomatic and supportive care and prevention of transmission to others by the fecal–oral route. Percy took acetaminophen 3 to 4 times a day for fever and arthralgias throughout his illness.

I. FATE OF AMINO ACID NITROGEN

A. Transamination Reactions

Transamination is the major process for removing nitrogen from amino acids. In most instances, the nitrogen is transferred as an amino group from the original amino acid to α-ketoglutarate, forming glutamate, whereas the original amino acid is converted to its corresponding α-keto acid (Fig. 38.3). For example, the amino acid aspartate can be transaminated to form its corresponding α-keto acid, oxaloacetate. In the process, the amino group is transferred to α-ketoglutarate, which is converted to its corresponding amino acid, glutamate.

All amino acids except lysine and threonine undergo transamination reactions. The enzymes catalyzing these reactions are known as transaminases or aminotransferases. For most of these reactions, α-ketoglutarate and glutamate serve as one of the α-keto acid–amino acid pairs. Pyridoxal phosphate is the cofactor, and the mechanism of the reaction is indicated in Figure 38.4.

Overall, in a transamination reaction, an amino group from one amino acid becomes the amino group of a second amino acid. Because these reactions are readily reversible, they can be used to remove nitrogen from amino acids or to transfer nitrogen to α-keto acids to form amino acids. Thus, they are involved both in amino acid degradation and in amino acid synthesis.

B. Removal of Amino Acid Nitrogen as Ammonia

Cells in the body and bacteria in the gut release the nitrogen of certain amino acids as ammonia or ammonium ion (NH_4^+) (Fig. 38.5). Because these two forms of nitrogen can be interconverted, the terms are sometimes used interchangeably. Ammonium ion releases a proton to form ammonia by a reaction with a pK of 9.3 (Fig. 38.6). Therefore, at physiologic pH, the equilibrium favors NH_4^+ by a factor of approximately 100/1 (see Chapter 4, the Henderson-Hasselbalch equation). However, it is important to note that NH_3 is also present in the body, because this is the form that can cross cell membranes. For example, NH_3 passes into the urine from kidney tubule cells and decreases the acidity of the urine by binding protons, forming NH_4^+. Once the NH_4^+ is formed, the compound can no longer freely diffuse across membranes.

Glutamate can be oxidatively deaminated by a reaction catalyzed by glutamate dehydrogenase that produces ammonium ion and α-ketoglutarate (Fig. 38.7). Either NAD^+ or $NADP^+$ can serve as the cofactor. This reaction, which occurs in the mitochondria of most cells, is readily reversible; it can incorporate ammonia

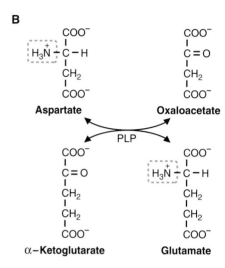

Fig. 38.3. Transamination. The amino group from one amino acid is transferred to another. Pairs of amino acids and their corresponding α-keto acids are involved in these reactions. α-ketoglutarate and glutamate are usually one of the pairs. The reactions, which are readily reversible, use pyridoxal phosphate (PLP) as a cofactor. The enzymes are called transaminases or aminotransferases. A. A generalized reaction. B. The aspartate transaminase reaction.

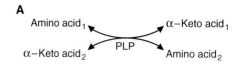

Whereas pyridoxal phosphate is used primarily for reactions involving amino acids, it is also required for the glycogen phosphorylase reaction, in which it acts as a general acid/base catalyst.

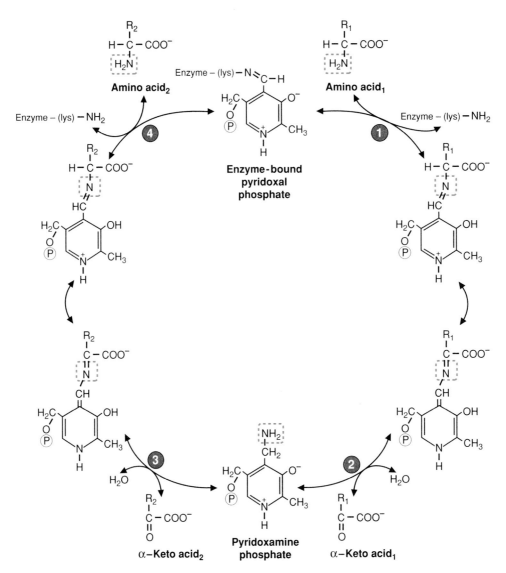

Fig. 38.4. Function of pyridoxal phosphate (PLP) in transamination reactions. The order in which the reactions occur is 1 to 4. Pyridoxal phosphate (enzyme-bound) reacts with amino acid₁, forming a Schiff base (a carbon–nitrogen double bond). After a shift of the double bond, α-keto acid₁ is released through hydrolysis of the Schiff base, and pyridoxamine phosphate is produced. Pyridoxamine phosphate then forms a Schiff base with α-keto acid₂. After the double bond shifts, amino acid₂ is released through hydrolysis of the Schiff base and enzyme-bound pyridoxal phosphate is regenerated. The net result is that the amino group from amino acid₁ is transferred to amino acid₂.

Glutamate dehydrogenase is one of three mammalian enzymes that can "fix" ammonia into organic molecules. The other two are glutamine synthetase and carbamoyl phosphate synthetase I.

into glutamate or release ammonia from glutamate. Glutamate can collect nitrogen from other amino acids as a consequence of transmination reactions and then release ammonia through the glutamate dehydrogenase reaction. This process provides one source of the ammonia that enters the urea cycle.

In addition to glutamate, a number of amino acids release their nitrogen as NH_4^+ (see Fig. 38.5). Histidine may be directly deaminated to form NH_4^+ and urocanate. The deaminations of serine and threonine are dehydration reactions that require pyridoxal phosphate and are catalyzed by serine dehydratase. Serine forms pyruvate, and threonine forms α-ketobutyrate. In both cases, NH_4^+ is released.

Glutamine and asparagine contain R group amides that may be released as NH_4^+ by deamidation. Asparagine is deamidated by asparaginase, yielding aspartate and NH_4^+. Glutaminase acts on glutamine, forming glutamate and NH_4^+. The glutaminase

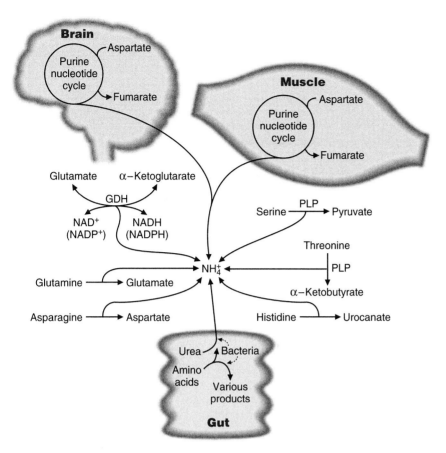

Fig. 38.5. Summary of the sources of NH_4^+ for the urea cycle. All of the reactions are irreversible except glutamate dehydrogenase (GDH). Only the dehydratase reactions, which produce NH_4^+ from serine and threonine, require pyridoxal phosphate as a cofactor. The reactions that are not shown occurring in the muscle or the gut can all occur in the liver, where the NH_4^+ generated can be converted to urea. The purine nucleotide cycle of the brain and muscle is further described in Chapter 41.

reaction is particularly important in the kidney, where the ammonium ion produced is excreted directly into the urine, where it forms salts with metabolic acids, facilitating their removal in the urine.

In muscle and brain, but not in liver, the purine nucleotide cycle allows NH_4^+ to be released from amino acids (see Fig. 38.5). Nitrogen is collected by glutamate from other amino acids by means of transamination reactions. Glutamate then transfers its amino group to oxaloacetate to form aspartate, which supplies nitrogen to the purine nucleotide cycle (see Chapter 41). The reactions of the cycle release fumarate and NH_4^+. The ammonium ion formed can leave the muscle in the form of glutamine.

Fig. 38.7. Reaction catalyzed by glutamate dehydrogenase. This reaction is readily reversible and can use either NAD^+ or $NADP^+$ as a cofactor. The oxygen on α-ketoglutarate is derived from H_2O.

Glutamate α-**Ketoglutarate**

Percy Veere's laboratory studies showed that his serum alanine transaminase (ALT) level was 294 units/L (reference range = 5–30), and his serum aspartate transaminase (AST) level was 268 units/L (reference range = 10–30). His serum alkaline phosphatase level was 284 units/L (reference range for an adult male = 40–125), and his serum total bilirubin was 9.6 mg/dL (reference range = 0.2–1.0). Bilirubin is a degradation product of heme, as described in Chapter 44.

Cellular enzymes such as AST, ALT, and alkaline phosphatase leak into the blood through the membranes of hepatic cells that have been damaged as a result of the inflammatory process. In acute viral hepatitis, the serum ALT level is often elevated to a greater extent than the serum AST level. Alkaline phosphatase, which is present on membranes between liver cells and the bile duct, is also elevated in the blood in acute viral hepatitis.

The rise in serum total bilirubin occurs as a result of the inability of the infected liver to conjugate bilirubin and of a partial or complete occlusion of the hepatic biliary drainage ducts caused by inflammatory swelling within the liver. In fulminant hepatic failure, the serum bilirubin level may exceed 20 mg/dL, a poor prognostic sign.

$$NH_4^+ \rightleftharpoons NH_3 + H^+$$
$$pK = 9.3$$

Fig. 38.6. Formation of ammonia from ammonium ion. Because the pK is 9.3, at physiologic pH, the concentration of NH_4^+ is almost 100 times that of NH_3.

Vitamin B_6 deficiency symptoms include dermatitis, a microcytic, hypochromic anemia, weakness, irritability, and, in some cases, convulsions. Xanthurenic acid (a degradation product of tryptophan) and other compounds appear in the urine because of an inability to completely metabolize amino acids. A decreased ability to synthesize heme from glycine may cause the microcytic anemia (see Chapter 44), and decreased decarboxylation of amino acids to form neurotransmitters (see Chapter 48) may explain the convulsions.

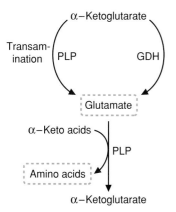

Fig. 38.8. Role of glutamate in amino acid synthesis. Glutamate transfers nitrogen by means of transamination reactions to α-keto acids to form amino acids. This nitrogen is either obtained by glutamate from transamination of other amino acids or from NH_4^+ by means of the glutamate dehydrogenase (GDH) reaction. PLP = pyridoxal phosphate.

Pyridoxal phosphate is derived from pyridoxine (vitamin B_6). Pyridoxal phosphate is the cofactor not only for transamination reactions but also for decarboxylations and a number of other reactions involving amino acids.

Pyridoxine (Vitamin B_6)

NAD^+
$NADH + H^+$

Pyridoxaldehyde

ATP
ADP

Pyridoxal phosphate (PLP)

In summary, NH_4^+ that enters the urea cycle is produced in the body by deamination or deamidation of amino acids (see Fig. 38.5). A significant amount of NH_4^+ is also produced by bacteria that live in the lumen of the intestinal tract. This ammonium ion enters the hepatic portal vein and travels to the liver.

C. Role of Glutamate in the Metabolism of Amino Acid Nitrogen

Glutamate plays a pivotal role in the metabolism of amino acids. It is involved in both synthesis and degradation.

Glutamate provides nitrogen for amino acid synthesis (Fig. 38.8). In this process, glutamate obtains its nitrogen either from other amino acids by transamination reactions or from NH_4^+ by the glutamate dehydrogenase reaction. Transamination reactions then serve to transfer amino groups from glutamate to α-keto acids to produce their corresponding amino acids.

When amino acids are degraded and urea is formed, glutamate collects nitrogen from other amino acids by transamination reactions. Some of this nitrogen is released as ammonia by the glutamate dehydrogenase reaction, but much larger amounts of ammonia are produced from the other sources shown in Figure 38.5. NH_4^+ is one of the two forms in which nitrogen enters the urea cycle (Fig. 38.9).

The second form of nitrogen for urea synthesis is provided by aspartate (see Fig. 38.9). Glutamate can be the source of the nitrogen. Glutamate transfers its amino group to oxaloacetate, and aspartate and α-ketoglutarate are formed.

D. Role of Alanine and Glutamine in Transporting Amino Acid Nitrogen to the Liver

Protein turnover and amino acid degradation occur in all tissues; however, the urea cycle enzymes are primarily active in the liver (the intestine expresses low levels of activity of these enzymes; see Chapter 42). Thus, a mechanism needs to be in place to transport amino acid nitrogen to the liver. Alanine and glutamine are the major carriers of nitrogen in the blood. Alanine is primarily exported by the muscle. Because the muscle is metabolizing glucose through glycolysis, pyruvate is available in the muscle. The pyruvate is transaminated by glutamate to form alanine, which travels to the liver (Fig. 38.10). The glutamate is formed by transamination of an amino acid that is being degraded. On arriving at the liver, alanine is transaminated to pyruvate, and the nitrogen will be used for urea synthesis. The pyruvate formed is used for gluconeogenesis and the glucose exported to the muscle for use as energy. This cycle of moving carbons and nitrogen between the muscle and liver is known as the glucose/alanine cycle.

Compounds that contain "glut" in their name have five carbons in a straight chain. At each end of the chain, the carbon is part of a carboxyl group. In glutamine, the carboxyl group has formed an amide, and in hydroxymethylglutaryl CoA (HMG-CoA), it has formed a thioester with coenzyme A.

Glutamine

Glutamate

α-Ketoglutarate

Hydroxymethyl-glutaryl CoA (HMG CoA)

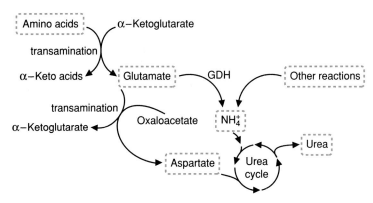

Fig. 38.9. Role of glutamate in urea production. Glutamate collects nitrogen from other amino acids by transamination reactions. This nitrogen can be released as NH_4^+ by glutamate dehydrogenase (GDH). NH_4^+ is also produced by other reactions (see Fig. 38.5). NH_4^+ provides one of the nitrogens for urea synthesis. The other nitrogen comes from aspartate and is obtained from glutamate by transamination of oxaloacetate.

Glutamine is synthesized from glutamate by the fixation of ammonia, requiring energy (adenosine triphosphate [ATP]) and the enzyme glutamine synthetase (Fig. 38.11), which is a cytoplasmic enzyme found in all cells. Under conditions of rapid amino acid degradation within a tissue, such that ammonia levels increase, the glutamate that has been formed from transamination reactions will accept another nitrogen molecule to form glutamine. The glutamine travels to the liver, kidney, or intestines, where glutaminase (see Fig. 38.11) will remove the amide nitrogen to form glutamate plus ammonia. In the kidney, the release of ammonia, and the formation of ammonium ion, serves to form salts with metabolic acids in the urine. In the intestine, the glutamine is used as a fuel (see Chapter 42). In the liver, the ammonia is used for urea biosynthesis.

Glutamine synthetase in liver is located in cells surrounding the portal vein. Its major role is to convert any ammonia that has escaped from urea production into glutamine, such that free ammonia does not leave the liver and enter the circulation.

II. UREA CYCLE

The normal human adult is in nitrogen balance; that is, the amount of nitrogen ingested each day, mainly in the form of dietary protein, is equal to the amount of nitrogen excreted. The major nitrogenous excretory product is urea, which exits from the body in the urine. This innocuous compound, produced mainly in the liver by the urea cycle, serves as the disposal form of ammonia, which is toxic, particularly to the brain and central nervous system. Normally, little ammonia (or NH_4^+) is present in the blood. The concentration ranges between

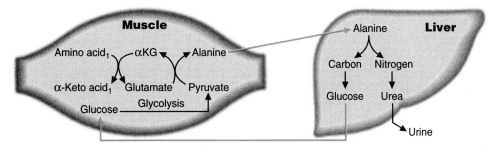

Fig. 38.10. The glucose/alanine cycle. Within the muscle, amino acid degradation leads to the transfer of nitrogens to α-ketoglutarate and pyruvate. The alanine formed travels to the liver, where the carbons of alanine are used for gluconeogenesis and the alanine nitrogen is used for urea biosynthesis. This could occur during exercise, when the muscle uses blood-borne glucose (see Chapter 47).

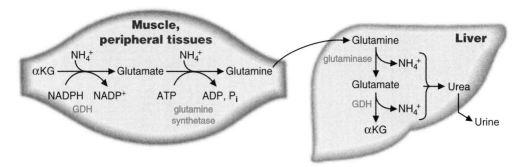

Fig. 38.11. Synthesis of glutamine in peripheral tissues and its transport to the liver. Within the liver, glutaminase converts glutamine to glutamate. Note how α-ketoglutarate can accept two molecules of ammonia to form glutamine. GDH = glutamate dehydrogenase.

Percy Veere's symptoms and laboratory abnormalities did not slowly subside over the next 6 weeks as they usually do in uncomplicated viral hepatitis A infections. Instead, his serum total bilirubin, ALT, AST, and alkaline phosphatase levels increased further. His vomiting became intractable, and his friend noted jerking motions of his arms (asterixis), facial grimacing, restlessness, slowed mentation, and slight disorientation. He was admitted to the hospital with a diagnosis of hepatic failure with incipient hepatic encephalopathy (brain dysfunction caused by accumulation of various toxins in the blood), a rare complication of acute type A viral hepatitis alone. The possibility of a superimposed acute hepatic toxicity caused by the use of acetaminophen was considered.

When ornithine transcarbamoylase (OTC) is deficient, the carbamoyl phosphate that normally would enter the urea cycle accumulates and floods the pathway for pyrimidine biosynthesis. Under these conditions, excess orotic acid (orotate), an intermediate in pyrimidine biosynthesis, is excreted in the urine. It produces no ill effects but is indicative of a problem in the urea cycle.

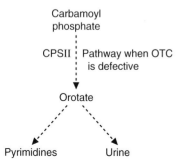

30 and 60 μM. Ammonia is rapidly removed from the blood and converted to urea by the liver. Nitrogen travels in the blood mainly in amino acids, particularly alanine and glutamine.

A. Reactions of the Urea Cycle

Nitrogen enters the urea cycle as NH_4^+ and aspartate (Fig. 38.12). NH_4^+ forms carbamoyl phosphate, which reacts with ornithine to form citrulline. Ornithine is the compound that both initiates and is regenerated by the cycle (similar to oxaloacetate in the TCA cycle). Aspartate reacts with citrulline, eventually donating its nitrogen for urea formation. Arginine is formed in two successive steps. Cleavage of arginine by arginase releases urea and regenerates ornithine.

1. SYNTHESIS OF CARBAMOYL PHOSPHATE

In the first step of the urea cycle, NH_4^+, bicarbonate, and ATP react to form carbamoyl phosphate (see Fig. 38.12). The cleavage of 2 ATPs is required to form the high-energy phosphate bond of carbamoyl phosphate. Carbamoyl phosphate synthetase I (CPSI), the enzyme that catalyzes this first step of the urea cycle, is found mainly in mitochondria of the liver and intestine. The Roman numeral suggests that another carbamoyl phosphate synthetase exists, and indeed, CPSII, located in the cytosol, produces carbamoyl phosphate for pyrimidine biosynthesis, using nitrogen from glutamine (see Chapter 41).

2. PRODUCTION OF ARGININE BY THE UREA CYCLE

Carbamoyl phosphate reacts with ornithine to form citrulline (see Fig. 38.12). The high- energy phosphate bond of carbamoyl phosphate provides the energy required for this reaction, which occurs in mitochondria and is catalyzed by ornithine transcarbamoylase. The product citrulline is transported across the mitochondrial membranes in exchange for cytoplasmic ornithine and enters the cytosol. The carrier for this transport reaction catalyzes an electroneutral exchange of the two compounds.

In the cytosol, citrulline reacts with aspartate, the second source of nitrogen for urea synthesis, to produce argininosuccinate (see Fig. 38.12). This reaction, catalyzed by argininosuccinate synthetase, is driven by the hydrolysis of ATP to adenosine monophosphate (AMP) and pyrophosphate. Aspartate is produced by transamination of oxaloacetate.

The urea cycle was proposed in 1932 by Hans Krebs and a medical student, Kurt Henseleit, based on their laboratory observations. It was originally called the Krebs-Henseleit cycle. Subsequently, Krebs used this concept of metabolic cycling to explain a second process that also bears his name, the Krebs (or TCA) cycle.

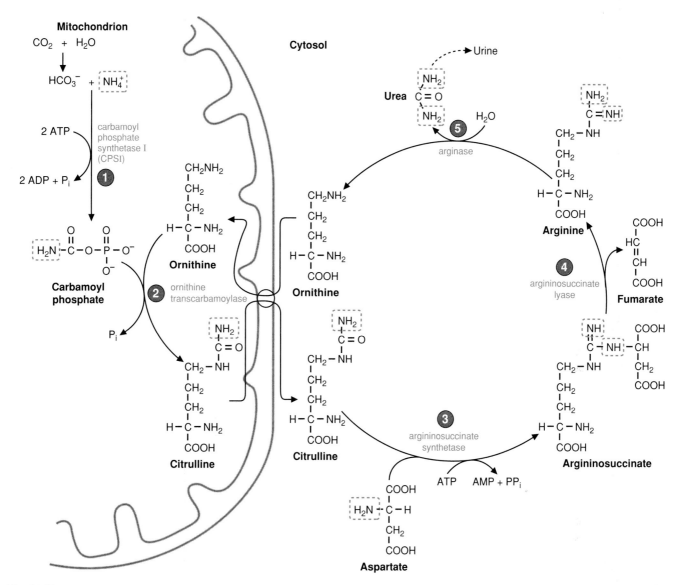

Fig. 38.12. Urea cycle. The steps of the cycle are numbered 1 to 5.

Argininosuccinate is cleaved by argininosuccinate lyase to form fumarate and arginine (see Fig. 38.12). Fumarate is produced from the carbons of argininosuccinate provided by aspartate. Fumarate is converted to malate (using cytoplasmic fumarase), which is used either for the synthesis of glucose by the gluconeogenic pathway or for the regeneration of oxaloacetate by cytoplasmic reactions similar to those observed in the TCA cycle (Fig. 38.13). The oxaloacetate that is formed is transaminated to generate the aspartate that carries nitrogen into the urea cycle. Thus, the carbons of fumarate can be recycled to aspartate.

3. CLEAVAGE OF ARGININE TO PRODUCE UREA

Arginine, which contains nitrogens derived from NH_4^+ and aspartate, is cleaved by arginase, producing urea and regenerating ornithine (see Fig. 38.12). Urea is produced from the guanidinium group on the side chain of arginine. The portion of arginine originally derived from ornithine is reconverted to ornithine.

The reactions by which citrulline is converted to arginine and arginine is cleaved to produce urea occur in the cytosol. Ornithine, the other product of the arginase

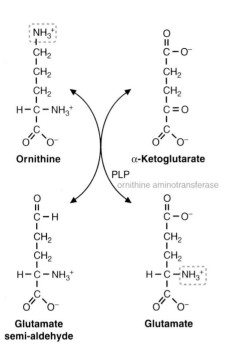

Fig. 38.14. The ornithine aminotransferase reaction. This is a reversible reaction dependent on pyridoxal phosphate, which normally favors ornithine degradation.

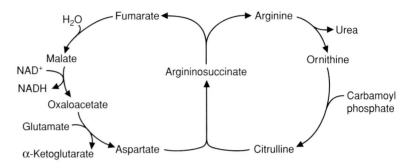

Fig. 38.13. The Krebs bicycle, indicating the common steps between the TCA and urea cycles. All reactions shown occur in the cytoplasm except for the synthesis of citrulline, which occurs within the mitochondria.

reaction, is transported into the mitochondrion in exchange for citrulline, where it can react with carbamoyl phosphate, initiating another round of the cycle.

B. Origin of Ornithine

Ornithine is an amino acid. However, it is not incorporated into proteins during the process of protein synthesis because no genetic codon exists for this amino acid. Although ornithine is normally regenerated by the urea cycle (one of the products of the arginase reaction), ornithine also can be synthesized de novo if needed. The reaction is an unusual transamination reaction catalyzed by ornithine aminotransferase under specific conditions in the intestine (Fig. 38.14). The usual direction of this reaction is the formation of glutamate semialdehyde, which is the first step of the degradation pathway for ornithine.

C. Regulation of the Urea Cycle

The human liver has a vast capacity to convert amino acid nitrogen to urea, thereby preventing toxic effects from ammonia, which would otherwise accumulate. In general, the urea cycle is regulated by substrate availability; the higher the rate of ammonia production, the higher the rate of urea formation. Regulation by substrate availability is a general characteristic of disposal pathways, such as the urea cycle, which remove toxic compounds from the body. This is a type of "feed-forward" regulation, in contrast to the "feedback" regulation characteristic of pathways that produce functional endproducts.

Two other types of regulation control the urea cycle: allosteric activation of CPSI by *N*-acetylglutamate (NAG) and induction/repression of the synthesis of urea cycle enzymes. NAG is formed specifically to activate CPSI; it has no other known function in mammals. The synthesis of NAG from acetyl CoA and glutamate is stimulated by arginine (Fig. 38.15). Thus, as arginine levels increase within the liver, two important reactions are stimulated. The first is the synthesis of NAG, which will increase the rate at which carbamoyl phosphate is produced. The second is to produce more ornithine (via the arginase reaction), such that the cycle can operate more rapidly.

The induction of urea cycle enzymes occurs in response to conditions that require increased protein metabolism, such as a high-protein diet or prolonged fasting. In both of these physiologic states, as amino acid carbon is converted to glucose, amino acid nitrogen is converted to urea. The induction of the synthesis of urea cycle enzymes under these conditions occurs even though the uninduced enzyme levels are far in excess of the capacity required. The ability of a high-protein diet to increase urea cycle enzyme levels is another type of "feed-forward" regulation.

The precise pathogenesis of the central nervous system (CNS) signs and symptoms that accompany liver failure (hepatic encephalopathy) in patients such as **Percy Veere** is not completely understood. These changes are, however, attributable in part to toxic materials that are derived from the metabolism of nitrogenous substrates by bacteria in the gut that circulate to the liver in the portal vein. These materials "bypass" their normal metabolism by the liver cells, however, because the acute inflammatory process of viral hepatitis severely limits the ability of liver cells to degrade these compounds to harmless metabolites. As a result, these toxins are "shunted" into the hepatic veins unaltered and eventually reach the brain through the systemic circulation ("portal-systemic encephalopathy").

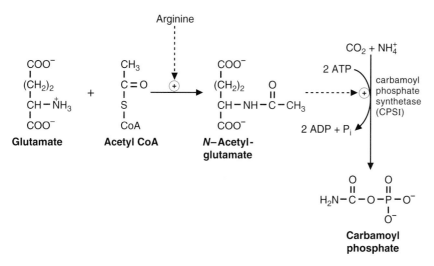

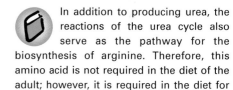

Fig. 38.15. Activation of carbamoyl phosphate synthetase I (CPSI). Arginine stimulates the synthesis of *N*-acetylglutamate, which activates CPSI.

D. Function of the Urea Cycle during Fasting

During fasting, the liver maintains blood glucose levels. Amino acids from muscle protein are a major carbon source for the production of glucose by the pathway of gluconeogenesis. As amino acid carbons are converted to glucose, the nitrogens are converted to urea. Thus, the urinary excretion of urea is high during fasting (Fig. 38.16). As fasting progresses, however, the brain begins to use ketone bodies, sparing blood glucose. Less muscle protein is cleaved to provide amino acids for gluconeogenesis, and decreased production of glucose from amino acids is accompanied by decreased production of urea (see Chapter 31).

The major amino acid substrate for gluconeogenesis is alanine, which is synthesized in peripheral tissues to act as a nitrogen carrier (see Fig. 38.10). Glucagon release, which is expected during fasting, stimulates alanine transport

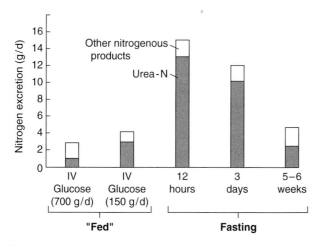

Fig. 38.16. Nitrogen excretion during fasting. Human subjects were initially given intravenous (IV) glucose as indicated, then fasted. Total nitrogen excretion was measured as well as the nitrogen in urea (dark area). Based on Ruderman NB, et al. Gluconeogenesis and its disorders in man. In: Hanson RW, Mehlman MA, eds. Gluconeogenesis: Its Regulation in Mammalian Species. New York: John Wiley, 1976:518.

 NH_4^+ is one of the toxins that results from the degradation of urea or proteins by intestinal bacteria and is not metabolized by the infected liver. The subsequent elevation of ammonia concentrations in the fluid bathing the brain causes depletion of tricarboxylic acid (TCA) cycle intermediates and ATP in the central nervous system. α-Ketoglutarate, a TCA cycle intermediate, combines with ammonia to form glutamate in a reaction catalyzed by glutamate dehydrogenase. Glutamate subsequently reacts with ammonia to form glutamine.

The absolute level of ammonia and its metabolites, such as glutamine, in the blood or cerebrospinal fluid in patients with hepatic encephalopathy correlates only roughly with the presence or severity of the neurologic signs and symptoms. γ-Aminobutyric acid (GABA), an important inhibitory neurotransmitter in the brain, is also produced in the gut lumen and is shunted into the systemic circulation in increased amounts in patients with hepatic failure. In addition, other compounds (such as aromatic amino acids, false neurotransmitters, and certain short-chain fatty acids) bypass liver metabolism and accumulate in the systemic circulation, adversely affecting central nervous system function. Their relative importance in the pathogenesis of hepatic encephalopathy remains to be determined.

In addition to producing urea, the reactions of the urea cycle also serve as the pathway for the biosynthesis of arginine. Therefore, this amino acid is not required in the diet of the adult; however, it is required in the diet for growth.

Urea is not cleaved by human enzymes. However, bacteria, including those in the human digestive tract, can cleave urea to ammonia and CO_2, using the enzyme urease. Urease is not produced by humans.

To some extent, humans excrete urea into the gut and saliva. Intestinal bacteria convert urea to ammonia. This ammonia, as well as ammonia produced by other bacterial reactions in the gut, is absorbed into the hepatic portal vein. It is normally extracted by the liver and converted to urea. Approximately one fourth of the total urea released by the liver each day is recycled by bacteria.

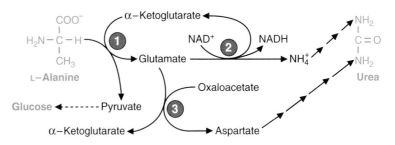

Fig. 38.17. Conversion of alanine to glucose and urea. 1. Alanine, the key gluconeogenic amino acid, is transaminated to form pyruvate, which is converted to glucose. The nitrogen, now in glutamate, can be released as NH_4^+ (2) or transferred to oxaloacetate to form aspartate (3). NH_4^+ and aspartate enter the urea cycle, which produces urea. In summary, the carbons of alanine form glucose and the nitrogens form urea. Two molecules of alanine are required to produce one molecule of glucose and one molecule of urea.

into the liver by activating the transcription of transport systems for alanine. Two molecules of alanine are required to generate one molecule of glucose. The nitrogen from the two molecules of alanine is converted to one molecule of urea (Fig. 38.17).

CLINICAL COMMENTS

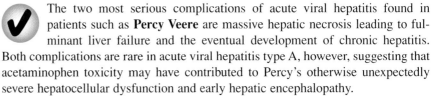

The two most serious complications of acute viral hepatitis found in patients such as **Percy Veere** are massive hepatic necrosis leading to fulminant liver failure and the eventual development of chronic hepatitis. Both complications are rare in acute viral hepatitis type A, however, suggesting that acetaminophen toxicity may have contributed to Percy's otherwise unexpectedly severe hepatocellular dysfunction and early hepatic encephalopathy.

Fortunately, bed rest, rehydration, parenteral nutrition, and therapy directed at decreasing the production of toxins that result from bacterial degradation of nitrogenous substrates in the gut lumen (e.g., administration of lactulose, which reduces gut ammonia levels by a variety of mechanisms, the use of enemas and antibiotics to decrease the intestinal flora, a low-protein diet) prevented **Percy Veere** from progressing to the later stages of hepatic encephalopathy. As with most patients who survive an episode of fulminant hepatic failure, recovery to his previous state of health occurred over the next 3 months. Percy's liver function studies returned to normal, and a follow-up liver biopsy showed no histologic abnormalities.

BIOCHEMICAL COMMENTS

Disorders of the urea cycle are dangerous because of the accumulation of ammonia in the circulation. Ammonia is toxic to the nervous system, and its concentration in the body must be carefully controlled. Under normal conditions, free ammonia is rapidly fixed into either α-ketoglutarate (by glutamate dehydrogenase, to form glutamate) or glutamate (by glutamine synthease, to form glutamine). The glutamine can be used by many tissues, including the liver; the glutamate donates nitrogens to pyruvate to form alanine, which travels to the liver. Within the liver, as the nitrogens are removed from their carriers, carbamoyl phosphate synthetase I fixes the ammonia into carbamoyl phosphate to initiate the urea cycle. However, when a urea cycle enzyme is defective, the cycle is interrupted, which leads to an accumulation of urea cycle intermediates before the block. Because of the block in the urea cycle, glutamine levels increase in the circulation, and because α-ketoglutarate is no longer being regenerated by removal of nitrogen from glutamine, the α-ketoglutarate levels are too low to fix more free ammonia, leading to elevated ammonia levels in the blood. So how does one reduce ammonia and glutamine levels in such patients?

The key to treating patients with urea cycle defects is to diagnose the disease early and then aggressively treat with compounds that can aid in nitrogen removal

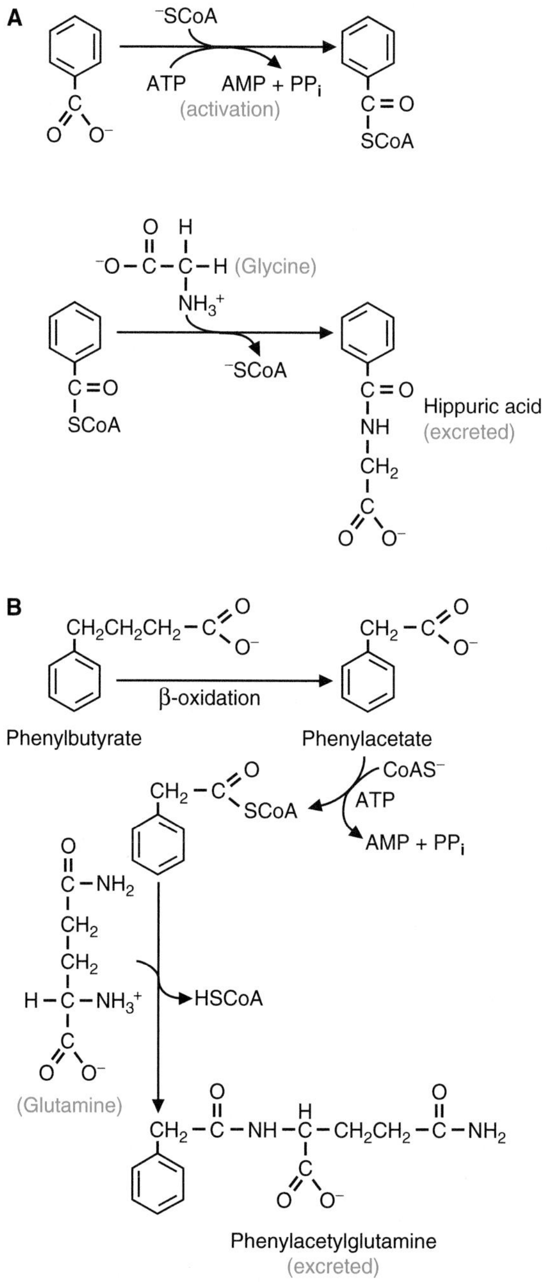

Fig. 38.18. The metabolism of benzoic acid (A) and phenylbutyrate (B), two agents used to reduce nitrogen levels in patients with urea cycle defects.

from the patient. Low-protein diets are essential to reduce the potential for excessive amino acid degradation. If the enzyme defect in the urea cycle comes after the synthesis of argininosuccinate, massive arginine supplementation has proved beneficial. Once argininosuccinate has been synthesized, the two nitrogen molecules destined for excretion have been incorporated into the substrate; the problem is that ornithine cannot be regenerated. If ornithine could be replenished to allow the cycle to continue, argininosuccinate could be used as the carrier for nitrogen excretion from the body. Thus, ingesting large levels of arginine leads to ornithine production by the arginase reaction, and nitrogen excretion via argininosuccinate in the urine can be enhanced.

Arginine therapy will not work for enzyme defects that exist in steps before the synthesis of argininosuccinate. For these disorders, drugs are used that form conjugates with amino acids. The conjugated amino acids are excreted, and the body then has to use its nitrogen to resynthesize the excreted amino acid. The two compounds most frequently used are benzoic acid and phenylbutyrate (the active component of pheylbutyrate is pheylacetate, its oxidation product. Phenylacetate has a bad odor, which makes it difficult to take orally). As indicated in Figure 38.18A, benzoic acid, after activation, reacts with glycine to form hippuric acid, which is excreted. As glycine is synthesized from serine, the body now uses nitrogens to synthesize serine, so more glycine can be produced. Phenylacetate (see Fig. 38.18B) forms a conjugate with glutamine, which is excreted. This conjugate removes two nitrogens per molecule and requires the body to resynthesize glutamine from glucose, thereby using another two nitrogen molecules.

Urea cycle defects are excellent candidates for treatment by gene therapy. This is because the defect only has to be repaired in one cell type (in this case, the hepatocyte), which makes it easier to target the vector carrying the replacement gene. Preliminary gene therapy experiments had been carried out on individuals with ornithine transcarbamolyase deficiency (the most common inherited defect in the urea cycle), but the experiments came to a halt when one of the patients died of a severe immunologic reaction to the vector used to deliver the gene. This incident has placed gene replacement therapy in the United States "on hold" for the foreseeable future.

Suggested Readings

Brusilow S, Horwich A. Urea cycle enzymes. In: Scriver CR, Beaudet AL, Valle D, Sly WS, et al., eds. The Metabolic and Molecular Bases of Inherited Disease, vol II, 8th Ed. New York: McGraw-Hill, 2001:1909–1963.

Marshall E. Gene therapy death prompts review of adenovirus vector. Science 1999;286:2244–2245.

Morris SM Jr. Regulation of enzymes of the urea cycle and arginine metabolism. Annu Rev Nutr 2002;22:87–105.

 REVIEW QUESTIONS—CHAPTER 38

1. Deficiency diseases have been described that involve each of the five enzymes of the urea cycle. Clinical manifestations may appear in the neonatal period. Infants with defects in the first four enzymes usually appear normal at birth, but after 24 hours progressively develop lethargy, hypothermia, and apnea. They have high blood ammonia levels, and the brain becomes swollen. One possible explanation for the swelling is the osmotic effect of the accumulation of glutamine in the brain produced by the reactions of ammonia with α-ketoglutarate and glutamate. Arginase deficiency is not as severe as deficiencies of the other urea cycle enzymes.

Given the following information about five newborn infants (identified as I to V) who appeared normal at birth but developed hyperammonemia after 24 hours, determine which urea cycle enzyme might be defective in each case (for each infant, choose from the same five answers, lettered A through E). All infants had low levels of blood urea nitrogen (BUN). (Normal citrulline levels are 10-20 μM.)

Infant	Urine Orotate	Blood Citrulline	Blood Arginine	Blood Ammonia
I	Low	Low	Low	High
II	-*	High (> 1,000 μM)	Low	High
III	-	-	High	Moderately high
IV	High	Low	Low	High
V	-	High (200 μM)	Low	High

* = Value not determined; low = below normal; high = above normal.

    (A) Carbamolyphosphate synthetase I
    (B) Ornithine transcarbamoylase
    (C) Argininosuccinate synthetase
    (D) Argininosuccinate lyase
    (E) Arginase

2.   The nitrogens in urea are directly derived from which of the following compounds?

    (A) Ornithine and carbamoyl phosphate
    (B) Ornithine and aspartate
    (C) Ornithine and glutamate
    (D) Carbamoyl phosphate and aspartate
    (E) Carbamoyl phosphate and glutamine
    (F) Aspartate and glutamine

3.   Which one of the following enzymes can fix ammonia into an organic molecule?

    (A) Alanine-pyruvate aminotransferase
    (B) Glutaminase
    (C) Glutamate dehydrogenase
    (D) Arginase
    (E) Argininosuccinate synthetase

4. Pyridoxal phosphate, which is required for transaminations, is also required for which of the following pathways?

    (A) Glycolysis
    (B) Gluconeogenesis
    (C) Glycogenolysis
    (D) TCA cycle
    (E) Fatty acid oxidation

5. The major regulated step of the urea cycle is which of the following?

    (A) Carbamoyl phosphate synthetase I
    (B) Ornithine transcarbamoylase
    (C) Argininosuccinate synthetase
    (D) Argininosuccinate lyase
    (E) Arginase

39 Synthesis and Degradation of Amino Acids

As a general rule, genetic codons exist for 20 amino acids. Only these 20 common amino acids are incorporated into proteins during the process of protein synthesis. Modifications to these amino acids occur after they are incorporated into proteins (such as the synthesis of hydroxyproline in collagen). The major exception to this rule is selenocysteine, which is an essential component of enzymes involved in scavenging free radicals (such as glutathione peroxidase-1; see Chapter 24). Selenocysteine has a selenium atom in the place of the oxygen atom in serine and is synthesized enzymatically in a reaction that requires adenosine triphosphate (ATP), selenium, and serine attached to a tRNA specific for selenocysteine. This reaction uses two high-energy bonds. The codon recognized by the tRNA-selenocysteine is a stop codon in the mRNA (UGA). The secondary structure of the mRNA allows the ribosomes and tRNA to understand which UGA is a stop codon and which requires the insertion of selenocysteine.

Because each of the 20 common amino acids has a unique structure, their metabolic pathways differ. Despite this, some generalities do apply to both the synthesis and degradation of all amino acids. These are summarized in the following sections. Because a number of the amino acid pathways are clinically relevant, we present most of the diverse pathways occurring in humans. However, we will be as succinct as possible.

Important coenzymes: *Pyridoxal phosphate (derived from vitamin B6) is the quintessential coenzyme of amino acid metabolism. In degradation, it is involved in the removal of amino groups, principally through **transamination reactions** and in donation of amino groups for various amino acid biosynthetic pathways. It is also required for certain reactions involving the carbon skeleton of amino acids.*
Tetrahydrofolate (FH$_4$) is a coenzyme used to transfer one-carbon groups at various oxidation states. FH$_4$ is used both in amino acid degradation (e.g., serine and histidine) and biosynthesis (e.g., glycine). Tetrahydrobiopterin (BH$_4$) is a cofactor required for ring hydroxylation reactions (e.g., phenylalanine to tyrosine).

Synthesis of the amino acids: *Eleven of the twenty common amino acids can be synthesized in the body (Fig. 39.1). The other nine are considered "essential" and must be obtained from the diet. Almost all of the amino acids that can be synthesized by humans are amino acids used for the synthesis of additional nitrogen-containing compounds. Examples include glycine, which is used for porphyrin and purine synthesis; glutamate, which is required for neurotransmitter and purine synthesis; and aspartate, which is required for both purine and pyrimidine biosynthesis.*

Nine of the eleven "nonessential" amino acids can be produced from glucose plus, of course, a source of nitrogen, such as another amino acid or ammonia. The other two nonessential amino acids, tyrosine and cysteine, require an essential amino acid for their synthesis (phenylalanine for tyrosine, and methionine for cysteine). The carbons for cysteine synthesis come from glucose; the methionine only donates the sulfur.

*The carbon skeletons of the 10 nonessential amino acids derived from glucose are produced from intermediates of **glycolysis** and the **tricarboxylic acid (TCA) cycle** (see Fig 39.1). Four amino acids (**serine, glycine, cysteine,** and **alanine**) are produced from glucose through components of the **glycolytic pathway**. TCA cycle intermediates (which can be produced from glucose) provide carbon for synthesis of the six remaining nonessential amino acids. α-Ketoglutarate is the precursor for the synthesis of glutamate, glutamine, proline, and arginine. Oxaloacetate provides carbon for the synthesis of aspartate and asparagine.*

*The regulation of individual amino acid biosynthesis can be quite complex, but the overriding feature is that the **pathways are feedback regulated** such that as the **concentration of free amino acid increases,** a key biosynthetic **enzyme is allosterically or transcriptionally inhibited.** Amino acid levels, however, are*

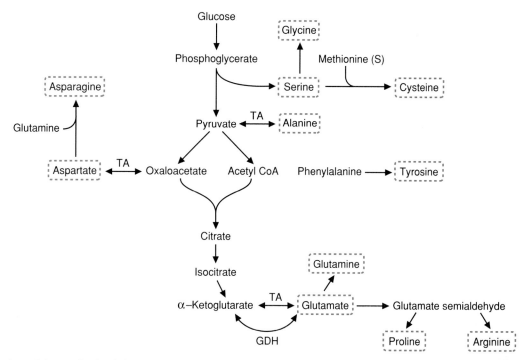

Fig. 39.1. Overview of the synthesis of the nonessential amino acids. The carbons of 10 amino acids may be produced from glucose through intermediates of glycolysis or the TCA cycle. The 11th nonessential amino acid, tyrosine, is synthesized by hydroxylation of the essential amino acid phenylalanine. Only the sulfur of cysteine comes from the essential amino acid methionine; its carbons and nitrogen come from serine. Transamination (TA) reactions involve pyridoxal phosphate (PLP) and another amino acid/α-keto acid pair.

always maintained at a level such that the aminoacyl-tRNA synthetases can remain active, and protein synthesis can continue.

Degradation of amino acids: *The **degradation pathways** for amino acids are, in general, **distinct from biosynthetic pathways**. This allows for separate regulation of the anabolic and catabolic pathways. Because protein is a fuel, almost every amino acid will have a degradative pathway that can generate NADH, which is used as an electron source for oxidative phosphorylation. However, the energy-generating pathway may involve direct oxidation, oxidation in the TCA cycle, conversion to glucose and then oxidation, or conversion to **ketone bodies,** which are then oxidized.*

*The fate of the carbons of the amino acids depends on the physiologic state of the individual and the tissue where the degradation occurs. For example, in the liver during fasting, the carbon skeletons of the amino acids produce glucose, ketone bodies, and CO_2. In the fed state, the liver can convert intermediates of amino acid metabolism to glycogen and triacylglycerols. Thus, the **fate of the carbons of the amino acids parallels that of glucose and fatty acids.** The **liver** is the only tissue that has all of the pathways of amino acid synthesis and degradation.*

*As amino acids are degraded, their **carbons** are converted to (a) CO_2, (b) compounds that produce **glucose** in the liver (pyruvate and the TCA cycle intermediates α-ketoglutarate, succinyl CoA, fumarate, and oxaloacetate), and (c) **ketone bodies** or their precursors (acetoacetate and acetyl CoA) (Fig. 39.2). For simplicity, amino acids are considered to be **glucogenic** if their carbon skeletons can be converted to a precursor of glucose and **ketogenic** if their carbon skeletons can be directly converted to acetyl CoA or acetoacetate. Some amino acids contain carbons that produce a glucose precursor and other carbons that produce acetyl CoA or acetoacetate. These amino acids are both glucogenic and ketogenic.*

*The amino acids synthesized from intermediates of glycolysis (**serine, alanine, and cysteine**) plus certain other amino acids (**threonine, glycine, and tryptophan**)*

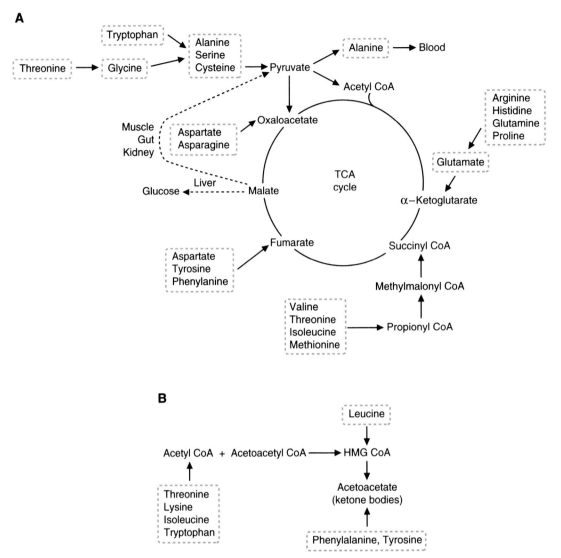

Fig. 39.2. Degradation of amino acids. A. Amino acids that produce pyruvate or intermediates of the TCA cycle. These amino acids are considered glucogenic because they can produce glucose in the liver. The fumarate group of amino acids produces cytoplasmic fumarate. Potential mechanisms whereby the cytoplasmic fumarate can be oxidized are presented in section III.C.1. B. Amino acids that produce acetyl CoA or ketone bodies. These amino acids are considered ketogenic.

produce **pyruvate** when they are degraded. The amino acids synthesized from TCA cycle intermediates (**aspartate, asparagines, glutamate, glutamine, proline, and arginine**) are reconverted to these intermediates during degradation. **Histidine** is converted to **glutamate** and then to the TCA cycle intermediate α-**ketoglutarate.** **Methionine, threonine, valine, and isoleucine** form **succinyl CoA**, and **phenylalanine** (after conversion to **tyrosine**) forms **fumarate.** Because pyruvate and the TCA cycle intermediates can produce glucose in the liver, these amino acids are glucogenic.

Some amino acids with carbons that produce glucose also contain other carbons that produce ketone bodies. **Tryptophan, isoleucine, and threonine** produce **acetyl CoA,** and **phenylalanine and tyrosine** produce **acetoacetate.** These amino acids are both glucogenic and ketogenic.

Two of the essential amino acids (**lysine and leucine**) are strictly **ketogenic.** They do not produce glucose, only acetoacetate and acetyl-CoA.

THE WAITING ROOM

Piquet Yuria, a 4-month-old female infant, emigrated from the Soviet Union with her French mother and Russian father 1 month ago. She was normal at birth but in the last several weeks was less than normally attentive to her surroundings. Her psychomotor maturation seemed delayed, and a tremor of her extremities had recently appeared. When her mother found her having gross twitching movements in her crib, she brought the infant to the hospital emergency room. A pediatrician examined Piquet and immediately noted a musty odor to the baby's wet diaper. A drop of her blood was obtained from a heel prick and used to perform a Guthrie bacterial inhibition assay using a special type of filter paper. This screening procedure was positive for the presence of an excess of phenylalanine in Piquet's blood.

Homer Sistine, a 14-year-old boy, had a sudden grand mal seizure (with jerking movements of the torso and head) in his eighth grade classroom. The school physician noted mild weakness of the muscles of the left side of Homer's face and of his left arm and leg. Homer was hospitalized with a tentative diagnosis of a cerebrovascular accident involving the right cerebral hemisphere, which presumably triggered the seizure.

Homer's past medical history was normal, except for slight mental retardation requiring placement in a special education group. He also had a downward partial dislocation of the lenses of both eyes for which he had had a surgical procedure (a peripheral iridectomy).

Homer's left-sided neurologic deficits cleared spontaneously within 3 days, but a computerized axial tomogram (CAT) showed changes consistent with a small infarction (damaged area caused by a temporary or permanent loss of adequate arterial blood flow) in the right cerebral hemisphere. A neurologist noted that Homer had a slight waddling gait, which his mother said began several years earlier and was progressing with time. Further studies confirmed the presence of decreased mineralization (decreased calcification) of the skeleton (called osteopenia if mild and osteoporosis if more severe) and high methionine and homocysteine but low cystine levels in the blood.

All of this information, plus the increased length of the long bones of Homer's extremities and a slight curvature of his spine (scoliosis), caused his physician to suspect that Homer might have an inborn error of metabolism.

I. THE ROLE OF COFACTORS IN AMINO ACID METABOLISM

Amino acid metabolism requires the participation of three important cofactors. Pyridoxal phosphate is the quintessential coenzyme of amino acid metabolism (see Chapter 38). All amino acid reactions requiring pyridoxal phosphate occur with the amino group of the amino acid covalently bound to the aldehyde carbon of the coenzyme (Fig. 39.3). The pyridoxal phosphate then pulls electrons away from the bonds around the α-carbon. The result is transamination, deamination, decarboxylation, β-elimination, racemization, and γ-elimination, depending on which enzyme and amino acid are involved.

The coenzyme FH_4 is required in certain amino acid pathways to either accept or donate a one-carbon group. The carbon can be in various states of oxidation. Chapter 40 describes the reactions of FH_4 in much more detail.

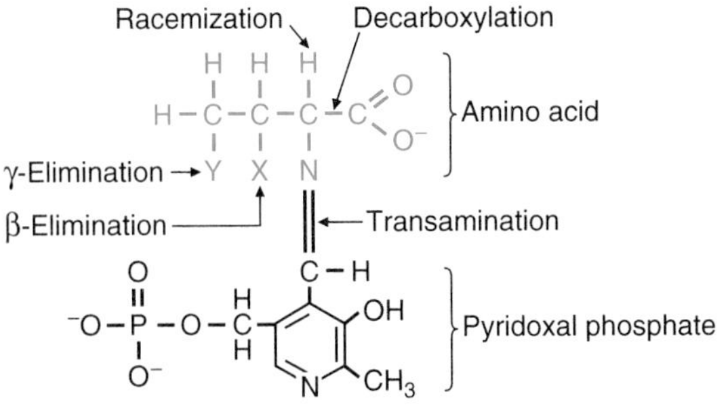

Fig. 39.3. Pyridoxal phosphate covalently attached to an amino acid substrate. The arrows indicate which bonds are broken for the various types of reactions in which pyridoxal phosphate is involved. The X and Y represent leaving groups that may be present on the amino acid (such as the hydroxyl group on serine or threonine).

The coenzyme BH_4 is required for ring hydroxylations. The reactions involve molecular oxygen, and one atom of oxygen is incorporated into the product. The second is found in water (see Chapter 24). BH_4 is important for the synthesis of tyrosine and neurotransmitters (see Chapter 48).

II. AMINO ACIDS DERIVED FROM INTERMEDIATES OF GLYCOLYSIS

Four amino acids are synthesized from intermediates of glycolysis: serine, glycine, cysteine, and alanine. Serine, which produces glycine and cysteine, is synthesized from 3-phosphoglycerate, and alanine is formed by transamination of pyruvate, the product of glycolysis (Fig. 39.4). When these amino acids are degraded, their carbon atoms are converted to pyruvate or to intermediates of the glycolytic/gluconeogenic pathway and, therefore, can produce glucose or be oxidized to CO_2.

A. Serine

In the biosynthesis of serine from glucose, 3-phosphoglycerate is first oxidized to a 2-keto compound (3-phosphohydroxypyruvate), which is then transaminated to form phosphoserine (Fig. 39.5). Phosphoserine phosphatase removes the phosphate, forming serine. The major sites of serine synthesis are the liver and kidney.

Serine can be used by many tissues and is generally degraded by transamination to hydroxypyruvate followed by reduction and phosphorylation to form 2-phosphoglycerate, an intermediate of gycolysis that forms PEP and, subsequently, pyruvate. Serine also can undergo β-elimination of its hydroxyl group, catalyzed by serine dehydratase, to form pyruvate.

Regulatory mechanisms maintain serine levels in the body. When serine levels fall, serine synthesis is increased by induction of 3-phosphoglycerate dehydrogenase and by release of the feedback inhibition of phosphoserine phosphatase (caused by higher levels of serine). When serine levels rise, synthesis of serine decreases because synthesis of the dehydrogenase is repressed and the phosphatase is inhibited (see Fig. 39.5).

B. Glycine

Glycine can be synthesized from serine and, to a minor extent, threonine. The major route from serine is by a reversible reaction that involves FH_4 and pyridoxal phosphate (Fig. 39.6). Tetrahydrofolate is a coenzyme that transfers one-carbon groups at different levels of oxidation. It is derived from the vitamin folate and is discussed in more detail in Chapter 40. The minor pathway for glycine production involves threonine degradation (this is an aldolase-like reaction because threonine contains a hydroxyl group located two carbons from the carbonyl group).

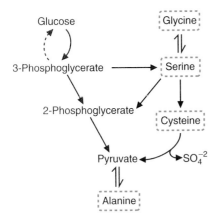

Fig. 39.4. Amino acids derived from intermediates of glycolysis. These amino acids can be synthesized from glucose. Their carbons can be reconverted to glucose in the liver.

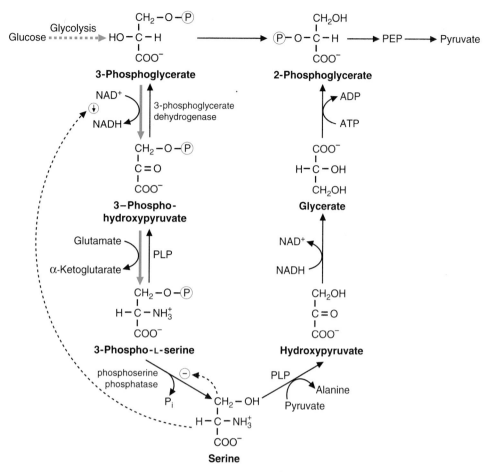

Fig. 39.5. The major pathway for serine synthesis from glucose is on the left, and for serine degradation on the right. Serine levels are maintained because serine causes repression (circled ↓) of 3-phosphoglycerate dehydrogenase synthesis. Serine also inhibits (circled -) phosphoserine phosphatase.

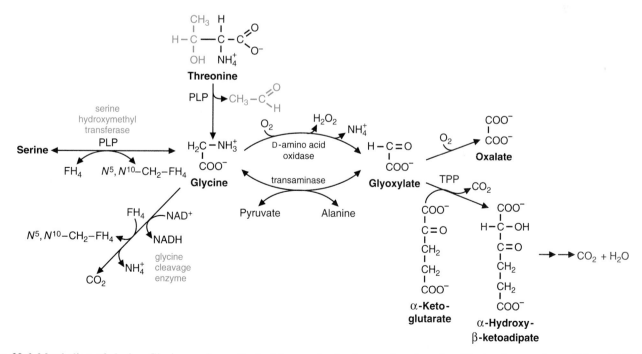

Fig. 39.6. Metabolism of glycine. Glycine can be synthesized from serine (major route) or threonine. Glycine forms serine or CO_2 and NH_4^+ by reactions that require tetrahydrofolate (FH_4). Glycine also forms glyoxylate, which is converted to oxalate or to CO_2 and H_2O.

Oxalate, produced from glycine or obtained from the diet, forms precipitates with calcium. Kidney stones (renal calculi) are often composed of calcium oxalate. A lack of the transaminase that can convert glyoxylate to glycine (see Fig 39.6) leads to the disease primary oxaluria type I (PH 1). This disease has a consequence of renal failure attributable to excessive accumulation of oxalate in the kidney.

Cystathionuria, the presence of cystathionine in the urine, is relatively common in premature infants. As they mature, cystathionase levels rise, and the levels of cystathionine in the urine decrease.

In adults, a genetic deficiency of cystathionase causes cystathionuria. Individuals with a genetically normal cystathionase can also develop cystathionuria from a dietary deficiency of pyridoxine (vitamin B6), because cystathionase requires the cofactor pyridoxal phosphate. No characteristic clinical abnormalities have been observed in individuals with cystathionase deficiency, and it is probably a benign disorder.

Cystinuria and cystinosis are disorders involving two different transport proteins for cystine, the disulfide formed from two molecules of cysteine. Cystinuria is caused by a defect in the transport protein that carries cystine, lysine, arginine, and ornithine into intestinal epithelial cells and that permits resorption of these amino acids by renal tubular cells. Cystine, which is not very soluble in the urine, forms renal calculi (stones). **Cal Kulis**, a patient with cystinuria, developed cystine stones (see Chapter 37).

Cystinosis is a rare disorder caused by a defective carrier that normally transports cystine across the lysosomal membrane from lysosomal vesicles to the cytosol. Cystine accumulates in the lysosomes in many tissues and forms crystals, impairing their function. Children with this disorder develop renal failure by 6–12 years of age.

Alanine aminotransferase (ALT) and aspartate amino transferase (AST) are released from the liver when liver cells are injured. Measurement of these two transaminases in the serum (ALT and AST) is one of the standard laboratory tests for liver damage caused by a variety of conditions.

The conversion of glycine to glyoxylate by the enzyme D-amino acid oxidase is a degradative pathway of glycine that is medically important. Once glyoxylate is formed, it can be oxidized to oxalate, which is sparingly soluble and tends to precipitate in kidney tubules, leading to kidney stone formation. Approximately 40% of oxalate formation in the liver comes from glycine metabolism. Dietary oxalate accumulation has been estimated to be a low contributor to excreted oxalate in the urine because of poor absorption of oxalate in the intestine.

Although glyoxalate can be transaminated back to glycine, this is not really considered a biosynthetic route for "new" glycine, because the primary route for glyoxylate formation is from glycine oxidation.

Generation of energy from glycine occurs through a dehydrogenase (glycine cleavage enzyme) that oxidizes glycine to CO_2, ammonia, and a carbon that is donated to FH_4.

C. Cysteine

The carbons and nitrogen for cysteine synthesis are provided by serine, and the sulfur is provided by methionine (Fig. 39.7). Serine reacts with homocysteine (which is produced from methionine) to form cystathionine. This reaction is catalyzed by cystathionine β-synthase. Cleavage of cystathionine by cystathionase produces cysteine and α-ketobutyrate, which forms succinyl CoA via propionyl CoA. Both cystathionine β-synthase (β-elimination) and cystathionase (γ-elimination) require PLP.

Cysteine inhibits cystathionine β-synthase and, therefore, regulates its own production to adjust for the dietary supply of cysteine. Because cysteine derives its sulfur from the essential amino acid methionine, cysteine becomes essential if the supply of methionine is inadequate for cysteine synthesis. Conversely, an adequate dietary source of cysteine "spares" methionine; that is, it decreases the amount that must be degraded to produce cysteine.

When cysteine is degraded, the nitrogen is converted to urea, the carbons to pyruvate, and the sulfur to sulfate, which has two potential fates (see Fig. 39.7; see also Chapter 43). Sulfate generation, in an aqueous media, is essentially generating sulfuric acid, and both the acid and sulfate need to be disposed of in the urine. Sulfate is also used in most cells to generate an activated form of sulfate known as PAPS (3′-phosphoadenosine 5′-phosphosulfate), which is used as a sulfate donor in modifying carbohydrates or amino acids in various structures (glycosaminoglycans) and proteins in the body.

The conversion of methionine to homocysteine and homocysteine to cysteine is the major degradative route for these two amino acids. Because this is the only degradative route for homocysteine, vitamin B6 deficiency or congenital cystathinone β-synthase deficiency can result in homocystinemia, which is associated with cardiovascular disease.

D. Alanine

Alanine is produced from pyruvate by a transamination reaction catalyzed by alanine aminotransaminase (ALT) and may be converted back to pyruvate by a reversal of the same reaction (see Fig. 39.4). Alanine is the major gluconeogenic amino acid because it is produced in many tissues for the transport of nitrogen to the liver.

III. AMINO ACIDS RELATED TO TCA CYCLE INTERMEDIATES

Two groups of amino acids are synthesized from TCA cycle intermediates; one group from α-ketoglutarate and one from oxaloacetate (see Fig. 39.2). During degradation, four groups of amino acids are converted to the TCA cycle intermediates α-ketoglutarate, oxaloacetate, succinyl CoA, and fumarate (see Fig. 39.3A).

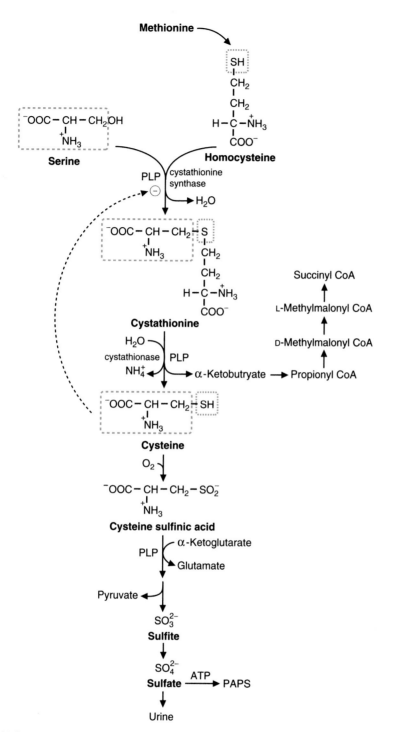

Fig. 39.7. Synthesis and degradation of cysteine. Cysteine is synthesized from the carbons and nitrogen of serine and the sulfur of homocysteine (which is derived from methionine). During the degradation of cysteine, the sulfur is converted to sulfate and either excreted in the urine or converted to PAPS (universal sulfate donor; 3′-phosphoadenosine 5′-phosphosulfate), and the carbons are converted to pyruvate.

Q: Homocysteine is oxidized to a disulfide, homocystine. To indicate that both forms are being considered, the term *homocyst(e)ine* is used.

Homocysteine

COO⁻   COO⁻
| |
H_3N^+— CH H_3N^+— CH
| |
CH_2 CH_2
| |
CH_2 CH_2
| |
SH   S
                         |
SH   S
| |
CH_2 CH_2
| |
CH_2 CH_2
| |
H — C — NH_3^+ H — C — NH_3^+
| |
COO⁻   COO⁻

Homocysteine   **Homocystine**

Because a colorimetric screening test for urinary homocystine was positive, the doctor ordered several biochemical studies on **Homer Sistine's** serum, which included tests for methionine, homocyst(e)ine (both free and protein-bound), cystine, vitamin B12, and folate. The level of homocystine in a 24-hour urine collection was also measured.

The results were as follows: the serum methionine level was 980 μM (reference range, <30); serum homocyst(e)ine (both free and protein bound) was markedly elevated; cystine was not detected in the serum; the serum B12 and folate levels were normal. A 24-hour urine homocystine level was elevated.

Based on these measurements, **Homer Sistine's** doctor concluded that he had homocystinuria caused by an enzyme deficiency. What was the rationale for this conclusion?

A: If the blood levels of methionine and homocysteine are very elevated and cystine is low, cystathionine β-synthase could be defective, but a cystathionase deficiency is also a possibility. With a deficiency of either of these enzymes, cysteine could not be synthesized, and levels of homocysteine would rise. Homocysteine would be converted to methionine by reactions that require B12 and tetrahydrofolate (see Chapter 40). In addition, it would be oxidized to homocystine, which would appear in the urine. The levels of cysteine (measured as its oxidation product cystine) would be low. A measurement of serum cystathionine levels would help to distinguish between a cystathionase or cystathionine β-synthase deficiency.

A. Amino Acids Related through α-Ketoglutarate/Glutamate

1. GLUTAMATE

The five carbons of glutamate are derived from α-ketoglutarate either by transamination or by the glutamate dehydrogenase reaction (see Chapter 38). Because α-ketoglutarate can be synthesized from glucose, all of the carbons of glutamate can be obtained from glucose (see Fig. 39.2). When glutamate is degraded, it is likewise converted back to α-ketoglutarate either by transamination or by glutamate dehydrogenase. In the liver, α-ketoglutarate leads to the formation of malate, which produces glucose via gluconeogenesis. Thus, glutamate can be derived from glucose and reconverted to glucose (Fig. 39.8).

Glutamate is used for the synthesis of a number of other amino acids (glutamine, proline, ornithine, and arginine) (see Fig. 39.8) and for providing the glutamyl moiety of glutathionine (γ-glutamyl-cysteinyl-glycine; see Biochemical Comments of Chapter 37). Glutathione is an important antioxidant, as has been described previously (see Chapter 24).

2. GLUTAMINE

Glutamine is produced from glutamate by glutamine synthetase, which adds NH_4^+ to the carboxyl group of the side chain, forming an amide (Fig. 39.9). This is one of only three human enzymes that can fix free ammonia into an organic molecule; the other two are glutamate dehydrogenase and carbamoyl-phosphate synthetase I (see Chapter 38). Glutamine is reconverted to glutamate by a different enzyme, glutaminase, which is particularly important in the kidney. The ammonia it produces enters the urine and can be used as an expendable cation to aid in the excretion of metabolic acids ($NH_3 + H^+ \rightarrow NH_4^+$).

3. PROLINE

In the synthesis of proline, glutamate is first phosphorylated and then converted to glutamate 5-semialdehyde by reduction of the side chain carboxyl group to an

```
        COO⁻
         |
        CH₂
         |
        CH₂
         |
   H—C—NH₃⁺
         |
        COO⁻
     Glutamate
```

NH_4^+ → NH_4^+

ATP — glutamine synthetase — ADP + P$_i$ glutaminase — H_2O

```
        NH₂
         +
        C=O
         |
        CH₂
         |
        CH₂
         |
   H—C—NH₃⁺
         |
        COO⁻
     Glutamine
```

Fig. 39.9. Synthesis and degradation of glutamine. Different enzymes catalyze the addition and the removal of the amide nitrogen of glutamine.

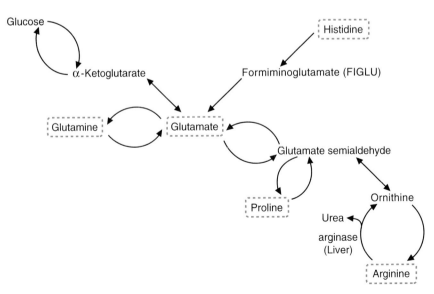

Fig. 39.8. Amino acids related through glutamate. These amino acids contain carbons that can be reconverted to glutamate, which can be converted to glucose in the liver. All of these amino acids except histidine can be synthesized from glucose.

aldehyde (Fig. 39.10). This semialdehyde spontaneously cyclizes (forming an internal Schiff base between the aldehyde and the α-amino group). Reduction of this cyclic compound yields proline. Hydroxyproline is only formed after proline has been incorporated into collagen (see Chapter 49) by the prolyl hydroxylase system, which uses molecular oxygen, iron, α-ketoglutarate, and ascorbic acid (vitamin C).

Proline is converted back to glutamate semialdehyde, which is reduced to form glutamate. The synthesis and degradation of proline use different enzymes even though the intermediates are the same. Hydroxyproline, however, has an entirely different degradative pathway (not shown). The presence of the hydroxyl group in hydroxyproline will allow an aldolase-like reaction to occur once the ring has been hydrolyzed, which is not possible with proline.

4. ARGININE

Arginine is synthesized from glutamate via glutamate semialdehyde, which is transaminated to form ornithine, an intermediate of the urea cycle (see Chapter 38 and Fig. 39.11). This activity (ornithine aminotransferase) appears to be greatest in the epithelial cells of the small intestine (see Chapter 42). The reactions of the urea cycle then produce arginine. However, the quantities of arginine generated by the urea cycle are adequate only for the adult and are insufficient to support growth. Therefore, during periods of growth, arginine becomes an essential amino acid. It is important to realize that if arginine is used for protein synthesis, the levels of ornithine will drop, thereby slowing the urea cycle. This will stimulate the formation of ornithine from glutamate.

Arginine is cleaved by arginase to form urea and ornithine. If ornithine is present in amounts in excess of those required for the urea cycle, it is transaminated to glutamate semialdehyde, which is reduced to glutamate. The conversion of an aldehyde to a primary amine is a unique form of a transamination reaction and requires pyridoxal phosphate (PLP).

5. HISTIDINE

Although histidine cannot be synthesized in humans, five of its carbons form glutamate when it is degraded. In a series of steps, histidine is converted to formiminoglutamate (FIGLU). The subsequent reactions transfer one carbon of FIGLU to the FH_4 pool (see Chapter 40) and release NH_4^+ and glutamate (Fig. 39.12).

B. Amino Acids Related to Oxaloacetate (Aspartate and Asparagine)

Aspartate is produced by transamination of oxaloacetate. This reaction is readily reversible, so aspartate can be reconverted to oxaloacetate (Fig. 39.13).

Asparagine is formed from aspartate by a reaction in which glutamine provides the nitrogen for formation of the amide group. Thus, this reaction differs from the synthesis of glutamine from glutamate, in which NH_4^+ provides the nitrogen. However, the reaction catalyzed by asparaginase, which hydrolyzes asparagine to NH_4^+ and aspartate, is analogous to the reaction catalyzed by glutaminase.

C. Amino Acids That Form Fumarate

1. ASPARTATE

Although the major route for aspartate degradation involves its conversion to oxaloacetate, carbons from aspartate can form fumarate in the urea cycle (see Chapter 38). This reaction generates cytosolic fumarate, which must be converted to malate (using cytoplasmic fumarase) for transport into the mitochondria for oxidative or anaplerotic purposes. An analogous sequence of reactions occurs in the purine nucleotide cycle. Aspartate reacts with inosine monophosphate (IMP) to

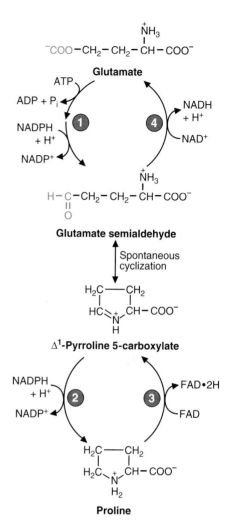

Fig. 39.10. Synthesis and degradation of proline. Reactions 1, 3, and 4 occur in mitochondria. Reaction 2 occurs in the cytosol. Synthesis and degradation involve different enzymes. The cyclization reaction (formation of a Schiff base) is nonenzymatic, i.e., spontaneous.

Certain types of tumor cells, particularly leukemic cells, require asparagine for their growth. Therefore, asparaginase has been used as an antitumor agent. It acts by converting asparagine to aspartate in the blood, decreasing the amount of asparagine available for tumor cell growth.

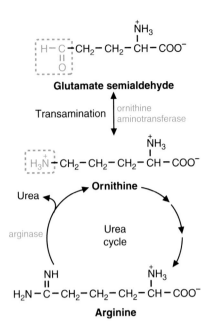

Glutamate semialdehyde

Transamination — ornithine aminotransferase

Ornithine

Urea

Urea cycle

arginase

Arginine

Fig. 39.11. Synthesis and degradation of arginine. The carbons of ornithine are derived from glutamate semialdehyde, which is derived from glutamate. Reactions of the urea cycle convert ornithine to arginine. Arginase converts arginine back to ornithine by releasing urea.

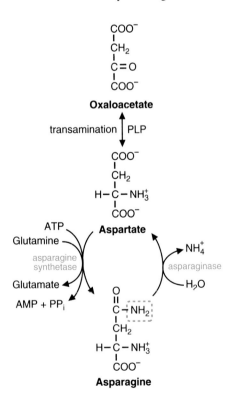

Oxaloacetate

transamination — PLP

ATP

Glutamine

asparagine synthetase

Glutamate

AMP + PP_i

Aspartate

NH_4^+

asparaginase

H_2O

Asparagine

Fig. 39.13. Synthesis and degradation of aspartate and asparagine. Note that the amide nitrogen of asparagine is derived from glutamine. (The amide nitrogen of glutamine comes from NH_4^+, see Fig. 39.9.)

form an intermediate (adenylosuccinate) which is cleaved, forming adenosine monophosphate (AMP) and fumarate (see Chapter 41).

2. PHENYLALANINE AND TYROSINE

Phenylalanine is converted to tyrosine by a hydroxylation reaction. Tyrosine, produced from phenylalanine or obtained from the diet, is oxidized, ultimately forming acetoacetate and fumarate. The oxidative steps required to reach this point are, surprisingly, not energy-generating. The conversion of fumarate to malate, followed by the action of malic enzyme, allows the carbons to be used for gluconeogenesis. The conversion of phenylalanine to tyrosine and the production of acetoacetate are considered further in section IV of this chapter.

D. Amino Acids That Form Succinyl CoA

The essential amino acids methionine, valine, isoleucine, and threonine are degraded to form propionyl-CoA. The conversion of propionyl CoA to succinyl CoA is common to their degradative pathways. Propionyl CoA is also generated from the oxidation of odd-chain fatty acids.

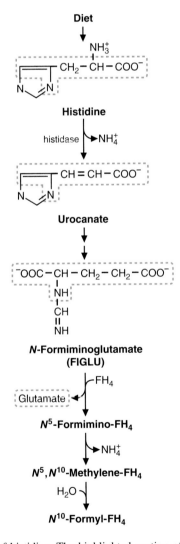

Diet

Histidine

histidase — NH_4^+

Urocanate

***N*-Formiminoglutamate (FIGLU)**

FH_4

Glutamate

***N*^5-Formimino-FH_4**

NH_4^+

***N*^5,*N*^10-Methylene-FH_4**

H_2O

***N*^10-Formyl-FH_4**

Fig. 39.12. Degradation of histidine. The highlighted portion of histidine forms glutamate. The remainder of the molecule provides one carbon for the tetrahydrofolate (FH_4) pool (see Chapter 40) and releases NH_4^+.

Propionyl CoA is carboxylated in a reaction that requires biotin and forms D-methylmalonyl CoA. The D-methylmalonyl CoA is racemized to L-methylmalonyl CoA, which is rearranged in a vitamin B12-requiring reaction to produce succinyl CoA, a TCA cycle intermediate (see Fig. 23.11).

1. METHIONINE

Methionine is converted to *S*-adenosylmethionine (SAM), which donates its methyl group to other compounds to form S-adenosylhomocysteine (SAH). SAH is then converted to homocysteine (Fig. 39.14). Methionine can be regenerated from homocysteine by a reaction requiring both FH_4 and vitamin B12 (a topic that is considered in more detail in Chapter 40). Alternatively, by reactions requiring PLP, homocysteine can provide the sulfur required for the synthesis of cysteine (see Fig. 39.7). Carbons of homocysteine are then metabolized to α-ketobutyrate, which undergoes oxidative decarboxylation to propionyl-CoA. The propionyl-CoA is then converted to succinyl CoA (see Fig. 39.14).

2. THREONINE

In humans threonine is primarily degraded by a PLP-requiring dehydratase to ammonia and α-ketobutyrate, which subsequently undergoes oxidative decarboxylation to form propionyl CoA, just as in the case for methionine (see Fig. 39.14).

The conversion of α-ketobutyrate to propionyl-CoA is catalyzed by either the pyruvate or branched-chain α-keto dehydrogenase enzymes.

Q: Homocystinuria is caused by deficiencies in the enzymes cystathionine β-synthase and cystathionase as well as by deficiencies of methyltetrahydrofolate (CH_3-FH_4) or of methyl-B12. The deficiencies of CH_3-FH_4 or of methyl-B12 are due either to an inadequate dietary intake of folate or B12 or to defective enzymes involved in joining methyl groups to tetrahydrofolate (FH_4), transferring methyl groups from FH_4 to B12, or passing them from B12 to homocysteine to form methionine (see Chapter 40).

Is **Homer Sistine's** homocystinuria caused by any of these problems?

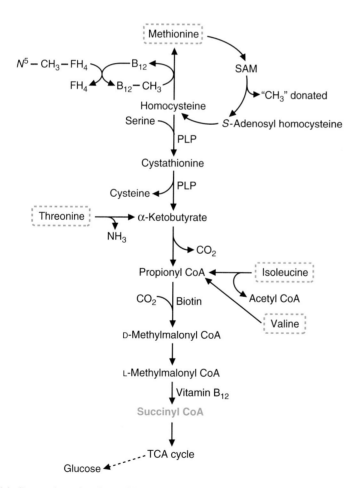

Fig. 39.14. Conversion of amino acids to succinyl CoA. The amino acids methionine, threonine, isoleucine, and valine, all of which form succinyl CoA via methylmalonyl CoA, are essential in the diet. The carbons of serine are converted to cysteine and do not form succinyl CoA by this pathway. SAM = *S*-adenosylmethionine.

Homer Sistine's methionine levels are elevated, and his B12 and folate levels are normal. Therefore, he does not have a deficiency of dietary folate or B12 or of the enzymes that transfer methyl groups from tetrahydrofolate to homocysteine to form methionine. In these cases, homocysteine levels are elevated but methionine levels are low.

A biopsy specimen from **Homer Sistine's** liver was sent to the hospital's biochemistry research laboratory for enzyme assays. Cystathionine β-synthase activity was reported to be 7% of that found in normal liver.

Thiamine deficiency will lead to an accumulation of α-keto acids in the blood because of an inability of pyruvate dehydrogenase, α-ketoglutarate dehydrogenase, and branched-chain α-keto acid dehydrogenase to catalyze their reactions (see Chapter 8). **Al Martini** had a thiamine deficiency resulting from his chronic alcoholism. His ketoacidosis resulted partly from the accumulation of these α-ketoacids in his blood and partly from the accumulation of ketone bodies used for energy production.

What compounds form succinyl CoA via propionyl CoA and methylmalonyl CoA?

In maple syrup urine disease, the branched-chain α-keto acid dehydrogenase that oxidatively decarboxylates the branched-chain amino acids is defective. As a result, the branched-chain amino acids and their α-keto analogs (produced by transamination) accumulate. They appear in the urine, giving it the odor of maple syrup or burnt sugar. The accumulation of α-keto analogs leads to neurologic complications. This condition is difficult to treat by dietary restriction, because abnormalities in the metabolism of three essential amino acids contribute to the disease.

3.   VALINE AND ISOLEUCINE

The branched-chain amino acids (valine, isoleucine, and leucine) are a universal fuel, and the degradation of these amino acids occurs at low levels in the mitochondria of most tissues, but the muscle carries out the highest level of branched-chain amino acid oxidation. The branched-chain amino acids make up almost 25% of the content of the average protein, so their use as fuel is quite significant. The degradative pathway for valine and isoleucine has two major functions, the first being energy generation and the second to provide precursors to replenish TCA cycle intermediates (anaplerosis). Valine and isoleucine, two of the three branched-chain amino acids, contain carbons that form succinyl CoA. The initial step in the degradation of the branched-chain amino acids is a transamination reaction. Although the enzyme that catalyzes this reaction is present in most tissues, the level of activity varies from tissue to tissue. Its activity is particularly high in muscle, however. In the second step of the degradative pathway, the α-keto analogs of these amino acids undergo oxidative decarboxylation by the α-keto acid dehydrogenase complex in a reaction similar in its mechanism and cofactor requirements to pyruvate dehydrogenase and α-ketoglutarate dehydrogenase (see Chapter 20). As with the first enzyme of the pathway, the highest level of activity for this dehydrogenase is found in muscle tissue. Subsequently, the pathways for degradation of these amino acids follow parallel routes (Fig. 39.15). The steps are analogous to those for β-oxidation of fatty acids so NADH and FAD(2H) are generated for energy production.

Valine and isoleucine are converted to succinyl CoA (see Fig. 39.14). Isoleucine also forms acetyl CoA. Leucine, the third branched-chain amino acid,

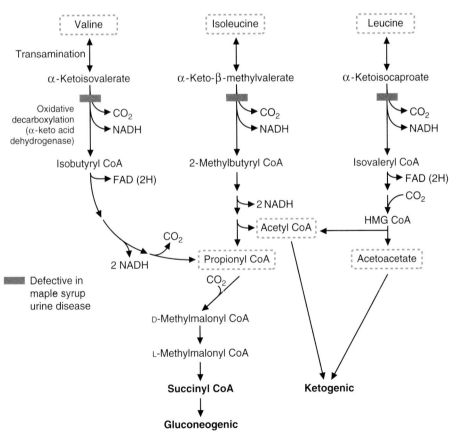

Fig. 39.15. Degradation of the branched-chain amino acids. Valine forms propionyl CoA. Isoleucine forms propionyl CoA and acetyl CoA. Leucine forms acetoacetate and acetyl CoA.

does not produce succinyl CoA. It forms acetoacetate and acetyl CoA and is strictly ketogenic .

IV. AMINO ACIDS THAT FORM ACETYL CoA AND ACETOACETATE

Seven amino acids produce acetyl CoA or acetoacetate and therefore are categorized as ketogenic. Of these, isoleucine, threonine, and the aromatic amino acids (phenylalanine, tyrosine, and tryptophan) are converted to compounds that produce both glucose and acetyl CoA or acetoacetate (Fig. 39.16). Leucine and lysine do not produce glucose; they produce acetyl CoA and acetoacetate.

A. Phenylalanine and Tyrosine

Phenylalanine is converted to tyrosine, which undergoes oxidative degradation (Fig. 39.17). The last step in the pathway produces both fumarate and the ketone body acetoacetate. Deficiencies of different enzymes in the pathway result in phenylketonuria, tyrosinemia, and alcaptonuria.

Phenylalanine is hydroxylated to form tyrosine by a mixed function oxidase, phenylalanine hydroxylase (PAH), which requires molecular oxygen and tetrahydrobiopterin (Fig. 39.18). The cofactor tetrahydrobiopterin is converted to quininoid dihydrobiopterin by this reaction. Tetrahydrobiopterin is not synthesized from a vitamin; it can be synthesized in the body from GTP. However, as is the case with other cofactors, the body contains limited amounts. Therefore, dihydrobiopterin must be reconverted to tetrahydrobiopterin for the reaction to continue to produce tyrosine.

 Alcaptonuria occurs when homogentisate, an intermediate in tyrosine metabolism, cannot be further oxidized because the next enzyme in the pathway, homogentisate oxidase, is defective. Homogentisate accumulates and auto-oxidizes, forming a dark pigment, which discolors the urine and stains the diapers of affected infants. Later in life, the chronic accumulation of this pigment in cartilage may cause arthritic joint pain.

 Transient tyrosinemia is frequently observed in newborn infants, especially those that are premature. For the most part, the condition appears to be benign, and dietary restriction of protein returns plasma tyrosine levels to normal. The biochemical defect is most likely a low level, attributable to immaturity, of 4-hydroxyphenylpyruvate dioxygenase. Because this enzyme requires ascorbate, ascorbate supplementation also aids in reducing circulating tyrosine levels.

Other types of tyrosinemia are related to specific enzyme defects (see Fig. 39.17). Tyrosinemia II is caused by a genetic deficiency of tyrosine aminotransferase (TAT) and may lead to lesions of the eye and skin as well as neurologic problems. Patients are treated with a low-tyrosine, low-phenylalanine diet.

Tyrosinemia I (also called tyrosinosis) is caused by a genetic deficiency of fumarylacetoacetate hydrolase. The acute form is associated with liver failure, a cabbagelike odor, and death within the first year of life.

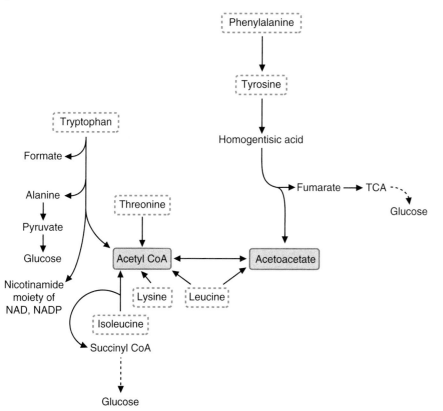

Fig. 39.16. Ketogenic amino acids. Some of these amino acids (tryptophan, phenylalanine, and tyrosine) also contain carbons that can form glucose. Leucine and lysine are strictly ketogenic; they do not form glucose.

 A: In addition to methionine, threonine, isoleucine, and valine (see Fig. 39.14), the last three carbons at the ω-end of odd-chain fatty acids, form succinyl CoA by this route (see Chapter 23)

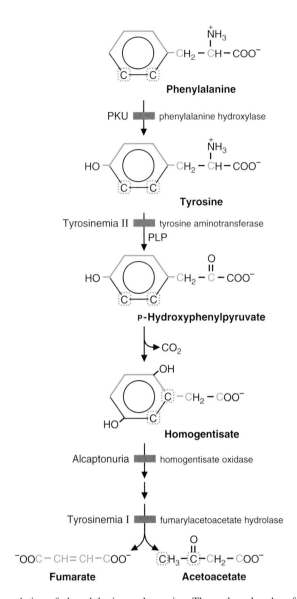

A small subset of patients with hyperphenylaninemia show an appropriate reduction in plasma phenylalanine levels with dietary restriction of this amino acid; however, these patients still develop progressive neurologic symptoms and seizures and usually die within the first 2 years of life ("malignant" hyperphenylaninemia). These infants exhibit normal phenylalanine hydroxylase (PAH) activity but have a deficiency in dihydropteridine reductase (DHPR), an enzyme required for the regeneration of tetrahydrobiopterin (BH_4), a cofactor of PAH (see Fig. 39.18). Less frequently, DHPR activity is normal but a defect in the biosynthesis of BH_4 exists. In either case, dietary therapy corrects the hyperphenylaninemia. However, BH_4 is also a cofactor for two other hydroxylations required in the synthesis of neurotransmitters in the brain: the hydroxylation of tryptophan to 5-hydroxytryptophan and of tyrosine to L-dopa (see Chapter 48). It has been suggested that the resulting deficit in central nervous system neurotransmitter activity is, at least in part, responsible for the neurologic manifestations and eventual death of these patients.

Fig. 39.17. Degradation of phenylalanine and tyrosine. The carboxyl carbon forms CO_2, and the other carbons form fumarate or acetoacetate as indicated. Deficiencies of enzymes (gray bars) result in the indicated diseases. PKU = phenylketonuria.

If the dietary levels of niacin and tryptophan are insufficient, the condition known as pellagra results. The symptoms of pellagra are dermatitis, diarrhea, dementia, and, finally, death. In addition, abnormal metabolism of tryptophan occurs in a vitamin B6 deficiency. Kynurenine intermediates in tryptophan degradation cannot be cleaved because kynureninase requires PLP derived from vitamin B6. Consequently, these intermediates enter a minor pathway for tryptophan metabolism that produces xanthurenic acid, which is excreted in the urine.

B. Tryptophan

Tryptophan is oxidized to produce alanine (from the non-ring carbons), formate, and acetyl CoA. Tryptophan is, therefore, both glucogenic and ketogenic (Fig. 39.19).

NAD and NADP can be produced from the ring structure of tryptophan. Therefore, tryptophan "spares" the dietary requirement for niacin. The higher the dietary levels of tryptophan, the lower the levels of niacin required to prevent symptoms of deficiency.

C. Threonine, Isoleucine, Leucine, and Lysine

As discussed previously, the major route of threonine degradation in humans is by threonine dehydratase (see section III.D.2.). In a minor pathway, threonine degradation by threonine aldolase produces glycine and acetyl CoA in the liver.

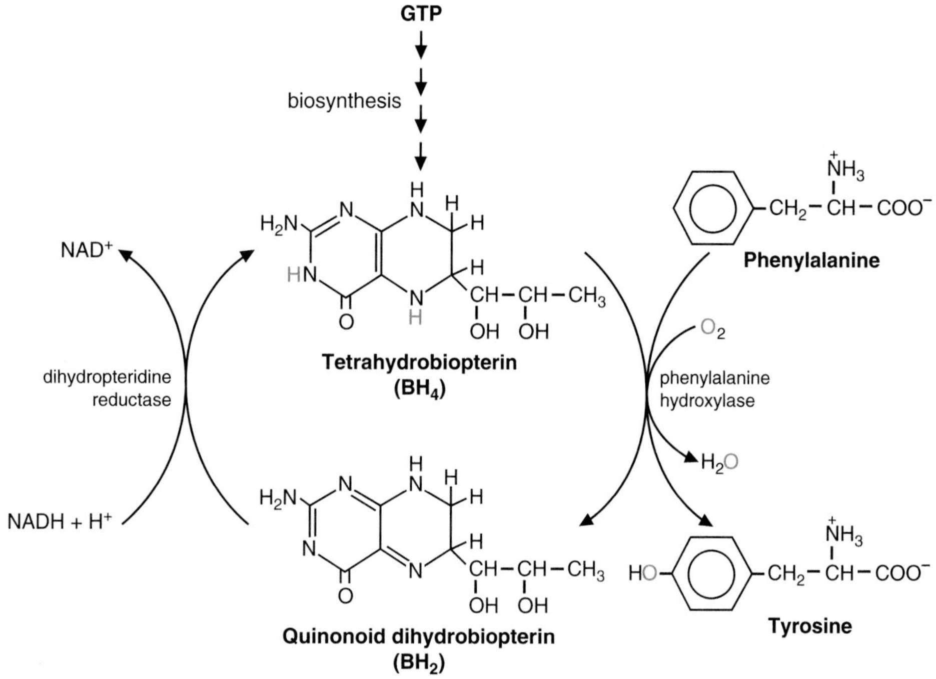

Fig. 39.18. Hydroxylation of phenylalanine. Phenylalanine hydroxylase (PAH) is a mixed-function oxidase; i.e., molecular oxygen (O_2) donates one atom to water and one to the product, tyrosine. The cofactor, tetrahydrobiopterin (BH_4), is oxidized to dihydrobiopterin (BH_2), and must be reduced back to BH_4 for the phenylalanine to continue forming tyrosine. BH_4 is synthesized in the body from GTP. PKU results from deficiencies of PAH (the classic form), dihydropteridine reductase, or enzymes in the biosynthetic pathway for BH_4.

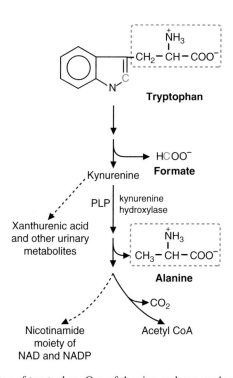

Fig. 39.19. Degradation of tryptophan. One of the ring carbons produces formate. The non-ring portion forms alanine. Kynurenine is an intermediate, which can be converted to a number of urinary excretion products (e.g., xanthurenate), degraded to CO_2 and acetyl CoA, or converted to the nicotinamide moiety of NAD and NADP, which also can be formed from the vitamin niacin.

On more definitive testing of **Piquet Yuria's** blood, the plasma level of phenylalanine was elevated at 18 mg/dL (reference range, <1.2). Several phenyl ketones and other products of phenylalanine metabolism, which give the urine a characteristic odor, were found in significant quantities in the baby's urine.

Phenylalanine

Transamination

Phenylpyruvate

CO_2

Phenylacetate

Phenyllactate

A liver biopsy was sent to the special chemistry research laboratory, where it was determined that the level of activity of phenylalanine hydroxylase (PAH) in Piquet's blood was less than 1% of that found in normal infants. A diagnosis of "classic" phenylketonuria (PKU) was made.

Until gene therapy allows substitution of the defective PAH gene with its normal counterpart in vivo, the mainstay of therapy in classic PKU is to maintain levels of phenylalanine in the blood between 3 and 12 mg/dL through dietary restriction of this essential amino acid.

Isoleucine produces both succinyl CoA and acetyl CoA (see section III.D.3.).

Leucine is purely ketogenic and produces hydroxymethylglutaryl CoA (HMG-CoA), which is cleaved to form acetyl CoA and the ketone body acetoacetate (see Figs. 39.15 and 39.16). Most of the tissues in which it is oxidized can use ketone bodies, with the exception of the liver. As with valine and isoleucine, leucine is a universal fuel, with its primary metabolism occurring in muscle.

Lysine cannot be directly transaminated at either of its two amino groups. Lysine is degraded by a complex pathway in which saccharopine, α-ketoadipate, and crotonyl CoA are intermediates. During the degradation pathway NADH and $FADH_2$ are generated for energy. Ultimately, lysine generates acetyl CoA (see Fig. 39.16) and is strictly ketogenic.

CLINICAL COMMENTS

Piquet Yuria. The overall incidence of hyperphenylalaninemia is approximately 100 per million births, with a wide geographic and ethnic variation. PKU occurs by autosomal recessive transmission of a defective PAH gene, causing accumulation of phenylalanine in the blood well above the normal concentration in young children and adults (less than 1–2 mg/dL). In the newborn, the upper limit of normal is almost twice this value. Values above 16 mg/dL are usually found in patients, such as **Piquet Yuria**, with "classic" PKU.

Patients with classic PKU usually appear normal at birth. If the disease is not recognized and treated within the first month of life, the infant gradually develops varying degrees of irreversible mental retardation (IQ scores frequently under 50), delayed psychomotor maturation, tremors, seizures, eczema, and hyperactivity. The neurologic sequelae may result in part from the competitive interaction of phenylalanine with brain amino acid transport systems and inhibition of neurotransmitter synthesis. These biochemical alterations lead to impaired myelin synthesis and delayed neuronal development, which result in the clinical picture in patients such as **Piquet Yuria**. Because of the simplicity of the test for PKU (elevated phenylalanine levels in the blood), all newborns in the United States are required to have a PKU test at birth. Early detection of the disease can lead to early treatment, and the neurologic consequences of the disease can be bypassed.

To restrict dietary levels of phenylalanine, special semisynthetic preparations such as Lofenalac or PKUaid are used in the United States. Use of these preparations reduces dietary intake of phenylalanine to 250–500 mg/day while maintaining normal intake of all other dietary nutrients. Although it is generally agreed that scrupulous adherence to this regimen is mandatory for the first decade of life, less consensus exists regarding its indefinite use. Evidence suggests, however, that without lifelong compliance with dietary restriction of phenylalanine, even adults will develop at least neurologic sequelae of PKU. A pregnant woman with PKU must be particularly careful to maintain satisfactory plasma levels of phenylalanine throughout gestation to avoid the adverse effects of hyperphenylalaninemia on the fetus.

Piquet's parents were given thorough dietary instruction, which they followed carefully. Although her pediatrician was not optimistic, it was hoped that the damage done to her nervous system before dietary therapy was minimal and that her subsequent psychomotor development would allow her to lead a relatively normal life.

Homer Sistine. The most characteristic biochemical features of the disorder affecting **Homer Sistine**, a cystathionine β-synthase deficiency, are the presence of an accumulation of both homocyst(e)ine and methionine in the blood. Because renal tubular reabsorption of methionine is highly efficient, this amino acid may not appear in the urine. Homocystine, the disulfide of homocysteine, is less efficiently reabsorbed, and amounts in excess of 1 mmol may be excreted in the urine each day.

In the type of homocystinuria in which the patient is deficient in cystathione β-synthase, the elevation in serum methionine levels is presumed to be the result of enhanced rates of conversion of homocysteine to methionine, caused by increased availability of homocysteine (see Fig. 39.14). In type II and type III homocystinuria, in which there is a deficiency in the synthesis of methyl cobalamin and of N^5-methyltetrahydrofolate, respectively (both required for the methylation of homocysteine to form methionine), serum homocysteine levels are elevated but serum methionine levels are low (see Fig. 39.14).

Acute vascular events are common in these patients. Thrombi (blood clots) and emboli (clots that have broken off and traveled to a distant site in the vascular system) have been reported in almost every major artery and vein as well as in smaller vessels. These clots result in infarcts in vital organs such as the liver, the myocardium (heart muscle), the lungs, the kidneys, and many other tissues. Although increased serum levels of homocysteine have been implicated in enhanced platelet aggregation and damage to vascular endothelial cells (leading to clotting and accelerated atherosclerosis), no generally accepted mechanism for these vascular events has yet emerged.

Treatment is directed toward early reduction of the elevated levels of homocysteine and methionine in the blood. In addition to a diet low in methionine, very high oral doses of pyridoxine (vitamin B6) have significantly decreased the plasma levels of homocysteine and methionine in some patients with cystathionine β-synthase deficiency. (Genetically determined "responders" to pyridoxine treatment make up approximately 50% of type I homocystinurics.) PLP serves as a cofactor for cystathionine β-synthase; however, the molecular properties of the defective enzyme that confer the responsiveness to B6 therapy are not known.

The terms *hypermethioninemia, homocystinuria* (or *-emia*), and *cystathioninuria* (or *-emia*) designate biochemical abnormalities and are not specific clinical diseases. Each may be caused by more than one specific genetic defect. For example, at least seven distinct genetic alterations can cause increased excretion of homocystine in the urine. A deficiency of cystathionine β-synthase is the most common cause of homocystinuria; more than 600 such proven cases have been studied.

 The pathologic findings that underlie the clinical features manifested by **Homer Sistine** are presumed (but not proved) to be the consequence of chronic elevations of homocysteine (and perhaps other compounds, e.g., methionine) in the blood and tissues. The zonular fibers that normally hold the lens of the eye in place become frayed and break, causing dislocation of the lens. The skeleton reveals a loss of bone ground substance (i.e., osteoporosis), which may explain the curvature of the spine. The elongation of the long bones beyond their normal genetically determined length leads to tall stature.

Animal experiments suggest that increased concentrations of homocysteine and methionine in the brain may trap adenosine as *S*-adenosylhomocysteine, diminishing adenosine levels. Because adenosine normally acts as a central nervous system depressant, its deficiency may be associated with a lowering of the seizure threshold as well as a reduction in cognitive function.

BIOCHEMICAL COMMENTS

Phenylketonuria. Many enzyme deficiency diseases have been discovered that affect the pathways of amino acid metabolism. These deficiency diseases have helped researchers to elucidate the pathways in humans, in whom experimental manipulation is, at best, unethical. These spontaneous mutations ("experiments" of nature), although devastating to patients, have resulted in an understanding of these diseases that now permit treatment of inborn errors of metabolism that were once considered to be untreatable.

Classic PKU is caused by mutations in the gene located on chromosome 12 that encodes the enzyme phenylalanine hydroxylase (PAH). This enzyme normally catalyzes the hydroxylation of phenylalanine to tyrosine, the rate-limiting step in the major pathway by which phenylalanine is catabolized.

In early experiments, sequence analysis of mutant clones indicated a single base substitution in the gene with a G to A transition at the canonical 5′ donor splice site of intron 12 and expression of a truncated unstable protein product. This protein lacked the C-terminal region, a structural change that yielded less than 1% of the normal activity of PAH.

Table 39.1. Genetic Disorders of Amino Acid Metabolism

Amino Acid Degradation Pathway	Missing Enzyme	Product That Accumulates	Disease	Symptoms
Phenylalanine	Phenylalanine hydroxylase	Phenylalanine	PKU (classical)	Mental retardation
	Dihydropteridine reductase	Phenylalanine	PKU (non-classical)	Mental retardation
	Homogentisate oxidase	Homogentisic acid	Alcaptonuria	Black urine, arthritis
	Fumarylacetoacetate hydrolase	Fumarylacetoacetate	Tyrosinemia I	Liver failure, death early
Tyrosine	Tyrosine aminotransferase	Tyrosine	Tyrosinemia II	Neurologic defects
	Cystathionase	Cystathionine	Cystathioninuria	Benign
Methionine	Cystathionine β-synthase	Homocysteine	Homocysteinemia	Cardiovascular complications and neurologic problems
Glycine	Glycine transaminase	Glyoxylate	Primary oxaluria type I	Renal failure due to stone formation
Branched-chain amino acids (leucine, isoleucine, valine)	Branched-chain α-keto acid dehydrogenase	α-Keto acids of the branched chain amino acids	Maple syrup urine disease	Mental retardation

Since these initial studies, DNA analysis has shown over 100 mutations (missense, nonsense, insertions, and deletions) in the PAH gene, associated with PKU and non-PKU hyperphenylalaninemia. That PKU is a heterogeneous phenotype is supported by studies measuring PAH activity in needle biopsy samples taken from the livers of a large group of patients with varying degrees of hyperphenylalaninemia. PAH activity varied from below 1% of normal in patients with classic PKU to up to 35% of normal in those with a non-PKU form of hyperphenylalaninemia (such as a defect in BH_4 production; see Chapter 48).

The genetic diseases affecting amino acid degradation that have been discussed in this chapter are summarized in Table 39.1.

Suggested References

Burton BK. Inborn errors of metabolism in infancy: a guide to diagnosis. Pediatrics 1998; 102:e69.

Mudd S, Levy H, Klaus, JP. Disorders of transsulfuration. In: Scriver CR, Beaudet AL, Sly WS, Valle D, eds. The Metabolic and Molecular Bases of Inherited Disease, vol. II, 8th Ed. New York: McGraw-Hill, 2001:2007–2056.

St. Joer ST, Howard BV, et al. Dietary protein and weight reduction. A statement for healthcare professionals from the nutrition committee of the Council on Nutrition, Physical Activity, and Metabolism of the American Heart Association. Circulation 2001;104:1869–1874.

Scriver C, Kaufman S,. Hyperphenylalanemia: Phenylalanine hydroxylase deficiency. In: Scriver CR, Beaudet AL, Sly WS, Valle D, eds. The Metabolic and Molecular Bases of Inherited Disease, vol. II, 8th Ed. New York: McGraw-Hill, 2001:1667–1724.

 REVIEW QUESTIONS—CHAPTER 39

1. If an individual has a vitamin B6 deficiency, which of the following amino acids could still be synthesized and be considered nonessential?

   (A) Tyrosine
   (B) Serine
   (C) Alanine
   (D) Cysteine
   (E) Aspartate

2. The degradation of amino acids can be classified into families, which are named after the end product of the degradative pathway. Which of the following is such an end product?

   (A) Citrate
   (B) Glyceraldehyde-3-phosphate
   (C) Fructose-6-phosphate
   (D) Malate
   (E) Succinyl-CoA

3. A newborn infant has elevated levels of phenylalanine and phenylpyruvate in her blood. Which of the following enzymes might be deficient in this baby?

   (A) Phenylalanine dehydrogenase
   (B) Phenylalanine oxidase
   (C) Dihydropteridine reductase
   (D) Tyrosine hydroxylase
   (E) Tetrahydrofolate synthase

4. Pyridoxal phosphate is required for which of the following reaction pathways or individual reactions?

   (A) Phenylalanine $\rightarrow$ tyrosine
   (B) Methionine $\rightarrow$ cysteine + α-ketobutyrate
   (C) Propionyl CoA $\rightarrow$ succinyl-CoA
   (D) Pyruvate $\rightarrow$ acetyl-CoA
   (E) Glucose $\rightarrow$ glycogen

5. A folic acid deficiency would interfere with the synthesis of which of the following amino acids from the indicated precursors?

   (A) Aspartate from oxaloacetate and glutamate
   (B) Glutamate from glucose and ammonia
   (C) Glycine from glucose and alanine
   (D) Proline from glutamate
   (E) Serine from glucose and alanine

40 Tetrahydrofolate, Vitamin B12, And S-Adenosylmethionine

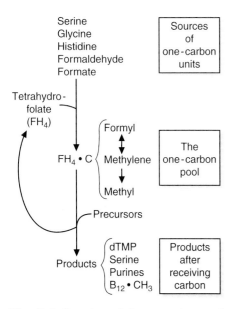

Fig. 40.1. Overview of the one-carbon pool. FH$_4$•C indicates tetrahydrofolate (FH$_4$) containing a one-carbon unit that is at the formyl, methylene, or methyl level of oxidation (see Fig. 40.3). The origin of the carbons is indicated, as are the final products after a one-carbon transfer.

Groups containing a single carbon atom can be transferred from one compound to another. These carbon atoms may be in a number of different oxidation states. The most oxidized form, CO_2, is transferred by biotin. One-carbon groups at lower levels of oxidation than CO_2 are transferred by reactions involving tetrahydrofolate (FH$_4$), vitamin B12, and S-adenosylmethionine (SAM).

Tetrahydrofolate: *Tetrahydrofolate, which is produced from the **vitamin folate**, is the primary one-carbon carrier in the body. This vitamin obtains one-carbon units from serine, glycine, histidine, formaldehyde, and formate (Fig. 40.1). While these carbons are attached to FH$_4$ they can be either oxidized or reduced. Because of this, folate can exist in a variety of chemical forms. Once a carbon has been reduced to the methyl level (methyl-FH$_4$), however, it cannot be re-oxidized. Collectively, these one-carbon groups attached to their carrier FH$_4$ are known as the **one-carbon pool**. The term folate is used to represent a water-soluble B-complex vitamin that functions in transferring single-carbon groups at various stages of oxidation.*

*The one-carbon groups carried by FH$_4$ are used for many biosynthetic reactions. For example, one-carbon units are transferred to the pyrimidine base of deoxyuridine monophosphate (**dUMP**) to form deoxythymidine monophosphate (**dTMP**), to the amino acid **glycine** to form **serine**, to precursors of the purine bases to produce carbons C2 and C8 of the **purine ring**, and to **vitamin B12**.*

Vitamin B12: *Vitamin B12 is involved in two reactions in the body. It participates in the rearrangement of the methyl group of L-methylmalonyl-CoA to form succinyl-CoA, and it transfers a methyl group, obtained from FH$_4$, to homocysteine, forming methionine.*

S-adenosylmethionine (SAM): *SAM, produced from methionine and adenosine triphosphate (ATP), transfers the methyl group to precursors forming a number of compounds, including creatine, phosphatidylcholine, epinephrine, melatonin, methylated nucleotides, and methylated DNA.*

Methionine metabolism is very dependent on both FH$_4$ and vitamin B12.
Homocysteine *is derived from methionine metabolism and can be converted back into methionine by using both methyl-FH$_4$ and vitamin B12. This is the only reaction in which methyl-FH$_4$ can donate the methyl group. If the enzyme that catalyzes this reaction is defective, or if vitamin B12 or FH$_4$ levels are insufficient, homocysteine will accumulate. Elevated homocysteine levels have been linked to cardiovascular and neurologic disease. A vitamin B12 deficiency can be brought about by the lack of **intrinsic factor**, a gastric protein required for the absorption of dietary B12. A consequence of vitamin B12 deficiency is the accumulation of methyl-FH$_4$ and a decrease in other folate derivatives. This is known as the*

methyl-trap hypothesis, *in which, because of the B12 deficiency, most of the carbons in the FH₄ pool are trapped in the methyl-FH₄ form, which is the most stable. The carbons cannot be released from the folate, because the one reaction in which they participate cannot occur because of the B12 deficiency. This will therefore lead to a functional folate deficiency, even though total levels of folate are normal. A folate deficiency (whether functional or actual) will lead to **megaloblastic anemia** caused by an inability of blood cell precursors to synthesize DNA and therefore to divide. This leads to large, partially replicated cells being released into the blood to attempt to replenish the cells that have died. Folate deficiencies also have been linked to an increased incidence of **neural-tube defects**, such as spina bifida, in mothers who become pregnant while folate deficient.*

THE WAITING ROOM

After resection of the cancer in his large intestine and completion of a course of postoperative chemotherapy with 5-fluorouracil (5-FU), **Colin Tuma** returned to his gastroenterologist for a routine follow-up colonoscopy. His colon was completely normal, with excellent healing at the site of the anastomosis. His physician expressed great optimism about a cure of Colin's previous malignancy but cautioned him about the need for regular colonoscopic examinations over the next few years.

Bea Twelvlow, a 75-year-old woman, went to see her physician because of a numbness and tingling in her arms. A diet history indicated a normal and healthy diet, but Bea was not taking any supplemental vitamin pills. Laboratory results indicated a slight elevation of methylmalonic acid, and this led the physician to suspect a vitamin B12 deficiency. Direct measurement of serum B12 levels did indicate a deficiency, but the results of a Schilling test were normal.

The initial laboratory profile, determined when **Jean Ann Tonich** first presented to her physician with evidence of early alcohol-induced hepatitis, included a hematologic analysis that showed that Jean Ann was anemic. Her hemoglobin was 11.0 g/dL (reference range = 12–16 for an adult female). The erythrocyte (red blood cell) count was 3.6 million cells/mm3 (reference range = 4.0–5.2 for an adult female). The average volume of her red blood cells (mean corpuscular volume, or MCV) was 108 fL (reference range = 80–100), and the hematology laboratory reported a striking variation in the size and shape of the red blood cells in a smear of her peripheral blood (see Chapter 44). The nuclei of the circulating granulocytic leukocytes had increased nuclear segmentation (polysegmented neutrophils). Because these findings are suggestive of a macrocytic anemia (in which blood cells are larger than normal), measurements of serum folate and vitamin B12 (cobalamin) levels were ordered.

I. TETRAHYDROFOLATE (FH₄)

A. Structure and Forms of FH₄

Folates exist in many chemical forms. The coenzyme form that functions in accepting one-carbon groups is tetrahydrofolate polyglutamate (Fig. 40.2), generally just referred to as tetrahydrofolate or FH₄. It has three major structural components, a bicyclic pteridine ring, para-aminobenzoic acid, and a polyglutamate tail consisting

The Schilling test involves the patient ingesting radioactive (Co⁶⁰) crystalline vitamin B12 after which a 24-hour urine sample is collected. The radioactivity in the urine sample is compared with the input radioactivity, and the difference represents the amount of B12 absorbed through the digestive tract.

Folate deficiencies frequently occur in individuals with chronic alcoholism. A number of factors are involved: inadequate dietary intake of folate; direct damage to intestinal cells and brush border enzymes, which interferes with absorption of dietary folate; a defect in the enterohepatic circulation, which reduces the absorption of folate; liver damage causing decreased hepatic production of plasma proteins; and interference with kidney resorption of folate.

Because of the possibility of a direct toxic effect of alcohol on hematopoietic tissues in **Jean Ann Tonich**, a bone marrow aspirate was performed. The aspirate contained a greater than normal number of red and white blood cell precursors, most of which were larger than normal. The large red blood cells are called megaloblasts.

These hematopoietic precursor cells when exposed to too little folate and/or vitamin B12 show slowed cell division, but cytoplasmic development occurs at a normal rate. Hence, the megaloblastic cells tend to be large, with an increased ratio of RNA to DNA. Megaloblastic erythroid progenitors are usually destroyed in the bone marrow (although some reach the circulation). Thus, marrow cellularity is often increased but production of red blood cells is decreased, a condition called "ineffective erythropoiesis."

Therefore, Jean Ann had a megaloblastic anemia, characteristic of a folate or B12 deficiency.

Jean Ann's serum folic acid level was 3.1 ng/mL (reference range = 6–15), and her serum B12 level was 154 pg/mL (reference range = 150–750). Her serum iron level was normal. It was clear, therefore, that Jean Ann's megaloblastic anemia was caused by a folate deficiency (although her B12 levels were in the low range of normal). The management of a pure folate deficiency in an alcoholic patient includes cessation of alcohol intake and a diet rich in folate.

The abbreviation fL stands for *femtoliters*. One fL is 10^{-12} milliliters (mL).

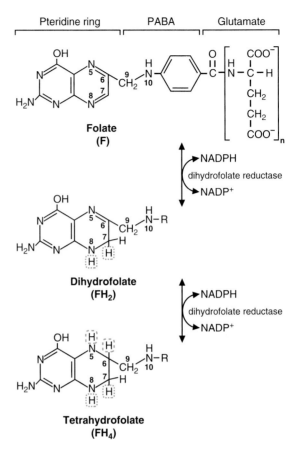

Fig. 40.2. Reduction of folate to tetrahydrofolate (FH_4). The same enzyme, dihydrofolate reductase, catalyzes both reactions. Multiple glutamate residues are added within cells ($n \sim 5$). Plants can synthesize folate, but humans cannot. Therefore, folate is a dietary requirement. R is the portion of the folate molecule shown to the right of N^{10}. The different precursors of FH_4 are indicated in the figure. PABA = para-aminobenzoic acid.

Sulfa drugs, which are used to treat certain bacterial infections, are analogs of para-aminobenzoic acid. They prevent growth and cell division in bacteria by interfering with the synthesis of folate. Because we cannot synthesize folate, sulfa drugs do not affect human cells in this way.

The current recommended dietary allowance (RDA) for folate equivalents is approximately 400 μg for adult men and women. In addition to being prevalent in green leafy vegetables, other good sources of this vitamin are liver, yeast, legumes, and some fruits. Protracted cooking of these foods, however, can destroy up to 90% of their folate content. A standard US diet provides 50 to 500 μg absorbable folate each day. Folate deficiency in pregnant women, especially during the month before conception and the month after, increases the risk of neural tube defects, such as spina bifida, in the fetus. To reduce the potential risk of neural tube defects for women capable of becoming pregnant, the recommendation is to take 400 μg of folic acid daily from a multivitamin pill. If the women has a history of having a child with a neural tube defect, this amount is increased to 4000 μg/day for the month before and the month after conception. Flour-containing products in the United States are now supplemented with folate to reduce the risk of neural tube defects in newborns.

of several glutamate residues joined in amide linkage. The one-carbon group that is accepted by the coenzyme and then transferred to another compound is bound to N^5, to N^{10}, or to both.

Different forms of folate may differ in the oxidation state of the one-carbon group, in the number of glutamate residues attached, or in the degree of oxidation of the pteridine ring. When the term *folate* or *folic acid* is applied to a specific chemical form, it is the most oxidized form of the pteridine ring (see Fig. 40.2). Folate is reduced to dihydrofolate and then to tetrahydrofolate by dihydrofolate reductase present in cells. Reduction is the favored direction of the reaction; therefore, most of the folate present in the body is present as the reduced coenzyme form, FH_4.

B. The Vitamin Folate

Folates are synthesized in bacteria and higher plants and ingested in green leafy vegetables, fruits, and legumes in our diet. The vitamin was named for its presence in green, leafy vegetables (foliage). Most of the dietary folate derived from natural food sources is present in the reduced coenzyme form. However, vitamin supplements and fortified foods contain principally the oxidized form of the pteridine ring.

As dietary folates pass into the proximal third of the small intestine, folate conjugases in the brush border of the lumen cleave off glutamate residues to produce the monoglutamate form of folate, which is then absorbed (see Fig. 40.2, upper structure, when n = 1). Within the intestinal cells, folate is converted principally to N^5-methyl FH_4, which enters the portal vein and goes to the liver. Smaller amounts of other forms of folate also follow this route.

The liver, which stores half of the body's folate, takes up much of the folate from the portal circulation; uptake may be through active transport or receptor-mediated endocytosis. Within the liver, FH_4 is reconjugated to the polyglutamate form before being used in reactions. A small amount of the folate is partially degraded, and the components enter the urine. A relatively large portion of the folate enters the bile and is subsequently reabsorbed (very similar to the fate of bile salts in the enterohepatic circulation).

N^5-Methyl-FH_4, the major form of folate in the blood, is loosely bound to plasma proteins, particularly serum albumin.

C. Oxidation and Reduction of the One-Carbon Groups of Tetrahydrofolate

One-carbon groups transferred by FH_4 are attached either to nitrogen N^5 or N^{10} or they form a bridge between N^5 and N^{10}. The collection of one-carbon groups attached to FH_4 is known as the one-carbon pool. While attached to FH_4, these one-carbon units can be oxidized and reduced (Fig. 40.3). Thus, reactions requiring a carbon at a particular oxidation state may use carbon from the one-carbon pool that was donated at a different oxidation state.

The individual steps for reduction of the one-carbon group are shown in Fig. 40.4. The most oxidized form is N^{10}-formyl FH_4. The most reduced form is N^5-methyl-FH_4. Once the methyl group is formed, it is *not readily reoxidized back to N^5, N^{10} methylene FH_4, and thus N^5-methyl-FH_4 will tend to accumulate in the cell.*

D. Sources of One-Carbon Groups Carried by FH_4

Carbon sources for the one-carbon pool include serine, glycine, formaldehyde, histidine, and formate (see Fig. 40.4). These donors transfer the carbons to folate at different oxidation states. Serine is the major carbon source of one-carbon groups in the human. Its hydroxymethyl group is transferred to FH_4 in a reversible reaction, catalyzed by the enzyme serine hydroxymethyltransferase. This reaction produces glycine and N^5, N^{10}-methylene-FH_4. Because serine can be synthesized from 3-phosphoglycerate, an intermediate of glycolysis, dietary carbohydrate can serve as a source of carbon for the one-carbon pool. The glycine that is produced may be further degraded by donation of a carbon to folate. Additional donors that form N^5, N^{10} methylene-FH_4 are listed in Table 40.1.

Table 40.1. One-Carbon Pool: Sources and Recipients of Carbon

Source[a]	Form of One-Carbon Donor Produced[b]	Recipient	Final Product
Formate	N^{10}-formyl-FH_4	Purine precursor	Purine (C2 and C8)
Serine Glycine Formaldehyde	N^5, N^{10} methylene FH_4	dUMP Glycine	dTMP Serine
N^5, N^{10} methylene FH_4	N^5-methyl FH_4	Vitamin B12	Methylcobalamin
Histidine	N^5-formimino FH_4 is converted to N^5, N^{10} methylene FH_4		
Choline	Betaine	Homocysteine	Methionine and Dimethylglycine
Methionine	S-adenosylmethionine (SAM)	Glycine (there are many others; see figure 40.9B)	N-methylglycine (sarcosine)

[a]The major source of carbon is serine.
[b]The carbon unit attached to FH_4 can be oxidized and reduced (see Fig. 40.3). At the methyl level, reoxidation does not occur.

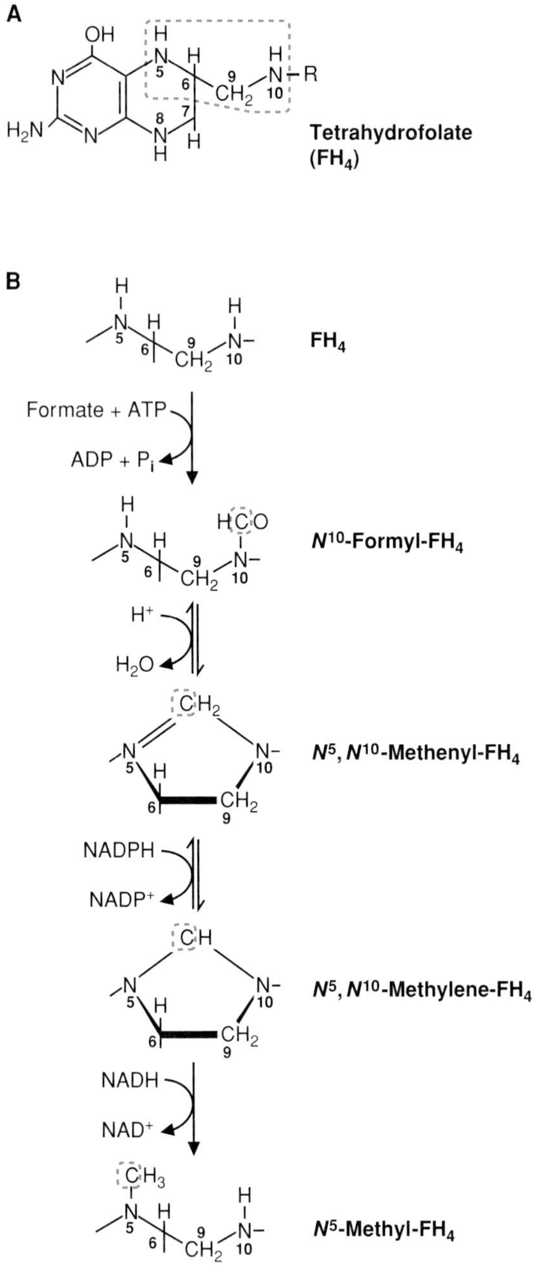

Fig. 40.3. One-carbon units attached to FH_4. A. The active form of FH_4. For definition of R, see Figure 40.2. B. Interconversions of one-carbon units of FH_4. Only the portion of FH_4 from N^5 to N^{10} is shown, which is indicated by the dashed line in Part A. After a formyl group forms a bridge between N^5 and N^{10}, two reductions can occur. Note that N^5-methyl-FH_4 cannot be reoxidized. The most oxidized form of FH_4 is at the top of the figure, whereas the most reduced form is at the bottom.

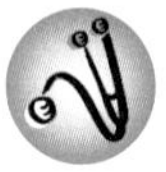

A deficiency of folate results in the accumulation of FIGLU, which is excreted in the urine. A histidine load test can be used for detecting folate deficiencies. Patients were given a test dose of histidine (a histidine load), and the amount of FIGLU that appeared in the urine was measured.

Histidine and formate provide examples of compounds that donate carbon at different oxidation levels (see Fig. 40.4). Degradation of histidine produces formiminoglutamate (FIGLU), which reacts with FH_4 to donate a carbon and nitrogen (generating N^5-formimino-FH_4), thereby releasing glutamate. Formate, produced from tryptophan oxidation, can react with FH_4 and generate N^{10}-formyl-FH_4, the most oxidized folate derivative.

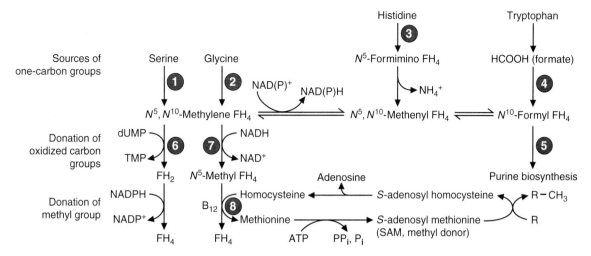

Fig. 40.4. Sources of carbon (reactions 1–4) for the FH$_4$ pool and the recipients of carbon (reactions 5–8) from the pool. See Figure 40.3 to view the FH$_4$ derivatives involved in each reaction.

E. Recipients of One-Carbon Groups

The one-carbon groups on FH$_4$ may be oxidized or reduced (see Fig. 40.3) and then transferred to other compounds (see Fig. 40.4 and Table 40.1). Transfers of this sort are involved in the synthesis of glycine from serine, the synthesis of the base thymine required for DNA synthesis, the purine bases required for both DNA and RNA synthesis, and the transfer of methyl groups to vitamin B12.

Because the conversion of serine to glycine is readily reversible, glycine can be converted to serine by drawing carbon from the one-carbon pool.

The nucleotide deoxythymidine monophosphate (dTMP) is produced from deoxyuridine monophosphate (dUMP) by a reaction in which dUMP is methylated to form dTMP (Fig. 40.5). The source of carbon is N^5, N^{10}-methylene FH$_4$. Two hydrogen atoms from FH$_4$ are used to reduce the donated carbon to the methyl level. Consequently, dihydrofolate (FH$_2$) is produced. Reduction of FH$_2$ by NADPH in a

FH$_4$ is required for the synthesis of deoxythymidine monophosphate and the purine bases used to produce the precursors for DNA replication. Therefore, FH$_4$ is required for cell division. Blockage of the synthesis of thymine and the purine bases either by a dietary deficiency of folate or by drugs that interfere with folate metabolism results in a decreased rate of cell division and growth.

A better understanding of the structure and function of the purine and pyrimidine bases and of folate metabolism led to the development of compounds having antimetabolic and antifolate action useful for treatment of neoplastic disease. For example, **Colin Tuma** was successfully treated for colon cancer with 5-fluorouracil (5-FU) (see Chapter 12 and Fig. 40.5). 5-FU is a pyrimidine analog, which is converted in cells to the nucleotide fluorodeoxyuridylate (FdUMP). FdUMP causes a "thymineless death," especially for tumor cells having a rapid turnover rate. It prevents the growth of cancer cells by blocking the thymidylate synthase reaction, i.e., the conversion of dUMP to dTMP.

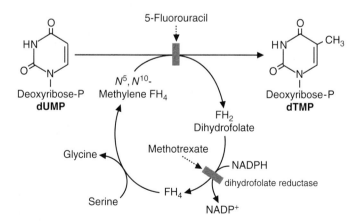

Fig. 40.5. Transfer of a one-carbon unit from N^5, N^{10} methylene FH$_4$ to dUMP to form dTMP. FH$_4$ is oxidized to FH$_2$ (dihydrofolate) in this reaction. FH$_2$ is reduced to FH$_4$ by dihydrofolate reductase and FH$_4$ is converted to N^5, N^{10} methylene FH$_4$ using serine as a carbon donor. Shaded bars indicate the steps at which the antimetabolites 5-fluorouracil (5-FU) and methotrexate act. 5-FU inhibits thymidylate synthase. Methotrexate inhibits dihydrofolate reductase.

Jean Ann Tonich's megaloblastic anemia was treated, in part, with folate supplements (see Clinical Comments). Within 48 hours of the initiation of folate therapy, megaloblastic or "ineffective" erythropoiesis usually subsides, and effective erythropoiesis begins.

A megaloblastic anemia is caused by a decrease in the synthesis of thymine and the purine bases. These deficiencies lead to an inability of hematopoietic (and other) cells to synthesize DNA and, therefore, to divide. Their persistently thwarted attempts at normal DNA replication, DNA repair, and cell division produce abnormally large cells (called megaloblasts) with abundant cytoplasm capable of RNA and protein synthesis, but with clumping and fragmentation of nuclear chromatin (see Chapter 44). Some of these large cells, although immature, are released early from the marrow in an attempt to compensate for the anemia. Thus, peripheral blood smears will also contain megaloblasts. Many of the large immature cells, however, are destroyed in the marrow and never reach the circulation.

The average daily diet in Western countries contains 5–30 μg vitamin B12, of which 1–5 μg is absorbed into the blood. (The RDA is 2.4 μg/day.) Total body content of this vitamin in an adult is approximately 2–5 mg, of which 1 mg is present in the liver. As a result, a dietary deficiency of B12 is uncommon and is only observed after a number of years on a diet deficient in this vitamin.

In spite of **Jean Ann Tonich's** relatively malnourished state because of chronic alcoholism, her serum cobalamin level was still within the low-to-normal range. If her undernourished state had continued, a cobalamin deficiency would eventually have developed.

reaction catalyzed by dihydrofolate reductase (DHFR) regenerates FH_4. This is the only reaction involving FH_4 in which the folate group is oxidized as the one-carbon group is donated to the recipient. Recall that DHFR is also required to reduce the oxidized form of the vitamin, which is obtained from the diet (see Fig. 40.2). Thus, DHFR is essential for both regenerating FH_2 in the tissues and from the diet. These reactions contribute to the effect of folate deficiency on DNA synthesis because dTMP is only required for the synthesis of DNA.

During the synthesis of the purine bases, carbons 2 and 8 are obtained from the one-carbon pool (see Chapter 41). N^{10}-Formyl-FH_4 provides both carbons. Folate deficiency would also hinder these reactions, contributing to an inability to replicate DNA because of the lack of precursors.

After the carbon group carried by FH_4 is reduced to the methyl level, it is transferred to vitamin B12. This is the only reaction through which the methyl group can leave FH_4 (recall that the reaction creating N^5-methyl FH_4 is not reversible).

II.   VITAMIN B12

A.   Structure and Forms of Vitamin B12

The structure of vitamin B12 (also known as cobalamin) is complex (Fig. 40.6). It contains a corrin ring, which is similar to the porphyrin ring found in heme. The corrin ring differs from heme, however, in that two of the four pyrrole rings are joined directly rather than by a methylene bridge. Its most unusual feature is the presence of cobalt, coordinated with the corrin ring (similar to the iron coordinated with the porphyrin ring). This cobalt can form a bond with a carbon atom. In the body, it reacts with the carbon of a methyl group, forming methylcobalamin, or with the 5′-carbon of 5′-deoxyadenosine, forming 5′-deoxyadenosylcobalamin (note that in this case the deoxy designation refers to the 5′ carbon, not the 2′ carbon as is the case in the sugar found in DNA). The form of B12 found in vitamin supplements is cyanocobalamin, in which a CN group is linked to the cobalt.

B.   Absorption and Transport of Vitamin B12

Although vitamin B12 is produced by bacteria, it cannot be synthesized by higher plants or animals. The major source of vitamin B12 is dietary meat, eggs, dairy products, fish, poultry, and seafood. The animals that serve as the source of these foods obtain B12 mainly from the bacteria in their food supply. The absorption of B12 from the diet is a complex process (Fig. 40.7).

Ingested B12 can exist in two forms, either free or bound to dietary proteins. If free, the B12 binds to proteins known as R-binders (haptocorrins, also known as transcobalamin I), which are secreted by the salivary glands and the gastric mucosa, in either the saliva or the stomach. If the ingested B12 is bound to proteins, it must be released from the proteins by the action of digestive proteases both in the stomach

Individuals with non-Hodgkin's lymphoma receive a number of drugs to treat the tumor, including the use of methotrexate. The structure of methotrexate is shown below.

Methotrexate

What compound does methotrexate resemble?

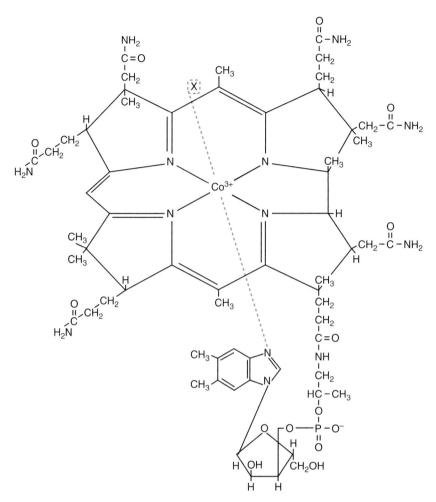

Fig. 40.6. Vitamin B12. X = 5′-deoxyadenosine in deoxyadenosylcobalamin; X = CH₃ in methylcobalamin; X = CN in cyanocobalamin (the commercial form found in vitamin tablets).

 Methotrexate has the same structure as folate except that it has an amino group on C4 and a methyl group on N10. Anticancer drugs such as methotrexate are folate analogs that act by inhibiting dihydrofolate reductase, thereby preventing the conversion of FH₂ to FH₄ (see Fig. 40.5). Thus, the cellular pools of FH₄ are not replenished, and reactions requiring FH₄ cannot proceed.

 Pernicious anemia, a deficiency of intrinsic factor, is a relatively common problem caused by malabsorption of dietary cobalamin. It may result from an inherited defect that leads to a decreased ability of gastric parietal cells to synthesize intrinsic factor or from partial resection of the stomach or of the ileum. Production of intrinsic factor often declines with age and may be low in elderly individuals. An alternative circumstance that leads to the development of a B12 deficiency is pancreatic insufficiency or a high intestinal pH, which would result from too little acid being produced by the stomach. Both of these conditions prevent the degradation of the R-binder-B12 complex; as a result, B12 will not be released from the R-binder protein and, therefore, cannot bind to intrinsic factor.

 How should vitamin B12 be administered to a patient with pernicious anemia?

and small intestine. Once the B12 is released from its bound protein, it will bind to the haptocorrins. In the small intestine, the pancreatic proteases digest the haptocorrins, and the released B12 then binds to intrinsic factor, a glycoprotein secreted by the parietal cells of the stomach when food enters the stomach. The intrinsic factor–B12 complex attaches to specific receptors in the terminal segment of the small intestine known as the ileum, after which the complex is internalized.

The B12 within the enterocyte complexes with transcobalamin II and then is released into circulation. The transcobalamin II–B12 complex delivers B12 to the tissues, which contain specific receptors for this complex. The liver takes up approximately 50% of the vitamin B12, and the remainder is transported to other tissues. The amount of the vitamin stored in the liver is large enough that 3 to 6 years pass before symptoms of a dietary deficiency occur.

C. Functions of Vitamin B12

Vitamin B12 is involved in two reactions in the body: the transfer of a methyl group from N⁵-methyl FH₄ to homocysteine to form methionine and the rearrangement of the methyl group of L-methylmalonyl CoA to form succinyl CoA (Fig. 40.8).

Tetrahydrofolate receives a one-carbon group from serine or from other sources. This carbon is reduced to the methyl level and transferred to vitamin B12, forming

Because the problem in pernicious anemia is a lack of intrinsic factor, which results in an inability to absorb vitamin B12 from the gastrointestinal tract, B12 cannot be administered orally to treat this condition. In the past, it was usually given by injection. An effective nasal spray containing B12 has recently been marketed, however, and its use precludes the need for lifelong injections of this vitamin.

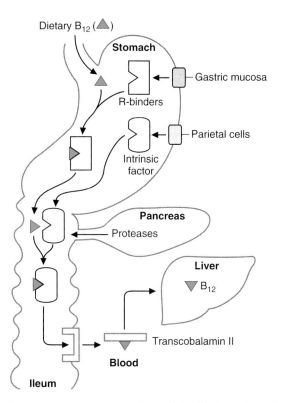

Fig. 40.7. Absorption, transport, and storage of vitamin B12. Dietary B12 binds to R-binders (haptocorrins) in the stomach and travels to the intestine, where the R-binders are destroyed by pancreatic proteases. The freed B12 then binds to intrinsic factor (IF). B12 is absorbed in the ileum and carried by called transcobalamins (TC) to the liver, where B12 is stored.

methyl-B12 (or methylcobalamin). Methylcobalamin transfers the methyl group to homocysteine, which is converted to methionine by the enzyme methionine synthase. Methionine can then be activated to SAM to transfer the methyl group to other compounds (Fig. 40.9).

Vitamin B12 also participates in the conversion of L-methylmalonyl CoA to succinyl CoA. In this case, the active form of the coenzyme is 5′-deoxyadenosylcobalamin. This reaction is part of the metabolic route for the conversion of carbons from valine, isoleucine, threonine, thymine, and the last three carbons of odd-chain fatty acids, all of which form propionyl CoA, to the TCA cycle intermediate succinyl CoA (see Chapter 39).

There are two major clinical manifestations of cobalamin (B12) deficiency. One such presentation is hematopoietic (caused by the adverse effects of a B12 deficiency on folate metabolism), and the other is neurologic (caused by hypomethylation in the nervous system).

The hemopoietic problems associated with a B12 deficiency are identical to those observed in a folate deficiency and, in fact, result from a folate deficiency secondary to (i.e., caused by) the B12 deficiency (i.e., the methyl trap hypothesis). As the FH$_4$ pool is exhausted, deficiencies of the tetrahydrofolate derivatives needed for purine and dTMP biosynthesis develop, leading to the characteristic megaloblastic anemia.

The classical clinical presentation of the neurologic dysfunction associated with a B12 deficiency includes symmetric numbness and tingling of the hands and feet, diminishing vibratory and position sense, and progression to a spastic gait disturbance. The patient may become somnolent or may become extremely irritable ("megaloblastic madness"). Eventually, blind spots in the central portions of the visual fields develop, accompanied by alterations in gustatory (taste) and olfactory (smell) function. This is believed to be caused by hypomethylation within the nervous system, brought about by an inability to recycle homocysteine to methionine and from there to S-adenosylmethionine. The latter is the required methyl donor in these reactions. The nervous system lacks the betaine pathway of methionine regeneration and is dependent on the B12 system. With a B12 deficiency, this pathway is inoperable in the nervous system.

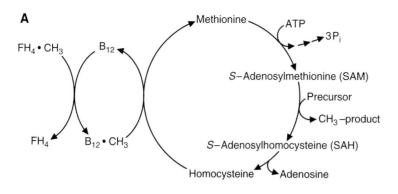

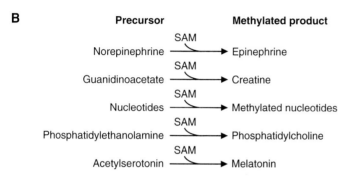

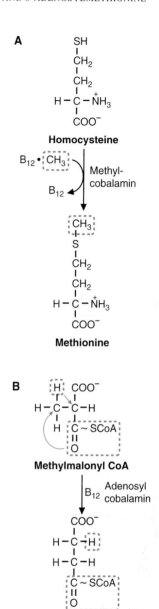

Fig. 40.9. Relationship between FH$_4$, B12, and SAM. A. Overall scheme. B. Some specific reactions requiring SAM.

III. *S*-ADENOSYLMETHIONINE

S-Adenosylmethionine (SAM) participates in the synthesis of many compounds that contain methyl groups. It is used in reactions that add methyl groups to either oxygen or nitrogen atoms in the acceptor (contrast that to folate derivatives, which can add one-carbon groups to sulfur or to carbon). As examples, SAM is required for the conversion of phosphatidylethanolamine to phosphatidylcholine, guanidinoacetate to creatine, norepinephrine to epinephrine, acetylserotonin to melatonin, and nucleotides to methylated nucleotides (see Fig. 40.9B). It is also required for the inactivation of catecholamines and serotonin (see Chapter 48). More than 35 reactions in humans require methyl donation from SAM.

SAM is synthesized from methionine and ATP. As with the activation of vitamin B12, ATP donates the adenosine. With the transfer of its methyl group, SAM forms *S*-adenosylhomocysteine, which is subsequently hydrolyzed to form homocysteine and adenosine.

Methionine, required for the synthesis of SAM, is obtained from the diet or produced from homocysteine, which accepts a methyl group from vitamin B12

Fig. 40.8. The two reactions involving vitamin B12 in humans.

Many health food stores now sell SAMe, a stabilized version of S-adenosylmethionine. SAMe has been hypothesized to relieve depression because the synthesis of certain neurotransmitters requires methylation by SAM (see Chapter 47). This has led to the hypothesis that by increasing SAM levels within the nervous system, the biosynthesis of these neurotransmitters will be accelerated. This in turn might alleviate the feelings of depression. There have been reports in the literature indicating that this may occur, but its efficacy as an antidepressant must be confirmed. The major questions that must be addressed include the stability of SAMe in the digestive system and the level of uptake of SAMe by cells of the nervous system.

(see Fig. 40.9A). Thus, the methyl group of methionine is regenerated. The portion of methionine that is essential in the diet is the homocysteine moiety. If we had an adequate dietary source of homocysteine, methionine would not be required in the diet. However, there is no good dietary source of homocysteine, whereas methionine is plentiful in the diet.

Homocysteine provides the sulfur atom for the synthesis of cysteine (see Chapter 39). In this case, homocysteine reacts with serine to form cystathionine, which is cleaved, yielding cysteine and α-ketobutyrate. The first reaction in this sequence is inhibited by cysteine. Thus, methionine, via homocysteine, is not used for cysteine synthesis unless the levels of cysteine in the body are lower than required for its metabolic functions. An adequate dietary supply of cysteine, therefore, can "spare" (or reduce) the dietary requirement for methionine.

IV. RELATIONSHIPS BETWEEN FOLATE, VITAMIN B12, AND SAM

A. The Methyl-Trap Hypothesis

If one analyzes the flow of carbon in the folate cycle, the equilibrium lies in the direction of the N^5-methyl FH_4 form. This appears to be the most stable form of carbon attached to the vitamin. However, in only one reaction can the methyl group be removed from N^5-methyl FH_4, and that is the methionine synthase reaction, which requires vitamin B12. Thus, if vitamin B12 is deficient, or if the methionine synthase enzyme is defective, N^5-methyl FH_4 will accumulate. Eventually most folate forms in the body will become "trapped" in the N^5-methyl form. A functional folate deficiency results because the carbons cannot be removed from the folate. The appearance of a functional folate deficiency caused by a lack of vitamin B12 is known as the "methyl-trap" hypothesis, and its clinical implications are discussed in following sections.

Other compounds involved in one-carbon metabolism are derived from degradation products of choline. Choline, an essential component of certain phospholipids, is oxidized to form betaine aldehyde, which is further oxidized to betaine (trimethylglycine). In the liver, betaine can donate a methyl group to homocysteine to form methionine and dimethyl glycine. This allows the liver to have two routes for homocysteine conversion to methionine. Under conditions in which SAM accumulates, glycine can be methylated to form sarcosine (N-methyl glycine). This route is used when methionine levels are high and excess methionine needs to be metabolized.

B. Hyperhomocysteinemia

Elevated homocysteine levels have been linked to cardiovascular and neurologic disease. Homocysteine levels can accumulate in a number of ways, which are related to both folic acid and vitamin B12 metabolism. Homocysteine is derived from S-adenosyl homocysteine, which arises when SAM donates a methyl group (Fig. 40.10). Because SAM is frequently donating methyl groups, there is a constant production of S-adenosyl homocysteine, which leads to a constant production of homocysteine. Recall from Chapter 39 that homocysteine has two biochemical fates. The homocysteine produced can either be remethylated to methionine or condensed with serine to form cystathionine. There are two routes to methionine production. The major one is methylation by N^5-methyl FH_4, requiring vitamin B12. The liver also contains a second pathway in which betaine (a degradation product of choline) can donate a methyl group to homocysteine to form methionine, but this is a minor pathway. The conversion of homocysteine to cystathionine requires pyridoxal phosphate. Thus, if an individual is deficient in vitamin B12, the conversion of homocysteine to methionine by the major route is inhibited. This will direct homocysteine to produce cystathionine, which eventually produces cysteine. As cysteine levels accumulate, the enzyme that makes cystathinonine undergoes feedback inhibition, and that pathway is also inhibited (see Fig. 40.10). This, overall, leads to an accumulation of homocysteine, which is released into the blood.

Homocysteine also accumulates in the blood if a mutation is present in the enzyme that converts N^5, N^{10} methylene FH_4 to N^5-methyl FH_4. When this occurs, the levels of N^5-methyl FH_4 are too low to allow homocysteine to be converted to methionine. The loss of this pathway, coupled with the feedback inhibition by cysteine on cystathionine formation, will also lead to elevated homocysteine levels in the blood.

A third way in which serum homocysteine levels can be elevated is by a mutated cystathinone-β-synthase or a deficiency in vitamin B6, the required cofactor for that enzyme. These defects block the ability of homocysteine to be converted to cystathionine, and the homocysteine that does accumulate cannot all be accommodated by conversion to methionine. Thus, an accumulation of homocysteine results.

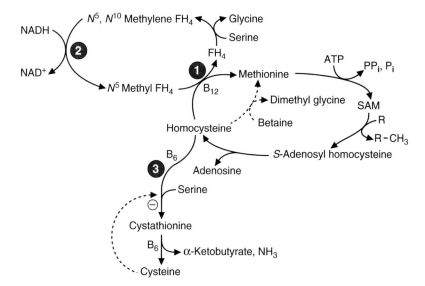

Fig. 40.10. Reaction pathways involving homocysteine. Defects in numbered enzymes (1 = methionine synthase, 2 = N^5, N^{10} methylene FH_4 reductase, 3 = cystathionine-β-synthase) lead to elevated homocysteine. Recall that as cysteine accumulates, there is feedback inhibition on cystathionine-β-synthase to stop further cysteine production.

C. Neural Tube Defects

Folate deficiency during pregnancy has been associated with an increased risk for neural tube defects in the developing fetus. This risk is significantly reduced if women take folic acid supplements periconceptually. The link between folate deficiency and neural tube defects was first observed in women with hyperhomocysteinemia brought about by a thermolabile variant of N^5, N^{10} methylene tetrahydrofolate reductase. This form of the enzyme, which results from a single nucleotide change (C to T) in position 677 of the gene encoding the protein, is less active at body temperature than at lower temperatures. This results in a reduced level of N^5-methyl tetrahydrofolate being generated and, therefore, an increase in the levels of homocysteine. Along with the elevated homocysteine, the women were also folate deficient. The folate deficiency and the subsequent inhibition of DNA synthesis leads to neural tube defects. The elevated homocysteine is one indication that such a deficit is present. These findings have led to the recommendation that women considering getting pregnant begin taking folate supplements before conception occurs, and for at least 1 month after conception. The Department of Agriculture has, in fact, mandated that folate be added to flour-containing products in the United States.

CLINICAL COMMENTS

 Jean Ann Tonich developed a folate deficiency and is on the verge of developing a cobalamin (vitamin B12) deficiency as a consequence of prolonged moderately severe malnutrition related to chronic alcoholism. Before folate therapy is started, the physician must ascertain that the megaloblastic anemia is not caused by a pure B12 deficiency or a combined deficiency of folate and B12.

If folate is given without cobalamin to a B12-deficient patient, the drug only partially corrects the megaloblastic anemia because it will "bypass" the methyl-folate trap and provide adequate FH_4 coenzyme for the conversion of dUMP to dTMP and for a resurgence of purine synthesis. As a result, normal DNA synthesis, DNA repair, and cell division occur. However, the neurologic syndrome, resulting from hypomethylation in nervous tissue, may progress unless the physician realizes that B12 supplementation is required. In Jean Ann's case, in which the serum B12 concentration was borderline low and in which the dietary history supported the possibility of a B12 deficiency, a combination of folate and B12 supplements is required to avoid this potential therapeutic trap.

 Colin Tuma continued to do well and faithfully returned for his regular colonoscopic examinations.

 Bea Twelvlow was diagnosed with an inability to absorb dietary B12 but not crystalline B12 (the Schilling test results were normal). One of the consequences of aging is a reduced acid production by the gastric mucosa (atrophic gastritis), which limits the ability of pepsin to work on dietary protein. A reduced pepsin efficiency would then reduce the amount of bound B12 released from dietary protein, as a result of which the B12 would be unavailable for absorption. Because Bea absorbs crystalline B12 without a problem, her condition can be easily treated by taking vitamin B12 supplements orally.

BIOCHEMICAL COMMENTS

Folate Deficiencies and DNA Synthesis. Folate deficiencies result in decreased availability of the deoxythymidine and purine nucleotides that serve as precursors for DNA synthesis. The decreased concentrations of these precursors affect not only the DNA synthesis that occurs during replication before cell division, but also the DNA synthesis that occurs as a step in the processes that repair damaged DNA.

Decreased methylation of deoxyuridine monophosphate (dUMP) to form deoxythymidine monophosphate (dTMP), a reaction that requires N^5, N^{10}-methylene tetrahydrofolate as a coenzyme (see Fig. 40.5), leads to an increase in the intracellular dUTP/dTTP ratio. This change causes a significant increase in the incorporation of uracil into DNA. Although much of this uracil can be removed by DNA repair enzymes, the lack of available dTTP blocks the step of DNA repair catalyzed by DNA polymerase. The result is fragmentation of DNA as well as blockade of normal DNA replication.

These abnormal nuclear processes are responsible for the clumping and polysegmentation seen in the nuclei of neutrophilic leukocytes in the bone marrow and in the peripheral blood of patients with a megaloblastic anemia caused either by a primary folate deficiency or one that is secondary to a B12 deficiency. The abnormalities in DNA synthesis and repair lead to an irreversible loss of the capacity for cell division and eventually to cell death.

Suggested References

Fenech M. The role of folic acid and vitamin B12 in genomic stability of human cells. Mutation Research 2000;475:57–67.

Herbert V. Folic acid. In: Shils ME, Olson JA, Shike M, Ross AC, eds. Modern Nutrition in Health and Disease. Philadelphia: Lippincott, Williams & Wilkins, 1999:433–446.

Selhub J. Homocysteine metabolism. Annu Rev Nutr 1999;19:217–246.

Van der Put NMJ, Van Straaten HWM, Trijbels FJM, Blom HJ. Folate, homocysteine and neural tube defects: An overview. Exp Biol Med 2001;226:243–270.

Weir DG, Scott JM. Vitamin B12 "cobalamin". In: Shils ME, Olson JA, Shike M, Ross AC, eds. Modern Nutrition in Health and Disease. Philadelphia: Lippincott, Williams & Wilkins, 1999:447–458.

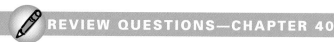

REVIEW QUESTIONS—CHAPTER 40

1. Which of the following reactions requires N^5, N^{10}-methylene FH$_4$ as a carbon donor?

    (A) Homocysteine to methionine
    (B) Serine to glycine
    (C) Betaine to dimethylglycine
    (D) dUMP to dTMP
    (E) The de novo biosynthesis of the purine ring

2. Propionic acid accumulation from amino acid degradation would result from a deficiency of which of the following vitamins?

    (A) Vitamin B6
    (B) Biotin
    (C) Folic acid
    (D) Vitamin B12
    (E) Vitamin B1
    (F) Vitamin B2

3. A dietary vitamin B12 deficiency can result from which of the following?

    (A) Excessive intrinsic factor production by the gastric parietal cells
    (B) Eating a diet high in animal protein
    (C) Pancreatic insufficiency
    (D) Increased absorption of folic acid
    (E) Inability to conjugate the vitamin with glutamic acid

4. Which of the following forms of tetrahydrofolate is required for the synthesis of methionine from homocysteine?

    (A) N^5, N^{10} -methylene tetrahydrofolate
    (B) N^5 -methyl tetrahydrofolate
    (C) N^5, N^{10} -methenyl tetrahydrofolate
    (D) N^{10} -formyl tetrahydrofolate
    (E) N^5 -formimino tetrahydrofolate

5. An alternative method to methylate homocysteine to form methionine is which of the following?

    (A) Using glycine and FH_4 as the methyl donor
    (B) Using dimethylglycine as the methyl donor
    (C) Using choline as the methyl donor
    (D) Using sarcosine as the methyl donor
    (E) Using betaine as the methyl donor

41 Purine and Pyrimidine Metabolism

Purines and pyrimidines are required for synthesizing **nucleotides** and **nucleic acids**. These molecules can be synthesized either from scratch, **de novo**, or **salvaged** from existing bases. Dietary uptake of purine and pyrimidine bases is low, because most of the ingested nucleic acids are metabolized by the intestinal epithelial cells.

The de novo pathway of purine synthesis is complex, consisting of 11 steps, and requiring 6 molecules of ATP for every purine synthesized. The precursors that donate components to produce purine nucleotides include **glycine, ribose 5-phosphate, glutamine, aspartate, carbon dioxide,** and **N^{10}-formyl FH₄** (Fig. 41.1). Purines are synthesized as **ribonucleotides**, with the initial purine synthesized being **inosine monophosphate (IMP).** Adenosine monophosphate (AMP) and guanosine monophosphate (GMP) are each derived from IMP in two-step reaction pathways.

The purine nucleotide salvage pathway allows free purine bases to be converted into nucleotides, nucleotides into nucleosides, and nucleosides into free bases. Enzymes included in this pathway are **AMP** and **adenosine deaminase, adenosine kinase, purine nucleoside phosphorylase, adenine phosphoribosyltransferase (APRT),** and **hypoxanthine guanine phosphoribosyltransferase (HGPRT).** Mutations in a number of these enzymes lead to serious diseases. Deficiencies in purine nucleoside phosphorylase and adenosine deaminase lead to **immunodeficiency disorders**. A deficiency in HGPRT leads to **Lesch-Nyhan syndrome.** The **purine nucleotide cycle,** in which aspartate carbons are converted to fumarate to replenish TCA cycle intermediates in working muscle, and the aspartate nitrogen is released as ammonia, uses components of the purine nucleotide salvage pathway.

Pyrimidine bases are first synthesized as the free base and then converted to a nucleotide. **Aspartate** and **carbamoyl phosphate** form all components of the pyrimidine ring. Ribose 5-phosphate, which is converted to phosphoribosyl pyrophosphate (PRPP), is required to donate the sugar phosphate to form a nucleotide. The first pyrimidine nucleotide produced is **orotate monophosphate (OMP).** The OMP is converted to **uridine monophosphate (UMP),** which will become the precursor for both **cytidine triphosphate (CTP)** and **deoxythymidine monophosphate (dTMP)** production.

The formation of deoxyribonucleotides requires **ribonucleotide reductase** activity, which catalyzes the reduction of ribose on nucleotide diphosphate substrates to 2'-deoxyribose. Substrates for the enzyme include adenosine diphosphate (ADP), guanosine diphosphate (GDP), cytidine diphosphate (CDP), and uridine diphosphate (UDP). Regulation of the enzyme is complex. There are two major allosteric sites. One controls the overall activity of the enzyme, whereas the other determines the substrate specificity of the enzyme. All deoxyribonucleotides are synthesized using this one enzyme.

The **regulation** of purine nucleotide biosynthesis occurs at four points in the pathway. The enzymes **PRPP synthetase, amidophosphoribosyl transferase, IMP**

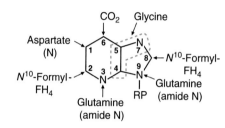

Fig. 41.1. Origin of the atoms of the purine base. FH_4 = tetrahydrofolate.

*dehydrogenase, and **adenylosuccinate synthetase** are regulated by allosteric modifiers, as they occur at key branch points through the pathway. Pyrimidine synthesis is regulated at the first committed step, which is the synthesis of cytoplasmic carbamoyl-phosphate, by the enzyme **carbamoyl phosphate synthetase II (CPS-II)**.*

*Purines, when degraded, cannot generate energy, nor can the purine ring be substantially modified. The end product of purine ring degradation is **uric acid**, which is excreted in the urine. Uric acid has a limited solubility, and if it were to accumulate, uric acid crystals would precipitate in tissues of the body with a reduced temperature (such as the big toe). This condition of acute painful inflammation of specific soft tissues and joints is called **gout**. Pyrimidines, when degraded, however, give rise to water-soluble compounds, such as urea, carbon dioxide, and water and do not lead to a disease state if pyrimidine catabolism is increased.*

THE WAITING ROOM

The initial acute inflammatory process that caused **Lotta Topaigne** to experience a painful attack of gouty arthritis responded quickly to colchicine therapy (see Chapter 10). Several weeks after the inflammatory signs and symptoms in her right great toe subsided, Lotta was placed on allopurinol, a drug that reduces uric acid synthesis. Her serum uric acid level gradually fell from a pretreatment level of 9.2 mg/dL into the normal range (2.5–8.0 mg/dL). She remained free of gouty symptoms when she returned to her physician for a follow-up office visit.

I. PURINES AND PYRIMIDINES

As has been seen in previous chapters of this text, nucleotides serve numerous functions in different reaction pathways. For example, nucleotides are the activated precursors of DNA and RNA. Nucleotides form the structural moieties of many coenzymes (examples include NADH, FAD, and coenzyme A). Nucleotides are critical elements in energy metabolism (ATP, GTP). Nucleotide derivatives are frequently activated intermediates in many biosyntheses. For example, UDP-glucose and CDP-diacylglycerol are precursors of glycogen and phosphoglycerides, respectively. S-Adenosylmethionine carries an activated methyl group. In addition, nucleotides act as second messengers in intracellular signaling (e.g., cAMP, cGMP). Finally, nucleotides and nucleosides act as metabolic allosteric regulators. Think about all of the enzymes that have been studied that are regulated by levels of ATP, ADP, and AMP.

Dietary uptake of purine and pyrimidine bases is minimal. The diet contains nucleic acids and the exocrine pancreas secretes deoxyribonuclease and ribonuclease, along with the proteolytic and lipolytic enzymes. This enables digested nucleic acids to be converted to nucleotides. The intestinal epithelial cells contain alkaline phosphatase activity, which will convert nucleotides to nucleosides. Other enzymes within the epithelial cells tend to metabolize the nucleosides to uric acid, or to salvage them for their own needs. Approximately 5% of ingested nucleotides will make it into the circulation, either as the free base or as a nucleoside. Because of the minimal dietary uptake of these important molecules, de novo synthesis of purines and pyrimidines is required.

II. PURINE BIOSYNTHESIS

The purine bases are produced de novo by pathways that use amino acids as precursors and produce nucleotides. Most de novo synthesis occurs in the liver (Fig. 41.2), and the nitrogenous bases and nucleosides are then transported to other tissues by red blood cells. The brain also synthesizes significant amounts of nucleotides. Because the de novo pathway requires six high-energy bonds per purine produced, a salvage pathway, which is used by many cell types, can convert free bases and nucleosides to nucleotides.

A. De Novo Synthesis of the Purine Nucleotides

1. SYNTHESIS OF IMP

As purines are built on a ribose base (see Fig. 41.2), an activated form of ribose is used to initiate the purine biosynthetic pathway. 5-Phosphoribosyl-1-pyrophosphate (PRPP) is the activated source of the ribose moiety. It is synthesized from ATP and ribose 5'-phosphate (Fig. 41.3), which is produced from glucose through the pentose phosphate pathway (see Chapter 29). The enzyme that catalyzes this reaction, PRPP synthetase, is a regulated enzyme (see section II.A.5); however, this step is not the committed step of purine biosynthesis. PRPP has many other uses, which are described as the chapter progresses.

In the first committed step of the purine biosynthetic pathway, PRPP reacts with glutamine to form phosphoribosylamine (Fig. 41.4). This reaction, which produces nitrogen 9 of the purine ring, is catalyzed by glutamine phosphoribosyl amidotransferase, a highly regulated enzyme.

In the next step of the pathway, the entire glycine molecule is added to the growing precursor. Glycine provides carbons 4 and 5 and nitrogen 7 of the purine ring (Fig. 41.5).

Subsequently, carbon 8 is provided by N^{10}-formyl FH$_4$, nitrogen 3 by glutamine, carbon 6 by CO_2, nitrogen 1 by aspartate, and carbon 2 by formyl tetrahydrofolate (see Fig. 41.1). Note that six molecules of ATP are required (starting with ribose 5-phosphate) to synthesize the first purine nucleotide, inosine monophosphate (IMP). This nucleotide contains the base hypoxanthine joined by an N-glycosidic bond from nitrogen 9 of the purine ring to carbon 1 of the ribose (Fig. 41.6).

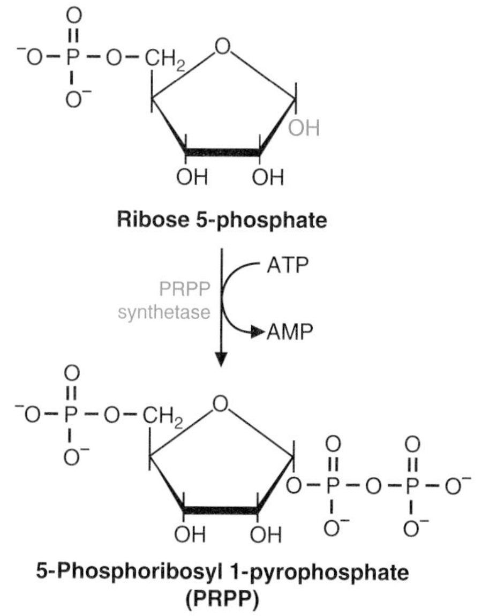

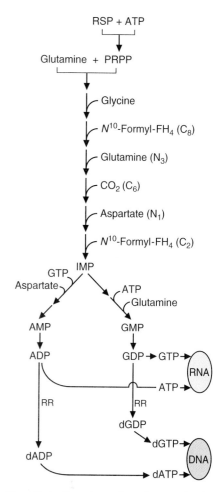

Fig. 41.2. Overview of purine production, starting with glutamine, ribose 5-phosphate, and ATP. The steps that require ATP are also indicated in this figure. RR = ribonucleotide reductase. FH$_4$ = tetrahydrofolate. PRPP = 5-phosphoribosyl 1-pyrophosphate.

Cellular concentrations of PRPP and glutamine are usually below their K$_m$ for glutamine phosphoribosyl amidotransferase. Thus, any situation which leads to an increase in their concentration can lead to an increase in de novo purine biosynthesis.

The base hypoxanthine is found in the anticodon of tRNA molecules (it is formed by the deamination of an adenine base). Hypoxanthine's role in tRNA is to allow wobble base-pairs to form, as the base hypoxanthine can base pair with adenine, cytosine, or uracil. The wobbling allows one tRNA molecule to potentially form base pairs with three different codons.

Ribose 5-phosphate

PRPP synthetase
ATP → AMP

5-Phosphoribosyl 1-pyrophosphate (PRPP)

Fig. 41.3. Synthesis of PRPP. Ribose 5-phosphate is produced from glucose by the pentose phosphate pathway.

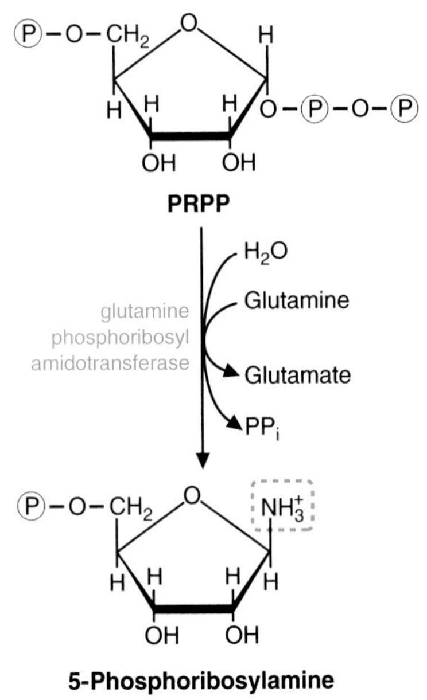

Fig. 41.4. The first step in purine biosynthesis. The purine base is built on the ribose moiety. The availability of the substrate PRPP is a major determinant of the rate of this reaction.

2.   SYNTHESIS OF AMP

IMP serves as the branchpoint from which both adenine and guanine nucleotides can be produced (see Fig. 41.2). Adenosine monophosphate (AMP) is derived from IMP in two steps (Fig. 41.7). In the first step, aspartate is added to IMP to form adenylosuccinate, a reaction similar to the one catalyzed by argininosuccinate synthetase in the urea cycle. Note how this reaction requires a high-energy bond, donated by GTP. Fumarate is then released from the adenylosuccinate by the enzyme adenylosuccinase to form AMP.

3.   SYNTHESIS OF GMP

GMP is also synthesized from IMP in two steps (Fig. 41.8). In the first step, the hypoxanthine base is oxidized by IMP dehydrogenase to produce the base xanthine and the nucleotide xanthosine monophosphate (XMP). Glutamine then donates the amide nitrogen to XMP to form GMP in a reaction catalyzed by GMP synthetase. This second reaction requires energy, in the form of ATP.

4.   PHOSPHORYLATION OF AMP AND GMP

AMP and GMP can be phosphorylated to the di- and triphosphate levels. The production of nucleoside diphosphates requires specific nucleoside monophosphate kinases, whereas the production of nucleoside triphosphates requires nucleoside diphosphate kinases, which are active with a wide range of nucleoside diphosphates. The purine nucleoside triphosphates are also used for energy-requiring processes in the cell and also as precursors for RNA synthesis (see Fig. 41.2).

5.   REGULATION OF PURINE SYNTHESIS

Regulation of purine synthesis occurs at several sites (Fig. 41.9). Four key enzymes are regulated: PRPP synthetase, amidophosphoribosyl transferase,

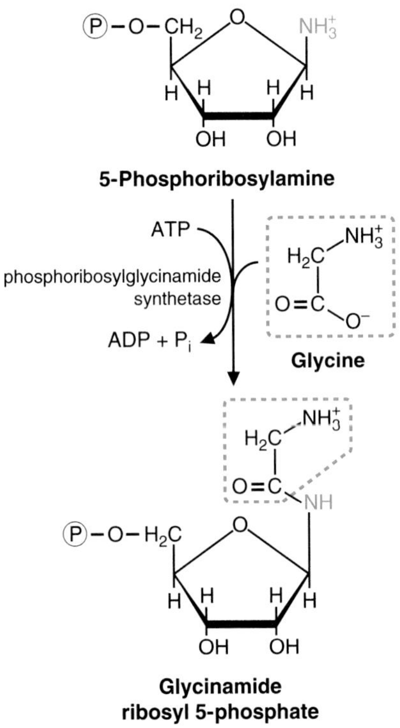

The aspartate to fumarate conversion also occurs in the urea cycle. In both cases, aspartate donates a nitrogen to the product, while the carbons of aspartate are released as fumarate.

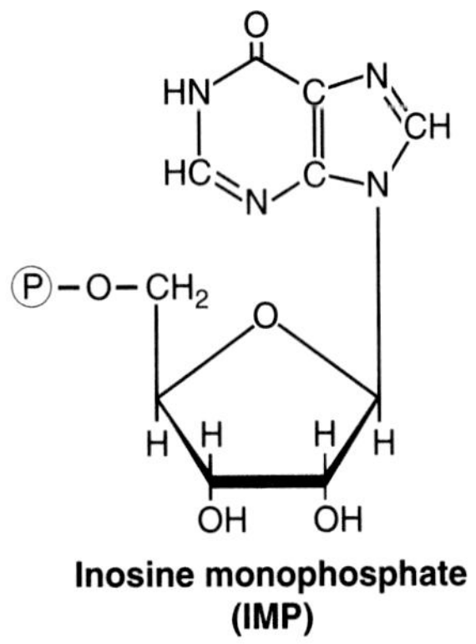

Fig. 41.5. Incorporation of glycine into the purine precursor. The ATP is required for the condensation of the glycine carboxylic acid group with the 1′-amino group of phosphoribosyl 1-amine.

**Inosine monophosphate
(IMP)**

Fig. 41.6. Structure of inosine monophosphate (IMP). The base is hypoxanthine.

adenylosuccinate synthetase, and IMP dehydrogenase. The first two enzymes regulate IMP synthesis; the last two regulate the production of AMP and GMP, respectively.

A primary site of regulation is the synthesis of PRPP. PRPP synthetase is negatively affected by GDP and, at a distinct allosteric site, by ADP. Thus, the simultaneous binding of an oxypurine (eg., GDP) and an aminopurine (eg., ADP) can occur with the result being a synergistic inhibition of the enzyme. This enzyme is not the committed step of purine biosynthesis; PRPP is also used in pyrimidine synthesis and both the purine and pyrimidine salvage pathways.

The committed step of purine synthesis is the formation of 5-phosphoribosyl 1-amine by glutamine phosphoribosyl amidotransferase. This enzyme is strongly inhibited by GMP and AMP (the end products of the purine biosynthetic pathway). The enzyme is also inhibited by the corresponding nucleoside di- and triphosphates, but under cellular conditions, these compounds probably do not play a central role in regulation. The active enzyme is a monomer of 133,000 daltons but is converted to an inactive dimer (270,000 daltons) by binding of the end products.

The enzymes that convert IMP to XMP and adenylosuccinate are both regulated. GMP inhibits the activity of IMP dehydrogenase, and AMP inhibits adenylosuccinate synthetase. Note that the synthesis of AMP is dependent on GTP (of which GMP is a precursor), whereas the synthesis of GMP is dependent on ATP (which is made from AMP). This serves as a type of positive regulatory mechanism to balance the pools of these precursors: when the levels of ATP are high, GMP will be

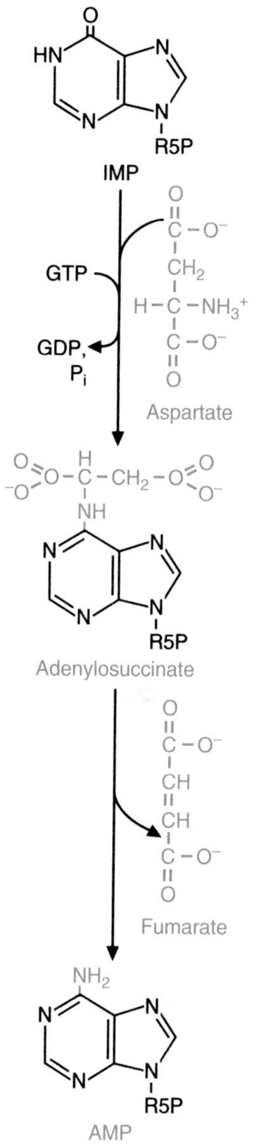

Fig. 41.7. The conversion of IMP to AMP. Note that GTP is required for the synthesis of AMP.

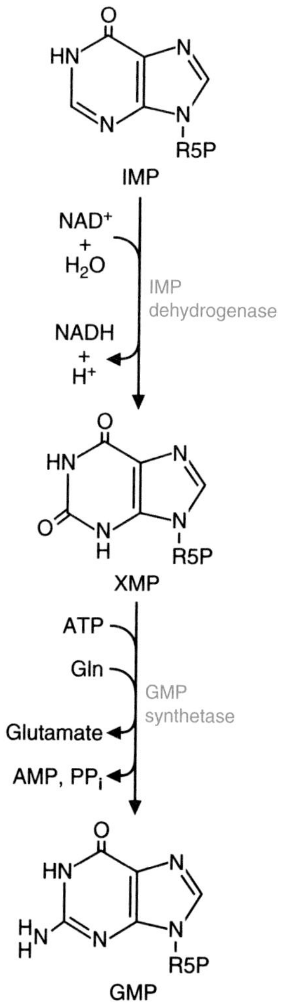

Fig. 41.8. The conversion of IMP to GMP. Note that ATP is required for the synthesis of GMP.

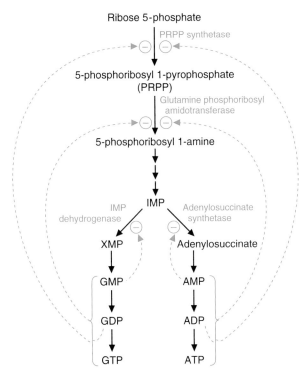

Fig. 41.9. The regulation of purine synthesis. PRPP synthetase has two distinct allosteric sites, one for ADP, the other for GDP. Glutamine phosphoribosyl amidotransferase contains adenine nucleotide and guanine nucleotide binding sites; the monophosphates are the most important, although the di- and tri-phosphates will also bind to and inhibit the enzyme. Adenylosuccinate synthetase is inhibited by AMP; IMP dehydrogenase is inhibited by GMP.

made; when the levels of GTP are high, AMP synthesis will take place. GMP and AMP act as negative effectors at these branch points, a classic example of feedback inhibition.

B. Purine Salvage Pathways

Most of the de novo synthesis of the bases of nucleotides occurs in the liver, and to some extent in the brain, neutrophils, and other cells of the immune system. Within the liver, nucleotides can be converted to nucleosides or free bases, which can be transported to other tissues via the red blood cell in the circulation. In addition, the small amounts of dietary bases or nucleosides that are absorbed also enter cells in this form. Thus, most cells can salvage these bases to generate nucleotides for RNA and DNA synthesis. For certain cell types, such as the lymphocytes, the salvage of bases is the major form of nucleotide generation.

The overall picture of salvage is shown in Figure 41.10. The pathways allow free bases, nucleosides, and nucleotides to be easily interconverted. The major enzymes required are purine nucleoside phosphorylase, phosphoribosyl transferases, and deaminases.

Purine nucleoside phosphorylase catalyzes a phosphorolysis reaction of the N-glycosidic bond that attaches the base to the sugar moiety in the nucleosides guanosine and inosine (Fig. 41.11). Thus, guanosine and inosine are converted to guanine and hypoxanthine, respectively, along with ribose 1-phosphate. The ribose 1-phosphate can be isomerized to ribose 5-phosphate, and the free bases then salvaged or degraded, depending on cellular needs.

 A deficiency in purine nucleoside phosphorylase activity leads to an immune disorder in which T-cell immunity is compromised. B-cell immunity, conversely, may be only slightly compromised or even normal. Children lacking this activity have recurrent infections, and more than half display neurologic complications. Symptoms of the disorder first appear at between 6 months and 4 years of age.

Free Bases **Nucleotides** **Nucleosides**

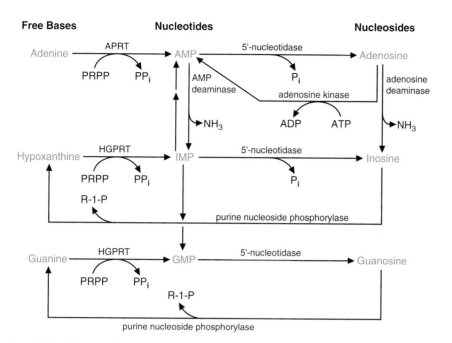

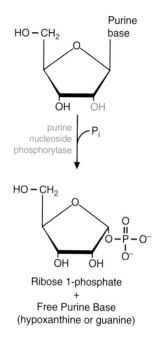

Fig. 41.10. Salvage of bases. The purine bases hypoxanthine and guanine react with PRPP to form the nucleotides inosine and guanosine monophosphate, respectively. The enzyme that catalyzes the reaction is hypoxanthine-guanine phosphoribosyltransferase (HGPRT). Adenine forms AMP in a reaction catalyzed by adenine phosphoribosyltransferase (APRT). Nucleotides are converted to nucleosides by 5′-nucleotidase. Free bases are generated from nucleosides by purine nucleoside phosphorylase. Deamination of the base adenine occurs with AMP and adenosine deaminase. Of the purines, only adenosine can be directly phosphorylated back to a nucleotide, by adenosine kinase.

Fig. 41.11. The purine nucleoside phosphorylase reaction, converting guanosine or inosine to ribose 1-phosphate plus the free bases guanine or hypoxanthine.

The phosphoribosyl transferase enzymes catalyze the addition of a ribose 5-phosphate group from PRPP to a free base, generating a nucleotide and pyrophosphate (Fig. 41.12). Two enzymes do this: adenine phosphoribosyl transferase (APRT) and hypoxanthine-guanine phosphoribosyl transferase (HGPRT). The reactions they catalyze are the same, differing only in their substrate specificity.

Adenosine and AMP can be deaminated by adenosine deaminase and AMP deaminase, respectively, to form inosine and IMP (see Fig. 41.10). Adenosine is also the only nucleoside to be directly phosphorylated to a nucleotide by adenosine kinase. Guanosine and inosine must be converted to free bases by purine nucleoside phosphorylase before they can be converted to nucleotides by HGPRT.

A portion of the salvage pathway that is important in muscle is the purine nucleotide cycle (Fig. 41.13). The net effect of these reactions is the deamination of aspartate to fumarate (as AMP is synthesized from IMP and then deaminated back to IMP by AMP deaminase). Under conditions in which the muscle must generate energy, the fumarate derived from the purine nucleotide cycle is used anaplerotically to replenish TCA cycle intermediates and to allow the cycle to operate at a high speed. Deficiencies in enzymes of this cycle lead to muscle fatigue during exercise.

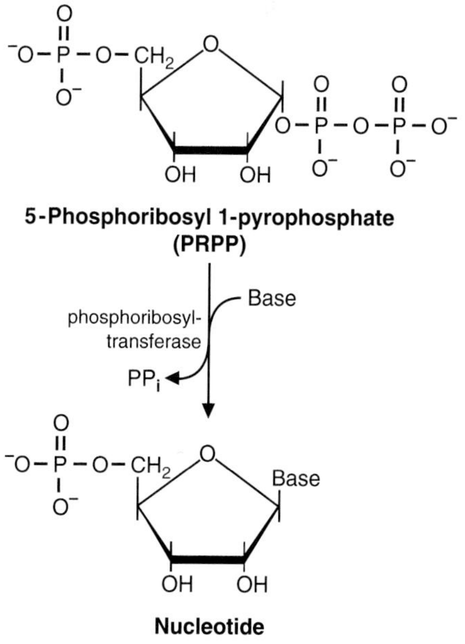

Lesch-Nyhan syndrome is caused by a defective hypoxanthine-guanine phosphoribosyltransferase (HGPRT) (see Fig. 41.12). In this condition, purine bases cannot be salvaged. Instead, they are degraded, forming excessive amounts of uric acid. Individuals with this syndrome suffer from mental retardation. They are also prone to chewing off their fingers and performing other acts of self-mutilation.

5-Phosphoribosyl 1-pyrophosphate (PRPP)

Nucleotide

Fig. 41.12. The phosphoribosyltransferase reaction. APRT uses the free base adenine; HGPRT can use either hypoxanthine or guanine as a substrate.

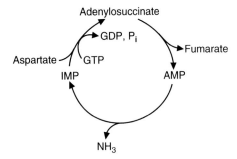

Fig. 41.13. The purine nucleotide cycle. Using a combination of biosynthetic and salvage enzymes, the net effect is the conversion of aspartate to fumarate plus ammonia, with the fumarate playing an anaplerotic role in the muscle.

In bacteria, aspartate transcarbamoylase is the regulated step of pyrimidine production. This is a very complex enzyme and was a model system for understanding how allosteric enzymes were regulated. In humans, however, this enzyme is not regulated.

III. SYNTHESIS OF THE PYRIMIDINE NUCLEOTIDES

A. De Novo Pathways

In the synthesis of the pyrimidine nucleotides, the base is synthesized first, and then it is attached to the ribose 5′-phosphate moiety (Fig. 41.14). The origin of the atoms of the ring (aspartate and carbamoyl-phosphate, which is derived from carbon dioxide and glutamine) is shown in Fig. 41.15. In the initial reaction of the pathway, glutamine combines with bicarbonate and ATP to form carbamoyl phosphate. This reaction is analogous to the first reaction of the urea cycle, except that it uses glutamine as the source of the nitrogen (rather than ammonia) and it occurs in the cytosol (rather than in mitochondria). The reaction is catalyzed by carbamoyl phosphate synthetase II, which is the regulated step of the pathway. The analogous reaction in urea synthesis is catalyzed by carbamoyl phosphate synthetase I, which is activated by *N*-acetylglutamate. The similarities and differences between these two carbamoyl phosphate synthetase enzymes is described in Table 41.1.

In the next step of pyrimidine biosynthesis, the entire aspartate molecule adds to carbamoyl phosphate in a reaction catalyzed by aspartate transcarbamoylase. The molecule subsequently closes to produce a ring (catalyzed by dihydroorotase), which is oxidized to form orotic acid (or its anion, orotate) through the actions of dihydroorotate dehydrogenase . The enzyme orotate phosphoribosyl transferase catalyzes the transfer of ribose 5-phosphate from PRPP to orotate, producing orotidine 5′-phosphate, which is decarboxylated by orotidylic acid dehydrogenase to form

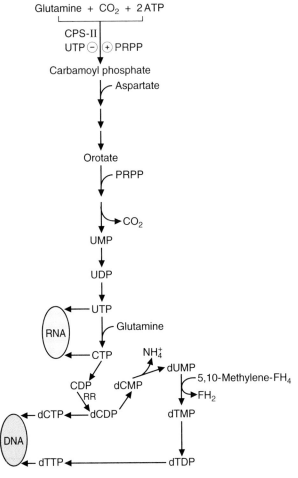

Fig. 41.14. Synthesis of the pyrimidine bases. CPSII = carbamoyl phosphate synthetase II. RR = ribonucleotide reductase; $\oplus$ = stimulated by; $\ominus$ = inhibited by; FH_2 and FH_4 = forms of folate.

Table 41.1. Comparison of Carbamoyl Phosphate Synthetases (CPSI and CPSII)

	CPS-I	CPS-II
Pathway	Urea cycle	Pyrimidine biosynthesis
Source of nitrogen	NH_4^+	Glutamine
Location	Mitochondria	Cytosol
Activator	N-Acetylglutamate	PRPP
Inhibitor	–	UTP

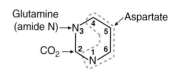

Fig. 41.15. The origin of the bases in the pyrimidine ring.

uridine monophosphate (UMP) (Fig. 41.16). In mammals, the first three enzymes of the pathway (carbamoyl phosphate synthetase II, aspartate transcarbamoylase, and dihydroorotase) are located on the same polypeptide, designated as CAD. The last two enzymes of the pathway are similarly located on a polypeptide known as UMP synthase (the orotate phosphoribosyl transferase and orotidylic acid dehydrogenase activities).

UMP is phosphorylated to UTP. An amino group, derived from the amide of glutamine, is added to carbon 4 to produce CTP by the enzyme CTP synthetase (this reaction cannot occur at the nucleotide monophosphate level). UTP and CTP are precursors for the synthesis of RNA (see Fig. 41.14). The synthesis of thymidine triphosphate (TTP) will be described in section IV.

B. Salvage of Pyrimidine Bases

Pyrimidine bases are normally salvaged by a two-step route. First, a relatively nonspecific pyrimidine nucleoside phosphorylase converts the pyrimidine bases to their respective nucleosides (Fig. 41.17). Notice that the preferred direction for this reaction is the reverse phosphorylase reaction, in which phosphate is being released and is not being used as a nucleophile to release the pyrimidine base from the nucleoside. The more specific nucleoside kinases then react with the nucleosides, forming nucleotides (Table 41.2). As with purines, further phosphorylation is carried out by increasingly more specific kinases. The nucleoside phosphorylase–nucleoside kinase route for synthesis of pyrimidine nucleoside monophosphates is relatively inefficient for salvage of pyrimidine bases because of the very low concentration of the bases in plasma and tissues.

Pyrimidine phosphorylase can use all of the pyrimidines but has a preference for uracil and is sometimes called uridine phosphorylase. The phosphorylase uses cytosine fairly well but has a very, very low affinity for thymine; therefore, a ribonucleoside containing thymine is almost never made in vivo. A second phosphorylase, thymine phosphorylase, has a much higher affinity for thymine and adds a deoxyribose residue (see Fig. 41.17).

Of the various ribonucleosides and deoxyribonucleoside kinases, one that merits special mention is *thymidine kinase* (TK). This enzyme is allosterically inhibited by dTTP. Activity of thymidine kinase in a given cell is closely related to the proliferative state of that cell. During the cell cycle, the activity of TK rises dramatically as cells enter S phase, and in general rapidly dividing cells have high levels of this enzyme. Radiolabeled thymidine is widely used for isotopic labeling of DNA, for example, in radioautographic investigations or to estimate rates of intracellular DNA synthesis.

 In hereditary orotic aciduria, orotic acid is excreted in the urine because the enzymes that convert it to uridine monophosphate, orotate phosphoribosyltransferase and orotidine 5'-phosphate decarboxylase, are defective (see Fig. 41.16). Pyrimidines cannot be synthesized, and, therefore, normal growth does not occur. Oral administration of uridine is used to treat this condition. Uridine, which is converted to UMP, bypasses the metabolic block and provides the body with a source of pyrimidines, as both CTP and dTMP can be produced from UMP.

Table 41.2. Salvage Reactions for Conversion of Pyrimidine Nucleosides to Nucleotides.

Enzyme	Reaction
Uridine-cytidine kinase	Uridine + ATP → UMP + ADP
	Cytidine + ATP → CMP + ADP
Deoxythymidine kinase	deoxythymidine + ATP → dTMP + ADP
Deoxycytidine kinase	Deoxycytidine + ATP → dCMP + ADP

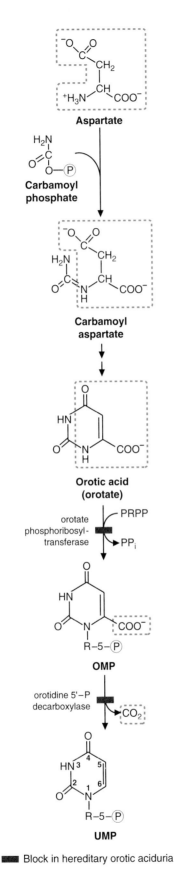

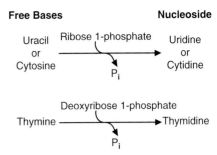

Fig. 41.17. Salvage reactions for pyrimidine nucleoside production. Thymine phosphorylase uses deoxyribose 1-phosphate as a substrate, such that ribothymidine is rarely formed.

Fig. 41.16. Conversion of carbamoyl phosphate and aspartate to UMP. The defective enzymes in hereditary orotic aciduria are indicated (■).

C. Regulation of De Novo Pyrimidine Synthesis

The regulated step of pyrimidine synthesis in humans is carbamoyl phosphate synthetase II. The enzyme is inhibited by UTP and activated by PRPP (see Fig. 41.14). Thus, as pyrimidines decrease in concentration (as indicated by UTP levels), CPS-II is activated and pyrimidines are synthesized. The activity is also regulated by the cell cycle. As cells approach S-phase, CPS-II becomes more sensitive to PRPP activation and less sensitive to UTP inhibition. At the end of S-phase, the inhibition by UTP is more pronounced, and the activation by PRPP is reduced. These changes in the allosteric properties of CPS-II are related to its phosphorylation state. Phosphorylation of the enzyme at a specific site by a MAP kinase leads to a more easily activated enzyme. Phosphorylation at a second site by the cAMP-dependent protein kinase leads to a more easily inhibited enzyme.

IV. THE PRODUCTION OF DEOXYRIBONUCLEOTIDES

For DNA synthesis to occur, the ribose moiety must be reduced to deoxyribose (Fig. 41.18). This reduction occurs at the dinucleotide level and is catalyzed by ribonucleotide reductase, which requires the protein thioredoxin. The deoxyribonucleoside diphosphates can be phosphorylated to the triphosphate level and used as precursors for DNA synthesis (see Figs. 41.2 and 41.14).

The regulation of ribonucleotide reductase is quite complex. The enzyme contains two allosteric sites, one controlling the activity of the enzyme and the other controlling the substrate specificity of the enzyme. ATP bound to the activity site activates the enzyme; dATP bound to this site inhibits the enzyme. Substrate specificity is more complex. ATP bound to the substrate site activates the reduction of pyrimidines (CDP and UDP), to form dCDP and dUDP. The dUDP is not used for DNA synthesis; rather, it is used to produce dTMP (see below). Once dTMP is produced, it is phosphorylated to dTTP, which then binds to the substrate site and induces the reduction of GDP. As dGTP accumulates, it replaces dTTP in the substrate site and allows ADP to be reduced to dADP. This leads to the accumulation of dATP, which will inhibit the overall activity of the enzyme. These allosteric changes are summarized in Table 41.3.

dUDP can be dephosphorylated to form dUMP, or, alternatively, dCMP can be deaminated to form dUMP. Methylene tetrahydrofolate transfers a methyl group to dUMP to form dTMP (see Figure 40.5). Phosphorylation reactions produce dTTP, a precursor for DNA synthesis and a regulator of ribonucleotide reductase.

V. DEGRADATION OF PURINE AND PYRIMIDINE BASES

A. Purine Bases

The degradation of the purine nucleotides (AMP and GMP) occurs mainly in the liver (Fig. 41.19). Salvage enzymes are used for most of these reactions. AMP is first deaminated to produce IMP (AMP deaminase). Then IMP and GMP are dephosphorylated (5'-nucleotidase), and the ribose is cleaved from the base by purine nucleoside phosphorylase. Hypoxanthine, the base produced by cleavage of IMP, is converted by xanthine oxidase to xanthine, and guanine is deaminated by

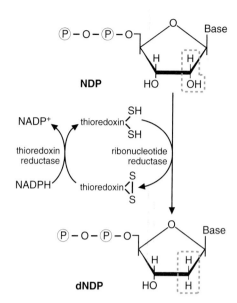

Fig. 41.18. Reduction of ribose to deoxyribose. Reduction occurs at the nucleoside diphosphate level. A ribonucleoside diphosphate (NDP) is converted to a deoxyribonucleoside diphosphate (dNDP). Thioredoxin is oxidized to a disulfide, which must be reduced for the reaction to continue producing dNDP. N = a nitrogenous base.

When ornithine transcarbamoylase is deficient (urea cycle disorder), excess carbamoyl phosphate from the mitochondria leaks into the cytoplasm. The elevated levels of cytoplasmic carbamoyl phosphate lead to pyrimidine production, as the regulated step of the pathway, the reaction catalyzed by carbamoyl synthetase II, is being bypassed. Thus, orotic aciduria results.

Q: Gout is caused by excessive uric acid levels in the blood and tissues. To determine whether a person with gout has developed this problem because of overproduction of purine nucleotides or because of a decreased ability to excrete uric acid, an oral dose of an ^{15}N-labeled amino acid is sometimes used. Which amino acid would be most appropriate to use for this purpose?

Table 41.3. Effectors of Ribonucleotide Reductase Activity

Preferred Substrate	Effector Bound to Overall Activity Site	Effector Bound to Substrate Specificity Site
None	dATP	Any nucleotide
CDP	ATP	ATP or dATP
UDP	ATP	ATP or dATP
ADP	ATP	dGTP
GDP	ATP	dTTP

A: The entire glycine molecule is incorporated into the precursor of the purine nucleotides. The nitrogen of this glycine also appears in uric acid, the product of purine degradation. ^{15}N-labeled glycine could be used, therefore, to determine whether purines are being overproduced.

Uric acid has a pK of 5.4. It is ionized in the body to form urate. Urate is not very soluble in an aqueous environment. The quantity in normal human blood is very close to the solubility constant.

Normally, as cells die, their purine nucleotides are degraded to hypoxanthine and xanthine, which are converted to uric acid by xanthine oxidase (see Fig. 41.15). Allopurinol (a structural analog of hypoxanthine) is a substrate for xanthine oxidase. It is converted to oxypurinol (also called alloxanthine), which remains tightly bound to the enzyme, preventing further catalytic activity (see Fig. 8.19). Thus, allopurinol is a suicide inhibitor. It reduces the production of uric acid and hence its concentration in the blood and tissues (e.g., the synovial lining of the joints in **Lotta Topaigne's** great toe). Xanthine and hypoxanthine accumulate, and urate levels decrease. Overall, the amount of purine being degraded is spread over three products rather than appearing in only one. Therefore, none of the compounds exceeds its solubility constant, precipitation does not occur, and the symptoms of gout gradually subside.

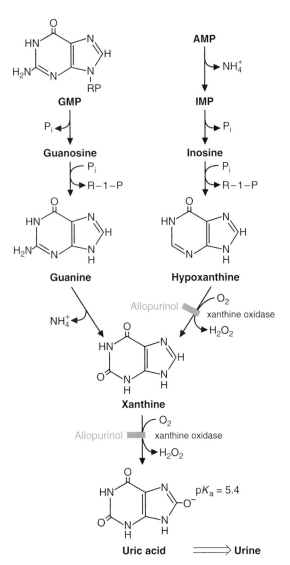

Fig. 41.19. Degradation of the purine bases. The reactions inhibited by allopurinol are indicated. A second form of xanthine oxidase exists that uses NAD^+ instead of O_2 as the electron acceptor.

the enzyme guanase to produce xanthine. The pathways for the degradation of adenine and guanine merge at this point. Xanthine is converted by xanthine oxidase to uric acid, which is excreted in the urine. Xanthine oxidase is a molybdenum-requiring enzyme that uses molecular oxygen and produces hydrogen peroxide (H_2O_2). Another form of xanthine oxidase exists that uses NAD^+ as the electron acceptor (see Chapter 24).

Note how little energy is derived from the degradation of the purine ring. Thus, it is to the cell's advantage to recycle and salvage the ring, because it costs energy to produce and not much is obtained in return.

B. Pyrimidine Bases

The pyrimidine nucleotides are dephosphorylated, and the nucleosides are cleaved to produce ribose 1-phosphate and the free pyrimidine bases cytosine, uracil, and thymine. Cytosine is deaminated, forming uracil, which is converted to CO_2, NH_4^+, and β-alanine. Thymine is converted to CO_2, NH_4^+, and β-aminoisobutyrate (Fig. 41.20). These products of pyrimidine degradation are excreted in the urine or converted to CO_2, H_2O, and NH_4^+ (which forms urea). They do not cause any problems for the body, in contrast to urate, which is produced from the purines and can precipitate, causing gout. As with the purine degradation pathway, little energy can be generated by pyrimidine degradation.

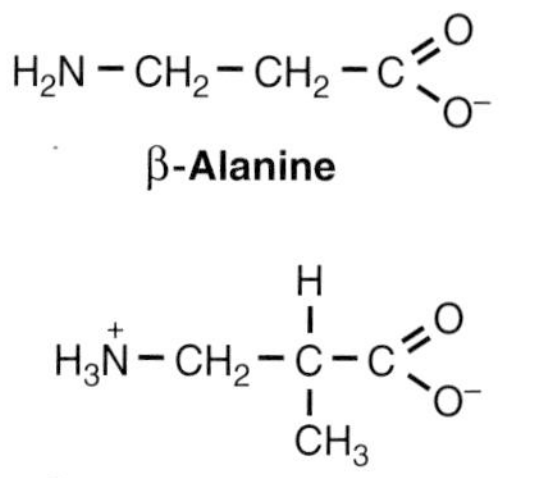

CLINICAL COMMENTS

Hyperuricemia in **Lotta Topaigne's** case arose as a consequence of over-production of uric acid. Treatment with allopurinol not only inhibits xan-thine oxidase, lowering the formation of uric acid with an increase in the excretion of hypoxanthine and xanthine, but also decreases the overall synthesis of purine nucleotides. Hypoxanthine and xanthine produced by purine degradation are salvaged (i.e., converted to nucleotides) by a process that requires the consumption of PRPP. PRPP is a substrate for the glutamine phosphoribosyl amidotransferase reaction that initiates purine biosynthesis. Because the normal cellular levels of PRPP and glutamine are below the K_m of the enzyme, changes in the level of either substrate can accelerate or reduce the rate of the reaction. Therefore, decreased levels of PRPP cause decreased synthesis of purine nucleotides.

BIOCHEMICAL COMMENTS

A deficiency in adenosine deaminase activity leads to severe combined immunodeficiency disease, or SCID. In the severe form of combined immunodeficiency, both T cells (which provide cell-based immunity, see Chapter 44) and B-cells (which produce antibodies) are deficient, leaving the individual without a functional immune system. Children born with this disorder lack a thymus gland and suffer from many opportunistic infections because of the lack of a functional immune system. Death results if the child is not placed in a sterile environment. Administration of polyethylene glycol–modified adenosine deaminase has been successful in treating the disorder, and the ADA gene was the first to be used in gene therapy in treating the disorder. The question that remains, however, is that even though all cells of the body are lacking ADA activity, why are the immune cells specifically targeted for destruction?

The specific immune disorder is not caused by any defect in purine salvage pathways, as children with Lesch-Nyhan syndrome have a functional immune system, although there are other major problems in those children. This suggests that perhaps the accumulation of precursors to ADA lead to toxic effects. Three hypotheses have been proposed and are outlined below.

In the absence of ADA activity, both adenosine and deoxyadenosine will accumulate. When deoxyadenosine accumulates, adenosine kinase can convert it to dAMP. Other kinases will allow dATP to then accumulate within the lymphocyte. Why specifically the lymphocyte? The other cells of the body are secreting the deoxyadenosine they cannot use, and it is accumulating in the circulation. As the lymphocytes are present in the circulation, they tend to accumulate this compound more so than cells not constantly present within the blood. As dATP accumulates, ribonucleotide reductase becomes inhibited, and the cells can no longer produce deoxyribonucleotides for DNA synthesis. Thus, when cells are supposed to grow and differentiate in response to cytokines, they cannot, and they die.

A second hypothesis suggests that the accumulation of deoxyadenosine in lymphocytes leads to an inhibition of S-adenosylhomocysteine hydrolase, the enzyme that converts S-adenosylhomocysteine to homocysteine and adenosine. This leads

Fig. 41.20. Water-soluble end products of pyrimidine degradation.

Once nucleotide biosynthesis and salvage was understood at the pathway level, it was quickly realized that one way to inhibit cell proliferation would be to block purine or pyrimidine synthesis. Thus, drugs were developed that would interfere with a cell's ability to generate precursors for DNA synthesis, thereby inhibiting cell growth. This is particularly important for cancer cells, which have lost their normal growth regulatory properties. Such drugs have been introduced previously with a number of different patients. **Colin Tuma** was treated with 5-fluorouracil, which inhibits thymidylate synthase (dUMP to TMP synthesis). **Arlyn Foma** was treated with methotrexate for his leukemia; methotrexate inhibits dihydrofolate reductase, thereby blocking the regeneration of tetrahydrofolate and de novo purine synthesis and thymidine synthesis. **Mannie Weitzels** was treated with hydroxyurea to block ribonucleotide reductase activity, with the goal of inhibiting DNA synthesis in the leukemic cells. Development of these drugs would not have been possible without an understanding of the biochemistry of purine and pyrimidine salvage and synthesis. Such drugs also affect rapidly dividing normal cells, which brings about a number of the side effects of chemotherapeutic regimens.

Table 41.4. Gene Disorders in Purine and Pyrimidine Metabolism

Disease	Gene defect	Metabolite that accumulates	Clinical symptoms
Gout	Multiple causes	Uric acid	Painful joints
Severe combined immunodeficiency disease (SCID)	Adenosine deaminase (purine salvage pathway)	Deoxyadenosine and derivatives thereof	Loss of immune system, including no T or B cells
Immunodeficiency disease	Purine nucleoside phosphorylase	Purine nucleosides	Partial loss of immune system; no T cells but B cells are present
Lesch-Nyhan syndrome	Hypoxanthine-guanine phosphoribosyltrans-ferase	Purines, uric acid	Mental retardation, self-mutilation
Hereditary orotic aciduria	UMP synthase	Orotic acid	Growth retardation

to hypo-methylation in the cell and an accumulation of S-adenosylhomocysteine. S-adenosylhomocysteine accumulation has been linked to the triggering of apoptosis.

The third hypothesis suggested is that elevated adenosine levels lead to inappropriate activation of adenosine receptors. Adenosine is also a signaling molecule, and stimulation of the adenosine receptors results in activation of protein kinase A and elevated cAMP levels in thymocytes. Elevated levels of cAMP in these cells triggers both apoptosis and developmental arrest of the cell.

Although it is still not clear which potential mechanism best explains the arrested development of immune cells, it is clear that elevated levels of adenosine and deoxyadenosine are toxic. The biochemical disorders of purine and pyrimidine metabolism discussed in this chapter are summarized in Table 41.4.

Suggested References

Becker MA. Hyperuricemia and gout. In: Scriver CR, Beaudet AL, Sly WS, Valle D, eds. The Metabolic and Molecular Bases of Inherited Disease, vol II, 8th Ed. New York: McGraw-Hill, 2001:2513–2535.

Hershfield MS, Mitchell BS. Immunodeficiency diseases caused by adenosine deaminase deficiency and purine nucleoside phosphorylase deficiency. In: Scriver CR, Beaudet AL, Sly WS, Valle D, eds. The Metabolic and Molecular Bases of Inherited Disease, vol II, 8th Ed. New York: McGraw-Hill, 2001:2585–2625.

Webster DR, Becroft DMO, Van Gennip AH, Van Kuilenberg ABP. Hereditary orotic aciduria and other disorders of pyrimidine metabolism. In: Scriver CR, Beaudet AL, Sly WS, Valle D, eds. The Metabolic and Molecular Bases of Inherited Disease, vol II, 8th Ed. New York: McGraw-Hill, 2001:2663–2702.

 REVIEW QUESTIONS—CHAPTER 41

1. Similarities between carbamoyl phosphate synthetase I and carbamoyl phosphate synthetase II include which ONE of the following?

(A) Carbon source
(B) Intracellular location
(C) Nitrogen source
(D) Regulation by N-acetyl glutamate
(E) Regulation by UMP

2. Gout can result from a reduction in activity of which one of the following enzymes?

    (A) Glutamine phosphoribosyl amidotransferase
    (B) Glucose 6-phosphatase
    (C) Glucose 6-phosphate dehydrogenase
    (D) PRPP synthetase
    (E) Purine nucleoside phosphorylase

3. Lesch-Nyhan syndrome is due to an inability to catalyze which of the following reactions?

    (A) Adenine to AMP
    (B) Adenosine to AMP
    (C) Guanine to GMP
    (D) Guanosine to GMP
    (E) Thymine to TMP
    (F) Thymidine to TMP

4. Allopurinol can be used to treat gout because of its ability to inhibit which one of the following reactions?

    (A) AMP to XMP
    (B) Xanthine to uric acid
    (C) Inosine to hypoxanthine
    (D) IMP to XMP
    (E) XMP to GMP

5. The regulation of ribonucleotide reductase is quite complex. Assuming that an enzyme deficiency leads to highly elevated levels of dGTP, what effect would you predict on the reduction of ribonucleotides to deoxyribonucleotides under these conditions?

    (A) Elevated levels of dCDP will be produced.
    (B) The formation of dADP will be favored.
    (C) AMP would begin to be reduced.
    (D) Reduced thioredoxin would become rate-limiting, thereby reducing the activity of ribonucleotide reductase.
    (E) Deoxy-GTP would bind to the overall activity site and inhibit the functioning of the enzyme.

42 Intertissue Relationships in the Metabolism of Amino Acids

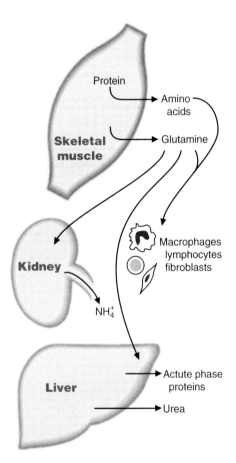

Fig. 42.1. Amino acid flux in sepsis and trauma. In sepsis and traumatic injury, glutamine and other amino acids are released from skeletal muscle for uptake by tissues involved in the immune response and tissue repair, such as macrophages, lymphocytes, fibroblasts, and the liver. Nitrogen excretion as urea and NH_4^+ results in negative nitrogen balance.

The body maintains a relatively large free amino acid pool in the blood, even during fasting. As a result, tissues have continuous access to individual amino acids for the synthesis of proteins and essential amino acid derivatives, such as neurotransmitters. The amino acid pool also provides the liver with **amino acid substrates** *for* **gluconeogenesis** *and provides several other cell types with a source of* **fuel.** *The* **free amino acid pool** *is derived from* **dietary amino acids** *and the* **turnover of proteins** *in the body. During an* **overnight fast** *and during* **hypercatabolic states,** *degradation of labile* **protein,** *particularly that in* **skeletal muscle,** *is the major source of free amino acids.*

The liver is the major site of amino acid metabolism in the body and the major site of **urea synthesis.** *The liver is also the major site of amino acid degradation. Hepatocytes partially oxidize most amino acids, converting the carbon skeleton to glucose, ketone bodies, or CO_2. Because ammonia is toxic, the liver converts most of the nitrogen from amino acid degradation to urea, which is excreted in the urine. The nitrogen derived from amino acid catabolism in other tissues is transported to the liver as* **alanine** *or* **glutamine** *and converted to urea.*

The **branched-chain amino acids,** *or BCAA (valine, isoleucine, and leucine) are oxidized principally in* **skeletal muscle** *and other tissues and not in the liver. In skeletal muscle, the carbon skeletons and some of the nitrogen are converted to glutamine, which is released into the blood. The remainder of the nitrogen is incorporated into alanine, which is taken up by the liver and converted to urea and glucose.*

The formation and release of glutamine from skeletal muscle and other tissues serves several functions. In the kidney, the NH_4^+ carried by glutamine is excreted into the urine. This process removes protons formed during fuel oxidation and helps to maintain the body's pH, especially during metabolic acidosis. **Glutamine** *also provides a* **fuel** *for the* **kidney** *and* **gut.** *In rapidly dividing cells (e.g., lymphocytes and macrophages), glutamine is required as a fuel, as a nitrogen donor for biosynthetic reactions, and as a substrate for protein synthesis.*

During conditions of **sepsis** *(the presence of various pathogenic organisms, or their toxins, in the blood or tissues),* **trauma, injury,** *or* **burns,** *the body enters a* **catabolic state** *characterized by a* **negative nitrogen balance** *(Fig. 42.1). Increased net protein degradation in skeletal muscle increases the availability of glutamine and other amino acids for cell division and protein synthesis in cells involved in the immune response and wound healing. In these conditions, an increased release of glucocorticoids from the adrenal cortex stimulates proteolysis.*

THE WAITING ROOM

Katta Bolic, a 62-year-old homeless woman, was found by a neighborhood child who heard Katta's moans coming from an abandoned building. The child's mother called the police, who took Katta to the hospital emergency room. The patient was semicomatose, incontinent of urine, and her clothes were stained with vomitus. She had a fever of 103°F, was trembling uncontrollably, appeared to be severely dehydrated, and had marked muscle wasting. Her heart rate was very rapid, and her blood pressure was low (85/46 mm Hg). Her abdomen was distended and without bowel sounds. She responded to moderate pressure on her abdomen with moaning and grimacing.

Blood was sent for a broad laboratory profile, and cultures of her urine, stool, throat, and blood were taken. Intravenous glucose, saline, and parenteral broad-spectrum antibiotics were begun. X-rays performed after her vital signs were stabilized suggested a bowel perforation. These findings were compatible with a diagnosis of a ruptured viscus (e.g., an infected colonic diverticulum that perforated, allowing colonic bacteria to infect the tissues of the peritoneal cavity, causing peritonitis). Further studies confirmed that a diverticulum had ruptured, and appropriate surgery was performed. All of the arterial blood cultures grew out *Escherichia coli*, indicating that Katta also had a Gram-negative infection of her blood (septicemia) that had been seeded by the proliferating organisms in her peritoneal cavity. Intensive fluid and electrolyte therapy and antibiotic coverage were continued. The medical team (surgeons, internists, and nutritionists) began developing a complex therapeutic plan to reverse Katta's severely catabolic state.

I. MAINTENANCE OF THE FREE AMINO ACID POOL IN BLOOD

The body maintains a relatively large free amino acid pool in the blood, even in the absence of an intake of dietary protein. The large free amino acid pool ensures the continuous availability of individual amino acids to tissues for the synthesis of proteins, neurotransmitters, and other nitrogen-containing compounds (Fig. 42.2). In a normal, well-fed, healthy individual, approximately 300 to 600 g body protein is degraded per day. At the same time, roughly 100 g protein is consumed in the diet per day, which adds additional amino acids. From this pool, tissues use amino acids for the continuous synthesis of new proteins (300–600 g) to replace those degraded. The continuous turnover of proteins in the body makes the complete complement of amino acids available for the synthesis of new and different proteins, such as antibodies. Protein turnover allows shifts in the quantities of different proteins produced in tissues in response to changes in physiologic state and continuously removes modified or damaged proteins. It also provides a complete pool of specific amino acids that can be used as oxidizable substrates; precursors for gluconeogenesis and for heme, creatine phosphate, purine, pyrimidine, and neurotransmitter synthesis; for ammoniagenesis to maintain blood pH levels; and for numerous other functions.

A. Interorgan Flux of Amino Acids in the Postabsorptive State

The fasting state provides an example of the interorgan flux of amino acids necessary to maintain the free amino acid pool in the blood and supply tissues with their required amino acids (Fig. 42.3). During an overnight fast, protein synthesis in the liver and other tissues continues, but at a diminished rate compared with the

The concentration of free amino acids in the blood is not nearly as rigidly controlled as blood glucose levels. The free amino acid pool in the blood is only a small part (0.5%) of the total amino acid pool in whole body protein. Because of the large skeletal muscle mass, approximately 80% of the body's total protein is in skeletal muscle. Consequently, the concentration of individual amino acids in the blood is strongly affected by the rates of protein synthesis and degradation in skeletal muscle, as well as the rate of uptake and utilization of individual amino acids for metabolism in liver and other tissues. For the most part, changes in the rate of protein synthesis and degradation take place over a span of hours.

 What changes in hormone levels and fuel metabolism occur during an overnight fast?

The hormonal changes that occur during an overnight fast include a decrease of blood insulin levels and an increase of glucagon relative to levels after a high-carbohydrate meal. Glucocorticoid levels also increase in the blood. These hormones coordinate the changes of fat, carbohydrate, and amino acid metabolism. Fatty acids are released from adipose triacylglycerols and are used as the major fuel by heart, skeletal muscle, liver, and other tissues. The liver converts some of the fatty acids to ketone bodies. Liver glycogen stores are diminished and gluconeogenesis becomes the major support of blood glucose levels for glucose-dependent tissues. The major precursors of gluconeogenesis include amino acids released from skeletal muscle, lactate, and glycerol.

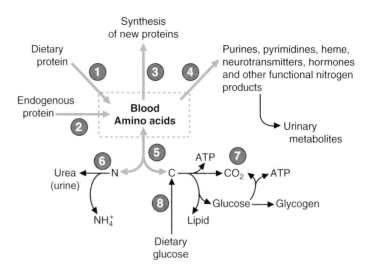

Fig. 42.2. Maintenance of the blood amino acid pool. Dietary protein (1) and degradation of endogenous protein (2) provide a source of essential amino acids (those that cannot be synthesized in the human). 3. The synthesis of new protein is the major use of amino acids from the free amino acid pool. 4. Compounds synthesized from amino acid precursors are essential for physiologic functions. Many of these compounds are degraded to N-containing urinary metabolites and do not return to the free amino acid pool. 5. In tissues, the nitrogen is removed from amino acids by transamination and deamination reactions. 6. The nitrogen from amino acid degradation appears in the urine primarily as urea or NH_4^+, the ammonium ion. Ammonia excretion is necessary to maintain the pH of the blood. 7. Amino acids are used as fuels either directly or after being converted to glucose by gluconeogenesis. 8. Some amino acids can be synthesized in the human, provided that glucose and a nitrogen source are available.

postprandial state. Net degradation of labile protein occurs in skeletal muscle (which contains the body's largest protein mass) and other tissues.

1. RELEASE OF AMINO ACIDS FROM SKELETAL MUSCLE DURING FASTING

The efflux of amino acids from skeletal muscle supports the essential amino acid pool in the blood (see Fig. 42.3). Skeletal muscle oxidizes the BCAA (valine, leucine, isoleucine) to produce energy and glutamine. The amino groups of the BCAA, and of aspartate and glutamate, are transferred out of skeletal muscle in alanine and glutamine. Alanine and glutamine account for approximately 50% of the total α-amino nitrogen released by skeletal muscle (Fig. 42.4).

The release of amino acids from skeletal muscle is stimulated during an overnight fast by the decrease of insulin and increase of glucocorticoid levels in the blood (see Chapters 31 and 43). Insulin promotes the uptake of amino acids and the general synthesis of proteins. The mechanisms for the stimulation of protein synthesis in human skeletal muscle are not all known, but probably include an activation of the A system for amino acid transport (a modest effect), a general effect on initiation of translation, and an inhibition of lysosomal proteolysis. The fall of blood insulin levels during an overnight fast results in net proteolysis and release of amino acids. As glucocorticoid release from the adrenal cortex increases, an induction of ubiquitin synthesis and an increase of ubiquitin-dependent proteolysis also occur.

2. AMINO ACID METABOLISM IN LIVER DURING FASTING

The major site of alanine uptake is the liver, which disposes of the amino nitrogen by incorporating it into urea (see Fig. 42.3). The liver also extracts free amino acids,

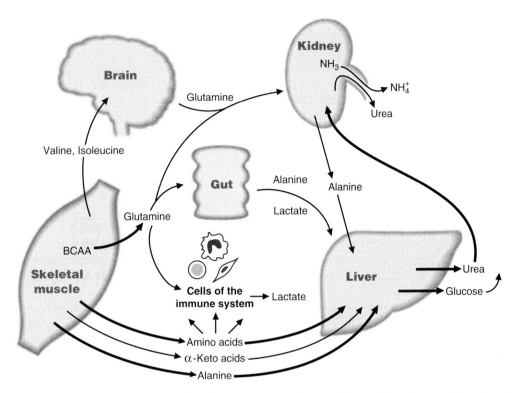

Fig. 42.3. Interorgan amino acid exchange after an overnight fast. After an overnight fast (the postabsorptive state), the utilization of amino acids for protein synthesis, for fuels, and for the synthesis of essential functional compounds continues. The free amino acid pool is supported largely by net degradation of skeletal muscle protein. Glutamine and alanine serve as amino group carriers from skeletal muscle to other tissues. Glutamine brings NH_4^+ to the kidney for the excretion of protons and serves as a fuel for the kidney, gut, and cells of the immune system. Alanine transfers amino groups from skeletal muscle, the kidney, and the gut to the liver, where they are converted to urea for excretion. The brain continues to use amino acids for neurotransmitter synthesis.

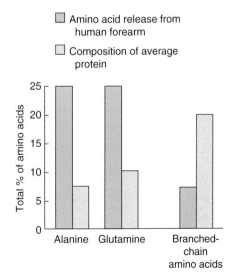

Fig. 42.4. Amino acid release from skeletal muscle. The arteriovenous difference (concentration in arterial blood minus the concentration in venous blood) across the human forearm has been measured for many amino acids. This graph compares the amount of alanine, glutamine, and BCAA released with their composition in the average protein. Alanine and glutamine represent a much higher percentage of total nitrogen released than originally present in the degraded protein, evidence that they are being synthesized in the skeletal muscle. The BCAA (leucine, valine, and isoleucine) are released in much lower amounts than those present in the degraded protein, evidence that they are being catabolized. Aspartate and glutamate also contribute nitrogen to the formation of alanine and glutamine

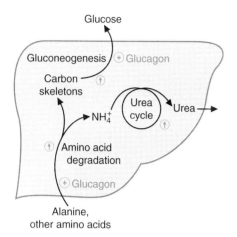

Fig. 42.5. Hormonal regulation of hepatic amino acid metabolism in the postabsorptive state. Circled + = glucagon-mediated activation of enzymes or proteins; circled ↑ = induction of enzyme synthesis mediated by glucagon and glucocorticoids. Induction of urea cycle enzymes occurs both during fasting and after a high-protein meal. Because many individuals in the United States normally have a high-protein diet, the levels of urea cycle enzymes may not fluctuate to any great extent.

Q: The body normally produces approximately 1 mmol of protons per kilogram of body weight per day. Nevertheless, the pH of the blood and extracellular fluid is normally maintained between 7.36 and 7.44. The narrow range is maintained principally by the bicarbonate (HCO_3^-), phosphate (HPO_4^-), and hemoglobin buffering systems, and by the excretion of an amount of acid equal to that produced. The excretion of protons by the kidney regenerates bicarbonate, which can be reclaimed from the glomerular filtrate.

The acids are produced from normal fuel metabolism. The major acid is carbonic acid, which is formed from water and CO_2 produced in the TCA cycle and other oxidative pathways. The oxidation of sulfur-containing amino acids (methionine and cysteine) ultimately produces sulfuric acid (H_2SO_4), which dissociates into $2H^+ + SO_4^{2-}$, and the protons and sulfate are excreted. The hydrolysis of phosphate esters produces the equivalent of phosphoric acid. What other acids produced during metabolism appear in the blood?

α-keto acids, and some glutamine from the blood. Alanine and other amino acids are oxidized and their carbon skeletons converted principally to glucose. Glucagon and glucocorticoids stimulate the uptake of amino acids into liver and increase gluconeogenesis and ureagenesis (Fig. 42.5). Alanine transport into the liver, in particular, is enhanced by glucagon. The induction of the synthesis of gluconeogenic enzymes by glucagon and glucocorticoids during the overnight fast correlates with an induction of many of the enzymes of amino acid degradation (e.g., tyrosine aminotransferase) and an induction of urea cycle enzymes (see Chapter 38). Urea synthesis also increases because of the increased supply of NH_4^+ from amino acid degradation in the liver.

3. METABOLISM OF AMINO ACIDS IN OTHER TISSUES DURING FASTING

Glucose, produced by the liver, is used for energy by the brain and other glucose-dependent tissues, such as erythrocytes. The muscle, under conditions of exercise, when the AMP-activated protein kinase is active, also oxidizes some of this glucose to pyruvate, which is used for the carbon skeleton of alanine (the glucose-alanine cycle; see Chapter 38).

Glutamine is generated in skeletal muscle from the oxidation of BCAA, and by the lungs and brain for the removal of NH_4^+ formed from amino acid catabolism or entering from the blood. The kidney, the gut, and cells with rapid turnover rates such as those of the immune system are the major sites of glutamine uptake (see Fig. 42.3). Glutamine serves as a fuel for these tissues, as a nitrogen donor for purine synthesis, and as a substrate for ammoniagenesis in the kidney. Much of the unused nitrogen from glutamine is transferred to pyruvate to form alanine in these tissues. Alanine then carries the unused nitrogen back to the liver.

The brain is glucose dependent, but, like many cells in the body, can use BCAA for energy. The BCAA also provide a source of nitrogen for neurotransmitter synthesis during fasting. Other amino acids released from skeletal muscle protein degradation also serve as precursors of neurotransmitters.

B. Principles Governing Amino Acid Flux between Tissues

The pattern of interorgan flux of amino acids is strongly affected by conditions that change the supply of fuels (for example, the overnight fast, a mixed meal, a high-protein meal) and by conditions that increase the demand for amino acids (metabolic acidosis, surgical stress, traumatic injury, burns, wound healing, and sepsis). The flux of amino acid carbon and nitrogen in these different conditions is dictated by several considerations:

1. Ammonia (NH_3) is toxic. Consequently, it is transported between tissues as alanine or glutamine. Alanine is the principal carrier of amino acid nitrogen from

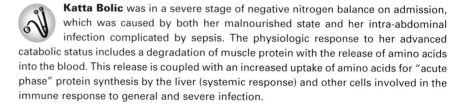

Katta Bolic was in a severe stage of negative nitrogen balance on admission, which was caused by both her malnourished state and her intra-abdominal infection complicated by sepsis. The physiologic response to her advanced catabolic status includes a degradation of muscle protein with the release of amino acids into the blood. This release is coupled with an increased uptake of amino acids for "acute phase" protein synthesis by the liver (systemic response) and other cells involved in the immune response to general and severe infection.

The differences in amino acid metabolism between tissues are dictated by the types and amounts of different enzyme and transport proteins present in each tissue and the ability of each tissue to respond to different regulatory messages (hormones and neural signals).

other tissues back to the liver, where the nitrogen is converted to urea and subsequently excreted into the urine by the kidneys. The amount of urea synthesized is proportional to the amount of amino acid carbon that is being oxidized as a fuel.

2. The pool of glutamine in the blood serves several essential metabolic functions (Table 42.1). It provides ammonia for excretion of protons in the urine as NH_4^+. It serves as a fuel for the gut, the kidney, and the cells of the immune system. Glutamine is also required by the cells of the immune system and other rapidly dividing cells in which its amide group serves as the source of nitrogen for biosynthetic reactions. In the brain, the formation of glutamine from glutamate and NH_4^+ provides a means of removing ammonia and of transporting glutamate between different cell types within the brain. The utilization of the blood glutamine pool is prioritized. During metabolic acidosis, the kidney becomes the predominant site of glutamine uptake, at the expense of glutamine utilization in other tissues. Conversly, during sepsis, in the absence of acidosis, cells involved in the immune response (macrophages, hepatocytes) become the preferential sites of glutamine uptake.

3. The BCAA (valine, leucine, and isoleucine) form a significant portion of the composition of the average protein and can be converted to tricarboxylic acid (TCA) cycle intermediates and used as fuels by almost all tissues. They are also the major precursors of glutamine. Except for the BCAA and alanine, aspartate, and glutamate, the catabolism of amino acids occurs principally in the liver.

4. Amino acids are major gluconeogenic substrates, and most of the energy obtained from their oxidation is derived from oxidation of the glucose formed from their carbon skeletons. A much smaller percentage of amino acid carbon is converted to acetyl CoA or to ketone bodies and oxidized. The utilization of amino acids for glucose synthesis for the brain and other glucose-requiring tissues is subject to the hormonal regulatory mechanisms of glucose homeostasis (see Chapters 31 and 36).

5. The relative rates of protein synthesis and degradation (protein turnover) determine the size of the free amino acid pools available for the synthesis of new proteins and for other essential functions. For example, the synthesis of new proteins to mount an immune response is supported by the net degradation of other proteins in the body.

II. UTILIZATION OF AMINO ACIDS IN INDIVIDUAL TISSUES

Because tissues differ in their physiologic functions, they have different amino acid requirements and contribute differently to whole body nitrogen metabolism. However, all tissues share a common requirement for essential amino acids for protein synthesis, and protein turnover is an ongoing process in all cells.

A. Kidney

One of the primary roles of amino acid nitrogen is to provide ammonia in the kidney for the excretion of protons in the urine. NH_4^+ is released from glutamine by glutaminase and by glutamate dehydrogenase, resulting in the formation of α-ketoglutarate (Fig. 42.6). α-Ketoglutarate is used as a fuel by the kidney and is oxidized to CO_2, converted to glucose for use in cells in the renal medulla, or converted to alanine to return ammonia to the liver for urea synthesis.

1. USE OF GLUTAMINE NITROGEN TO BUFFER URINE

The rate of glutamine uptake from the blood and its utilization by the kidney depends principally on the amount of acid that must be excreted to maintain a normal pH in the blood. During a metabolic acidosis, the excretion of NH_4^+ by the kidney increases severalfold (Table 42.2). Because glutamine nitrogen provides

Table 42.1. Functions of Glutamine

Protein synthesis
Ammoniagenesis for proton excretion
Nitrogen donor for synthesis of:
  Purines
  Pyrimidines
  NAD^+
  Amino sugars
  Asparagine
  Other compounds
Glutamate donor for synthesis of:
  Glutathione
  GABA
  Ornithine
  Arginine
  Proline
  Other compounds

The ability to convert 4-carbon intermediates of the TCA cycle to pyruvate is required for oxidation of both BCAA and glutamine. This sequence of reactions requires PEP carboxykinase, or decarboxylating malate dehydrogenase (malic enzyme). Most tissues have one, or both, of these enzymes.

Lactic acid is produced from glucose and amino acid metabolism. The ketone bodies (acetoacetate and β-hydroxybutyrate) produced during fatty acid oxidation are also acids. Many α-keto acids, formed from transamination reactions, are also found in the blood.

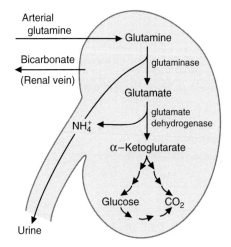

Fig. 42.6. Renal glutamine metabolism. Renal tubule cells preferentially oxidize glutamine. During metabolic acidosis, it is the major fuel for the kidney. Conversion of glutamine to α-ketoglutarate generates NH_4^+. Ammonium ion excretion helps to buffer systemic acidemia.

Table 42.2. Excretion of Compounds in the Urine

Component	g/24 hr	Nitrogen (mmol)
H_2O	1,000	–
SO_4^{-2}	2–5	–
PO_4^{-2}	2–5	–
K^+	1–2	–
Urea	12–20	400–650
Creatinine	1–1.8	25–50
Uric acid	0.2–0.8	4–16
NH_4^+	0.2–1	11–55
	(up to 10 in acidosis)	(up to 550 in acidosis)

approximately two thirds of the NH_4^+ excreted by the kidney, glutamine uptake by the kidney also increases. Renal glutamine utilization for proton excretion takes precedence over the requirements of other tissues for glutamine.

Ammonia increases proton excretion by providing a buffer for protons that are transported into the renal tubular fluid (which is transformed into urine as it passes through the tubules of the kidney) (Fig. 42.7). Specific transporters in the membranes of the renal tubular cells transport protons from these cells into the tubular lumen in exchange for Na^+. The protons in the tubular fluid are buffered by

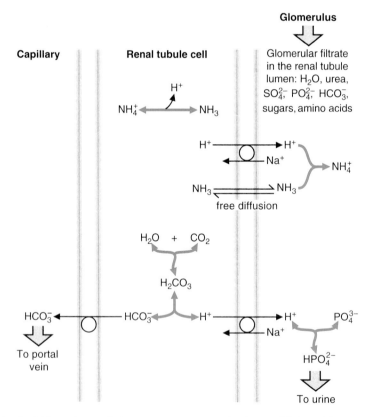

Fig. 42.7. Ammonia excretion by the kidney. Ammonia increases proton excretion by combining with a proton to form ammonium ion in the renal tubular fluid, which is transformed into urine as it passes through the tubules of the kidney. As blood is filtered in the capillary bed of the glomerulus, urea, sugars, amino acids, ions, and H_2O enter the renal tubular fluid (glomerular filtrate). As this fluid passes through a progression of tubules (the proximal convoluted tubule, the loop of Henle, the distal convoluted tubule, and the collecting duct) on its way to becoming urine, various components are reabsorbed or added to the filtrate by the epithelial cells lining the tubules. Specific transporters in the membranes of the renal tubule cells transport protons into the tubule lumen in exchange for Na^+ so that the glomerular filtrate becomes more acidic as it is transformed into urine. The protons in the tubule fluid are buffered by phosphate, by bicarbonate, and by NH_3. The ammonia, which is uncharged, is able to diffuse through the membrane of the renal tubule cells into the urine. As it combines with a proton in the urine, it forms NH_4^+, which cannot be transported back into the cells. The removal of protons as NH_4^+ decreases the requirement for bicarbonate excretion to buffer the urine.

Table 42.3. Major Fuel Sources for the Kidney

	% of Total CO_2 Formed in Different Physiologic States		
Fuel	Normal	Acidosis	Fasted
Lactate	45	20	15
Glucose[a]	25	20	0
Fatty acids	15	20	60
Glutamine	15	40	25

[a]Glucose used in the renal medulla is produced in the renal cortex.

phosphate, by bicarbonate, and by ammonia. Ammonia (NH_3), which is uncharged, enters the urine by free diffusion through the cell membrane. As it combines with a proton in the fluid, it forms ammonium ion (NH_4^+), which cannot be transported back into the cells and is excreted in the urine.

2. GLUTAMINE AS A FUEL FOR THE KIDNEY

Glutamine is used as a fuel by the kidney in the normal fed state and, to a greater extent, during fasting and metabolic acidosis (Table 42.3). The carbon skeleton forms α-ketoglutarate, which is oxidized to CO_2, converted to glucose, or released as the carbon skeleton of serine or alanine (Fig. 42.8). α-Ketoglutarate can be converted to oxaloacetate by TCA cycle reactions, and oxaloacetate is converted to phospho-enolpyruvate (PEP) by PEP carboxykinase. PEP can then be converted to pyruvate and subsequently acetyl CoA, alanine, serine, or glucose. The glucose is used principally by the cells of the renal medulla, which have a relatively high dependence on anaerobic glycolysis because of their lower oxygen supply and mitochondrial capacity. The lactate released from anaerobic glycolysis in these cells is taken up and oxidized in the renal cortical cells, which have a higher mitochondrial capacity and a greater blood supply.

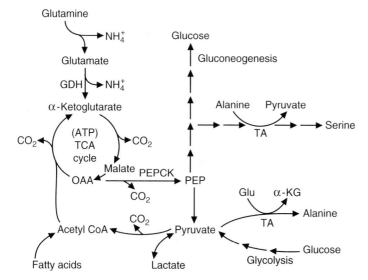

Fig. 42.8. Metabolism of glutamine and other fuels in the kidney. To completely oxidize glutamate carbon to CO_2, it must enter the TCA cycle as acetyl CoA. Carbon entering the TCA cycle as α-Ketoglutarate (α-KG) exits as oxaloacetate and is converted to phosphoenolpyruvate (PEP) by PEP carboxykinase. PEP is converted to pyruvate, which may be oxidized to acetyl CoA. PEP also can be converted to serine, glucose, or alanine. GDH = glutamate dehydrogenase; PEPCK = phosphoenolpyruvate carboxykinase; TA = transaminase; OAA = oxaloacetate.

B. Skeletal Muscle

Skeletal muscle, because of its large mass, is a major site of protein synthesis and degradation in the human. After a high-protein meal, insulin promotes the uptake of certain amino acids and stimulates net protein synthesis. The insulin stimulation of protein synthesis is dependent on an adequate supply of amino acids to undergo protein synthesis. During fasting and other catabolic states, a net degradation of skeletal muscle protein and release of amino acids occur (see Fig. 42.3). The net degradation of protein affects functional proteins, such as myosin, which are sacrificed to meet more urgent demands for amino acids in other tissues. During sepsis, degradation of skeletal muscle protein is stimulated by the glucocorticoid cortisol. The effect of cortisol is exerted through the activation of ubiquitin-dependent proteolysis. During fasting, the decrease of blood insulin levels and the increase of blood cortisol levels increase net protein degradation.

Skeletal muscle is a major site of glutamine synthesis, thereby satisfying the demand for glutamine during the postabsorptive state, during metabolic acidosis, and during septic stress and trauma. The carbon skeleton and nitrogen of glutamine are derived principally from the metabolism of BCAA. Amino acid degradation in skeletal muscle is also accompanied by the formation of alanine, which transfers amino groups from skeletal muscle to the liver in the glucose-alanine cycle.

1. OXIDATION OF BRANCHED-CHAIN AMINO ACIDS IN SKELETAL MUSCLE

The BCAA play a special role in muscle and most other tissues because they are the major amino acids that can be oxidized in tissues other than the liver. However, all tissues can interconvert amino acids and TCA cycle intermediates through transaminase reactions, i.e., alanine $\leftrightarrow$ pyruvate, aspartate $\leftrightarrow$ oxaloacetate, and α-ketoglutarate $\leftrightarrow$ glutamate. The first step of the pathway, transamination of the BCAA to α-keto acids, occurs principally in brain, heart, kidney, and skeletal muscles. These tissues have a high content of BCAA transaminase relative to the low levels in liver. The α-keto acids of the BCAA are then either released into the blood and taken up by liver, or oxidized to CO_2 or glutamine within the muscle or other tissue (Fig. 42.9). They can be oxidized by all tissues that contain mitochondria.

The oxidative pathways of the BCAA convert the carbon skeleton to either succinyl CoA or acetyl CoA (see Chapter 39 and Fig. 42.9). The pathways generate NADH and FAD(2H) for ATP synthesis before the conversion of carbon into intermediates of the TCA cycle, thus providing the muscle with energy without loss of carbon as CO_2. Leucine is "ketogenic" in that it is converted to acetyl CoA and acetoacetate. Skeletal muscle, adipocytes, and most other tissues are able to use these products and, therefore, directly oxidize leucine to CO_2. The portion of isoleucine converted to acetyl CoA is also oxidized directly to CO_2. For the portion of valine and isoleucine that enters the TCA cycle as succinyl CoA to be completely oxidized to CO_2, it must first be converted to acetyl CoA. To form acetyl CoA, succinyl CoA is oxidized to malate in the TCA cycle, and malate is then converted to pyruvate by malic enzyme (malate + $NADP^+ \rightarrow$ pyruvate + NADPH + H^+) (see Fig. 42.9). Pyruvate can then be oxidized to acetyl CoA. Alternatively, pyruvate can form alanine or lactate.

2. CONVERSION OF BRANCHED-CHAIN AMINO ACIDS TO GLUTAMINE

The major route of valine and isoleucine catabolism in skeletal muscle is to enter the TCA cycle as succinyl CoA and exit as α-ketoglutarate to provide the carbon skeleton for glutamine formation (see Fig. 42.9). Some of the glutamine and CO_2 that is formed from net protein degradation in skeletal muscle may also arise from

Q: When the carbon skeleton of alanine is derived from glucose, the efflux of alanine from skeletal muscle and its uptake by liver provide no net transfer of amino acid carbon to the liver for gluconeogenesis. However, some of the alanine carbon is derived from sources other than glucose. Which amino acids can provide carbon for alanine formation? (Hint: See Fig. 42.9.)

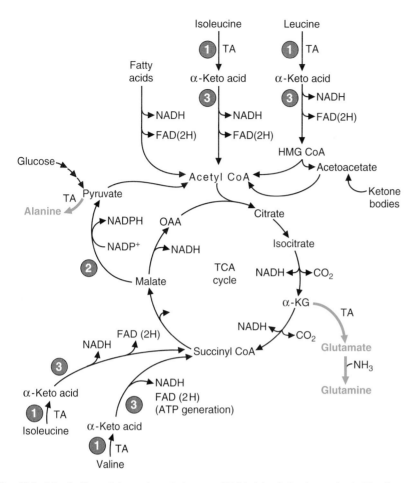

Fig. 42.9. Metabolism of the carbon skeletons of BCAA in skeletal muscle. 1. The first step in the metabolism of BCAA is transamination (TA). 2. Carbon from valine and isoleucine enters the TCA cycle as succinyl CoA and is converted to pyruvate by decarboxylating malate dehydrogenase (malic enzyme). 3. The oxidative pathways generate NADH and FAD(2H) even before the carbon skeleton enters the TCA cycle. The rate-limiting enzyme in the oxidative pathways is the α-keto acid dehydrogenase complex. The carbon skeleton also can be converted to glutamate and alanine, shown in blue.

the carbon skeletons of aspartate and glutamate. These amino acids are transaminated and become part of the pool of 4-carbon intermediates of the TCA cycle.

Glutamine nitrogen is derived principally from the BCAA (Fig. 42.10). The α-amino group arises from transamination reactions that form glutamate from α-ketoglutarate, and the amide nitrogen is formed from the addition of free ammonia to glutamate by glutamine synthetase. Free ammonia in skeletal muscle arises principally from the deamination of glutamate by glutamate dehydrogenase or from the purine nucleotide cycle.

In the purine nucleotide cycle (Fig. 42.11), the deamination of AMP to IMP releases NH_4^+. AMP is resynthesized with amino groups provided from aspartate. The aspartate amino groups can arise from the BCAA through transamination reactions. The fumarate can be used to replenish TCA cycle intermediates.

3. GLUCOSE-ALANINE CYCLE

The nitrogen arising from the oxidation of BCAA in skeletal muscle can also be transferred back to the liver as alanine in the glucose-alanine cycle (Fig. 42.12, see also Fig. 41.13). The amino group of the BCAA is first transferred to α-ketoglutarate

A: Some of the alanine released from skeletal muscle is derived directly from protein degradation. The carbon skeletons of valine, isoleucine, aspartate, and glutamate, which are converted to malate and oxaloacetate in the TCA cycle, can be converted to pyruvate and subsequently transaminated to alanine. The extent to which these amino acids contribute carbon to alanine efflux differs between different types of muscles in the human. These amino acids also may contribute to alanine efflux from the gut.

The purine nucleotide cycle is found in skeletal muscle and brain but is absent in liver and many other tissues. One of its functions in skeletal muscle is to respond to the rapid utilization of ATP during exercise. During exercise, the rapid hydrolysis of ATP increases AMP levels, resulting in an activation of AMP deaminase (see Fig. 42.11). As a consequence, the cellular concentration of IMP increases and ammonia is generated. IMP, like AMP, activates muscle glycogen phosphorylase during exercise (see Chapter 22). The ammonia that is generated may help to buffer the increased lactic acid production occurring in skeletal muscles during strenuous exercise.

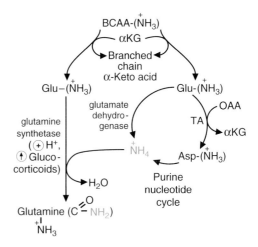

Fig. 42.10. Formation of glutamine from the amino groups of BCAA. The BCAA are first transaminated with α-ketoglutarate to form glutamate and the branched chain α-keto acids. The glutamate nitrogen can then follow either of two paths leading to glutamine formation. TA = transamination; OAA = oxaloacetate; α-KG = α-ketoglutarate.

to form glutamate and then transferred to pyruvate to form alanine by sequential transamination reactions. The pyruvate arises principally from glucose via the glycolytic pathway. The alanine released from skeletal muscle is taken up principally by the liver, where the amino group is incorporated into urea, and the carbon skeleton can be converted back to glucose through gluconeogenesis. Although the amount of alanine formed varies with dietary intake and physiologic state, the transport of nitrogen from skeletal muscle to liver as alanine occurs almost continuously throughout our daily fasting–feeding cycle.

C. Gut

Amino acids are an important fuel for the intestinal mucosal cells after a protein-containing meal and in catabolic states such as fasting or surgical trauma (Fig. 42.13). During fasting, glutamine is one of the major amino acids used by the gut. The principal fates of glutamine carbon in the gut are oxidation to CO_2 and conversion to the carbon

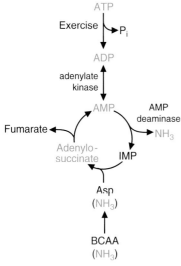

Fig. 42.11. Purine nucleotide cycle. In skeletal muscle, the purine nucleotide cycle can convert the amino groups of the BCAA to NH_3, which is incorporated into glutamine. The compounds containing the amino group released in the purine nucleotide cycle are shown in blue.

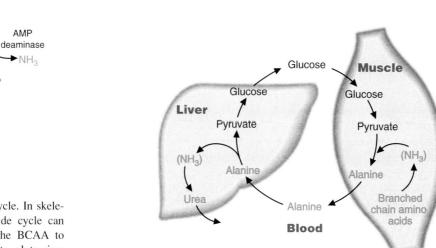

Fig. 42.12. Glucose-alanine cycle. The pathway for transfer of the amino groups from BCAA in skeletal muscle to urea in the liver is shown in blue.

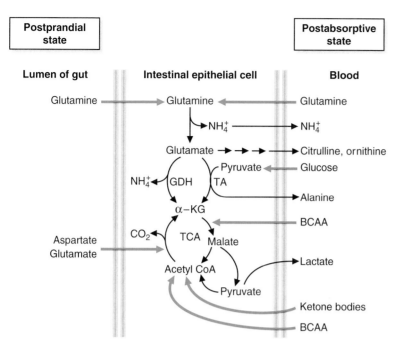

Fig. 42.13. Amino acid metabolism in the gut. The pathways of glutamine metabolism in the gut are the same whether it is supplied by the diet (postprandial state) or from the blood (postabsorptive state). Cells of the gut also metabolize aspartate, glutamate, and BCAA. Glucose is converted principally to the carbon skeleton of alanine. α-KG = α-ketoglutarate; GDH = glutamate dehydrogenase; TA = transaminase.

skeletons of lactate, citrulline, and ornithine. The gut also oxidizes BCAA. Nitrogen derived from amino acid degradation is converted to citrulline, alanine, NH_4^+, and other compounds that are released into the blood and taken up by the liver. Although most of the carbon in this alanine is derived from glucose, the oxidation of glucose to CO_2 is not a major fuel pathway for the gut. Fatty acids are also not a significant source of fuel for the intestinal mucosal cells, although they do use ketone bodies.

After a protein meal, dietary glutamine is a major fuel for the gut, and the products of glutamine metabolism are similar to those seen in the postabsorptive state. The gut also uses dietary aspartate and glutamate, which enter the TCA cycle. Colonocytes (the cells of the colon) also use short-chain fatty acids, derived from bacterial action in the lumen.

The importance of the gut in whole body nitrogen metabolism arises from the high rate of division and death of intestinal mucosal cells and the need to continuously provide these cells with amino acids to sustain the high rates of protein synthesis required for cellular division. Not only are these cells important for the uptake of nutrients, but they maintain a barrier against invading bacteria from the gut lumen and are, therefore, part of our passive defense system. As a result of these important functions, the intestinal mucosal cells are supplied with the amino acids required for protein synthesis and fuel oxidation at the expense of the more expendable skeletal muscle protein.

D. Liver

The liver is the major site of amino acid metabolism. It is the major site of amino acid catabolism and converts most of the carbon in amino acids to intermediates of the TCA cycle or the glycolytic pathway (which can be converted to glucose or oxidized to CO_2), or to acetyl CoA and ketone bodies. The liver is also the major site for urea synthesis. It can take up both glutamine and alanine and convert the

The intestine contains the enzymes for the urea cycle, but the V_{max} for argininosuccinate synthetase and argininosuccinate lyase are very low, suggesting that the primary role of the urea cycle enzymes in the gut is to produce citrulline from the carbons of glutamine (glutamine → glutamate → glutamate semialdehyde → ornithine → citrulline). The citrulline is released in the circulation for use by the liver.

Glutamine utilization by the gut is diminished by a metabolic acidosis compared with the postabsorptive or postprandial states. During metabolic acidosis, the uptake of glutamine by the kidney is increased, and blood glutamine levels decrease. As a consequence, the gut takes up less glutamine.

nitrogen to urea for disposal (see Chapter 38). Other pathways in the liver provide it with an unusually high amino acid requirement. The liver synthesizes plasma proteins, such as serum albumin, transferrin, and the proteins of the blood coagulation cascade. It is a major site for the synthesis of nonessential amino acids, the conjugation of xenobiotic compounds with glycine, the synthesis of heme and purine nucleotides, and the synthesis of glutathione.

E. Brain and Nervous Tissue

1. AMINO ACID POOL AND NEUROTRANSMITTER SYNTHESIS

A major function of amino acid metabolism in neural tissue is the synthesis of neurotransmitters. More than 40 compounds are believed to function as neurotransmitters, and all of these contain nitrogen derived from precursor amino acids. They include amino acids, which are themselves neurotransmitters (e.g., glutamate, glycine), the catecholamines derived from tyrosine (dopamine and norepinephrine), serotonin (derived from tryptophan), GABA (derived from glutamate), acetylcholine (derived from choline synthesized in the liver and acetyl CoA), and many peptides. In general, neurotransmitters are formed in the presynaptic terminals of axons and stored in vesicles until released by a transient change in electrochemical potential along the axon. Subsequent catabolism of some of the neurotransmitter results in the formation of a urinary excretion product. The rapid metabolism of neurotransmitters requires the continuous availability of a precursor pool of amino acids for de novo neurotransmitter synthesis (see Chapter 47).

2. METABOLISM OF GLUTAMINE IN THE BRAIN

The brain is a net glutamine producer owing principally to the presence of glutamine synthetase in astroglial cells (see Chapter 47). Glutamate and aspartate are synthesized in these cells, using amino groups donated by the BCAA (principally valine) and TCA cycle intermediates formed from glucose and from the carbon skeletons of BCAA (Fig. 42.14) The glutamate is converted to glutamine by glutamine synthetase, which incorporates NH_4^+ released from deamination of amino acids and deamination of AMP in the purine nucleotide cycle in the brain. This glutamine may efflux from the brain, carrying excess NH_4^+ into the blood, or serve as a precursor of glutamate in neuronal cells.

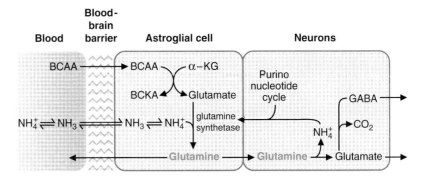

Fig. 42.14. Role of glutamine in the brain. Glutamine serves as a nitrogen transporter in the brain for the synthesis of many different neurotransmitters. Different neurons convert glutamine to γ-aminobutyric acid (GABA) or to glutamate. Glutamine also transports excess NH_4^+ from the brain into the blood. BCKA = branched-chain keto acids; α-KG = α-ketoglutarate.

Glutamine synthesized in the astroglial cells is a precursor of glutamate (an excitatory neurotransmitter) and GABA (an inhibitory neurotransmitter) in the neuronal cells (see Fig. 42.14). It is converted to glutamate by a neuronal glutaminase isozyme. In GABAergic neurons, glutamate is then decarboxylated to GABA, which is released during excitation of the neuron. GABA is one of the neurotransmitters that is recycled; a transaminase converts it to succinaldehyde, which is then oxidized to succinate. Succinate enters the TCA cycle.

III. CHANGES IN AMINO ACID METABOLISM WITH DIETARY AND PHYSIOLOGIC STATE

The rate and pattern of amino acid utilization by different tissues change with dietary and physiologic state. Two such states, the postprandial period following a high-protein meal and the hypercatabolic state produced by sepsis or surgical trauma, differ from the postabsorptive state with respect to the availability of amino acids and other fuels and the levels of different hormones in the blood. As a result, the pattern of amino acid utilization is somewhat different.

A. A High-Protein Meal

After the ingestion of a high-protein meal, the gut and the liver use most of the absorbed amino acids (Fig. 42.15). Glutamate and aspartate are used as fuels by the gut, and very little enters the portal vein. The gut also may use some BCAA. The liver takes up 60 to 70% of the amino acids present in the portal vein. These amino acids, for the most part, are converted to glucose in the gluconeogenic pathway.

After a pure protein meal, the increased levels of dietary amino acids reaching the pancreas stimulate the release of glucagon above fasting levels, thereby increasing amino acid uptake into liver and stimulating gluconeogenesis. Insulin release is also stimulated, but not nearly to the levels found after a high-carbohydrate meal.

During hyperammonemia, ammonia (NH_3) can diffuse into the brain from the blood. The ammonia is able to inhibit the neural isozyme of glutaminase, thereby decreasing additional ammonia formation in the brain and inhibiting the formation of glutamate and its subsequent metabolism to GABA. This effect of ammonia might contribute to the lethargy associated with the hyperammonemia found in patients with hepatic disease.

The levels of transthyretin (binds to vitamin A and thyroid hormones in the blood) and serum albumin in the blood may be used as indicators of the degree of protein malnutrition. In the absence of hepatic disease, decreased levels of these proteins in the blood indicate insufficient availability of amino acids to the liver for synthesis of serum proteins.

Q: In what ways does liver metabolism after a high-protein meal resemble liver metabolism in the fasting state?

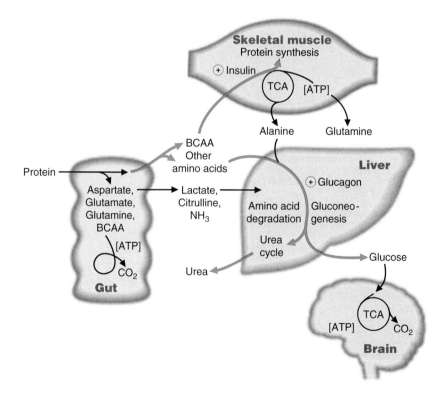

Fig. 42.15. Flux of amino acids after a high-protein meal.

A: Both of these dietary states are characterized by an elevation of glucagon. Glucagon stimulates amino acid transport into the liver, stimulates gluconeogenesis through decreasing levels of fructose 2,6-bisphosphate, and induces the synthesis of enzymes in the urea cycle, the gluconeogenic pathway, and the pathways for degradation of some of the amino acids.

The Atkins high-protein diet is based on the premise that ingesting high-protein, low-carbohydrate meals will keep circulating insulin levels low, such that energy storage is not induced, and glucagon release will point the insulin/glucagon ratio to energy mobilization, particularly fatty acid release from the adipocyte and oxidation by the tissues. The lack of energy storage, coupled with the loss of fat, leads to weight loss.

In general, the insulin released after a high-protein meal is sufficiently high that the uptake of BCAA into skeletal muscle and net protein synthesis is stimulated, but gluconeogenesis in the liver is not inhibited. The higher the carbohydrate content of the meal, the higher the insulin/glucagon ratio and the greater the shift of amino acids away from gluconeogenesis into biosynthetic pathways in the liver such as the synthesis of plasma proteins.

Most of the amino acid nitrogen entering the peripheral circulation after a high-protein meal or a mixed meal is present as the BCAA. Because the liver has low levels of transaminases for these amino acids, it cannot oxidize them to a significant extent, and they enter the systemic circulation. The BCAA are slowly taken up by skeletal muscle and other tissues. These peripheral nonhepatic tissues use the amino acids derived from the diet principally for net protein synthesis.

B. Hypercatabolic States

Surgery, trauma, burns, and septic stress are examples of hypercatabolic states characterized by increased fuel utilization and a negative nitrogen balance (Fig. 42.16). The mobilization of body protein, fat, and carbohydrate stores serves to maintain normal tissue function in the presence of a limited dietary intake, as well as to support the energy and amino acid requirements for the immune response and wound healing. The negative nitrogen balance that occurs in these hypercatabolic states

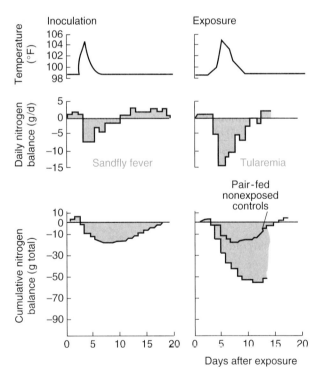

Fig. 42.16. Negative nitrogen balance during infection. The effects of experimentally induced infections on nitrogen balance were determined in human volunteers. After inoculation with sandfly fever, increased amino acid catabolism produced a negative nitrogen balance. A few days after exposure, the daily nitrogen balance became positive until the volunteers returned to their original state. Experiments with patients exposed to tularemia showed that the negative nitrogen balance was much larger than could be expected from a decreased appetite alone. Volunteers who ate the same amount of food as the infected individuals (pair-fed nonexposed controls) had a much smaller cumulative negative nitrogen balance than the infected volunteers. From Beisel WR. Am J Clin Nutr 1977;30:1236–1247. © 1977 American Society for Clinical Nutrition.

results from an accelerated protein turnover and an increased rate of net protein degradation, primarily in skeletal muscle.

The catabolic state of sepsis (acute, generalized, febrile infection) is one of enhanced mobilization of fuels and amino acids to provide the energy and precursors required by cells of the immune system, host defense mechanisms, and wound healing. The amino acids must provide the substrates for new protein synthesis and cell division. Glucose synthesis and release are enhanced to provide fuel for these cells, and the patient may become mildly hyperglycemic.

In these hypercatabolic states, skeletal muscle protein synthesis decreases, and protein degradation increases. Oxidation of BCAA is increased and glutamine production enhanced. Amino acid uptake is diminished. Cortisol is the major hormonal mediator of these responses, although certain cytokines may also have direct effects on skeletal muscle metabolism. As occurs during fasting and metabolic acidosis, increased levels of cortisol stimulate ubiquitin-mediated proteolysis, induce the synthesis of glutamine synthetase, and enhance release of amino acids and glutamine from the muscle cells.

The amino acids released from skeletal muscle during periods of hypercatabolic stress are used in a prioritized manner, with the cellular components of the immune system receiving top priority. For example, the uptake of amino acids by the liver for the synthesis of acute phase proteins, which are part of the immune system, is greatly increased. Conversely, during the early phase of the acute response, the synthesis of other plasma proteins (e.g., albumin) is decreased. The increased availability of amino acids and the increased cortisol levels also stimulate gluconeogenesis, thereby providing fuel for the glucose-dependent cells of the immune system (e.g., lymphocytes). An increase of urea synthesis accompanies the acceleration of amino acid degradation.

The increased efflux of glutamine from skeletal muscle during sepsis serves several functions (see Fig. 42.1). It provides the rapidly dividing cells of the immune system with an energy source. Glutamine is available as a nitrogen donor for purine synthesis, for NAD^+ synthesis, and for other biosynthetic functions essential to growth and division of the cells. An increased production of metabolic acids may accompany stress such as sepsis, so there is an increased utilization of glutamine by the kidney.

Under the influence of elevated levels of glucocorticoids, epinephrine, and glucagon, fatty acids are mobilized from adipose tissue to provide alternate fuels for other tissues and spare glucose. Under these conditions, fatty acids are the major energy source for skeletal muscle, and glucose uptake is decreased. These changes may lead to a mild hyperglycemia.

 The degree of the body's hypercatabolic response depends on the severity and duration of the trauma or stress. After an uncomplicated surgical procedure in an otherwise healthy patient, the net negative nitrogen balance may be limited to about 1 week. The mild nitrogen losses are usually reversed by dietary protein supplementation as the patient recovers. With more severe traumatic injury or septic stress, the body may catabolize body protein and adipose tissue lipids for a prolonged period, and the negative nitrogen balance may not be corrected for weeks.

 Katta Bolic's severe negative nitrogen balance was caused by both her malnourished state and her intra-abdominal infection complicated by sepsis. The systemic and diverse responses the body makes to insults such as an acute febrile illness are termed the "acute phase response." An early event in this response is the stimulation of phagocytic activity (see Fig. 42.17). Stimulated macrophages release cytokines, which are regulatory proteins that stimulate the release of cortisol, insulin, and growth hormone. Cytokines also directly mediate the acute phase response of the liver and skeletal muscle to sepsis.

CLINICAL COMMENTS

The clinician can determine whether a patient such as **Katta Bolic** is mounting an acute phase response to some insult, however subtle, by determining whether several unique acute phase proteins are being secreted by the liver. C-reactive protein, so named because of its ability to interact with the C-polysaccharide of pneumococci, and serum amyloid A protein, a precursor of the amyloid fibril found in secondary amyloidosis, are elevated in patients undergoing the acute phase response and as compared with healthy individuals. Other proteins normally found in the blood of healthy individuals are present in increased concentrations in patients undergoing an acute phase response. These include haptoglobin, certain protease inhibitors, complement components, ceruloplasmin, and fibrinogen. The elevated concentration of these proteins in the blood increases the erythrocyte sedimentation rate (ESR), another laboratory measure of the presence of an acute phase response.

To determine the ESR, the patients' blood is placed vertically in a small-bore glass tube. The speed with which the red blood cells sediment toward the bottom of the tube depends on what percentage of the red blood cells clump together and, thereby, become more dense. The degree of clumping is directly correlated with the presence of one or more of the first-phase proteins listed previously. These proteins interfere with what is known as the zeta-potential of the red blood cells, which normally prevents the red blood cells from clumping. Because many different proteins can individually alter the zeta-potential, the ESR is a nonspecific test for the presence of acute inflammation.

The weight loss often noted in septic patients is primarily caused by a loss of appetite resulting from the effect of certain cytokines on the medullary appetite center. Other causes include increased energy expenditure from fever and enhanced muscle proteolysis.

BIOCHEMICAL COMMENTS

  After a catabolic insult such as injury, trauma, infection, or cancer, the interorgan flow of glutamine and fuels is dramatically altered. Teleologically, the changes in metabolism that occur give first priority to cells that are part of the immune system. Evidence suggests that the changes in glutamine and

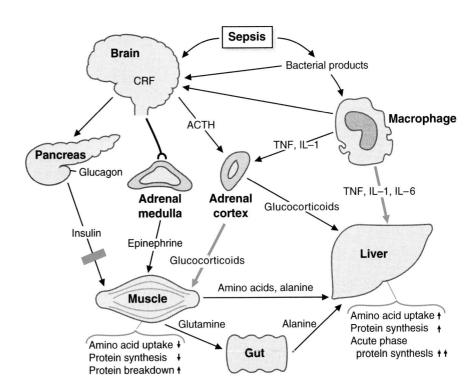

Fig. 42.17. Cytokines and hormones mediate amino acid flux during sepsis. Bacterial products act on macrophages to stimulate the release of cytokines and on the brain to stimulate the sympathoadrenal response. The result is a stimulation of the release of the insulin counterregulatory hormones, epinephrine, glucagon, and glucocorticoids. The glucocorticoid cortisol may be the principal mediator of net muscle protein degradation during sepsis. Hepatic protein synthesis, particularly that of acute phase proteins, is stimulated both by cortisol and cytokines. Amino acid metabolism in the gut is also probably affected by glucocorticoids and cytokines. Because of the release of the counterregulatory hormones, muscle and other tissues become resistant to insulin action, as indicated by the bar on the figure. Adapted with permission from Fisher J. Am J Surg 1991;161:270.

fuel metabolism are mediated by the insulin counterregulatory hormones, such as cortisol and epinephrine, and several different cytokines (see Chapter 11 for a review of cytokines). Cytokines appear to play a more important role than hormones during sepsis, although they exert their effects, in part, through hormones (Fig. 42.17). Although cytokines can be released from a variety of cells, macrophages are the principal source during trauma and sepsis.

Two cytokines that are important in sepsis are interleukin-1 (IL-1) and tumor necrosis factor (TNF). IL-1 and TNF affect amino acid metabolism both through regulation of the release of glucocorticoids and through direct effects on tissues. Although cytokines are generally considered to be paracrine, with their effects being exerted over cells in the immediate vicinity, TNF and IL-1 increase in the blood during sepsis. Other cytokines, such as IL-6, also may be involved.

During sepsis, TNF, IL-1, and possibly other cytokines, bacterial products, or mediators act on the brain to stimulate the release of glucocorticoids from the adrenal cortex (a process mediated by adrenocorticotropic hormone [ACTH]), epinephrine from the adrenal medulla, and both insulin and glucagon from the pancreas. Although insulin is elevated during sepsis, the tissues exhibit an insulin resistance that is similar to that of the non–insulin-dependent diabetes mellitus patient, possibly resulting from the elevated levels of the insulin counterregulatory hormones (glucocorticoids, epinephrine, and glucagon). Changes in the rate of acute phase protein synthesis are mediated, at least in part, by effects of TNF, IL-1, and IL-6 on the synthesis of groups of proteins in the liver.

Hypercatabolic states may be accompanied by varying degrees of insulin resistance caused, in part, by the release of counterregulatory hormones into the blood. Thus, patients with diabetes mellitus may require higher levels of exogenous insulin during sepsis.

Suggested References

Abcouwer SF, Bode BP, Souba WW. Glutamine as a metabolic intermediate. In: Fischer JE, ed. Nutrition and Metabolism of the Surgical Patient. 2nd Ed. Boston: Little, Brown & Company, 1996:353–384.

Abumrad NN, Williams P, Frexes-Steed M, et al. Inter-organ metabolism of amino acids in vivo. Diabetes Metabol Rev 1989;5:213–226.

Bessey PQ. Metabolic response to trauma and infection. In: Fischer JE, ed. Nutrition and Metabolism of the Surgical Patient. 2nd Ed. Boston: Little, Brown & Company, 1996:1577–1600.

Fischer J, Hasselgren P-O. Cytokines and glucocorticoids in the regulation of the "hepato-skeletal muscle axis" in sepsis. Am J Surg 1991:161:266–271.

Newsholme P, Procopio J, Lima, MMR, Pithon-Curu TC, Cori R. Glutamine and glutamate—their central role in cell metabolism and function. Cell Biochem Funct 2003;21:1–9.

Wolfe RR. Effects of insulin on muscle tissue. Curr Opin Clin Nutr Metab Care 2000;3:67–71.

REVIEW QUESTIONS—CHAPTER 42

1. Which of the profiles indicated below would occur within 2 hours after eating a meal very high in protein and low in carbohydrates?

	Blood glucagon levels	Liver gluconeogenesis	BCAA oxidation in muscle
(A)	↓	↓	↑
(B)	↑	↓	↑
(C)	↓	↑	↑
(D)	↑	↑	↑
(E)	↓	↓	↓
(F)	↑	↓	↓
(G)	↓	↑	↓
(H)	↑	↑	↓

2. The gut uses glutamine as an energy source, but can also secrete citrulline, synthesized from the carbons of glutamine. Which of the following compounds is an obligatory intermediate in this conversion (consider only the carbon atoms of glutamine while answering this question)?

    (A) Aspartate
    (B) Succinyl CoA
    (C) Glutamate
    (D) Serine
    (E) Fumarate

3. The signal that indicates to muscle that protein degradation needs to be initiated is which of the following?

    (A) Insulin
    (B) Glucagon
    (C) Epinephrine
    (D) Cortisol
    (E) Glucose

4. The skeletal muscles convert BCAA carbons to glutamine for export to the rest of the body. An obligatory intermediate, which carries carbons originally from the BCAA, in the conversion of BCAA to glutamine, is which of the following?

    (A) Urea
    (B) Pyruvate
    (C) Lactate
    (D) Isocitrate
    (E) Phosphoenolpyruvate

5. An individual in sepsis would display which of the following metabolic patterns?

	Nitrogen balance	Gluconeogenesis	Fatty acid oxidation
(A)	Positive	↑	↑
(B)	Negative	↑	↑
(C)	Positive	↑	↓
(D)	Negative	↑	↓
(E)	Positive	↓	↑
(F)	Negative	↓	↓

Tissue Metabolism

Although many of the pathways described previously are present in all tissues of the body, many tissues also carry out specialized functions and contain unique biochemical pathways. This section describes a number of such tissues and, in some cases, how the tissues interact with the rest of the body to coordinate their functions.

The previous chapters of this text have focused primarily on insulin and glucagon as the major mediators for regulating metabolic pathways; however, a large number of other hormones also regulate the storage and utilization of metabolic fuels (see Chapter 43). These hormones primarily counteract the effects of insulin and are called counter-regulatory hormones. They include growth hormone; thyroid hormone; glucocorticoids, such as cortisol; small peptides, such as the somatostatins; and small molecules, such as the catecholamines. Growth hormone works, in part, by inducing the synthesis of the insulin-like growth factors. These hormones can exert their effects rapidly (through covalent modification of selected enzymes) or long-term (through alterations in the rate of synthesis of selected enzymes). The interplay of these hormones with insulin and glucagon is discussed, as are the synthesis, secretion, and conditions leading to secretion of each hormone.

The proteins and cells in the blood form their own tissue system (see Chapter 44). All blood cells are derived from a common precursor, the stem cell, in the bone marrow. Different cytokine signals trigger differentiation of a particular blood cell lineage. For example, when there is a decreased supply of oxygen to the tissues, the kidney responds by releasing erythropoietin. This hormone specifically stimulates the production of red blood cells.

The red blood cell has limited metabolic functions, owing to its lack of internal organelles. Its main function is to deliver oxygen to the tissues through the binding of oxygen to hemoglobin. When the number of red blood cells is reduced, an anemia is said to have developed. This can be attributable to many causes, including nutritional deficiencies or mutations (hereditary anemias). The morphology of the red blood cell can sometimes aid in distinguishing between the various types of anemia.

Red blood cell metabolism is geared toward preserving the ability of these cells to transport oxygen, as well as to regulate oxygen binding to hemoglobin. Glycolysis provides energy and NADH to protect the oxidation state of the heme-bound iron. The hexose monophosphate shunt pathway generates NADPH to protect red blood cell membranes from oxidation. Heme synthesis, which uses succinyl CoA and glycine for all of the carbon and nitrogen atoms in the structure, occurs in the precursors of red blood cells. Inherited defects in heme synthesis lead to a class of diseases known as the porphyrias. Because the red blood cell normally passes through the very narrow capillaries, its membrane must be easily deformable. This deformability is, in part, attributable to the complex cytoskeletal structure that surrounds the erythrocyte. Mutations in these structural proteins can lead to less deformable cells. This, in turn, can result in a hemolytic anemia.

Among other functions, the hematologic system is responsible for hemostasis as well as for maintaining a constant blood volume (see Chapter 45). A tear in the wall of a vessel can lead to blood loss, which, when extensive, can be fatal. Repairing vessel damage, whether internal or external, is accomplished by a complicated series of zymogen activations of circulating blood proteins resulting in the formation of a fibrin clot (the coagulation cascade). Platelets play a critical role in hemostasis not only through their release of procoagulants but through their ability to form aggregates within the thrombus (clot) as well. Clots function as a plug, allowing vessel walls to repair and preventing further blood loss. Conversely, inappropriate clot formation in vessels that supply blood to vital organs or tissues can have devastating consequences, such as an acute cerebral or myocardial infarction. Because clotting must be tightly controlled, intricate mechanisms exist that regulate this important hematologic function.

The liver is an altruistic organ that provides multiple services for other tissues (see Chapter 46). It supplies glucose and ketone bodies to the rest of the body when fuel stores are limiting. It disposes of ammonia as urea when amino acid degradation occurs. It is the site of detoxification of xenobiotics, and it synthesizes many of the proteins found in the blood. The liver synthesizes fatty acids and cholesterol and distributes them to other tissues in the form of very-low-density lipoprotein (VLDL). The liver also synthesizes bile acids for fat digestion in the intestine. The liver recycles cholesterol and triglyceride through its uptake of intermediate density lipoprotein (IDL), chylomicron and VLDL remnants, and low-density lipoprotein (LDL) particles. Because of its protective nature and its strategic location between the gut and the systemic circulation, the liver has "first crack" at all compounds that enter the blood through the enterohepatic circulation. Thus, xenobiotic compounds can be detoxified as they enter the liver before they have a chance to reach other tissues.

Muscle cells contain unique pathways that allow them to store energy as creatine phosphate and to closely regulate their use of fatty acids as an energy source (see Chapter 47). The adenosine monophosphate (AMP)-activated protein kinase is an important regulator of muscle energy metabolism. Muscle is comprised of different types of contractile fibers that derive their energy from different sources. For example, the slow-twitch type I fibers use oxidative energy pathways, whereas the type II fast-twitch fibers use the glycolytic pathway for their energy requirements.

The nervous system consists of various cell types that are functionally interconnected so as to allow efficient signal transmission throughout the system (see Chapter 48). The cells of the central nervous system are protected from potentially toxic compounds by the blood-brain barrier, which restricts entry of compounds into the nervous system (ammonia, however, is a notable exception). The brain cells communicate with each other and with other organs, through the synthesis of neurotransmitters and neuropeptides. Many of the neurotransmitters are derived from amino acids, most of which are synthesized within the nerve cell. Because the pathways of amino acid and neurotransmitter biosynthesis require cofactors (such as pyridoxal phosphate, thiamine pyrophosphate, and vitamin B12), deficiencies of these cofactors can lead to neuropathies (dysfunction of specific neurons within the nervous system).

Because of the restrictions imposed by the blood-brain barrier, the brain also must synthesize its own lipids. An adequate supply of lipids is vital to the central nervous system because they are constituents of the myelin sheath that surrounds the neurons and allows them to conduct impulses normally. The neurodegenerative disorders, such as multiple sclerosis, are a consequence of varying degrees of demyelination of the neurons.

Connective tissue, which consists primarily of fibroblasts, produces extracellular matrix materials that surround cells and tissues, determining their appropriate position within the organ (see Chapter 49). These materials include structural proteins (collagen and elastin), adhesive proteins (fibronectin), and glycosaminoglycans (heparan sulfate, chondroitin sulfate). The unique structures of the proteins and carbohydrates found within the extracellular matrix allow tissues and organs to carry out their many functions. A loss of these supportive and barrier functions of connective tissue sometimes leads to significant clinical consequences, such as those that result from the microvascular alterations that lead to blindness or renal failure, or peripheral neuropathies in patients with diabetes mellitus.

43 Actions of Hormones That Regulate Fuel Metabolism

Many hormones affect fuel metabolism, including those that regulate appetite as well as those that influence absorption, transport, and oxidation of foodstuffs. The major hormones that influence nutrient metabolism and their actions on muscle, liver, and adipose tissue are listed in Table 43.1.

*   *Insulin is the major anabolic hormone. It promotes the storage of nutrients as glycogen in liver and muscle, and as triacylglycerols in adipose tissue. It also stimulates the synthesis of proteins in tissues such as muscle. At the same time, insulin acts to inhibit fuel mobilization.*

*   *Glucagon is the major counterregulatory hormone. The term counterregulatory means that its actions are generally opposed to those of insulin (contrainsular). The major action of glucagon is to mobilize fuel reserves by stimulating glycogenolysis and gluconeogenesis. These actions ensure that glucose will be available to glucose-dependent tissues between meals.*

*   *Epinephrine, norepinephrine, cortisol, somatostatin, and growth hormone also have contrainsular activity. Thyroid hormone also must be classified as an insulin counterregulatory hormone because it increases the rate of fuel consumption and also increases the sensitivity of the target cells to other insulin counterregulatory hormones.*

Insulin and the counterregulatory hormones exert two types of metabolic regulation (see Chapter 26). The first type of control occurs within minutes to hours of the hormone–receptor interaction and usually results from changes in the catalytic activity or kinetics of key preexisting enzymes, caused by phosphorylation or dephosphorylation of these enzymes. The second type of control involves regulation of the synthesis of key enzymes by mechanisms that stimulate or inhibit transcription and translation of mRNA. These processes are slow and require hours to days.

THE WAITING ROOM

Otto Shape, now a third-year medical student, was assigned to do a history and physical examination on a newly admitted 47-year-old patient named **Corti Solemia**. Mr. Solemia had consulted his physician for increasing weakness and fatigue and was found to have a severely elevated serum glucose level. While examining the patient, Otto noted marked redness of the patient's facial skin as well as reddish-purple stripes (striae) in the skin of the patient's lower abdomen and thighs. The patient's body fat was unusually distributed in that it appeared to be excessively

Table 43.1. Major Hormones that Regulate Fuel Metabolism

Hormones	Muscle			Liver						Adipose Tissue	
	Glucose Uptake	Glucose Utilization	Protein Synthesis	Glucose Output	Ketogenesis	Gluconeogenesis	Glycogenolysis	Glycogenesis	Protein Synthesis	Fat Synthesis	Lipolysis
Anabolic hormone											
Insulin	↑↑	↑↑	↑↑	↓↓	↓↓	↓↓	↓↓	↑	↑	↑↑	↓↓
Counterregulatory hormones[a]											
Glucagon	–	–	–	↑↑	↑	↑	↑↑	↓	–	–	↑ (at large doses)
Epinephrine and norepinephrine	–	↑	–	↑↑	–	↑	↑↑ (initial)	↑↓	–	–	↑↑
Glucocorticoid	↓	↓	↓	↑	↑	↑ (mainly permissive)	–	↑	↑	–	↑ (permissive)
Growth hormone	↓ (weakly)	↓ (weakly)	↑	↑	↑	↑	–	–	↑	–	↑ (mainly permissive)
Thyroid hormone	–	↑	↑	↑	↑	↑	–	–	–	–	↑ (permissive)
Somatostatin[b]	–	–	–	–	–	–	–	–	–	–	–

[a] Hormones with actions that are generally opposed to those of insulin.

[b] Somatostatin's effects on metabolism are indirect via suppression of secretion of insulin, glucagon, growth hormone, and thyroid hormone and by effects on gastric acid secretion, gastric emptying time, and pancreatic exocrine secretion (see text).

deposited centrally in his face, neck, upper back, chest and abdomen, while the distal portions of his arms and legs appeared to be almost devoid of fat. The patient's skin appeared thinned, and large bruises were present over many areas of his body, for which Mr. Solemia had no explanation. The neurologic examination showed severe muscle weakness, especially in the proximal arms and legs, where the muscles seemed atrophied.

Sam Atotrope, a 42-year-old jeweler, noted increasingly severe headaches behind his eyes sometimes associated with a "flash of light" in his visual fields. At times his vision seemed blurred, making it difficult to perform some of the intricate work required of a jeweler. He consulted his ophthalmologist, who was impressed with the striking change in Sam's facial features that had occurred since he last saw the patient 5 years earlier. The normal skin creases in Sam's face had grown much deeper, his skin appeared to be thickened, his nose and lips appeared more bulbous, and his jaw seemed more prominent. The doctor also noted that Sam's hands appeared bulky, and his voice had deepened. An eye examination showed that Sam's optic nerves appeared slightly atrophied, and there was a loss of the upper outer quadrants of his visual fields.

I. PHYSIOLOGIC EFFECTS OF INSULIN

The effects of insulin on fuel metabolism and substrate flux were considered in many of the earlier chapters of this book, particularly in Chapter 26. Insulin stimulates the storage of glycogen in liver and muscle and the synthesis of fatty acids and triacylglycerols and their storage in adipose tissue. In addition, insulin stimulates the synthesis in various tissues of more than 50 proteins, some of which contribute to the growth of the organism. In fact, it is difficult to separate the effects of insulin on cell growth from those of a family of proteins known as the somatomedins or the insulin-like growth factors I and II (IGF-I and IGF-II) (see Section III.B.6. of this chapter).

Finally, insulin has paracrine actions within the pancreatic islet cells. When insulin is released from the β cells, it suppresses glucagon release from the α cells.

II. PHYSIOLOGIC EFFECTS OF GLUCAGON

Glucagon is one of several counterregulatory (contrainsular) hormones. It is synthesized as part of a large precursor protein, proglucagon. Proglucagon is produced in the α cells of the islets of Langerhans in the pancreas and in the L cells of the intestine. It contains a number of peptides linked in tandem: glicentin-related peptide, glucagon, glucagon-related peptide 1 (GLP-1), and glucagon-related peptide 2 (GLP-2). Proteolytic cleavage of proglucagon releases various combinations of its constituent peptides. Glucagon is cleaved from proglucagon in the pancreas and constitutes 30 to 40% of the immunoreactive glucagon in the blood. The remaining immunoreactivity is caused by other cleavage products of proglucagon released from the pancreas and the intestine. Pancreatic glucagon has a plasma half-life of 3 to 6 minutes and is removed mainly by the liver and kidney.

Glucagon promotes glycogenolysis, gluconeogenesis, and ketogenesis by stimulating the generation of cyclic adenosine monophosphate (cAMP) in target cells. The liver is the major target organ for glucagon, in part because the concentrations of this hormone bathing the liver cells in the portal blood are higher than in the peripheral circulation. Portal vein levels of glucagon may reach concentrations as high as 500 pg/mL.

Finally, glucagon stimulates insulin release from the β cells of the pancreas. Whether this is a paracrine effect or an endocrine effect has not been established. The pattern of blood flow in the pancreatic islet cells is believed to bathe the β cells first and then the α-cells. Therefore, the β cells may influence α-cell function by an endocrine mechanism, whereas the influence of β-cell hormone on α-cell function is more likely to be paracrine.

III. PHYSIOLOGIC EFFECTS OF OTHER COUNTERREGULATORY HORMONES

A. Somatostatin

1. BIOCHEMISTRY

Preprosomatostatin, a 116–amino acid peptide, is encoded on the long arm of chromosome 3. Somatostatin (SS-14), a cyclic peptide with a molecular weight of 1,600, is produced from the 14 amino acids at the C-terminus of this precursor molecule. SS-14 was first isolated from the hypothalamus and named for its ability to inhibit the release of growth hormone (GH, somatotropin) from the anterior pituitary. It also inhibits the release of insulin. In addition to the hypothalamus, somatostatin is also secreted from the D cells (δ cells) of the pancreatic islets, many areas of the central nervous system outside of the hypothalamus, and in gastric and duodenal mucosal cells. SS-14 predominates in the central nervous system (CNS) and is the sole form secreted by the δ cells of the pancreas. In the gut, however, prosomatostatin (SS-28), which has 14 additional amino acids extending from the C-terminal portion of the precursor, makes up 70 to 75% of the immunoreactivity (the amount of hormone that reacts with antibodies to SS-14). The prohormone SS-28 is 7 to 10 times more potent in inhibiting the release of GH and insulin than is SS-14.

2. SECRETION OF SOMATOSTATIN

The secretagogues for somatostatin are similar to those that cause secretion of insulin. The metabolites that increase somatostatin release include glucose, arginine, and leucine. The hormones that stimulate somatostatin secretion include glucagon, vasoactive intestinal polypeptide (VIP), and cholecystokinin (CCK). Insulin, however, does not directly influence somatostatin secretion.

3. PHYSIOLOGIC EFFECTS OF SOMATOSTATIN

Five somatostatin receptors have been identified and characterized, all of which are members of the G protein–coupled receptor superfamily. Four of the five receptors do not distinguish between SS-14 and SS-28. Somatostatin binds to its plasma membrane receptors on target cells. These "activated" receptors interact with inhibitory G proteins of adenylate cyclase. As a result, the production of cAMP is inhibited, and protein kinase A is not activated. This inhibitory effect suppresses secretion of GH and thyroid-stimulating hormone (TSH) from the anterior pituitary gland as well as the secretion of insulin and glucagon from the pancreatic islets. If one were to summarize the action of somatostatin in one phrase, it would be "somatostatin inhibits the secretion of many other hormones." As such, it acts to regulate the effects of those other hormones. In addition to these effects on hormones that regulate fuel metabolism, somatostatin also reduces nutrient absorption from the gut by prolonging gastric emptying time (through a decrease in the secretion of gastrin, which reduces gastric acid secretion), by diminishing pancreatic exocrine secretions (i.e., digestive enzymes, bicarbonate, and water), and by decreasing visceral blood flow. Thus, somatostatin exerts a broad, albeit indirect, influence on nutrient absorption and, therefore, the utilization of fuels.

Somatostatin and its synthetic analogs are used clinically to treat a variety of secretory neoplasms such as GH-secreting tumors of the pituitary. Such tumors can cause gigantism if growth hormone is secreted in excess before the closure of the

---

Tolbutamide, a sulfonylurea drug that increases insulin secretion, also increases the secretion of pancreatic somatostatin.

In addition to its effects on normal GH secretion, somatostatin also suppresses the pathologic increase in GH that occurs in acromegaly (caused by a GH-secreting pituitary tumor), diabetes mellitus, and carcinoid tumors (tumors that secrete serotonin). Somatostatin also suppresses the basal secretion of TSH, TRH, insulin, and glucagon. The hormone also has a suppressive effect on a wide variety of nonendocrine secretions.

The major limitation in the clinical use of native somatostatin is its short half-life of less than 3 minutes in the circulation. Analogs of native somatostatin, however, have been developed that are resistant to degradation and, therefore, have a longer half-life. One such analog is octreotide, an octapeptide variant of somatostatin with a half-life of approximately 110 minutes.

growth centers of the ends of long bones or acromegaly if excess growth hormone is chronically secreted after the closure of these centers (as in **Sam Atrope**).

B. Growth Hormone

1. BIOCHEMISTRY

Growth hormone is a polypeptide that, as its name implies, stimulates growth. Many of its effects are mediated by insulin-like growth factors (IGFs, also known as somatomedins) that are produced by cells in response to the binding of GH to its cell membrane receptors (see Section 6 below). However, GH also has direct effects on fuel metabolism.

Human growth hormone is a water-soluble 22-kDa polypeptide with a plasma half-life of 20 to 50 minutes. It is composed of a single chain of 191 amino acids having two intramolecular disulfide bonds (Fig. 43.1). The gene for GH is located on chromosome 17. It is secreted by the somatotroph cells (the cells that synthesize and release GH) present in the lateral areas of the anterior pituitary. GH is structurally related to human prolactin and to human chorionic somatomammotropin (hCS) from the placenta, a polypeptide that stimulates growth of the developing fetus. Yet the hCS peptide has only 0.1% of the growth-inducing potency of GH. Growth hormone is the most abundant trophic hormone in the anterior pituitary, being present in concentrations of 5 to 15 mg per gram of tissue. The other anterior pituitary hormones are present in microgram-per-gram of tissue quantities.

The actions of GH can be classified as those that occur as a consequence of the hormone's direct effect on target cells and those that occur indirectly through the ability of GH to generate other factors, particularly IGF-I.

The IGF-I–independent actions of GH are exerted primarily in hepatocytes. GH administration is followed by an early increase in the synthesis of 8 to 10 proteins, among which are IGF-I, α_2-macroglobulin, and the serine protease inhibitors Spi 2.1 and Spi 2.3. Expression of the gene for ornithine decarboxylase, an enzyme active in polyamine synthesis (and, therefore, in the regulation of cell proliferation), is also significantly increased by GH.

Muscle and adipocyte cell membranes contain GH receptors that mediate direct, rapid metabolic effects on glucose and amino acid transport as well as on lipolysis. These receptors use associated cytoplasmic tyrosine kinases for signal transduction (such as the janus kinases; see Chapter 11, section III.C.). For example, in adipose tissue, GH has acute insulinlike effects followed by increased lipolysis, inhibition of lipoprotein lipase, stimulation of hormone-sensitive lipase, decreased glucose transport, and decreased lipogenesis. In muscle, GH causes increased amino acid transport, increased nitrogen retention, increased fat-free (lean) tissue, and increased energy expenditure. GH also has growth-promoting effects. GH receptors

 An MRI scan of **Sam Atotrope's** brain showed a macroadenoma (a tumor greater than 10 mm in diameter) in the pituitary gland, with superior extension that compressed the optic nerve as it crossed above the sella turcica, causing his visual problems. The skeletal and visceral changes noted by the ophthalmologist are characteristic of acromegalic patients with chronically elevated serum levels of GH and IGF-I.

Therapeutic alternatives for acromegaly caused by a GH-secreting tumor of the anterior pituitary gland include lifelong medical therapy with the somatostatin analog octreotide or the GH receptor antagonist pegvisomant. Other therapeutic options include stereotactic radiation therapy or surgical resection of the neoplasm. If the excessive secretion of GH is controlled successfully, some of the visceral or soft tissue changes of acromegaly may slowly subside to varying degrees. The skeletal changes, however, cannot be reversed.

 The ophthalmologist ordered a morning fasting serum GH level on **Sam Atotrope**, which was elevated at 56 ng/mL (normal = 0–5 ng/mL)

 Sam Atotrope was given an oral dose of 100 g glucose syrup. This dose would suppress serum GH levels to less than 2 ng/mL in normal subjects, but not in patients with acromegaly who have an autonomously secreting pituitary tumor making GH. Because Sam's serum GH level was 43 ng/mL after the oral glucose load, a diagnosis of acromegaly was made. The patient was referred to an endocrinologist for further evaluation.

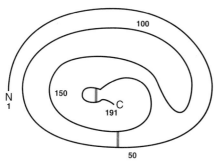

Human growth hormone

Fig. 43.1. Structure of human growth hormone. From Murray, RK, et al, Harper's Biochemistry, 23rd Ed. Stamford, CT: Appleton & Lange, 1993:502.

GH not only stimulates IGF-I gene expression in the liver but in a number of extrahepatic tissues as well. In acromegalics, rising levels of IGF-I cause a gradual generalized increase in skeletal, muscular, and visceral growth. As a consequence, a diffuse increase occurs in the bulk of all tissues (enlargement = "megaly") especially in the "acral" (most peripheral) tissues of the body, such as the face, the hands, and the feet, hence the term "acromegaly."

Sam Atotrope's coarse facial features and bulky hands are typical of patients with acromegaly.

are present on a variety of tissues in which GH increases IGF-I gene expression. The subsequent rise in IGF-I levels contributes to cell multiplication and differentiation by autocrine or paracrine mechanisms. These, in turn, lead to skeletal, muscular, and visceral growth. These actions are accompanied by a direct anabolic influence of GH on protein metabolism with a diversion of amino acids from oxidation to protein synthesis and a shift to a positive nitrogen balance.

2. CONTROL OF SECRETION OF GROWTH HORMONE

Although the regulation of GH secretion is complex, the major influence is hormonal (Fig. 43.2). The pulsatile pattern of GH secretion reflects the interplay of two hypothalamic regulation peptides. Release is stimulated by growth hormone–releasing hormone (GHRH, also called somatocrinin). The structure of GHRH was identified in 1982 (Fig. 43.3). It exists as both a 40– and a 44–amino acid peptide encoded on chromosome 20 and produced exclusively in cells of the arcuate nucleus. Its C-terminal leucine residue is amidated. Full biologic activity of this releasing hormone resides in the first 29 amino acids of the N-terminal portion of the molecule. GHRH interacts with specific receptors on the plasma membranes of the somatotrophs. The intracellular signaling mechanisms that result in GH synthesis and release appear to be multiple, as cAMP and calcium-calmodulin both stimulate GH release.

Conversely, GH secretion is suppressed by growth hormone release-inhibiting hormone (GHRIH, also called somatostatin, which has already been discussed). In addition, IGF-I, produced primarily in the liver in response to the action of GH on hepatocytes, feeds back negatively on the somatotrophs to limit GH secretion. Other physiologic factors (e.g., exercise and sleep) and many pathologic factors control its release (Table 43.2).

In addition, GH release is modulated by plasma levels of all of the metabolic fuels, including proteins, fats, and carbohydrates. A rising level of glucose in the blood normally suppresses GH release, whereas hypoglycemia increases GH

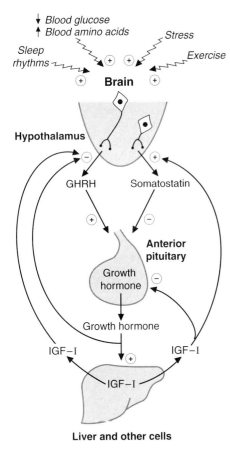

Fig. 43.2. Control of growth hormone secretion. Various factors stimulate the release of GHRH from the hypothalamus. The hypothalamus also releases somatostatin in response to other stimuli. GHRH stimulates and somatostatin inhibits the release of growth hormone from the anterior pituitary. Growth hormone causes the release of IGF-I from liver and other tissues. IGF-I inhibits GHRH release and stimulates somatostatin release.

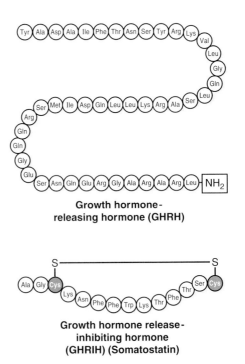

Growth hormone-releasing hormone (GHRH)

Growth hormone release-inhibiting hormone (GHRIH) (Somatostatin)

Fig. 43.3. Structures of growth hormone–releasing hormone (GHRH) and growth hormone release-inhibiting hormone (GHRIH, also called somatostatin). GHRH has an amide at the C-terminal.

Table 43.2. Some Factors Affecting Growth Hormone Secretion

	Stimulate	**Suppress**
Physiologic	Low blood glucose after meals	High blood glucose after meals
	High blood amino acids after meals	High blood fatty acids
	Exercise	
	Sleep	
	Stress	
Pharmacologic	GHRH	Somatostatin
	Estrogens	Progesterone
	α-Adrenergic agonists	α-Adrenergic antagonists
	β-Adrenergic antagonists	β-Adrenergic agonists
	Dopamine agonists	Dopamine antagonists
	Serotonin precursors	
	K⁺ infusion	Growth hormone and IGF-I
Pathologic	Starvation	Obesity
	Anorexia nervosa	Hypothyroidism
	Ectopic GHRH production	Hyperthyroidism
	Acromegaly	
	Chronic renal failure	
	Hypoglycemia	

secretion in normal subjects. Amino acids, such as arginine, stimulate release of GH when their concentrations rise in the blood. Rising levels of fatty acids may blunt the GH response to arginine or a rapidly dropping blood glucose level. However, prolonged fasting, in which fatty acids are mobilized in an effort to spare protein, is associated with a rise in GH secretion. Some of the physiologic, pharmacologic, and pathologic influences on GH secretion are given in Table 43.2.

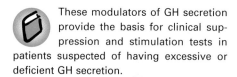 These modulators of GH secretion provide the basis for clinical suppression and stimulation tests in patients suspected of having excessive or deficient GH secretion.

3.   EFFECTS OF GROWTH HORMONE ON ENERGY METABOLISM

GH affects the uptake and oxidation of fuels in adipose tissue, muscle, and liver and indirectly influences energy metabolism through its actions on the islet cells of the pancreas. In summary, GH increases the availability of fatty acids, which are oxidized for energy. This and other effects of GH spare glucose and protein; that is, GH indirectly decreases the oxidation of glucose and amino acids (Fig. 43.4).

While **Sam Atotrope** was trying to decide which of the major alternatives for the treatment of his growth hormone (GH)–secreting pituitary tumor to choose, he noted progressive fatigue and the onset of increasing urinary frequency associated with a marked increase in thirst. In addition, he had lost 4 lb over the course of the last 6 weeks in spite of a good appetite. His physician suspected that Mr. Atotrope had developed diabetes mellitus, perhaps related to the chronic hypersecretion of GH. This suspicion was confirmed when Sam's serum glucose level, drawn before breakfast, was reported to be 236 mg/dL.

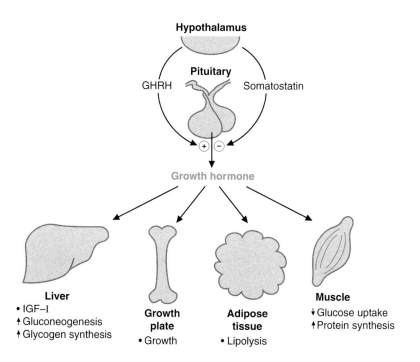

Fig. 43.4. Anabolic effects of growth hormone on various tissues.

As a result of the metabolic effects of GH, the clinical course of acromegaly may be complicated by impaired glucose tolerance or even overt diabetes mellitus, as occurred with **Sam Atotrope**.

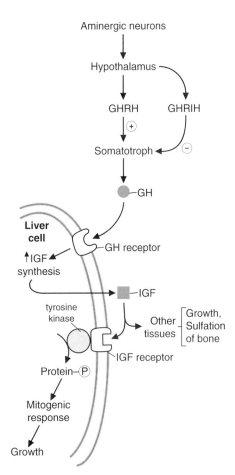

Fig 43.5. Production and action of IGFs. The hypothalamus produces growth hormone–releasing hormone (GHRH), which stimulates somatotrophs in the anterior pituitary to release growth hormone (GH). Growth hormone release-inhibiting hormone (GHRIH) inhibits GH release. GH binds to cell surface receptors and stimulates IGF production and release by liver and other tissues. IGF binds to cell surface receptors and stimulates the phosphorylation of proteins that cause mitosis and growth.

High levels of circulating IGF-1 has been linked to the development of breast, prostate, colon, and lung cancer. Additionally, experimental modulation of IGF-1 receptor activity can alter the growth of different types of tumor cells. Current research is aimed at targeting the interaction of IGF-1 and its receptor to reduce tumor cell proliferation.

4. EFFECTS OF GROWTH HORMONE ON ADIPOSE TISSUE

Growth hormone increases the sensitivity of the adipocyte to the lipolytic action of the catecholamines and decreases its sensitivity to the lipogenic action of insulin. These actions lead to the release of free fatty acids and glycerol into the blood to be metabolized by the liver. GH also decreases esterification of fatty acids, thereby reducing triacylglycerol synthesis within the fat cell. Recent evidence suggests that GH may impair glucose uptake by both fat and muscle cells by a postreceptor inhibition of insulin action.

5. EFFECTS OF GROWTH HORMONE ON MUSCLE

The lipolytic effects of GH increase free fatty acid levels in the blood bathing muscle. These fatty acids are preferentially used as fuel, indirectly suppressing glucose uptake by muscle cells. Through the effects on glucose uptake, the rate of glycolysis is proportionately reduced.

GH increases the transport of amino acids into muscle cells, providing substrate for protein synthesis. Through a separate mechanism, GH increases the synthesis of DNA and RNA. The positive effect on nitrogen balance is reinforced by the protein-sparing effect of GH-induced lipolysis that makes fatty acids available to muscle as an alternative fuel source.

6. EFFECTS OF GROWTH HORMONE ON THE LIVER

When plasma insulin levels are low, as in the fasting state, GH enhances fatty acid oxidation to acetyl CoA. This effect in concert with the increased flow of fatty acids from adipose tissue enhances ketogenesis. The increased amount of glycerol reaching the liver as a consequence of enhanced lipolysis acts as a substrate for gluconeogenesis.

Hepatic glycogen synthesis is also stimulated by GH in part because of the increased gluconeogenesis in the liver. Finally, glucose metabolism is suppressed by GH at several steps in the glycolytic pathway.

A major effect of GH on liver is to stimulate production and release of IGFs. The IGFs are also known as somatomedins. The two somatomedins in humans share structural homologies with proinsulin, and both have substantial insulin-like growth activity; hence the designations, insulin-like growth factor I (human IGF-I, or somatomedin-C) and insulin-like growth factor II (human IGF-II, or somatomedin A). IGF-I is a single-chain basic peptide having 70 amino acids, and IGF-II is slightly acidic with 67 amino acids. These two peptides are identical to insulin in half of their residues. In addition, they contain a structural domain that is homologous to the C-peptide of proinsulin.

A broad spectrum of normal cells respond to high doses of insulin by increasing thymidine uptake and initiating cell propagation. In most instances, IGF-I causes the same response as insulin in these cells but at significantly smaller, more physiologic concentrations. Thus, the IGFs are more potent than insulin in their growth-promoting actions.

Evidence suggests that the IGFs exert their effects through either an endocrine or a paracrine/autocrine mechanism. IGF-I appears to stimulate cell propagation and growth by binding to specific IGF-I receptors on the plasma membrane of target cells, rather than binding to GH receptors (Fig. 43.5).

Like insulin, the intracellular portion of the plasma membrane receptor for IGF-I (but not IGF-II) has intrinsic tyrosine kinase activity. The fact that the receptors for insulin and a number of other growth factors have intrinsic tyrosine kinase activity indicates that tyrosine phosphorylation initiates the process of cellular replication and growth. Subsequently, a chain of kinases is activated, which include a number of proto-oncogene products (see Chapters 11 and 18).

Most cells of the body have mRNA for IGF, but the liver has the greatest concentration of these messengers, followed by kidney and heart. The synthesis of IGF-I is regulated, for the most part, by GH, whereas hepatic production of IGF-II is independent of GH levels in the blood.

C. Catecholamines (Epinephrine, Norepinephrine, Dopamine)

The catecholamines belong to a family of bioamines and are secretory products of the sympathoadrenal system, which are required for the body to adapt to a great variety of acute and chronic stresses. Epinephrine (80–85% of stored catecholamines) is synthesized primarily in the cells of the adrenal medulla, whereas norepinephrine (15–20% of stored catecholamines) is synthesized and stored not only in the adrenal medulla but also in various areas of the central nervous system (CNS) and in the nerve endings of the adrenergic nervous system. Dopamine, another catecholamine, acts primarily as a neurotransmitter and has little effect on fuel metabolism.

The first total chemical synthesis of epinephrine was accomplished by F. Stolz et al in 1904. In 1950, Earl Sutherland was the first to demonstrate that epinephrine (and glucagon) induces glycogenolysis. This marked the beginning of our understanding of the molecular mechanisms through which hormones act.

1. SYNTHESIS OF THE CATECHOLAMINES

Tyrosine is the precursor of the catecholamines. The pathway for the biosynthesis of these molecules is described in Chapter 48.

2. SECRETION OF THE CATECHOLAMINES

Secretion of epinephrine and norepinephrine from the adrenal medulla is stimulated by a variety of stresses, including pain, hemorrhage, exercise, hypoglycemia, and hypoxia. Release is mediated by stress-induced transmission of nerve impulses emanating from adrenergic nuclei in the hypothalamus. These impulses stimulate the release of the neurotransmitter acetylcholine from preganglionic neurons that innervate the adrenomedullary cells. Acetylcholine depolarizes the plasma membranes of these cells, allowing the rapid entry of extracellular calcium (Ca^{2+}) into the cytosol. Ca^{2+} stimulates the synthesis and release of epinephrine and norepinephrine from the chromaffin granules into the extracellular space by exocytosis.

3. PHYSIOLOGIC EFFECTS OF EPINEPHRINE AND NOREPINEPHRINE

The catecholamines act through two major types of receptors on the plasma membrane of target cells, the α-adrenergic and the β-adrenergic receptors (see Chapter 26, section IV.C).

The actions of epinephrine and norepinephrine in the liver, the adipocyte, the skeletal muscle cell, and the α and β cells of the pancreas directly influence fuel metabolism (Fig. 43.6). These catecholamines are counterregulatory hormones that have metabolic effects directed toward mobilization of fuels from their storage sites for oxidation by cells to meet the increased energy requirements of acute and chronic stress. They simultaneously suppress insulin secretion, which ensures that fuel fluxes will continue in the direction of fuel utilization rather than storage as long as the stressful stimulus persists.

In addition, norepinephrine works as a neurotransmitter and affects the sympathetic nervous system in the heart, lungs, blood vessels, bladder, gut, and other

In patients suspected of having a neoplasm of the adrenal medulla that is secreting excessive quantities of epinephrine or norepinephrine (a pheochromocytoma), either the catecholamines themselves (epinephrine, norepinephrine, and dopamine) or their metabolites (the metanephrines and vanillylmandelic acid, VMA) may be measured in a 24-hour urine collection, or the level of catecholamines in the blood may be measured. A patient who has consistently elevated levels in the blood or urine should be considered to have a pheochromocytoma, particularly if the patient has signs and symptoms of catecholamine excess, such as excessive sweating, palpitations, tremulousness, and hypertension.

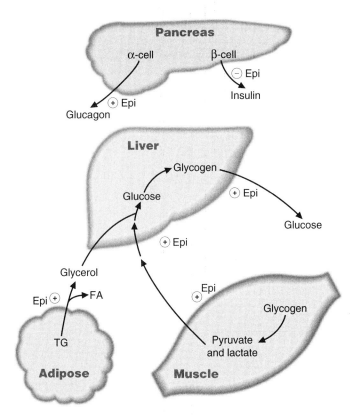

Fig. 43.6. Effects of epinephrine on fuel metabolism and pancreatic endocrine function. Epinephrine (Epi) stimulates glycogen breakdown in muscle and liver, gluconeogenesis in liver, and lipolysis in adipose tissue. Epinephrine further reinforces these effects because it increases the secretion of glucagon, a hormone that shares many of the same effects as epinephrine. Epi also inhibits insulin release but stimulates glucagon release from the pancreas.

Q: A relatively rare form of secondary hypertension (high blood pressure) is caused by a catecholamine-secreting neoplasm of the adrenal medulla, known as a pheochromocytoma. Patients with the tumor periodically secrete large amounts of epinephrine and norepinephrine into the bloodstream. Symptoms related to this secretion include a sudden and often severe increase in blood pressure, heart palpitations, a throbbing headache, and inappropriate and diffuse sweating. In addition, chronic hypersecretion of these catecholamines may lead to impaired glucose tolerance or even overt diabetes mellitus. Describe the actions of these hormones that lead to the significant rise in glucose levels.

Glucocorticoids, such as cortisol, were named for their ability to raise blood glucose levels. These steroids are among the "counterregulatory" hormones that protect the body from insulin-induced hypoglycemia.

organs. These effects of catecholamines on the heart and blood vessels serve to increase cardiac output and systemic blood pressure, hemodynamic changes that facilitate the delivery of blood borne fuels to metabolically active tissues.

Epinephrine has a short half-life in the blood and to be effective pharmacologically must be administered parenterally. It may be used clinically to support the beating of the heart, to dilate inflamed bronchial muscles, and even to decrease bleeding from organs during surgery.

4.   METABOLISM AND INACTIVATION OF CATECHOLAMINES

Catecholamines have a relatively low affinity for both α- and β-receptors. After binding, the catecholamine disassociates from its receptor quickly, causing the duration of the biologic response to be brief. The free hormone is degraded in several ways, as outlined in Chapter 48.

D. Glucocorticoids

1.   BIOCHEMISTRY

Cortisol (hydrocortisone) is the major physiologic glucocorticoid (GC) in humans, although corticosterone also has some glucocorticoid activity. The biosynthesis of steroid hormones and their basic mechanism of action has been described in Chapters 34 and 17.

2.   SECRETION OF GLUCOCORTICOIDS

The synthesis and secretion of cortisol is controlled by a cascade of neural and endocrine signals linked in tandem in the cerebrocortical-hypothalamic-pituitary-adrenocortical axis. Cerebrocortical signals to the midbrain are initiated in the cerebral cortex by "stressful" signals such as pain, hypoglycemia, hemorrhage, and exercise (Fig. 43.7). These nonspecific "stresses" elicit the production of monoamines in the cell bodies of neurons of the midbrain. Those that stimulate the synthesis and release of corticotropin-releasing hormone (CRH) are acetylcholine and serotonin. These neurotransmitters then induce the production of CRH by neurons originating in the paraventricular nucleus. These neurons discharge CRH into the hypothalamico-hypophyseal portal blood. CRH is delivered through these portal vessels to specific receptors on the cell membrane of the adrenocorticotropic hormone (ACTH)-secreting cells of the anterior pituitary gland (corticotrophs). This hormone–receptor interaction causes ACTH to be released into the general circulation to eventually interact with specific receptors for ACTH on the plasma membranes of cells in the zona fasciculata and zona reticulosum of the adrenal cortex. The major trophic influence of ACTH on cortisol synthesis is at the level of the conversion of cholesterol to pregnenolone, from which the adrenal steroid hormones are derived (see Chapter 34 for the biosynthesis of the steroid hormones).

Cortisol is secreted from the adrenal cortex in response to ACTH. The concentration of free (unbound) cortisol that bathes the CRH-producing cells of the hypothalamus and the ACTH-producing cells of the anterior pituitary acts as a negative feedback signal that has a regulatory influence on the release of CRH and ACTH (see Fig. 43.7). High cortisol levels in the blood suppress CRH and ACTH secretion, and low cortisol levels stimulate secretion. In severe stress, however, the negative feedback signal on ACTH secretion exerted by high cortisol levels in the blood is overridden by the stress-induced activity of the higher portions of the axis (see Fig. 43.7).

The effects of glucocorticoids on fuel metabolism in liver, skeletal muscle, and adipose tissue are outlined in Table 43.1 and in Figure 43.8. Their effects on other tissues are diverse and, in many instances, essential for life. Some of the nonmetabolic actions of GCs are listed in Table 43.3.

3.   EFFECTS OF GLUCOCORTICOIDS

Glucocorticoids have diverse actions that affect most tissues of the body. At first glance, some of these effects may appear to be contradictory (such as inhibition of

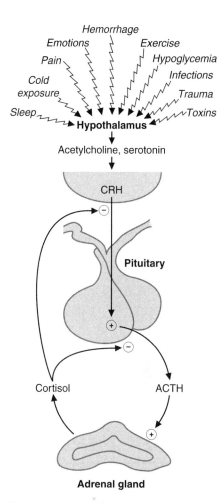

Fig. 43.7. Regulation of cortisol secretion. Various factors act on the hypothalamus to stimulate the release of corticotrophin-releasing hormone (CRH). CRH stimulates the release of ACTH from the anterior pituitary, which stimulates the release of cortisol from the adrenal cortex. Cortisol inhibits the release of CRH and ACTH.

 The catecholamines are counterregulatory hormones that mobilize fuels from their storage sites for oxidation in target cells to meet the increased energy requirements that occur during acute or chronic stress, or, in this case, the release of catecholamines by a tumor in the adrenal medulla. These actions provide the liver, for example, with increased levels of substrate needed for gluconeogenesis. Although in normal individuals most of the glucose generated through this mechanism is oxidized, blood glucose levels rise in the process. In addition, the catecholamines suppress insulin secretion to ensure that fuels will continue to flow in the direction of utilization rather than storage under these circumstances. Hence, blood glucose levels may rise in patients who have a pheochromocytoma.

When Otto was writing his list of differential diagnoses to explain the clinical presentation of **Corti Solemia**, he suddenly thought of a relatively rare endocrine disorder that could explain all of the presenting signs and symptoms. He made a provisional diagnosis of excessive secretion of cortisol secondary to an excess secretion of ACTH (Cushing's "disease") or by a primary increase of cortisol production by an adrenocortical tumor (Cushing's syndrome).

Otto suggested that resting, fasting plasma cortisol and ACTH levels be measured at 8:00 the next morning. These studies showed that Mr. Solemia's morning plasma ACTH and cortisol levels were both significantly above the reference range. Therefore, Otto concluded that Mr. Solemia probably had a tumor that was producing ACTH autonomously (i.e., not subject to normal feedback inhibition by cortisol). The high plasma levels of ACTH were stimulating the adrenal cortex to produce excessive amounts of cortisol. Additional laboratory and imaging studies indicated that the hypercortisolemia was caused by a benign ACTH-secreting adenoma of the anterior pituitary gland (Cushing's "disease").

Table 43.3. Some Nonmetabolic Physiologic Actions of Glucocorticoids

On electrolyte and water balance:
  Increase sodium and water retention (1/3,000 the potency of aldosterone)
  Increase renal glomerular filtration rate to maintain water excretion rate
  Suppress arginine vasopressin (ADH) release from posterior pituitary (?)

On cardiovascular system:
  Indirect effect of glucocorticoid actions on sodium and water metabolism (above)
  Maintain volume of microcirculation to tissues (cardiac output)
  Maintain normal vasomotor response to vasoconstricting agents

On skeletal muscle:
  Maintain muscle function by providing normal microcirculation to muscle
  Influence muscle mass by enhancing protein catabolism and suppressing protein synthesis

On central nervous system:
  Indirect
    Maintain normal cerebral microcirculation
  Direct
    Influence mood, behavior
    Influence sensitivity of special senses to stimuli
    Suppress CRH, ACTH, and ADH secretion

On formed elements in blood:
  Increase red blood cell mass and granulocyte proliferation
  Decrease lymphocyte, monocyte, and basophil proliferation

Anti-inflammatory actions:
  Inhibit early inflammatory process (i.e., edema, fibrin deposition, capillary dilation, leuko
    cyte migration, and phagocytic action)
  Inhibit late inflammatory process (proliferation of capillaries and fibroblasts, deposition of
    collagen, and, later, scar formation)

Immune suppressant actions (of questionable significance at physiologic levels):
  Prevent manifestations of humoral and cellular immunity
  Interfere with production of cytokines needed for immune competence via cell-to-cell
    communication

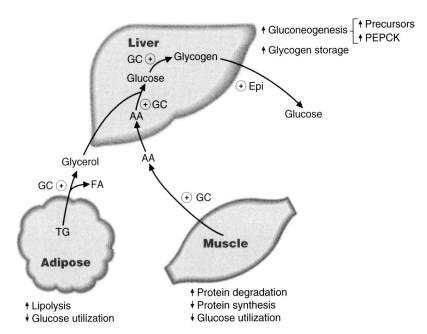

Fig. 43.8. Effects of glucocorticoids (GC) on fuel metabolism. Glucocorticoids stimulate lipolysis in adipose tissue and the release of amino acids from muscle protein. In liver, glucocorticoids stimulate gluconeogenesis and the synthesis of glycogen. The breakdown of liver glycogen is stimulated by epinephrine.

glucose uptake by certain tissues), but taken together they promote survival in times of stress.

In many tissues, GCs inhibit DNA, RNA, and protein synthesis and stimulate the degradation of these macromolecules. In response to chronic stress, GCs act to make fuels available, so that when the acute alarm sounds and epinephrine is released, the organism can fight or flee. When GCs are elevated, glucose uptake by the cells of many tissues is inhibited, lipolysis occurs in peripheral adipose tissue, and proteolysis occurs in skin, lymphoid cells, and muscle. The fatty acids that are released are oxidized by the liver for energy, and the glycerol and amino acids serve in the liver as substrates for the production of glucose, which is converted to glycogen and stored. The alarm signal of epinephrine stimulates liver glycogen breakdown, making glucose available as fuel to combat the acute stress.

The mechanism by which GCs exert these effects involves binding of the steroid to intracellular receptors, interaction of the steroid-receptor complex with GC response elements on DNA, transcription of genes, and synthesis of specific proteins (see Chapter 16, section III.C.2.). In some cases, the specific proteins responsible for the GC effect are known (e.g., the induction of phosphoenolpyruvate carboxykinase that stimulates gluconeogenesis). In other cases, the proteins responsible for the GC effect have not yet been identified.

E. Thyroid Hormone

1. BIOCHEMISTRY

The secretory products of the thyroid acinar cells are tetraiodothyronine (thyroxine, T_4) and triiodothyronine (T_3). Their structures are shown in Figure 43.9. The basic steps in the synthesis of T_3 and T_4 in these cells involve the transport or trapping of iodide from the blood into the thyroid acinar cell against an electrochemical gradient; the oxidation of iodide to form an iodinating species; the iodination of tyrosyl residues on the protein, thyroglobulin, to form iodotyrosines; and the coupling of residues of monoiodo- and diiodotyrosine in thyroglobulin to form residues of T_3 and T_4 (Fig. 43.10). Proteolytic cleavage of thyroglobulin releases free T_3 and T_4. The steps in thyroid hormone synthesis are stimulated by thyroid-stimulating hormone (TSH), a glycoprotein produced by the anterior pituitary.

Iodide transport from the blood into the thyroid acinar cell is accomplished through an energy-requiring, iodide-trapping mechanism that is poorly defined but may involve the Na^+,K^+-ATPase coupled to a cotransporter for Na^+ and iodide in the plasma membrane of the acinar cell.

Otto was now able to explain the mechanism for most of **Corti Solemia's** signs and symptoms. For example, Otto knew the metabolic explanation for the patient's hyperglycemia. Some of Mr. Solemia's muscle wasting and weakness were caused by the catabolic effect of hypercortisolemia on protein stores, such as those in skeletal muscle, to provide amino acids as precursors for gluconeogenesis. This catabolic action also resulted in the degradation of elastin, a major supportive protein of the skin, as well as an increased fragility of the walls of the capillaries of the cutaneous tissues. These changes resulted in the easy bruisability and the torn subcutaneous tissues of the lower abdomen, which resulted in red striae or stripes. The plethora (redness) of Mr. Solemia's facial skin was also caused in part by the thinning of the skin as well as by a cortisol-induced increase in the bone marrow production of red blood cells, which enhanced the "redness" of the subcutaneous tissues.

Q: If **Corti Solemia's** problem had been caused by a neoplasm of the adrenal cortex, what would his levels of blood ACTH and cortisol have been?

Normally, the thyroid gland secretes 80–100 μg T_4 and approximately 5 μg T_3 per day. The additional 22–25 μg T_3 "produced" daily is the result of the deiodination of the 5'-carbon of T_4 in peripheral tissues. T_3 is believed to be the predominant biologically active form of thyroid hormone in the body.

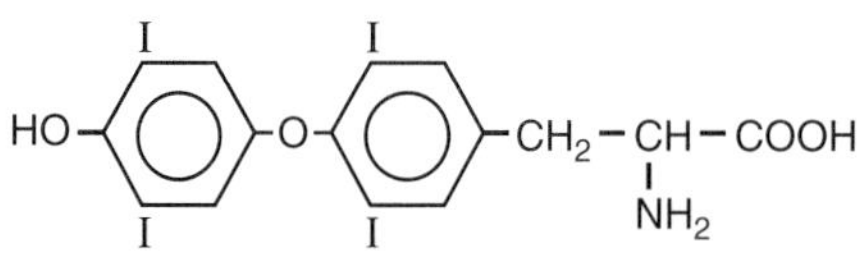

The "central" deposition of fat in patients, such as **Corti Solemia,** with Cushing's "disease" or syndrome is not readily explained because GCs actually cause lipolysis in adipose tissue. The increased appetite caused by an excess of GC and the lipogenic effects of the hyperinsulinemia that accompanies the GC-induced chronic increase in blood glucose levels have been suggested as possible causes. Why the fat is deposited centrally under these circumstances, however, is not understood. This central deposition leads to the development of a large fat pad at the center of the upper back ("buffalo hump"), to accumulation of fat in the cheeks and jowls ("moon facies") and neck area, as well as a marked increase in abdominal fat. Simultaneously, there is a loss of adipose and muscle tissue below the elbows and knees, exaggerating the appearance of "central obesity" in Cushing's "disease" or syndrome.

Approximately 35% of T_4 is deiodinated at the 5' position to form T_3, and 43% is deiodinated at the 5 position to form the inactive "reverse" T_3. Further deiodination or oxidative deamination leads to formation of compounds that have no biologic activity.

3,5,3',5'–Tetraiodothyronine (T_4)

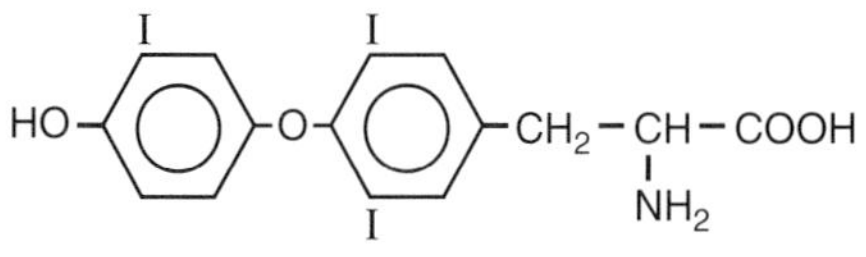

3,5,3'–Triiodothyronine (T_3)

Fig. 43.9. Thyroid hormones, T_3 and T_4.

A: If **Corti Solemia's** problem had resulted from primary hypersecretion of cortisol by a neoplasm of the adrenal cortex, his blood cortisol levels would have been elevated. The cortisol would have acted on the CRH-producing cells of the hypothalamus and the ACTH-secreting cells of the anterior pituitary by a negative feedback mechanism to decrease ACTH levels in the blood.

Because his cortisol and ACTH levels were both high, Mr. Solemia's tumor was most likely in the pituitary gland or possibly in neoplastic extrapituitary tissue that was secreting ACTH "ectopically." (Ectopic means that the tumor or neoplasm is producing and secreting a substance that is not ordinarily made or secreted by the tissue from which the tumor developed.) Mr. Solemia's tumor was in the anterior pituitary, not in an extrapituitary ACTH-producing site.

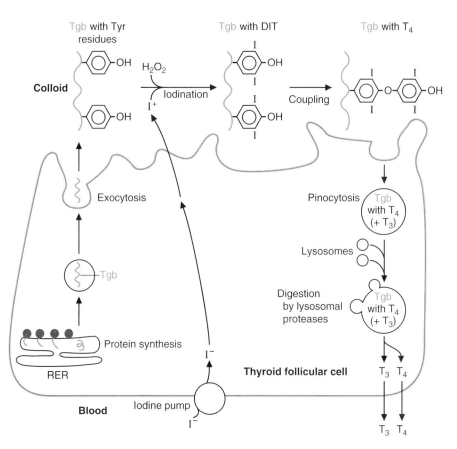

Fig. 43.10. Synthesis of the thyroid hormones (T_3 and T_4). The protein thyroglobulin (Tgb) is synthesized in thyroid follicular cells and secreted into the colloid. Iodination and coupling of tyrosine residues in Tgb produce T_3 and T_4 residues, which are released from Tgb by pinocytosis (endocytosis) and lysosomal action. The coupling of a monoiodotyrosine with a diiodotyrosine (DIT) to form triiodothyronine (T_3) is not depicted here.

The iodide concentrating or trapping process present in the plasma membrane of thyroid acinar cells creates iodide levels within the thyroid cell that are several hundredfold greater than those in the blood, depending on the current size of the total body iodide pool and the present need for new hormone synthesis.

In areas of the world in which the soil is deficient in iodide, hypothyroidism is prevalent. The thyroid gland enlarges (forms a goiter) in an attempt to produce more thyroid hormone. In the United States, table salt (NaCl) enriched with iodide (iodized salt) is used to prevent hypothyroidism caused by iodine deficiency.

The thyroid gland is unique in that it has the capacity to store large amounts of hormone as amino acid residues in thyroglobulin within its colloid space. This storage accounts for the low overall turnover rate of T_3 and T_4 in the body.

The rate of iodide transport is influenced by the absolute concentration of iodide within the thyroid cell. An internal autoregulatory mechanism decreases transport of iodide into the cell when the intracellular iodide concentration exceeds a certain threshold and increases transport when intracellular iodide falls below this threshold level.

The oxidation of intracellular iodide is catalyzed by thyroid peroxidase (located at the apical border of the thyroid acinar cell) in what may be a two-electron oxidation step forming I^+ (iodinium ion). Iodinium ion may react with a tyrosine residue in the protein thyroglobulin to form a tyrosine quinoid and then a 3'-monoiodotyrosine (MIT) residue. It has been suggested that a second iodide is added to the ring by similar mechanisms to form a 3,5-diiodotyrosine (DIT) residue. Because iodide is added to these organic compounds, iodination is also referred to as the "organification of iodide."

The biosynthesis of thyroid hormone proceeds with the coupling of an MIT and a DIT residue to form a triiodothyronine (T_3) residue or of two DIT residues to form a tetraiodothyronine (T_4) residue. T_3 and T_4 are stored in the thyroid follicle as amino acid residues in thyroglobulin. Under most circumstances, the T_4/T_3 ratio in thyroglobulin is approximately 13:1.

The plasma half-life of T_4 is approximately 7 days, and that of T_3 is 1 to 1.5 days. These relatively long plasma half-lives result from binding of T_3 and T_4 to several transport proteins in the blood. Of these transport proteins, thyroid-binding globulin (TBG) has the highest affinity for these hormones and carries approximately 70% of bound T_3 and T_4. Only 0.03% of total T_4 and 0.3% of total T_3 in the blood are in the unbound state. This free fraction of hormone has biologic activity because it is the only form that is capable of diffusing across target cell membranes to interact with intracellular receptors. The transport proteins, therefore, serve as a large reservoir of hormone that can release additional free hormone as the metabolic need arises.

The thyroid hormones are degraded in liver, kidney, muscle, and other tissues by deiodination, which produces compounds with no biologic activity.

2. SECRETION OF THYROID HORMONE

The release of T_3 and T_4 from thyroglobulin is controlled by thyroid-stimulating hormone (TSH) from the anterior pituitary. TSH stimulates the endocytosis of thyroglobulin to form endocytic vesicles within the thyroid acinar cells (see Fig. 43.10). Lysosomes fuse with these vesicles, and lysosomal proteases hydrolyze thyroglobulin, releasing free T_4 and T_3 into the blood in a 10:1 ratio. In various tissues, T_4 is deiodinated, forming T_3, which is the active form of the hormone.

TSH is synthesized in the thyrotropic cells of the anterior pituitary. Its secretion is primarily regulated by a balance between the stimulatory action of hypothalamic thyroid-releasing hormone (TRH) and the inhibitory (negative feedback) influence of thyroid hormone (primarily T_3) at levels above a critical threshold in the blood bathing the pituitary thyrotrophs. TSH secretion occurs in a circadian pattern, a surge beginning late in the afternoon and peaking before the onset of sleep. In addition, TSH is secreted in a pulsatile fashion with intervals of 2 to 6 hours between peaks.

TSH stimulates all phases of thyroid hormone synthesis by the thyroid gland, including iodide trapping from the plasma, organification of iodide, coupling of monoiodotyrosine and diiodotyrosine, endocytosis of thyroglobulin, and proteolysis of thyroglobulin to release triiodothyronine (T_3) and tetraiodothyronine (T_4) (see Fig. 43.10). In addition, the vascularity of the thyroid gland increases as TSH stimulates hypertrophy and hyperplasia of the thyroid acinar cells.

The predominant mechanism of action of TSH is mediated by binding of TSH to its specific receptor on the plasma membrane of the thyroid acinar cell, leading to an increase in the concentration of cytosolic cAMP. Recent evidence indicates, however, that TSH also increases the cellular levels of inositol trisphosphate and diacylglycerol, causing a rise in cytosolic Ca^{2+} within the thyroid cell.

The large protein thyroglobulin, which contains T_3 and T_4 in peptide linkage, is stored extracellularly in the colloid that fills the central space of each thyroid follicle. Each of the biochemical reactions that leads to the release and eventual secretion of T_3 and T_4, such as those that lead to their formation in thyroglobulins, is TSH-dependent. Rising levels of serum TSH stimulate the endocytosis of stored thyroglobulin into the thyroid acinar cell. Lysosomal enzymes then cleave T_3 and T_4 from thyroglobulin. T_3 and T_4 are secreted into the bloodstream in response to rising levels of TSH.

As the free T_3 level in the blood bathing the thyrotrophs of the anterior pituitary gland rises, the feedback loop is closed. Secretion of TSH is inhibited until the free T_3 levels in the systemic circulation fall just below a critical level, which once again signals the release of TSH. This feedback mechanism ensures an uninterrupted supply of biologically active free T_3 in the blood (Fig. 43.11). High levels of T_3 also inhibit the release of TRH from the hypothalamus.

3. PHYSIOLOGIC EFFECTS OF THYROID HORMONE

Only those physiologic actions of thyroid hormone that influence fuel metabolism are considered here. It is important to stress the term *physiologic*, because the effects of supraphysiologic concentrations of thyroid hormone on fuel metabolism may not be simple extensions of their physiologic effects. In general, the following

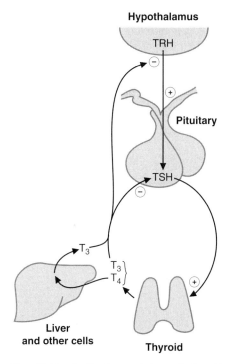

Fig. 43.11. Feedback regulation of thyroid hormone levels. TRH from the hypothalamus stimulates the release of TSH from the anterior pituitary, which stimulates the release of T_3 and T_4 from the thyroid. T_4 is converted to T_3 in the liver and other cells. T_3 and T_4 inhibit the release of TSH from the anterior pituitary and of TRH from the hypothalamus.

Q: A patient presents with the following clinical and laboratory profile: the serum free and total T_3 and T_4 and the serum TSH levels are elevated, but the patient has symptoms of mild hypothyroidism, including a diffuse, palpable goiter. What single abnormality in the pituitary-thyroid-thyroid hormone target cell axis would explain all of these findings?

A generalized (i.e., involving all of the target cells for thyroid hormone in the body), but incomplete resistance of cells to the actions of thyroid hormone could explain the profile of the patient. In Refetoff's disorder, a mutation in the portion of the gene that encodes the ligand binding domain of the β-subunit of the thyroid hormone receptor protein causes a relative resistance to the suppressive action of thyroid hormone on the secretion of TSH by the thyrotrophs of the anterior pituitary gland. Therefore, the gland releases more TSH than normal into the blood. The elevated level of TSH causes an enlargement of the thyroid gland (goiter) as well as an increase in the secretion of thyroid hormone into the blood. As a result, the serum levels of both T_3 and T_4 rise in the blood. The increase in the secretion of thyroid hormone may or may not be adequate to fully compensate for the relative resistance of the peripheral tissues to thyroid hormone. If the compensatory increase in the secretion of thyroid hormone is inadequate, the patient may develop the signs and symptoms of hypothyroidism.

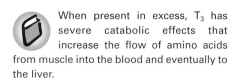

When present in excess, T_3 has severe catabolic effects that increase the flow of amino acids from muscle into the blood and eventually to the liver.

comments apply to the effects of thyroid hormone on energy metabolism in individuals with normal thyroid hormone levels in the blood.

i. Effects of Thyroid Hormone on The Liver

Several of the actions of thyroid hormone affect carbohydrate and lipid metabolism in the liver. Thyroid hormone increases glycolysis and cholesterol synthesis and increases the conversion of cholesterol to bile salts. Through its action of increasing the sensitivity of the hepatocyte to the gluconeogenic and glycogenolytic actions of epinephrine, T_3 indirectly increases hepatic glucose production (permissive or facilitatory action). Because of its ability to sensitize the adipocyte to the lipolytic action of epinephrine, T_3 increases the flow of fatty acids to the liver and thereby indirectly increases hepatic triacylglycerol synthesis. The concurrent increase in the flow of glycerol to the liver (as a result of increased lipolysis) further enhances hepatic gluconeogenesis.

ii. Effects of Thyroid Hormone on The Adipocyte

T_3 has an amplifying or facilitatory effect on the lipolytic action of epinephrine on the fat cell. Yet thyroid hormone has a bipolar effect on lipid storage, because it increases the availability of glucose to the fat cell, which serves as a precursor for fatty acid and glycerol 3-phosphate synthesis. The major determinant of the rate of lipogenesis, however, is not T_3, but rather the amount of glucose and insulin available to the adipocyte for triacylglycerol synthesis.

iii. Effects of Thyroid Hormone on Muscle

In physiologic concentrations, T_3 increases glucose uptake by muscle cells. It also stimulates protein synthesis, and, therefore, growth of muscle, through its stimulatory actions on gene expression.

In physiologic concentrations, thyroid hormone sensitizes the muscle cell to the glycogenolytic actions of epinephrine. Glycolysis in muscle is increased by this action of T_3.

iv. Effects of Thyroid Hormone on The Pancreas

Thyroid hormone increases the sensitivity of the β cells of the pancreas to those stimuli that normally promote insulin release and is required for optimal insulin secretion.

4. CALORIGENIC EFFECTS OF THYROID HORMONE

The oxidation of fuels converts approximately 25% of the potential energy present in the foods ingested by humans to ATP. This relative inefficiency of the human "engine" leads to the production of heat as a consequence of fuel utilization. This inefficiency, in part, allows homeothermic animals to maintain a constant body temperature in spite of rapidly changing environmental conditions. The acute response to cold exposure is shivering, which is probably secondary to increased activity of the sympathetic nervous system in response to this "stressful" stimulus.

Thyroid hormone participates in this acute response by sensitizing the sympathetic nervous system to the stimulatory effect of cold exposure. The ability of T_3 to increase heat production is related to its effects on the pathways of fuel oxidation, which both generate ATP and release energy as heat. The effects of T_3 on the sympathetic nervous system increase the release of norepinephrine. Norepinephrine stimulates the uncoupling protein thermogenin in brown adipose tissue (BAT), resulting in increased heat production from the uncoupling of oxidative phosphorylation (see Chapter 21). Very little residual brown fat persists in normal adult human beings, however.

Norepinephrine also increases the permeability of BAT and skeletal muscle to sodium. Because an increase of intracellular Na^+ is potentially toxic to cells, Na^+,K^+-ATPase is stimulated to transport Na+ out of the cell in exchange for K^+. The increased hydrolysis of ATP by Na^+,K^+-ATPase stimulates the oxidation of fuels and the regeneration of more ATP and heat from oxidative phosphorylation. Over a longer time course, thyroid hormone also increases the level of Na^+,K^+-ATPase and many of the enzymes of fuel oxidation. Because even at normal room temperature ATP utilization by Na^+,K^+-ATPase accounts for 20% or more of our basal metabolic rate (BMR), changes in its activity can cause relatively large increases in heat production.

Thyroid hormone also may increase heat production by stimulating ATP utilization in futile cycles (in which reversible ATP-consuming conversions of substrate to product and back to substrate use fuels and, therefore, produce heat).

F. Gastrointestinal-Derived Hormones Affecting Fuel Metabolism

In addition to insulin and the counterregulatory hormones discussed, a variety of peptides synthesized in the endocrine cells of the pancreatic islets, or the cells of the enteric nervous system, or the endocrine cells of the stomach, small bowel and large bowel, as well as certain cells of the central and peripheral nervous system, influence fuel metabolism directly. Some of these peptides and their tissue of origin, their actions on fuel metabolism, and the factors that stimulate (or suppress) their secretion are listed in Table 43.4. In addition to these peptides, others such as gastrin, motilin, pancreatic polypeptide (PP), peptide YY (PYY), and secretin may also influence fuel metabolism but by indirect effects on the synthesis or secretion of insulin or the counterregulatory hormones (Table 43.5). For example, gastrin induces gastric acid secretion, which ultimately affects nutrient absorption and metabolism. Motilin, secreted by enteroendocrine M cells of the proximal small bowel, stimulates gastric and pancreatic enzyme secretion, which, in turn, influences nutrient digestion. Pancreatic polypeptide (PP) from the pancreatic islets reduces gastric emptying and slows upper intestinal motility. Peptide YY (PYY) from the alpha cells in the mature pancreatic islets inhibits gastric acid secretion. Finally, secretin, produced by the enteroendocrine S cells in the proximal small bowel, regulates pancreatic enzyme secretion and inhibits gastrin release and gastric acid secretion. Although not directly influencing fuel metabolism, these "gut" hormones have a significant impact on how ingested nutrients are digested and prepared for absorption. If digestion or absorption of fuels is altered through a disturbance in the delicate interplay of all of the peptides, fuel metabolism will be altered as well.

Several of these gastrointestinal peptides such as GLP-1 and GIP do not act as direct insulin secretagogues when blood glucose levels are normal but do so after a meal large enough to cause an increase in the blood glucose concentration.

The release of these peptides may explain why the modest postprandial increase in serum glucose seen in normal subjects has a relatively robust stimulatory effect on insulin release, whereas a similar glucose concentration in vitro elicits a significantly smaller increase in insulin secretion. Likewise, this effect (certain factors potentiating insulin release), known as the "incretin effect," could account for the greater beta cell response seen after an oral glucose load as opposed to that seen after the administration of glucose intravenously.

 In hypothyroid patients, insulin release may be suboptimal, although glucose intolerance on this basis alone is uncommon.

In hyperthyroidism, the degradation and the clearance of insulin are increased. These effects, plus the increased demand for insulin caused by the changes in glucose metabolism, may lead to varying degrees of glucose intolerance in these patients (a condition called metathyroid diabetes mellitus). The patient with uncomplicated hyperthyroidism, however, rarely develops significant diabetes mellitus.

Table 43.4. Gastrointestinal-Derived Hormones Directly Affecting Fuel Metabolism

Hormone	Primary Cell/ Tissue of Origin	Actions	Secretory Stimuli (and Inhibitors)
Amylin	Pancreatic beta cell, endocrine cells of stomach and small intestine	1. Inhibits arginine-stimulated and postprandial glucagon secretion 2. Inhibits insulin secretion	Co-secreted with insulin in response to oral nutrients
Calcitonin gene-related peptide (CGRP)	Enteric neurons and enteroendocrine cells of the rectum	Inhibits insulin secretion	Oral glucose intake and gastric acid secretion
Galanin	Nervous system, pituitary, neurons of gut, pancreas, thyroid, and adrenal gland	Inhibits secretion of insulin, somatostatin, enteroglucagon, pancreatic polypeptide, and others	Intestinal distension
Gastric inhibitory polypeptide/ glucose-dependent insulinotropic polypeptide (GIP)	Neuroendocrine K cells of duodenum and proximal jejunum	1. Increases insulin release via an "incretin" effect 2. Regulates glucose and lipid metabolism	Oral nutrient ingestion, especially long-chain fatty acids
Gastrin-releasing peptide (GRP)	Enteric nervous system and pancreas	Stimulates release of cholecystokinin; GIP, gastrin, glucagon, GLP-1, GLP-2, and somatostatin	
Ghrelin	Central nervous system, stomach, small intestine, and colon	Stimulates growth hormone release	Fasting
Glucagon	Pancreatic alpha cell, central nervous system	Primary counter-regulatory hormone that restores glucose levels in hypoglycemic state (increases glycogenolysis and gluconeogenesis as well as protein-lipid flux in liver and muscle)	Neural and humoral factors released in response to hypoglycemia
Glucagon-like peptide-1 (GLP-1)	Enteroendocrine L cells in ileum, colon, and central nervous system	1. Enhances glucose disposal after meals by inhibiting glucagon secretion and stimulating insulin secretion 2. Acts through second messengers in beta cells to increase sensitivity of these cells to glucose (an incretin)	1. Oral nutrient ingestion 2. Vagus nerve 3. GRP and GIP 4. Somatostatin inhibits secretion
Glucagon-like peptide-2 (GLP-2)	The same as for GLP-1	Stimulates intestinal hexose transport	Same as GLP-1
Neuropeptide Y	Central and peripheral nervous system, pancreatic islet cells	Inhibits glucose-stimulated insulin secretion	Oral nutrient ingestion and activation of sympathetic nervous system
Neurotensin (NT)	Small intestinal N cells (especially ileum), enteric nervous system, adrenal gland, pancreas	In brain, modulates dopamine neurotransmission and anterior pituitary secretions	1. Luminal lipid nutrients 2. GRP 3. Somatostatin inhibits secretion
Pituitary adenylate cyclase activating peptide (PACAP)	Brain, lung, and enteric nervous system	Stimulates insulin and catecholamine release	Activation of central nervous system
Somatostatin	Central nervous system, pancreatic delta cells, and enteroendocrine delta cells	1. Inhibits secretion of insulin, glucagon and PP (islets), and gastrin, secretin, GLP-1, and GLP-2 (in gut) 2. Reduces carbohydrate absorption from gut lumen	1. Luminal nutrients 2. GLP-1 3. GIP 4. PACAP 5. VIP 6. Beta-adrenergic stimulation
Vasoactive intestinal peptide (VIP)	Widely expressed in the central and peripheral nervous systems	May regulate release of insulin and pancreatic glucagon	1. Mechanical stimulation of gut 2. Activation of central and peripheral nervous systems

Table 43.5. Gastrointestinal-Derived Hormones Indirectly Affecting Fuel Metabolism

Hormone	Primary Cell/ Tissue of Origin	Actions	Secretory Stimuli (and Inhibitors)
Cholecystokinin (CCK)	Enteroendocrine I cells, enteric nerves, others	1. Inhibits proximal gastric motility 2. Increases antral and pyloric contractions 3. Regulates nutrient-stimulated enzyme secretion and gallbladder contraction 4. Increases postprandial satiety	1. Oral nutrient ingestion 2. GGRP and bombesin from gut
Gastrin	Enteroendocrine G cells of the stomach, duodenal bulb, and other cells	Induces gastric acid secretion	1. Luminal contents, especially aromatic amino acids, calcium, coffee, and ethanol 2. Vagus nerve stimulation; activation of beta-adrenergic and GABA neurons 3. Somatostatin inhibits secretion
Motilin	Enteroendocrine M cells in upper small bowel and other cells	1. Induces phase III contractions in stomach 2. Stimulates gastric secretion and pancreatic enzyme secretion 3. Induces gallbladder contraction	4. Duodenal alkalinization 5. Gastric distension 6. Secretion suppressed by nutrients in duodenum
Pancreatic polypeptide (PP)	Endocrine cells in periphery of islets in the head of the pancreas	1. Reduces CCK-mediated gastric acid secretion 2. Increases intestinal transit time (slows motility)	Stimulated by intraluminal nutrients, hypoglycemia, and vagal nerve stimulation
Peptide YY (PYY)	Enteroendocrine cells, developing pancreas; alpha cells in mature islets	1. Inhibits both gastric acid secretion and gastric motility 2. Slows intestinal motility 3. Inhibits pancreatic exocrine secretion	1. Oral nutrient ingestion 2. Bile acids and fatty acids 3. Amino acids in colon
Secretin	Enteroendocrine S cells in upper small bowel	1. Stimulates pancreatic and biliary bicarbonate and water secretion 2. Regulates pancreatic enzyme secretion 3. Inhibits postprandial gastric emptying, gastrin release, and gastric acid secretion	1. Gastric acid, bile salts, fatty acids, peptides, and ethanol 2. Somatostatin inhibits secretion
Tachykinins	Neurons localized in the submucous and myenteric plexuses; enterochromaffin cells in gut epithelium	1. Regulates vasomotor and gastrointestinal smooth muscle contraction 2. Mucus secretion and water absorption	Direct and indirect activation of neurons in submucosa and myenteric plexuses in gut epithelium
Thyrotropin-releasing hormone (TRH)	Enteric nervous system, colon, G cells of stomach, and pancreatic beta cell	1. Suppresses hormone-stimulated gastric acid secretion 2. Inhibits cholesterol synthesis within the intestinal mucosa	In the stomach, histamine and serotonin stimulate secretion

G. Neural Factors Controlling Insulin and Counter-regulatory Hormone Secretion

Although beyond the scope of this text, the gastrointestinal neuroendocrine system is briefly described with regard to its effects on fuel metabolism. The pancreatic islet cells are innervated by both the adrenergic and the cholinergic limbs of the autonomic nervous system. Although stimulation of both the sympathetic and the parasympathetic systems increases glucagon secretion, insulin secretion is increased by vagus nerve fibers and suppressed by sympathetic fibers via the alpha-adrenoreceptors. Evidence also suggests that the sympathetic nervous system indirectly regulates pancreatic beta cell function through stimulation or suppression of the secretion of somatostatin, beta$_2$-adrenergic receptor number, and the neuropeptides, neuropeptide Y and galanin.

A tightly controlled interaction between the hormonal and neural factors that control nutrient metabolism is necessary to maintain normal fuel and, hence, energy homeostasis.

To establish the diagnosis of a secretory tumor of an endocrine gland, one must first demonstrate that basal serum levels of the hormone in question are regularly elevated. More importantly, one must show that the hypersecretion of the hormone (and, hence, its elevated level in the peripheral blood) cannot be adequately inhibited by "maneuvers" that are known to suppress secretion from a normally functioning gland (i.e., one must show that the hypersecretion is "autonomous").

To ensure that both the basal and the postsuppression levels of the specific hormone to be tested will reflect the true secretory rate of the suspected endocrine tumor, all of the known factors that can stimulate the synthesis of the hormone must be eliminated. For GH, for example, the secretagogues (stimulants to secretion) include nutritional factors; the patient's level of activity, consciousness, and stress; and certain drugs. GH secretion is stimulated by a high-protein meal or by a low level of fatty acids or of glucose in the blood. Vigorous exercise, stage III–IV sleep, psychological and physical stress, and levodopa, clonidine, and estrogens also increase GH release.

The suppression test used to demonstrate the autonomous hypersecretion of GH involves giving the patient an oral glucose load and, subsequently, measuring GH levels. A sudden rise in blood glucose suppresses serum GH to 2 ng/mL or less in normal subjects, but not in patients with active acromegaly.

If one attempts to demonstrate autonomous hypersecretion of GH in a patient suspected of having acromegaly, therefore, before drawing the blood for both the basal (pre-glucose load) serum GH level and the post-glucose load serum GH level, one must be certain that the patient has not eaten for 6–8 hours, has not done vigorous exercise for at least 4 hours, remains fully awake during the entire testing period (in a nonstressed state to the extent possible), and has not taken any drugs known to increase GH secretion for at least 1 week.

Under these carefully controlled circumstances, if both the basal and postsuppression serum levels of the suspect hormone are elevated, one can conclude that autonomous hypersecretion is probably present. At this point, localization procedures (such as an MRI of the pituitary gland in an acromegalic suspect) are performed to further confirm the diagnosis.

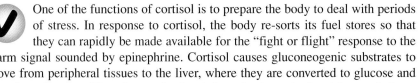

One of the functions of cortisol is to prepare the body to deal with periods of stress. In response to cortisol, the body re-sorts its fuel stores so that they can rapidly be made available for the "fight or flight" response to the alarm signal sounded by epinephrine. Cortisol causes gluconeogenic substrates to move from peripheral tissues to the liver, where they are converted to glucose and stored as glycogen. The release of epinephrine stimulates the breakdown of glycogen, increasing the supply of glucose to the blood. Thus fuel becomes available for muscle to fight or flee.

Cushing's "disease," the cause of **Corti Solemia's** current problems, results from prolonged hypersecretion of ACTH from a benign pituitary tumor. ACTH stimulates the adrenal cortex to produce cortisol, and blood levels of this steroid hormone rise.

Other nonpituitary causes of Cushing's syndrome, however, include a primary tumor of the adrenal cortex secreting excessive amounts of cortisol directly into the bloodstream. This disorder also can result from the release of ACTH from secretory nonendocrine nonpituitary neoplasms ("ectopic" ACTH syndrome). Cushing's syndrome is often caused by excessive doses of synthetic GCs used to treat a variety of disorders because of their potent anti-inflammatory effects (iatrogenic Cushing's syndrome).

The diabetogenic potential of chronically elevated GH levels in the blood is manifest by the significant incidence of diabetes mellitus (25%) and impaired glucose tolerance (33%) in patients with acromegaly, such as **Sam Atotrope**. Yet, under normal circumstances, physiologic concentrations of GH (as well as cortisol and thyroid hormone) have a facilitatory or permissive effect on the quantity of insulin released in response to hyperglycemia and other insulin secretagogues. This "proinsular" effect is probably intended to act as a "brake" to dampen any potentially excessive "contrainsular" effects that increments in GH and the other counterregulatory hormones exert.

BIOCHEMICAL COMMENTS

Most hormones are present in body fluids in picomolar to nanomolar amounts, requiring highly sensitive assays to determine their concentration in the blood or urine. Radioimmunoassays (RIAs), developed in the 1960s, use an antibody, generated in animals, against a specific antigen (the hormone to be measured). Determining the concentration of the hormone in the sample involves incubating the plasma or urine sample with the antibody and then quantifying the level of antigen–antibody complex formed during the incubation by one of several techniques.

The classic RIA uses very high-affinity antibodies, which have been fixed (immobilized) on the inner surface of a test tube, a Teflon bead, or a magnetized particle. A standard curve is prepared, using a set amount of the antibody and various known concentrations of the unlabeled hormone to be measured. In addition to a known concentration of the unlabeled hormone, each tube contains the same small, carefully measured amount of radiolabeled hormone. The labeled hormone and the unlabeled hormone compete for binding to the antibody. The higher the amount of unlabeled hormone in the sample, the less radiolabeled hormone is bound. A standard curve is plotted (Fig. 43.12). The unknown sample from the patient's blood or urine, containing the unlabeled hormone to be measured, is incubated with the immobilized antibody in the presence of the same small, carefully measured amount of radiolabeled hormone. The amount of radiolabeled hormone bound to the antibody is determined, and the standard curve is used to quantitate the amount of unlabeled hormone in the patient sample.

The same principle is used in immunoradiometric assays (IRMAs), but with this technique the antibody, rather than the antigen to be measured, is radiolabeled.

The sensitivity of RIAs can be enhanced using a "sandwich technique." This method uses two different monoclonal antibodies (antibodies generated by a single clone of plasma cells rather than multiple clones), each of which recognizes a different specific portion of the hormone's structure. The first antibody, attached to a solid support matrix such as a plastic culture dish, binds the hormone to be assayed. After exposure of the patient sample to this first antibody, the excess plasma is washed away, and the second antibody (which is radiolabeled) is then incubated with the first antibody–hormone complex. The amount of binding of the second (labeled) antibody to the first complex is proportional to the concentration of the hormone in the sample.

The sandwich technique can be improved even further if the second antibody is attached to an enzyme, such as alkaline phosphatase. The enzyme rapidly converts an added colorless substrate into a colored product, or a nonfluorescent substrate into a highly fluorescent product. These changes can be quantitated if the degree of change in color or fluorescence is proportional to the amount of hormone present in the patient sample. Less than a nanogram (10^{-9} g) of a protein can be measured by such an enzyme-linked immunosorbent assay (ELISA).

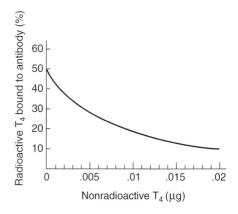

Fig. 43.12. Standard curve for a radioimmunoassay. A constant amount of radioactive T_4 is added to a series of tubes, each of which contains a different amount of nonradioactive T_4. The amount of radioactive hormone that binds to an antibody specific for the hormone is measured and plotted against the nonradioactive hormone concentration. When more nonradioactive T_4 is present in the tube, less radioactive T_4 binds to the antibody.

References

Bloomgarden ZT. Fat metabolism and diabetes: 2003 American Diabetes Association Postgraduate Course. Diabetes Care, 2003 (July);26:2198–2203.

Davis SN, Shavers C, Costa F, Mosqueda-Garcia R. Role of cortisol in the pathogenesis of deficient counterregulation after antecedent hypoglycemia in normal humans. J Clin Invest 1996; 98:680–691.

Goodman HM. Hormonal regulation of fuel metabolism. In: Basic Medical Endocrinology. New York: Raven Press, 1994:203–224.

Itani SI, Ruderman NB, Schmieder F, Boden G. Lipid-induced insulin resistance in human muscle is associated with changes in diacylglycerol, protein kinase C, and I kappa B-α. Diabetes 2002; 51:2005–2011.

Laurent D, Peterson KF, Russell RR, et al. Effect of epinephrine on muscle glycogenolysis and insulin-stimulated muscle glycogen synthesis in humans. Am J Physiol 1998;274:E130–E138.

Cryer PE. Glucose homeostasis and hypoglycemia. In: Larsen PF, Kronenberg HM, Melmed S, Polonsky KS, eds. Williams Textbook of Endocrinology, 10th Ed. Philadelphia: Saunders Publishing, 2003;1585–1591.

Zander M., Madsbad S, Madsen JL, Holst JJ. Effect of 6-week course of glucagon-like peptide one on glycemic conrol, insulin sensitivity, and beta cell function in type 2 diabetes. Lancet 2002;359:824–830.

 REVIEW QUESTIONS—CHAPTER 43

1. As a third-year medical student, you examine your first patient. You find that he is 52 years old, has a round face, acne, and a large hump of fat on the back of his neck. He complains that he is too weak to mow his lawn. His fasting blood glucose level is 170 mg/dL (reference range = 80–100 mg/dL). Plasma cortisol levels are 62 μg/mL (reference range = 3–31 μg/mL). Plasma ACTH levels are 0 pg/mL (reference range = 0–100 pg/mL).

   Based on the information given above, if the patient's problem is attributable to a single cause, the most likely diagnosis is which of the following?

   (A) Non–insulin-dependent diabetes mellitus
   (B) Insulin-dependent diabetes mellitus
   (C) A secretory tumor of the anterior pituitary
   (D) A secretory tumor of the posterior pituitary
   (E) A secretory tumor of the adrenal cortex

2. A woman was scheduled for a growth hormone suppression test. If each of the following events occurred the morning of the test, which one of the events would be most likely to cause a decrease in growth hormone levels?

    (A) She ate four large doughnuts for breakfast.
    (B) She was on estrogen replacement therapy and took her tablets after breakfast.
    (C) While unlocking her car, she was chased by the neighbor's vicious dog.
    (D) She fell asleep at the start of the test and slept soundly until it was completed 1.5 hours later.
    (E) She forgot to eat her breakfast before the test.

3. A dietary deficiency of iodine would lead to which of the following?

    (A) A direct effect on the synthesis of thyroglobulin on ribosomes
    (B) An increased secretion of thyroid stimulatory hormone (TSH)
    (C) Decreased production of thyrotropin releasing hormone (TRH)
    (D) Increased heat production
    (E) Weight loss

4. A woman whose thyroid gland was surgically removed was treated with 0.10 mg thyroxine daily (tablet form). After 3 months of treatment, serial serum TSH levels ranged between 10 and 15 MIU/mL (reference range = 0.3 – 5.0 MIU/mL). She complained of fatigue, weight gain, and hoarseness. Her dose of thyroid hormone should be adjusted in which direction?

    (A) Increased
    (B) Decreased
    (C) Remain the same

The next question is based on the following scenario:

A patient complains of nervousness, palpitations, sweating, and weight loss without loss of appetite, and has a goiter. Suspecting a defect in thyroid function, the physician orders a total serum T_4. The test is performed by radioimmunoassay. The standard curve for the assay, which measures T_4 in 0.1 mL serum, is shown in Fig. 43.12. Normal levels of T_4 = 4–10 μg/dL. In an assay of 0.1 mL of the patient's serum, 15% of the radioactive T_4 was bound by the antibody.

5. According to the radioimmunoassay, the approximate blood level of T_4 is is which of the following?

    (A) 0.015 μg/dL
    (B) 0.15 μg/dL
    (C) 15 μg/dL
    (D) 20 μg/dL
    (E) 30 μg/dL

44 The Biochemistry of the Erythrocyte and other Blood Cells

*The cells of the blood are classified as **erythrocytes, leukocytes,** or **thrombocytes.** The erythrocytes (**red cells**) carry oxygen to the tissues and are the most numerous cells in the blood. The leukocytes (**white cells**) are involved in defense against infection, and the thrombocytes (**platelets**) function in blood clotting. All of the cells in the blood can be generated from hematopoietic stem cells in the bone marrow on demand. For example, in response to infection, leukocytes secrete **cytokines** called **interleukins** that stimulate the production of additional leukocytes to fight the infection. Decreased supply of oxygen to the tissues signals the kidney to release **erythropoietin**, a hormone that stimulates the production of red cells.*

*The red cell has limited metabolic function, owing to its lack of internal organelles. **Glycolysis** is the main energy-generating pathway, with lactate production regenerating NAD^+ for glycolysis to continue. The NADH produced in glycolysis is also used to reduce the ferric form of hemoglobin, **methemoglobin**, to the normal ferrous state. Glycolysis also leads to a side pathway in which **2,3 bisphosphoglycerate** is produced, which is a major allosteric effector for oxygen binding to hemoglobin. The **hexose monophosphate shunt** pathway generates **NADPH** to protect red cell membrane lipids and proteins from oxidation, through regeneration of reduced glutathione. **Heme synthesis** occurs in the precursors of red cells and is a complex pathway that originates from succinyl-CoA and glycine. Mutations in any of the steps of heme synthesis lead to a group of diseases known collectively as **porphyrias**.*

*The red cell membrane must be highly deformable to allow it to travel throughout the capillary system in the body. This is because of a complex **cytoskeletal** structure that consists of the major proteins **spectrin, ankyrin,** and **band 3 protein**. Mutations in these proteins lead to improper formation of the membrane cytoskeleton, ultimately resulting in malformed red cells, **spherocytes**, in the circulation. Spherocytes have a shortened life span, leading to loss of blood cells.*

*When the body does not have sufficient red cells, the patient is said to be **anemic**. Anemia can result from many causes. **Nutritional deficiencies** of iron, **folate**, or **vitamin B12** prevent the formation of adequate numbers of red cells. **Mutations** in the genes that encode red cell metabolic **enzymes, membrane structural proteins,** and **globins** cause **hereditary anemias**. The appearance of red cells on a blood smear frequently provides clues to the cause of an anemia. Because the mutations that give rise to hereditary anemias also provide some protection against malaria, hereditary anemias are some of the most common genetic diseases known.*

*The human alters globin gene expression during development, a process known as **hemoglobin switching**. The switch between expression of one gene to another is regulated by transcription factor binding to the promoter regions of these genes. Current research is attempting to reactivate fetal hemoglobin genes to combat sickle-cell disease and thalassemia.*

THE WAITING ROOM

Anne Niemick, who has β^+ thalassemia, complains of pain in her lower spine (see Chapters 14 and 15). A quantitative computed tomogram (CT) of the vertebral bodies of the lumbar spine shows evidence of an area of early spinal cord compression in the upper lumbar region. She is suffering from severe anemia, resulting in stimulation of production of red blood cell precursors (the erythroid mass) from the stem cells in her bone marrow. This expansion of marrow volume causes compression of tissues in this area, which, in turn, causes pain. Local irradiation is considered, as is a program of regular blood transfusions to maintain the oxygen-carrying capacity of circulating red blood cells. The results of special studies related to the genetic defect underlying her thalassemia are pending, although preliminary studies have shown that she has elevated levels of fetal hemoglobin, which, in part, moderates the manifestations of her disease. **Anne Niemick's** parents have returned to the clinic to discuss the results of these tests.

Spiro Site is a 21-year-old college student who complains of feeling tired all the time. Two years previously he had had gallstones removed, which consisted mostly of bilirubin. His spleen is palpable, and jaundice is evidenced by yellowing of the whites of his eyes. His hemoglobin was low (8 g/dL; reference value 13.5–17.5 gm/dL). A blood smear showed dark, rounded, abnormally small red cells called spherocytes as well as an increase in the number of circulating immature red blood cells known as reticulocytes.

I. CELLS OF THE BLOOD

The blood, together with the bone marrow, makes up the organ system that makes a significant contribution to achieving **homeostasis,** the maintenance of the normal composition of the body's internal environment. Blood can be considered a liquid tissue consisting of water, proteins, and specialized cells. The most abundant cell in the blood is the **erythrocyte** or red blood cell, which transports oxygen to the tissues and contributes to buffering of the blood through the binding of protons by hemoglobin (see section IV of this chapter, and the material in Chapter 4, section IV.D.2., and Chapter 7, section VII). Red blood cells lose all internal organelles during the process of differentiation. The white blood cells (**leukocytes**) are nucleated cells present in blood that function in the defense against infection. The platelets (**thrombocytes**), which contain cytoplasmic organelles but no nucleus, are involved in the control of bleeding by contributing to normal thrombus (clot) formation within the lumen of the blood vessel. The average concentration of these cells in the blood of normal individuals is presented in Table 44.1.

Table 44.1. Normal Values of Blood Cell Concentrations in Adults

Cell Type	Mean (cells/mm³)
Erythrocytes	5.2×10^6 (men); 4.6×10^6 women
Neutrophils	4,300
Lymphocytes	2,700
Monocytes	500
Eosinophils	230
Basophils	40

A. Classification and Functions of Leukocytes and Thrombocytes

The leukocytes can be classified either as polymorphonuclear leukocytes (granulo-cytes) or mononuclear leukocytes, depending on the morphology of the nucleus in these cells. The mononuclear leukocyte has a rounded nucleus, whereas the poly-morphonuclear leukocytes have a multilobed nucleus.

1. THE GRANULOCYTES

The granulocytes, so named because of the presence of secretory granules visible on staining, are the **neutrophils, eosinophils,** and **basophils**. When these cells are activated in response to chemical stimuli, the vesicle membranes fuse with the cell plasma membrane, resulting in the release of the granule contents (**degranulation**). The granules contain many cell-signaling molecules that mediate inflammatory processes. The granulocytes, in addition to displaying segmented nuclei (are poly-morphonuclear), can be distinguished from each other by their staining properties (caused by different granular contents) in standard hematologic blood smears; neu-trophils stain pink, eosinophils stain red, and basophils stain blue.

Neutrophils are phagocytic cells that rapidly migrate to areas of infection or tis-sue damage. As part of the response to acute infection, neutrophils engulf foreign bodies, and destroy them, in part, by initiating the respiratory burst (see Chapter 24). The respiratory burst creates oxygen radicals that rapidly destroy the foreign material found at the site of infection.

A primary function of eosinophils is to destroy parasites such as worms. The eosinophilic granules are lysosomes containing hydrolytic enzymes and cationic proteins, which are toxic to parasitic worms. Eosinophils have also been implicated in asthma and allergic responses, although their exact role in the development of these disorders is still unknown, and this is an active area of research.

Basophils, the least abundant of the leukocytes, participate in hypersensitivity reactions, such as allergic responses. Histamine, produced by the decarboxylation of histidine, is stored in the secretory granules of basophils. Release of histamine during basophil activation stimulates smooth muscle cell contraction and increases vascular permeability. The granules also contain enzymes such as proteases, β-glucuronidase, and lysophospholipase. These enzymes degrade microbial structures and assist in the remodeling of damaged tissue.

2. MONONUCLEAR LEUKOCYTES

The mononuclear leukocytes consist of various classes of lymphocytes and the monocytes. Lymphocytes are small, round cells originally identified in lymph fluid. These cells have a high ratio of nuclear volume to cytoplasmic volume and are the primary antigen (foreign body)-recognizing cells. There are three major types of lymphocytes: T cells, B cells, and NK cells. The precursors of T cells (thymus-derived lymphocytes) are produced in the bone marrow and then migrate to the thymus, where they mature before being released to the circulation. Several subclasses of T cells exist. These subclasses are identified by different surface membrane proteins, the presence of which correlate with the function of the sub-class. Lymphocytes that mature in the bone marrow are the B cells, which secrete antibodies in response to antigen binding. The third class of lymphocytes are the natural killer cells (NK cells), which target virally infected and malignant cells for destruction.

Circulatory monocytes are the precursors of tissue macrophages. Macrophages (large eater) are phagocytic cells that enter inflammatory sites and consume microorganisms and necrotic host cell debris left behind by granulocyte attack of the foreign material. Macrophages in the spleen play an important role in maintaining

Table 44.2. Normal Hemoglobin Levels in Blood (g/dL)

Adult	
Males	13.5–17.5
Females	11.5–15.5
Children	
Newborns	15.0–21.0
3–12 mo.	9.5–12.5
1 yr to puberty	11.0–13.5

Other measurements used to classify the type of anemia present include the mean corpuscular volume (MCV) and the mean corpuscular hemoglobin concentration (MCHC). The MCV is the average volume of the red blood cell, expressed in femto (10^{-15}) liters. Normal MCV range from 80 to 100 fL. The MCHC is the average concentration of hemoglobin in each individual erythrocyte, expressed in g/L. The normal range is 32 to 37; a value of less than 32 would indicate hypochromic cells. Thus, microcytic, hypochromic red blood cells have an MCV of less than 80 and an MCHC of less than 32. Macrocytic, normochromic cells have an MCV of greater than 100, with an MCHC between 32 and 37.

The trace amounts of 2,3 BPG found in cells other than erythrocytes is required for the phosphoglycerate mutase reaction of glycolysis, in which 3-phosphoglycerate is isomerized to 2-phosphoglycerate. As the 2,3 BPG is regenerated during each reaction cycle, it is only required in catalytic amounts.

the oxygen-delivering capabilities of the blood by removing damaged red blood cells that have a reduced oxygen-carrying capacity.

3. THE THROMBOCYTES

Platelets are heavily granulated disc-like cells that aid in intravascular clotting. Like the erythrocyte, platelets lack a nucleus. Their function is discussed in the following chapter. Platelets arise by budding of the cytoplasm of megakaryocytes, multinucleated cells that reside in the bone marrow.

B. Anemia

The major function of erythrocytes is to deliver oxygen to the tissues. To do this, a sufficient concentration of hemoglobin in the red blood cells is necessary for efficient oxygen delivery to occur. When the hemoglobin concentration falls below normal values (Table 44.2), the patient is classified as anemic. Anemias can be categorized based on red cell size and hemoglobin concentration. Red cells can be of normal size (normocytic), small (microcytic), or large (macrocytic). Cells containing a normal hemoglobin concentration are termed normochromic; those with decreased concentration are hypochromic. This classification system provides important diagnostic tools (Table 44.3) that enable one to properly classify, diagnose, and treat the anemia.

II. ERYTHROCYTE METABOLISM

A. The Mature Erythrocyte

To best understand how the erythrocyte can carry out its major function, a discussion of erythrocyte metabolism is required. Mature erythrocytes contain no intracellular organelles, so the metabolic enzymes of the red blood cell are limited to those found in the cytoplasm. In addition to hemoglobin, the cytosol of the red blood cell contains enzymes necessary for the prevention and repair of damage done by reactive oxygen species (see Chapter 24) and the generation of energy (Fig. 44.1). Erythrocytes can only generate adenosine triphosphate (ATP) by glycolysis (see Chapter 22). The ATP is used for ion transport across the cell membrane (primarily Na^+, K^+, and Ca^{+2}), the phosphorylation of membrane proteins, and the priming reactions of glycolysis. Erythrocyte glycolysis also uses the Rapaport-Luebering shunt to generate 2,3-bisphosphoglycerate (2,3-BPG). Red cells contain 4 to 5 mM 2,3-BPG, compared with trace amounts in other cells. As discussed in more detail in Section IV, 2,3-BPG is a modulator of oxygen binding to hemoglobin that stabilizes the deoxy form of hemoglobin, thereby facilitating the release of oxygen to the tissues.

To bind oxygen, the iron of hemoglobin must be in the ferrous (+2) state. Reactive oxygen species can oxidize the iron to the ferric (+3) state, producing

Table 44.3. Classification of the Anemias on the Basis of Red Cell Morphology

Red Cell Morphology	Functional Deficit	Possible Causes
Microcytic, hypochromic	Impaired hemoglobin synthesis	Iron deficiency, thalassemia mutation, lead poisoning
Macrocytic, normochromic	Impaired DNA synthesis	B12 or folic acid deficiency, erythroleukemia
Normocytic, normochromic	Red cell loss	Acute bleeding, sickle cell disease, red cell metabolic defects, red cell membrane defects

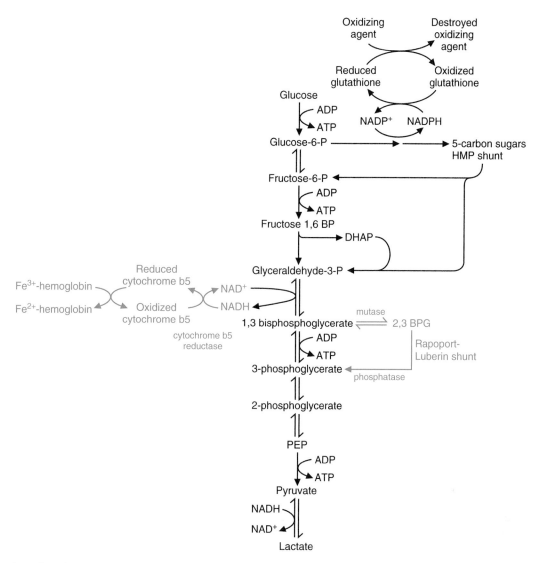

Fig. 44.1. Overview of erythrocyte metabolism. Glycolysis is the major pathway, with branches for the hexose monophosphate shunt (for protection against oxidizing agents) and the Rapoport-Luebering shunt (which generates 2,3 bisphosphoglycerate, which moderates oxygen binding to hemoglobin). The NADH generated from glycolysis can be used to reduce methemoglobin (Fe^{+3}) to normal hemoglobin (Fe^{+2}), or to convert pyruvate to lactate, such that NAD^+ can be regenerated and used for glycolysis. Pathways unique to the erythrocyte are indicated in blue.

methemoglobin. Some of the NADH produced by glycolysis is used to regenerate hemoglobin from methemoglobin by the NADH-cytochrome b_5 methemoglobin reductase system. Cytochrome b_5 reduces the Fe^{+3} of methemoglobin. The oxidized cytochrome b_5 is then reduced by a flavin-containing enzyme, cytochrome b_5 reductase (also called methemoglobin reductase), using NADH as the reducing agent.

An inherited deficiency in pyruvate kinase leads to hemolytic anemia (an anemia caused by the destruction of red blood cells; hemoglobin values typically drop to 4 to 10 g/dL in this condition). Because the amount of ATP formed from glycolysis is decreased by 50%, red blood cell ion transporters cannot function effectively. The red blood cells tend to gain Ca^{2+} and lose K^+ and water. The water loss increases the intracellular hemoglobin concentration. With the increase in intracellular hemoglobin concentration, the internal viscosity of the cell is increased to the point that the cell becomes rigid and, therefore, more susceptible to damage by shear forces in the circulation. Once damaged, the red blood cells are removed from circulation, leading to the anemia. However, the effects of the anemia are frequently moderated by the twofold to threefold elevation in 2,3-BPG concentration that results from the blockage of the conversion of phosphoenol pyruvate to pyruvate. Because 2,3-BPG binding to hemoglobin decreases the affinity of hemoglobin of oxygen, the red blood cells that remain in circulation are highly efficient in releasing their bound oxygen to the tissues.

Congenital methemoglobinemia, the presence of excess methemoglobin, is found in people with an enzymatic deficiency in cytochrome b_5 reductase or in people who have inherited hemoglobin M. In hemoglobin M, a single amino acid substitution in the heme-binding pocket stabilizes the ferric (Fe^{+3}) oxygen. Individuals with congenital methemoglobinemia appear cyanotic but have few clinical problems. Methemoglobinemia can be acquired by ingestion of certain oxidants such as nitrites, quinones, aniline, and sulfonamides. Acquired methemoglobinemia can be treated by the administration of reducing agents, such as ascorbic acid or methylene blue.

G6PD deficiency is the most common enzyme deficiency known in humans, probably, in part, because individuals with G6PD deficiency are resistant to malaria. The resistance to malaria counterbalances the deleterious effects of the deficiency. G6PD-deficient red cells have a shorter life span and are more likely to lyse under conditions of oxidative stress. When soldiers during the Korean War were given the antimalarial drug primaquine prophylactically, approximately 10% of the soldiers of African ancestry developed a spontaneous anemia. Because the gene for G6PD is found on the X chromosome, these men had only one copy of a variant G6PD gene

All known G6PD variant genes contain small in-frame deletions or missense mutations. The corresponding proteins, therefore, have decreased stability or lowered activity, leading to a reduced half-life or lifespan for the red cell. No mutations have been found that result in complete absence of G6PD. Based on studies with knockout mice, those mutations would be expected to result in embryonic lethality.

Heme, which is red, is responsible for the color of red blood cells and of muscles that contain a large number of mitochondria.

Chlorophyll, the major porphyrin in plants, is similar to heme, except that it is coordinated with magnesium rather than iron, and it contains different substituents on the rings, including a long-chain alcohol (phytol). As a result of these structural differences, chlorophyll is green.

Approximately 5 to 10% of the glucose metabolized by red blood cells is used to generate NADPH by way of the hexose monophosphate shunt. The NADPH is used to maintain glutathione in the reduced state. The glutathione cycle is the red blood cell's chief defense against damage to proteins and lipids by reactive oxygen species (see Chapter 24).

The enzyme that catalyzes the first step of the hexose monophosphate shunt is glucose-6-phosphate dehydrogenase (G6PD). The lifetime of the red blood cell correlates with G6PD activity. Lacking ribosomes, the red blood cell cannot synthesize new G6PD protein. Consequently, as the G6PD activity decreases, oxidative damage accumulates, leading to lysis of the erythrocyte. When red blood cell lysis (hemolysis) substantially exceeds the normal rate of red blood cell production, the number of erythrocytes in the blood drops below normal values, leading to a **hemolytic anemia.**

B. The Erythrocyte Precursor Cells and Heme Synthesis

1. HEME STRUCTURE

Heme consists of a porphyrin ring coordinated with an atom of iron (Fig. 44.2). Four pyrrole rings are joined by methionyl bridges (—CH—) to form the porphyrin ring (see Fig. 7.12). Eight side chains serve as substituents on the porphyrin ring, two on each pyrrole. These side chains may be acetyl (A), propionyl (P), methyl (M), or vinyl (V) groups. In heme, the order of these groups is M V M V M P P M. This order, in which the position of the methyl group is reversed on the fourth ring, is characteristic of the porphyrins of the type III series, the most abundant in nature.

Heme is the most common porphyrin found in the body. It is complexed with proteins to form hemoglobin, myoglobin, and the cytochromes (see Chapters 7 and 21), including cytochrome P450 (see Chapter 24).

2. SYNTHESIS OF HEME

Heme is synthesized from glycine and succinyl CoA (Fig. 44.3), which condense in the initial reaction to form δ-aminolevulinic acid (δ-ALA) (Fig 44.4). The enzyme that catalyzes this reaction, δ-ALA synthase, requires the participation of pyridoxal phosphate, as the reaction is an amino acid decarboxylation reaction (glycine is decarboxylated; see Chapter 39).

The next reaction of heme synthesis is catalyzed by δ-ALA dehydratase, in which two molecules of δ-ALA condense to form the pyrrole, porphobilinogen (Fig. 44.5). Four of these pyrrole rings condense to form a linear chain and then a series of porphyrinogens. The side chains of these porphyrinogens initially contain

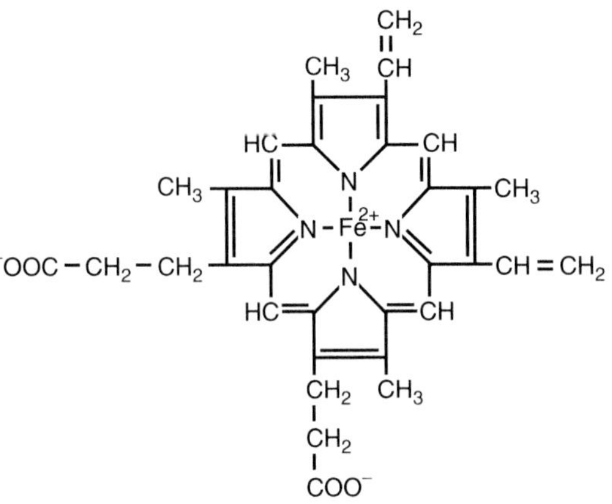

Fig. 44.2. Structure of heme. The side chains can be abbreviated as MVMVMPPM. M = methyl (CH_3); V = vinyl (—CH=CH$_2$); P = propionyl (—CH$_2$—CH$_2$—COO$^-$).

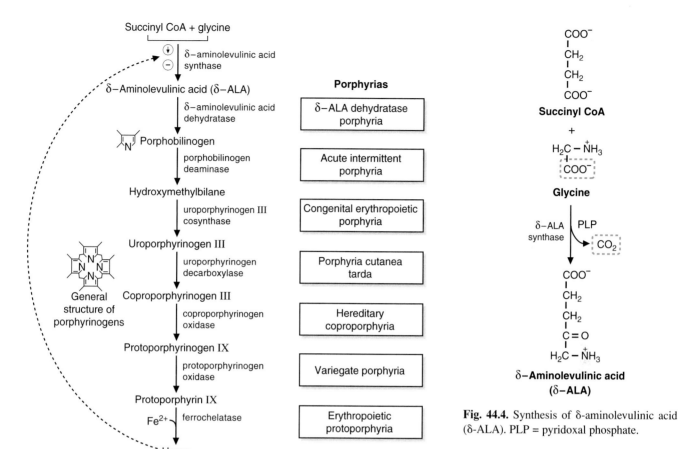

Fig. 44.3. Synthesis of heme. To produce one molecule of heme, 8 molecules each of glycine and succinyl CoA are required. A series of porphyrinogens are generated in sequence. Finally, iron is added to produce heme. Heme regulates its own production by repressing the synthesis of δ-aminolevulinic acid (δ-ALA) synthase (circled ↓) and by directly inhibiting the activity of this enzyme (circled −). Deficiencies of enzymes in the pathway result in a series of diseases known as porphyrias (listed on the right, beside the deficient enzyme).

Fig. 44.4. Synthesis of δ-aminolevulinic acid (δ-ALA). PLP = pyridoxal phosphate.

acetyl (A) and propionyl (P) groups. The acetyl groups are decarboxylated to form methyl groups. Then the first two propionyl side chains are decarboxylated and oxidized to vinyl groups, forming a protoporphyrinogen. The methylene bridges are subsequently oxidized to form protoporphyrin IX (see Fig. 44.3).

In the final step of the pathway, iron (as Fe^{2+}) is incorporated into protoporphyrin IX in a reaction catalyzed by ferrochelatase (also known as heme synthase).

3. SOURCE OF IRON

Iron, which is obtained from the diet, has a Recommended Dietary Allowance (RDA) of 10 mg for men and postmenopausal women, and 15 mg for premenopausal women. The average American diet contains 10 to 50 mg of iron. However, only 10 to 15% is normally absorbed, and iron deficiencies are fairly common.

Q: Pyridoxine (vitamin B6) deficiencies are often associated with a microcytic, hypochromic anemia. Why would a B6 deficiency result in small (microcytic), pale (hypochromic) red blood cells?

δ-ALA dehydratase, which contains zinc, and ferrochelatase are inactivated by lead. Thus, in lead poisoning, δ-ALA and protoporphyrin IX accumulate, and the production of heme is decreased. Anemia results from a lack of hemoglobin, and energy production decreases because of the lack of cytochromes for the electron transport chain.

Porphyrias are a group of rare inherited disorders resulting from deficiencies of enzymes in the pathway for heme biosynthesis (see Fig. 44.3). Intermediates of the pathway accumulate and may have toxic effects on the nervous system that cause neuropsychiatric symptoms. When porphyrinogens accumulate, they may be converted by light to porphyrins, which react with molecular oxygen to form oxygen radicals. These radicals may cause severe damage to the skin. Thus, individuals with excessive production of porphyrins are photosensitive. The scarring and increased growth of facial hair seen in some porphyrias may have contributed to the development of the werewolf legends.

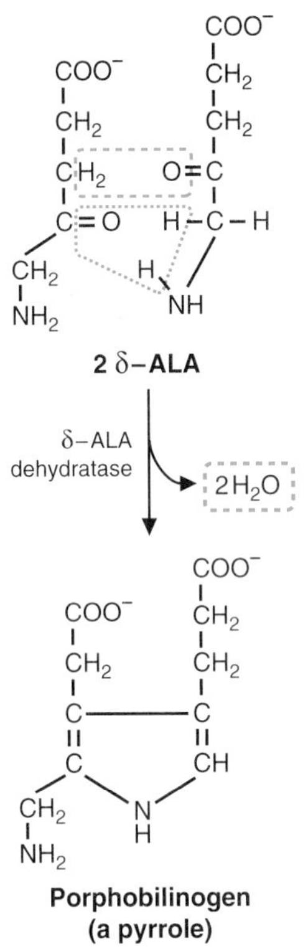

2 δ–ALA

δ–ALA
dehydratase

2H₂O

**Porphobilinogen
(a pyrrole)**

Fig. 44.5. Two molecules of δ-ALA condense to form porphobilinogen.

In a B6 deficiency, the rate of heme production is slow because the first reaction in heme synthesis requires pyridoxal phosphate (see Fig. 44.4). Thus, less heme is synthesized, causing red blood cells to be small and pale. Iron stores are usually elevated.

The iron lost by adult males (approximately 1 mg/day) by desquamation of the skin and in bile, feces, urine, and sweat is replaced by iron absorbed from the diet. Men are not as likely to suffer from iron deficiencies as premenopausal adult women, who also lose iron during menstruation and who must supply iron to meet the needs of the growing fetus during a pregnancy. If a man eating a Western diet has iron-deficiency anemia, his physician should suspect bleeding from the gastrointestinal tract due to ulcers or colon cancer.

Although spinach has been touted as a wonderful source of iron (mostly by the cartoon character Popeye), this iron is not readily absorbed because spinach has a high content of phytate (inositol with a phosphate group attached to each of its 6 hydroxyl groups).

The iron in meats is in the form of heme, which is readily absorbed. The non-heme iron in plants is not as readily absorbed, in part because plants often contain oxalates, phytates, tannins, and other phenolic compounds that chelate or form insoluble precipitates with iron, preventing its absorption. Conversely, vitamin C (ascorbic acid) increases the uptake of non-heme iron from the digestive tract. The uptake of iron is also increased in times of need by mechanisms that are not yet understood. Iron is absorbed in the ferrous (Fe^{2+}) state (Fig. 44.6), but is oxidized to the ferric state by a ferroxidase known as ceruloplasmin (a copper-containing enzyme) for transport through the body.

Because free iron is toxic, it is usually found in the body bound to proteins (see Fig. 44.6). Iron is carried in the blood (as Fe^{3+}) by the protein apotransferrin, with which it forms a complex known as transferrin. Transferrin is usually only one-third saturated with iron. The total iron-binding capacity of blood, mainly due to its content of transferrin, is approximately 300 μg/dL.

Storage of iron occurs in most cells but especially those of the liver, spleen, and bone marrow. In these cells, the storage protein, apoferritin, forms a complex with iron (Fe^{3+}) known as ferritin. Normally, little ferritin is present in the blood. This amount increases, however, as iron stores increase. Therefore, the amount of ferritin in the blood is the most sensitive indicator of the amount of iron in the body's stores.

Iron can be drawn from ferritin stores, transported in the blood as transferrin, and taken up via receptor-mediated endocytosis by cells that require iron (e.g., by reticulocytes that are synthesizing hemoglobin). When excess iron is absorbed from the diet, it is stored as hemosiderin, a form of ferritin complexed with additional iron that cannot be readily mobilized.

4.   REGULATION OF HEME SYNTHESIS

Heme regulates its own synthesis by mechanisms that affect the first enzyme in the pathway, δ-ALA synthase (see Fig. 44.3). Heme represses the synthesis of this enzyme, and also directly inhibits the activity of the enzyme (an allosteric modifier). Thus, heme is synthesized when heme levels fall. As heme levels rise, the rate of heme synthesis decreases.

Heme also regulates the synthesis of hemoglobin by stimulating synthesis of the protein globin. Heme maintains the ribosomal initiation complex for globin synthesis in an active state (see Chapter 15).

5.   DEGRADATION OF HEME

Heme is degraded to form bilirubin, which is conjugated with glucuronic acid and excreted in the bile (Fig. 44.7). Although heme from cytochromes and myoglobin also undergoes conversion to bilirubin, the major source of this bile pigment is hemoglobin. After red blood cells reach the end of their lifespan (approximately 120 days), they are phagocytosed by cells of the reticuloendothelial system. Globin is cleaved to its constituent amino acids, and iron is returned to the body's iron stores. Heme is oxidized and cleaved to produce carbon monoxide and biliverdin (Fig. 44.8). Biliverdin is reduced to bilirubin, which is transported to the liver complexed with serum albumin.

In the liver, bilirubin is converted to a more water-soluble compound by reacting with UDP-glucuronate to form bilirubin monoglucuronide, which is converted to the diglucuronide (see Fig. 30.5). This conjugated form of bilirubin is excreted into the bile.

Drugs, such as phenobarbital, induce enzymes of the drug metabolizing systems of the endoplasmic reticulum that contain cytochrome P450. Because heme is used for synthesis of cytochrome P450, free heme levels will fall and δ-ALA synthase will be induced to increase the rate of heme synthesis.

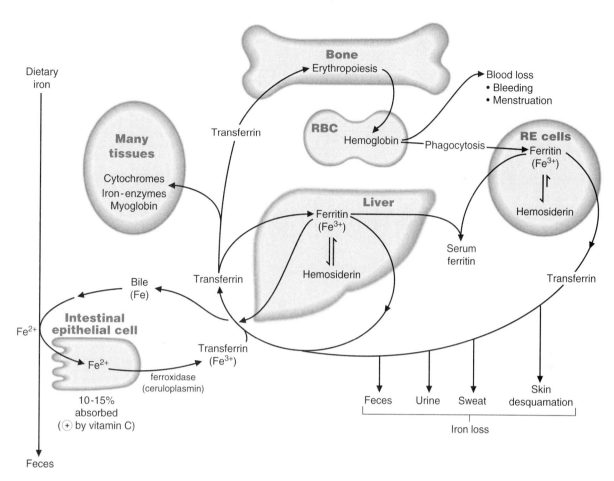

Fig. 44.6. Iron metabolism. Iron is absorbed from the diet, transported in the blood in transferrin, stored in ferritin, and used for the synthesis of cytochromes, iron-containing enzymes, hemoglobin, and myoglobin. It is lost from the body with bleeding and sloughed-off cells, sweat, urine, and feces. Hemosiderin is the protein in which excess iron is stored. Small amounts of ferritin enter the blood and can be used to measure the adequacy of iron stores. RE = reticuloendothelial.

In the intestine, bacteria deconjugate bilirubin diglucuronide and convert the bilirubin to urobilinogens (see Fig. 44.7). Some urobilinogen is absorbed into the blood and excreted in the urine. However, most of the urobilinogen is oxidized to urobilins, such as stercobilin, and excreted in the feces. These pigments give feces their brown color.

 In an iron deficiency, what characteristics would blood exhibit?

III. THE RED BLOOD CELL MEMBRANE

Under the microscope, the red blood cell appears to be a red disc with a pale central area (biconcave disc) (Fig.44.9). The biconcave disc shape (as opposed to a spherical shape) serves to facilitate gas exchange across the cell membrane. The membrane proteins that maintain the shape of the red blood cell also allow the red blood cell to traverse the capillaries with very small luminal diameters to deliver oxygen to the tissues. The interior diameters of many capillaries are smaller than the approximately 7.5-μm diameter of the red cell. Furthermore, in passing through the kidney, red blood cells traverse hypertonic areas that are up to six times the normal isotonicity, and back again, causing the red cell to shrink and expand during its travels. The spleen is the organ responsible for determining the viability of the red blood cells. Erythrocytes pass through the spleen 120 times per day. The elliptical passageways through the spleen are approximately 3 μm in diameter, and

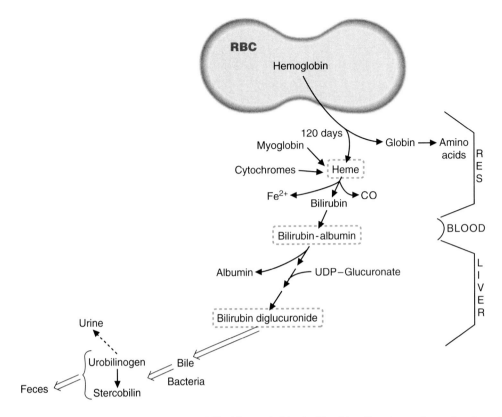

Fig. 44.7. Overview of heme degradation. Heme is degraded to bilirubin, carried in the blood by albumin, conjugated to form the diglucuronide in the liver, and excreted in the bile. The iron is returned to the body's iron stores. RES = reticuloendothelial system: RBC = red blood cells.

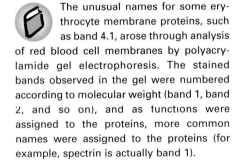

Iron deficiency would result in a microcytic, hypochromic anemia. Red blood cells would be small and pale. In contrast to a vitamin B6 deficiency, which also results in a microcytic, hypochromic anemia, iron stores are low in an iron-deficiency anemia.

The unusual names for some erythrocyte membrane proteins, such as band 4.1, arose through analysis of red blood cell membranes by polyacrylamide gel electrophoresis. The stained bands observed in the gel were numbered according to molecular weight (band 1, band 2, and so on), and as functions were assigned to the proteins, more common names were assigned to the proteins (for example, spectrin is actually band 1).

normal red cells traverse them in approximately 30 seconds. Thus, to survive in the circulation, the red cell must be highly deformable. Damaged red cells that are no longer deformable become trapped in the passages in the spleen, where they are destroyed by macrophages. The reason for the erythrocyte's deformability lies in its shape and in the organization of the proteins that make up the red blood cell membrane.

The surface area of the red cell is approximately 140 μm^2, which is greater than the surface of a sphere needed to enclose the contents of the red cell (98 μm^2). The presence of this extra membrane and the cytoskeleton that supports it allows the red cell to be stretched and deformed by mechanical stresses as the cell passes through narrow vascular beds. On the cytoplasmic side of the membrane, proteins form a two-dimensional lattice that gives the red cell its flexibility (Fig. 44.10). The major proteins are spectrin, actin, band 4.1, band 4.2, and ankyrin. Spectrin, the major protein, is a heterodimer composed of α and β subunits wound around each other. The dimers self-associate at the heads. At the opposite end of the spectrin dimers, actin and band 4.1 bind near to each other. Multiple spectrins can bind to each actin filament, resulting in a branched membrane cytoskeleton.

The spectrin cytoskeleton is connected to the membrane lipid bilayer by ankyrin, which interacts with β-spectrin and the integral membrane protein, band 3. Band 4.2 helps to stabilize this connection. Band 4.1 anchors the spectrin skeleton with the membrane by binding the integral membrane protein glycophorin C and the actin complex, which has bound multiple spectrin dimers.

When the red blood cell is subjected to mechanical stress, the spectrin network rearranges. Some spectrin molecules become uncoiled and extended; others

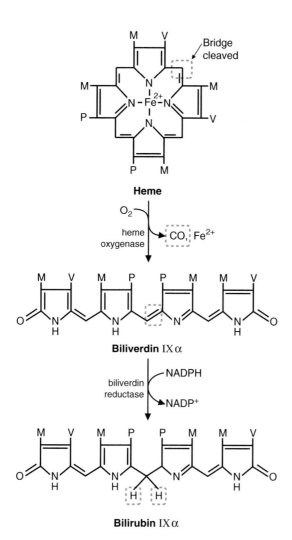

Heme

Biliverdin IXα

Bilirubin IXα

Fig. 44.8. Conversion of heme to bilirubin. A methylene bridge in heme is cleaved, releasing carbon monoxide (CO) and iron. Then, the center methylene bridge is reduced.

become compressed, thereby changing the shape of the cell, but not its surface area.

The mature erythrocyte cannot synthesize new membrane proteins or lipids. However, membrane lipids can be freely exchanged with circulating lipoprotein lipids. The glutathione system protects the proteins and lipids from oxidative damage.

IV. AGENTS THAT AFFECT OXYGEN BINDING

The major agents that affect oxygen binding to hemoglobin are shown in Figure 44.11.

A. 2,3-Bisphosphoglycerate

2,3-Bisphosphoglycerate (2,3-BPG) is formed in red blood cells from the glycolytic intermediate 1,3-bisphosphoglycerate, as indicated in Figure 44.1. 2,3-BPG binds to hemoglobin in the central cavity formed by the four subunits, increasing the energy required for the conformational changes that facilitate the binding of oxygen. Thus, 2,3-BPG lowers the affinity of hemoglobin for oxygen. Therefore, oxygen is less readily bound (i.e., more readily released in tissues) when hemoglobin contains 2,3-BPG.

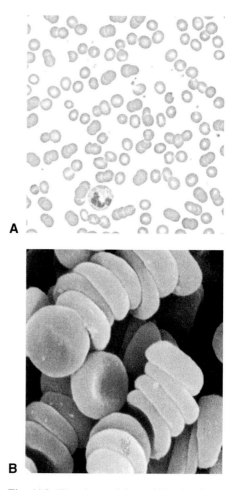

A

B

Fig. 44.9. The shape of the red blood cell. A. Wright-stained cells, displaying the pale staining in the center. Three leukocytes also are present in the preparation. The magnification is 350×. B. Scanning electron micrograph, showing the biconcave disc structure of the cells. The stacks of erythrocytes in this preparation (collected from a blood tube) is not unusual. The magnification is 28,000×. These photographs were obtained, with permission, from Ross et al, Histology, A Text and Atlas with Cell and Molecular Biology, 4th Ed. Philadelphia: Lippincott, 2003:216–217.

 Defects in erythrocyte cytoskeletal proteins lead to hemolytic anemia. Shear stresses in the circulation result in the loss of pieces of the red cell membrane. As the membrane is lost, the red blood cell becomes more spherical and loses its deformability. As these cells become more spherical, they are more likely to lyse in response to mechanical stresses in the circulation, or to be trapped and destroyed in the spleen.

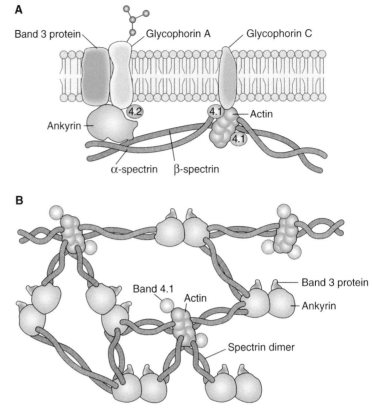

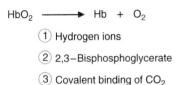

(1) Hydrogen ions

(2) 2,3–Bisphosphoglycerate

(3) Covalent binding of CO_2

Fig. 44.11. Agents that affect oxygen binding by hemoglobin. Binding of hydrogen ions, 2,3 bisphosphoglycerate, and carbon dioxide to hemoglobin decrease its affinity for oxygen.

Fig. 44.10. A generalized view of the erythrocyte cytoskeleton. A. The major protein, spectrin, is linked to the plasma membrane either through interactions with ankyrin and band 3, or with actin, band 4.1, and glycophorin. Other proteins in this complex, but not shown, are tropomyosin and adducin. B. A view from inside the cell, looking up at the cytoskeleton. This view displays the cross-linking of the spectrin dimers to actin and band 3 anchor sites.

B. Proton Binding (Bohr effect)

The binding of protons by hemoglobin lowers its affinity for oxygen (Fig. 44.12), contributing to a phenomenon known as the Bohr effect (Fig. 44.13). The pH of the blood decreases as it enters the tissues (and the proton concentration rises) because the CO_2 produced by metabolism is converted to carbonic acid by the reaction catalyzed by carbonic anhydrase in red blood cells. Dissociation of carbonic acid produces protons that react with several amino acid residues in hemoglobin, causing conformational changes that promote the release of oxygen.

In the lungs, this process is reversed. Oxygen binds to hemoglobin, causing a release of protons, which combine with bicarbonate to form carbonic acid. This decrease of protons causes the pH of the blood to rise. Carbonic anhydrase cleaves the carbonic acid to H_2O and CO_2, and the CO_2 is exhaled. Thus, in tissues in which the pH of the blood is low because of the CO_2 produced by metabolism, oxygen is released from hemoglobin. In the lungs, where the pH of the blood is higher because CO_2 is being exhaled, oxygen binds to hemoglobin.

C. Carbon Dioxide

Although most of the CO_2 produced by metabolism in the tissues is carried to the lungs as bicarbonate, some of the CO_2 is covalently bound to hemoglobin (Fig. 44.14). In the tissues, CO_2 forms carbamate adducts with the N-terminal amino groups of deoxyhemoglobin and stabilizes the deoxy conformation. In the

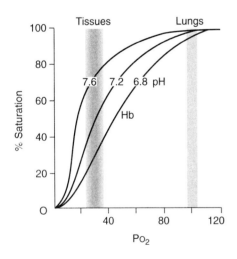

Fig. 44.12. Effect of pH on oxygen saturation curves. As the pH decreases, the affinity of hemoglobin for oxygen decreases, producing the Bohr effect.

A

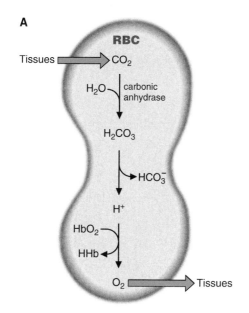

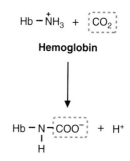

Carbamate of hemoglobin

Fig. 44.14. Binding of CO_2 to hemoglobin. CO_2 forms carbamates with the N-terminal amino groups of Hb chains. Approximately 15% of the CO_2 in blood is carried to the lungs bound to Hb. The reaction releases protons, which contribute to the Bohr effect. The overall effect is the stabilization of the deoxy form of hemoglobin.

B

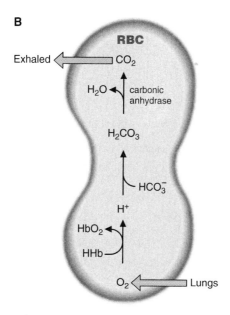

Fig. 44.13. Effect of H^+ on oxygen binding by hemoglobin (Hb). A. In the tissues, CO_2 is released. In the red blood cell, this CO_2 forms carbonic acid, which releases protons. The protons bind to Hb, causing it to release oxygen to the tissues. B. In the lungs, the reactions are reversed. O_2 binds to protonated Hb, causing the release of protons. They bind to bicarbonate (HCO_3^-), forming carbonic acid, which is cleaved to water and CO_2, which is exhaled.

lungs, where the pO_2 is high, oxygen binds to hemoglobin and this bound CO_2 is released.

V. HEMATOPOIESIS

The various types of cells (lineages) that make up the blood are constantly being produced in the bone marrow. All cell lineages are descended from hematopoietic stem cells, cells that are renewable throughout the life of the host. The population of hematopoietic stem cells is quite small. Estimates vary between 1 to 10 per 10^5 bone marrow cells. In the presence of the appropriate signals, hematopoietic stem

 Populations of hematopoietic cells enriched with stem cells can be isolated by fluorescence activated cell sorting, based on the expression of specific cell surface markers. Increasing the population of stem cells in cells used for a bone marrow transplantation increases the chances of success of the transplantation.

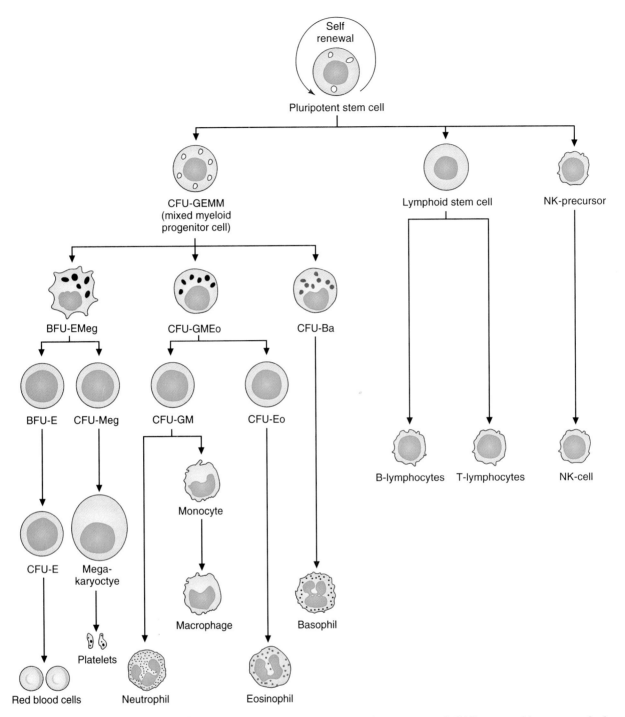

Fig. 44.15. The hematopoietic tree. All blood cells arise from the self-renewing pluripotent stem cell. Different cytokines are required at each step for these events to occur. CFU = colony-forming unit; BFU = burst-forming unit.

 Leukemias, malignancies of the blood, arise when a differentiating hematopoietic cell does not complete its developmental program but remains in an immature, proliferative state. Leukemias have been found in every hematopoietic lineage.

cells proliferate, differentiate, and mature into any of the types of cells that make up the blood (Figure 44.15).

Hematopoietic differentiation is hierarchical. The number of fates a developing blood cell may adopt becomes progressively restricted. Hematopoietic progenitors are designated colony-forming unit–lineage, or colony-forming unit–erythroid (CFU-E). Progenitors that form very large colonies are termed burst-forming units.

A. Cytokines and Hematopoiesis

Developing progenitor cells in the marrow grow in proximity with marrow stromal cells. These include fibroblasts, endothelial cells, adipocytes, and macrophages. The stromal cells form an extracellular matrix and secrete growth factors that regulate hematopoietic development.

The hematopoietic growth factors have multiple effects. An individual growth factor may stimulate proliferation, differentiation, and maturation of the progenitor cells and also may prevent apoptosis. These factors also may activate various functions within the mature cell. Some hematopoietic growth factors act on multiple lineages, whereas others have more limited targets.

Most hematopoietic growth factors are recognized by receptors belonging to the cytokine receptor superfamily. Binding of ligand to receptor results in receptor aggregation, which induces phosphorylation of Janus kinases (JAKs). The JAKs are a family of cytoplasmic tyrosine kinases that are active when phosphorylated (see Chapter 11, section III.C., and Fig. 11.15). The activated JAKs then phosphorylate the cytokine receptor. Phosphorylation of the receptor creates docking regions where additional signal transduction molecules bind, including members of the signal transducer and activator of transcription (STAT) family of transcription factors. The JAKs phosphorylate the STATs, which dimerize and translocate to the nucleus, where they activate target genes. Additional signal transduction proteins bind to the phosphorylated cytokine receptor, leading to activation of the Ras/Raf/MAP kinase pathways. Other pathways are also activated, some of which lead to an inhibition of apoptosis (see Chapter 18).

The response to cytokine binding is usually transient because the cell contains multiple negative regulators of cytokine signaling. The family of **s**ilencer **o**f **c**ytokine **s**ignaling (SOCS) proteins are induced by cytokine binding. One member of the family binds to the phosphorylated receptor and prevents the docking of signal transduction proteins. Other SOCS proteins bind to JAKs and inhibit them. Whether SOCS inhibition of JAKs is a consequence of steric inhibition or whether SOCS recruit phosphatases that then dephosphorylate the JAKs (Figure 44.16) is uncertain.

SHP-1 is a tyrosine phosphatase found primarily in hematopoietic cells that is necessary for proper development of myeloid and lymphoid lineages. Its function is to dephosphorylate JAK2, thereby inactivating it.

STATs are also inactivated. The **p**rotein **i**nhibitors of **a**ctivated **S**TAT (PIAS) family of proteins bind to phosphorylated STATs and prevent their dimerization or promote the dissociation of STAT dimers. STATs also may be inactivated by dephosphorylation, although the specific phosphatases have not yet been identified, or by targeting activated STATs for proteolytic degradation.

B. Erythropoiesis

The production of red cells is regulated by the demands of oxygen delivery to the tissues. In response to reduced tissue oxygenation, the kidney releases the hormone erythropoietin, which stimulates the multiplication and maturation of erythroid progenitors. The progression along the erythroid pathway begins with the stem cell and passes through the mixed myeloid progenitor cell, (CFU-GEMM, colony-forming unit–granulocyte, erythroid, monocyte, megakaryocyte), burst-forming unit–erythroid (BFU-E), colony-forming unit–erythroid (CFU-E), and to the first recognizable red cell precursor, the normoblast. Each normoblast undergoes four more cycles of cell division. During these four cycles, the nucleus becomes smaller and more condensed. After the last division, the nucleus is extruded. The red cell at this state is called a reticulocyte. Reticulocytes still retain ribosomes and mRNA and are capable of synthesizing hemoglobin. They are released from the bone marrow and circulate for 1 to 2 days. Reticulocytes mature in the spleen, where the ribosomes and mRNA are lost (Fig. 44.17).

Bone marrow cells can be cultured in semisolid media with the addition of the appropriate growth factors. After 14 to 18 days in culture, colonies of blood cells can be seen. The type (lineage) of these cells can be determined based on morphological or staining properties. Most colonies will be of single lineage, indicating descent from a hematopoietic progenitor that was committed to a lineage. Occasionally a multilineage colony will be obtained, indicating that it was derived from a more primitive hematopoietic progenitor.

In X-linked severe combined immunodeficiency disease (SCID), the most common form of SCID, circulating T lymphocytes are not formed, and B lymphocytes are not active. The affected gene encodes the gamma chain of the interleukin 2 receptor. Mutant receptors are unable to activate JAK3, and the cells are unresponsive to the cytokines that stimulate growth and differentiation. Recall also that adenosine deaminase deficiency (see Chapter 41), which is not X-linked, also leads to a form of SCID, but for different reasons.

Families have been identified whose members have a mutant erythropoietin (epo) receptor that is unable to bind SHP-1. Erythropoietin is the hematopoietic cytokine that stimulates production of red blood cells. Individuals with the mutant epo receptor have a higher than normal percentage of red blood cells in the circulation, because the mutant epo receptor cannot be deactivated by SHP-1. Erythropoietin causes sustained activation of JAK2 and STAT 5 in this case.

Perturbed JAK/STAT signaling is associated with development of lymphoid and myeloid leukemias, severe congenital neutropenia, a condition in which levels of circulating neutrophils are severely reduced, and Fanconi anemia, which is characterized by bone marrow failure and increased susceptibility to malignancy.

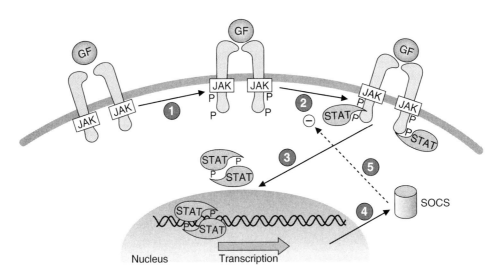

Fig. 44.16. Cytokine signaling through the JAK/STAT pathway. 1. Cytokine binding to receptors initiates dimerization and activation of the JAK kinase, which phosphorylates the receptor on tyrosine residues. 2. STAT proteins bind to the activated receptors and are themselves phosphorylated. 3. Phosphorylated STAT proteins dimerize, travel to the nucleus, and initiate gene transcription. 4. One of the proteins whose synthesis is stimulated by STATs is SOCS (**s**uppressor **o**f **c**ytokine **s**ignaling), which inhibits further activation of STAT proteins (circle 5) by a variety of mechanisms.

C. Nutritional Anemias

Each person produces approximately 10^{12} red blood cells per day. Because so many cells must be produced, nutritional deficiencies in iron, vitamin B12, and folate prevent adequate red blood cell formation. The physical appearance of the cells in the case of a nutritional anemia frequently provides a clue as to the nature of the deficiency.

In the case of iron deficiency, the cells are smaller and paler than normal. The lack of iron results in decreased heme synthesis, which in turn affects globin synthesis. Maturing red cells following their normal developmental program divide until their hemoglobin has reached the appropriate concentration. Iron- (and hemoglobin-) deficient developing red blood cells continue dividing past their normal stopping point, resulting in small (microcytic) red cells. The cells are also pale because of the lack of hemoglobin, as compared with normal cells (thus, a pale, microcytic anemia results).

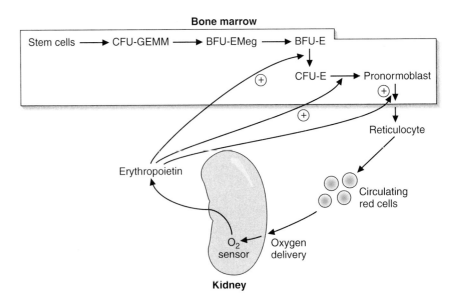

Fig. 44.17. Erythropoietin stimulation of erythrocyte maturation. The abbreviations are described in the text.

Deficiencies of folate or vitamin B12 can cause megaloblastic anemia, in which the cells are larger than normal. Folate and B12 are required for DNA synthesis (see Chapters 40 and 41). When these vitamins are deficient, DNA replication and nuclear division do not keep pace with the maturation of the cytoplasm. Consequently, the nucleus is extruded before the requisite number of cell divisions has taken place, and the cell volume is greater than it should be, and fewer blood cells are produced.

VI. HEMOGLOBINOPATHIES, HEREDITARY PERSISTENCE OF FETAL HEMOGLOBIN, AND HEMOGLOBIN SWITCHING

A. Hemoglobinopathies: Disorders in the Structure or Amount of the Globin Chains

More than 700 different mutant hemoglobins have been discovered. Most arise from a single base substitution, resulting in a single amino acid replacement. Many have been discovered during population screenings and are not clinically significant. However, in patients with hemoglobin S (HbS, sickle cell anemia), the most common hemoglobin mutation, the amino acid substitution has a devastating effect in the homozygote (see **Will Sichel** in Chapter 6). Another common hemoglobin variant, HbC, results from a glu to lys replacement in the same position as the HbS mutation. This mutation has two effects. It promotes water loss from the cell by activating the K^+ transporter by an unknown mechanism, resulting in a higher than normal concentration of hemoglobin within the cell. The amino acid replacement also substantially lowers the hemoglobin solubility in the homozygote, resulting in a tendency of the mutant hemoglobin to precipitate within the red cell, although, unlike sickle cells, the cell does not become deformed. Homozygotes for the HbC mutation have a mild hemolytic anemia. Heterozygous individuals are clinically unaffected.

B. Thalassemias

For optimum function, the hemoglobin α and β-globin chains must have the proper structure and be synthesized in a 1:1 ratio. A large excess of one subunit over the other results in the class of diseases called thalassemias. These anemias are clinically very heterogeneous, as they can arise by multiple mechanisms. Like sickle cell anemia, the thalassemia mutations provide resistance to malaria in the heterozygous state.

Hemoglobin single amino acid replacement mutations that give rise to a globin subunit of decreased stability is one mechanism by which thalassemia arises. More common, however, are mutations that result in decreased synthesis of one subunit. Alpha thalassemias usually arise from complete gene deletions. Two copies of the α-globin gene are found on each chromosome 16, for a total of 4 α-globin genes per precursor cell. If one copy of the gene is deleted, the size and hemoglobin concentration of the individual red blood cells is minimally reduced. If two copies are deleted, the red blood cells are of decreased size (microcytic) and reduced hemoglobin concentration (hypochromic). However, the individual is usually not anemic. The loss of three α-globin genes causes a moderately severe microcytic hypochromic anemia (hemoglobin 7–10 g/dL) with splenomegaly (enlarged spleen). The absence of four α-globin genes (hydrops fetalis) is usually fatal in utero.

There are two ways in which an individual could have two α-globin genes deleted. In one case, one copy of chromosome 16 could have both α-globin genes deleted, whereas the other copy had two functional α genes. In the second case, both chromosomes could have lost one of their two copies of the α-globin gene. The former possibility is more common among Asians; the latter among Africans.

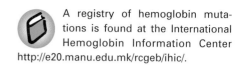

A registry of hemoglobin mutations is found at the International Hemoglobin Information Center http://e20.manu.edu.mk/rcgeb/ihic/.

A complication of sickle cell disease is an increased formation of gallstones. A sickle cell crisis accompanied by the intravascular destruction of red blood cells (hemolysis) experienced by patients with sickle cell disease, such as **Will Sichel**, increases the amount of unconjugated bilirubin that is transported to the liver. If the concentration of this unconjugated bilirubin exceeds the capacity of the hepatocytes to conjugate it to the more soluble diglucuronide through interaction with hepatic UDP-glucuronate, both the total and the unconjugated bilirubin levels would rise in the blood. More unconjugated bilirubin would be secreted by the liver into the bile. The increase in unconjugated bilirubin (which is not very water-soluble) results in its precipitation within the gallbladder lumen, leading to the formation of pigmented (calcium bilirubinate) gallstones.

HbC is found in high frequency in West Africa, in regions with a high frequency of HbS. Consequently, compound heterozygotes for HbS and HbC are not uncommon both in some African regions and among African-Americans. HbS/HbC individuals have significantly more hematopathology than individuals with sickle cell trait (HbA/HbS). Polymerization of deoxygenated HbS is dependent on the HbS concentration within the cell. The presence of HbC in the compound heterozygote increases the HbS concentration by stimulating K^+ and water efflux from the cell. Because the HbC globin is produced more slowly than HbA or HbS, the proportion of HbS tends to be higher in HbS/HbC cells than in the cells of individuals with sickle cell trait (HbS/HbA). The way in which multiple mutations ameliorate or exacerbate hematologic diseases has provided insights into the molecular mechanisms of hemoglobin function and developmental regulation.

The difference in amino acid composition between the β-chains of HbA and γ-chains of HbF results in structural changes that cause HbF to have a lower affinity for 2,3-BPG than adult hemoglobin (HbA) and, thus, a greater affinity for oxygen. Therefore, the oxygen released from the mother's hemoglobin (HbA) is readily bound by HbF in the fetus. Thus, the transfer of oxygen from the mother to the fetus is facilitated by the structural difference between the hemoglobin molecule of the mother and that of the fetus.

Individuals with sickle cell anemia or beta thalassemia (usually) have intact γ-globin loci. If a way could be found to reactivate the γ-globin loci (the drug hydroxyurea is a potential candidate for this), it would be an attractive therapeutic option for the treatment of these diseases.

An additional source of variation in the levels of fetal hemoglobin is the FCP (**F**-cell **p**roducing) locus on the short arm of the X chromosome in a region thought not to be susceptible to X inactivation. Both normal individuals and individuals with hemoglobinopathies vary in the amount of hemoglobin F they produce. In studies of normal individuals, a high level of hemoglobin F appears to be inherited as an X-linked dominant trait. The FCP locus is responsible for a substantial amount of the variation in Hemoglobin F seen among sickle cell patients. The protein encoded at the FCP locus has not been identified; current speculations are that it is a transcription factor involved in the regulation of the globin locus.

As discussed in Chapter 14, beta thalassemia is a very heterogeneous genetic disease. Insufficient β-globin synthesis can result from deletions, promoter mutations, and splice junction mutations. Heterozygotes for β^+ (some globin chain synthesis) or β null (β^0, no globin chain synthesis) are generally asymptomatic, though they typically have microcytic, hypochromic red blood cells and may have a mild anemia. β^+/β^+ homozygotes have an anemia of variable severity, β^+/β^0 compound heterozygotes tend to be more severely affected, and β^0/β^0 homozygotes have severe disease. In general, diseases of β chain deficiency are more severe than diseases of α chain deficiency. Excess β chains form a homotetramer, hemoglobin H (HbH), which is useless for delivering oxygen to the tissues because of its high oxygen affinity. As red blood cells age, HbH will precipitate in the cells, forming inclusion bodies. Red blood cells with inclusion bodies have a shortened life span, because they are more likely to be trapped and destroyed in the spleen. Excess α chains are unable to form a stable tetramer. However, excess α chains precipitate in erythrocytes at every developmental stage. The α chain precipitation in erythroid precursors results in their widespread destruction, a process called ineffective erythropoiesis. The precipitated α chains also damage red blood cell membranes through the heme-facilitated lipid oxidation by reactive oxygen species. Both lipids and proteins, particularly band 4.1, are damaged.

C. Hereditary Persistence of Fetal Hemoglobin

Fetal hemoglobin (HbF), the predominant hemoglobin of the fetal period, consists of two alpha chains and two gamma chains, whereas adult Hb consists of two alpha and two beta chains. The process that regulates the conversion of HbF to HbA is called hemoglobin switching. Hb switching is not 100%; most individuals continue to produce a small amount of HbF throughout life. However, some people, who are clinically normal, produce abnormally high levels (up to 100%) of fetal hemoglobin (Hemoglobin F) in place of HbA. Patients with hemoglobinopathies such as β-thalassemia or sickle cell anemia frequently have less severe illnesses if their levels of fetal hemoglobin are elevated. One goal of much research on hemoglobin switching is to discover a way to reactivate transcription of the γ-globin genes to compensate for defective β-globin synthesis. Individuals who express fetal hemoglobin past birth have hereditary persistence of fetal hemoglobin (HPFH).

1. NON-DELETION FORMS OF HPFH

The non-deletion forms of HPFH are those that derive from point mutations in the Aγ and Gγ promoters. When these mutations are found with sickle cell or beta thalassemia mutations, they have an ameliorating effect on the disease, because of the increased production of gamma chains.

2. DELETION FORMS OF HPFH

In deletion HPFH, both the entire delta and beta genes have been deleted from one copy of chromosome 11 and only HbF can be produced. In some individuals the fetal globins remain activated after birth, and enough HbF is produced that the individuals are clinically normal. Other individuals with similar deletions that remove the entire delta and beta genes do not produce enough fetal hemoglobin to compensate for the deletion and are considered to have $\delta^0\beta^0$ thalassemia. The difference between these two outcomes is believed to be the site at which the deletions end within the β-globin gene cluster. In deletion HPFH, powerful enhancer sequences 3' of the β-globin gene are resituated because of the deletion such that they activate the gamma promoters. In individuals with $\delta^0\beta^0$ thalassemia, the enhancer sequences have not been relocated such that they can interact with the gamma promoters.

D. Hemoglobin Switching: A Developmental Process Controlled by Transcription Factors

In humans, embryonic megaloblasts (the embryonic red blood cell is large and is termed a "blast" because it retains its nucleus) are first produced in the yolk sac approximately 15 days after fertilization. After 6 weeks, the site of erythropoiesis shifts to the liver. The liver and to a lesser extent the spleen are the major sites of fetal erythropoiesis. In the last few weeks before birth, the bone marrow begins producing red blood cells. By 8 to 10 weeks after birth, the bone marrow is the sole site of erythrocyte production. The composition of the hemoglobin also changes with development, because both the α-globin locus and the β-globin locus have multiple genes that are differentially expressed during development (Figure 44.18).

E. Structure and Transcriptional Regulation of the Alpha and Beta Globin Gene Loci

The α-globin locus on chromosome 16 contains the embryonic ζ (zeta) gene and two copies of the alpha gene, α_2 and α_1. The β-globin locus on chromosome 11 contains the embryonic ε gene, two copies of the fetal β-globin gene G_γ and A_γ

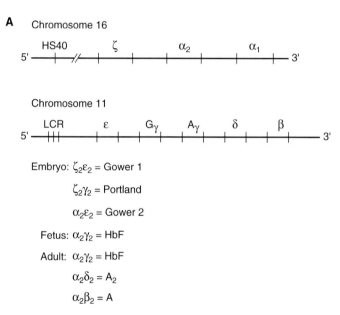

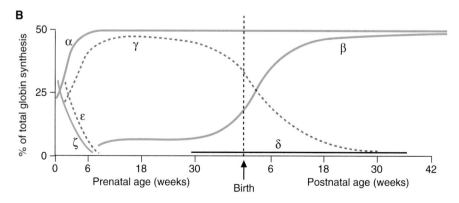

Fig 44.18. Globin gene clusters and expression during development. A. The globin gene clusters with the α genes on chromosome 16 and the β genes on chromosome 11. LCR = locus control region. B. The switching of globin chain synthesis during development.

(which differ by one amino acid), and two adult genes, δ and β. The order of the genes along the chromosome parallels the order of expression of the genes during development (see Fig. 44.18). The embryonic hemoglobins are $\zeta_2\epsilon_2$ (Gower 1), $\zeta_2\gamma_2$ (Portland), and $\alpha_2\gamma_2$ (Gower 2). Fetal hemoglobin is predominantly $\alpha_2G_{\gamma2}$. The major adult species is $\alpha_2\beta_2$ (hemoglobin A); the minor adult species is $\alpha_2\delta_2$ (hemoglobin A_2). The fetal hemoglobin found in adult cells is $\alpha_2A_{\gamma2}$. The timing of hemoglobin switching is controlled by a developmental clock not significantly altered by environmental conditions and is related to changes in expression of specific transcription factors. Premature newborns convert from HbF to HbA on schedule with their gestational ages.

CLINICAL COMMENTS

Spiro Site's red blood cells are deficient in spectrin. This deficiency impairs the ability of his erythrocytes to maintain the redundant surface area necessary to maintain deformability. Mechanical stresses in the circulation cause progressive loss of pieces of membrane. As membrane components are lost, **Spiro Site's** red blood cells become spherical and unable to deform. His spleen is enlarged because of the large number of red blood cells that have become trapped within it. His erythrocytes are lysed by mechanical stresses in the circulation and by macrophages in the spleen. Consequently, this hemolytic process results in an anemia. His gallstones were the result of the large amounts of bilirubin that were produced and stored in the gallbladder as a result of the hemolysis. The abnormally rounded red cells seen on a blood smear are characteristic of hereditary spherocytosis.

Mutations in the genes for ankyrin, β-spectrin, or band 3 account for three quarters of the cases of hereditary spherocytosis, whereas mutations in the genes for α-spectrin or band 4.2 account for the remainder. The result of defective synthesis of any of the membrane cytoskeletal proteins results in improper formation of the membrane cytoskeleton. Excess membrane proteins are catabolized, resulting in a net deficiency of spectrin. **Spiro Site** underwent a splenectomy. Because the spleen was the major site of destruction of his red blood cells, his anemia significantly improved after surgery. He was discharged with the recommendation to take a folate supplement daily. It was explained to Mr. Site that because the spleen plays a major role in protection against certain bacterial agents, he would require immunizations against pneumococcus, meningococcus, and Haemophilus influenzae type b.

Anne Niemick was found to be a compound heterozygote for mutations in the β-globin gene. On one gene, a mutation in position 6 of intron 1 converted a T to a C. The presence of this mutation, for unknown reasons, raises HbF production. The other β-globin gene had a mutation in position 110 of exon 1 (a C to T mutation). Both β-globin chains have reduced activity, but combined with the increased expression of HbF, results in a β^+ thalassemia.

BIOCHEMICAL COMMENTS

How is hemoglobin switching controlled? Although there are still many unanswered questions, some of the molecular mechanisms have been identified. The α-globin locus covers ~100 kb. The major regulatory element, HS 40, is a nuclease-sensitive region of DNA that lies $5'$ of the ζ gene (see Fig. 44.18). HS 40 acts as an erythroid-specific enhancer that interacts with the upstream regulatory regions of the ζ and α genes, and stimulates their transcription. The region immediately $5'$ of the ζ gene contains the regulatory sequences responsible for silencing ζ gene transcription. However, the exact sequences and transcription factors responsible for this silencing have not yet been identified. Even after silencing, low levels of

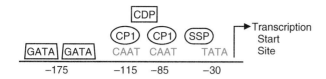

Fig. 44.19. The γ-globin gene promoter indicating some of the transcription factor binding sites associated with hereditary persistence of fetal hemoglobin.

ζ gene transcripts are still produced after the embryonic period; however, they are not translated. This is because both the ζ globin and α-globin transcripts have regions that bind to a messenger ribonucleoprotein (mRNP) stability-determining complex. Binding to this complex prevents the mRNA from being degraded. The α-globin messenger RNA has a much higher affinity for the mRNP than the ζ-globin message, which leads to the ζ-globin message being rapidly degraded.

The β-globin locus covers ~100 kb. From 5 to 25 kb upstream of the ε gene is the locus control region (LCR), containing five DNAse hypersensitive sites. The LCR is necessary for the function of the β-globin locus. It maintains the chromatin of the entire locus in an active configuration and acts as an enhancer and entry point for the factors that transcribe the genes of the β-globin locus. One model of the control of hemoglobin switching postulates that proteins bound at the promoters of the ε–, γ–, and β-globin genes compete to interact with the enhancers of the LCR.

Each gene in the β-globin locus has individual regulatory elements—a promoter, silencers, or enhancers that control its developmental regulation. The promoters controlling the γ and β-globin genes have been intensively studied because of their clinical relevance.

The ε-globin gene, like the ζ globin gene, has silencers in the 5′ regulatory region. Binding of proteins to these regions turns off the ε gene.

The proximal region of the γ-globin gene promoter has multiple transcription factor binding sites (Fig. 44.19). Many HPFH mutations map to these transcription factor–binding sites, either by destroying a site or by creating a new one, but the exact mechanisms are still not understood. Two sites that appear to be significant in the control of hemoglobin switching are the stage selector protein binding (SSP) site and the CAAT box region. When the SSP complex is bound to the promoter, the γ-globin gene has a competitive advantage over the β-globin promoter for interaction with the LCR. A second transcription factor, Sp1, also binds at the SSP-binding site, where it may act as a repressor, and competition between these two protein complexes for the SSP-binding site helps to determine the activity of the γ-globin gene. A similar mechanism appears to be operating at the CAAT box. CP1, thought to be a transcription activator, binds at the CAAT box. CAAT displacement protein (CDP) is a repressor that binds at the CAAT site and displaces CP1. Part of the mechanism of hemoglobin switching appears to be the binding of repressors at the ε-globin and γ-globin upstream regulatory regions.

The β-globin gene also has binding sites for multiple transcription factors in its regulatory regions. Mutations that affect binding of transcription factors can produce thalassemia by reducing the activity of the β-globin promoter. There is also an enhancer 3′ of the poly A signal that seems to be required for stage-specific activation of the β-globin promoter.

 Transgenic mice are an invaluable tool for studying the roles of transcription factors in developmental processes in general and hemoglobin switching in particular. Transgenic mice were created with mutations in the silencer regions of the ε-globin genes. These mice continued to express the ε-globin gene into adulthood.

Suggested References

Krebs DL, Hilton DJ. SOCS proteins: negative regulators of cytokine signaling. Stem Cells 2001;19:378–387.

Stamatoyannopoulos G, Grosveld F. Hemoglobin switching. In: Stamatoyannopoulos G, Majerus PW, Perlmutter, RM Varmus H, eds. The Molecular Basis of Blood Diseases. 3rd Ed. Philadelphia: WB Saunders, 2001:135–182

Ward AC, Touw I, Yoshimura A. The Jak-Stat pathway in normal and perturbed hematopoiesis. Blood 2000;95:19–29.

Weatherall DJ. The thalassemias In: Stamatoyannopoulos G, Majerus PW, Perlmutter, RM Varmus H, eds. The Molecular Basis of Blood Diseases. 3rd Ed. Philadelphia: WB Saunders, 2001:183–226.

 REVIEW QUESTIONS—CHAPTER 44

1. A compensatory mechanism to allow adequate oxygen delivery to the tissues at high altitudes, where oxygen concentrations are low, would be which of the following?

    (A) An increase in 2,3-bisphosphoglycerate synthesis by the red cell
    (B) A decrease in 2,3-bisphosphoglycerate synthesis by the red cell
    (C) An increase in hemoglobin synthesis by the red cell
    (D) A decrease in hemoglobin synthesis by the red cell
    (E) Decreasing the blood pH

2. A 2-year-old boy of normal weight and height is brought to a clinic because of excessive fatigue. Blood work indicates an anemia, with microcytic hypochromic red cells. The boy lives in a 100-year-old apartment building and has been caught ingesting paint chips. His parents indicate that the child eats a healthy diet and takes a Flintstones vitamin supplement every day. His anemia is most likely attributable to a deficiency in which of the following?

    (A) Iron
    (B) B12
    (C) Folate
    (D) Heme
    (E) B6

3. Drugs are being developed that will induce the transcription of globin genes, which are normally silent in patients affected with sickle cell disease. A good target gene for such therapy in this disease would be which of the following?

    (A) The α1 gene
    (B) The α2 gene
    (C) The γ gene
    (D) The β gene
    (E) The ζ gene

4. A mature blood cell that lacks a nucleus is which of the following?

    (A) Lymphocyte
    (B) Basophil
    (C) Eosinophil
    (D) Platelet
    (E) Neutrophil

5. A family has two children, one with a mild case of thalassemia, and a second with a severe case of thalassemia, requiring frequent blood transfusions as part of the treatment plan. One parent is of Mediterranean descent, the other is of Asian descent. Neither parent exhibits clinical signs of thalassemia. Both children express 20% of the expected level of β-globin; the more severely affected child expresses normal levels of α-globin, whereas the less severely affected child only expresses 50% of the normal levels of α-globin. Why is the child who has a deficiency in α-globin expression less severely affected?

    (A) Thalassemia is caused by a mutation in the α gene, and the more severely affected child expresses more of it.
    (B) The less severely affected child must be synthesizing the ζ gene to make up for the deficiency in a α chain synthesis.
    (C) The more severely affected child also has HPFH.
    (D) The more severely affected child produces more inactive globin tetramers than the less severely affected child.
    (E) Thalassemia is caused by an iron deficiency, and when the child is synthesizing normal levels of α-globin there is insufficient iron to populate all of the heme molecules synthesized.

45 Blood Plasma Proteins, Coagulation and Fibrinolysis

The blood is the body's main transport system. Although the transport and delivery of oxygen to the cells of the tissues is carried out by specialized cells, other vital components such as nutrients, metabolites, electrolytes, and hormones, are all carried in the noncellular fraction of the blood, the **plasma***. Some components, such as glucose, are dissolved in the plasma; others, for example, lipids and steroid hormones, are bound to carrier proteins for transport. The* **osmotic pressure** *of the plasma proteins regulates the distribution of water between the blood and the tissues. Plasma proteins in conjunction with platelets maintain the integrity of the circulatory system through the process of clotting.*

Blood normally circulates through endothelium-lined blood vessels. When a blood vessel is severed, a **blood clot** *(called* **a thrombus,** *which is formed by the process of* **thrombosis***) forms as part of* **hemostasis***, the physiologic response that stops bleeding. Blood clots also form to repair damage to the endothelial lining, in which components of the* **subendothelial layer** *become accessible to plasma proteins.*

In hemostasis and thrombosis, a primary hemostatic plug, consisting of **aggregated platelets** *and a* **fibrin clot***, forms at the site of injury. Platelets are attached to the subendothelial layer of the vessel principally through the protein* **von Willebrand factor,** *and are activated to bind fibrinogen.* **Fibrinogen** *binds the platelets to each other to form a platelet aggregate. The platelet aggregate is rapidly covered with layers of* **fibrin***, which are formed from fibrinogen by the proteolytic enzyme* **thrombin***.*

Injury to the endothelium and exposure of **tissue factor** *on the* **subendothelial layer** *to plasma proteins also activate the blood coagulation cascade, which ultimately activates thrombin and* **Factor XIII***. Factor XIII* **cross-links** *strands of polymerized fibrin monomers to form a stable clot (the* **secondary hemostatic plug***). The blood coagulation cascade consists of a series of enzymes (such as* **Factor X***), which are inactive until proteolytically cleaved by the preceding enzyme in the cascade. Other proteins (* **Factor V** *and* **Factor VIII***) serve as binding proteins, which assemble factor complexes at the site of injury.* **Ca^{2+}** *and* γ-**carboxyglutamate** *residues in the proteins (formed by a vitamin K–dependent process in the liver) attach the factor complexes to* **phospholipids** *exposed on platelet membranes. Consequently, thrombus formation is rapidly accelerated and localized to the site of injury.*

Regulatory mechanisms *within the blood coagulation cascade and* **antifibrinolytic mechanisms** *prevent random coagulation within blood vessels that might obstruct blood flow. Impairments in these mechanisms lead to thrombosis.*

THE WAITING ROOM

 Sloe Klotter, a 6-month-old male infant, was brought to his pediatrician's office with a painful, expanding mass in his right upper thigh that was first noted just hours after he fell down three uncarpeted steps in his home. The child appeared to be in severe distress.

An x-ray showed no fractures, but a soft tissue swelling, consistent with a hematoma (bleeding into the tissues), was noted. Sloe's mother related that soon after he began to crawl, his knees occasionally became swollen and seemed painful.

The pediatrician suspected a disorder of coagulation. A screening coagulation profile suggested a possible deficiency of Factor VIII, a protein involved in the formation of blood clots. Sloe's plasma Factor VIII level was found to be only 3% of the average level found in normal subjects. A diagnosis of hemophilia A was made.

I. PLASMA PROTEINS MAINTAIN PROPER DISTRIBUTION OF WATER BETWEEN BLOOD AND TISSUES

When the cells are removed from the blood, the remaining plasma is composed of water, nutrients, metabolites, hormones, electrolytes, and proteins. Plasma has essentially the same electrolyte composition as other extracellular fluids and constitutes approximately 25% of the body's total extracellular fluid. The plasma proteins serve a number of functions, which include maintaining the proper distribution of water between the blood and the tissues, transporting nutrients, metabolites, and hormones throughout the body, defending against infection, and maintaining the integrity of the circulation through clotting. Many diseases alter the amounts of plasma proteins produced and, hence, their concentration in the blood. These changes can be determined by electrophoresis of plasma proteins over the course of a disease.

A. Body Fluid Maintenance between Tissues and Blood

As the arterial blood enters the capillaries, fluid moves from the intravascular space into the interstitial space (that surrounding the capillaries) because of what are known as Starling's forces. The hydrostatic pressure in the arteriolar end of the capillaries (~37 mm Hg) exceeds the sum of the tissue pressure (~1 mm Hg) and the osmotic pressure of the plasma proteins (~25 mm Hg). Thus, water tends to leave the capillaries and enter extravascular spaces. At the venous end of the capillaries, the hydrostatic pressure falls to approximately 17 mm Hg while the osmotic pressure and the tissue pressure remain constant, resulting in movement of fluid back from the extravascular (interstitial) spaces and into the blood. Thus, most of the force bringing water back from the tissues is the osmotic pressure mediated by the presence of proteins in the plasma.

B. The Major Serum Protein, Albumin

As indicated in Table 45.1, the liver produces a number of transport or binding proteins and secretes them into the blood. The major protein synthesized is albumin, which constitutes approximately 60% of the total plasma protein, but because of its relatively small size (69 kDa) is thought to contribute 70 to 80% of the total osmotic pressure of the plasma. Albumin, like most plasma proteins, is a glycoprotein and is a carrier of free fatty acids, calcium, zinc, steroid hormones, copper, and bilirubin.

The hydrostatic pressure in an arteriole is the force that "pushes" fluid out of the capillary and into the interstitial spaces. The plasma protein osmotic pressure, plus the tissue pressure, is the force that "pulls" water from interstitial spaces into the venular side of the capillary. Thus, if the hydrostatic pressure is greater than the osmotic pressure, fluid will leave the circulation; if it is less, fluid will enter the circulation.

In cases of severe protein malnutrition (kwashiorkor), the concentration of the plasma proteins decreases, as a result of which the osmotic pressure of the blood decreases. As a result, fluid is not drawn back to the blood and instead accumulates in the interstitial space (edema). The distended bellies of famine victims are the result of fluid accumulation in the extravascular tissues because of the severely decreased concentration of plasma proteins, particularly albumin. Albumin synthesis decreases fairly early under conditions of protein malnutrition.

Table 45.1. Specific Plasma Binding Proteins Synthesized in the Liver

Ceruloplasmin	Binds copper; appears to be more important as a copper storage pool than as a transport protein; integrates iron and copper homeostasis
Corticosteroid-binding globulin	Binds cortisol
Haptoglobin	Binds extracorpuscular heme
Lipoproteins	Transport cholesterol and fatty acids
Retinol-binding protein	Binds vitamin A
Sex hormone–binding globulin	Binds estradiol and testosterone
Transferrin	Transports iron
Transthyretin	Binds thyroxine (T_4); also forms a complex with retinol-binding protein

Many drugs also bind to albumin, which may have important pharmacologic implications. For example, when a drug binds to albumin, such binding will likely lower the effective concentration of that drug and may lengthen its lifetime in the circulation. Drug dosimetry may need to be recalculated if a patient's plasma protein concentration is abnormal.

II. THE PLASMA CONTAINS PROTEINS THAT AID IN IMMUNE DEFENSE

Two different sets of proteins aid in the immune response, the immunoglobulins and the complement proteins. The immunoglobulins are secreted by a subset of differentiated B lymphocytes termed plasma cells and bind antigens at binding sites formed by the hypervariable regions of the proteins (see Chapter 7). Once the antibody–antigen complex is formed, it must be cleared from the circulation. The complement system participates in this function. The complement system consisting of approximately 20 proteins becomes activated in either of two ways. The first is interaction with antigen–antibody complexes, and the second, specific for bacterial infections, is through interaction of bacterial cell polysaccharides with complement protein C3b. Activation of the complement system by either trigger results in a proteolytic activation cascade of the proteins of the complement system, resulting in the release of biologically active peptides or polypeptide fragments. These peptides mediate the inflammatory response, attract phagocytic cells to the area, initiate degranulation of granulocytes, and promote clearance of antigen–antibody complexes.

Protease inhibitors in plasma serve to carefully control the inflammatory response. Activated neutrophils release lysosomal proteases from their granules that can attack elastin, the various types of collagen, and other extracellular matrix proteins. The plasma proteins α1-antiproteinase (α1-antitrypsin) and α2-macroglobulin limit proteolytic damage by forming noncovalent complexes with the proteases, thereby inactivating them. However, the product of neutrophil myeloperoxidase, HOCl, inactivates the protease inhibitors, thereby insuring that the proteases are active at the site of infection.

III. PLASMA PROTEINS MAINTAIN THE INTEGRETY OF THE CIRCULATORY SYSTEM

Blood is lost from the circulation when the endothelial lining of the blood vessels is damaged and the vessel wall is partly or wholly severed. When this occurs, the subendothelial cell layer is exposed, consisting of the basement membrane of the endothelial cells and smooth muscle cells. In response to the damage, a barrier (the hemostatic plug, a fibrin clot), initiated by platelet binding to the damaged area, is formed at the site of injury. Regulatory mechanisms limit clot formation to the site of injury and control its size and stability. As the vessel heals, the clot is degraded (fibrinolysis). Plasma proteins are required for these processes to occur.

In spite of the importance of albumin in the maintenance of osmotic pressure in the blood, individuals lacking albumin (analbuminemia) have only moderate edema. Apparently, the concentration of other plasma proteins is increased to compensate for the lack of albumin. The frequency of analbuminemia is less than one per million individuals.

α1-Antiproteinase (AAP) is the main serine protease inhibitor of human plasma. Individuals with a point mutation in exon 5 of the AAP gene, which results in a single amino acid substitution in the protein, have diminished secretion of AAP from the liver. These individuals are at increased risk for developing emphysema. When neutrophils degranulate in the lungs as part of the body's defense against microorganisms, insufficient levels of AAP are present to neutralize the elastase and other proteases released. The excess proteolytic activity damages lung tissue, leading to loss of alveolar elasticity and emphysema.

Methionine 358 of AAP is necessary for AAP binding to the proteases. Oxidation of this methionine destroys AAP's protease-binding capacity. Cigarette smoke oxidizes Met-358, thereby increasing the risk for emphysema.

A. Formation of the Hemostatic Plug

1. THE PLATELET

Platelets are non-nucleated cells present in the blood whose major role is to form mechanical plugs at the site of vessel injury and to secrete regulators of the clotting process and vascular repair. In the absence of platelets, leakage of blood from vents in small vessels is common.

In the nonactivated platelet (a platelet not involved in forming a clot), the plasma membrane invaginates extensively into the interior of the cell, forming an open membrane (canalicular) system. Because the plasma membrane contains receptors and phospholipids that accelerate the clotting process, the canalicular structure substantially increases the membrane surface area potentially available for clotting reactions. The platelet interior contains microfilaments and an extensive actin/myosin system. Platelet activation in response to endothelial injury causes Ca^{2+}-dependent changes in the contractile elements, which, in turn, substantially change the architecture of the plasma membrane. Long pseudopodia are generated, increasing the surface area of the membrane as clot formation is initiated.

Platelets contain three types of granules. The first are electron-dense granules, which contain calcium, adenosine diphosphate (ADP), adenosine triphosphate (ATP), and serotonin. The second type of granule is the α granule, which contains a heparin antagonist (heparin interferes with blood clotting; see biochemical comments), platelet-derived growth factor, β-thromboglobulin, fibrinogen, von Willebrand factor (vWF), and other clotting factors. The third type of granule is the lysosomal granule, which contains hydrolytic enzymes. During activation, the contents of these granules, which modulate platelet aggregation and clotting, are secreted.

2. PLATELET ACTIVATION

Three fundamental mechanisms are involved in platelet function during blood coagulation: adhesion, aggregation, and secretion. Adhesion sets off a series of reactions termed platelet activation, which leads to platelet aggregation and secretion of platelet granule contents.

The adhesion step refers primarily to the platelet–subendothelial interaction that occurs when platelets initially adhere to the sites of blood vessel injury (Fig. 45.1). Blood vessel injury exposes collagen, subendothelial matrix-bound vWF, and other matrix components. vWF is a protein synthesized in endothelial cells and megakaryocytes, and is located in the subendothelial matrix, in specific platelet granules, in the circulation bound to Factor VIII. The platelet cell membrane contains glycoproteins (GPs) that bind to collagen and to vWF, causing the platelet

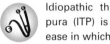 Platelets are derived from megakaryocytes in the bone marrow. Megakaryocytes differentiate from the hematopoietic stem cell. As the megakaryocyte matures, it undergoes synchronous nuclear replication without cellular division, to form a cell with a multilobed nucleus and enlarged cytoplasm. At approximately the 8-nucleus stage, the cytoplasm becomes granular, and the platelets are budded off the cytoplasm. A single megakaryocyte gives rise to approximately 4,000 platelets.

Idiopathic thrombocytopenic purpura (ITP) is an autoimmune disease in which antibodies to platelet glycoproteins are produced. Antibody binding to platelets results in their clearance by the spleen. An early symptom of the disorder is the appearance of small red spots on the skin (petechial hemorrhages) caused by blood leakage from capillaries. Minor damage to vascular endothelial cells is constantly being caused by mechanical forces related to blood flow. In patients with ITP, few platelets are available to repair the damage.

Von Willebrand factor is a large multimeric glycoprotein with a subunit molecular weight of 220,000 daltons. Its size in the circulation ranges between 500 and 20,000 kDa, and its role in circulation is to stabilize Factor VIII and protect it from degradation. The high-molecular-weight forms are concentrated in the endothelium of blood vessels and are released in response to stress hormones and endothelial damage. High-molecular-weight vWF released by the endothelium is cleaved by a specific metalloprotease in the serum, reducing the size of the circulating vWF. Large vWF multimers are more effective at forming complexes with platelets than are small vWF multimers.

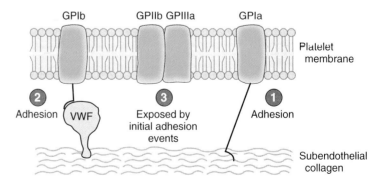

Fig. 45.1. Adhesion of platelets to the subendothelial cell layer. 1. GPIa initially binds to the exposed collagen, which results in changes in the three-dimensional configuration of the complex, allowing GPIb to bind to vWF (2). 3. This second binding event exposes the GPIIb/GPIIIa complex, which also can bind to vWF and fibrinogen.

to adhere to the subendothelium. Binding to collagen by GPIa (integrin α2β1) causes the platelet to change its shape from a flat disc to a spherical cell. The latter extrudes long pseudopods, which promote platelet/platelet interactions. Binding of subendothelial vWF by GPIb causes changes in the platelet membrane that expose GPIIb/IIIa (integrin αIIbβ3) binding sites to fibrinogen and vWF.

The initial adherence of platelets sets off a series of reactions (platelet activation) that results in more platelets being recruited and aggregated at the site of injury. After initial adherence, some of the platelets release the contents of their dense granules and their α granules, with ADP release being of particular importance because ADP is a potent platelet activator. ADP released from the platelets and from damaged red blood cells binds to a receptor on the platelet membrane, which leads to the further unmasking of GPIIb/IIIa binding sites. Aggregation of platelets cannot take place without ADP stimulation, because ADP induces swelling of the activated platelets, promoting platelet/platelet contact and adherence.

Fibrinogen is a protein that circulates in the blood and is also found in platelet granules. It consists of two triple helices held together with disulfide bonds. (Fig.45.2) Binding of fibrinogen to activated platelets is necessary for aggregation,

 vWF deficiency is the most common cause of inherited bleeding disorders. Both platelet adherence and the clotting cascade are affected because levels of Factor VIII are low. In the absence of vWF, Factor VIII is rapidly cleared from the system. The vWF gene is large, covering approximately 180 kb, and contains 52 exons. Multiple mutations are known, with varying clinical presentations.

 Defects in GPIb cause a bleeding disorder known as Bernard-Soulier syndrome. Platelet aggregation is affected, because of the inability of GPIb to adhere to subendothelial vWF.

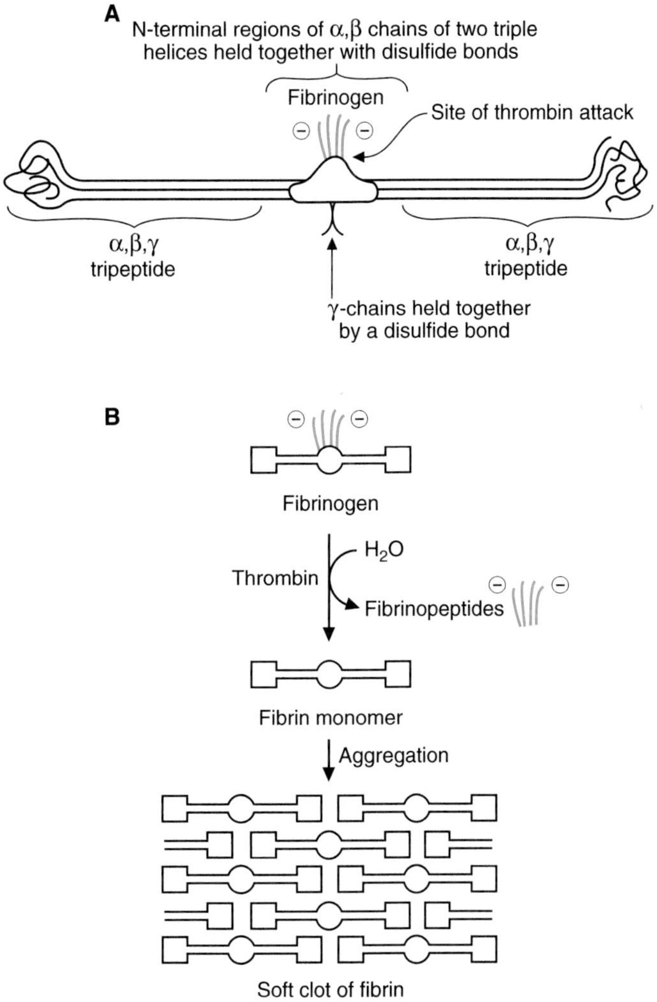

A

N-terminal regions of α,β chains of two triple helices held together with disulfide bonds

Fibrinogen

⊖ ⦀ ⊖

Site of thrombin attack

α,β,γ
tripeptide

α,β,γ
tripeptide

γ-chains held together
by a disulfide bond

B

⊖ ⦀ ⊖

Fibrinogen

Thrombin

H₂O

Fibrinopeptides ⊖ ⦀ ⊖

Fibrin monomer

Aggregation

Soft clot of fibrin

Fig. 45.2. Cleavage of fibrinogen results in clot formation. A. Fibrinogen, the precursor protein of fibrin, is formed from two triple helices joined together at their N-terminal ends. The α, β peptides are held together by disulfide bonds, and the γ-peptides are joined to each other by disulfide bonds. The terminal α, β peptide regions, shown in blue, contain negatively charged glutamate and aspartate residues that repel each other and prevent aggregation. B. Thrombin, a serine protease, cleaves the terminal portions of fibrinogen containing negative charges. The fibrin monomers can then aggregate and form a "soft" clot. The soft clot is then subsequently cross-linked by another enzyme.

Thrombotic thrombocytopenic purpura (TTP) is a disease characterized by the formation in the circulation of microclots (microthrombi) consisting of aggregated platelets. The microthrombi collect in the microvasculature and damage red blood cells, resulting in hemolytic anemia. They also damage vascular endothelium, exposing collagen and releasing high-molecular-weight vWF, promoting more platelet aggregation. The subsequent depletion of platelets renders the patient susceptible to internal hemorrhage. Mortality in untreated TTP can approach 90%.

Familial TTP is associated with mutations in the vWF-specific metalloprotease, although not all individuals with defective protease develop TTP. Sporadic cases of TTP are associated with the development of an antibody to the metalloprotease.

In response to collagen and thrombin, platelets release vasoconstrictors. Serotonin is released from the dense granules of the platelets, and the synthesis of thromboxane A2 is stimulated. This will reduce blood flow to the damaged area. Platelet-derived growth factor, which stimulates proliferation of vascular cells, is also released into the environment surrounding the damage.

The utilization of an active site serine to cleave a peptide bond is common to a variety of enzymes referred to as serine proteases. Serine proteases are essential for activating the formation of a blood clot from fibrin. Fibrin and many of the other proteins involved in blood coagulation are present in the blood as inactive precursors or zymogens, which must be activated by proteolytic cleavage. Thrombin, the serine protease that converts fibrinogen to fibrin, has the same aspartate-histidine-serine catalytic triad found in chymotrypsin and trypsin.

Thrombin is activated by proteolytic cleavage of its precursor protein, prothrombin. The sequence of proteolytic cleavages leading to thrombin activation requires Factor VIII, the blood-clotting protein deficient in **Sloe Klotter.**

providing, in part, the mechanism by which platelets adhere to one another. Cleavage of fibrinogen by thrombin (a protease that is activated by the coagulation cascade) produces fibrin monomers that polymerize and, together with platelets, form a "soft clot". Thrombin itself is a potent activator of platelets, through binding to a specific receptor on the platelet surface.

B. The Blood Coagulation Cascade

Thrombus (clot) formation is enhanced by thrombin activation, which is mediated by the complex interaction that constitutes the blood coagulation cascade. This cascade (Fig. 45.3) consists primarily of proteins that serve as enzymes or cofactors, which function to accelerate thrombin formation and localize it at the site of injury. These proteins are listed in Table 45.2. All of these proteins are present in the plasma as proproteins (zymogens). These precursor proteins are activated by cleavage of the polypeptide chain at one or more sites. The key to successful and appropriate thrombus formation is the regulation of the proteases that activate these zymogens.

The proenzymes (Factors VII, XI, IX, X, XII, and prothrombin) are serine proteases that, when activated by cleavage, cleave the next proenzyme in the cascade. Because of the sequential activation, a great acceleration and amplification of the response is achieved. That cleavage and activation have occurred is indicated by the addition of an "a" to the name of the proenzyme (e.g., Factor IX is cleaved to form the active Factor IXa).

The cofactor proteins (tissue factor, Factors V and VIII) serve as binding sites for other factors. Tissue factor is not related structurally to the other blood coagulation cofactors and is an integral membrane protein that does not require cleavage for active function. Factors V and VIII serve as procofactors, which, when activated by cleavage, function as binding sites for other factors.

Two additional proteins that are considered part of the blood coagulation cascade, protein S and protein C, are regulatory proteins. Only protein C is regulated by proteolytic cleavage, and when activated, is itself a serine protease.

C. The Process of Blood Coagulation

Activation of the blood coagulation cascade is triggered by the reaction of plasma proteins with the subendothelium at the same time that platelets are adhering to the subendothelial layer. Historically, two different pathways were discovered, one dependent on external stimuli (such as blunt trauma, which initiates the extrinsic pathway) and one using internal stimuli (the intrinsic pathway). As our understanding of blood clotting has expanded, it has become obvious that these distinctions are no longer correct, because there is overlap between the pathways, but the terms have persisted in the description of the pathways.

In the case of external trauma, damaged tissues present tissue factor to the blood at the injured site, thereby triggering the extrinsic phase of blood coagulation. Circulating Factor VII binds to tissue factor, which autocatalyzes its own activation to Factor VIIa. Factor VIIa then activates Factor X (to Xa) in the extrinsic pathway and Factor IX (to IXa) in the intrinsic pathway. Factor IXa, as part of the intrinsic pathway, also activates Factor X. Therefore, activation of both the extrinsic and intrinsic pathways result in the conversion of Factor X to Factor Xa. All of these conversions require access to membranes and calcium; the platelet membrane, which had adhered to the damaged site, is used as a scaffold for the activation reactions to occur. The γ-carboxylated clotting proteins are chelated to membrane surfaces via electrostatic interactions with calcium and negatively charged phospholipids of the platelet membrane. The protein cofactors VIIIa and Va serve as sites for assembling enzyme–cofactor complexes on the platelet surface, thereby accelerating and localizing the reaction. The result is thrombin formation, which augments its own formation by converting Factors V, VIII, and XI into activated cofactors and

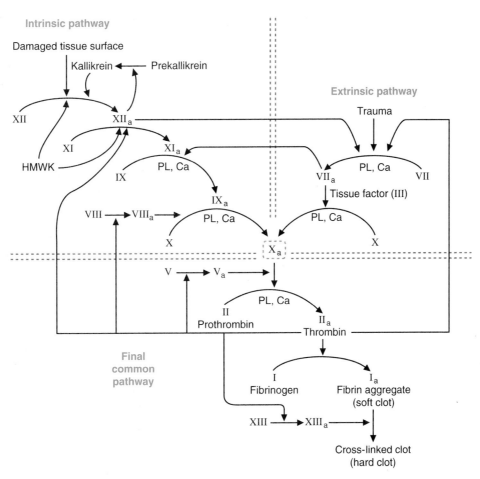

Fig. 45.3. Blood coagulation cascade. Activation of clot formation occurs through two separate but interlocking pathways, termed the intrinsic and extrinsic pathways. The intrinsic pathway is activated when plasma proteins react with the exposed subendothelium of the damaged blood vessel. Platelets and vWF bind to the exposed subendothelium, and the platelets, in turn, bind fibrinogen. The extrinsic pathway is activated by tissue factor. The reactions designated by "PL, Ca" are occurring through cofactors bound to phospholipids (PL) on the cell surface in a Ca^{2+}-coordination complex. Factors XIIa, XIa, IXa, VIIa, Xa, and thrombin are serine proteases. Note the positive feedback regulation of thrombin on the activation of proteases earlier in the cascade sequence. HMWK = high-molecular-weight kininogen.

Table 45.2. Proteins of Blood Coagulation

Coagulation Factors		
Factor	**Descriptive Name**	**Function/Active Form**
I	Fibrinogen	Fibrin
II	Prothrombin	Serine protease
III	Tissue factor	Receptor and cofactor
IV	Ca^{+2}	Cofactor
V	Proaccelerin, labile factor	Cofactor
VII	Proconvertin	Serine protease
VIII	Antihemophilia factor A	Cofactor
IX	Antihemophilia factor B, Christmas factor	Serine protease
X	Stuart-Prower factor	Serine protease
XI	Plasma thromboplastin antecedent	Serine protease
XII	Hageman (contact) factor	Serine protease
XIII	Fibrin stabilizing factor	Ca^{2+}-dependent transglutaminase
Prekallikrein		Serine protease
High-molecular-weight kininogen		Cofactor
Regulatory Proteins		
Thrombomodulin	Endothelial cell receptor, binds thrombin	
Protein C	Activated by thrombomodulin-bound thrombin; is a serine protease	
Protein S	cofactor; binds activated protein C	

The initial activation of prothrombin to thrombin is slow, because the activator cofactors, Factors VIIIa and Va, are only present in small amounts. However, once a small amount of thrombin is activated, it will accelerate its own production by cleaving Factors V and VIII to their active forms.

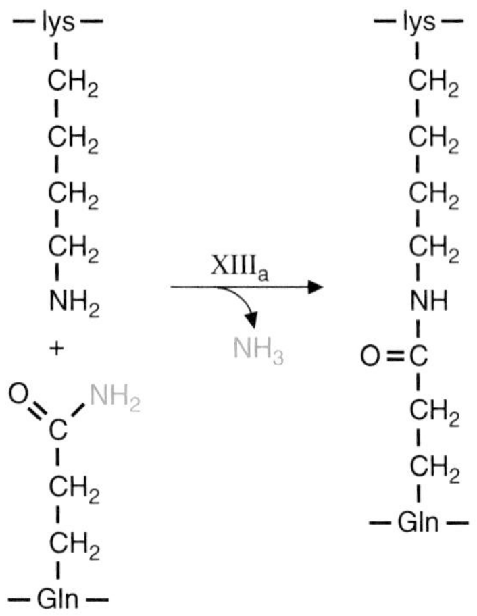

Fig. 45.4. The transamidation reaction catalyzed by Factor XIIIa, transglutaminase. This reaction cross-links fibrin monomers, allowing "hard" clots to form.

stimulating platelet degranulation. Note that these factors are in the intrinsic pathway. The intrinsic pathway is thought to sustain the coagulation response initiated by the extrinsic pathway. The major substrate of thrombin is fibrinogen, which is hydrolyzed to form fibrin monomers that undergo spontaneous polymerization to form the fibrin clot. This is considered a "soft" clot because the fibrin monomers are not cross-linked. Cross-linking requires Factor XIIIa, which is activated by thrombin cleavage of Factor XIII.

1. CROSS-LINKING OF FIBRIN

Factor XIIIa catalyzes a transamidation reaction between Gln and Lys side chains on adjacent fibrin monomers. The covalent cross-linking takes place in three dimensions, creating a strong network of fibers resistant to mechanical and proteolytic damage. This network of fibrin fibers traps the aggregated platelets and other cells, forming the clot that plugs the vent in the vascular wall. (Fig. 45.4) Factor XIIIa is the only enzyme in the blood coagulation cascade that is not a serine protease.

2. KALLIKREIN AND HIGH-MOLECULAR-WEIGHT KININOGEN (HMWK)

The classical intrinsic pathway begins with the assembly of prekallikrein, high-molecular-weight kininogen (HMWK), Factor XII, and Factor XI on a negatively charged surface, presumably an endothelial cell in vivo (see Fig. 45.3). High-molecular-weight kininogen is a glycoprotein that binds prekallikrein and aids in its assembly on the endothelial cell. Prekallikrein is the zymogen form of a serine protease. Factor XII autoactivates, forming Factor XIIa, which converts prekallikrein to kallikrein. Kallikrein then enhances the activation of Factor XII, which leads to the activation of Factors XI and VII.

How important these steps are in the initiation of the coagulation cascade is unknown. Individuals lacking HMWK, prekallikrein, or Factor XII do not suffer from bleeding disorders. Under usual conditions, activation of Factor VII with subsequent activation of Factors IX and X is thought to be sufficient to activate the coagulation pathway.

3. FACTOR COMPLEXES

In several of the essential steps in the blood coagulation cascade, the activated protease is bound in a complex attached to the surface of the platelets that have aggregated at the site of injury. Factors VII, IX, X, and prothrombin contain a domain in which one or more glutamate residues are carboxylated to γ-carboxyglutamate in a reaction requiring vitamin K (Fig 45.5). Prothrombin and Factor X both contain 10 or more γ-carboxyglutamate residues that bind Ca^{2+}. Ca^{2+} forms a coordination complex with the negatively charged platelet membrane phospholipids and the γ-carboxyglutamates, thereby localizing the complex assembly and thrombin formation to the platelet surface.

Cofactor Va contains a binding site for both Factor Xa and prothrombin, the zymogen substrate of Factor Xa. On binding to the Factor Va–platelet complex, prothrombin undergoes a conformational change, rendering it more susceptible to enzymatic cleavage. Binding of Factor Xa to the Factor Va–prothrombin–platelet complex allows the prothrombin-to-thrombin conversion. Complex assembly accelerates the rate of this conversion 10,000- to 15,000-fold as compared with non–complex formation.

Factor VIIIa forms a similar type of complex on the surface of activated platelets, but binds Factor IXa and its zymogen substrate, Factor X. Tissue factor works slightly differently because it is an integral membrane protein. However, once exposed by injury, it also binds Factor VIIa and initiates complex formation.

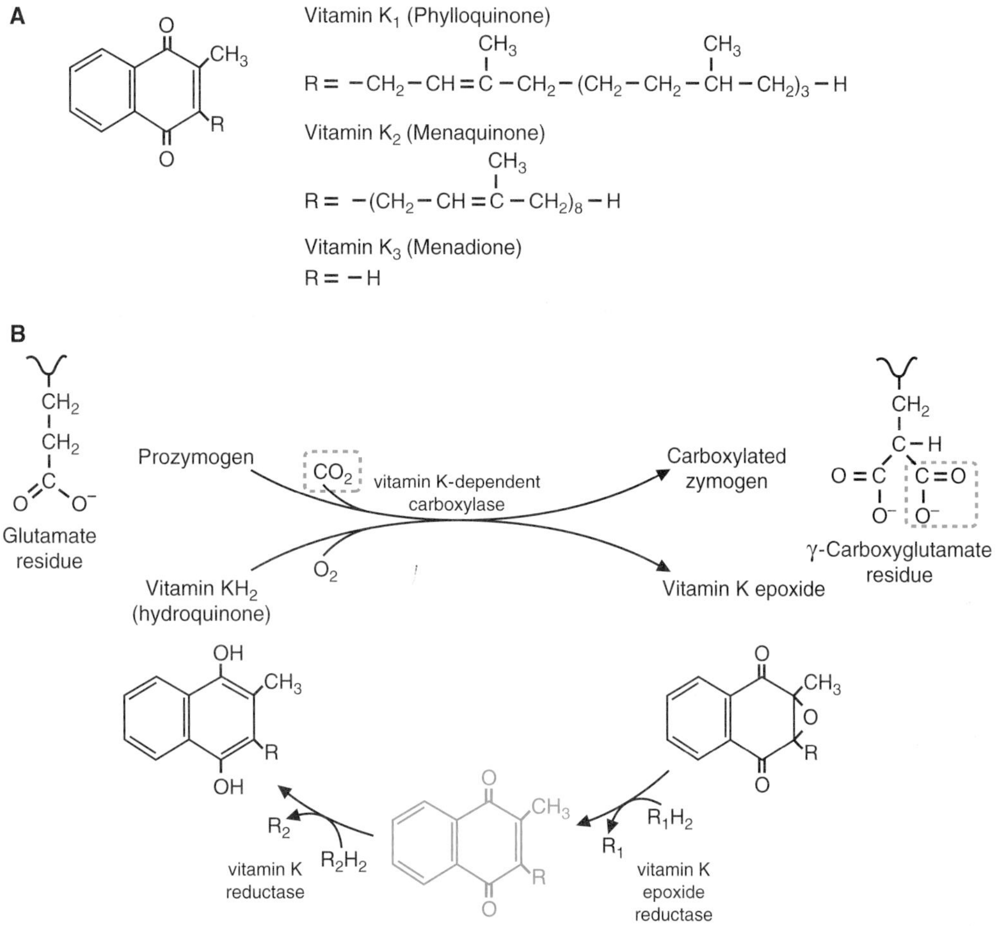

Fig. 45.5. A. Structures of vitamin K derivatives. Phylloquinone is found in green leaves, and intestinal bacteria synthesize menaquinone. Humans will convert menadione to a vitamin K active form. B. Vitamin K–dependent formation of γ-carboxyglutamate residues. Thrombin, Factor VII, Factor IX, and Factor X are bound to their phospholipid activation sites on cell membranes by Ca^{2+}. The vitamin K–dependent carboxylase, which adds the extra carboxyl group, uses a reduced form of vitamin K (KH_2) as the electron donor and converts vitamin K to an epoxide. Vitamin K epoxide is reduced, in two steps, back to its active form by the enzymes vitamin K epoxide reductase and vitamin K reductase.

Complex assembly has two physiologically important consequences. First, it enhances the rate of thrombin formation by as much as several hundred thousand-fold, enabling the clot to form rapidly enough to preserve hemostasis. Secondly, such explosive thrombin formation is localized to the site of vascular injury at which the negatively charged phospholipids are exposed. From our knowledge of the location of such phospholipids in cellular and subcellular organelle membranes, these surface-binding sites are only exposed at an injury site in which cell rupture exposes the internal membrane surface (recall that certain phospholipids only face the cytoplasm; if these lipids are now exposed to the environment, substantial cell damage must have occurred).

4. VITAMIN K REQUIREMENT FOR BLOOD COAGULATION

The formation of the γ-carboxyglutamate residues on blood coagulation factors takes place in the hepatocyte before release of the protein. Within the hepatocyte, vitamin K (which is present in the quinone form) is reduced to form vitamin KH_2 by a microsomal quinone reductase (see Fig.45.5). Vitamin KH_2 is a cofactor for carboxylases that add a carboxyl group to the appropriate glutamate residues in the proenzyme to form the carboxylated proenzyme (e.g., prothrombin). In the same

Warfarin (Coumadin®) is a slow- and long-acting blood anticoagulant with a structure resembling that of vitamin K. The structural similarity allows the compound to compete with vitamin K and prevent γ-carboxylation of glutamate residues in Factors II, VII, IX, X, and proteins C and S. The noncarboxylated blood clotting protein precursors increase in both the blood and plasma, but they are unable to promote blood coagulation because they cannot bind calcium and thus cannot bind to their phospholipid membrane sites of activation.

Warfarin

Warfarin is a commonly used rat poison and thus is occasionally encountered in emergency departments in cases of accidental poisoning. It is effective as a rat poison because it takes many hours to develop pathologic symptoms, which allows one poisoned trap to kill more than one rat.

Deficiency in the amount or functionality of protein C or protein S increases the risk for venous thromboembolism. Homozygous individuals for these mutations do not survive the neonatal period unless given replacement therapy.

In European populations, a point mutation in the Factor V gene (Factor V Leiden) causes the replacement of an arg with a gln in the preferred site for cleavage by activated protein C, rendering Factor Va Leiden resistant to APC. Heterozygous individuals have a sixfold to eightfold increased risk of deep vein thromboses, and homozygous individuals have a 30- to 140-fold increased risk. The Factor V Leiden mutation does not appear to be associated with increased risk for arterial thrombosis, such as myocardial infarction, except in young women who smoke.

Genetic studies suggest that the Factor V Leiden mutation arose after the separation of the European, Asian, and African populations. The frequency of this variant indicates that it conferred some selective advantage at one time. In the developed world, inherited APC resistance is the most prevalent risk factor for familial thrombotic disease.

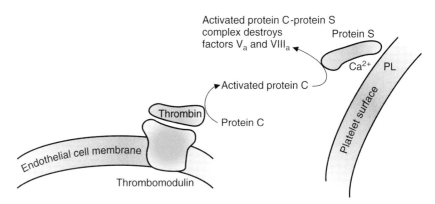

Fig. 45.6. Anti-thrombotic effects of thrombin. Thrombin, bound to thrombomodulin on the endothelial cell surface, activates protein C. Activated protein C, in complex with protein S, binds to the platelet membrane, and the activated complex destroys Factors Va and VIIIa, thereby inhibiting the coagulation cascade.

reaction, vitamin K is converted to vitamin K epoxide. To recover active vitamin KH_2, vitamin K is first reduced to the quinone form by vitamin K epoxide reductase, and then to the active hydroquinone form.

D. Regulation through Feedback Amplification and Inhibition

Once the formation of the clot (thrombus) begins, clot formation is accelerated in an almost explosive manner by a number of processes collectively termed feedback amplification.

1. THE ROLE OF THROMBIN IN REGULATION

Thrombin has both a prothrombotic regulatory role (feedback amplification) and an antithrombotic regulatory role (feedback inhibition). The prothrombotic action is initiated when thrombin stimulates its own formation by activating Factors V, VIII, and XI, thereby accelerating the rate of clot formation (see Fig. 45.3). Thrombin also promotes clot formation by activating platelet aggregation, stimulating the release of Factor VIII from vWF, and cleaving Factor XIII to Factor XIIIa.

Antithrombotic effects of thrombin result from its binding to an endothelial cell receptor called thrombomodulin (Fig. 45.6). Thrombomodulin abolishes the clotting function of thrombin and allows thrombin to activate protein C, which has anticoagulant effects.

2. PROTEINS S AND C

Protein C and its cofactor protein S serve to suppress the activity of the coagulation cascade. After activation, protein C forms a complex with protein S. Protein S anchors the activated protein C complex (APC) to the clot through Ca^{++}/γ-carboxyglutamate binding to platelet phospholipids. The APC destroys the active blood coagulation cofactors Factor VIIIa and Factor Va by proteolytic cleavage, decreasing the production of thrombin. The APC also stimulates endothelial cells to increase secretion of the prostaglandin PGI_2, which reduces platelet aggregation.

3. SERPINS

Many proteases of the blood coagulation enzyme system are serine proteases. Because uncontrolled proteolytic activity would be destructive, modulating mechanisms control and limit intravascular proteolysis. The serpins (**ser**ine **p**rotease **in**hibitors) are a group of naturally occurring inhibitory proteins present in the plasma at high concentration (approximately 10% of the plasma proteins are serpins). Eight major inhibitors have been found that share a common mechanism of action and inhibit proteases involved in coagulation and clot dissolution (fibrinolysis). Each inhibitor possesses a reactive site that appears to be an ideal substrate for a specific serine protease and thus acts as a trap for that protease. The bound serine protease attacks a peptide bond located at a critical amino acid residue within the serpin and forms a tight enzyme–inhibitor complex.

The activity of thrombin is controlled by the serpin antithrombin III (ATIII). Regulation of blood coagulation at the level of thrombin is critical because this enzyme affects the pathways of both coagulation and fibrinolysis (see section F). One molecule of ATIII irreversibly inactivates one molecule of thrombin through reaction of an arginine residue in ATIII with the active-site serine residue of thrombin. ATIII–thrombin complex formation is markedly enhanced in the presence of heparin. Heparin is a glycosaminoglycan (see Chapter 49) found in the secretory granules of mast cells and in the loose connective tissue around small vascular beds. Heparin binds to lysyl residues on ATIII and dramatically accelerates its rate of binding to thrombin. This is because of an allosteric alteration in ATIII such that the position of the critical arginine residue of ATIII is more readily available for interaction with thrombin. The formation of the ATIII–thrombin complex releases the heparin molecule so that it can be reused, and therefore, the function of heparin is catalytic. Thrombin that is attached to a surface, for example, to thrombomodulin on the endothelial cell membrane, is no longer participating in clot formation and is not readily attacked by ATIII or the ATIII–heparin complex. The ATIII–heparin complex also can inactivate the serine protease Factors XIIIa, XIa, IXa and Xa, but has no effect on Factor VIIa or activated protein C.

E. Thromboresistance of Vascular Endothelium

Endothelial cells of blood vessels provide a selectively permeable barrier between the circulating blood and the tissues. The normal endothelial cell lining neither activates coagulation nor supports platelet adhesion; thus, it is called a nonthrombogenic surface. The thromboresistance of normal vascular endothelium is contributed to by several properties. Endothelial cells are highly negatively charged, a feature that may repel the negatively charged platelets. Endothelial cells synthesize prostaglandin I_2 (PGI_2) and nitric oxide, vasodilators and powerful inhibitors of platelet aggregation. PGI_2 synthesis is stimulated by thrombin, epinephrine, and local vascular injury. Endothelial cells also synthesize two cofactors that each inhibit the action of thrombin, thrombomodulin and heparan sulfate. Heparan sulfate is a glycosaminoglycan similar to heparin that potentiates antithrombin III, but not as efficiently. The inactivation of thrombin is accelerated by heparan sulfate present on the endothelial cell surface. Thus, the intact endothelium has the capability of modifying thrombin action and inhibiting platelet aggregation.

F. Fibrinolysis

After successful formation of a hemostatic plug, further propagation of the clot must be prevented. This is accomplished in part by switching off blood coagulation and in part by turning on fibrinolysis. Fibrinolysis involves the degradation of fibrin in a clot by plasmin, a serine protease that is formed from its zymogen, plasminogen. Plasminogen is a circulating serum protein that has a high affinity for fibrin, promoting the incorporation of plasminogen in the developing clot. The activity of plasminogen is mediated by proteins known as plasminogen activators. The conversion of plasminogen to plasmin by plasminogen activators can occur both in the liquid phase of the blood and at the clot surface; however, the latter process is by

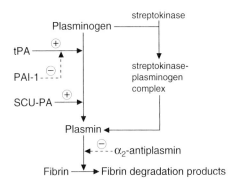

Fig. 45.7. Regulation of plasmin activation. Plasminogen can be activated by either t-PA or scu-PA (+). PAI-1 blocks t-PA action (−). Streptokinase binding to plasminogen allows autocatalysis to form plasmin. Circulating α2-antiplasmin blocks (−) the activity of any soluble plasmin that may be in the blood.

Both streptokinase and t-PA have been approved for the treatment of myocardial infarction. Both reduce mortality. Although there are more side effects associated with the use of streptokinase, it is substantially cheaper than t-PA.

far more efficient. Activated protein C (APC), in addition to turning off the blood coagulation cascade, also stimulates the release of plasminogen activator from tissues (t-PA, tissue plasminogen activator) and simultaneously inactivates an inhibitor of plasminogen activator, PAI-1.

Plasminogen activator release can lead to plasmin formation in the circulation. However, the circulating plasmin is rapidly inactivated by binding with α2-antiplasmin, a circulating protease inhibitor. Clot-bound plasmin is not readily inactivated by α-antiplasmin. Thus, plasminogen binding to fibrin facilitates its activation to plasmin, protects it from blood serpins, and localizes it on the fibrin substrate for subsequent efficient proteolytic attack. This mechanism allows for dissolution of fibrin in pathologic thrombi or oversized hemostatic plugs, and at the same time prevents degradation of fibrinogen in the circulating blood.

Two endogenous plasminogen activators are most important; both are synthesized in a variety of cells. Tissue plasminogen activator (t-PA) is chiefly produced by the vascular endothelial cells, has a high binding affinity for fibrin, and plays a major role in fibrinolysis. Single-chain urokinase (scu-PA), is synthesized in most cells and tissues and has a moderate affinity for fibrin. Streptokinase, the bacterial exogenous plasminogen activator from β-hemolytic streptococci, is not an enzyme but an allosteric modifier of human plasminogen that allows an autocatalytic reaction such that plasmin is formed. In vivo, physical stress, hypoxia, and large numbers of low-molecular-weight organic compounds promote increased synthesis and release of t-PA and scu-PA from tissues into the blood. The balance between release of plasminogen activators, the availability of fibrin, and inhibitors of the activators and plasmin determines regulation of the fibrinolytic response, as indicated in Figure 45.7.

G. Regulation of Fibrinolysis

Anti-activators regulate interaction of plasminogen in blood with plasminogen activators in a dynamic equilibrium. Even if minute amounts of plasmin are generated (e.g., after release of vascular plasminogen activator after stress), the enzyme is probably inactivated by antiplasmin. On activation of the blood coagulation system, a fibrin clot is formed, which not only strongly binds t-PA and plasminogen from blood but also accelerates the rate of plasmin activation. The clot-bound plasmin is protected from inhibitors while attached to fibrin. The enzyme is inactivated by α2-antiplasmin and α2-macroglobulin after proteolytic dissolution of fibrin and its liberation into the liquid phase of blood. Thus, the fibrin network catalyzes both initiation and regulation of fibrinolysis.

CLINICAL COMMENTS

Sloe Klotter has hemophilia A, the most frequently encountered serious disorder of blood coagulation in humans, occurring in 1 in every 10,000 males. The disease is transmitted with an X-linked pattern of inheritance.

The most common manifestations of hemophilia A are those caused by bleeding into soft tissues (hematomas) such as muscle or into body spaces such as the peritoneal cavity or the lumen of the gastrointestinal tract. When bleeding occurs repeatedly into joints (hemarthrosis), the joint may eventually become deformed and immobile.

In the past, bleeding episodes have been managed primarily by administration of Factor VIII, sometimes referred to as antihemophilia cofactor. Unfortunately, the concentration of Factor VIII in plasma is quite low (0.3 nM compared with 8,800 nM for fibrinogen), requiring that it be prepared from multiple human donors. Before donor screening and virus inactivation procedures during preparation essentially eliminated transmission with blood transfusions, more than 50% of hemophiliac patients treated with Factor VIII during the 1980s in Western Europe or North America became infected with HIV. Recombinant Factor VIII is now available for clinical use.

Another X-linked bleeding disorder is hemophilia B, which is caused by mutations in the gene for Factor IX. Lack of Factor IX activity leads to an inability to convert prothrombin to thrombin, and impaired clotting.

BIOCHEMICAL COMMENTS

A number of drugs have been developed that inhibit the blood coagulation cascade. Such drugs are useful in cases in which patients develop spontaneous thrombi, which, if left untreated, would result in a fatal pulmonary embolism. There are three major classes of such drugs; the heparins, vitamin K antagonists, and specific inhibitors of thrombin.

Heparin will bind to and activate ATIII, which leads to thrombin inactivation. ATIII also blocks the activity of Factors VIIIa, IXa, Xa, and XIa. Heparin can be administered in either of two forms: unfractionated, or high-molecular-weight (HMW) heparin, and fractionated, or low-molecular-weight (LMW) heparin. HMW heparin is a heterogenous mixture of glycosaminoglycans, with an average chain length of 45 monosaccharides with an average molecular weight of 15 kDa (the range is 3–30 kDa). LMW heparins are fragments of HMW heparin, containing fewer than 18 monosaccharides with an average molecular weight of 4 to 5 kDa.

HMW heparin will bind to plasma proteins and cell surfaces in addition to its prime target, ATIII. Because different individuals synthesize different levels of plasma proteins, the use of this form of heparin as an anticoagulant requires constant monitoring of the patient to ensure that the correct dosage has been given such that spontaneous thrombi do not develop, but not so much that spontaneous bleeding occurs. LMW heparin has fewer nonspecific interactions than HMW heparin, and its effects are easier to predict on patients, so that constant monitoring is not required.

A major complication of heparin therapy is heparin-induced thrombocytopenia (HIT, excessive blood clotting with a reduction in the number of circulating platelets). This unexpected result of heparin treatment is caused by heparin binding to a platelet protein, platelet factor 4 (PF4), which induces a conformational change in PF4 such that the immune system believes the complex is foreign. Thus, antibodies are developed against the heparin–PF4 complex. When the antibodies bind to the platelets, the platelets become activated, and thrombi develop. Treatment consists of removing the heparin and using a different form of anti-thrombotic agent.

The classic vitamin K antagonist is warfarin. Warfarin acts by blocking the vitamin K reductase enzymes required to regenerate active vitamin K (see Fig. 45.5). This results in reduced γ-carboxylation of Factors II, VII, IX, and X. In the absence of γ-carboxylation, the factors cannot bind calcium nor form the complexes necessary for the coagulation cascade to be initiated. However, warfarin also blocks the activity of proteins S and C, so both blood clotting and the regulation of clotting are impaired by warfarin administration.

Both heparin and warfarin therapy suffer from their lack of specificity, so drugs specific for single steps in the blood coagulation pathway have been sought and identified. Analysis of heparin potentiation of Factor Xa binding to ATIII showed that a unique pentasaccharide sequence was required. An appropriate pentasaccharide, named fondaparinux, was developed that would specifically enhance ATIII interactions with Factor Xa (Fig. 45.8). Fondaparinux stimulates the binding of ATIII to Factor Xa by 300-fold and is specific for Factor Xa inhibition. Fondaparinux does not affect thrombin or platelet activity, and it is not an activating agent of platelets. Because fondaparinux does not bind to PF4, HIT is not a complication with this therapy.

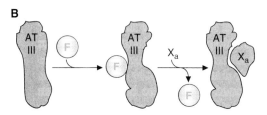

Fig. 45.8. A. Structure of fondaparinux. B. Mechanism of fondaparinux action. The drug (shown in blue) binds to ATIII, which induces a conformational change such that Factor Xa can now bind to ATIII. Once Factor Xa binds, and is inactivated, the drug is released and can activate another molecule of ATIII.

Direct thrombin inhibitors are based on the hirudin molecules, which were initially discovered in leeches and other blood-sucking organisms. These organisms would not be able to feed if the blood clotted at the site of the puncture wound, so the organisms secrete thrombin inhibitors to prevent clotting from occurring. Hirudin treatment itself is dangerous in that formation of the hirudin–thrombin complex is irreversible, and use of the drug requires constant monitoring of the patient. Thus, to overcome this problem, rational drug design based on the hirudin structure was used, and a synthetic 20–amino acid peptide known as bivalirudin was synthesized. This agent has a high binding affinity and specificity for thrombin although its effects on thrombin are transient (not irreversible), making this a safer agent for long-term use.

Suggested References

Bauer KA. Selective inhibition of coagulation factors: advances in antithrombotic therapy. Seminars in Thrombosis and Hemostasis 2002;28:15–24.

Robetorye RS, Rodgers GM. Update on selected inherited venous thrombotic disorders. Am J Hematol 2001;68:256–268.

 REVIEW QUESTIONS—CHAPTER 45

1. The edema observed in patients with non-calorie protein malnutrition is due to which of the following?

   (A) Loss of muscle mass
   (B) Ingestion of excess carbohydrates
   (C) Increased fluid uptake
   (D) Reduced protein synthesis in the liver
   (E) Increased ketone body production

2. A recent surgery patient receiving warfarin therapy was found to be bleeding internally. The clotting process is impaired in this patient primarily because of which of the following?

   (A) Inability of the liver to synthesize clotting factors
   (B) A specific inhibition of Factor XIII activation
   (C) An inability to form clotting factor complexes on membranes
   (D) A reduction of plasma calcium levels
   (E) An enhancement of protein C activity

3. An inactivating mutation in which of the following proenzymes would be expected to lead to thrombosis, uncontrolled blood clotting?

   (A) Factor XIII
   (B) Prothrombin
   (C) Protein C
   (D) Factor VIII
   (E) Tissue factor

4. Classical hemophilia A results in an inability to directly activate which of the following factors?

   (A) Factor II
   (B) Factor IX
   (C) Factor X
   (D) Protein S
   (E) Protein C

5. Hemophilia B results in an inability to directly activate which of the following factors?

   (A) Factor II
   (B) Factor IX
   (C) Factor X
   (D) Protein S
   (E) Protein C

46 Liver Metabolism

*The liver is strategically interposed between the general circulation and the digestive tract. It receives 20 to 25% of the volume of blood leaving the heart each minute (the cardiac output) through the portal vein (which delivers absorbed nutrients and other substances from the gastrointestinal tract to the liver) and through the hepatic artery (which delivers blood from the general circulation back to the liver). Potentially toxic agents absorbed from the gut or delivered to the liver by the hepatic artery must pass through this **metabolically active organ** before they can reach the other organs of the body. The liver's relatively large size (approximately 3% of total body weight) allows extended residence time within the liver for nutrients to be properly metabolized as well as for potentially harmful substances to be detoxified and prepared for excretion into the urine or feces. Among other functions, therefore, the liver, along with the kidney and gut, is an **excretory organ**, equipped with a broad spectrum of detoxifying mechanisms. It has the capacity, for example, to carry out **metabolic conversion pathways** as well as **secretory systems** that allow the excretion of potentially toxic compounds. Concurrently, the liver contains highly specific and selective **transport mechanisms** for essential nutrients that are required not only to sustain its own energy but to provide physiologically important substrates for the systemic needs of the organism. In addition to the myriad of transport processes within the sinusoidal and canalicular plasma membrane sheets (see below), intracellular hepatocytic transport systems exist in organelles such as **endosomes, mitochondria, lysosomes,** as well as the **nucleus**. The sequential transport steps carried out by these organelles include (1) **uptake**, (2) **intracellular binding and sequestration**, (3) **metabolism**, (4) **sinusoidal secretion**, and (5) **biliary excretion**. The rate of hepatobiliary transport is determined, in part, by the rate of activity of each of these steps. The overall transport rate is also determined by such factors as hepatic blood flow, plasma protein binding, and the rate of canalicular reabsorption. The various aspects of the major metabolic processes performed by the liver have been discussed in greater detail elsewhere in this text. These sources are referred to as the broad spectrum of the liver's contributions to overall health and disease are described.*

THE WAITING ROOM

 Jean Ann Tonich's family difficulties continued, and, in spite of a period of sobriety lasting 6 months, she eventually started drinking increasing amounts of gin again in an effort to deal with her many anxieties. Her appetite for food declined slowly as well. She gradually withdrew from much of the social support system that her doctors and friends had attempted to build during her efforts for rehabilitation. Upper mid-abdominal pain became almost constant, and she noted an increasing girth and distention of her abdomen. Early one morning, she was awakened in excruciating pain in her upper abdomen. She vomited dark-brown "coffee ground" material followed by copious amounts of bright red blood. She called a friend, who rushed her to the hospital emergency room.

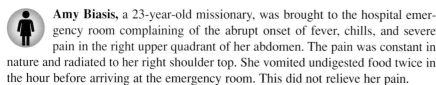 **Amy Biasis,** a 23-year-old missionary, was brought to the hospital emergency room complaining of the abrupt onset of fever, chills, and severe pain in the right upper quadrant of her abdomen. The pain was constant in nature and radiated to her right shoulder top. She vomited undigested food twice in the hour before arriving at the emergency room. This did not relieve her pain.

Her medical history indicated that, while serving as a missionary in western Belise, Central America, 2 months earlier, she had a 3-day illness that included fever, chills, and mild but persistent diarrhea. A friend of Amy's there, a medical missionary, had given her an unidentified medication for 7 days. Amy's diarrhea slowly resolved, and she felt well again until her current abdominal symptoms began.

On physical examination, she appeared toxic and had a temperature of 101°F. She was sweating profusely. Her inferior anterior liver margin was palpable three fingerbreadths below the right rib cage, suggestive of an enlarged liver. The liver edge was rounded and tender. Gentle first percussion of the lower posterior right rib cage caused severe pain. Routine laboratory studies were ordered, and a computed tomogram (CT) of the upper abdomen was scheduled to be done immediately.

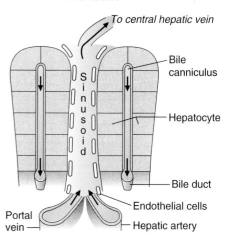

Liver lobule

Fig. 46.1. Schematic view of liver anatomy.

I. LIVER ANATOMY

The human liver consists of two lobes, each containing multiple lobules and sinusoids. The liver receives 75% of its blood supply from the portal vein, which carries blood returning to the heart from the small intestine, stomach, pancreas and spleen. The remaining 25% of the liver's blood supply is arterial, carried to the liver by the hepatic artery.

Blood from both the portal vein and hepatic artery empty into a common conduit, mixing their contents as they enter the liver sinusoids (Fig. 46.1). The sinusoids are expandable vascular channels that run through the hepatic lobules. They are lined with endothelial cells that have been described as "leaky" because, as blood flows through the sinusoids, the contents of the plasma have relatively free access to the hepatocytes, which are located on the other side of the endothelial cells.

The liver is also an exocrine organ, secreting bile into the biliary drainage system. The hepatocytes secrete bile into the bile canniculus, whose contents flow parallel to that in the sinusoids but in the opposite direction. The canniculi empty into the bile ducts. The lumina of the bile ducts then fuse, forming the common bile duct. The common duct then releases bile into the duodenum. Some of the liver's effluent is stored in the gallbladder and discharged into the duodenum postprandially to aid in digestion.

The entire liver surface is covered by a capsule of connective tissue that branches and extends throughout the liver. This capsule provides support for the blood vessels, lymphatic vessels, and bile ducts that permeate the liver. In addition, this connective tissue sheet subdivides the liver lobes into the smaller lobules.

II. LIVER CELL TYPES

The primary cell type of the liver is the hepatocyte. Hepatocytes, also known as the hepatic parenchymal cells, form the liver lobules. Eighty percent of the liver volume is composed of hepatocytes, but only 60% of the total number of cells in the liver are hepatocytes. The other 40% of the cells are the nonparenchymal cells, which constitute the lining cells of the walls of the sinusoids. The lining cells comprise the endothelial cells, Kupffer cells, and hepatic stellate cells. In addition, intrahepatic lymphocytes, which include pit cells (liver-specific natural killer cells) are also present in the sinusoidal lining.

A. Hepatocytes

The hepatocyte is the cell that carries out the many functions of the liver. Almost all pathways of metabolism are represented in the hepatocyte and these pathways are controlled through the actions of hormones that bind to receptors located on the plasma membrane of their cells. Although normally quiescent cells with low turnover and a long life span, hepatocytes can be stimulated to grow if damage occurs to other cells in the liver. The liver mass has a relatively constant relationship to the total body mass of adult individuals. Deviation from the normal or optimal ratio (caused, for example, by a partial hepatectomy or significant hepatic cell death or injury) is rapidly corrected by hepatic growth caused by a proportional increase in hepatocyte replication.

The reports of **Amy Biasis'** initial laboratory studies showed an elevation in her serum hepatic transaminases, her serum alkaline phosphatases, as well as her serum total bilirubin level.

B. Endothelial Cells

The sinusoidal endothelial cells constitute the lining cells of the sinusoid. Unlike endothelial cells in other body tissues, these cells contain fenestrations with a mean diameter of 100 nm. They do not, therefore, form a tight basement membrane barrier between themselves and the hepatocytes. In this way, they allow for free diffusion of small molecules to the hepatocytes but not of particles the size of chylomicrons (chylomicron remnants, however, which are smaller than chylomicrons, do have free passage to the hepatocyte). The endothelial cells are capable of endocytosing many ligands and also may secrete cytokines when appropriately stimulated. Because of their positioning, lack of tight junctions, and absence of a tight basement membrane, the liver endothelial cells do not present a significant barrier against the movement of the contents of the sinusoids into hepatocytes. Their fenestrations or pores further promote the free passage of blood components through this membrane into the liver parenchymal cells.

C. Kupffer Cells

These cells are located within the sinusoidal lining. They contain almost one quarter of all the lysosomes of the liver. The Kupffer cells are tissue macrophages with both endocytotic and phagocytic capacity. They phagocytose many substances such as denatured albumin, bacteria, and immune complexes. They protect the liver from gut-derived particulate materials and bacterial products. On stimulation by immunomodulators, these cells secrete potent mediators of the inflammatory response and play a role in liver immune defense through the release of cytokines that lead to the inactivation of substances considered foreign to the organism. The Kupffer cells also remove damaged erythrocytes from the circulation.

D. Hepatic Stellate Cells

The stellate cells are also called perisinusoidal or Ito cells. There are approximately 5 to 20 of these cells per 100 hepatocytes. The stellate cells are lipid-filled cells (the primary storage site for vitamin A). They also control the turnover of hepatic connective tissue and extracellular matrix and regulate the contractility of the sinusoids. When cirrhosis of the liver is present, the stellate cells are stimulated by various signals to increase their synthesis of extracellular matrix material. This, in turn, diffusely infiltrates the liver, eventually interfering with the function of the hepatocytes.

E. Pit Cells

The hepatic pit cells, also known as liver-associated lymphocytes, are natural killer cells, which are a defense mechanism against the invasion of the liver by potentially toxic agents, such as tumor cells or viruses.

III. MAJOR FUNCTIONS OF THE LIVER

A. The Liver Is a Central Receiving and Recycling Center for the Body

The liver can carry out a multitude of biochemical reactions. This is necessary because of its role in constantly monitoring, recycling, modifying, and distributing all of the various compounds absorbed from the digestive tract and delivered to the liver. If any portion of an ingested compound is potentially useful to that organism, the liver will retrieve this portion and convert it to a substrate that can be used by hepatic and nonhepatic cells. At the same time, the liver removes many of the toxic compounds that are ingested or produced in the body and targets them for excretion in the urine or in the bile.

As mentioned previously, the liver receives nutrient-rich blood from the enteric circulation through the portal vein; thus, all of the compounds that enter the blood from the digestive tract pass through the liver on their way to other tissues. The enterohepatic circulation allows the liver first access to nutrients to fulfill specific functions (such as the synthesis of blood coagulation proteins, heme, purines, and pyrimidines) and first access to ingested toxic compounds (such as ethanol) and to such potentially harmful metabolic products (such as NH_4^+ produced from bacterial metabolism in the gut).

In addition to the blood supply from the portal vein, the liver receives oxygen-rich blood through the hepatic artery; this arterial blood mixes with the blood from the portal vein in the sinusoids. This unusual mixing process gives the liver access to various metabolites produced in the periphery and secreted into the peripheral circulation, such as glucose, individual amino acids, certain proteins, iron–transferrin complexes, and waste metabolites as well as potential toxins produced during substrate metabolism. As mentioned, fenestrations in the endothelial cells, combined with gaps between the cells, the lack of a basement membrane between the endothelial cells and the hepatocytes, and low portal blood pressure (which results in slow blood flow) contribute to the efficient exchange of compounds between sinusoidal blood and the hepatocyte and clearance of unwanted compounds from the blood. Thus, large molecules targeted for processing, such as serum proteins and chylomicron remnants, can be removed by hepatocytes, degraded, and their components recycled. Similarly, newly synthesized molecules, such as very-low-density lipoprotein (VLDL) and serum proteins, can be easily secreted into the blood. In addition, the liver can convert all of the amino acids found in proteins into glucose, fatty acids, or ketone bodies. The secretion of VLDL by the liver not only delivers excess calories to adipose tissue for storage of fatty acids in triacylglycerol, but it also delivers phospholipids and cholesterol to tissues that are in need of these compounds for synthesis of cell walls as well as other functions. The secretion of glycoproteins by the liver is accomplished through the liver's gluconeogenic capacity as well as its access to a variety of dietary sugars to form the oligosaccharide chains, as well as its access to dietary amino acids with which is synthesizes proteins. Thus, the liver has the capacity to carry out a large number of biosynthetic reactions. It has the biochemical wherewithal to synthesize a myriad of compounds from a broad spectrum of precursors. At the same time, the liver metabolizes compounds into biochemically useful products. Alternatively, it has the ability to degrade and excrete those compounds presented to it that cannot be further used by the body.

The CT scan of **Amy Biasis'** upper abdomen showed an elevated right hemidiaphragm as well as several cystic masses in her liver, the largest of which was located in the superior portion of the right lobe. Her clinical history as well as her history of possible exposure to various parasites while working in a part of Belize, Central America, that is known to practice substandard sanitation, prompted her physicians to order a titer of serum antibodies against the parasite *Entamoeba histolytica* in addition to measuring serum antibodies against other invasive parasites.

A knowledge of functional characteristics of liver cells has been used to design diagnostic agents that can be used to determine the normalcy of specific biochemical pathways of the hepatocytes. These "tailor-made" pharmaceuticals can be designed to be taken up by one or more of the available transport mechanisms available to the liver. For example, receptor-related endocytic processes can be used as targets to probe specific receptor-mediated transport functions of the liver cells. The asialoglycoprotein receptor, also known as the hepatic-binding protein, has been used in this diagnostic approach. The substrate $^{99}T_c{}^m$-galactosyl-neoglycoalbumin (NGA) was developed as a specific ligand for selective uptake via this specific hepatic receptor. The timing and extent of the assimilation of this probe into the hepatocytes, as determined by imaging the liver at precise intervals after the administration of this isotope, yields an estimate of hepatic blood flow as well as the transport capacity of this specific hepatic transporter protein.

Antibody titers against *Entamoeba histolytica* by use of an enzyme immunoassay were strongly reactive in **Amy Biasis'** blood. A diagnosis of **amoebiasis** was made. Her physicians started nitroimidazole amoebicides intravenously in a dose of 500 mg every 6 hours for 10 days. By the third day of treatment, Amy began to feel noticeably better. Her physicians told her that they expected a full clinical response in 95% of patients with amoebic liver abscesses treated in this way, although her multiple hepatic abscesses adversely affected her prognosis to a degree.

Table 46.1. Examples of Enzymes Used in Biotransformation of Xenobiotic Compounds

Acetyltransferase
Amidase-esterase
Dehydrogenase
Flavin-containing mono-oxygenase
Glutathione-S-transferase
Methyl transferase
Mixed-function oxidase
Reductase
Sulfotransferase
UDP-glucosyltransferase
UDP-glucuronosyltransferase

Each of the liver cells described contains specialized transport and uptake mechanisms for enzymes, infectious agents, drugs, and other xenobiotics that specifically target these substances to certain liver cell types. These are accomplished by linking these agents covalently by way of biodegradable bonds to their specific carrier. The latter then determines the particular fate of the drug by using specific cell recognition, uptake, transport, and biodegradation pathways.

B. Inactivation and Detoxification of Xenobiotic Compounds and Metabolites

Xenobiotics are compounds that have no nutrient value (cannot be used by the body for energy requirements) and are potentially toxic. They are present as natural components of foods or they may be introduced into foods as additives or through processing. Pharmacologic and recreational drugs are also xenobiotic compounds. The liver is the principal site in the body for the degradation of these compounds. Because many of these substances are lipophilic, they are oxidized, hydroxylated, or hydrolyzed by enzymes in phase I reactions. Phase I reactions introduce or expose hydroxyl groups or other reactive sites that can be used for conjugation reactions (the phase II reactions). The conjugation reactions add a negatively charged group such as glycine or sulfate to the molecule. Many xenobiotic compounds will be transformed through several different pathways. A general scheme of inactivation is shown in Figure 46.2.

The conjugation and inactivation pathways are similar to those used by the liver to inactivate many of its own metabolic waste products. These pathways are intimately related to the biosynthetic cascades that exist in the liver. The liver can synthesize the precursors that are required for conjugation and inactivation reactions from other compounds. For example, sulfation is used by the liver to clear steroid hormones from the circulation. The sulfate used for this purpose can be obtained from the degradation of cysteine or methionine.

The liver, kidney, and intestine are the major sites in the body for biotransformation of xenobiotic compounds. Many xenobiotic compounds contain aromatic rings (such as benzopyrene in tobacco smoke) or heterocyclic ring structures (such as the nitrogen-containing rings of nicotine or pyridoxine) that we are unable to degrade or recycle into useful components. These structures are hydrophobic, causing the molecules to be retained in adipose tissue unless they are sequestered by the liver, kidney, or intestine for biotransformation reactions. Sometimes, however, the phase I and II reactions backfire, and harmless hydrophobic molecules are converted to toxins or potent chemical carcinogens.

1. CYTOCHROME P450 AND XENOBIOTIC METABOLISM

The toxification/detoxification of xenobiotics is accomplished through the activity of a group of enzymes with a broad spectrum of biologic activity. Some examples of enzymes involved in xenobiotic transformation are described in Table 46.1. Of the wide variety of enzymes that are involved in xenobiotic metabolism, only the cytochrome P450–dependent monooxygenase system is discussed here. The cytochrome P450–dependent monooxygenase enzymes are determinants in oxidative, peroxidative, and reductive degradation of exogenous (chemicals, carcinogens, and pollutants, etc.) and endogenous (steroids, prostaglandins,

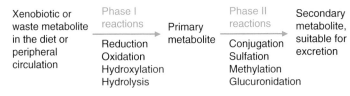

Fig. 46.2. General scheme of xenobiotic detoxification.

retinoids, etc.) substances. The key enzymatic constituents of this system are the flavo protein NADPH-cytochrome P450 oxidoreductase and cytochrome P450 (Fig. 46.3). The latter is the terminal electron acceptor and substrate-binding site of the microsomal mixed-function oxidase complex, a very versatile catalytic system. The system got its name in 1962, when Omura and Sato found a pigment with unique spectral characteristics derived from liver microsome of rabbits. When reduced and complexed with carbon monoxide, it exhibited a spectral absorbance maximum at 450 nm.

The major role of the cytochrome P450 enzymes (see Chapter 25) is to oxidize substrates and introduce oxygen to the structure. Similar reactions can be carried out by other flavin monoxygenases that do not contain cytochrome P450.

The cytochrome P450 enzyme family contains at least 100 to 150 different isozymes with at least 40% sequence homology. These isozymes have different but overlapping specificities. The human enzymes are generally divided into six major subfamilies, and each of these is further subdivided. For example, in the naming of the principal enzyme involved in the oxidation of ethanol to acetaldehyde, CYP2E1, the CYP denotes the cytochrome P450 family, the 2 denotes the subfamily, the E denotes ethanol, and the 1 denotes the specific isozyme.

The CYP3A4 isoform accounts for 60% of CYP450 enzymes in the liver and 70% of cytochrome enzymes in gut wall enterocytes. It metabolizes the greatest number of drugs in humans. Specific drugs are substrates for CYP3A4. The concomitant ingestion of two CYP3A4 substrates could potentially induce competition for the binding site, which, in turn, could alter the blood levels of these two agents. The drug with the highest affinity for the enzyme would be preferentially metabolized, whereas the metabolism (and degradation) of the other drug would be reduced. The latter drug's concentration in the blood would then rise.

Moreover, many substances or drugs impair or inhibit the activity of the CYP3A4 enzyme, thereby impairing the body's ability to metabolize a drug. The lipid-lowering agents known as the statins (HMGCoA reductase inhibitors) require CYP3A4 for degradation. Appropriate drug treatment and dosing takes into account the normal degradative pathway of the drug. However, grapefruit juice is a potent inhibitor of CYP3A4-mediated drug metabolism. Evidence suggests that if a statin is regularly taken with grapefruit juice, its level in the blood may increase as much as 15-fold. This marked increase in plasma concentration could increase the muscle and liver toxicity of the statin in question. because side effects of the statins appear to be dose-related.

The cytochrome P450 isozymes all have certain features in common:

1. They all contain cytochrome P450, oxidize the substrate, and reduce oxygen.
2. They all have a flavin-containing reductase subunit that uses NADPH, and not NADH, as a substrate.
3. They are all found in the smooth endoplasmic reticulum and are referred to as microsomal enzymes (for example, CYP2E1 is also referred to as the microsomal ethanol oxidizing system, MEOS).
4. They are all bound to the lipid portion of the membrane, probably to phosphatidylcholine.
5. They are all inducible by the presence of their own best substrate and somewhat less inducible by the substrates for other P450 isozymes.
6. They all generate a reactive free radical compound as an intermediate in the reaction.

2. EXAMPLES OF CYTOCHROME P450 DETOXIFICATION REACTIONS

i. Vinyl Chloride

The detoxification of vinyl chloride provides an example of effective detoxification by a P450 isozyme (ethanol detoxification was previously discussed in Chapter 25). Vinyl chloride is used in the synthesis of plastics and can cause angiosarcoma in the liver of exposed workers. It is activated in a phase I reaction to a reactive epoxide by

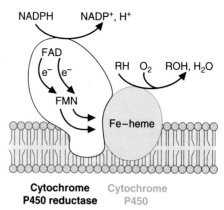

Fig. 46.3. General structure of the P450 enzymes. O_2 binds to the P450 Fe-heme in the active site and is activated to a reactive form by accepting electrons. The electrons are donated by the cytochrome P450 reductase, which contains an FAD plus an FMN or Fe-S center to facilitate the transfer of single electrons from NADPH to O_2. The P450 enzymes involved in steroidogenesis have a somewhat different structure. For CYP2E1, RH is ethanol (CH_3CH_2OH), and ROH is acetaldehyde (CH_3COH).

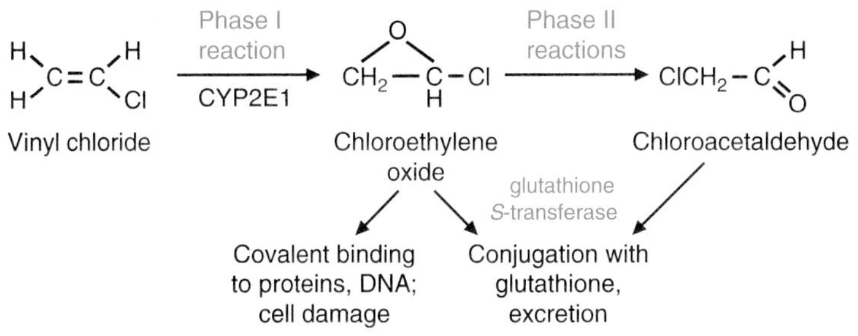

Fig. 46.4. Detoxification of vinyl chloride.

a hepatic P450 isozyme (CYP2E1), which can react with guanine in DNA or other cellular molecules. However, it also can be converted to chloroacetate, conjugated with reduced glutathione, and excreted in a series of phase II reactions (Fig. 46.4).

ii.   Aflatoxin B1

Aflatoxin B1 is an example of a compound that is made more toxic by a cytochrome P450 reaction (CYP2A1). Current research suggests that ingested aflatoxin B1 in contaminated food (it is produced by a fungus [*Aspergillus flavus*] that grows on peanuts that may have been stored in damp conditions) is directly involved in hepatocarcinogenesis in humans by introducing a G>T mutation into the *p53* gene. Aflatoxin is metabolically activated to its 8,9 epoxide by two different isozymes of cytochrome P450. The epoxide modifies DNA by forming covalent adducts with guanine residues. In addition, the epoxide can combine with lysine residues within proteins and thus is also a hepatotoxin.

iii.   Acetaminophen

Acetaminophen (Tylenol) is an example of a xenobiotic that is metabolized by the liver for safe excretion; however, it can be toxic if ingested in high doses. The pathways for acetaminophen metabolism are shown in Fig. 46.5 As shown in the

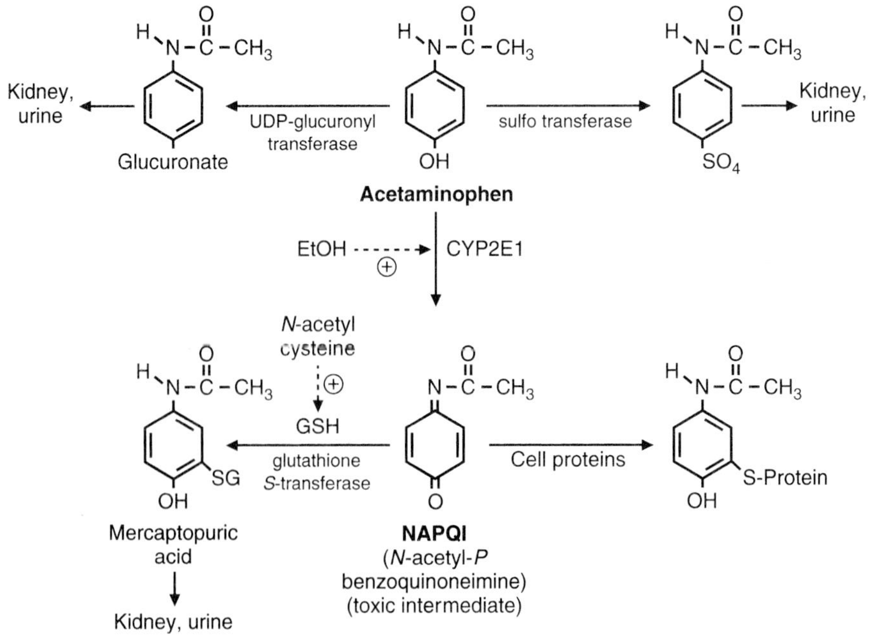

Fig. 46.5. Pathways of acetaminophen detoxification. N-acetyl cysteine stimulates the production of glutathione, thereby reducing the levels of NAPQI, which can damage cellular proteins. Ethanol upregulates CYP2E1 activity (the MEOS).

figure, acetaminophen can be glucuronylated or sulfated for safe excretion by the kidney. However, a cytochrome P450 enzyme produces the toxic intermediate N-acetyl-p-benzoquinoneimine (NAPQI), which can be excreted safely in the urine after conjugation with glutathione.

NAPQI is a dangerous and unstable metabolite that can damage cellular proteins and lead to death of the hepatocyte. Under normal conditions, when acetaminophen is taken in the correct therapeutic amounts, less than 10% of the drug forms NAPQI, an amount that can be readily handled by the glutathione detoxifying system (phase II reactions). However, when taken at doses that are potentially toxic, the sulfotransferase and glucuronyl transferase systems are overwhelmed, and more acetaminophen is metabolized through the NAPQI route. When this occurs, the levels of glutathione in the hepatocyte are insufficient to detoxify NAPQI, and hepatocyte death can result.

The enzyme that produces NAPQI, CYP2E1, is induced by alcohol (see Chapter 25, MEOS). Thus, individuals who chronically abuse alcohol have an increased sensitivity to acetaminophen toxicity, because a higher percentage of acetaminophen metabolism is directed toward NAPQI, as compared with an individual with low levels of CYP2E1. Therefore, even recommended therapeutic doses of acetaminophen can be toxic to these individuals.

An effective treatment for acetaminophen poisoning involves the use of N-acetyl cysteine. This compound supplies cysteine as a precursor for increased glutathione production, which, in turn, enhances the phase II reactions, which reduces the levels of the toxic intermediate.

C. Regulation of Blood Glucose Levels

One of the primary functions of the liver is to maintain blood glucose concentrations within the normal range. The manner in which the liver accomplishes this has been the subject of previous chapters (26, 31, and 36). In brief, the pancreas monitors blood glucose levels and secretes insulin when blood glucose levels rise and glucagon when such levels decrease. These hormones initiate regulatory cascades that affect liver glycogenolysis, glycogen synthesis, glycolysis, and gluconeogenesis. In addition, sustained physiologic increases in growth hormone, cortisol, and catecholamine secretion help to sustain normal blood glucose levels during fasting.

Numerous other factors, beside insulin and glucagon, can affect liver glucose metabolism, as has been described in Chapter 43.

When blood glucose levels drop, glycolysis and glycogen synthesis are inhibited, and gluconeogenesis and glycogenolysis are activated. Concurrently, fatty acid oxidation is activated to provide energy for glucose synthesis. During an overnight fast, blood glucose levels are primarily maintained by glycogenolysis and, if gluconeogenesis is required, the energy (6 ATP are required to produce one molecule of glucose from two molecules of pyruvate) is obtained by fatty acid oxidation. On insulin release, the opposing pathways are activated such that excess fuels can be stored either as glycogen or fatty acids. The pathways are regulated by the activation or inhibition of two key kinases, the cyclic adenosine monophosphate (cAMP)-dependent protein kinase, and the AMP-activated protein kinase (see Fig. 36.11 for a review of these pathways). Recall that the liver can export glucose because it is one of only two tissues that express glucose-6-phosphatase.

D. Synthesis and Export of Cholesterol and Triacylglycerol

When food supplies are plentiful, hormonal activation leads to fatty acid, triacylglycerol, and cholesterol synthesis. A high dietary intake and intestinal absorption of cholesterol will compensatorily reduce the rate of hepatic cholesterol synthesis, in which case the liver acts as a recycling depot for sending excess dietary cholesterol to the peripheral tissue when needed as well as accepting cholesterol from these tissues when required. The pathways of cholesterol metabolism were discussed in Chapter 34.

E. Ammonia and the Urea Cycle

The liver is the primary organ for synthesizing urea and, as such, is the central depot for the disposition of ammonia in the body. Ammonia groups travel to the liver on glutamine and alanine, and the liver converts these ammonia nitrogens to urea for excretion in the urine. The reactions of the urea cycle were discussed in Chapter 38.

Table 46.2 lists some of the important nitrogen-containing compounds that are primarily synthesized or metabolized by the liver.

F. Ketone Body Formation

The liver is the only organ that can produce ketone bodies, yet it is one of the few that cannot use these molecules for energy production. Ketone bodies are produced when the rate of glucose synthesis is limited (i.e., substrates for gluconeogenesis are limited), and fatty acid oxidation is occurring rapidly. Ketone bodies can cross the blood-brain barrier and become a major fuel for the nervous system under conditions of starvation. Ketone body synthesis and metabolism have been described in Chapter 23.

G. Nucleotide Biosynthesis

The liver can synthesize and salvage all ribonucleotides and deoxyribonucleotides for other cells to use. Certain cells have lost the capacity to produce nucleotides de

Table 46.2. Nitrogen-Containing Products Produced by the Liver

Product	Precursors	Tissues	Function
Creatine	Arginine, glycine, and S-adenosyl methionine (SAM)	Liver	Forms creatine phosphate in muscle for energy storage. Excreted as creatinine.
Glutathione	Glutamate, cysteine, glycine	All tissues but highest use in the liver	Protection against free radical injury by reduction of hydrogen peroxide and lipid peroxides. In liver and kidney forms mercapturic acids.
Purines	Glycine, glutamine, aspartate, carbon dioxide, tetrahydrofolate, PRPP	Liver, small amounts in brain and cells of the immune system	Adenine and guanine nucleosides and nucleotides. DNA, RNA, and coenzymes, and energy-transferring nucleotides.
Pyrimidines	Aspratate, glutamine, carbon dioxide	Liver, small amounts in brain and cells of the immune system	Uracil, thymine and cytosine
Sialic acid (NANA), other amino sugars	Glutamine	Most cells	In the liver, synthesis of oligosaccharide chains on secreted proteins. Most cells, glycoproteins, proteoglycans, and glycolipids.
Sulfated compounds	Cysteine	Liver and kidney produce sulfate	Many cells use sulfate in blood for formation of PAPS, which transfers sulfate to proteoglycans, drugs, and xenobiotics
Taurine	Cysteine	Liver	Conjugated bile salts
Glycocholic acid, and glycocheno-Deoxycholic acid	Glycine, bile salts	Liver	Conjugated bile salts are excreted into the bile and assist in the absorption of lipids and fat-soluble vitamins through the formation of micelles
Sphingosine	Serine and palmitoyl CoA	Liver, brain, and other tissues	Precursor of sphingolipids found in myelin and other membranes
Heme	Glycine and succinyl CoA	Liver, bone marrow	Heme from liver is incorporated into cytochromes. Heme from bone marrow is incorporated into hemoglobin.
Glycine conjugates of xenobiotic compounds	Glycine, medium-size hydrophobic carboxylic acids	Liver, kidney	Inactivation and targeting toward urinary excretion
Niacin	Tryptophan, glutamine	Liver	NAD, NADP coenzymes for oxidation reactions
One-carbon methyl donors for tetrahydrofolate and SAM	Glycine, serine, histidine, methionine	Most cells, but highest in liver	Choline, phosphatidylcholine, purine and pyrimidine synthesis, inactivation of waste metabolites and xenobiotics through methylation.

novo but can use the salvage pathways to convert free bases to nucleotides. The liver can secrete free bases into the circulation for these cells to use for this purpose. Nucleotide synthesis and degradation are discussed in Chapter 41.

H. Synthesis of Blood Proteins

The liver is the primary site of the synthesis of circulating proteins such as albumin and the clotting factors. When liver protein synthesis is compromised, the protein levels in the blood are reduced. Hypoproteinemia may lead to edema because of a decrease in the protein-mediated osmotic pressure in the blood. This, in turn, causes plasma water to leave the circulation and enter (and expand) the interstitial space, causing edema.

Most circulating plasma proteins are synthesized by the liver. Therefore, the hepatocyte has a well-developed endoplasmic reticulum, Golgi system, and cellular cytoskeleton, all of which function in the synthesis, processing, and secretion of proteins. The most abundant plasma protein produced by the liver is albumin, which represents 55 to 60% of the total plasma protein pool. Albumin serves as a carrier for a large number of hydrophobic compounds, such as fatty acids, steroids, hydrophobic amino acids, vitamins, and pharmacologic agents. It is also an important osmotic regulator in the maintenance of normal plasma osmotic pressure. The other proteins synthesized by the liver are, for the most part, glycoproteins. They function in hemostasis, transport, protease inhibition, and ligand binding, as well as secretogogues for hormone release. The acute phase proteins that are part of the immune response and the body's response to many forms of "injury" are also synthesized in the liver. Table 46.3 lists some of the proteins and their functions.

I. The Synthesis of Glycoproteins and Proteoglycans

The liver, because it is the site of synthesis of most of the blood proteins (including the glycoproteins), has a high requirement for the sugars that go into the oligosaccharide portion of glycoproteins (The synthesis of glycoproteins is discussed in Chapter 30.). These include mannose, fructose, galactose, and amino sugars.

One of the intriguing aspects of the hepatic biosynthetic pathways that use carbohydrate in the synthesis of these compounds is that the liver is not dependent on either dietary glucose or hepatic glucose to generate the precursor intermediates for these pathways. This is because the liver can generate carbohydrates from dietary amino acids (which enter gluconeogenesis generally as pyruvate or an intermediate of the TCA cycle), lactate (generated from anaerobic glycolysis in other tissues), and glycerol (generated by the release of free fatty acids from the adipocyte). Of course, if dietary carbohydrate is available, the liver can use that source as well.

Most of the sugars secreted by the liver are O-linked, that is, the carbohydrate is attached to the protein at its anomeric carbon through a glucosidic link to the –OH of a serine or a threonine residue. This is in contrast to the N-linked arrangement in which there is an N-glycosyl link to the amide nitrogen of an asparagine residue (Fig. 46.6). A particularly important O-linked sugar is N-acetylneuraminic acid (NANA or sialic acid), a nine-carbon sugar that is synthesized from fructose-6-phosphate and phosphoenolpyruvate (see Fig. 30.8). As circulating proteins age,

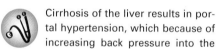 Cirrhosis of the liver results in portal hypertension, which because of increasing back pressure into the esophageal veins promotes the development of dilated thin-walled esophageal veins (varices). At the same time, synthesis of blood coagulation proteins by the liver and required vitamin K–dependent reactions are greatly diminished (resulting in a prolonged prothrombin time; which, in turn, increases clotting time). When the esophageal varices rupture, massive bleeding into the thoracic or abdominal cavity as well as the stomach may occur. Much of the protein content of the blood entering the gastrointestinal tract is metabolized by intestinal bacteria, releasing ammonium ion, which enters the portal vein. Because hepatocellular function has been compromised, the urea cycle capacity is inadequate, and the ammonium ion enters the peripheral circulation, thereby contributing to hepatic encephalopathy (brain toxicity due to elevated ammonia levels).

Table 46.3. A Partial List of Proteins Synthesized in the Liver

Type of Protein	Examples
Blood coagulation	Blood coagulation factors: fibrinogen, prothrombin, Factors V, VII, IX and X. Also α-2 macroglobulin.
Metal-binding proteins	Transferrin (iron), ceruloplasmin (copper), haptoglobin (heme), hemopexin (heme)
Lipid transport	Apoprotein B-100, apoprotein A-1
Protease inhibitor	α1-Antitrypsin

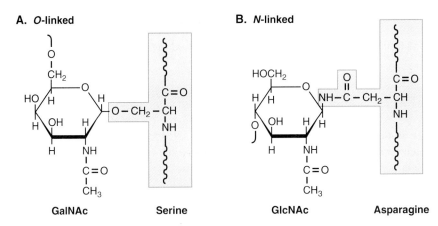

Fig. 46.6. The general configuration of O-linked and N-linked glycoproteins.

NANA (sialic acid) residues are lost from the serum proteins. This change signals their removal from the circulation and their eventual degradation. An asialoglycoprotein receptor on the liver cell surface binds such proteins, and the receptor–ligand complex is endocytosed and transported to the lysosomes. The amino acids from the degraded protein are then recycled within the liver.

J. The Pentose Phosphate Pathway

The major functions of the pentose phosphate pathway (see Chapter 29) are the generation of NADPH and five-carbon sugars. All cell types, including the red blood cell, can carry out this pathway because they need to generate NADPH so that the activity of glutathione reductase, the enzyme that catalyzes the conversion of oxidized glutathione (GSSG) back to reduced glutathione (GSH) can be maintained. Without the activity of this enzyme, the protection against free radical injury is lost. All cells also need this pathway for the generation of ribose, especially those cells that are dividing rapidly or have high rates of protein synthesis.

The liver has a much greater demand for NADPH than do most other organs. It uses NADPH for the biosynthesis of fatty acids and cholesterol, which the liver must make to produce phospholipids, and for the synthesis of VLDL and bile salts. It also uses NADPH for other biosynthetic reactions, such as that of proline synthesis. NADPH is also used by mixed-function oxidases such as cytochrome P450 that are involved in the metabolism of xenobiotics and of a variety of pharmaceuticals. Because the liver participates in so many reactions capable of generating free radicals, the liver uses more glutathione and NADPH to maintain glutathione reductase and catalase activity than any other tissue. Consequently, the concentration of glucose-6-phosphate dehydrogenase (the rate-limiting and regulated enzyme in the pentose phosphate pathway) is high in the liver, and the rate of flux through this pathway may be as high as 30% of the rate of flux through glycolysis.

IV. FUELS FOR THE LIVER

The reactions used to modify and inactivate dietary toxins and waste metabolites are energy requiring, as are the reactions used by anabolic (biosynthetic) pathways such as gluconeogenesis and fatty acid synthesis. Thus, the liver has a high energy requirement and consumes approximately 20% of the total oxygen used by the body. The principle forms in which energy is supplied to these reactions is the high-energy phosphate bonds of adenosine triphosphate (ATP), uridine triphosphate (UTP), and guanosine triphosphate (GTP), reduced NADPH, and acyl-CoA thioesters. The energy for the formation of these compounds is obtained directly

Table 46.4. Major Fates of Carbohydrates in the Liver

- Storage as Glycogen
- Glycolysis to pyruvate
  - Followed by oxidation to carbon dioxide in the TCA cycle
  - Precursors for the synthesis of glycerol-3-phosphate (the backbone of triacylglycerols and other glyceolipids), sialic acid, and serine
  - Entry into the TCA cycle and exit as citrate, followed by conversion to acetyl CoA, malonyl CoA, and entry into fatty acid synthesis and secretion as VLDL
    - Synthesis of phospholipids and other lipids from triacylglycerols
- Conversion to mannose, sialic acid, and other sugars necessary for the synthesis of oligosaccharides for glycoproteins, including those secreted into blood
- Synthesis of acid sugars for proteoglycan synthesis and formation of glucuronides
- Oxidation in the pentose phosphate pathway for the formation of NADPH (necessary for biosynthetic reactions such as fatty acid synthesis, glutathione reduction, and other NADPH-utilizing detoxification reactions)

from oxidative metabolism, the TCA cycle, or the electron transport chain and oxidative phosphorylation. After a mixed meal containing carbohydrate, the major fuels used by the liver are glucose, galactose, and fructose. If ethanol is consumed, the liver is the major site of ethanol oxidation, yielding principally acetate and then acetyl CoA. During an overnight fast, fatty acids become the major fuel for the liver. They are oxidized to carbon dioxide or ketone bodies. The liver also can use all of the amino acids as fuels, converting many of them to glucose. The urea cycle disposes of the ammonia that is generated from amino acid oxidation.

A. Carbohydrate Metabolism in the Liver

After a carbohydrate-containing meal, glucose, galactose, and fructose enter the portal circulation and flow to the liver. This organ serves as the major site in the body for the utilization of dietary galactose and fructose. It metabolizes these compounds by converting them to glucose and intermediates of glycolysis. Their fate is essentially the same as that of glucose (Table 46.4).

B. Glucose as a Fuel

The entry of glucose into the liver is dependent on a high concentration of glucose in the portal vein after a high-carbohydrate meal. Because the K_m for both the glucose transporter (GLUT2) and glucokinase is so high (approximately 10 mM), glucose will enter the liver principally after its concentration rises to 10 to 40 mM in the portal blood and not at the lower 5-mM concentration in the hepatic artery. The increase in insulin secretion that follows a high-carbohydrate meal will promote the conversion of glucose to glycogen. In addition, the rate of glycolysis will be increased (PFK-2 is active; thus, PFK-1 is activated by fructose-2, 6 bisphosphate) such that acetyl CoA can be produced for fatty acid synthesis (acetyl CoA carboxylase will be activated by citrate; see Chapter 33). Thus, after a high-carbohydrate meal, the liver uses glucose as its major fuel, while activating the pathways for glycogen and fatty acid synthesis.

The rate of glucose utilization by the liver is determined, in part, by the level of activity of glucokinase. Glucokinase activity is regulated by a glucokinase regulatory protein (RP, Fig. 46.7), which is located in the nucleus. In the absence of glucose, glucokinase is partially sequestered within the nucleus, bound to RP, in an inactive form. High concentrations of fructose 6-phosphate promote the interaction of glucokinase with RP, whereas high levels of either glucose or fructose 1-phosphate block glucokinase from binding to RP and promote the dissociation of the complex. Thus, as glucose levels rise in the cytoplasm and nucleus (because of increased blood glucose levels after a meal, for example), there is a significant enhancement of glucose phosphorylation as glucokinase is released from the nucleus, travels to the cytoplasm, and phosphorylates glucose.

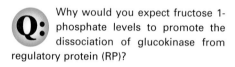

Q: Why would you expect fructose 1-phosphate levels to promote the dissociation of glucokinase from regulatory protein (RP)?

The role of glucokinase RP is very complex. Mice that have been genetically engineered to no longer express the RP (a knockout mouse) display reduced levels of total glucokinase activity in the liver. This is attributable to the finding that RP is important in the post-transcriptional processing of the mRNA for glucokinase. In the absence of RP, less glucokinase is produced. These mice, therefore, have no glucokinase in the nucleus, a reduced cytoplasmic glucokinase content, and inefficient glucose phosphorylation in the liver when glucose levels rise.

A: Fructose-1-phosphate is produced from fructose metabolism. The major dietary source of fructose, the ingestion of which would lead to increased fructose 1-phosphate levels, is sucrose. Sucrose is a disaccharide of glucose and fructose. Thus, an elevation of fructose 1-phosphate usually indicates an elevation of glucose levels as well.

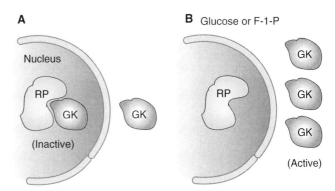

Fig. 46.7. Regulation of glucokinase by regulatory protein (RP). RP is localized to the nucleus, and in the absence of glucose or presence of fructose 6-phosphate, most glucokinase is translocated to the nucleus and binds RP. This leads to the formation of the inactive form of glucokinase. When glucose or fructose-1-phosphate levels rise, glucokinase is released from RP. It then translocates to the cytoplasm and actively converts glucose to glucose 6-phosphate.

The major regulatory step for liver glycolysis is the PFK-1 step. Even under fasting conditions, the ATP concentration in the liver (approximately 2.5 mM) is sufficiently high to inhibit PFK-1 activity. Thus, liver glycolysis is basically controlled by modulating the levels of fructose 2,6-bisphosphate, the product of the PFK-2 reaction. As fructose 2,6-bisphosphate levels increase (which would occur in the presence of insulin) the rate of glycolysis increases; when glucagon levels increase and protein kinase A is activated such that PFK-2 is phosphorylated and inactive, glycolysis will slow down, and gluconeogenesis will be enhanced (see Chapters 22 and 31).

C. Lipid Metabolism

Long-chain fatty acids are a major fuel for the liver during periods of fasting, when they are released from adipose tissue triacylglycerols and travel to the liver as fatty acids bound to albumin.

Within the liver, they bind to fatty acid–binding proteins and are then activated on the outer mitochondrial membrane, the peroxisomal membrane, and the smooth endoplasmic reticulum by fatty acyl CoA synthetases. The fatty acyl group is transferred from CoA to carnitine for transport through the inner mitochondrial membrane, where it is reconverted back into fatty acyl CoA and oxidized to acetyl CoA in the β-oxidation spiral (see Chapter 23).

The enzymes in the pathways of fatty acid activation and β-oxidation (the synthetases, the carnitine acyltransferases, and the dehydrogenases of β-oxidation) are somewhat specific for the length of the fatty acid carbon chain. The chain length specificity is divided into enzymes for long-chain fatty acids (C20 to approximately C12), medium-chain (approximately C12 to C4), and short-chain (C4–C2). The major lipids oxidized in the liver as fuels are the long-chain fatty acids (palmitic, stearic, and oleic acids), because these are the lipids that are synthesized in the liver, are the major lipids ingested from meat or dairy sources, and are the major form of fatty acids present in adipose tissue triacylglycerols. The liver, as well as many other tissues, uses fatty acids as fuels when the concentration of the fatty acid–albumin complex is increased in the blood.

1. MEDIUM-CHAIN LENGTH FATTY ACID OXIDATION

The liver and certain cells in the kidney are the major sites for the oxidation of medium-chain-length fatty acids. These fatty acids usually enter the diet of infants in maternal milk as medium-chain-length triacylglycerols (MCT). In the intestine, the MCT are hydrolyzed by gastric lipase, bile salt–dependent lipases, and pancreatic lipase more readily than long-chain triacylglycerols. Within the enterocytes, they are neither reconverted to triacylglycerols nor incorporated into chylomicrons. Instead, they are directly released into the portal circulation (fatty acids of approximately 8-carbon chain lengths or less are water-soluble). In the liver, they diffuse through the inner mitochondrial membrane and are activated to acyl CoA derivatives by medium-chain-length fatty acid activating enzyme (MMFAE), a family of similar isozymes present only in liver and kidney. The medium-chain fatty acyl-CoA is then oxidized by the normal route, beginning with medium-chain-length acyl CoA dehydrogenase (MCAD; see Chapter 23).

2. PEROXISOMAL OXIDATION OF VERY-LONG-CHAIN FATTY ACIDS

Peroxisomes are present in greater number in the liver than in other tissues. Liver peroxisomes contain the enzymes for the oxidation of very-long-chain fatty acids such as C24:0 and phytanic acid, for the cleavage of the cholesterol side chain necessary for the synthesis of bile salts, for a step in the biosynthesis of ether lipids, and for several steps in arachidonic acid metabolism. Peroxisomes also contain catalase and are capable of detoxifying hydrogen peroxide.

Very-long-chain fatty acids of C20 to C26 or greater are activated to CoA derivatives by very-long-chain acyl CoA synthetase present in the peroxisomal membrane. The very-long-chain acyl CoA derivatives are then oxidized in liver peroxisomes to the 8-carbon octanoyl CoA level. In contrast to mitochondrial β-oxidation, the first enzyme in peroxisomal β-oxidation introduces a double bond and generates hydrogen peroxide instead of FAD(2H). The remainder of the cycle, however, remains the same, releasing NADH and acetyl CoA. Peroxisomal catalase inactivates the hydrogen peroxide, and the acetyl CoA can be used in biosynthetic pathways such as those of cholesterol and dolichol synthesis.

The octanoyl CoA that is the end-product of peroxisomal oxidation leaves the peroxisomes and the octanoyl group is transferred through the inner mitochondrial membrane by medium-chain-length acylcarnitine transferase. In the mitochondria, it enters the regular β-oxidation pathway, beginning with medium-chain-length acyl CoA dehydrogenase (MCAD).

3. PEROXISOME PROLIFERATOR ACTIVATED RECEPTORS

The peroxisome proliferator activated receptors (PPAR) play an important role in liver metabolism. These receptors obtained their name from the finding that certain agonists were able to induce the proliferation of peroxisomes in liver. These agonists included hypolipidemic agents, nonsteroidal anti-inflammatory agents, and environmental toxins. The receptors that bind these agents, the PPAR, are members of a nuclear receptor family and, when activated, stimulate new gene transcription. Within the liver, the major form of PPAR directly regulates the activity of genes that are involved in fatty acid uptake and β- and ω-oxidation of fatty acids.

There are three major PPAR isoforms, α, δ/β, and γ,. The major form found in the liver is the α form. Fatty acids are an endogenous ligand for PPAR α, such that when the level of fatty acids in the circulation is increased (with a concurrent increase in the fatty acid content of hepatocytes), there is increased gene transcription for those proteins involved in regulating fatty acid metabolism (Table 46.5). Genetically altered mice have been generated that lack PPAR α. These "knockout" mice exhibit no abnormal phenotype when fed a normal diet. When fasted, however, or when fed a high-fat diet, these mice develop severe fatty infiltration of the liver. The inability to increase the rate of fatty acid oxidation in this organ leads to excessive fatty acid buildup in the hepatocytes. It also leads to an insufficient energy supply with which to make glucose (leading to hypoglycemia) as well as an inability to

Medium-chain triglycerides (MCT) are important components of nutritional supplements used in patients with digestive disorders. They therefore can be employed as an easily absorbed source of calories in patients who have a gastrointestinal (GI) disorder that may result in malabsorption of nutrients. These diseases include pancreatic insufficiency, intraluminal bile salt deficiency due to cholestatic liver disease, biliary obstruction, ileal disease or resection, and disease causing obstruction of intestinal lymphatics. Remember, however, that MCT do not contain polyunsaturated fatty acids that can be used for synthesis of eicosanoids (see Chapter 35).

Zellweger's (cerebrohepatorenal) syndrome occurs in individuals with a rare inherited absence of peroxisomes in all tissues. Patients accumulate C26-C38 polyenoic acids in brain tissue owing to defective peroxisomal oxidation of the very-long-chain fatty acids synthesized in the brain for myelin formation. In liver, bile acid and ether lipid synthesis are affected, as is the oxidation of very-long-chain fatty acids.

Table 46.5. Genes Regulated by Activation of PPAR-α

Fatty acid transport proteins
The mitochondrial and peroxisomal enzymes of fatty acid oxidation
Carnitine palmitoyl transferase I
HMG-CoA synthase
Apoprotein CIII (suppression)

The fibrates (e.g., clofibrate) are a class of drugs that bind to PPARs to elicit changes in lipid metabolism. They are typically prescribed for individuals with elevated triglyceride levels because they increase the rate of triglyceride oxidation. This, in turn, leads to a reduction in serum tri-acylglycerol levels. Fibrates, through PPAR-α stimulation, also suppress apoprotein CIII synthesis and stimulate LPL activity. Apo CIII normally inhibits LPL activity, so by reducing CIII synthesis overall, LPL activity is increased. Apo CIII also blocks apoprotein E on IDL particles, causing the IDL particles to accumulate because they cannot be taken up by the apo E receptor in the liver. The suppression of apo CIII levels allows more IDL to be endocytosed, thereby also reducing circulating triacylglycerol levels.

 Reye's syndrome is characterized clinically by vomiting with signs of progressive central nervous system damage. In addition, there are signs of hepatic injury and hypoglycemia. There is mitochondrial dysfunction with decreased activity of hepatic mitochondrial enzymes. Hepatic coma may occur as serum ammonia levels rise. It is epidemiologically associated with the consumption of aspirin by children during a viral illness, but it may occur in the absence of exposure to salicylates. The incidence in the United States has decreased dramatically since the 1980s, when parents were made aware of the dangers of giving aspirin to children to reduce fever. Reye's syndrome is not necessarily confined to children. In patients who die of this disease, the liver at autopsy shows swollen and disrupted mitochondria and extensive accumulation of lipid droplets with fatty vacuolization of cells in both the liver and the renal tubules.

produce ketone bodies. In normal fasted mice or mice fed a high-fat diet, fatty acids would eventually stimulate their own oxidation, via peroxisome proliferation and by induction of other enzymes needed for their oxidation. The knockout mice cannot make these compensations.

4. XENOBIOTICS METABOLIZED AS FATTY ACIDS

The liver uses the pathways of fatty acid metabolism to detoxify very hydrophobic and lipid-soluble xenobiotics that, like fatty acids, either have carboxylic acid groups or can be metabolized to compounds that contain carboxylic acids. Benzoate and salicylate are examples of xenobiotics that are metabolized in this way. Benzoate is naturally present in plant foods and is added to foods such as sodas as a preservative. Its structure is similar to salicylic acid (which is derived from the degradation of aspirin). Salicylic acid and benzoate are similar in size to medium-chain-length fatty acids and are activated to an acyl CoA derivative by MMFAE (Fig. 46.8). The acyl group is then conjugated with glycine, which targets the compound for urinary excretion. The glycine derivatives of salicylate and benzoate are called salicylurate and hippurate, respectively. Salicylurate is the major urinary metabolite of aspirin in humans. Benzoate has been administered to treat hyperammonemia associated with congenital defects, because urinary hippurate excretion tends to lower the free ammonia pool. Aspirin cannot be used for this purpose because it is toxic in the large doses required

5. THE METABOLISM OF LIPIDS IN LIVER DISEASE

Chronic parenchymal liver disease is associated with relatively predictable changes in plasma lipids and lipoproteins. Some of these changes are related to a reduction in the activity of lethicin cholesterol acyltransferase (LCAT). This plasma enzyme is synthesized and glycosylated in the liver; then enters the blood, where it catalyzes the transfer of a fatty acid from the 2-position of lecithin to the 3β-OH group of free cholesterol to produce cholesterol ester and lysolecithin. As expected, in severe parenchymal liver disease, in which LCAT activity is decreased, plasma levels of cholesterol ester are reduced and free cholesterol levels normal or increased.

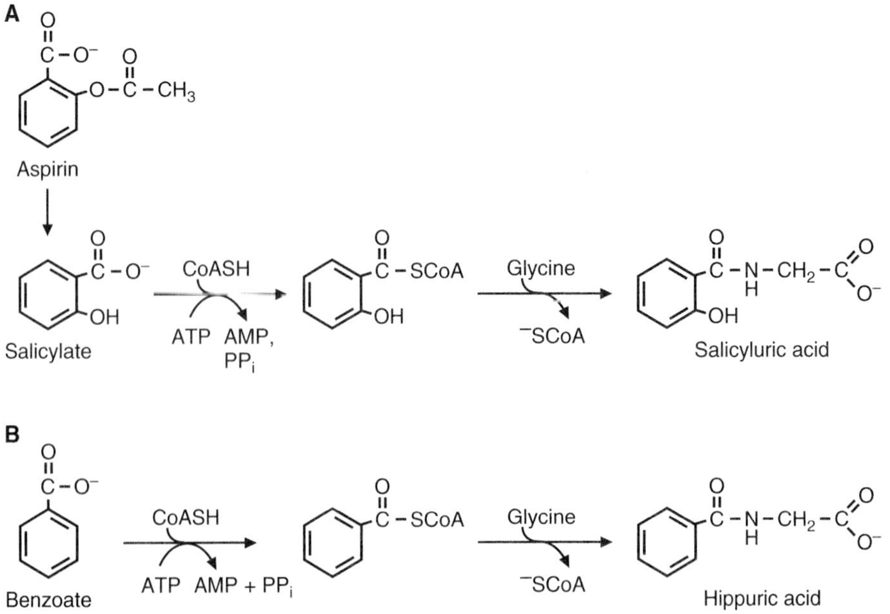

Fig. 46.8. Benzoate and salicylate metabolism.

Plasma triacylglycerols are normally cleared by peripheral lipases (lipoprotein lipase or LPL and hepatic triglyceride lipase or HTGL). Because the activities of both LPL and HTGL are reduced in patients with hepatacellular disease, a relatively high level of plasma triacylglycerols may be found in both acute and chronic hepatitis, in patients with cirrhosis of the liver, and in patients with other diffuse hepatocellular disorders.

With low LCAT activity and the elevated triacylglycerol level described, low-density lipoprotein (LDL) particles have an abnormal composition. They are relatively triacylglycerol rich and cholesterol ester poor.

High-density lipoprotein (HDL) metabolism may be abnormal in chronic liver disease as well. For example, because the conversion of HDL$_3$ (less antiatherosclerotic) to HDL$_2$ (more antiatherosclerotic) is catalyzed by LCAT, the reduced activity of LCAT in patients with cirrhosis leads to a decrease in the HDL$_2$:HDL$_3$ ratio. Conversely, the conversion of HDL$_2$ to HDL$_3$ requires hepatic lipases. If the activity of this lipase is reduced, one would expect an elevation in the HDL$_2$:HDL$_3$ ratio. Because the HDL$_2$:HDL$_3$ ratio is usually elevated in cirrhosis, the lipase deficiency appears to be the more dominant of the two mechanisms. These changes may result in an overall increase in serum total HDL levels. How this affects the efficiency of the reverse cholesterol transport mechanism and the predisposition to atherosclerosis is not fully understood.

With regard to triacylglycerol levels in patients with severe parenchymal liver disease, the hepatic production of the triacylglycerol-rich, very-low-density lipoprotein (VLDL) particle is impaired. Yet the total level of plasma triacylglycerols remains relatively normal because the LDL particle in such patients is triacylglycerol-rich, for reasons that have not been fully elucidated.

Non-esterified fatty acid (NEFA) levels are elevated in patients with cirrhosis. This change might be expected because basal hepatic glucose output is low in these patients. As a result, more NEFA are presumably required (via increased lipolysis) to meet the fasting energy requirements of peripheral tissues.

D. Amino Acid Metabolism in the Liver

The liver is the principle site of amino acid metabolism in humans. It essentially balances the free amino acid pool in the blood through the metabolism of amino acids supplied by the diet after a protein-containing meal and through metabolism of amino acids supplied principally by skeletal muscles during an overnight fast. In an adult who is no longer growing linearly, the total protein content of the body on a daily basis is approximately constant, such that the net degradation of amino acids (either to other compounds or used for energy) is approximately equal to the amount consumed. The key points concerning hepatic amino acid metabolism are the following:

1. The liver contains all the pathways for catabolism of all of the amino acids and can oxidize most of the carbon skeletons to carbon dioxide. A small proportion of the carbon skeletons are converted to ketone bodies. The liver also contains the pathways for converting amino acid carbon skeletons to glucose (gluconeogenesis) that can be released into the blood.
2. Because the liver is the principle site of amino acid catabolism, it also contains the urea cycle, the pathway that converts toxic ammonium ion to nontoxic urea. The urea is then excreted in the urine.
3. After a mixed or high-protein meal, the gut uses dietary aspartate, glutamate, and glutamine as a fuel (during fasting the gut uses glutamine from the blood as a major fuel). Thus, the ingested acidic amino acids do not enter the general circulation. The nitrogen from gut metabolism of these amino acids is passed to the liver as citrulline or ammonium ion via the portal vein.
4. The branched-chain amino acids (valine, leucine, and isoleucine) can be used by most cell types as a fuel, including cells of the gut and skeletal muscle. After a

high-protein meal, most of the branched-chain amino acids are not oxidized by the liver (because of very low activity of the branched-chain amino acid transaminase) and instead enter the peripheral circulation to be used as a fuel by other tissues or for protein synthesis (these amino acids are essential amino acids). The liver does, however, take up whatever amino acids it needs to carry out its own protein synthesis.

5. Most tissues transfer the amino acid nitrogen to the liver to dispose of as urea. They, therefore, produce either alanine (from the pyruvate–glucose–alanine cycle, in skeletal muscle, kidney, and intestinal mucosa) or glutamine (skeletal muscle, lungs, neural tissues) or serine (kidney), which are released into the blood and taken up by the liver.

6. The liver uses amino acids for the synthesis of proteins that it requires as well as for the synthesis of proteins to be used elsewhere. For example, the liver uses the carbon skeletons and nitrogens of amino acids for the synthesis of nitrogen-containing compounds such as heme, purines, and pyrimidines. The amino acid precursors for these compounds are all nonessential, because they can be synthesized in the liver.

E. Amino Acid Metabolism in Liver Disease

The concentration of amino acids in the blood of patients with liver disease is often elevated. This change is, in part, attributable to a significantly increased rate of protein turnover (general catabolic effect seen in severely ill patients) as well as to impaired amino acid uptake by the diseased liver. It is unlikely that the increased levels are due to degradation of liver protein and the subsequent release of amino acids from the failing hepatocyte into the blood. This is true because the total protein content of the liver is only approximately 300 g. To account for the elevated amino acid levels in the blood, the entire protein content of the liver would have to be degraded within 6 to 8 hours to account for the increased protein turnover rates found. Because 18 to 20 times more protein is present in skeletal muscle (greater mass), the muscle is probably the major source of the elevated plasma levels of amino acids seen in catabolic states such as cirrhosis of the liver.

In cirrhotic patients, such as **Jean Ann Tonich**, the fasting blood α-amino nitrogen level is elevated as a result of reduced clearance. Urea synthesis is reduced as well.

The plasma profile of amino acids in cirrhosis characteristically shows an elevation in aromatic amino acids, phenylalanine and tyrosine, and in free tryptophan and methionine. The latter changes may be caused by impaired hepatic utilization of these amino acids as well as to portosystemic shunting. Although the mechanism is not known, a reduction in fasting plasma levels of the branched-chain amino acids (BCAA) is also seen in cirrhotic patients. These findings, however, must be interpreted with caution because most of the free amino acid pool in humans is found in the intracellular space. Therefore, changes seen in their plasma concentrations do not necessarily reflect their general metabolic fate. Yet the elevation in aromatic amino acids and the suppression of the level of BCAAs in the blood of cirrhotics have been implicated in the pathogenesis of hepatic encephalopathy.

V. DISEASES OF THE LIVER

Diseases of the liver can be clinically and biochemically devastating, because no other organ can compensate for the loss of the multitude of functions that the liver normally performs. Alcohol-induced liver disease has been discussed in Chapter 25. A number of diseases can lead to hepatic fibrosis (see Biochemical Comments)

 Unlike **Amy Biasis**, whose hepatic amoebic disorder was more localized (abscesses), **Jean Anne Tonich** had a diffuse hepatic disease, known as alcohol-induced cirrhosis (historically referred to as "Laennec's cirrhosis"). The latter is characterized by diffuse fine scarring, a fairly uniform loss of hepatic cells, and the formation of small regenerative nodules (sometimes referred to as "micronodular cirrhosis"). With continued alcohol intake, fibroblasts and activated stellate cells deposit collagen at the site of persistent injury. This leads to the formation of weblike septa of connective tissue in periportal and pericentral zones. These eventually connect portal triads and central veins. With further exposure to alcohol, the liver shrinks and then becomes nodular and firm as "end-stage" cirrhosis develops. Unless successfully weaned from alcohol, these patients eventually die of liver failure. **Amy Biasis,** however, can probably look forward to enjoying normal liver function after successful amoebicidal therapy without evidence of residual hepatic scarring.

and cirrhosis. When this occurs to a great enough extent, liver function becomes inadequate for life. Signs and symptoms of liver disease include elevated levels of the enzymes alanine aminotransferase (ALT) and aspartate aminotransferase (AST) in the plasma (due to hepatocyte injury or death with a consequent release of these enzymes into the blood), jaundice (an accumulation of bilirubin in the blood caused by inefficient bilirubin glucuronidation by the liver; see Chapter 45), increased clotting times (the liver has difficulty producing clotting factors for secretion), edema (reduced albumin synthesis by the liver leads to a reduction in osmotic pressure in the blood), and hepatic encephalopathy (reduced urea cycle activity leading to excessive levels of ammonia and other toxic compounds in the central nervous system).

Alanine aminotransferase and aspartate aminotransferase are the modern versions of older names. ALT was formally known as serum glutamic pyruvate transaminase (SPGT), and AST was formally known as serum glutamic oxaloacetic transaminase (SGOT).

CLINCAL COMMENTS

Patients with cirrhosis of the liver who have no known genetic propensity to glucose intolerance, such as **Jean Ann Tonich**, tend to have higher blood glucose levels than do normal subjects in both fasting and fed states. The mechanisms that may increase glucose levels in the fasting state include a reduction in the metabolic clearance rate of glucose by 25 to 40% compared with normal subjects. This reduction in glucose clearance results, in part, from increased oxidation of fatty acids and ketone bodies and the consequent decrease in glucose oxidation by peripheral tissues in cirrhosis patients. This is suggested by the discovery that plasma non-esterified fatty acid (NEFA) levels are high in many patients with hepatocellular dysfunction, in part because of decreased hepatic clearance of NEFA and in part because of increased adipose tissue lipolysis. Another possible explanation for the reduction in whole body glucose utilization in cirrhotic patients relates to the finding that ketone body production is increased in some patients with cirrhosis. This could lead to enhanced utilization of ketone bodies for fuel by the central nervous system in such patients, thereby reducing the need for glucose oxidation by the highly metabolically active brain.

After glucose ingestion (fed state), many patients with liver disease have abnormally elevated blood glucose levels ("hepatogenous diabetes"). Using World Health Organization (WHO) criteria, 60 to 80% of cirrhotic patients have varying degrees of glucose intolerance, and overt diabetes mellitus occurs 2 to 4 times as often in cirrhotics than it does in subjects without liver disease. The proposed mechanisms include a degree of insulin resistance in peripheral tissues; however, as the cirrhotic process progresses, they develop a marked impairment of insulin secretion as well. Although the mechanisms are not well understood, this decrease in insulin secretion leads to increased hepatic glucose output (leading to fasting hyperglycemia) and reduced suppression of hepatic glucose output after meals, leading to postprandial hyperglycemia as well. If the patient has an underlying genetic predisposition to diabetes mellitus, the superimposition of the mechanisms outlined above will lead to an earlier and more significant breakdown in glucose tolerance in these specific patients.

BIOCHEMICAL COMMENTS

Extensive and progressive fibrosis of the hepatic parenchyma leads to cirrhosis of the liver, a process that has many causes. The development of fibrosis requires the activities of hepatic stellate cells, cytokines, proteases, and protease inhibitors.

A major change that occurs when fibrosis is initiated is that the normally "sparse" or "leaky" basement membrane between the endothelial cells and the hepatocyte is replaced with a high-density membrane containing fibrillar collagen. This occurs because of both an increased synthesis of a different type of collagen than is normally produced and a reduction in the turnover rate of existing extracellular matrix components.

The supportive tissues of the normal liver contain an extracellular matrix that, among other proteins, includes type IV collagen (which does not form fibers), glycoproteins, and proteoglycans. After a sustained insult to the liver, a threefold to eightfold increase occurs in extracellular matrix components, some of which contain fibril-producing collagen (types I and III), glycoproteins, and proteoglycans. The accumulation of these fibril-producing compounds leads to a loss of endothelial cell fenestrations and, therefore, a loss of the normal sieve-like function of the basement membranes. These changes interfere with normal transmembrane metabolic exchanges between the blood and hepatocytes.

The hepatic stellate cell is the source of the increased and abnormal collagen production. These cells are activated by growth factors whose secretion is induced by injury to the hepatocytes or endothelial cells. Growth factors involved in cellular activation include TGF-β1 (which is derived from the endothelial cells, Kupffer cells, and platelets) and platelet-derived growth factor (PDGF) and epidermal growth factor (EGF) from platelets. The release of PDGF stimulates stellate cell proliferation and, in the process, increases their synthesis and release of extracellular matrix materials and remodeling enzymes. These enzymes include matrix metalloproteinases (MMPs) and tissue inhibitors of MMPs, as well as converting (activating) enzymes. This cascade leads to the degradation of the normal extracellular matrix and replacement with a much denser and more rigid type of matrix material. These changes are, in part, the result of an increase in the activity of tissue inhibitors of MMP's for the new collagen relative to the original collagen in the extracellular matrix.

One consequence of the increasing stiffness of the hepatic vascular channels through which hepatic blood must flow is a greater resistance to the free flow of blood through the liver as a whole. Resistance to intrahepatic blood flow is also increased by a loss of vascular endothelial cell fenestrations, loss of free space between the endothelial cells and the hepatocytes (space of Disse), and even loss of vascular channels per se. This increased vascular resistance leads to an elevation in intrasinusoidal fluid pressure. When this intrahepatic (portal) hypertension reaches a critical threshold, the shunting of portal blood away from the liver (portosystemic shunting) further contributes to hepatic dysfunction. If the portal hypertension cannot be reduced, portal blood will continue to bypass the liver and return to the heart through the normally low-pressure esophageal veins. When this increasing intraesophageal venous pressure becomes severe enough, the walls of these veins thin dramatically and expand to form varices, which may suddenly burst, causing life-threatening esophageal variceal hemorrhage. This is a potentially fatal complication of cirrhosis of the liver.

Suggested Reading

Berger J, Moller DE. The mechanism of action of PPARs. Annu Rev Med 2002;53:409–435.

Gibson DM, Harris RA. Liver metabolism, in Metabolic Regulation in Mammals. New York: Francis, Inc, 2002:177–210.

Sherlock S, Dooley J. Hepatic cirrhosis, in Diseases of the Liver and Biliary System, Chapter 21. Malden, MA: Blackwell Science, 2002:365–380.

Meijer DKF, Jansen PLM, Groothuis GMM. Hepatobiliary disposition and targeting of drugs and genes, in Oxford Textbook of Clinical Hepatology, vol 1, 2nd Ed. New York: Oxford Medical Publications, 1999.

1. Drinking grapefruit juice while taking statins can lead to potentially devastating side effects. This is due to a component of grapefruit juice doing which of the following?

   (A) Interfering with hepatic uptake of statins
   (B) Accelerating the conversion of the statin to a more toxic form
   (C) Inhibiting the inactivation of statins
   (D) Upregulating the HMG CoA reductase
   (E) Downregulating the HMG CoA reductase

2. Which one of the following characteristics of cytochrome P450 enzymes is correct?

   (A) They are all found in the Golgi apparatus and are referred to as microsomal enzymes.
   (B) They all contain a flavin-containing reductase unit that uses NADH and not NADPH as a source of electrons.
   (C) They are all inducible by oxygen, which binds to the iron of the cytochrome.
   (D) They all oxidize the substrate on which they act.
   (E) They all generate a free radical compound as final products of the reaction.

3. Fairly predictable changes occur in the various metabolic pathways of lipid metabolism in patients with moderately advanced hepatocellular disease. Which one of the following changes would you expect to see under these conditions?

   (A) The activity of plasma lecithin cholesterol acyltransferase (LCAT) is increased.
   (B) Serum cholesterol esters are increased.
   (C) Hepatic triglyceride lipase (HTGL) activity is increased.
   (D) Serum triacylglycerol levels are increased.
   (E) Serum nonesterified fatty acid levels are decreased.

4. After a 2-week alcoholic binge, **Jean Ann Tonich** ingested some Tylenol to help her with a severe headache. She took three times the suggested dose because of the severity of the pain. However, within 24 hours Jean Ann became very lethargic, vomited frequently, and developed severe abdominal pain. The symptoms Jean Ann is experiencing are attributable to a reaction to the Tylenol due to which of the following?

   (A) The hypoglycemia experienced by the patient
   (B) Ethanol-induced inhibition of Tylenol metabolism
   (C) The hyperglycemia experienced by the patient
   (D) Ethanol-induced acceleration of Tylenol metabolism
   (E) Acetaminophen inhibition of VLDL secretion by the liver

5. An individual displays impaired glucose tolerance; blood glucose levels remain elevated after a meal for a longer time than is normal, although they do eventually go down to fasting levels. The patient has a normal release of insulin from the pancreas in response to elevated blood glucose levels. Fibroblasts obtained from the patient display normal levels of insulin binding to its receptor, and normal activation of the intrinsic tyrosine kinase activity associated with the insulin receptor. Analysis of glucose 6-phosphate formation within the fibroblasts, however, indicated a much slower rate of formation than in fibroblasts obtained from a normal control. A possible mutation that could lead to these results is which of the following?

   (A) A decrease in the K_m of glucokinase
   (B) An increase in the V_{max} of glucokinase
   (C) A nonfunctional glucokinase regulatory protein
   (D) An increase in hexokinase activity
   (E) A decrease in hexokinase activity

47 Metabolism of Muscle at Rest and During Exercise

*There are three types of muscle cells: **smooth**, **skeletal**, and **cardiac**. In all types of muscle, contraction occurs via an actin/myosin sliding filament system, which is regulated by oscillations in **intracellular calcium levels**.*

*Muscle cells use stored glycogen and circulating glucose, fatty acids, and amino acids as energy sources. Muscle glycolysis is regulated differently from the liver, with the key difference being the regulation of **phosphofructokinase-2 (PFK-2)**. Muscle PFK-2 is not inhibited by phosphorylation; cardiac PFK-2 is actually activated by an insulin-stimulated protein kinase. Thus, under conditions in which liver PFK-2 is inactive, and glycolysis is running slowly, muscle glycolysis is either unaffected, or even stimulated, depending on the isoform of PFK-2 being expressed.*

*Although muscle cells do not synthesize fatty acids, they do contain an isozyme of **acetyl CoA carboxylase (ACC-2)** to regulate the **rate of fatty acid oxidation**. ACC-2 produces malonyl CoA, which inhibits carnitine palmitoyl transferase I, thereby blocking fatty acid entry into the mitochondria. Muscle also contains **malonyl CoA decarboxylase**, which catalyzes the conversion of malonyl CoA to acetyl CoA and carbon dioxide. Thus, both the synthesis and degradation of malonyl CoA is carefully regulated in muscle cells to balance glucose and fatty acid oxidation. Both allosteric and covalent means of regulation are employed. Citrate activates ACC-2, and phosphorylation of ACC-2 by the adenosine monophosphate (AMP)-activated protein kinase inhibits ACC-2 activity. Phosphorylation of malonyl CoA decarboxylase by the AMP-activated protein kinase activates the enzyme, further enhancing fatty acid oxidation when energy levels are low.*

*Muscles use **creatine phosphate** to store high-energy bonds. Creatine is derived from arginine and glycine in the kidney, and the guanidinoacetate formed is methylated (using S-adenosyl methionine) in the liver to form creatine. The enzyme **creatine phosphokinase (CPK)** then catalyzes the reversible transfer of a high-energy phosphate from adenosine triphosphate (ATP) to creatine, forming creatine-phosphate and adenosine diphosphate (ADP). Creatine phosphate is unstable and spontaneously cyclizes to form **creatinine**, which is excreted in the urine. The spontaneous production of creatinine occurs at a constant rate and is proportional to body muscle mass. Thus, the amount of creatinine excreted each day (the creatinine clearance rate) is constant and can be used as an indicator of the normalcy of the excretory function of the kidneys.*

*Skeletal muscle cells can be subdivided into **type I** and **type II fibers**. Type I fibers are **slow-twitch** fibers that use primarily **oxidative metabolism** for energy, whereas the type II fibers (**fast-twitch**) use **glycolysis** as their primary energy-generating pathway.*

*****Glucose transport** into muscle cells can be stimulated during exercise because of the activity of the **AMP-activated protein kinase**. Fatty acid uptake into exercising muscle is dependent on the levels of circulating fatty acids, which are increased by **epinephrine** release.*

THE WAITING ROOM

Rena Felya, a 9-year-old girl, complained of a severe pain in her throat and difficulty in swallowing. She had chills, sweats, headache, and a fever of 102.4° F. When her symptoms persisted for several days, her mother took her to the pediatrician, who found diffuse erythema (redness) in her posterior pharynx (throat) with yellow exudates (patches) on her tonsils. Large, tender lymph nodes were present under her jaw on both sides of her neck. A throat culture was taken, and therapy with penicillin was begun.

Although the sore throat and fever improved, 8 days after the onset of the original infection, Rena's eyes and legs became swollen and her urine suddenly turned the color of "Coca-Cola." Her blood pressure was elevated. Protein and red blood cells were found in her urine. Her serum creatinine level was elevated at 1.8 mg/dL (reference range = 0.3–0.7 for a child). Because the throat culture grew out group A β-hemolytic streptococci, the doctor ordered a Streptozyme test. This test was positive for antibodies to streptolysin O and several other streptococcal antigens. As a result, a diagnosis of acute poststreptococcal glomerulonephritis was made. Supportive therapy, including bed rest and treatment for hypertension, was initiated.

I. MUSCLE CELL TYPES

Muscle consists of three different types: skeletal, smooth, and cardiac (Fig. 47.1). The metabolism of each is similar, but the functions of the muscle are quite different.

A. Skeletal Muscle

Skeletal muscles are those muscles that are attached to bone and facilitate the movement of the skeleton. Skeletal muscles are found in pairs, which are responsible for opposing, coordinated directions of motion on the skeleton. The muscles appear striated under the microscope, and are controlled voluntarily (you think about moving a specific muscle group, and then it happens).

Skeletal muscle cells are long, cylindrical fibers that run the length of the muscle. The fibers are multinucleated because of cell fusion during embryogenesis. The cell membrane surrounding the fibers is called the sarcolemma, and the sarcoplasm is the intracellular milieu, which contains the proteins, organelles, and contractile apparatus of the cell. The sarcoplasmic reticulum is analogous to the endoplasmic reticulum in other cell types and is an internal membrane system that runs throughout the length of the muscle fiber. Another membrane structure, the transverse tubules (T-tubules), are thousands of invaginations of the sarcolemma that tunnel from the surface toward the center of the muscle fiber to make contact with the terminal cisterns of the sarcoplasmic reticulum. Because the T tubules are open to the outside of the muscle fiber and filled with extracellular fluid, the muscle action potential that propagates along the surface of the muscle fiber's sarcolemma travels into the T tubules and to the sarcoplasmic reticulum.

The striations in skeletal muscle are attributable to the presence and organization of myofibrils in the cells. Myofibrils are thread-like structures consisting of thin and thick filaments. The contractile proteins actin and myosin are contained within the filaments; myosin within the thick filaments, actin within the thin filaments. The sliding of these filaments relative to each other, using myosin-catalyzed ATP hydrolysis as an energy source, allows for the contraction and relaxation of the muscle (see Fig. 19.4).

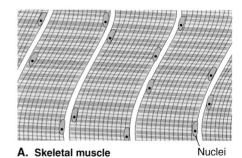

A. Skeletal muscle   Nuclei

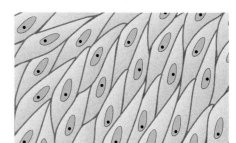

B. Smooth muscle

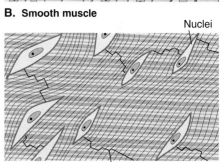

Nuclei

C. Cardiac muscle   Intercalated disks

Fig. 47.1. Structures of the three different muscle types. Smooth Cardiac. Adapted from Basic Histology, Text and Atlas, Junqueira and Carneiro, 10th Ed. Lange, McGraw-Hill, 2002.

Duchenne's muscular dystrophy is caused by the absence of the protein dystrophin, which is a structural protein located in the sarcolemma. Dystrophin is required to maintain the integrity of the sarcolemma, and when absent leads to a loss of muscle function, caused by breakdown of the sarcolemma. The gene is X-linked, and mutations that lead to Duchenne's muscular dystrophy generally result from large deletions of the gene, such that dystrophin is absent from the membrane. Becker's muscular dystrophy, a milder form of disease, is caused by point mutations in the dystrophin gene. In Becker's muscular dystrophy, dystrophin is present in the sarcolemma, but in a mutated form.

Muscle fibers can be classified as either fast-twitch or slow-twitch. The slow-twitch fibers, or type I fibers (also called slow-oxidative), contain large amounts of mitochondria and myoglobin (giving them a red color), utilize respiration and oxidative phosphorylation for energy, and are relatively resistant to fatigue. Compared with fast-twitch fibers, their glycogen content is low. The slow-twitch fibers develop force slowly but maintain contractions longer than fast-twitch muscle.

The fast-twitch fibers, or type II, can be subdivided as type IIa or IIb. Type IIb fibers (also called fast-glycolytic) have few mitochondria and low levels of myoglobin (hence, they appear white). They are rich in glycogen and use glycogenolysis and glycolysis as their primary energy source. These muscles are prone to fatigue, because a continued reliance on glycolysis to produce ATP leads to an increase in lactic acid levels, resulting in a drop in the intracellular pH. As the pH drops, the ability of the muscle to produce ATP also diminishes. However, fast-twitch muscle can develop greater forces than slow-twitch muscle, such that contractions occur more rapidly. Type IIa fibers (also called fast-oxidative glycolytic) have properties of both type I and IIb fibers and thus display functional characteristics of both fiber types. The properties of types I, IIa, and IIb fibers are summarized in Table 47.1.

Muscles are a mixture of the different fiber types, but depending on the function a muscle could have a preponderance of one fiber type over another. Type I fibers are found in postural muscles such as the psoas in the back musculature or the soleus in the leg. The percentage of type I to type II will vary with the muscle. The triceps, which functions phasically, has 32.6% type I, whereas the soleus, which functions tonically, has 87.7% type I. Type II fibers are more prevalent in the large muscles of the limbs that are responsible for sudden, powerful movements. Extraocular muscles would also have more of these fibers than type I.

B. Smooth Muscle Cells

Smooth muscle cells are found in the digestive system, blood vessels, bladder, airways, and uterus. The cells have a spindle shape with a central nucleus (see Fig. 47.1B). The designation of smooth refers to the fact that these cells, which contain a single nucleus, display no striations under the microscope. The contraction of smooth muscle is controlled involuntarily (the cells contract and relax without any conscious attempt to have them do so; examples of smooth muscle activity include moving food

Table 47.1. Properties of Muscle Fiber Types

Type I Fibers	Type II Fibers	
	Type IIa	Type IIb
• Slow-twitch (slow speed of contraction)	• Intermediate-twitch (fast speed of contraction)	• Fast-twitch (fast speed of contraction)
• Slow-oxidative (low glycogen content)	• Fast-oxidative glycolytic fibers (intermediate glycogen levels)	• Fast-glycolytic (high glycogen content)
• High myoglobin content (appear red)	• Intermediate fiber diameter	• Low myoglobin content (appear white)
• Small fiber diameter	• High myoglobin content (appear red)	• Low mitochondrial content
• Increased concentration of capillaries surrounding muscle (greater oxygen delivery)	• Increased oxidative capacity on training	• Limited aerobic metabolism
	• Intermediate resistance to fatigue	• Large fiber diameter
• High capacity for aerobic metabolism		• More sensitive to fatigue as compared with other fiber types
• High resistance to fatigue		• Least efficient use of energy, primarily glycolytic
• Used for prolonged, aerobic exercise		• Used for sprinting and resistance tasks

along the digestive tract, altering the diameter of the blood vessels, and expelling urine from the bladder). In contrast to skeletal muscle, these cells have the ability to maintain tension for extended periods, and do so efficiently, with a low use of energy.

C. Cardiac Muscle Cells

The cardiac cells are similar to skeletal muscle in that they are striated (contain fibers), but like smooth muscle cells they are regulated involuntarily (we do not have to think about making our heart beat). The cells are quadrangular in shape (see Fig. 47.1C) and form a network with multiple other cells through tight membrane junctions and gap junctions. The multicellular contacts allow the cells to act as a common unit and to contract and relax synchronously. Cardiac muscle cells are designed for endurance and consistency. They depend on aerobic metabolism for their energy needs because they contain many mitochondria and very little glycogen. These cells thus generate only a small amount of their energy from glycolysis using glucose derived from glycogen.

II. NEURONAL SIGNALS TO MUSCLE

For an extensive review of how muscle contracts or a detailed view of the signaling to allow muscle contraction, consult a medical physiology book. Only a brief overview is presented here.

The nerve–muscle cell junction is called the neuromuscular junction (Fig. 47.2). When appropriately stimulated, the nerve cell releases acetylcholine at the junction, which binds to acetylcholine receptors on the muscle membrane. This binding stimulates the opening of sodium channels on the sarcolemma. The massive influx of sodium ions results in the generation of an action potential in the sarcolemma at the edges of the motor end plate of the neuromuscular junction. The action potential sweeps across the surface of the muscle fiber and down the transverse tubules to the sarcoplasmic reticulum, where it initiates the release of calcium from its lumen, via the ryanodine receptor (Fig. 47.3). The calcium ion binds to troponin, resulting in a conformational change in the troponin–tropomyosin complexes such that they move away from the myosin-binding sites on the actin. When the binding site becomes available, the myosin head attaches to the myosin-binding site on the actin. The binding is followed by a conformational change (pivoting) in the myosin head, which shortens the sarcomere. After the pivoting, ATP binds the myosin head, which detaches from the actin and is available to bind another myosin-binding site on the

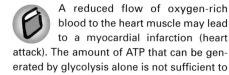 A reduced flow of oxygen-rich blood to the heart muscle may lead to a myocardial infarction (heart attack). The amount of ATP that can be generated by glycolysis alone is not sufficient to meet the energy requirements of the contracting heart.

The ryanodine receptors are calcium release channels found in the endoplasmic reticulum and sarcoplasmic reticulum of muscle cells. One type of receptor can be activated by a depolarization signal (depolarization-induced calcium release). Another receptor type is activated by calcium ions (calcium-induced calcium release). The proteins received their name because they bind ryanodine, a toxin obtained from the stem and roots of the plant *Ryania speciosa*. Ryanodine inhibits sarcoplasmic reticulum calcium release, and acts as a paralytic agent. It was first used commercially in insecticides.

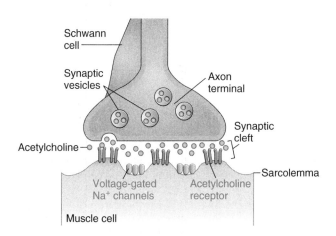

Fig. 47.2. The neuromuscular junction. When appropriately stimulated, the synaptic vesicles, containing acetylcholine, fuse with the axonal membrane and release acetylcholine into the synaptic cleft. The acetylcholine binds to its receptors on the muscle cells, which will initiate signaling for muscle contraction.

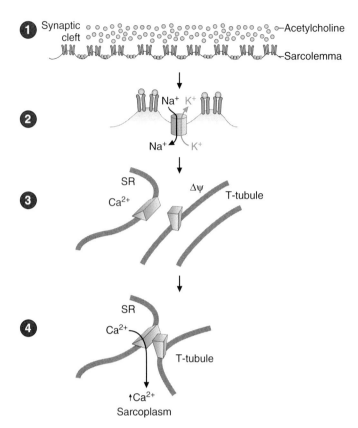

Fig. 47.3. Events leading to sarcoplasmic reticulum calcium release in skeletal muscle. 1. Acetylcholine, released at the synaptic cleft, binds to acetylcholine receptors on the sarcolemma, leading to a change of conformation of the receptors such that they now act as an ion pore. This allows sodium to enter the cell and potassium to leave. 2. The membrane polarization that results from these ion movements is transmitted throughout the muscle fiber by the T-tubule system. 3. A receptor in the T-tubules (the dihydropyridine receptor, DHPR) is activated by membrane polarization (a voltage-gated activation) such that activated DHPR physically binds to and activates the ryanodine receptor in the sarcoplasmic reticulum (depolarization-induced calcium release). 4. The activation of the ryanodine receptor, which is a calcium channel, leads to calcium release from the SR into the sarcoplasm. In cardiac muscle, activation of DHPR leads to calcium release from the T-tubules, and this small calcium release is responsible for the activation of the cardiac ryanodine receptor (calcium-induced calcium release) to release large amounts of calcium into the sarcoplasm.

Acetylcholine levels in the neuromuscular junction are rapidly reduced by the enzyme acetylcholinesterase. A number of nerve gas poisons act to inhibit acetylcholinesterase (such as sarin and VX), such that muscles are continuously stimulated to contract. This leads to blurred vision, bronchoconstriction, seizures, respiratory arrest, and death. The poisons are covalent modifiers of acetylcholinesterase; therefore, recovery from exposure to such poisons requires the synthesis of new enzyme. A new generation of acetylcholinesterase inhibitors, which act reversibly (i.e., they do not form covalent bonds with the enzyme), are now being used to treat dementia, in particular dementia as brought about by Alzheimer's disease.

actin. As long as calcium ion and ATP remain available, the myosin heads will repeat this cycle of attachment, pivoting, and detachment (Fig. 47.4). This movement requires ATP, and when ATP levels are low (such as occurs during ischemia), the ability of the muscle to relax or contract is compromised. As the calcium release channel closes, the calcium is pumped back into the sarcoplasmic reticulum against its concentration gradient by use of the energy-requiring protein SERCA (sarcoplasmic reticulum Ca^{2+} ATPase), and contraction stops. This basic process occurs in all muscle cell types, with some slight variations between cell types.

III. GLYCOLYSIS AND FATTY ACID METABOLISM IN MUSCLE CELLS

The pathways of glycolysis and fatty acid oxidation in muscle are the same as has been previously described (see Chapters 22 and 23). The difference between muscles and other tissues is how these pathways are regulated.

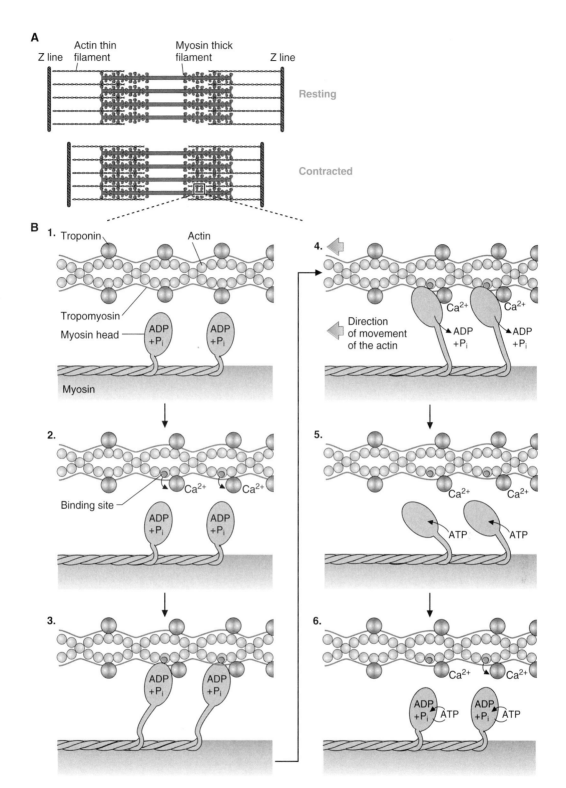

Fig. 47.4. An overview of muscle contraction. A. Muscle contraction. During muscle contraction, the myosin head binds to the actin thin filament. A pivoting of the myosin head toward the center of the sarcomere pulls the Z-lines closer together, with subsequent shortening of the sarcomere. B. A closer look at myosin–actin interactions. 1. A resting sarcomere. The troponin–tropomyosin complex is blocking the myosin-binding sites on the actin. The myosin head is already energized to power a contraction. 2. Exposure of the active site. After calcium binding to troponin, a conformational change in the troponin molecule pulls the troponin away from the binding site. 3. Cross-bridge attachment. Once the binding sites on the actin are exposed, the myosin head binds to it. 4. Myosin head pivoting. After cross-bridge attachment, the energy stored in the myosin head is released, and the myosin head pivots toward the center of the sarcomere (power stroke). Now the ADP and phosphate bound to the myosin head are released. 5. Detachment of the cross-bridge. Now a molecule of ATP binds to the myosin head with simultaneous detachment of the myosin head from the binding site on the actin molecule. 6. Reactivation of the myosin head. The ATPase activity of the myosin head hydrolyzes the ATP into ADP and phosphate. The energy released from the hydrolysis of this high-energy bond is used to re-energize the myosin head, and the entire cycle can be repeated as long as calcium is present and there are sufficient ATP reserves.

ACC-1 is the isozyme of acetyl-coA carboxylase, which is used to synthesize malonyl-CoA for fatty acid synthesis. Muscle cells do not synthesize fatty acids; however, they do carefully regulate the oxidation of fatty acids through the synthesis and destruction of malonyl-CoA. ACC-1 is a cytosolic protein, whereas ACC-2 is mitochondrial, closely linked to CPT-I in the outer mitochondrial membrane. Mice that have been bred to lack ACC-2 have a 50% reduction of fat stores as compared with "normal" mice. This was shown to be attributable to a 30% increase in skeletal muscle fatty acid oxidation because of the dysregulation of CPT-I, because malonyl CoA could not be produced to regulate the rate at which fatty acid oxidation occurred.

Under conditions in which ketone bodies are produced, fatty acid levels in the plasma are also elevated. Because the heart preferentially burns fatty acids as a fuel rather than the ketone bodies produced by the liver, the ketone bodies are spared for use by the nervous system.

Phosphofructokinase 2 (PFK-2) is negatively regulated by phosphorylation in the liver (the enzyme that catalyzes the phosphorylation is the cyclic adenosine monophosphate [cAMP]–dependent protein kinase). However, in skeletal muscle, PFK-2 is not regulated by phosphorylation. This is because the skeletal muscle isozyme of PFK-2 lacks the regulatory serine residue, which is phosphorylated in the liver. However, the cardiac isozyme of PFK-2 is phosphorylated and activated by a kinase cascade initiated by insulin. This allows the heart to activate glycolysis and to use blood glucose when blood glucose levels are elevated.

Fatty acid uptake by muscle requires the participation of fatty acid–binding proteins and the usual enzymes of fatty acid oxidation. Fatty acyl-CoA uptake into the mitochondria is controlled by malonyl-CoA, which is produced by an isozyme of acetyl-coA carboxylase (ACC-2; the ACC-1 isozyme is found in liver and adipose tissue and is used for fatty acid biosynthesis). ACC-2 is inhibited by phosphorylation by the AMP-activated protein kinase (AMP-PK) such that when energy levels are low the levels of malonyl CoA will drop, allowing fatty acid oxidation by the mitochondria. In addition, muscle cells also contain the enzyme malonyl CoA decarboxylase, which is activated by phosphorylation by the AMP-PK. Malonyl CoA decarboxylase converts malonyl CoA to acetyl CoA, thereby relieving the inhibition of carnitine palmitoyl transferase I (CPT-I) and stimulating fatty acid oxidation (Fig. 47.5). Muscle cells do not synthesize fatty acids; the presence of acetyl CoA carboxylase in muscle is exclusively for regulatory purposes.

IV. FUEL UTILIZATION IN CARDIAC MUSCLE

A. Normal Conditions

The heart primarily uses fatty acids (60–80%), lactate, and glucose (20–40%) as its energy sources. Ninety-eight percent of cardiac ATP is generated by oxidative means; 2% is derived from glycolysis. The lactate used by the heart is taken up by a monocarboxylate transporter in the cell membrane that is also used for the transport of ketone bodies. However, ketone bodies are not a preferred fuel for the heart, because the heart prefers to use fatty acids.

Lactate is generated by red blood cells and working skeletal muscle. When the lactate is used by the heart, it is oxidized to carbon dioxide and water, following the

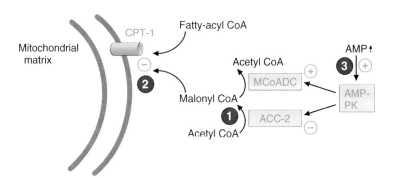

Fig. 47.5. Regulation of fatty acyl CoA entry into muscle mitochondria. 1. Acetyl CoA carboxylase-2 (ACC-2) converts acetyl CoA to malonyl CoA, which inhibits carnitine palmitoyl transferase I (CPT-I), thereby blocking fatty acyl CoA entry into the mitochondria. 2. However, as energy levels drop, AMP levels rise because of the activity of the adenylate kinase reaction. 3. The increase in AMP levels activates the AMP-activated protein kinase (AMP-PK), which phosphorylates and inactivates ACC-2, and also phosphorylates and activates malonyl CoA decarboxylase (MCoADC). The decarboxylase converts malonyl CoA to acetyl CoA, thereby relieving the inhibition of CPT-1, and allowing fatty acyl CoA entry into the mitochondria. This allows the muscle to generate ATP via the oxidation of fatty acids.

pathway lactate to pyruvate, pyruvate to acetyl-coA, acetyl CoA oxidation in the TCA cycle, and ATP synthesis through oxidative phosphorylation. An alternative fate for lactate is its utilization in the reactions of the Cori cycle in the liver.

Glucose transport into the cardiocyte occurs via both GLUT1 and GLUT4 transporters, although approximately 90% of the transporters are GLUT4. Insulin stimulates an increase in the number of GLUT4 transporters in the cardiac cell membrane, as does myocardial ischemia. This ischemia-induced increase in GLUT4 transporter number is additive to the effect of insulin on the translocation of GLUT4 transporters to the plasma membrane.

Fatty acid uptake into cardiac muscle is similar to that for other muscle cell types and requires fatty acid–binding proteins and carnitine palmitoyl transferase I for transfer into the mitochondria. Fatty acid oxidation in cardiac muscle cells is regulated by altering the activities of ACC-2 and malonyl CoA decarboxylase.

B. Ischemic Conditions

When blood flow to the heart is interrupted, the heart switches to anaerobic metabolism. The rate of glycolysis increases, but the accumulation of protons (via lactate formation) is detrimental to the heart. Ischemia also increases the levels of free fatty acids in the blood and, surprisingly, when oxygen is reintroduced to the heart, the high rate of fatty acid oxidation in the heart is detrimental to the recovery of the damaged heart cells. Fatty acid oxidation occurs so rapidly that NADH accumulates in the mitochondria, leading to a reduced rate of NADH shuttle activity, an increased cytoplasmic NADH level, and lactate formation, which generates more protons. In addition, fatty acid oxidation increases the levels of mitochondrial acetyl CoA, which inhibits pyruvate dehydrogenase, leading to cytoplasmic pyruvate accumulation and lactate production. As lactate production increases and the intracellular pH of the heart drops, it is more difficult to maintain ion gradients across the sarcolemma. ATP hydrolysis is required to repair these gradients, which are essential for heart function. However, the use of ATP for gradient repair reduces the amount of ATP available for the heart to use in contraction, which, in turn, compromises the ability of the heart to recover from the ischemic event.

 A new class of drugs, known as partial fatty acid oxidation (pFOX) inhibitors, are being developed to reduce the extensive fatty acid oxidation in heart after an ischemic episode (the prototype drug is ranolazine). The reduction in fatty acid oxidation induced by the drug will allow glucose oxidation to occur and reduce lactate buildup in the damaged heart muscle. Other possible targets of such drugs, which have yet to be developed, include ACC-2, malonyl CoA decarboxylase, and carnitine palmitoyl transferase I.

V. FUEL UTILIZATION IN SKELETAL MUSCLE

Skeletal muscles use many fuels to generate ATP. The most abundant immediate source of ATP is creatine phosphate. ATP also can be generated from glycogen stores either anaerobically (generating lactate) or aerobically, in which case pyruvate is converted to acetyl CoA for oxidation via the TCA cycle. All human skeletal muscles have some mitochondria and thus are capable of fatty acid and ketone body oxidation. Skeletal muscles are also capable of completely oxidizing the carbon skeletons of alanine, aspartate, glutamate, valine, leucine, and isoleucine, but not other amino acids. Each of these fuel oxidation pathways plays a somewhat unique role in skeletal muscle metabolism.

A. ATP and Creatine Phosphate

ATP is not a good choice as a molecule to store in quantity for energy reserves. Many reactions are allosterically activated or inhibited by ATP levels, especially those that generate energy. Muscle cells solve this problem by storing high-energy phosphate bonds in the form of creatine phosphate. When energy is required, creatine phosphate will donate a phosphate to ADP, to regenerate ATP for muscle contraction (Fig. 47.6).

Creatine synthesis begins in the kidney and is completed in the liver. In the kidney, glycine combines with arginine to form guanidinoacetate. In this reaction, the guanidinium group of arginine (the group that also forms urea), is transferred to

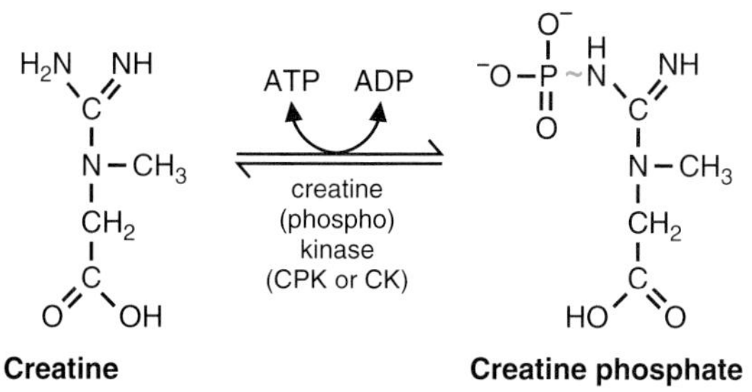

Fig. 47.6. The creatine phosphokinase reaction. The high-energy bond is the unusual nitrogen–phosphate bond, as indicated by the blue squiggle.

glycine, and the remainder of the arginine molecule is released as ornithine. Guanidinoacetate then travels to the liver, where it is methylated by S-adenosyl methionine to form creatine (Fig 47.7).

The creatine formed is released from the liver and travels through the bloodstream to other tissues, particularly skeletal muscle, heart, and brain, where it reacts with ATP to form the high-energy compound creatine phosphate (see Fig. 47.6). This reaction, catalyzed by creatine phosphokinase (CK, also abbreviated as CPK), is reversible. Therefore, cells can use creatine phosphate to regenerate ATP.

Creatine phosphate serves as a small reservoir of high-energy phosphate that can readily regenerate ATP from ADP. As a result, it plays a particularly important role in muscle during exercise. It also carries high-energy phosphate from

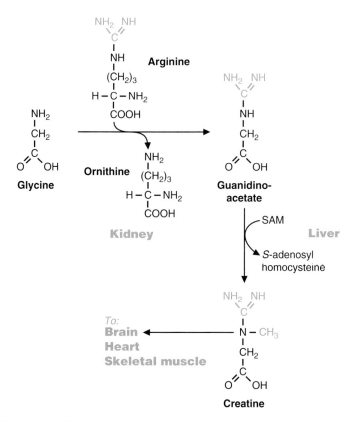

Fig. 47.7. The synthesis of creatine from arginine, glycine, and S-adenosyl methionine. Synthesis originates in the kidney and is completed in the liver.

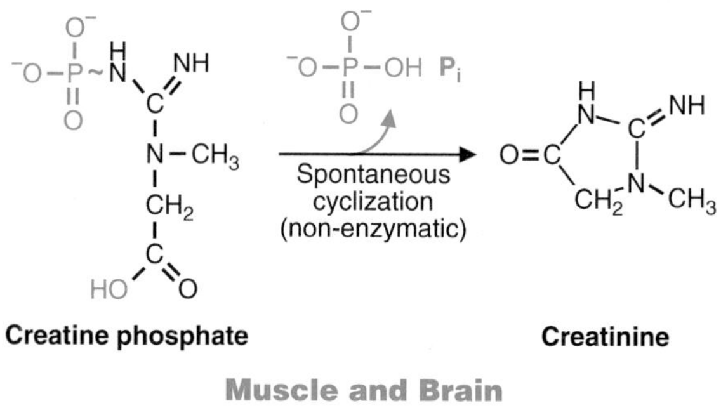

Fig. 47.8. The spontaneous production of creatinine from creatine phosphate.

mitochondria, where ATP is synthesized, to myosin filaments, where ATP is used for muscle contraction.

Creatine phosphate is an unstable compound. It spontaneously cyclizes, forming creatinine (Fig. 47.8). Creatinine cannot be further metabolized and is excreted in the urine. The amount of creatinine excreted each day is constant and depends on body muscle mass. Therefore, it can be used as a gauge for determining the amounts of other compounds excreted in the urine as well as an indicator of renal excretory function. The daily volume of urine is determined by such factors as the volume of blood reaching the renal glomeruli and the amount of renal tubular fluid reabsorbed from the tubular urine back into the interstitial space of the kidneys over time. At any given moment, the concentration of a compound in a single urine specimen does not give a good indication of the total amount that is being excreted on a daily basis. However, if the concentration of the compound is divided by the concentration of creatinine, the result provides a better indication of the true excretion rate.

B. Fuel Utilization at Rest

Muscle fuel utilization at rest is dependent on the serum levels of glucose, amino acids, and fatty acids. If blood glucose and amino acids are elevated, glucose will be converted to glycogen, and branched-chain amino acid metabolism will be high. Fatty acids will be used for acetyl CoA production and will satisfy the energy needs of the muscle under these conditions.

There is a balance between glucose oxidation and fatty acid oxidation, which is regulated by citrate. When the muscle cell has adequate energy, citrate leaves the mitochondria and activates ACC-2, which produces malonyl CoA. The malonyl CoA inhibits carnitine palmitoyl transferase-1, thereby reducing fatty acid oxidation by the muscle. Malonyl CoA decarboxylase is also inactive, because the AMP-PK is not active in the fed state. Thus, the muscle regulates its oxidation of glucose and fatty acids in part through monitoring of cytoplasmic citrate levels.

C. Fuel Use during Starvation

As blood glucose levels drop, insulin levels drop. This reduces the levels of GLUT4 transporters in the muscle membrane, and glucose use by muscle drops significantly. This conserves glucose for use by the nervous system and red blood cells. In cardiac muscle, PFK-2 is phosphorylated and activated by insulin. The lack of insulin results in a reduced use of glucose by these cells as well. Pyruvate dehydrogenase is inhibited by the high levels of acetyl CoA and NADH being produced by fatty acid oxidation.

Fatty acids become the muscle's preferred fuel under starvation conditions. The AMP-PK is active because of lower than normal ATP levels, ACC-2 is inhibited, and malonyl CoA decarboxylase is activated, thereby retaining full activity of CPT-1.

Each kidney normally contains approximately one million glomerular units. Each unit is supplied by arterial blood via the renal arteries and acts as a "filter." Metabolites such as creatinine leave the blood by passing through pores or channels in the glomerular capillaries and enter the fluid within the proximal kidney tubule for eventual excretion in the urine. When functionally intact, these glomerular tissues are impermeable to all but the smallest of proteins. When acutely inflamed, however, this barrier function is lost, and albumin and other proteins may appear in the urine.

The marked inflammatory changes in the glomerular capillaries that accompany poststreptococcal glomerulonephritis significantly reduce the flow of blood to the filtering surfaces of these vessels. As a result, creatinine, urea, and other circulating metabolites that are filtered into the urine at a normal rate (the glomerular filtration rate or GFR) in the absence of kidney disease now fail to reach the filters, and, therefore, they accumulate in the plasma.

These changes explain **Rena Felya's** laboratory profile during her acute inflammatory glomerular disease.

Muscle and brain cells contain large amounts of creatine phosphokinase (CK), and damage to these cells causes the enzyme to leak into the blood. Serum CK is measured to diagnose and evaluate patients who have had strokes and heart attacks. The presence of 5% or more of the CK in the blood as the muscle isoform is indicative of a heart attack (see Chapters 8 and 9).

Recall that in prolonged starvation muscle proteolysis is induced to provide substrates for gluconeogenesis by the liver. This does not, however, alter the use of fatty acids by the muscle for its own energy needs under these conditions.

The lack of glucose reduces the glycolytic rate, and glycogen synthesis does not occur because of the inactivation of glycogen synthase by epinephrine-stimulated phosphorylation.

D. Fuel Utilization during Exercise

The rate of ATP utilization in skeletal muscle during exercise can be as much as 100 times greater that that in resting skeletal muscles; thus, the pathways of fuel oxidation must be rapidly activated during exercise to respond to the much greater demand for ATP. ATP and creatine phosphate would be rapidly used up if they were not continuously regenerated. The synthesis of ATP occurs from glycolysis (either aerobic or anaerobic) and oxidative phosphorylation (which requires a constant supply of oxygen).

Anaerobic glycolysis is especially important as a source of ATP in three conditions. The first is during the initial period of exercise before exercise-stimulated increase in blood flow and substrate and oxygen delivery begin, allowing aerobic processes to occur. The second condition in which anaerobic glycolysis is important is exercise by muscle containing predominately fast-twitch glycolytic muscle fibers, because these fibers have low oxidative capacity and generate most of their ATP through glycolysis. The third condition is during strenuous activity, when the ATP demand exceeds the oxidative capacity of the tissue, and the increased ATP demand is met by anaerobic glycolysis.

1. ANAEROBIC GLYCOLYSIS AT THE ONSET OF EXERCISE

During rest, most of the ATP required in all types of muscle fibers is obtained from aerobic metabolism. However, as soon as exercise begins, the demand for ATP increases. The amount of ATP present in skeletal muscle could sustain exercise for only 1.2 seconds if not regenerated, and the amount of phosphocreatine could sustain exercise for only 9 seconds if it were not regenerated. It takes longer than 1 minute for the blood supply to exercising muscle to increase significantly due to vasodilation, and therefore oxidative metabolism of blood-borne glucose and fatty acids cannot increase rapidly at the onset of exercise. Thus, for the first few minutes of exercise, the conversion of glycogen to lactate provides a considerable portion of the ATP requirement.

2. ANAEROBIC GLYCOLYSIS IN THE TYPE IIB FAST-TWITCH GLYCOLYTIC FIBER

Although the human has no muscles that consist entirely of this fiber type, many animals do. Examples are white abdominal muscles of fish and the pectoral muscle of game birds (turkey white meat). These muscles contract rapidly and vigorously (the fast twitch refers to the time to peak tension), but only for short periods. Thus, they are used for activities such as flight in birds and sprinting and weight-lifting in humans.

In such muscles, the glycolytic capacity is high because the enzymes of glycolysis are present in large amounts (thus, the overall V_{max} [maximum velocity] is large). The levels of hexokinase, however, are low, so very little circulating glucose is used. The low levels of hexokinase in fast-twitch glycolytic fibers prevent the muscle from drawing on blood glucose to meet this high demand for ATP, thus avoiding hypoglycemia. Glucose 6-phosphate, formed from glycogenolysis, further inhibits hexokinase. The tissues rely on endogenous fuel stores (glycogen and creatine phosphate) to generate ATP, following the pathway of glycogen breakdown to glucose 1-phosphate, the conversion of glucose 1-phosphate to glucose 6-phosphate, and the metabolism of glucose 6-phosphate to lactate. Thus, anaerobic glycolysis is the main source of ATP during exercise of these muscle fibers.

3. ANAEROBIC GLYCOLYSIS FROM GLYCOGEN

Glycogenolysis and glycolysis during exercise are activated together because both PFK-1 (the rate-limiting enzyme of glycolysis) and glycogen phosphorylase b (the inhibited form of glycogen phosphorylase) are allosterically activated by AMP.

AMP is an ideal activator because its concentration is normally kept low by the adenylate kinase (also called myokinase in muscle) equilibrium [2 ADP ↔ AMP + ATP]. Thus, whenever ATP levels decrease slightly, the AMP concentration increases manyfold (Fig. 47.9)

Starting from a molecule of glucose 1-phosphate derived from glycogenolysis, three ATP molecules are produced in anaerobic glycolysis, as compared with 32 to 34 moles of ATP in aerobic glycolysis. To compensate for the low ATP yield of anaerobic glycolysis, fast-twitch glycolytic fibers have a much higher content of glycolytic enzymes, and the rate of glucose 6-phosphate utilization is more than 12 times as fast as slow-twitch fibers.

Muscle fatigue during exercise generally results from a lowering of the pH of the tissue to approximately 6.4. Both aerobic and anaerobic metabolism lowers the pH. Both the lowering of pH and lactate production can cause pain.

Metabolic fatigue also can occur once muscle glycogen is depleted. Muscle glycogen stores are used up in less than 2 minutes of anaerobic exercise. If you do pushups, you can prove this to yourself. The muscle used in pushups, a high-strength exercise, is principally fast-twitch glycolytic fibers. Time yourself from the start of your pushups. No matter how well you have trained, you probably cannot do pushups for as long as 2 minutes. Furthermore, you will feel the pain as the muscle pH drops as lactate production continues.

The regulation of muscle glycogen metabolism is complex. Recall that glycogen degradation in muscle is not sensitive to glucagon (muscles lack glucagon receptors), so there is little change in muscle glycogen stores during overnight fasting or long-term fasting, if the individual remains at rest. Glycogen synthase is inhibited during exercise but can be activated in resting muscle by the release of insulin after a high-carbohydrate meal. Unlike the liver form of glycogen phosphorylase, the muscle isozyme contains an allosteric site for AMP binding. When AMP binds to muscle glycogen phosphorylase b, the enzyme is activated even though it is not phosphorylated. Thus, as muscle begins to work and the myosin-ATPase hydrolyzes existing ATP stores to ADP, AMP will begin to accumulate (due to the myokinase reaction), and glycogen degradation will be enhanced. The activation of muscle glycogen phosphorylase b is further enhanced by the release of Ca^{2+} from the sarcoplasmic reticulum, which occurs when muscles are stimulated to contract. The increase in sarcoplasmic Ca^{2+} also leads to the allosteric activation of glycogen phosphorylase kinase (through binding to the calmodulin subunit of the enzyme), which phosphorylates muscle glycogen phosphorylase b, fully activating it. And, finally, during intense exercise, epinephrine release stimulates the activation of adenylate cyclase in muscle cells, thereby activating the

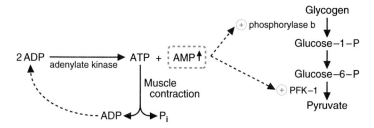

Fig. 47.9. Activation of muscle glycogenolysis and glycolysis by AMP. As muscle contracts, ATP is converted to ADP and P_i. In the adenylate kinase reaction, two ADP react to form ATP and AMP. The ATP is used for contraction. As AMP accumulates, it activates glycogenolysis and glycolysis.

cAMP-dependent protein kinase (see Fig. 28.10). Protein kinase A phosphorylates and fully activates glycogen phosphorylase kinase such that continued activation of muscle glycogen phosphorylase can occur. The hormonal signal is slower than the initial activation events triggered by AMP and calcium (Fig. 47.10).

4. ANAEROBIC GLYCOLYSIS DURING HIGH-INTENSITY EXERCISE

Once exercise begins, the electron transport chain, the TCA cycle, and fatty acid oxidation are activated by the increase of ADP and the decrease of ATP. Pyruvate dehydrogenase remains in the active, nonphosphorylated state as long as NADH can be reoxidized in the electron transport chain and acetyl CoA can enter the TCA cycle. However, even though mitochondrial metabolism is working at its maximum capacity, additional ATP may be needed for very strenuous, high-intensity exercise. When this occurs, ATP is not being produced rapidly enough to meet the muscle's needs, and AMP begins to accumulate. Increased AMP levels activate PFK-1 and glycogenolysis, thereby providing additional ATP from anaerobic glycolysis (the additional pyruvate

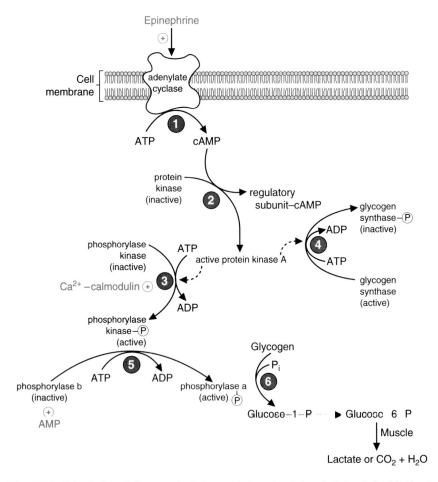

Fig. 47.10. Stimulation of glycogenolysis in muscle by epinephrine. 1. Epinephrine binding to its receptor leads to the activation of adenylate cyclase, which increases cAMP levels. 2. cAMP binds to the regulatory subunits of protein kinase A, thereby activating the catalytic subunits. 3. Active protein kinase A phosphorylates and activates phosphorylase kinase. Phosphorylase kinase also can be activated partially by the Ca^{2+}-calmodulin complex as Ca^{2+} levels increase as muscles contract. 4. Protein kinase A phosphorylates and inactivates glycogen synthase. 5. Active phosphorylase kinase converts glycogen phosphorylase b to glycogen phosphorylase a. 6. Glycogen degradation forms glucose 1-phosphate, which is converted to glucose 6-phosphate, which enters the glycolytic pathway for energy production.

produced does not enter the mitochondria but rather is converted to lactate such that glycolysis can continue). Thus, under these conditions, most of the pyruvate formed by glycolysis enters the TCA cycle whereas the remainder is reduced to lactate to regenerate NAD$^+$ for continued use in glycolysis.

5. FATE OF LACTATE RELEASED DURING EXERCISE

The lactate that is released from skeletal muscles during exercise can be used by resting skeletal muscles or by the heart, a muscle with a large amount of mitochondria and very high oxidative capacity. In such muscles, the NADH/NAD$^+$ ratio will be lower than in exercising skeletal muscle, and the lactate dehydrogenase reaction will proceed in the direction of pyruvate formation. The pyruvate that is generated is then converted to acetyl CoA and oxidized in the TCA cycle, producing energy by oxidative phosphorylation.

The second potential fate of lactate is that it will return to the liver through the Cori cycle, where it will be converted to glucose (see Fig. 22.10).

VI. MILD AND MODERATE-INTENSITY LONG-TERM EXERCISE

A. Lactate Release Decreases with Duration of Exercise

Mild to moderate-intensity exercise can be performed for longer periods than can high-intensity exercise. This is because of the aerobic oxidation of glucose and fatty acids, which generates more energy per fuel molecule than anaerobic metabolism, and which also produces acid at a slower rate than anaerobic metabolism. Thus, during mild and moderate-intensity exercise, the release of lactate diminishes as the aerobic metabolism of glucose and fatty acids becomes predominant.

B. Blood Glucose as a Fuel

At any given time during fasting, the blood contains only approximately 5 g glucose, enough to support a person running at a moderate pace for a few minutes. Therefore, the blood glucose supply must be constantly replenished. The liver performs this function by processes similar to those used during fasting. The liver produces glucose by breaking down its own glycogen stores and by gluconeogenesis. The major source of carbon for gluconeogenesis during exercise is, of course, lactate, produced by the exercising muscle, but amino acids and glycerol are also used (Fig. 47.11). Epinephrine released during exercise stimulates liver glycogenolysis and gluconeogenesis by causing cAMP levels to increase.

During long periods of exercise, blood glucose levels are maintained by the liver through hepatic glycogenolysis and gluconeogenesis. The amount of glucose that the liver must export is greatest at higher work loads, in which case the muscle is using a greater proportion of the glucose for anaerobic metabolism. With increasing duration of exercise, an increasing proportion of blood glucose is supplied by gluconeogenesis. However, for up to 40 minutes of mild exercise, glycogenolysis is mainly responsible for the glucose output of the liver. However, after 40 to 240 minutes of exercise, the total glucose output of the liver decreases. This is caused by the increased utilization of fatty acids, which are being released from adipose tissue triacylglycerols (stimulated by epinephrine release). Glucose uptake by the muscle is stimulated by the increase in AMP levels and the activation of the AMP-activated protein kinase, which stimulates the translocation of GLUT4 transporters to the muscle membrane.

The hormonal changes that direct the increased hepatic glycogenolysis, hepatic gluconeogenesis, and adipose tissue include a decrease in insulin and an increase in glucagon, epinephrine, and norepinephrine. Plasma levels of growth hormone, cortisol, and thyroid-stimulating hormone (TSH) also increase and may make a contribution to

Q: If **Otto Shape** runs at a pace at which his muscles require approximately 500 Calories per hour, how long could he run on the amount of glucose that is present in circulating blood? Assume the blood volume is 5 liters.

Remember from Chapter 1 that a food Calorie is equivalent to 1 kcal of energy. One gram of glucose can give rise to 4 kcal of energy, so at a rate of consumption of 500 Calories per hour we have the following:

(500 Calories/hr) × (1 gram glucose/4 Calories energy) × (1 hour/60 minutes) = 2 grams of glucose/min.

Thus, Otto must use 2 grams of glucose per minute to run at his current pace. In the fasting state, blood glucose levels are approximately 90 mg/dL, or 900 mg/L. Because blood volume is estimated at 5 liters, Otto has 4.5 grams glucose available. If not replenished, that amount of glucose would only support 2.5 minutes of running, at 2 grams glucose per minute.

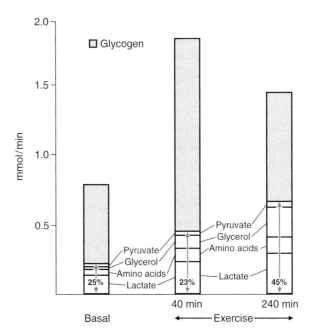

Fig. 47.11. Production of blood glucose by the liver from various precursors during rest and during prolonged exercise. The shaded area represents the contribution of liver glycogen to blood glucose, and the open area represents the contribution of gluconeogenesis. From Wahren J, et al. In: Howald H, Poortmans JR, eds. Metabolic Adaptation to Prolonged Physical Exercise. Cambridge, MA: Birkhauser, 1973:148.

fuel mobilization as well (see Chapter 43). The activation of hepatic glycogenolysis occurs through glucagon and epinephrine release. Hepatic gluconeogenesis is activated by the increased supply of precursors (lactate, glycerol, amino acids, and pyruvate), the induction of gluconeogenic enzymes by glucagon and cortisol (this only occurs in prolonged exercise), and the increased supply of fatty acids to provide the ATP and NADH needed for gluconeogenesis and the regulation of gluconeogenic enzymes.

C. Free Fatty Acids as a Source of ATP

The longer the duration of the exercise, the greater the reliance of the muscle on free fatty acids for the generation of ATP (Fig. 47.12). Because ATP generation from

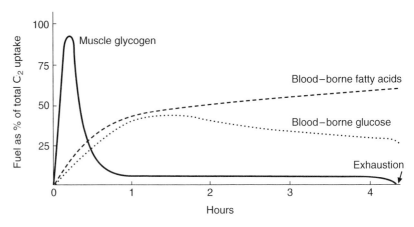

Fig. 47.12. Fuels used during exercise. The pattern of fuel utilization changes with the duration of the exercise. From Felig P, et al. Endocrinology & Metabolism. New York: McGraw-Hill, 1981:796.

free fatty acids depends on mitochondria and oxidative phosphorylation, long-distance running uses muscles that are principally slow-twitch oxidative fibers, such as the gastrocnemius. It is also important to realize that resting skeletal muscle uses free fatty acids as a principle fuel. At almost anytime except the postprandial state (right after eating), free fatty acids are the preferred fuel for skeletal muscle.

The preferential utilization of fatty acids over glucose as a fuel in skeletal muscle depends on the following factors:

1. The availability of free fatty acids in the blood, which depends on their release from adipose tissue triacylglycerols by hormone-sensitive lipase. During prolonged exercise, the small decrease of insulin, and increases of glucagon, epinephrine and norepinephrine, cortisol, and possibly growth hormone all activate adipocyte tissue lipolysis.
2. Inhibition of glycolysis by products of fatty acid oxidation. Pyruvate dehydrogenase activity is inhibited by acetyl CoA, NADH, and ATP, all of which are elevated as fatty acid oxidation proceeds. As AMP levels drop, and ATP levels rise, PFK-1 activity is decreased (see Chapter 22).
3. Glucose transport may be reduced during long-term exercise. Glucose transport into skeletal muscles via the GLUT 4 transporter is greatly activated by either insulin or exercise. During long-term exercise, the effect of falling insulin levels or increased fatty acid levels may counteract the stimulation of glucose transport by the exercise itself.
4. Ketone body oxidation also increases during exercise. Their utilization as a fuel is dependent on their rate of production by the liver. Ketone bodies are, however, never a major fuel for skeletal muscle (muscles prefer free fatty acids).
5. Acetyl-CoA carboxylase (isozyme ACC-2) must be inactivated for the muscle to use fatty acids. This occurs as the AMP-PK is activated and phosphorylates ACC-2, rendering it inactive.

D. Branched-Chain Amino Acids

Branched-chain amino acid oxidation has been estimated to supply a maximum of 20% of the ATP supply of resting muscle. Oxidation of branched-chain amino acids in muscle serves two functions. The first is the generation of ATP, and the second is the synthesis of glutamine, which effluxes from the muscle. The highest rates of branched-chain amino acid oxidation occur under conditions of acidosis, in which there is a higher demand for glutamine to transfer ammonia to the kidney and to buffer the urine as ammonium ion during proton excretion. Recall that glutamine synthesis occurs from the carbon skeletons of branched-chain amino acid oxidation (valine and isoleucine) after the initial five steps of the oxidative pathway.

E. The Purine Nucleotide Cycle

Exercise increases the activity of the purine nucleotide cycle, which converts aspartate to fumarate plus ammonia (see Fig. 41.13). The ammonia is used to buffer the proton production and lactate production from glycolysis, and the fumarate is recycled and can form glutamine.

F. Acetate

Acetate is an excellent fuel for skeletal muscle. It is treated by the muscle as a very-short-chain fatty acid. It is activated to acetyl CoA in the cytosol and then transferred into the mitochondria via acetylcarnitine transferase, an isozyme of carnitine palmitoyl transferase. Sources of acetate include the diet (vinegar is acetic acid) and acetate produced in the liver from alcohol metabolism. Certain commercial power bars for athletes contain acetate.

VII. METABOLIC EFFECTS OF TRAINING ON MUSCLE METABOLISM

The effect of training depends, to some extent, on the type of training. In general, training increases the muscle glycogen stores and increases the number and size of mitochondria. The fibers thus increase their capacity for generation of ATP from oxidative metabolism and their ability to use fatty acids as a fuel. The winners in marathon races seem to use muscle glycogen more efficiently than others.

Training to improve strength, power, and endurance of muscle performance is called resistance training. Its goal is to increase the size of the muscle fibers (hypertrophy of the muscle). Muscle fibers can develop a maximal force of 3 to 4 kg/cm^2 of muscle area. Thus, if one can increase their muscle size from 80 to 120 cm^2, the maximal resistance that could be lifted would increase from 240 to 360 kg. Hypertrophy occurs by increased protein synthesis in the muscle and a reduction in existing protein turnover.

CLINICAL COMMENTS

Poststreptococcal glomerulonephritis (PSGN) may follow pharyngeal or cutaneous infection with one of a limited number of "nephritogenic" strains of group A β-hemolytic streptococci. The pathogenesis of PSGN involves a host immune (antibody) response to one or more of the enzymes secreted by the bacterial cells. The antigen–antibody complexes are deposited on the tissues of glomerular units, causing a local acute inflammatory response. Hypertension may occur as a consequence of sodium and water retention caused by an inability of the inflamed glomerular units to filter sodium and water into the urine. Proteinuria is usually mild if the immune response is self-limited.

Overall, one of the most useful clinical indicators of glomerular filtration rate in both health and disease is the serum creatinine concentration. The endogenous production of creatinine, which averages approximately 15 mg/kg of body weight per day, is correlated with muscle mass and, therefore, tends to be constant for a given individual if renal function is normal. Any rise in serum creatinine in patients such as **Rena Felya,** therefore, can be assumed to result from decreased excretion of this metabolite into the urine. The extent of the rise in the blood is directly related to the severity of the pathologic process involving the glomerular units within the kidneys.

BIOCHEMICAL COMMENTS

The SERCA pump is a transmembrane protein of 110 kDa present in several different isoforms throughout the body. Three genes encode SERCA proteins, designated SERCA1, SERCA2, and SERCA3. The SERCA1 gene produces two alternatively spliced transcripts, SERCA1a and SERCA1b. SERCA1b is expressed in the fetal and neonatal fast-twitch skeletal muscles, and is replaced by SERCA1a in adult fast-twitch muscle. The SECA2 gene also undergoes alternative splicing, producing the SERCA2a and SERCA2b isoforms. The SERCA2b isoform is expressed in all cell types and is associated with inositol trisphosphate (IP$_3$)-regulated calcium stores. SERCA2a is the primary isoform expressed in cardiac tissue. SERCA3 produces at least five different alternatively spliced isoforms, which are specifically expressed in different tissues.

SERCA2a plays an important role in cardiac contraction and relaxation. Contraction is initiated by the release of calcium from intracellular stores, whereas relaxation occurs as the calcium is re-sequestered in the sarcoplasmic reticulum, in part mediated by the SERCA2a protein. The SERCA2a pump is regulated, in part, by its association with the protein phospholamban (PLN). PLN is a pentameric molecule consisting of five identical subunits of molecular weight 22,000 Daltons. PLN associates with SERCA2a in the sarcoplasmic reticulum and reduces its pumping activity. Because new contractions cannot occur until cytosolic calcium has been re-sequestered into the sarcoplasmic reticulum, a reduction in SERCA2a activity increases the relaxation time. However, when called on, the heart can increase its rate of contractions by inhibiting the activity of phospholamban. This is accomplished by phosphorylation of phospholamban by protein kinase A (PKA). Epinephrine release stimulates the heart to beat faster. This occurs through epinephrine binding to its receptor, activating a G protein, which leads to adenylyl cyclase activation, elevation of cAMP levels, and activation of protein kinase A. PKA phosphorylates PLN, thereby reducing its association with SERCA2a and relieving the inhibition of pumping activity. This results in reduced relaxation times and more frequent contractions.

Mutations in PLN lead to cardiomyopathies, primarily an autosomal dominant form of dilated cardiomyopathy. This mutation leads to an arginine in place of cysteine at position 9 in PLN, which forms an inactive complex with PKA and blocks PKA phosphorylation of PLN. Individuals with this form of PLN develop cardiomyopathy in their teens. In this condition, the cardiac muscle does not pump well (because of the constant inhibition of SERCA2a), and becomes enlarged (dilated). Because of the poor pumping action of the heart, fluid can build up in the lungs. The pulmonary congestion results in a sense of breathlessness (left heart failure). Eventually, progressive left heart failure leads to fluid accumulation in other tissues and organs of the body, such as the legs and ankles (right heart failure).

Suggested References

Dyck JRB, Lopaschuk GD. Malonyl CoA control of fatty acid oxidation in the ischemic heart. J Mol Cell Cardiol 2002;34:1099–1109.

Gibson DM, Harris RA. Muscle Metabolism in Metabolic Regulation in Mammals. New York: Taylor and Francis, 2002: 123–154.

MacLennan DH, Kranias EG. Phospholamban: a crucial regulator of cardiac contractility. Nature Review, Molecular Cell Biology 2003;4:566–577.

REVIEW QUESTIONS—CHAPTER 47

1. The process of stretching before exercise has which of the following biochemical benefits?

    (A) Stimulates the release of epinephrine
    (B) Activates glycolysis in the liver
    (C) Increases blood flow to the muscles
    (D) Activates glycolysis in the muscles
    (E) Stimulates glycogenolysis in the liver

2. The major metabolic fuel for participating in a prolonged aerobic exercise event is which of the following?

    (A) Liver glycogen
    (B) Muscle glycogen
    (C) Brain glycogen
    (D) Adipose triacylglycerol
    (E) Red blood cell–produced lactate

3. A 24-hour urine collection showed that an individual's excretion of creatinine was much lower than normal. Decreased excretion of creatinine could be caused by which of the following?

   (A) A decreased dietary intake of creatine
   (B) A higher than normal muscle mass resulting from weight lifting
   (C) A genetic defect in the enzyme that converts creatine phosphate to creatinine
   (D) Kidney failure
   (E) A vegetarian diet

4. In the biosynthetic pathways for the synthesis of heme, creatine, and guanine, which one of the following amino acids directly provides carbon atoms that appear in the final product?

   (A) Serine
   (B) Aspartate
   (C) Cysteine
   (D) Glutamate
   (E) Glycine

5. In skeletal muscle, increased hydrolysis of ATP during muscular contraction leads to which of the following?

   (A) A decrease in the rate of palmitate oxidation to acetyl CoA
   (B) A decrease in the rate of NADH oxidation by the electron transport chain
   (C) The activation of PFK-1
   (D) An increase in the proton gradient across the inner mitochondrial membrane.
   (E) The activation of glycogen synthase

48 Metabolism of the Nervous System

*The nervous systems consists of various cell types. The most abundant cell in the nervous system is the **glial cell**, which consists of **astrocytes** and **oligodendrocytes** in the **central nervous system**, and **Schwann cells** in the **peripheral nervous system**. These cells provide support for the neurons and synthesize the protective **myelin sheath** that surrounds the axons emanating from the neurons. **Microglial cells** in the nervous system act as immune cells, destroying and ingesting foreign organisms that enter the nervous system. The interface between the brain parenchyma and the cerebrospinal fluid compartment is formed by the **ependymal cells**, which line the cavities of the brain and spinal cord. These cells use their cilia to allow for the circulation of the **cerebrospinal fluid** (CSF), which bathes the cells of the central nervous system.*

*The cells of the brain are separated from free contact with the rest of the body by the **blood-brain barrier**. The capillaries of the brain exhibit features, such as tight endothelial cell junctions, that restrict their permeability to metabolites in the blood. This protects the brain from compounds that might be toxic or otherwise interfere with nerve impulse transmission. It also affects the entry of precursors for brain metabolic pathways such as fuel metabolism and neurotransmitter synthesis.*

*Neurotransmitters can be divided structurally into two categories: **small nitrogen-containing neurotransmitters** and **neuropeptides**. The small nitrogen-containing neurotransmitters are generally synthesized in the **presynaptic terminal** from amino acids and intermediates of glycolysis and the TCA cycle. They are retained in storage vesicles until the neuron is depolarized. The **catecholamine** neurotransmitters (**dopamine, norepinephrine, and epinephrine**) are derived from tyrosine. **Serotonin** is synthesized from **tryptophan**. **Acetylcholine** is synthesized from **choline**, which can be supplied from the diet or is synthesized and stored as part of **phosphatidylcholine**. **Glutamate** and its neurotransmitter derivative, **γ-aminobutyric acid (GABA)**, are derived from α-ketoglutarate in the TCA cycle. **Glycine** is synthesized in the brain from **serine**. The synthesis of the neurotransmitters is regulated to correspond to the rate of depolarization of the individual neurons. A large number of cofactors are required for the synthesis of neurotransmitters, and deficiencies of **pyridoxal phosphate**, **thiamine-pyrophosphate**, and **vitamin B12** result in a variety of neurologic dysfunctions.*

*Brain metabolism has a high **requirement for glucose and oxygen. Deficiencies of either (hypoglycemia or hypoxia)** affect brain function because they influence adenosine triphosphate (ATP) production and the supply of precursors for neurotransmitter synthesis. **Ischemia** elicits a condition in which increased **calcium levels, swelling, glutamate excitotoxicity,** and **nitric oxide** generation affect brain function, and can lead to a stroke. The generation of **free radicals** and abnormalities in nitric oxide production are important players in the pathogenesis of a variety of **neurodegenerative** diseases.*

Because of the restrictions posed by the blood-brain barrier to the entry of a variety of substances into the central nervous system, the brain generally synthesizes and

881

*degrades its own lipids. Essential fatty acids can enter the brain, but the more common fatty acids do not. The turnover of lipids at the synaptic membrane is very rapid, and the neuron must replace those lipids lost during exocytosis. The glial cells produce the **myelin** sheath, which is composed primarily of lipids. These lipids are of a different composition than those of the neuronal cells. Because there is considerable lipid synthesis and turnover in the brain, this organ is sensitive to **disorders of peroxisomal function** (Refsum's disease; interference in very-long-chain fatty acid oxidation and α-oxidation) and **lysosomal diseases** (mucopolysaccharidoses; inability to degrade complex lipids and glycolipids).*

THE WAITING ROOM

Katie Colamin, a 34-year-old dress designer, developed alarming palpitations of her heart while bending forward to pick up her cat. She also developed a pounding headache and sweated profusely. After 5 to 10 minutes, these symptoms subsided. One week later, her aerobic exercise instructor, a registered nurse, noted that Katie grew very pale and was tremulous during exercise. The instructor took Katie's blood pressure, which was 220 mm Hg systolic (normal, up to 120 at rest) and 132 mm Hg diastolic (normal, up to 80 at rest). Within 15 minutes, Katie recovered, and her blood pressure returned to normal. The instructor told Katie to see her physician the next day.

The doctor told Katie that her symptom complex coupled with severe hypertension strongly suggested the presence of a tumor in the medulla of one of her adrenal glands (a pheochromocytoma) that was episodically secreting large amounts of catecholamines, such as norepinephrine (noradrenaline) and epinephrine (adrenaline). Her blood pressure was normal until moderate pressure to the left of her umbilicus caused Katie to suddenly develop a typical attack, and her blood pressure rose rapidly. She was immediately scheduled for a magnetic resonance imaging (MRI) study of her adrenal glands. The MRI showed a 3.5 × 2.8 × 2.6 cm mass in the left adrenal gland, with imaging characteristics typical of a pheochromocytoma.

Ivan Applebod's brother, **Evan Applebod,** was 6 feet tall and weighed 425 pounds. He had only been successful in losing weight once in his life, in 1977. Evan's weight was not usually a concern for him, but in 1997 he had become concerned when it became difficult for him to take walks or go fishing because of joint pain in his knees. He was also suffering from symptoms suggestive of a peripheral neuropathy, manifest primarily as tingling in his legs. He had failed in all previous dieting attempts and was desperate now to lose weight. The physician placed Evan on a new drug, Redux, which had just been approved for use as a weight loss agent, and a slightly restricted low-fat, low-calorie diet. In 4 months, Evan's weight dropped from 425 pounds to 335 pounds, his total cholesterol dropped from 250 to 185, and his serum triglycerides dropped from 375 to 130. However, Redux was withdrawn from the market by its manufacturer late in 1997 because of its toxicity. Evan was then placed on Prozac, a drug used primarily as an antidepressant and less commonly as an appetite suppressant.

I. CELL TYPES OF THE NERVOUS SYSTEM

The nervous system consists of neurons, the cells that transmit signals, and supporting cells, the neuroglia. The neuroglia consists of oligodendrocytes and astrocytes (collectively known as glial cells), microglial cells, ependymal cells, and Schwann cells. The neuroglia are designed to support and sustain the neurons and do so by surrounding neurons and holding them in place, supplying nutrients and oxygen to the neurons, insulating neurons so their electrical signals are more rapidly propagated, and cleaning up any debris that enters the nervous system. The central nervous system (CNS) consists of the brain and spinal cord. This system integrates all signals emanating from the peripheral nervous system (PNS). The PNS is composed of all neurons lying outside of the CNS.

A. Neurons

Neurons consist of a cell body (soma) from which long (axons) and short (dendrites) extensions protrude. Dendrites receive information from the axons of other neurons, whereas the axons transmit information to other neurons. The axon–dendrite connection is known as a synapse (Fig. 48.1). Most neurons contain multiple dendrites, each of which can receive signals from multiple axons. This configuration allows a single neuron to integrate information from multiple sources. Although neurons also contain just one axon, most axons branch extensively and distribute information to multiple targets (divergence). The neurons transmit signals by changes in the electrical potential across their membrane. Signaling across a synapse requires the release of neurotransmitters that, when bound to their specific receptors, initiate an electrical signal in the receiving or target cell. Neurons are terminally differentiated cells and, as such, have little capability for division. Because of this, injured neurons have a limited capacity to repair themselves and frequently undergo apoptosis (programmed cell death) when damaged.

B. Neuroglial Cells

1. ASTROCYTES

The astrocytes are found in the CNS and are star-shaped cells that provide physical and nutritional support for neurons. During development of the CNS, the astrocytes guide neuronal migration to their final adult position and form a matrix that keeps neurons in place. These cells serve several functions, including the ability to phagocytose debris left behind by cells, to provide lactate (from glucose metabolism) as

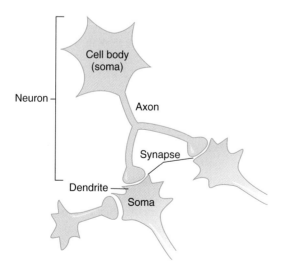

Fig. 48.1. A neuron consists of a cell body (soma) with short extensions (dendrites) and a long extension (axon). The axon–dendrite interface is the synapse. A soma may receive input from multiple axons.

a carbon source for the neurons, and to control the brain extracellular ionic environment Astrocytes help to regulate the content of the extracellular fluid (ECF) by taking up, processing, and metabolizing nutrients and waste products.

2. OLIGODENDROCYTES

The oligodendrocyte provides the myelin sheath that surrounds the axon, acting as an "insulation" for many of the neurons in the CNS. The myelin sheath consists of a lipid–protein covering of the axons (see section V.B. for a description of the composition and synthesis of the myelin sheath). Oligodendrocytes can form myelin sheaths around multiple neurons in the CNS by sending out processes that bind to the axons on target neurons. The speed with which a neuron conducts its electrical signal (action potential) is directly proportional to the degree of myelination. Oligodendrocytes, along with the astrocytes, form a supporting matrix for the neurons. Oligodendrocytes have a limited capacity for mitosis, and if damaged, do not replicate. If this occurs, demyelination of the axons may occur, resulting in abnormalities in signal conduction along that axon (see Biochemical Comments).

3. SCHWANN CELLS

Peripheral axons can regenerate if Schwann cells are available to guide the growth of the axon. There is a synergistic interaction between the Schwann cells, secreted growth factors, and the axon that allows the axons to reconnect to its appropriate target.

Schwann cells are the supporting cells of the PNS. Like oligodendrocytes, Schwann cells form myelin sheaths around the axons, but unlike the oligodendrocytes, Schwann cells only myelinate one axon. Schwann cells also clean up cellular debris in the PNS.

4. MICROGLIAL CELLS

These are the smallest type of glial cells in the nervous system. They serve as immunologically responsive cells similar to the action of macrophages in the circulation. Microglial cells destroy invading microorganisms and phagocytose cellular debris.

5. EPENDYMAL CELLS

The ependymal cells are ciliated cells that line the cavities (ventricles) of the CNS and the spinal cord. In some areas of the brain, the ependymal cells are functionally specialized to elaborate and secrete cerebrospinal fluid (CSF) into the ventricular system. The beating of the ependymal cilia allow for efficient circulation of the CSF throughout the CNS. The CSF acts as both a shock absorber protecting the CNS from mechanical trauma and a system for the removal of metabolic wastes. The CSF can be aspirated from the spinal canal and analyzed to determine whether disorders of CNS function, with their characteristic CSF changes, are present.

For many years, it had been believed that damaged neurons in the CNS could not regenerate, for it was thought that there were no pluripotent stem cells (cells that could differentiate into various cell types found in the CNS) in the CNS. However, recent data suggest that cells found within the ependymal layer can act as neural stem cells, which under appropriate stimulation can regenerate neurons. Such a finding opens up a large number of potential treatments for diseases that alter neuronal cell function.

II. THE BLOOD-BRAIN BARRIER

A. Capillary Structure

In the capillary beds of most organs, a rapid passage of molecules occurs from the blood through the endothelial wall of the capillaries into the interstitial fluid. Thus, the composition of interstitial fluid resembles that of blood, and specific receptors or transporters in the plasma membrane of the cells being bathed by the interstitial fluid may directly interact with amino acids, hormones, or other compounds from the blood. In the brain, transcapillary movement of substrates in the peripheral circulation into the brain is highly restricted by the blood-brain barrier. This barrier limits the accessibility of blood-borne toxins and other potentially harmful compounds to the neurons of the CNS.

The blood-brain barrier begins with the endothelial cells that form the inner lining of the vessels supplying blood to the CNS (Fig. 48.2). Unlike the endothelial cells of other organs, these cells are joined by tight junctions that do not permit the movement of polar molecules from the blood into the interstitial fluid bathing the neurons. They also lack mechanisms for transendothelial transport that are present in other capillaries of the body. These mechanisms include fenestrations ("windows" or pores that span the endothelial lining and permit the rapid movement of molecules across membranes) or transpinocytosis (vesicular transport from one side of the endothelial cell to another).

The endothelial cells actively, as well as passively, serve to protect the brain. Because they contain a variety of drug-metabolizing enzyme systems similar to the drug-metabolizing enzymes found in the liver, the endothelial cells can metabolize neurotransmitters and toxic chemicals and, therefore, form an enzymatic barrier to entry of these potentially harmful substances into the brain. They actively pump hydrophobic molecules that diffuse into endothelial cells back into the blood (especially xenobiotics) with P-glycoproteins, which act as transmembranous, ATP-dependent efflux pumps. Although lipophilic substances, water, oxygen, and carbon dioxide can readily cross the blood-brain barrier by passive diffusion, other molecules depend on specific transport systems. Differential transporters on the luminal and abluminal endothelial membranes can transport compounds into, as well as out of, the brain.

Further protection against the free entry of blood-borne compounds into the CNS is provided by a continuous collagen-containing basement membrane that completely surrounds the capillaries. The basement membrane appears to be surrounded by the foot processes of astrocytes. Thus, compounds must pass through endothelial cell membranes, the enzymatic barrier in the endothelial cells, the basement membrane, and possibly additional cellular barriers formed by the astrocytes to reach the neurons in the brain.

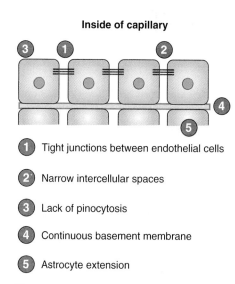

Inside of capillary

1. Tight junctions between endothelial cells
2. Narrow intercellular spaces
3. Lack of pinocytosis
4. Continuous basement membrane
5. Astrocyte extension

Fig. 48.2. The blood-brain barrier. Compounds in the blood cannot freely pass into the brain; they must traverse the endothelial cells, basement membrane, and astrocytes, by use of specific carriers to gain access to the brain. Very lipophilic molecules may pass through all of these membranes in the absence of a carrier.

B. Transport through the Blood-Brain Barrier

Many nonpolar substances, such as drugs and inert gases, probably diffuse through the endothelial cell membranes. A large number of other compounds are transported through the endothelial capillaries by facilitative transport, whereas others, such as nonessential fatty acids, cannot cross the blood-brain barrier. Essential fatty acids, however, are transported across the barrier.

1. FUELS

Glucose, which is the principle fuel of the brain, is transported through both endothelial membranes by facilitated diffusion via the GLUT-1 transporter (see Fig. 27.4). GLUT-3 transporters present on the neurons then allow the neurons to transport the glucose from the ECF. Glial cells express GLUT-1 transporters. Although the rate of glucose transport into the ECF normally exceeds the rate required for energy metabolism by the brain, glucose transport may become rate-limiting as blood glucose levels fall below the normal range. Thus, individuals begin to experience hypoglycemic symptoms at approximately 60 mg/dL, as the glucose levels are reduced to the K_m, or below the K_m values of the GLUT-1 transporters in the endothelial cells of the barrier.

Monocarboxylic acids, including L-lactate, acetate, pyruvate, and the ketone bodies acetoacetate and β-hydroxybutyrate, are transported by a separate stereospecific system that is slower than the transport system for glucose. During starvation, when the level of ketone bodies in the blood is elevated, this transporter is upregulated. Ketone bodies are important fuels for the brain of both the adult and the neonate during prolonged starvation (greater than 48 hours).

 A number of disorders of glucose transport across the blood-brain barrier are known. The most common of these is facilitated glucose transporter protein type 1 (GLUT1) deficiency syndrome. In this disorder, GLUT1 transporters are impaired, which results in a low glucose concentration in the CSF (a condition known as hypoglycorrhachia). A diagnostic indication of this disorder is that in the presence of normal blood glucose levels the ratio of CSF glucose to blood glucose levels is less than 0.4. Clinical features are variable but include seizures, developmental delay, and a complex motor disorder. These symptoms are the result of inadequate glucose levels within the brain. The disorder can be treated by prescribing a ketogenic diet (high-fat, low-carbohydrate). This will force the patient to produce ketone bodies, which are easily transported into the CNS and can spare the brain's requirement for glucose as an energy source.

The finding that the large, neutral amino acids (LNAA) have a common carrier system across the blood-brain barrier suggests that if one amino acid is in excess, it can, by competitive inhibition, result in a lower transport of the other amino acids. This suggests that the mental retardation that results from untreated PKU and maple syrup urine disease (see Chapter 39) may be attributable to the high levels of either phenylalanine or branched-chain amino acids in the blood. These high levels overwhelm the LNAA carrier, such that excessive levels of the damaging amino acid enter the CNS. In support of this theory is the finding that treatment of PKU patients with large doses of LNAA lacking phenylalanine resulted in a decrease of phenylalanine levels in the CSF and brain, with an improvement in their cognitive functions as well.

2. AMINO ACIDS AND VITAMINS

Large neutral amino acids (LNAA, such as phenylalanine, leucine, tyrosine, isoleucine, valine, tryptophan, methionine, and histidine) rapidly enter the CSF via a single amino acid transporter. (L-[leucine preferring]-system amino acid transporter). Many of these compounds are essential in the diet and must be imported for protein synthesis or as precursors of neurotransmitters. Because a single transporter is involved, these amino acids compete with each other for transport into the brain.

The entry of small neutral amino acids, such as alanine, glycine, proline, and γ-aminobutyrate (GABA), is markedly restricted because their influx could dramatically change the content of neurotransmitters (see section III). They are synthesized in the brain, and some are transported out of the CNS and into the blood via the A-(alanine-preferring)-system carrier. Vitamins have specific transporters through the blood-brain barrier as they do in most tissues.

3. RECEPTOR-MEDIATED TRANSCYTOSIS

Certain proteins, such as insulin, transferrin, and insulin-like growth factors, cross the blood-brain barrier by receptor-mediated transcytosis. Once the protein binds to its membrane receptor, the membrane containing the receptor–protein complex is endocytosed into the endothelial cell to form a vesicle. It is released on the other side of the endothelial cell. Absorptive-mediated transcytosis also can occur. It differs from receptor-mediated transcytosis in that the protein binds nonspecifically to the membrane and not to a distinct receptor.

III. SYNTHESIS OF SMALL NITROGEN-CONTAINING NEUROTRANSMITTERS

Molecules that serve as neurotransmitters fall into two basic structural categories: (1) small nitrogen-containing molecules, and (2) neuropeptides. The major small nitrogen-containing molecule neurotransmitters include glutamate, γ-aminobutyric acid (GABA), glycine, acetylcholine, dopamine, norepinephrine, serotonin, and histamine. Additional neurotransmitters that fall into this category include epinephrine, aspartate, and nitric oxide. In general, each neuron synthesizes only those neurotransmitters that it uses for transmission through a synapse or to another cell. The neuronal tracts are often identified by their neurotransmitter; for example, a dopaminergic tract synthesizes and releases the neurotransmitter dopamine.

Neuropeptides are usually small peptides, which are synthesized and processed in the CNS. Some of these peptides have targets within the CNS (such as endorphins, which bind to opioid receptors and block pain signals), whereas others are released into the circulation to bind to receptors on other organs (such as growth hormone and thyroid-stimulating hormone). Many neuropeptides are synthesized as a larger precursor, which is then cleaved to produce the active peptides. Until recently, the assumption was that a neuron only synthesized and released a single neurotransmitter. More recent evidence suggests that a neuron may contain (1) more than one small molecule neurotransmitter, (2) more than one neuropeptide neurotransmitter, or (3) both types of neurotransmitters. The differential release of the various neurotransmitters is the result of the neuron altering its frequency and pattern of firing.

A. General Features of Neurotransmitter Synthesis

A number of features are common to the synthesis, secretion, and metabolism of most small nitrogen-containing neurotransmitters (Table 48.1). Most of these neurotransmitters are synthesized from amino acids, intermediates of glycolysis and the TCA cycle, and O_2 in the cytoplasm of the presynaptic terminal. The rate of synthesis is

Table 48.1. Features Common to Neurotransmitters[a]

- Synthesis from amino acid and common metabolic precursors usually occurs in the cytoplasm of the presynaptic nerve terminal. The synthetic enzymes are transported by fast axonal transport from the cell body, where they are synthesized, to the presynaptic terminal.
- The synthesis of the neurotransmitter is regulated to correspond to the rate of firing of the neuron, both acutely and through long-term enhancement of synaptic transmission.
- The neurotransmitter is actively taken up into storage vesicles in the presynaptic terminal.
- The neurotransmitter acts at a receptor on the postsynaptic membrane.
- The action of the neurotransmitter is terminated through reuptake into the presynaptic terminal, diffusion away from the synapse, or enzymatic inactivation. The enzymatic inactivation may occur in the postsynaptic terminal, the presynaptic terminal, or an adjacent astrocyte or microglial cell.
- The blood-brain barrier affects the supply of precursors for neurotransmitter synthesis.

[a]Not all neurotransmitters exhibit all of these features. Nitric oxide is an exception to most of these generalities. Some neurotransmitters (epinephrine, serotonin, and histamine) are also secreted by cells other than neurons. Their synthesis and secretion by non-neuronal cells follows other principles.

generally regulated to correspond to the rate of firing of the neuron. Once synthesized, the neurotransmitters are transported into storage vesicles by an ATP-requiring pump linked with the proton gradient. Release from the storage vesicle is triggered by the nerve impulse that depolarizes the postsynaptic membrane and causes an influx of Ca^{2+} ions through voltage-gated calcium channels. The influx of Ca^{2+} promotes fusion of the vesicle with the synaptic membrane and release of the neurotransmitter into the synaptic cleft. The transmission across the synapse is completed by binding of the neurotransmitter to a receptor on the postsynaptic membrane (Fig. 48.3).

The action of the neurotransmitter is terminated through reuptake into the presynaptic terminal, uptake into glial cells, diffusion away from the synapse, or enzymatic inactivation. The enzymatic inactivation may occur in the postsynaptic terminal, the presynaptic terminal or an adjacent astrocyte microglia cell, or in endothelial cells in the brain capillaries.

Drugs have been developed that block neurotransmitter uptake into storage vesicles. Reserpine, which blocks catecholamine uptake into vesicles, had been used as an antihypertensive and antiepileptic drug for many years, but it was noted that a small percentage of patients on the drug became depressed and even suicidal. Animals treated with reserpine showed signs of lethargy and poor appetite, similar to depression in humans. Thus, a link was forged between monoamine release and depression in humans.

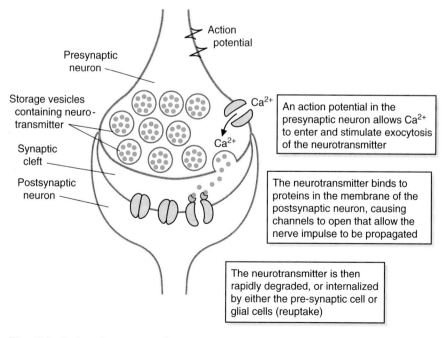

Fig. 48.3. Action of neurotransmitters.

Not all neurotransmitters exhibit all of these features. Nitric oxide, because it is a gas, is an exception to most of these generalities. Some neurotransmitters are synthesized and secreted by both neurons and other cells (e.g., epinephrine, serotonin, histamine).

B. Dopamine, Norepinephrine, and Epinephrine

1. SYNTHESIS OF THE CATECHOLAMINE NEUROTRANSMITTERS

These three neurotransmitters are synthesized in a common pathway from the amino acid L-tyrosine. Tyrosine is supplied in the diet or is synthesized in the liver from the essential amino acid phenylalanine by phenylalanine hydroxylase (see Chapter 39). The pathway of catecholamine biosynthesis is shown in Figure 48.4.

The first and rate-limiting step in the synthesis of these neurotransmitters from tyrosine is the hydroxylation of the tyrosine ring by tyrosine hydroxylase, a tetrahydrobiopterin (BH_4)-requiring enzyme. The product formed is dihydroxyphenylalanine or DOPA. The phenyl ring with two adjacent OH groups is a catechol, and hence dopamine, norepinephrine, and epinephrine are called catecholamines.

The second step in catecholamine synthesis is the decarboxylation of DOPA to form dopamine. This reaction, like many decarboxylation reactions of amino acids, requires pyridoxal phosphate. Dopaminergic neurons (neurons using dopamine as a neurotransmitter) stop the synthesis at this point, because these neurons do not synthesize the enzymes required for the subsequent steps.

Neurons that secrete norepinephrine synthesize it from dopamine in a hydroxylation reaction catalyzed by dopamine β-hydroxylase (DBH). This enzyme is present only within the storage vesicles of these cells. Like tyrosine hydroxylase, it is a mixed-function oxidase that requires an electron donor. Ascorbic acid (vitamin C) serves as the electron donor and is oxidized in the reaction. Copper (Cu^{2+}) is a bound cofactor required for the electron transfer.

Although the adrenal medulla is the major site of epinephrine synthesis, it is also synthesized in a few neurons that use epinephrine as a neurotransmitter. These neurons contain the above pathway for norepinephrine synthesis and in addition contain the enzyme that transfers a methyl group from SAM to norepinephrine to form epinephrine. Thus, epinephrine synthesis is dependent on the presence of adequate levels of B12 and folate (see Chapter 40).

2. STORAGE AND RELEASE OF CATECHOLAMINES

Ordinarily, only low concentrations of catecholamines are free in the cytosol, whereas high concentrations are found within the storage vesicles. Conversion of tyrosine to L-DOPA and that of L-DOPA to dopamine occurs in the cytosol. Dopamine is then taken up into the storage vesicles. In norepinephrine-containing neurons, the final β-hydroxylation reaction occurs within the vesicles.

The catecholamines are transported into vesicles by the protein VMAT2 (vesicle membrane transporter 2) (Fig. 48.5). The vesicle transporters contain 12 transmembrane domains and are homologous to a family of bacterial drug resistance transporters, including the P-glycoprotein. The mechanism that concentrates the catecholamines in the storage vesicles is an ATP-dependent process linked to a proton pump (secondary active transport). Protons are pumped into the vesicles by a vesicular-ATPase (v-ATPase). The protons then exchange for the positively charged catecholamine via the transporter VMAT2. The influx of the catecholamine is thus driven by the H^+ gradient across the membrane. The intravesicular concentration of catecholamines is approximately 0.5 M, roughly 100 times the cytosolic concentration. In the vesicles, the catecholamines exist in a complex with ATP and acidic proteins known as chromogranins.

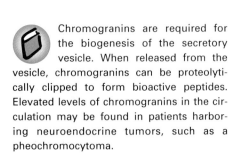

Chromogranins are required for the biogenesis of the secretory vesicle. When released from the vesicle, chromogranins can be proteolytically clipped to form bioactive peptides. Elevated levels of chromogranins in the circulation may be found in patients harboring neuroendocrine tumors, such as a pheochromocytoma.

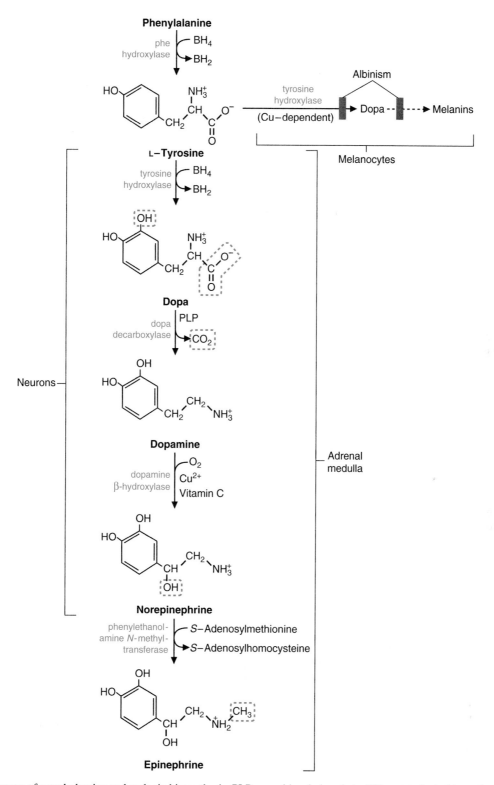

Fig. 48.4. The pathways of catecholamine and melanin biosynthesis. PLP = pyridoxal phosphate. BH$_4$ = tetrahydrobiopterin. The shaded boxes indicate the enzymes, which, when defective, lead to albinism.

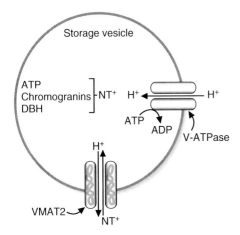

In albinism, either the copper-dependent tyrosine hydroxylase of melanocytes (which is distinct from the tyrosine hydroxylase found in the adrenal medulla) or other enzymes that convert tyrosine to melanins may be defective. Individuals with albinism suffer from a lack of pigment in the skin, hair, and eyes, and they are sensitive to sunlight.

Fig. 48.5. Transport of catecholamines into storage vesicles. This is a secondary active transport based on the generation of a proton gradient across the vesicular membrane. NT+ = positively charged neurotransmitter (catecholamine); DBH = dopamine β-hydroxylase; VMAT2 = vesicle membrane transporter 2; V-ATPase = vesicular ATPase.

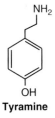

Tyramine is a degradation product of tyrosine that can lead to headaches, palpitations, nausea and vomiting, and elevated blood pressure if present in large quantities. Tyramine mimics norepinephrine and binds to norepinephrine receptors, stimulating them. Tyramine is inactivated by MAO-A, but if a person is taking an MAO inhibitor, foods containing tyramine should be avoided.

Tyramine

The vesicles play a dual role: they maintain a ready supply of catecholamines at the nerve terminal that is available for immediate release, and they mediate the process of release. When an action potential reaches the nerve terminal, Ca^{2+} channels open, allowing an influx of Ca^{2+}, which promotes the fusion of vesicles with the neuronal membrane. The vesicles then discharge their soluble contents, including the neurotransmitters, ATP, chromogranins, and DBH, into the extraneuronal space by the process of exocytosis. In some cases, the catecholamines affect other neurons. In other cases, they circulate in the blood and initiate responses in peripheral tissues.

3. INACTIVATION AND DEGRADATION OF CATECHOLAMINE NEUROTRANSMITTERS

The action of catecholamines is terminated through reuptake into the presynaptic terminal and diffusion away from the synapse. Degradative enzymes are present in the presynaptic terminal, and in adjacent cells, including glial cells and endothelial cells.

Two of the major reactions in the process of inactivation and degradation of catecholamines are catalyzed by monamine oxidase (MAO) and catechol-O-methyltransferase (COMT). MAO is present on the outer mitochondrial membrane of many cells and oxidizes the carbon containing the amino group to an aldehyde, thereby releasing ammonium ion (Fig. 48.6). In the presynaptic terminal, MAO inactivates catecholamines that are not protected in storage vesicles. (Thus, drugs that deplete storage vesicles indirectly increase catecholamine degradation.) There are two isoforms of MAO with different specificities of action: MAO-A preferentially deaminates norepinephrine and serotonin, whereas MAO-B acts on a wide spectrum of phenylethylamines (phenylethyl refers to a –CH₂- group linked to a phenyl ring). MAO in the liver and other sites protects against the ingestion of dietary biogenic amines such as the tyramine found in many cheeses.

COMT is also found in many cells, including the erythrocyte. It works on a broad spectrum of extraneuronal catechols and those that have diffused away from the synapse. COMT transfers a methyl group from SAM to a hydroxyl group on the catecholamine or its degradation product (see Fig. 48.6). Because the inactivation reaction requires SAM, it is indirectly dependent on vitamins B12 and folate. The action of MAO and COMT can occur in almost any order, thereby resulting in a large number of degradation products and intermediates, many of which appear in the urine. Cerebrospinal homovanillylmandelic acid (HVA) is an indicator of dopamine degradation. Its concentration is decreased in the brain of patients with Parkinson's disease.

Katie Colamin's doctor ordered plasma catecholamine (epinephrine, norepinephrine, and dopamine) levels and also had Katie collect a 24-hour urine specimen for the determination of catecholamines and their degradation products. All of these tests showed unequivocal elevations of these compounds in Katie's blood and urine. Katie was placed on phenoxybenzamine, an α₁- and α₂-adrenergic receptor antagonist that blocks the pharmacologic effect of the elevated catecholamines on these receptors. After ruling out evidence to suggest metastatic disease to the liver or other organs (in case Katie's tumor was malignant), the doctor referred Katie to a surgeon with extensive experience in adrenal surgery.

The catecholamines exert their physiologic and pharmacologic effects by circulating in the bloodstream to target cells whose plasma membranes contain catecholamine receptors. This interaction initiates a biochemical cascade leading to responses that are specific for different types of cells. Patients such as **Katie Colamin** experience palpitations, excessive sweating, hypertensive headaches, and a host of other symptoms when a catecholamine-producing tumor of the adrenal medulla suddenly secretes supraphysiologic amounts of epinephrine or norepinephrine into the venous blood draining the neoplasm.

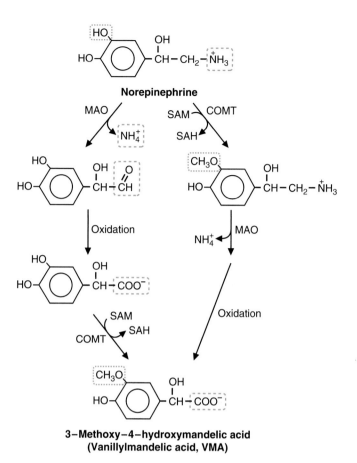

**3–Methoxy–4–hydroxymandelic acid
(Vanillylmandelic acid, VMA)**

Fig. 48.6. Inactivation of catecholamines. Methylation and oxidation may occur in any order. Methylated and oxidized derivatives of norepinephrine and epinephrine are produced, and 3-methoxy-4-hydroxymandelic acid is the final product. These compounds are excreted in the urine. MAO = monoamine oxidase; COMT = catechol O-methyltransferase; SAM = S-adenosylmethionine; SAH = S-adenosylhomocysteine.

4. REGULATION OF TYROSINE HYDROXYLASE

Efficient regulatory mechanisms coordinate the synthesis of catecholamine neurotransmitters with the rate of firing. Tyrosine hydroxylase, the first committed step and rate-limiting enzyme in the pathway, is regulated by feedback inhibition that is coordinated with depolarization of the nerve terminal. Tyrosine hydroxylase is inhibited by free cytosolic catecholamines that compete at the binding site on the enzyme for the pterin cofactor (tetrahydrobiopterin, BH_4; see Chapter 39).

Depolarization of the nerve terminal activates tyrosine hydroxylase. Depolarization also activates a number of protein kinases (including protein kinase C, protein kinase A [the cAMP-dependent protein kinase] and CAM kinases [Ca^{2+}-calmodulin–dependent kinases]) that phosphorylate tyrosine hydroxylase. These activation steps result in an enzyme that binds BH_4 more tightly, making it less sensitive to end-product inhibition.

In addition to these short-term regulatory processes, a long-term process involves alterations in the amounts of tyrosine hydroxylase and dopamine β-hydroxylase present in nerve terminals. When sympathetic neuronal activity is increased for a prolonged period, the amounts of mRNA coding for tyrosine hydroxylase and dopamine β-hydroxylase are increased in the neuronal perikarya (the cell body of the neuron). The increased gene transcription may be the result of phosphorylation of CREB (cAMP response element binding protein; see Chapter 26) by

In addition to the catecholamines, serotonin is also inactivated by monoamine oxidase. The activity of a number of antipsychotic drugs are based on inhibiting MAO. The first generation of drugs (exemplified by iproniazid, which was originally developed as an antituberculosis drug and was found to induce mood swings in patients) were irreversible inhibitors of both the A and B forms of MAO. Although leading to a reduction in the severity of depression (by maintaining higher levels of serotonin), these drugs suffered from the "cheese" effect. Cheese and other foods that are processed over long periods (such as red wine) contain tyramine. Usually tyramine is inactivated by MAO-A, but if an individual is taking an MAO inhibitor, tyramine levels will increase. Tyramine induces the release of norepinephrine from storage vesicles, which leads to potentially life-threatening hypertensive episodes. When it was realized that MAO existed in two forms, selective irreversible inhibitors were developed; examples include clorgyline for MAO-A, and deprenyl for MAO-B. Deprenyl has been used to treat Parkinson's disease (which is caused by a lack of dopamine, which is also inactivated by MAO). Deprenyl, however, is not an antidepressant. Clorgyline is an antidepressant but suffers from the "cheese" effect. This led to the development of the third generation of MAO inhibitors, which are reversible inhibitors of the enzyme, as typified by moclobemide. Moclobemide is a specific, reversible inhibitor of MAO-A and is effective as an antidepressant. More importantly, because of the reversible nature of the drug, the "cheese" effect is not observed, because as tyramine levels increase, they displace the drug from MAO, and the tyramine is safely inactivated.

protein kinase A or by other protein kinases. CREB then binds to the CRE (cAMP response element) in the promoter region of the gene (similar to the mechanism for the induction of gluconeogenic enzymes in the liver). The newly synthesized enzyme molecules are then transported down the axon to the nerve terminals. The concentration of dopamine decarboxylase in the terminal does not appear to change in response to neuronal activity.

C. Metabolism of Serotonin

The pathway for the synthesis of serotonin from tryptophan is very similar to the pathway for the synthesis of norepinephrine from tyrosine (Fig. 48.7). The first enzyme of the pathway, tryptophan hydroxylase, uses an enzymic mechanism similar to that of tyrosine and phenylalanine hydroxylase and requires BH_4 to hydroxylate the ring structure of tryptophan. The second step of the pathway is a decarboxylation reaction

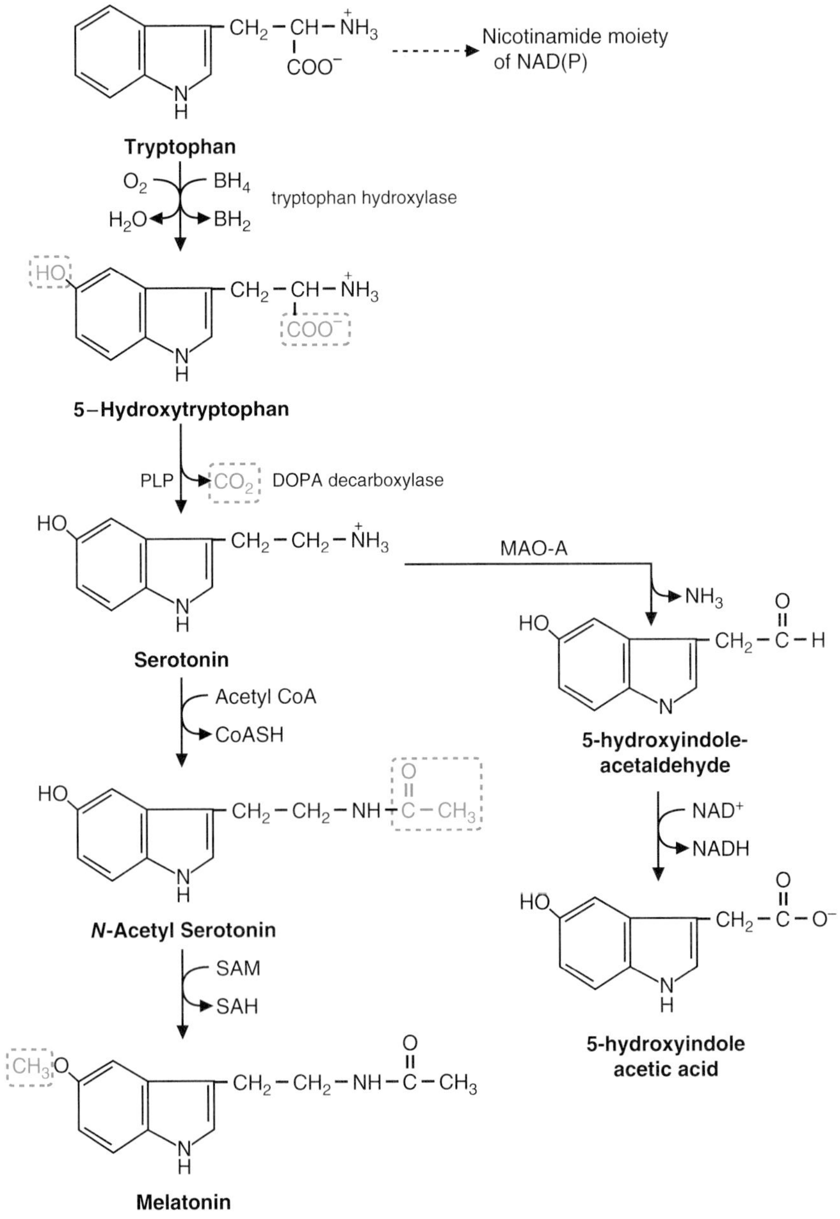

Fig. 48.7. Synthesis and inactivation of serotonin.

catalyzed by the same enzyme that decarboxylates DOPA. Serotonin, like the catecholamine neurotransmitters, can be inactivated by MAO.

The neurotransmitter melatonin is also synthesized from tryptophan (see Fig. 48.7). Melatonin is produced in the pineal gland in response to the light–dark cycle, its level in the blood rising in a dark environment. It is probably through melatonin that the pineal gland conveys information about light–dark cycles to the body, organizing seasonal and circadian rhythms. Melatonin also may be involved in regulating reproductive functions.

D. Metabolism of Histamine

Within the brain, histamine is produced both by mast cells and by certain neuronal fibers. Mast cells are a family of bone marrow–derived secretory cells that store and release high concentrations of histamine. They are prevalent in the thalamus, hypothalamus, dura mater, leptomeninges, and choroid plexus. Histaminergic neuronal cell bodies in the human are found in the tuberomamillary nucleus of the posterior basal hypothalamus. The fibers project into nearly all areas of the CNS, including the cerebral cortex, the brainstem, and spinal cord.

Histamine is synthesized from histidine in a single enzymatic step. The enzyme histidine decarboxylase requires pyridoxal phosphate, and its mechanism is very similar to that of DOPA decarboxylase (Fig. 48.8).

Like other neurotransmitters, newly synthesized neuronal histamine is stored within the nerve terminal vesicle. Depolarization of nerve terminals activates the exocytotic release of histamine by voltage-dependent as well as a calcium-dependent mechanism.

Once released from neurons, histamine is thought to activate both postsynaptic and presynaptic receptors. Unlike other neurotransmitters, histamine does not appear to be recycled into the presynaptic terminal to any great extent. However, astrocytes have a specific high-affinity uptake system for histamine and may be the major site of the inactivation and degradation of this monoamine.

The first step in the inactivation of histamine in the brain is methylation (see Fig. 48.8). The enzyme histamine methyltransferase transfers a methyl group from SAM to a ring nitrogen of histamine to form methylhistamine. The second step is oxidation by MAO-B, followed by an additional oxidation step. In peripheral tissues, histamine undergoes deamination by diamine oxidase, followed by oxidation to a carboxylic acid (see Fig. 48.8).

E. Acetylcholine

1. SYNTHESIS

The synthesis of acetylcholine from acetyl CoA and choline is catalyzed by the enzyme choline acetyltransferase (ChAT) (Fig. 48.9). This synthetic step occurs in the presynaptic terminal. The compound is stored in vesicles and later released through calcium-mediated exocytosis. Choline is taken up by the presynaptic terminal from the blood via a low-affinity transport system (high K_m) and from the synaptic cleft via a high-affinity transport mechanism (low K_m). It is also derived from the hydrolysis of phosphatidylcholine (and possibly sphingomyelin) in membrane lipids. Thus, membrane lipids may form a storage site for choline, and their hydrolysis, with the subsequent release of choline, is highly regulated.

 It is believed that the vitamin B12 requirement for choline synthesis contributes to the neurologic symptoms of vitamin B12 deficiency. The methyl groups for choline synthesis are donated by SAM, which is converted to S-adenosylhomocysteine in the reaction. Recall that formation of SAM through recycling of homocysteine requires both tetrahydrofolate and vitamin B12 (unless extraordinary amounts of methionine are available to bypass the B12-dependent methionine synthase step).

 Evan Applebod was placed on Redux, which increased the secretion of serotonin. Serotonin has been implicated in many processes, including mood control and appetite regulation. When serotonin levels are low, increased appetite, or depression, or both can occur. Thus, drugs that can increase serotonin levels may be able to control appetite and depression. Redux was a second-generation drug developed from fenfluramine, a known appetite suppressant. When first used, fenfluramine could not be resolved between two distinct optical isomers (d versus l). The l-isomer induced sleepiness, so to counteract this effect fenfluramine was often given with phentermine, which elevated epinephrine levels to counteract the drowsiness (the combination of drugs was known as fen/phen). Once the two isomers of fenfluramine could be resolved, Redux, dexfenfluramine, was developed. Because levels of serotonin have been linked to mood, many antidepressant drugs were developed that affect serotonin levels. The first of these were the MAO inhibitors; a second class are the tricyclics, and the third class are known as the SSRI (selective serotonin reuptake inhibitors). The SSRI block reuptake of serotonin from the synapse, leading to an elevated response to serotonin. Redux acted both as an SSRI but also increased the secretion of serotonin, leading to elevated levels of this compound in the synapse. None of the other drugs that affect serotonin levels have this effect.

Histamine elicits a number of effects on different tissues. Histamine is the major mediator of the allergic response and when released from mast cells (a type of white blood cell found in tissues) leads to vasodilation and an increase in the permeability of blood vessel walls. This leads to the allergic symptoms of a runny nose and watering eyes. When histamine is released in the lungs, the airways constrict in an attempt to reduce the intake of the allergic material. The ultimate result of this, however, is bronchospasm, which can lead to difficulty in breathing. In the brain, histamine is an excitatory neurotransmitter. Antihistamines block histamine from binding to its receptor. In the tissues, this will counteract histamine's effect on vasodilation and blood vessel wall permeability, but in the brain the effect is to cause drowsiness. The new generation of "non-drowsy" antihistamines have been modified such that they cannot pass through the blood-brain barrier. Thus, the effects on the peripheral tissues are retained with no effect on CNS histamine response.

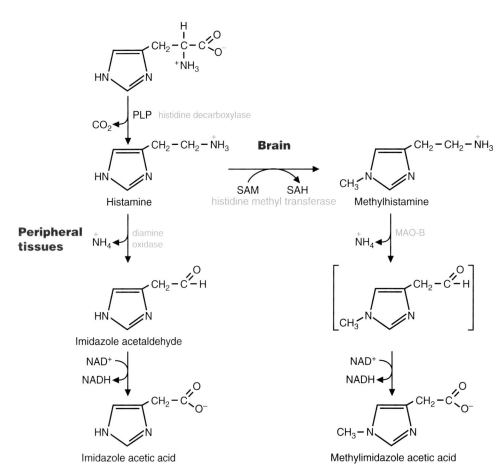

Fig. 48.8. Synthesis and inactivation of histamine; note the different pathways for brain and peripheral tissues. SAM = S-adenosylmethionine; SAH = S-adenosylhomocysteine.

Choline is a common component of the diet but also can be synthesized in the human as part of the pathway for the synthesis of phospholipids (see Chapter 33). The only route for choline synthesis is via the sequential addition of three methyl groups from SAM to the ethanolamine portion of phosphatidylethanolamine to form phosphatidylcholine. Phosphatidylcholine is subsequently hydrolyzed to release choline or phosphocholine. Conversion of phosphatidylethanolamine to phosphatidylcholine occurs in many tissues, including liver and brain. This conversion is B6- and B12-dependent.

The acetyl group used for acetylcholine synthesis is derived principally from glucose oxidation to pyruvate and decarboxylation of pyruvate to form acetyl

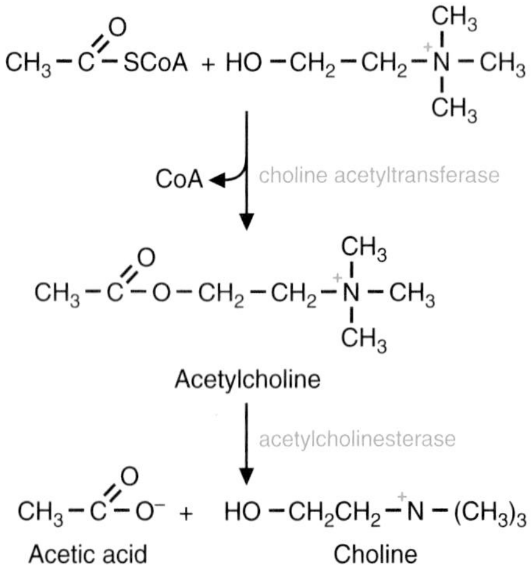

Fig. 48.9. Acetylcholine synthesis and degradation.

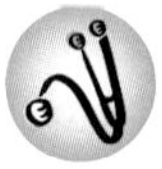

The supply of choline in the brain can become rate-limiting for acetylcholine synthesis, and supplementation of the diet with lecithin (phosphatidylcholine) has been used to increase brain acetylcholine in patients suffering from tardive dyskinesia (often persistent involuntary movements of the facial muscles and tongue). The neonate has a very high demand for choline, for both brain lipid synthesis (phosphatidylcholine and sphingomyelin) and acetylcholine biosynthesis. High levels of phosphatidylcholine in the maternal milk and a high activity of a high-affinity transport system through the blood-brain barrier for choline in the neonate help to maintain brain choline concentrations. The fetus also has a high demand for choline, and there is a high-affinity transport system for choline across the placenta. The choline is derived from maternal stores, maternal diet, and synthesis primarily in the maternal liver. Because choline synthesis is dependent on folate and vitamin B12, the high fetal demand may contribute to the increased maternal requirement for both vitamins during pregnancy.

CoA via the pyruvate dehydrogenase reaction. This is because neuronal tissues have only a limited capacity to oxidize fatty acids to acetyl CoA so that glucose oxidation is the major source of acetyl groups. Pyruvate dehydrogenase is found only in mitochondria. The acetyl group is probably transported to the cytoplasm as part of citrate, which is then cleaved in the cytosol to form acetyl CoA and oxaloacetate.

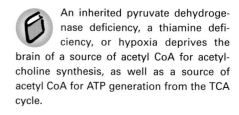 An inherited pyruvate dehydrogenase deficiency, a thiamine deficiency, or hypoxia deprives the brain of a source of acetyl CoA for acetylcholine synthesis, as well as a source of acetyl CoA for ATP generation from the TCA cycle.

2. INACTIVATION OF ACETYLCHOLINE

Acetylcholine is inactivated by acetylcholinesterase, which is a serine esterase that forms a covalent bond with the acetyl group. The enzyme is inhibited by a wide range of compounds (pharmacologic drugs and neurotoxins) that form a covalent bond with this reactive serine group. Neurotoxins such as Sarin (the gas used in Japanese subways by a terrorist group) and the nerve gas in the movie "The Rock" work through this mechanism. Acetylcholine is the major neurotransmitter at the neuromuscular junctions; inability to inactivate this molecule leads to constant activation of the nerve–muscle synapses, a condition that leads to varying degrees of paralysis.

F. Glutamate and GABA

1. SYNTHESIS OF GLUTAMATE

Glutamate functions as an excitatory neurotransmitter within the central nervous system, leading to the depolarization of neurons. Within nerve terminals, glutamate is generally synthesized de novo from glucose rather than taken up from the blood because its plasma concentration is low and it does not readily cross the blood-brain barrier.

Glutamate is primarily synthesized from the TCA cycle intermediate α-ketoglutarate (Fig. 48.10). This can occur via either of two routes. The first is via the enzyme glutamate dehydrogenase, which reduces α-ketoglutarate to glutamate, thereby incorporating free ammonia into the carbon backbone. The ammonia pool is provided by amino acid /neurotransmitter degradation or by diffusion of ammonia across the blood-brain barrier. The second route is through transamination reactions in which an amino group is transferred from other amino acids to α-ketoglutarate to form glutamate. Glutamate also can be synthesized from glutamine, using glutaminase. The glutamine is derived from glial cells as described in section F.2.

Like other neurotransmitters, glutamate is stored in vesicles, and its release is Ca^{2+} -dependent. It is removed from the synaptic cleft by high-affinity uptake systems present in nerve terminals and glial cells.

The β-cells of the pancreas also express glutamate decarboxylase (GAD), and patients with type 1 diabetes express autoantigens against pancreatic GAD. Studies in a mouse model of type 1 diabetes have implicated GAD as a key autoantigen. If GAD expression is blocked in these mice by use of genetic tricks, diabetes does not develop. As usual, what occurs in the human condition is not as straightforward as it appears to be in animals, but there is a relationship between pancreatic GAD expression and the cause of type 1 diabetes in humans.

2. GABA

GABA (γ-aminobutyric acid) is the major inhibitory neurotransmitter in the central nervous system. Its functional significance is far-reaching, and altered GABA-ergic function plays a role in many neurologic and psychiatric disorders.

GABA is synthesized by the decarboxylation of glutamate (see Fig. 48.10) in a single step catalyzed by the enzyme glutamic acid decarboxylase (GAD). GABA is recycled in the central nervous system by a series of reactions called the GABA shunt, which conserves glutamate and GABA (see Fig. 48.10).

Much of the uptake of GABA occurs in glial cells. The GABA shunt in glial cells produces glutamate, which is converted to glutamine and transported out of the glial cells to neurons, where it is converted back to glutamate. Glutamine thus serves as a transporter of glutamate between cells in the CNS (see Chapter 42). Glial cells lack GAD and cannot synthesize GABA.

Tiagabine is a drug that inhibits the reuptake of GABA from the synapse, and it has been used to treat epilepsy as well as other convulsant disorders. Because GABA is an inhibitory neurotransmitter in the brain, its prolonged presence can block neurotransmission by other agents, thereby reducing the frequency of convulsions.

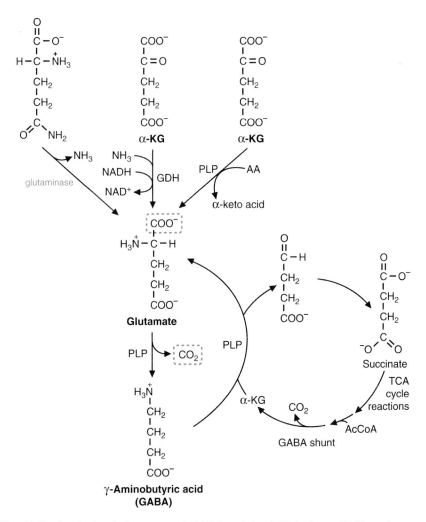

Fig. 48.10. Synthesis of glutamate and GABA and the GABA shunt. GDH = glutamate dehydrogenase; PLP = pyridoxal phosphate.

G. Other Amino Acid Neurotransmitters

1.   ASPARTATE

Aspartate, like glutamate, is an excitatory neurotransmitter, but it functions in far fewer pathways. It is synthesized from the TCA cycle intermediate oxaloacetate via transamination reactions. Like glutamate synthesis, aspartate synthesis uses oxaloacetate that must be replaced through anaplerotic reactions. Aspartate cannot pass through the blood-brain barrier.

2.   GLYCINE

Glycine is the major inhibitory neurotransmitter in the spinal cord. Most of the glycine in neurons is synthesized de novo within the nerve terminal from serine by the enzyme serine hydroxymethyltransferase, which requires folic acid. Serine, in turn, is synthesized from the intermediate 3-phosphoglycerate in the glycolytic pathway. The action of glycine is probably terminated via uptake by a high-affinity transporter.

3.   CONVERSION OF ARGININE TO NITRIC OXIDE

Nitric oxide (NO) is a biologic messenger in a variety of physiologic responses, including vasodilation, neurotransmission, and the ability of the immune system to kill tumor cells and parasites. NO is synthesized from arginine in a reaction catalyzed by NO synthase (see Fig. 24.10).

NO synthase exists as tissue-specific forms of two families of enzymes. The form present in macrophages is responsible for the overproduction of NO, leading to its cytotoxic actions on parasites and tumor cells. The enzyme present in nervous tissue, vascular endothelium, platelets, and other tissues is responsible for the physiologic responses to NO such as vasodilation and neural transmission. In target cells, NO activates a soluble guanylate cyclase, which results in increased cellular levels of cGMP (3′, 5′-cyclic GMP)(Fig. 48.11). In smooth muscle cells, cGMP, like cAMP, activates one or more protein kinases, which are responsible for the relaxation of smooth muscle and the subsequent dilation of vessels. NO stimulates penile erection by acting as a neurotransmitter, stimulating smooth muscle relaxation that permits the corpus cavernosum to fill with blood. Nitric oxide can readily cross cell membranes because it is a gas. As a result, its effect may not necessarily be limited to the neuron that synthesizes it (Fig. 48.12). There is ample evidence that NO may function as a retrograde messenger that can influence neurotransmitter release from the presynaptic terminal after diffusing from the postsynaptic neuron (where it is synthesized). There is also evidence supporting retrograde messenger roles for both arachidonic acid and carbon monoxide in the CNS.

IV. METABOLIC ENCEPHALOPATHIES AND NEUROPATHIES

The brain has an absolute dependence on the blood for its supply of glucose and oxygen. It uses approximately 20% of the oxygen supply of the body. During the developmental period and during prolonged fasting, ketone bodies can be used as a fuel, but they cannot totally substitute for glucose. Glucose is converted to pyruvate in glycolysis, and the pyruvate is oxidized in the TCA cycle. Anaerobic glycolysis, with a yield of 2 ATPs/glucose, cannot sustain the ATP requirement of the brain, which can be provided only by the complete oxidation of glucose to CO_2, which yields approximately 32 ATPs/glucose. However, during periods of mild hypoglycemia or mild hypoxia, decreased neurotransmitter synthesis contributes as much, if not more, to the development of symptoms as does an absolute deficiency of ATP for energy needs.

A. Hypoglycemic Encephalopathy

Hypoglycemia is sometimes encountered in medical conditions such as malignancies producing insulin, insulin-like growth factors, or chronic alcoholism. Early clinical signs in hypoglycemia reflect the appearance of physiologic protective mechanisms initiated by hypothalamic sensory nuclei such as sweating, palpitations, anxiety, and hunger. If unheeded, these symptoms give way to a more serious CNS disorder progressing through confusion and lethargy to seizures and eventually coma. Prolonged hypoglycemia can lead to irreversible brain damage.

During the progression of hypoglycemic encephalopathy, as blood glucose falls below 2.5 mM (45 mg/dL), the brain attempts to use internal substrates such as glutamate and TCA cycle intermediates as fuels. Because the pool size of these substrates is quite small, they are quickly depleted. If blood glucose levels continue to fall below 1 mM (18 mg/dL), ATP levels become depleted.

As the blood glucose drops from 2.5 to 2.0 mM (45 to 36 mg/dL, before EEG changes are observed), the symptoms appear to arise from decreased synthesis of neurotransmitters in particular regions of the brain rather than a global energy deficit. Figure 48.13 summarizes the relationship between the oxidation of glucose in glycolysis and the provision of precursors for the synthesis of neurotransmitters in different types of neurons.

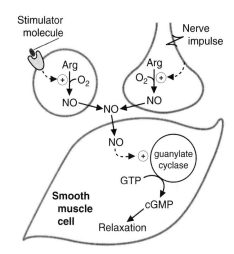

Fig. 48.11. Action of nitric oxide (NO) in vasodilation. The synthesis of NO occurs in response to a stimulator binding to a receptor on some cells or to a nerve impulse in neurons. NO enters smooth muscle cells, stimulating guanylate cyclase to produce cGMP, which causes smooth muscle cell relaxation. When the smooth muscle cells relax, blood vessels dilate.

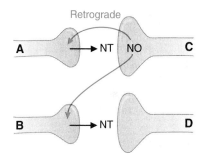

Fig. 48.12. NO as a retrograde messenger. Cell A releases a neurotransmitter, which stimulates cell C to produce NO. NO, being a gas, can diffuse back and regulate cell A's production and release of neurotransmitters. NO can also diffuse to cell B, and to stimulate cell B to produce a different neurotransmitter to elicit a response from cell D. NT = neurotransmitter.

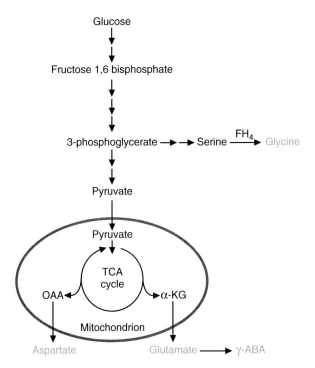

Fig. 48.13. Glucose metabolism leading to the synthesis of the neurotransmitters glycine, aspartate, glutamate, and GABA. As blood glucose levels drop and brain glucose levels diminish, synthesis of these neurotransmitters may be compromised.

As hypoglycemia progresses below 1 mM (18 mg/dL), and high-energy phosphate levels are depleted, the EEG becomes isoelectric, and neuronal cell death ensues. As is the case in some other metabolic encephalopathies, cell death is not global in distribution; rather, certain brain structures, in particular hippocampal and cortical structures, are selectively vulnerable to hypoglycemic insult. Pathophysiologic mechanisms responsible for neuronal cell death in hypoglycemia include the involvement of glutamate excitotoxicity. Glutamate excitotoxicity occurs when the cellular energy reserves are depleted. The failure of the energy-dependent reuptake pumps results in a buildup of glutamate in the synaptic cleft and overstimulation of the postsynaptic glutamate receptors. The prolonged glutamate receptor activation leads to prolonged opening of the receptor ion channel and the influx of lethal amounts of Ca^{+2} ion, which can activate cytotoxic intracellular pathways in the postsynaptic neuron.

B. Hypoxic Encephalopathy

Experimental studies with human volunteers show that cerebral energy metabolism remains normal when mild to moderate hypoxia (partial pressure of oxygen, or $PaO_2 = 25$–40 mm Hg) results in severe cognitive dysfunction. The diminished cognitive function is believed to result from impaired neurotransmitter synthesis. In mild hypoxia, cerebral blood flow increases to maintain oxygen delivery to the brain. In addition, anaerobic glycolysis is accelerated, resulting in maintenance of ATP levels. This occurs, however, at the expense of an increase of lactate production and a fall of pH. Acute hypoxia ($PaO_2 \leq 20$ mm Hg) generally results in a coma.

Hypoxia can result from insufficient oxygen reaching the blood (e.g., at high altitudes), severe anemia (e.g., iron deficiency), or a direct insult to the oxygen-utilizing capacity of the brain (e.g., cyanide poisoning). All forms of hypoxia result in diminished neurotransmitter synthesis. Inhibition of pyruvate dehydrogenase diminishes acetylcholine synthesis, which is acutely sensitive to hypoxia. Glutamate and

GABA synthesis, which depend on a functioning TCA cycle, are decreased as a result of elevated NADH levels, which inhibit TCA cycle enzymes. NADH levels are increased when oxygen is unavailable to accept electrons from the electron transport chain and NADH cannot be converted back into NAD^+. Even the synthesis of catecholamine neurotransmitters may be decreased because the hydroxylase reactions require O_2.

C. The Relationship Between Glutamate Synthesis and the Anaplerotic Pathways of Pyruvate Carboxylase and Methylmalonyl CoA Mutase

Synthesis of glutamate removes α-ketoglutarate from the TCA cycle, thereby decreasing the regeneration of oxaloacetate in the TCA cycle. Because oxaloacetate is necessary for the oxidation of acetyl CoA, oxaloacetate must be replaced by anaplerotic reactions. There are two major types of anaplerotic reactions: (1) pyruvate carboxylase and (2) the degradative pathway of the branched-chain amino acids, valine and isoleucine, which contribute succinyl CoA to the TCA cycle. This pathway uses B12 (but not folate) in the reaction catalyzed by methylmalonyl CoA mutase.

V. LIPID SYNTHESIS IN THE BRAIN AND PERIPHERAL NERVOUS SYSTEM

A number of features of lipid synthesis and degradation in the nervous system distinguish it from most other tissues. The first is that the portion of the neuronal cell membrane involved in synaptic transmission has a unique role and a unique composition. At the presynaptic terminal, the lipid composition is rapidly changing as storage vesicles containing the neurotransmitter fuse with the cell membrane and release their contents. Portions of the membrane are also lost as endocytotic vesicles. On the postsynaptic terminal, the membrane contains the receptors for the neurotransmitter as well as a high concentration of membrane signaling components, such as phosphatidylinositol. A second important feature of brain lipid metabolism is that the blood-brain barrier restricts the entry of nonessential fatty acids such as palmitate, which are released from adipose tissue or present in the diet. Conversely, essential fatty acids are taken up by the brain. Because of these considerations, the brain is constantly synthesizing those lipids (cholesterol, fatty acids, glycosphingolipids, and phospholipids), which it needs for various neurologic functions. Neuronal signaling also requires that non-neuronal glial cells synthesize myelin, a multilayered membrane that surrounds the axons of many neurons. Myelin is lipid rich and has a different lipid composition than the neuronal membranes. The white matter in the brain contains significantly more myelin than the gray matter; it is the presence of myelin sheaths that is responsible for the characteristic color differences that exist between the two types of brain tissue.

A. Brain Lipid Synthesis and Oxidation

Because the blood-brain barrier significantly inhibits the entry of certain fatty acids and lipids into the CNS, virtually all lipids found there must be synthesized within the CNS. The exceptions are the essential fatty acids (linoleic and linolenic acid), which do enter the brain, where they are elongated or further desaturated. The uptake of fatty acids into the CNS is insufficient to meet the energy demands of the CNS; hence the requirement for aerobic glucose metabolism. Thus, cholesterol, glycerol, and sphingolipids, glycosphingolipids, and cerebrosides are all synthesized using pathways previously discussed in this text. Of particular note is that very-long-chain fatty acids are synthesized in the brain, where they play a major role in myelin formation.

Oxidation and turnover of brain lipids occurs as described previously in the text (see Chapter 23). Peroxisomal fatty acid oxidation is important in the brain because the brain contains very-long-chain fatty acids and phytanic acid (from the diet), both of which are oxidized in the peroxisomes by α-oxidation. Thus, disorders that affect peroxisome biogenesis (such as Refsum's disease) severely affect brain cells because of the inability to metabolize both branched-chain and very-long-chain fatty acids. If there is a disorder in which the degradation of glycosphingolipids or mucopolysaccharides is reduced, lysosomes in brain cells will become engorged with partially digested glycolipids, leading to varying degrees of neurologic dysfunction.

B. Myelin Synthesis

A rapid rate of nerve conduction in the peripheral and central motor nerves depends on the formation of myelin, a multilayered lipid and protein structure that is formed from the plasma membrane of glial cells. In the peripheral nervous system, the Schwann cell is responsible for myelinating one portion of an axon of one nerve cell. The Schwann cell does this by wrapping itself around the axon multiple times such that a multilayered sheath of membrane surrounds the axon. In the central nervous system, the oligodendrocyte is responsible for myelination. Unlike the Schwann cell, oligodendrocytes can myelinate portions of numerous axons (up to 40), and do so by extending a thin process that wraps around the axon multiple times Thus, CNS axons are only surrounded by the membranes of oligodendrocytes, whereas axons in the PNS are surrounded by the entire Schwann cell. A generalized view of myelination is depicted in Figure 48.14. To maintain the myelin structure, the oligodendrocyte synthesizes 4 times its own weight in lipids per day.

1. MYELIN LIPIDS

As the plasma membrane of the glial cell is converted into myelin, the lipid composition of the brain changes (Table 48.2). The lipid-to-protein ratio is greatly increased, as is the content of sphingolipids. The myelin is a tightly packed structure,

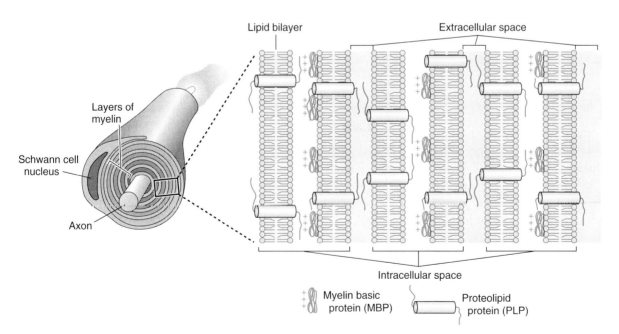

Fig. 48.14. A composite diagram indicating a Schwann cell that has wrapped around a portion of an axon, forming the myelin sheath. The expansion represents a portion of the myelin sheath. CNS myelin is shown, although it is similar to PNS myelin except that Po would take the place of PLP (proteolipid protein). Recall that there are multiple layers of membrane surrounding the axon; PLP protrudes into the extracellular space and aids in compaction of the membranes through hydrophobic interactions. MBPs help to stabilize the structure from within the membrane.

Table 48.2. Protein and Lipid Composition of CNS Myelin and Human Brain

Substance[a]	Myelin	White Matter	Gray Matter
Protein	30.0	39.0	55.3
Lipid	70.0	54.9	32.7
Cholesterol	27.7	27.5	22.0
Cerebroside	22.7	19.8	5.4
Sulfatide	3.8	5.4	1.7
Total galactolipid	27.5	26.4	7.3
Ethanolamine phosphatides	15.6	14.9	22.7
Phosphatidylcholine	11.2	12.8	26.7
Sphingomyelin	7.9	7.7	6.9
Phosphatidylserine	4.8	7.9	8.7
Phosphatidylinositol	0.6	0.9	2.7
Plasmalogens	12.3	11.2	8.8
Total phospholipids	43.1	45.9	69.5

[a]Protein and lipid figures in percent dry weight; all others in percent total lipid weight
Data from W. Norton, in Siegel GJ, Albers RW, Agranoff BW, Katzman R, eds. Basic Neurochemistry, 3rd Ed. Boston: Little Brown & Co, 1981:77.

and there are significant hydrophobic interactions between the lipids and proteins to allow this to occur. Cerebrosides constitute approximately 16% of total myelin lipid and are almost completely absent from other cell-type membrane lipids. The predominant cerebroside, galactosylcerebroside, has a single sugar attached to the hydroxyl group of the sphingosine. In contrast, sphingomyelin, which one might guess is the predominant lipid of myelin, is present in roughly the same low concentration in all membranes. Galactocerebrosides pack more tightly together than phosphatidylcholine; the sugar, although polar, carries no positively charged amino group or negatively charged phosphate. The brain synthesizes very-long-chain fatty acids (greater than 20 carbons long); these long uncharged side chains develop strong hydrophobic associations, allowing a close packing of the myelin sheath. The high cholesterol content of the membrane also contributes to the tight packing, although the myelin proteins are also required to complete the tightness of the packing process.

2. MYELIN STRUCTURAL PROTEINS

The layers of myelin are held together by protein/lipid and protein/protein interactions, and any disruption can lead to demyelination of the membrane (see Biochemical Comments). Although numerous proteins are found in both the CNS and PNS, only the major proteins are discussed here. The major proteins in the CNS and PNS are different. In the CNS, two proteins constitute between 60 and 80% of the total proteins—proteolipid protein (PLP) and myelin basic proteins (MBP). The PLP is a very hydrophobic protein that forms large aggregates in aqueous solution and is relatively resistant to proteolysis. Its molecular weight, based on sequence analysis, is 30,000 Daltons. PLP is highly conserved in sequence amongst species. Its role is thought to be one of promoting the formation and stabilization of the multilayered myelin structure.

The MBPs are a family of proteins. Unlike PLP, MBPs are easily extracted from the membrane and are soluble in aqueous solution. The major MBP has no tertiary structure and has a molecular weight of 15,000 Daltons. MBP is located on the cytoplasmic face of myelin membranes. Antibodies directed against MBPs elicit experimental allergic encephalomyelitis (EAE), which has become a model system for understanding multiple sclerosis, a demyelinating disease. A model of how PLP and MBPs aid in stabilizing myelin is shown in Figure 48.14.

In the PNS, the major myelin protein is Po, a glycoprotein that accounts for greater than 50% of the PNS myelin protein content. The molecular weight of Po is 30,000, the same as PLP. Po is thought to play a similar structural role in maintaining myelin structure, as does PLP in the CNS. Myelin basic proteins are also found in the PNS, with some similarities and differences to the MBPs found in the CNS. The major PNS-specific MBP has been designated P2.

CLINICAL COMMENTS

 Catecholamines affect nearly every tissue and organ in the body. Their integrated release from nerve endings of the sympathetic (adrenergic) nervous system plays a critical role in the reflex responses we make to sudden changes in our internal and external environment. For example, under stress, catecholamines appropriately increase heart rate, blood pressure, myocardial (heart muscle) contractility, and conduction velocity of the heart.

Episodic, inappropriate secretion of catecholamines in pharmacologic amounts, such as occurs in patients with pheochromocytomas, like **Katie Colamin,** causes an often alarming array of symptoms and signs of a hyperadrenergic state.

Most of the signs and symptoms related to catecholamine excess can be masked by phenoxybenzamine, a long-acting α_1- and α_2-adrenergic receptor antagonist, combined with a β_1- and β_2-adrenergic receptor blocker such as propranolol. Pharmacologic therapy alone is reserved for patients with inoperable pheochromocytomas (e.g., patients with malignant tumors with metastases and patients with severe heart disease). Because of the sudden, unpredictable, and sometimes life-threatening discharges of large amounts of catecholamines from these tumors, definitive therapy involves surgical resection of the neoplasms(s) after appropriate preoperative preparation of the patient with the agents mentioned above. Katie's tumor was resected without intraoperative or postoperative complications. After surgery, she remained free of symptoms, and her blood pressure decreased to normal levels.

 Evan Applebod, after stopping Redux, was placed on Prozac, an antidepressant that acts as a specific serotonin reuptake inhibitor (SSRI) but does not lead to increased synthesis or secretion of serotonin, as did dexfenfluramine in Redux. Thus, the mechanism of action of these two drugs is different, even if the end result (elevated levels of serotonin) is the same. Unfortunately, Prozac did not work as well for Mr. Applebod as did Redux, and he regained his 100 pounds within a year after switching medications. Redux was withdrawn from the market by its manufacturer because of reports of heart valve abnormalities in a small percentage of patients who had taken either phen/fen or Redux. Since then, the FDA has banned the use of Redux for weight loss because of the undesirable side effects. Other treatments, such as orlistat, a partial inhibitor of dietary fatty acid absorption from the gastrointestinal tract, are being tried in an effort to effect weight loss safely in patients like **Evan Applebod**.

BIOCHEMICAL COMMENTS

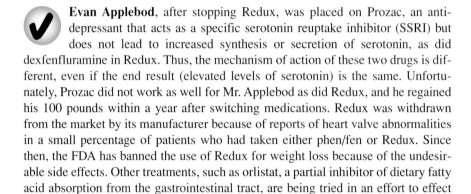 The importance of myelin in nerve transmission is underscored by the wide variety of demyelinating diseases, all of which lead to neurologic symptoms. The best known disease in this class is multiple sclerosis (MS). MS can be a progressive disease of the CNS in which demyelination of CNS neurons is the key anatomic and pathologic finding. The cause of MS has yet to be determined, although it is believed that an event occurs that triggers the formation of autoimmune antibodies directed against components of the nervous system. This

event could be a bacterial or viral infection that stimulates the immune system to fight off the invaders. Unfortunately, this stimulus may also trigger the autoimmune response that leads to the antibody-mediated demyelinating process. The unusual geographic distribution of MS is of interest. Patients are concentrated in northern and southern latitudes, yet its incidence is almost nil at the equator. Clinical presentation of MS varies widely. Most commonly it is a mild disease that has few or no obvious clinical manifestations. At the other end of the spectrum is a rapidly progressive and fatal disease. The most well-known presentation is the relapsing-remitting type. In this type, early in the course of the disease, the natural history is one of exacerbations, followed by remission. Eventually the CNS cannot repair the damage that has accumulated through the years, and remissions occur less and less frequently. Available treatments for MS target the relapsing-remitting type of disease.

The primary injury to the CNS in MS is the loss of myelin in the white matter, which interferes with nerve conduction along the demyelinated area (the insulator is lost). The CNS compensates by stimulating the oligodendrocyte to remyelinate the damaged axon, and when this occurs, remission is achieved. Often remyelination leads to a slowing in conduction velocity because of a reduced myelin thickness (speed is proportional to myelin thickness) or a shortening of the internodal distances (the action potential has to be propagated more times). Eventually, when it becomes too difficult to remyelinate large areas of the CNS, the neuron adapts by upregulating and redistributing along its membrane ion pumps, to allow nerve conductance along demyelinated axons. Eventually this adaptation also fails, and the disease progresses.

Treatment of MS is now based on blocking the action of the immune system. Because antibodies directed against cellular components appear to be responsible for the progression of the disease (regardless of how the autoantibodies were first generated), agents that interfere with immune responses have had various levels of success in keeping patients in remission for extended periods.

Other demyelinating diseases also exist, and their cause is much more straightforward. These are relatively rare disorders. In all of these diseases, there is no fully effective treatment for the patient. Inherited mutations in Po (the major PNS myelin protein) leads to a version of Charcot-Marie-Tooth polyneuropathy syndrome. The inheritance pattern for this disease is autosomal dominant, indicating that the expression of one mutated allele will lead to expression of the disease. Mutations in PLP (the major myelin protein in the CNS) lead to Pelizaeus-Merzbacher disease and X-linked spastic paraplegia type 2 disease. These diseases display a wide range of phenotypes, from a lack of motor development and early death (most severe) to mild gait disturbances. The phenotype displayed depends on the precise location of the mutation within the protein. An altered function of either Po or PLP leads to demyelination and its subsequent clinical manifestations.

Suggested Readings

Herndon RM. Multiple Sclerosis: Immunology, Pathology, and Pathophysiology. New York: Demos Medical Publishing, 2003.

Lupski JR, Garcia CA. Charcot-Marie-Tooth peripheral neuropathies and related disorders. In: Scriver CR, Beaudet AL, Valle D, Sly WS, et al eds. The Metabolic and Molecular Bases of Inherited Disease, vol II, 8th Ed. New York: McGraw-Hill, 2001:5759–5788.

Siegel G, Agranoff B, Albers RW, Molinoff P, eds. Basic Neurochemistry, 4th Ed. New York: Raven Press, 1989.

Webster RA, ed. Neurotransmitters, Drugs and Brain Function. London: John Wiley and Sons Ltd, 2001.

1. A patient with a tumor of the adrenal medulla experienced palpitations, excessive sweating, and hypertensive headaches. His urine contained increased amounts of vanillylmandelic acid. His symptoms are probably caused by an overproduction of which of the following?

   (A) Acetylcholine
   (B) Norepinephrine and epinephrine
   (C) DOPA and serotonin
   (D) Histamine
   (E) Melatonin

2. The two lipids found in highest concentration in myelin are which of the following?

   (A) Cholesterol and cerebrosides such as galactosylceramide
   (B) Cholesterol and phosphatidylcholine
   (C) Galactosylceramide sulfatide and sphingomyelin
   (D) Plasmalogens and sphingomyelin
   (E) Triacylglycerols and lecithin

3. Myelin basic protein can best be described by which of the following?

   (A) It is synthesized in Schwann cells, but not in oligodendrocytes.
   (B) It is a transmembrane protein found only in peripheral myelin.
   (C) It attaches the two extracellular leaflets together in central myelin.
   (D) It contains basic amino acid residues that bind the negatively charged extracellular sides of the myelin membrane together.
   (E) It contains lysine and arginine residues that bind the negatively charged intracellular sides of the myelin membrane together.

4. A patient presented with dysmorphia and cerebellar degeneration. Analysis of his blood indicated elevated levels of phytanic acid and very-long-chain fatty acids, but no elevation of palmitate. His symptoms are consistent with a defect in an enzyme involved in which of the following?

   (A) α-Oxidation
   (B) Mitochondrial β-oxidation
   (C) Transport of enzymes into lysosomes
   (D) Degradation of mucopolysaccharides
   (E) Elongation of fatty acids

5. One of the presenting symptoms of vitamin B6 deficiency is dementia. This may result from an inability to synthesize serotonin, norepinephrine, histamine, and GABA from their respective amino acid precursors. This is because B6 is required for which type of reaction?

   (A) Hydroxylation
   (B) Transamination
   (C) Deamination
   (D) Decarboxylation
   (E) Oxidation

49 The Extracellular Matrix and Connective Tissue

*Many of the cells in tissues are embedded in an **extracellular matrix** that fills the spaces between cells and binds cells and tissue together. In so doing, the extracellular matrix aids in determining the shape of tissues as well as the nature of the partitioning between tissue types. In the skin, loose connective tissue beneath epithelial cell layers consists of an extracellular matrix in which fibroblasts, blood vessels, and other components are distributed (Fig 49.1). Other types of connective tissue, such as tendon and cartilage, consist largely of extracellular matrix, which is principally responsible for their structure and function. This matrix also forms the sheetlike **basal laminae**, or basement membranes, on which layers of epithelial cells rest, and which act as supportive tissue for muscle cells, adipose cells, and peripheral nerves.*

*Basic components of the extracellular matrix include fibrous structural proteins, such as **collagens**, **proteoglycans** containing long glycosaminoglycan chains attached to a protein backbone, and **adhesion proteins** linking components of the matrix to each other and to cells.*

*These **fibrous structural proteins** are composed of repeating elements that form a linear structure. **Collagens**, **elastin**, and **laminin** are the principal structural proteins of connective tissue.*

*__Proteoglycans__ consist of a core protein covalently attached to many long, linear chains of **glycosaminoglycans**, which contain repeating disaccharide units. The repeating disaccharides usually contain a **hexosamine** and a **uronic acid,** and these sugars are frequently **sulfated**. Synthesis of the proteoglycans starts with the attachment of a sugar to a serine, threonine, or asparagine residue of the protein. Additional sugars, donated by **UDP-sugar precursors**, add sequentially to the nonreducing end of the molecule.*

*Proteoglycans, such as glycoproteins and glycolipids, are **synthesized in the endoplasmic reticulum (ER)** and the **Golgi complex**. The glycosaminoglycan chains of proteoglycans are **degraded by lysosomal enzymes** that cleave one sugar at a time from the nonreducing end of the chain. An inability to degrade proteoglycans leads to a set of diseases known as the **mucopolysaccharidoses**.*

*__Adhesion proteins, such as fibronectin and laminin,__ are extracellular glycoproteins that contain separate distinct binding domains for proteoglycans, collagen, and fibrin. These domains allow these adhesion proteins to bind the various components of the extracellular matrix. They also contain specific binding domains for specific cell surface receptors known as the **integrins**. These integrins bind to **fibronectin** on the external surface, span the plasma membrane of cells, and adhere to proteins, which, in turn, bind to the intracellular **actin** filaments of the **cytoskeleton**. Integrins also provide a mechanism for signaling between cells via both internal signals as well as through signals generated via the extracellular matrix.*

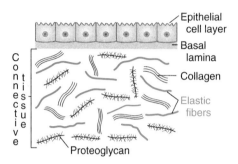

Fig. 49.1. An overview of connective tissue extracellular matrix. Supporting the epithelial cell layer is a basal lamina, beneath which are collagen, elastic fibers, and proteoglycans. The cell types present in connective tissue, such as fibroblasts and macrophages, have been removed from the diagram for clarity.

905

*Cell movement within the extracellular matrix requires remodeling of the various components of the matrix. This is accomplished by a variety of **matrix metalloproteinases (MMPs)** and regulators of the MMPs, **tissue inhibitors of matrix metalloproteinases (TIMPs)**. Dysregulation of this delicate balance of the regulators of cell movement allows cancer cells to travel to other parts of the body (**metastasize**) as well as to spread locally to contiguous tissues.*

THE WAITING ROOM

Sis Lupus (first introduced in Chapter 14) noted a moderate reduction in pain and swelling in the joints of her fingers when she was taking a 6-week course of high-dose prednisone, an anti-inflammatory steroid. As the dose of this drug was tapered to minimize its long-term side effects, however, the pain in the joints of her fingers returned, and, for the first time, her left knee became painful, swollen, and warm to the touch. Her rheumatologist described to her the underlying inflammatory tissue changes that her systemic lupus erythematosus (SLE) was causing in the joint tissues.

Ann Sulin complained of a declining appetite for food as well as severe weakness and fatigue. The reduction in her kidneys' ability to maintain normal daily total urinary net acid excretion contributed to her worsening metabolic acidosis. This plus her declining ability to excrete nitrogenous waste products, such as creatinine and urea, into her urine ("azotemia") are responsible for many of her symptoms. Her serum creatinine level was rising steadily. As it approached a level of 5 mg/dL, she developed a litany of complaints caused by the multisystem dysfunction associated with her worsening metabolic acidosis, retention of nitrogenous waste products, and so forth ("uremia"). Her physicians discussed with Ann the need to consider peritoneal dialysis or hemodialysis.

I. COMPOSITION OF THE EXTRACELLULAR MATRIX

A. Fibrous Proteins

1. COLLAGEN

Collagen, a family of fibrous proteins, is produced by a variety of cell types but principally by fibroblasts (cells found in interstitial connective tissue), muscle cells, and epithelial cells. Type I collagen [collagen(I)], the most abundant protein in mammals, is a fibrous protein that is the major component of connective tissue. It is found in the extracellular matrix (ECM) of loose connective tissue, bone, tendons, skin, blood vessels, and the cornea of the eye. Collagen(I) contains approximately 33% glycine and 21% proline and hydroxyproline. Hydroxyproline is an amino acid produced by posttranslational modification of peptidyl proline residues (see Chapter 7, section V.C., for an earlier introduction to collagen).

Procollagen(I), the precursor of collagen(I), is a triple helix composed of three polypeptide (pro-α) chains that are twisted around each other, forming a rope-like structure. Polymerization of collagen(I) molecules forms collagen fibrils, which provide great tensile strength to connective tissues (Fig. 49.2). The individual polypeptide chains each contain approximately 1,000 amino acid residues. The three polypeptide chains of the triple helix are linked by interchain hydrogen bonds.

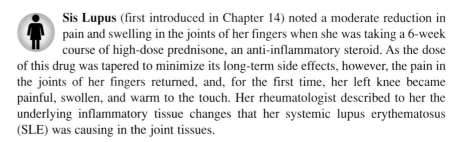

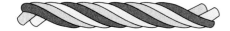
Fig. 49.2. The triple helix of collagen.

Each turn of the triple helix contains three amino acid residues, such that every third amino acid is in close contact with the other two strands in the center of the structure. Only glycine, which lacks a side chain, can fit in this position, and indeed, every third amino acid residue of collagen is glycine. Thus, collagen is a polymer of (Gly-X-Y) repeats, where Y is frequently proline or hydroxyproline, and X is any other amino acid found in collagen.

Procollagen(I) is an example of a protein that undergoes extensive posttranslational modifications. Hydroxylation reactions produce hydroxyproline residues from proline residues and hydroxylysine from lysine residues. These reactions occur after the protein has been synthesized (Fig. 49.3) and require vitamin C (ascorbic acid) as a cofactor of the enzymes, for example, prolyl hydroxylases and lysyl hydroxylase. Hydroxyproline residues are involved in hydrogen bond formation that helps to stabilize the triple helix, whereas hydroxylysine residues are the sites of attachment of disaccharide moieties (galactose-glucose).

The side chains of lysine residues also may be oxidized to form the aldehyde, allysine. These aldehyde residues produce covalent cross-links between collagen molecules (Fig. 49.4). An allysine residue on one collagen molecule reacts with the amino group of a lysine residue on another molecule, forming a covalent Schiff base that is converted to more stable covalent cross-links. Aldol condensation also may occur between two allysine residues, which forms the structure lysinonorleucine.

The role of carbohydrates in collagen structure is still controversial. The hydroxyproline residues in collagen are required for stabilization of the triple helix by hydrogen bond formation. In the absence of vitamin C (scurvy), the melting temperature of collagen can drop from 42°C to 24°C, because of the loss of interstrand hydrogen bond formation from the lack of hydroxyproline residues.

i. Types of Collagen

At least 19 different types of collagen have been characterized (Table 49.1). Although each type of collagen is found only in particular locations in the body, more than one type may be present in the ECM at a given location. The various types of collagen can be classified as fibril-forming (types I, II, III, V, and XI), network-forming (types IV, VIII and X), those that associate with fibril surfaces (types IX, XII, and XIV), those that are transmembrane proteins (types XIII and XVII), endostatin-forming (types XV and XVIII), and those that form periodic beaded filaments (type VI).

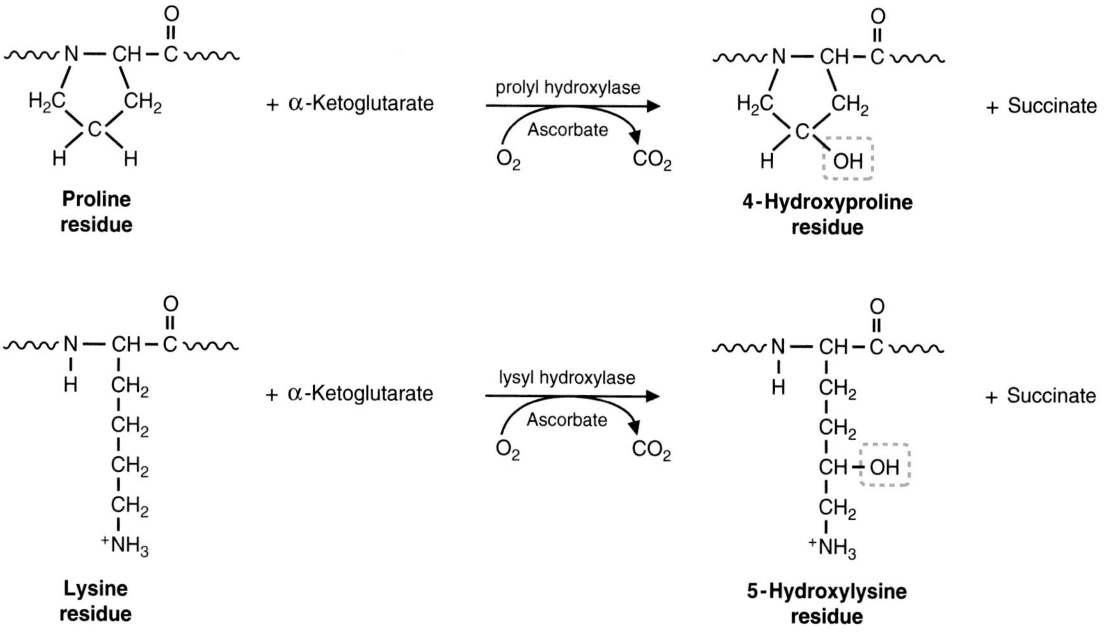

Fig. 49.3. Hydroxylation of proline and lysine residues in collagen. Proline and lysine residues within the collagen chains are hydroxylated by reactions that require vitamin C.

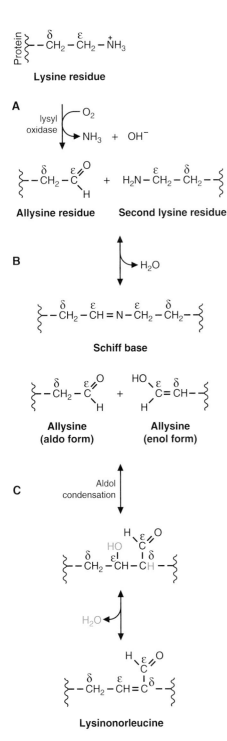

Fig. 49.4. Formation of cross-links in collagen. A. Lysine residues are oxidized to allysine (an aldehyde). Allysine may react with an unmodified lysine residue to form a Schiff base (B), or two allysine residues may undergo an aldol condensation (C).

Table 49.1. Types of Collagen

Collagen Type	Gene	Structural Details	Localization
I	Col1A1-Col1A2	Fibrils	Skin, tendon, bone, cornea
II	Col2A1	Fibrils	Cartilage, vitreous humour
III	Col3A1	Fibrils	Skin, muscle, associates with type I collagen
IV	Col4A1–Col4A6	Nonfibrillar, mesh collagen	All basal laminae (basement membranes)
V	Col5A1-Col5A3	Small fibers, N-terminal globular domains	Associates with type I collagen in most interstitial tissues
VI	Col6A1-Col6A3	Microfibrils, with both N and C-terminal globular domains	Associates with type I collagen in most interstitial tissues
VII	Col7A1	An anchoring collagen	Epithelial cells; dermal–epidermal junction
VIII	Col8A1-Col8A2	Nonfibrillar, mesh collagen	Cornea, some endothelial cells
IX	Col9A1-Col9A3	Fibril-associated collagens with interrupted triple helices (FACIT); N-terminal globular domain	Associates with type II collagen in cartilage and vitreous humour
X	Col10A1	Nonfibrillar, mesh collagen, with C-terminal globular domain	Growth plate, hypertrophic and mineralizing cartilage
XI	Col11A1-Col11A3	Small fibers	Cartilage, vitreous humor
XII	Col12A1	FACIT	Interacts with types I and II collagen in soft tissues
XIII	Col13A1	Transmembrane collagen	Cell surfaces, epithelial cells
XIV	Col14A1	FACIT	Soft tissue
XV	Col15A1	Endostatin-forming collagen	Endothelial cells
XVI	Col16A1	Other	Ubiquitous
XVII	Col17A1	Transmembrane collagen	Epidermal cell surface
XVIII	Col18A1	Endostatin-forming	Endothelial cells
XIX	Col19A1	Other	Ubiquitous

See the text for descriptions of the differences in types of collagen.

All collagens contain three polypeptide chains with at least one stretch of triple helix. The non–triple helical domains can be short (such as in the fibril-forming collagens) or can be rather large, such that the triple helix is actually a minor component of the overall structure (examples are collagen types XII and XIV). The FACIT (fibril-associated collagens with interrupted triple helices, collagen types IX, XII, and XIV) collagen types associate with fibrillar collagens, without themselves forming fibers. The endostatin-forming collagens are cleaved at their C-terminus to form endostatin, an inhibitor of angiogenesis. The network-forming collagens (type IV) form a mesh-like structure, because of large (approximately 230 amino acids) noncollagenous domains at the carboxy-terminal (Fig. 49.5). And finally, a number of collagen types are actually transmembrane proteins (XIII and XVII) found on epithelial or epidermal cell surfaces, which play a role in a number of cellular processes, including adhesion of components of the ECM to cells embedded within it.

Types I, II, and III collagens form fibrils that assemble into large insoluble fibers. The fibrils (see below) are strengthened through covalent cross-links between lysine residues on adjacent fibrils. The arrangement of the fibrils gives individual tissues their distinct characteristics. Tendons, which attach muscles to bones, contain collagen

Endostatins block angiogenesis (new blood vessel formation) by inhibiting endothelial cell migration. Because endothelial cell migration and proliferation are required to form new blood vessels, inhibiting this action blocks angiogenesis. Tumor growth is dependent on a blood supply; inhibiting angiogenesis can reduce tumor cell proliferation.

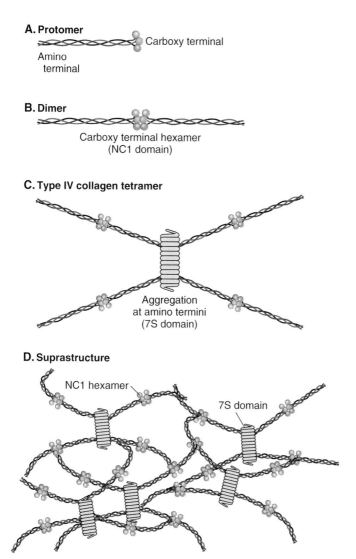

A. Protomer

Amino terminal — Carboxy terminal

B. Dimer

Carboxy terminal hexamer (NC1 domain)

C. Type IV collagen tetramer

Aggregation at amino termini (7S domain)

D. Suprastructure

NC1 hexamer   7S domain

Fig. 49.5. Type IV collagen contains a globular carboxy-terminal domain (A), which forms tropocollagen dimers (hexamers of collagen, B). Four dimers associate at the amino-terminal domains to form a 7S domain (C), and the tetramers form a lattice (D), which provides structural support to the basal lamina.

fibrils aligned parallel to the long axis of the tendon, thus giving the tendon tremendous tensile strength.

The types of collagen that do not form fibrils perform a series of distinct roles. Fibril-associated collagens bind to the surface of collagen fibrils and link them to other matrix-forming components. The transmembrane collagens form anchoring fibrils that link components of the extracellular matrix to underlying connective tissue. The network-forming collagens (type IV) form a flexible collagen that is part of the basement membrane and basal lamina that surround many cells.

ii. Synthesis and Secretion of Collagen

Collagen is synthesized within the endoplasmic reticulum as a precursor known as preprocollagen. The presequence acts as the signal sequence for the protein and is cleaved, forming procollagen within the endoplasmic reticulum. From there it is transported to the Golgi apparatus (Table 49.2). Three procollagen molecules associate through formation of intrastrand disulfide bonds at the carboxy-terminus; once

 One type of osteogenesis imperfecta (OI) is caused by a mutation in a gene that codes for collagen. The phenotype of affected individuals varies greatly, depending on the location and type of mutation. See the Biochemical Comments for more information concerning this type of OI.

Table 49.2. Steps Involved in Collagen Biosynthesis

Location	Process
Rough endoplasmic reticulum	Synthesis of preprocollagen; insertion of the procollagen molecule into the lumen of the ER
Lumen of the ER	Hyroxylation of proline and lysine residues; glycosylation of selected hydroxylysine residues
Lumen of ER and Golgi apparatus	Self-assembly of the tropocollagen molecule, initiated by disulfide bond formation in the carboxy-terminal extensions; triple helix formation
Secretory vesicle	Procollagen prepared for secretion from cell
Extracellular	Cleavage of the propeptides, removing the amino- and carboxy-terminal extensions, and self-assembly of the collagen molecules into fibrils, and then fibers

these disulfides are formed, the three molecules can align properly to initiate formation of the triple helix. The triple helix forms from the carboxy-end toward the amino-end, forming tropocollagen. The tropocollagen contains a triple helical segment between two globular ends, the amino- and carboxy-terminal extensions. The tropocollagen is secreted from the cell, the extensions are removed using extracellular proteases, and the mature collagen takes its place within the ECM. The individual fibrils of collagen line up in a highly ordered fashion to form the collagen fiber.

2. ELASTIN

Elastin is the major protein found in elastic fibers, which are located in the ECM of connective tissue of smooth muscle cells, endothelial and microvascular cells, chondrocytes, and fibroblasts. Elastic fibers allow tissues to expand and contract; this is of particular importance to blood vessels, which must deform and reform repeatedly in response to the changes in intravascular pressure that occur with the contraction of the left ventricle of the heart. It is also important for the lungs, which stretch each time a breath is inhaled and return to their original shape with each exhalation. In addition to elastin, the elastic fibers contain microfibrils, which are composed of a number of acidic glycoproteins, the major ones being fibrillin-1 and fibrillin-2.

i. Tropoelastin

Elastin has a highly cross-linked, insoluble, amorphous structure. Its precursor, tropoelastin, is a molecule of high solubility, which is synthesized on the rough endoplasmic reticulum (RER) for eventual secretion. Tropoelastin contains two types of alternating domains. The first domain consists of a hydrophilic sequence rich in lysine and alanine residues. The second domain consists of a hydrophobic sequence rich in valine, proline, and glycine, which frequently occur in repeats of VPGVG or VGGVG. The protein contains approximately 16 regions of each domain, alternating throughout the protein (Fig. 49.6).

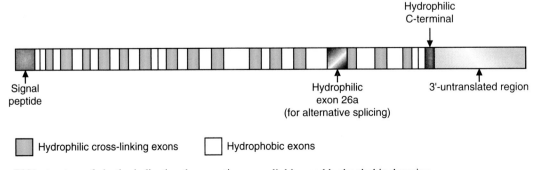

Fig. 49.6. The cDNA structure of elastin, indicating the repeating cross-linking and hydrophobic domains.

On secretion from the cell, the tropoelastin is aligned with the microfibrils, and lysyl oxidase initiates the reactions that cross-link elastin molecules, using lysine residues within the hydrophilic alternating domains in the proteins. This cross-linking reaction is the same as that which occurs in collagen. In this reaction, 2, 3, or 4 lysine residues are cross-linked to form a stable structure. The net result of the cross-linking is the generation of a fibrous mesh that encircles the cells.

ii. Elastic Properties of Elastin

Elastic fibers have the ability to stretch and then to reform without requiring an obvious energy source to do so. The mechanism by which this stretching and relaxing actively occurs is still controversial but does relate to the basic principles of protein folding described in Chapter 7. When the elastic fibers are stretched (such as when a breath is taken in and the lung fills up with air), the amorphous elastin structure is stretched. This stretching exposes the repeating hydrophobic regions of the molecule to the aqueous environment. This, in turn, leads to a decrease in the entropy of water, because the water molecules need to rearrange to form cages about each hydrophobic domain. When this stretching force within the lung is removed (e.g., when the subject exhales), the elastin takes on its original structure because of the increase in entropy that occurs because the water no longer needs to form cages about hydrophobic domains. Thus, the hydrophobic effect is the primary force that allows this stretched structure to reform. Elastin is inherently stable, with a half-life of up to 70 years.

3. LAMININ

After type IV collagen, laminin is the most abundant protein in basal laminae. Laminin provides additional structural support for the tissues through its ability to bind to type IV collagen, to other molecules present in the ECM, and to cell surface–associated proteins (the integrins, see section D).

i. Laminin Structure

Laminin is a heterotrimeric protein shaped, for the most part, like a cross (Fig. 49.7). The trimer is composed of α, β, and γ subunits. There are five possible α proteins (designated α1–α5), three different versions of the β subunit (β1–β3), and three different γ forms (γ1 – γ3). Thus, there is a potential for the formation of as many as 45 different combinations of these three subunits. However, only 12 have been discovered (designated laminins 1–12). Laminin 1, composed of α1β1γ1, is typical of this class of proteins. The major feature of the laminin structure is a coiled α-helix, which joins the three subunits together and forms a rigid rod. All three chains have extensions at the amino-terminal end. Only the α chain has a significant carboxy-terminal extension past the rod-like structure. It is the laminin extensions that allow laminin to bind to other components within the ECM and to provide stability for the structure. Components of the ECM that are bound by laminin include collagen, sulfated lipids, and proteoglycans.

ii. Laminin Biosynthesis

Like other secreted proteins, laminin is synthesized with a leader sequence targeting the three chains to the endoplasmic reticulum. Chain association occurs within the Golgi apparatus before secretion from the cell. After laminin is secreted by the cell, the amino terminal extensions promote self-association, as well as the binding to other ECM components. Disulfide linkages are formed to stabilize the trimer, but there is much less posttranslational processing of laminin than there is of collagen and elastin.

Supravalvular aortic stenosis (SVAS) results from an insufficiency of elastin in the vessel wall, leading to a narrowing of the large elastic arteries. Current theory suggests that the levels of elastin in the vessel walls may regulate the number of smooth muscle cell rings that encircle the vessel. If the levels of elastin are low, smooth muscle hypertrophy results, leading to a narrowing and stenosis of the artery.

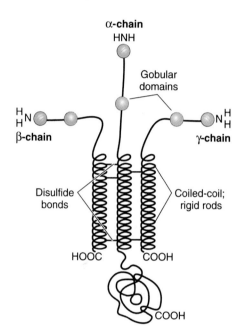

Fig. 49.7. The structure of laminin.

Defects in the structures of laminin 5 or laminin 6 (proteins that contribute to the cohesion of the dermis and epidermis) lead to the disorder referred to as junctional epidermolysis bullosa (JEB). In this disorder, there can be severe spontaneous blistering of the skin and mucous membranes. A severe form of the disease, JEB gravis, is often fatal early in life. Death occurs as a result of epithelial blistering of the respiratory, digestive, and genitourinary systems.

Congenital muscular dystrophy (CMD) results from a defect in laminin 2, which is a component of the bridge that links the muscle cell cytoskeleton to the extracellular matrix. Lack of this bridge triggers muscle cell apoptosis, which results in weakened muscles.

The ECM is not simply a glue that holds cells together; it also serves to keep cells from moving to other locations and to prevent large molecules and other particles, such as microorganisms, from reaching contiguous and distant cells. This confining property of the matrix is medically important. For example, infections spread, in part, because the infectious agent alters the "containing" capacity of the ECM. Cancer cells that metastasize (migrate to other tissues) can do so only by altering the integrity of the matrix. Diseases such as rheumatoid arthritis (an autoimmune destruction of articular and periarticular tissues) and osteoarthritis (degenerative joint disease often associated with aging) involve damage to the functional capacity of the matrix. Alterations in the structural characteristics of the matrix of the renal glomerulus may allow proteins to be excreted into the urine, an indication of inexorable decline in renal function. Genetic defects may cause components of the matrix to be structurally and functionally abnormal, resulting in connective tissue disorders such as the Ehlers-Danlos syndrome (caused by a number of mutations that affect specific collagen genes) and Marfan's syndrome (a defect in the protein, fibrillin, in which over 330 different mutations, many of which give rise to different phenotypes, have been identified). Deficiencies of lysosomal enzymes involved in normal degradation of molecules of the matrix result in diseases such as the mucopolysaccharidoses.

The principal components of the matrix of cartilage are collagen and proteoglycans, both of which are produced and degraded by the chondrocytes that are embedded in this matrix. An autoimmune attack on articular proteins alters the balance between cartilage degradation and formation. The resulting loss of cartilage organization accompanied by an inflammatory response is responsible for the symptoms experienced by **Sis Lupus**.

The collagen component forms a network of fine fibrils that give shape to the cartilage. The proteoglycans embedded in the cartilage are responsible for its compressibility and its deformability.

B. Proteoglycans

The fibrous structural proteins of the ECM are embedded in gels formed from proteoglycans. Proteoglycans consist of polysaccharides called glycosaminoglycans (GAG) linked to a core protein. The GAGs are composed of repeating units of disaccharides. One sugar of the disaccharide is either N-acetylglucosamine or N-acetylgalactosamine, and the second is usually acidic (either glucuronic acid or iduronic acid). These sugars are modified by the addition of sulfate groups to the parent sugar. A proteoglycan may contain more than 100 GAG chains and consist of up to 95% oligosaccharide by weight.

The negatively charged carboxylate and sulfate groups on the proteoglycan bind positively charged ions and form hydrogen bonds with trapped water molecules, thereby creating a hydrated gel. The gel provides a flexible mechanical support to the ECM. The gel also acts as a filter that allows the diffusion of ions (e.g., Ca^{2+}), H_2O, and other small molecules, but slows diffusion of proteins and movement of cells. Hyaluronan is the only GAG that occurs as a single long polysaccharide chain and is the only GAG that is not sulfated.

1. STRUCTURE AND FUNCTION OF THE PROTEOGLYCANS

Proteoglycans are found in interstitial connective tissues, for example, the synovial fluid of joints, the vitreous humor of the eye, arterial walls, bone, cartilage, and cornea. They are major components of the ECM in these tissues. The proteoglycans interact with a variety of proteins in the matrix, such as collagen and elastin, fibronectin (which is involved in cell adhesion and migration), and laminin.

Proteoglycans are proteins that contain many chains of GAGs (formerly called mucopolysaccharides). Glycosaminoglycans are long, unbranched polysaccharides composed of repeating disaccharide units (Fig. 49.8). The repeating disaccharides usually contain an iduronic or uronic acid and a hexosamine and are frequently sulfated. Consequently, they carry a negative charge, are hydrated, and act as lubricants. After synthesis, proteoglycans are secreted from cells; thus, they function extracellularly. Because the long, negatively charged glycosaminoglycan chains repel each other, the proteoglycans occupy a very large space and act as "molecular sieves," determining which substances enter or leave cells (Table 49.3). Their properties also give resilience and a degree of flexibility to substances such as cartilage, permitting compression and reexpansion of the molecule to occur.

At least seven types of glycosaminoglycans exist, which differ in the monosaccharides present in their repeating disaccharide units—chondroitin sulfate, dermatan sulfate, heparin, heparin sulfate, hyaluronic acid, and keratan sulfates I and II. Except for hyaluronic acid, the glycosaminoglycans are linked to proteins, usually attached covalently to serine or threonine residues (Fig. 49.9). Keratan sulfate I is attached to asparagine.

2. SYNTHESIS OF THE PROTEOGLYCANS

The protein component of the proteoglycans is synthesized on the ER. It enters the lumen of this organelle, where the initial glycosylations occur. UDP-sugars serve as

 The long polysaccharide side chains of the proteoglycans in cartilage contain many anionic groups. This high concentration of negative charges attracts cations that create a high osmotic pressure within cartilage, drawing water into this specialized connective tissue and placing the collagen network under tension. At equilibrium, the resulting tension balances the swelling pressure caused by the proteoglycans. The complementary roles of this macromolecular organization give cartilage its resilience. Cartilage can thus withstand the compressive load of weight bearing and then reexpand to its previous dimensions when that load is relieved.

Table 49.3. Some Specific Functions of the Glycosaminoglycans and Proteoglycans

Glycosaminoglycan	Function
Hyaluronic acid	Cell migration in: Embryogenesis Morphogenesis Wound healing
Chondroitin sulfate proteoglycans	Formation of bone, cartilage, cornea
Keratan sulfate proteoglycans	Transparency of cornea
Dermatan sulfate proteoglycans	Transparency of cornea Binds LDL to plasma walls
Heparin	Anticoagulant (binds antithrombin III) Causes release of lipoprotein lipase from capillary walls
Heparan sulfate (syndecan)	Component of skin fibroblasts and aortic wall; commonly found on cell surfaces

the precursors that add sugar units, one at a time, first to the protein and then to the nonreducing end of the growing carbohydrate chain (Fig. 49.10). Glycosylation occurs initially in the lumen of the ER and subsequently in the Golgi complex. Glycosyltransferases, the enzymes that add sugars to the chain, are specific for the sugar being added, the type of linkage that is formed, and the sugars already present in the chain. Once the initial sugars are attached to the protein, the alternating action of two glycosyltransferases adds the sugars of the repeating disaccharide to the growing glycosaminoglycan chain. Sulfation occurs after addition of the sugar. 3′-Phosphoadenosine 5′-phosphosulfate (PAPS), also called active sulfate, provides the sulfate groups (see Fig. 33.34). An epimerase converts glucuronic acid residues to iduronic acid residues.

After synthesis, the proteoglycan is secreted from the cell. Its structure resembles a bottle brush, with many glycosaminoglycan chains extending from the core protein (Fig. 49.11). The proteoglycans may form large aggregates, noncovalently attached by a "link" protein to hyaluronic acid (Fig. 49.12). The proteoglycans interact with the adhesion protein, fibronectin, which is attached to the cell membrane protein integrin. Cross-linked fibers of collagen also associate with this complex, forming the ECM (Fig. 49.13).

 The functional properties of a normal joint depend, in part, on the presence of a soft, well-lubricated, deformable, and compressible layer of cartilaginous tissue covering the ends of the long bones that constitute the joint.

In **Sis Lupus'** case, the pathologic process that characterizes SLE disrupted the structural and functional integrity of her articular (joint) cartilage.

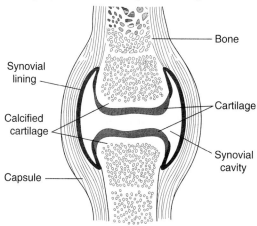

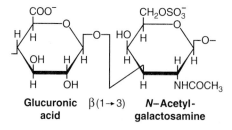

Hyaluronate

Glucuronic   β(1→3)   **N–Acetyl-**
acid   **glucosamine**

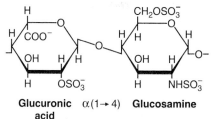

Chondroitin 6–sulfate

Glucuronic   β(1→3)   **N–Acetyl-**
acid   **galactosamine**

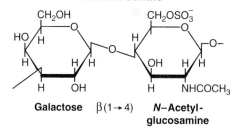

Heparin

Glucuronic   α(1→4)   **Glucosamine**
acid

Keratan sulfate

Galactose   β(1→4)   **N–Acetyl-**
                 glucosamine

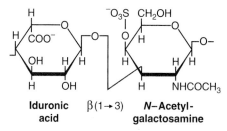

Dermatan sulfate

Iduronic   β(1→3)   **N–Acetyl-**
acid   **galactosamine**

Fig. 49.8. Repeating disaccharides of some glycosaminoglycans. These repeating disaccharides usually contain an *N*-acetylated sugar and a uronic acid, which usually is glucuronic acid or iduronic acid. Sulfate groups are often present but are not included in the sugar names in this figure.

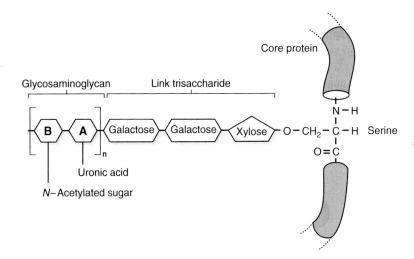

Fig. 49.9. Attachment of glycosaminoglycans to proteins. The sugars are linked to a serine or threonine residue of the protein. A and B represent the sugars of the repeating disaccharide.

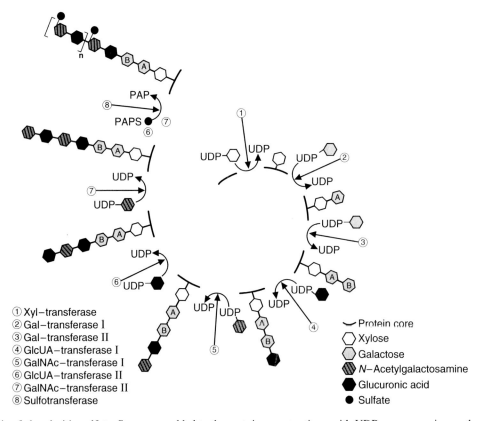

Fig. 49.10. Synthesis of chondroitin sulfate. Sugars are added to the protein one at a time, with UDP-sugars serving as the precursors. Initially a xylose residue is added to a serine in the protein. Then two galactose residues are added, followed by a glucuronic acid (GlcUA) and an N-acetylglucosamine (GalNAc). Subsequent additions occur by the alternating action of two enzymes that produce the repeating disaccharide units. One enzyme (6) adds GlcUA residues, and the other (7) adds GalNAc. As the chain grows, sulfate groups are added by phosphoadenosine phosphosulfate (PAPS). Modified from Roden L. In: Fishman WH, ed. Metabolic Conjugation and Metabolic Hydrolysis, vol II. Orlando, FL: Academic Press, 1970:401.

Table 49.4. Defective Enzymes in the Mucopolysaccharidoses

Disease	Enzyme Deficiency	Accumulated Products
Hunter	Iduronate sulfatase	Heparan sulfate, Dermatan sulfate
Hurler + Scheie	α-L-Iduronidase	Heparan sulfate, Dermatan sulfate
Maroteaux-Lamy	N-Acetylgalactosamine sulfatase	Dermatan sulfate
Mucolipidosis VII	β-Glucuronidase	Heparan sulfate, Dermatan sulfate
Sanfilippo A	Heparan sulfamidase	Heparan sulfate
Sanfilippo B	N-Acetylglucosaminidase	Heparan sulfate
Sanfilippo D	N-Acetylglucosamine 6-sulfatase	Heparin sulfate

These disorders share many clinical features, although there are significant variations between disorders, and even within a single disorder, based on the amount of residual activity remaining. In most cases, multiple organ systems are affected (with bone and cartilage being a primary target). For some disorders, there is significant neuronal involvement, leading to mental retardation.

3. DEGRADATION OF PROTEOGLYCANS

Lysosomal enzymes degrade proteoglycans, glycoproteins, and glycolipids, which are brought into the cell by the process of endocytosis. Lysosomes fuse with the endocytic vesicles, and lysosomal proteases digest the protein component. The carbohydrate component is degraded by lysosomal glycosidases.

Lysosomes contain both endoglycosidases and exoglycosidases. The endoglycosidases cleave the chains into shorter oligosaccharides. Then exoglycosidases, specific for each type of linkage, remove the sugar residues, one at a time, from the nonreducing ends.

Deficiencies of lysosomal glycosidases cause partially degraded carbohydrates from proteoglycans, glycoproteins, and glycolipids to accumulate within membrane-enclosed vesicles inside cells. These "residual bodies" can cause marked enlargement of the organ with impairment of its function.

In the clinical disorder known as the mucopolysaccharidoses (caused by accumulation of partially degraded glycosaminoglycans), deformities of the skeleton may occur (Table 49.4). Mental retardation often accompanies these skeletal changes.

II. INTEGRINS

Integrins are the major cellular receptors for ECM proteins and provide a link between the internal cytoskeleton of cells (primarily the actin microfilament system) and extracellular proteins, such as fibronectin, collagen, and laminin. Integrins

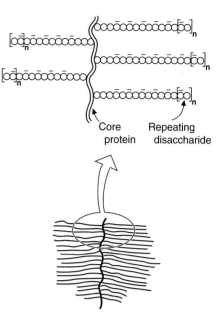

Fig. 49.11. "Bottle-brush" structure of a proteoglycan, with a magnified segment.

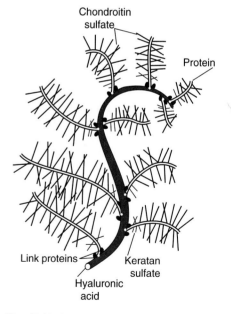

Fig. 49.12. Proteoglycan aggregate.

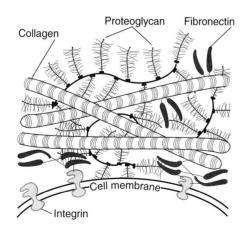

Fig. 49.13. Interactions between the cell membrane and the components of the extracellular matrix.

consist of an α and a β subunit. There are 18 distinct α and eight distinct β gene products. Twenty-four unique α/β dimers have been discovered. Mice have been genetically engineered to be unable to express many of the integrin genes (one gene at a time), and the phenotypes of these knockout mice vary from embryonic lethality (the α5 gene is an example) to virtually no observable defects (as exemplified by the α1 gene). In addition to anchoring the cell's cytoskeleton to the ECM, thereby providing a stable environment in which the cell can reside, the integrins are also involved in a wide variety of cell signaling options.

Certain integrins, such as those associated with white blood cells, are normally inactive because the white cell must circulate freely in the bloodstream. However, if an infection occurs, cells located in the area of the infection release cytokines, which activate the integrins on the white blood cells, allowing them to bind to vascular endothelial cells (leukocyte adhesion) at the site of infection. Leukocyte adhesion deficiency (LAD) is a genetic disorder that results from mutations in the β2 integrin such that leukocytes cannot be recruited to the sites of infection. Conversely, drugs are now being developed to block either the β2 or α4 integrins (on lymphocytes) to treat inflammatory and autoimmune disorders by interfering with the normal white cell response to cytokines.

Integrins can be activated by "inside-out" mechanisms, whereby intracellular signaling events activate the molecule, or "outside-in" mechanisms, in which a binding event with the extracellular portion of the molecule initiates intracellular signaling events. For those integrins that bind cells to ECM components, activation of specific integrins can result in migration of the affected cell through the ECM. This mechanism is operative during growth, during cellular differentiation, and in the process of metastasis of malignant cells to neighboring tissues.

III. ADHESION PROTEINS

Adhesion proteins are found in the ECM and link integrins to ECM components. Adhesion proteins, of which fibronectin is a prime example, are large multidomain proteins that allow binding to many different components simultaneously. In addition to integrin binding sites, fibronectin contains binding sites for collagen and glycosaminoglycans. As the integrin molecule is bound to intracellular cytoskeletal proteins, the adhesion proteins provide a bridge between the actin cytoskeleton of the cell and the cells' position within the ECM. Loss of adhesion protein capability can lead to either physiologic or abnormal cell movement. Alternative splicing of fibronectin allows many different forms of this adhesion protein to be expressed, including a soluble form (versus cell-associated forms), which is found in the plasma. The metabolic significance of these products remains to be determined.

IV. MATRIX METALLOPROTEINASES

The ECM contains a series of proteases known as the matrix metalloproteinases, or MMPs. These are zinc-containing proteases that use the zinc to appropriately position water to participate in the proteolytic reaction. At least 23 different types of human MMPs exist, and they cleave all proteins found in the ECM, including collagen and laminin.

A propeptide is present in newly synthesized MMPs that contains a critical cysteine residue. The cysteine residue in the propeptide binds to the zinc atom at the active site of the protease and prevents the propeptide from exhibiting proteolytic activity. Removal of the propeptide is required to activate the MMPs. Once activated, certain MMPs can activate other forms of MMP.

Regulation of MMP activity is quite complex. These regulatory processes include transcriptional regulation, proteolytic activation, inhibition by the circulating protein α2-macroglobulin, and regulation by a class of inhibitors known as

Fibronectin was first discovered as a large, external transformation-sensitive protein (LETS), which was lost when fibroblasts were transformed into tumor cells. Many tumor cells secrete less than normal amounts of adhesion protein material, which allows for more movement within the extracellular milieu. This, in turn, increases the potential for the tumor cells to leave their original location and take root at another location within the body (metastasis).

Because MMPs degrade extracellular matrix (ECM) components, their expression is important to allow cell migration and tissue remodeling during growth and differentiation. In addition, many growth factors bind to ECM components and, as a bound component, do not exhibit their normal growth-promoting activity. Destruction of the ECM by the MMPs releases these growth factors, thereby allowing them to bind to cell surface receptors to initiate growth of tissues. Thus, coordinated expression of the MMPs is required for appropriate cell movement and growth. Cancer cells that metastasize require extensive ECM remodeling and usually use MMP activity to spread throughout the body.

tissue inhibitors of metalloproteinases, or TIMPs. It is important that the synthesis of TIMPs and MMPs be coordinately regulated, because dissociation of their expression can facilitate various clinical disorders, such as certain forms of cancer and atherosclerosis.

CLINICAL COMMENTS

Articular cartilage is a living tissue with a turnover time determined by a balance between the rate of its synthesis and that of its degradation (Fig. 49.14). The chondrocytes that are embedded in the matrix of intra-articular cartilage participate in both its synthesis and its enzymatic degradation. The latter occurs as a result of cleavage of proteoglycan aggregates by enzymes produced and secreted by the chondrocytes.

In SLE, the condition that affects **Sis Lupus,** this delicate balance is disrupted in favor of enzymatic degradation, leading to dissolution of articular cartilage and, with it, the loss of its critical cushioning functions. The underlying mechanisms responsible for this process in SLE include the production of antibodies directed against specific cellular proteins in cartilage as well as in other intra-articular tissues. The cellular proteins thus serve as the "antigens" to which these antibodies react. In this sense, SLE is an "autoimmune" disease because antibodies are produced by the host that attack "self" proteins. This process excites the local release of cytokines such as interleukin-1 (IL-1), which increases the proteolytic activity of the chondrocytes, causing further loss of articular proteins such as the proteoglycans. The associated inflammatory cascade is responsible for **Sis Lupus'** joint pain.

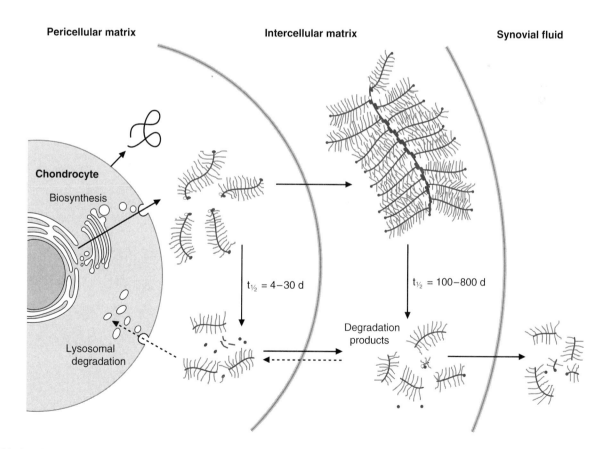

Fig. 49.14. Synthesis and degradation of proteoglycans by chondrocytes. From Cohen RD, et al. The Metabolic Basis of Acquired Disease, vol 2. London: Bailliere Tindall, 1990:1859.

The microvascular complications of both type 1 and type 2 diabetes mellitus involve the small vessels of the retina (diabetic retinopathy), the renal glomerular capillaries (diabetic nephropathy), and the vessels supplying blood to the peripheral nerves (autonomic neuropathy). The lack of adequate control of **Ann Sulin's** diabetic state over many years caused a progressive loss of the filtering function of the approximately one-and-one-half million glomerular capillary–mesangial units that are present in her kidneys.

Chronic hyperglycemia is postulated to be a major metabolic initiator or inducer of diabetic microvascular disease, including those renal glomerular changes that often lead to end-stage renal disease ("glucose toxicity").

For a comprehensive review of the four postulated molecular mechanisms by which chronic hyperglycemia causes these vascular derangements, the reader is referred to an excellent review by Sheetz and King (see suggested references).

Regardless of which of the postulated mechanisms (increased flux through the aldose reductase or polyol pathway [see Chapter 30], the generation of advanced glycosylation end products [AGEs], the generation of reactive oxygen intermediates [see Chapter 24], or excessive activation of protein kinase C [see Chapter 18]) will eventually be shown to be the predominant causative mechanism, each can lead to the production of critical intracellular and extracellular signaling molecules (e.g., cytokines). These, in turn, can cause pathologic changes within the glomerular filtration apparatus that reduce renal function. These changes include: (1) increased synthesis of collagen, type IV, fibronectin, and some of the proteoglycans, causing the glomerular basement membrane (GBM; Fig. 49.15) to become diffusely thickened throughout the glomerular capillary network. This membrane thickening alters certain specific filtration properties of the GBM, preventing some of the metabolites that normally enter the urine from the glomerular capillary blood (via the fenestrated capillary endothelium) from doing so (a decline in glomerular filtration rate or GFR). As a result, these potentially toxic substances accumulate in the blood and contribute to the overall clinical presentation of advancing uremia. In spite of the

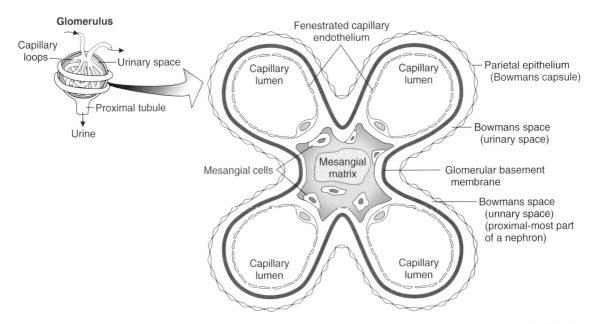

Fig. 49.15. A cross-section of a normal renal glomerulus showing four capillary tufts delivering blood to the glomerulus for filtration across the fenestrated capillary endothelium then through the glomerular basement membrane into the Bowman's space to form urine. The urine then enters the proximal tubule of the nephron. This filtration removes potentially toxic metabolic end products from the blood. The mesangium, by contracting and expanding, controls the efficiency of these filtering and excretory functions by regulating the hydraulic filtration pressures within the glomerulus. An intact basement membrane must be present to maintain the integrity of the filtering process.

thickening of the GBM, this membrane becomes "leaky" for some macromolecules (e.g., albumin) that normally do not enter the urine from the glomerular capillaries (microalbuminuria). Suggested mechanisms for this increased permeability or leakiness include reduced synthesis of the specific proteoglycan, heparan sulphate, as well as increased basement membrane production of vascular endothelium growth factor (VEGF), a known angiogenic and permeability factor; and expansion of the extracellular matrix in the mesangium. The mesangium consists of specialized tissue containing collagen, proteoglycans, and other macromolecules that surround the glomerular capillaries and that, through its gel-like and sieving properties, determine, in part, the glomerular capillary hydraulic filtration pressure as well as the functional status of the capillary endothelium–mesangial glomerular basement membrane filtration apparatus (see Fig. 49.15). As the mesangial tissue expands, the efficiency of glomerular filtration diminishes proportionately. The cause of these mesangial changes is, in part, the consequence of increased expression of certain growth factors, especially transforming growth factor β (TGF-β) and connective tissue growth factor (CTGF). Current therapeutic approaches in patients with early diabetic nephropathy include the use of antibodies that neutralize TGF-β.

BIOCHEMICAL COMMENTS

Osteogenesis imperfecta (OI) is a heterogenous group of diseases that have in common a defect in collagen production. This defect can be either of two types: The first type is associated with a reduction in the synthesis of normal collagen (due to a gene deletion or splice-site mutation). The second type is associated with the synthesis of a mutated form of collagen. Most of the mutations have a dominant-negative effect, leading to an autosomal dominant mode of transmission.

In the second type of OI, many of the known mutations involve substitutions of another amino acid for glycine. This results in an unstable collagen molecule, because glycine is the only amino acid that can fit between the other two chains within the triple helix of collagen. If the mutation is near the carboxy-terminal of the molecule, the phenotype of the disease is usually more severe than if the mutation is near the amino-terminal end (recall that triple helix formation proceeds from the carboxy- to the amino-terminal end of the molecule). Of interest are mutations that replace glycine with either serine or cysteine. Such mutations are more stable than expected, because of the hydrogen-bonding capabilities of serine and the ability of cysteine to form disulfide bonds. Both would aid in preventing the strands of the triple helix from unwinding.

Children with OI can be treated with a class of compounds known as bisphosphonates, which consist of two phosphates linked by a carbon or nitrogen bridge (thus, they are analogs of pyrophosphate, in which the two phosphates are linked by oxygen). Normal bone remodeling is the result of a coordinated "coupling" between osteoclast activity (cells that resorb bone) and osteoblast activity (cells that form bone). In OI, bone resorption outpaces bone formation because osteoclast activity is enhanced (perhaps because of the reduced levels of normal collagen present to act as nucleating sites for bone formation). This leads to a net loss of bone mass and fragility of the skeleton. Bisphosphonates inhibit osteoclast action with the potential to increase bone mass and its tensile strength.

Suggested References

Bosman FT, Stamenhovic I. Functional structure and composition of the extracellular matrix. J Pathol 2003;200:423–428.

Byers PH. Disorders of collagen biosynthesis and structure. In: Scriver CR, Beaudet AL, Valle D, Sly WS, et al., eds. The Metabolic and Molecular Bases of Inherited Disease, vol IV, 8th Ed. New York: McGraw-Hill, 2001:5241–5286.

Hynes RO. Integrins: biodirectional allosteric signalling machines. Cell 2002;110:673–687.

Neufeld EF, Muenzer J. The mucopolysaccharidoses. In: Scriver CR, Beaudet AL, Valle D, Sly WS, et al., eds. The Metabolic and Molecular Bases of Inherited Disease, vol. IV, 8th Ed. New York: McGraw-Hill, 2001:3421–3452.

Sheetz MJ, King GL. Molecular understanding of hyperglycemia's adverse effects for diabetic complications. JAMA 2002;288(20):2579–2588.

 REVIEW QUESTIONS—CHAPTER 49

1. Individuals who develop scurvy suffer from sore and bleeding gums and loss of teeth. This is due, in part, to the synthesis of a defective collagen molecule. The step that is affected in collagen biosynthesis attributable to scurvy is which of the following?

    (A) The formation of disulfide bonds, which initiates tropocollagen formation
    (B) The formation of lysyl cross-links between collagen molecules
    (C) Secretion of tropocollagen into the extracellular matrix
    (D) The formation of collagen fibrils
    (E) The hydroxylation of proline residues, which stabilizes the collagen structure

2. The underlying mechanism that allows elastin to exhibit elastic properties (expand and contract) is which of the following?

    (A) Proteolysis during expansion, and resynthesis during contraction
    (B) Breaking of disulfide bonds during expansion, reformation of these bonds during contraction
    (C) A decrease in entropy during expansion, and an increase in entropy during contraction
    (D) The breaking of salt bridges during expansion, and reformation of the salt bridges during contraction
    (E) Hydroxylation of elastin during expansion, and decarboxylation of elastin during contraction

3. The underlying mechanism by which glycosaminoglycans allow for the formation of a gel-like substance in the extracellular matrix in which of the following?

    (A) Charge attraction between glycosaminoglycan chains
    (B) Charge repulsion between glycosaminoglycan chains
    (C) Hydrogen bonding between glycosaminoglycan chains
    (D) Covalent cross-linking between glycosaminoglycan chains
    (E) Hydroxylation of adjacent glycosaminoglycan chains

4. The movement of tumor cells from their site of origin to other locations within the body requires the activity of which of the following proteins?

    (A) Collagen
    (B) Laminin
    (C) Proteoglycans
    (D) Elastin
    (E) Matrix metalloproteinases

5. Fibronectin is frequently absent in malignant fibroblast cells. One of the major functions of fibronectin is which of the following?

    (A) To inhibit the action of matrix metalloproteinases
    (B) To coordinate collagen deposition within the extracellular matrix
    (C) To fix the position of cells within the extracellular matrix
    (D) To regulate glycosaminoglycan production
    (E) To extend glycosaminoglycan chains using nucleotide sugars

Appendix

ANSWERS

Chapter 1

1. **The answer is B.** In the process of respiration, O_2 is consumed and fuels are oxidized to CO_2 and H_2O. The energy from the oxidation reactions is used to generate ATP from ADP and P_i. However, a small amount of energy is also released as heat (thus, C is incorrect). Although fuels can be stored as triacylglycerols, this is not part of respiration (thus, A is incorrect). Respiration is a catabolic pathway (fuels are degraded), as opposed to an anabolic pathway (compounds combine to make larger molecules) (thus, E is incorrect).

2. **The answer is D.** The caloric content per gram of a fuel is the amount of energy that can be obtained from oxidizing the fuel. It is lower for carbohydrates and proteins than for fats because proteins and carbohydrates contain more oxygen and are already partially oxidized (thus, A, B, and C are incorrect). The caloric content of a fuel is principally a property of its chemical structure and our ability to oxidize that structure and generate ATP; there is little difference between children and adults.

3. **The answer is A.** The resting metabolic rate (RMR) is the calories being expended by a recently awakened resting person who has fasted 12 to 18 hours and is at 20°C. It is equivalent to the energy expenditure of our major organs and resting skeletal muscle. Women generally have a lower RMR per kilogram body weight because more of their body weight is usually metabolically inactive adipose tissue. Children have a higher RMR per kilogram body weight because more of their body weight is metabolically active organs such as the brain. The RMR increases in a cold environment because more energy is being expended to generate heat. The RMR is not equivalent to our daily energy expenditure (DEE), which includes RMR, physical activity, and diet-induced thermogenesis.

4. **The answer is D.** The recommended daily allowance of a nutrient is determined from the EAR + 2 SD, and should meet the needs for 97 to 98% of the healthy population. It is therefore a reasonable goal for the intake of a healthy individual. The EAR is the amount that prevents development of established signs of deficiency in 50% of the healthy population. Although data with laboratory animals have been used to establish deficiency symptoms, RDAs are based on data collected on nutrient ingestion by humans.

5. **The answer is B.** The recommended total fat intake is less than 30% of total calories. His total caloric consumption was 4,110 kcal/day (carbohydrate, $4 \times 585 = 2,340$ kcal; protein $150 \times 4 = 600$ kcal; fat, $95 \times 9 = 855$ kcal; alcohol, $45 \times 7 = 315$ kcal.) (Thus, A is incorrect). His fat intake was 21% ($855 \div 4110$) of his total caloric intake. His alcohol intake was 7.7% ($315 \div 4110$) (thus, C is incorrect). His protein intake was well above the RDA of 0.8 g/kg body weight (thus, D is incorrect). His RMR is roughly 24 kcal/day per kilogram body weight, or 2,880 kcal/day (it will actually be less because he is obese and has a greater proportion of metabolically inactive tissue than the average 70-kg man). His daily energy expenditure is approximately 3,744 kcal/day ($1.3 \times 2,880$) or less. Thus, his intake is greater than his expenditure, and he is in positive caloric balance and is gaining weight (thus, E is incorrect).

Chapter 2

1. **The answer is E.** During digestion of a mixed meal, starch and other carbohydrates, proteins, and dietary triacylglycerols are broken into their monomeric units (carbohydrates into simple monosaccharides; protein into amino acids; triacylglycerols into fatty acids and glycerol.) Glucose is the principal sugar in dietary carbohydrates, and thus it increases in the blood. Amino acids and monosaccharides enter the portal vein and go to the liver first. After digestion of fats and absorption of the fatty acids, most fatty acids are converted back into triacylglycerols and subsequently into chylomicrons by intestinal cells. Chylomicrons go through lymphatic vessels and then blood principally to adipose tissue.

2. **The answer is C.** After a high carbohydrate meal, glucose is the major fuel for most tissues, including skeletal muscle and adipose tissue. The increase in blood glucose levels stimulates the release of insulin, not glucagon. Insulin stimulates the transport of glucose in skeletal muscle and

adipose tissue, not brain. Liver, not skeletal muscle, converts glucose to fatty acids. Although the red blood cell uses glucose as its only fuel at all times, it generates ATP from conversion of glucose to lactate, not CO_2.

3. **The answer is A.** Amino acids from digestion of dietary protein are transported to the liver, where they are used for precursors of nitrogen-containing compounds, such as nonessential amino acids and serum proteins. They also can be converted to glucose and fatty acids in liver cells (hepatocytes). Hepatocytes are the only cells containing the pathways for degradation of all amino acids, as well as the pathways for synthesis of glucose and fatty acids from amino acids. Fatty acids synthesized in the liver are eventually deposited as adipose tissue fat. Unused amino groups are converted to urea in the liver to prevent ammonia toxicity. Amino acids are not excreted in the urine of a healthy individual.

4. **The answer is B.** Chylomicrons are the lipoprotein particles formed in intestinal epithelial cells from dietary fats, and they principally contain triacylglycerols formed from components of dietary triacylglycerols. A decreased intake of calories in general would include a decreased consumption of fat, carbohydrate, and protein, which might not lower chylomicron levels. Dietary cholesterol, although found in chylomicrons, is not their principal component.

5. **The answer is A.** His BMI is in the obese range, with large abdominal fat deposits. He needs to decrease his intake of total calories, because an excess of calories ingested as carbohydrate, fat, or protein results in deposition of triacylglycerols in adipose tissue. If he keeps his total caloric intake the same, substitution of one type of food for another will help very little with weight loss. (However, a decreased intake of fat may be advisable for other reasons.) Limited food diets, such as the ice cream and sherry diet, or a high-protein diet of shrimp, work if they decrease appetite and therefore ingestion of total calories.

Chapter 3

1. **The answer is A.** By 24 hours after a meal, hepatic (liver) gluconeogenesis is the major source of blood glucose because hepatic glycogen stores have been nearly depleted. Muscle and other tissues lack an enzyme necessary to convert glycogen or amino acids to glucose (thus, B is incorrect). The liver is the only significant source of blood glucose. Glucose is synthesized in the liver from amino acids (provided by protein degradation), from glycerol (provided by hydrolysis of triacylglycerols in adipose tissue), and from lactate (provided by anaerobic glycolysis in red blood cells and other tissues). Glucose cannot be synthesized from fatty acids or ketone bodies (thus, D and E are incorrect).

2. **The answer is D.** The conversion of ammonia to urea (the urea cycle) occurs to a significant extent only in the liver. Thus, the liver is able to dispose of toxic ammonia that is produced when it converts amino acid carbon skeletons to glucose. Although the liver has the largest glycogen stores per gram of tissue, most cells have glycogen deposits. Muscle mass is so large that muscle is a significant glycogen store (thus, A is incorrect). Most tissues (with the exception of the brain and tissues without mitochondria such as the red blood cell) oxidize fatty acids during overnight fasting (thus, B is incorrect). The liver synthesizes ketone bodies but lacks an enzyme necessary to oxidize them (thus, C is incorrect). It generally oxidizes glucose to CO_2, or converts it to fatty acids and not to lactate.

3. **The answer is C.** The major change during prolonged fasting is that as muscles decrease their use of ketone bodies, ketone bodies increase enormously in the blood and are used by brain as a fuel. However, even during starvation, glucose is still required by the brain, which cannot oxidize fatty acids to an appreciable extent (thus, D is incorrect). Red blood cells can use only glucose as a fuel (thus, B is incorrect). Because the brain, red blood cells, and certain other tissues are glucose dependent, the liver continues to synthesize glucose, and blood glucose levels are maintained at only slightly less than fasting levels (thus, A is incorrect). Adipose tissue stores are 135,000 kcal and are not depleted in a well-nourished individual after 1 week of fasting (thus, E is incorrect).

4. **The answer is A.** Decreased serum albumin could have a number of causes, including hepatic disease (which decreases the ability of the liver to synthesize serum proteins), protein malnutrition, marasmus, or diseases affecting the ability of the intestine to digest protein and absorb the amino acids. However, his BMI is in the healthy range (thus, B and D are incorrect). His normal creatinine–height index (CHI) indicates that he has not lost muscle mass and therefore is not suffering from protein malnutrition (thus, B, C, D, and E are incorrect).

5. **The answer is C.** His protein intake of 150 kcal is approximately 37 g protein (150 kcal ÷ 4 kcal/g = 37 g), below the RDA for protein (thus, A is incorrect). His carbohydrate intake of 150 kcal is below the glucose requirements of his brain and red blood cells (approximately 150 g/day, see Chap. 2) (thus, B is incorrect). Therefore, he will be breaking down muscle protein to synthesize glucose for the brain and other glucose-dependent tissues and adipose tissue mass to supply fatty acids for muscle and tissues able to oxidize fatty acids. Because he will be breaking down muscle protein to amino acids, and converting the nitrogen from both these amino acids and his dietary amino acids to urea, his nitrogen excretion will be greater than his intake, and he will be in negative nitrogen

balance (thus, D is incorrect). He is not likely to develop hypoglycemia while he is able to supply gluconeogenic precursors.

Chapter 4

1. **The answer is A.** The pH is the negative log of the hydrogen ion concentration ($[H^+]$). Thus, at a pH of 7.5, $[H^+]$ is $10^{-7.5}$, and at pH 6.5 it is $10^{-6.5}$. The $[H^+]$ has changed by a factor of $10^{-6.5}/10^{-7.5}$, which is 10^1, or 10. Any decrease of 1 pH unit is a 10-fold increase of $[H^+]$, or a 10-fold decrease of $[OH^-]$. A shift in the concentration of buffer anions has definitely occurred, but the change in pH reflects the increase in hydrogen ion concentration in excess of that absorbed by buffers.

2. **The answer is C.** Buffers, by definition, tend to keep the pH of a solution constant, absorbing protons if an acid is added to the solution, and releasing protons if a base is added to the solution. Because they must have the ability to dissociate or re-associate a proton, they work best at the pH at which they are 50% dissociated, the pK_a (B and D are incorrect). Buffers cannot be composed of strong acids or strong bases because strong acids and bases are fully dissociated in solution (thus, A is incorrect). The higher the buffer concentration, the better the buffer works because it can absorb or dissociate more protons (thus, E is incorrect).

3. **The answer is B.** NH_3 is a weak base, which associates with a proton to produce the ammonium ion ($NH_3 + H^+ \rightarrow NH_4^+$), which has a pK_a of 9.5. Thus, at pH 7.4, most of the ammonia will be present as ammonium ion. The absorption of hydrogen ions tends to increase, not decrease, the pH of the blood (thus, A is incorrect). With the decrease of hydrogen ions, carbonic acid dissociates to produce more bicarbonate ($H_2CO_3 \rightarrow HCO_3^- + H^+$) and more CO_2 will go toward carbonic acid (thus, C is incorrect). Kussmaul's respiration, an increased expiration of CO_2, occurs under an acidosis, the opposite condition.

4. **The answer is C.** Vomiting expels the strong acid gastric acid (HCl). As cells in the stomach secrete more HCl, they draw on H^+ ions in interstitial fluid and blood, thereby tending to increase blood pH and cause an alkalosis. The other conditions tend to produce an acidosis (thus, A, B, D, and E are incorrect). Lactic acid is a weak acid secreted into the blood by muscles during exercise. A patient with increased ketone body production can exhibit a decrease in pH because the ketone bodies acetoacetate and β-hydroxybutyrate are dissociated acids. As bicarbonate in the intestinal lumen is lost in the watery diarrhea, more bicarbonate is secreted by intestinal cells. As intestinal cells produce bicarbonate, more H^+ is also generated ($H_2CO_3 \rightarrow HCO_3^- + H^+$). While the bicarbonate produced by these cells is released into the intestinal lumen,

the protons accumulate in blood, resulting in an acidosis. Hypercatabolism (see E), an increased rate of catabolism, generates additional CO_2, which produces more acid ($CO_2 + H_2O \rightarrow H_2CO_3 \rightarrow HCO_3^- + H^+$).

5. **The answer is B.** Methylmalonic acid contains two carboxylic acid groups and is therefore a weak acid. According to the Henderson-Hasselbalch equation, the carboxylic acid groups are 50% dissociated at their pK_as (thus, C is incorrect). Carboxylic acid groups usually have pK_as between 2 and 5, so that this acid would be nearly fully dissociated at a blood pH of 7.4 and cannot buffer intracellularily at neutral pH (thus, D and E are incorrect). (Although you do not need to know anything about methylmalonate to answer this question, methylmalonate is an organic acid generated in patients with a problem in metabolism of methylmalonyl CoA, such as a deficiency in vitamin B_{12}. Its acidity may contribute to the development of symptoms involving the nervous system. Its appearance in the urine can be classified as an organic aciduria).

Chapter 5

1. **The answer is D.** Water-soluble compounds are polar (contain an uneven distribution of charge) so that the more positive portion of the molecule hydrogen bonds (shares electrons) with the oxygen of water, and the more negative portion of the molecule hydrogen bonds with the hydrogens of water. Water-soluble compounds need not contain a full negative or positive charge (thus, C and D are incorrect), and generally contain oxygen or nitrogen, in addition to carbon and hydrogen (see A). Large C-H portions of a molecule, such as an aromatic ring, are nonpolar and contribute to the water-insolubility of a molecule (see E).

2. **The answer is E.** The compound contains an OH group, which should appear in the name as an "ol" or a "hydroxy" group. All answers fit this criterion. The structure also contains a carboxylate group (COO^-), which should appear in the name as an "ate" or "acid". Only D and E fit this criterion. Counting backwards from the carboxylate group (carbon 1), the 2nd carbon is α, the 3rd is β, and the 4th carbon, containing the hydroxyl group, is γ. Thus, the compound is γ-hydroxybutyrate. "A," "B," and "C" can also be eliminated because "meth" denotes a single carbon, "eth" denotes two carbons, and the "ene" in ethylene denotes a double bond.

3. **The answer is B.** The term "glycosidic bond" refers to a *covalent* bond formed between the anomeric carbon of one sugar, when it is in a ring form, and a hydroxyl group or nitrogen of another compound (see Fig. 5.17) (Thus, A, D, and E are incorrect). Disaccharides can be linked through their anomeric carbons, but not polysaccharides, because there would be no anomeric carbon left to form a link with the next sugar in the chain (thus, C is incorrect).

4. **The answer is A.** Triglycerides (triacylglycerols) are composed of a glycerol backbone to which 3 fatty acids ("tri") are attached (see Fig. 5.20). The carboxylic acid group of each fatty acid forms an ester with one of the three –OH groups on glycerol; thus, the fatty acid is an "acyl" group. Sphingolipids, in contrast, contain one fatty acyl group and one group derived from a fatty acid, attached to a group derived from serine (see Fig. 5.22).

5. **The answer is B.** Sphingolipids contain a ceramide group, which is sphingosine with an attached fatty acid. They do not contain a glycerol moiety (thus, A is incorrect). However, different sphingolipids have different substituents on the CH_2OH group of ceramide. For example, sphingomyelin contains phosphorylcholine, and gangliosides contain NANA (thus, C and D are incorrect). No known sphingolipids contain a steroid (E).

Chapter 6

1. **The answer is D.** In hydrogen bonds, a hydrogen atom is shared between two electron-rich groups, such as oxygen or nitrogen. Thus, the nitrogen in the peptide bond may share its hydrogen with the oxygen in an aspartate carboxyl group, which will be negatively charged at a pH of 7.4. Leucine is nonpolar and cannot participate in hydrogen bonding (thus, A is incorrect) and aspartyl and glutamyl residues are both negatively charged (thus, B is incorrect). Bonds between two fully charged groups are electrostatic bonds, not hydrogen bonds (thus, C is incorrect). Sulfhydryl groups do not participate in hydrogen bonding.

2. **The answer is A.** The peptide backbone contains only carbon and nitrogen atoms covalently linked in a chain. The amide nitrogen of one amino acid (N) is covalently attached to the α-carbon of the same amino acid (C), which is covalently linked to the carboxyl carbon (C) of that amino acid, which forms a peptide bond with the nitrogen of the next amino acid (N).

3. **The answer is A.** Arginine is a *basic* amino acid that has a positively charged side chain at neutral pH. It therefore can form tight electrostatic bonds with negatively charged *asp* and *glu* side chains in insulin. The α-carboxylic acid groups at the N-terminals of proteins are bound through peptide bonds (thus, B is incorrect). The arginine side chain is not hydrophobic, and it cannot form disulfide bonds because it has no sulfhydryl group (thus C and D are incorrect). Its basic group is a guanidino group that cannot form peptide bonds (see E).

4. **The answer is B.** Only these amino acids have side chain hydroxyl groups. As a general rule, serine–threonine protein kinases form one group of protein kinases, and tyrosine protein kinases form another.

5. **The answer is E.** In a single individual, the primary structures of enzymes catalyzing the same reaction may differ between cellular compartments, or between different cell types, or they may differ from enzymes produced at a different stage of development (thus, A and B are incorrect). Paralogs have somewhat different amino acid structures and different functions. Members of a homologous family have somewhat different structures and are related only by their evolution from the same ancestral gene.

Chapter 7

1. **The answer is B.** The regular repeating structure of an α-helix is possible because it is formed by hydrogen bonds within the peptide backbone of a single strand. Thus, α-helices can be formed from a variety of primary structures. However, proline cannot accommodate the bends for an α-helix because the atoms involved in the peptide backbone are part of a ring structure, and glycine cannot provide the space-filling required for a stable structure.

2. **The answer is C.** Globular proteins fold into a sphere-like structure with their hydrophilic residues on the outside to interact with water (hence, A is incorrect) and their hydrophobic residues on the inside away from water (thus, B is incorrect). Secondary structures are formed by hydrogen bonding, not hydrophobic bonding (thus, D is incorrect). Disulfide bonds are rare in globular proteins and are not needed to maintain a stable structure (thus, E is incorrect).

3. **The answer is D.** When an α-helix is formed, all side chains face the outside of the helix, which is the hydrophobic environment of the lipid membrane. Thus, the side chains should be hydrophobic. Of the amino acids listed, only leucine fits the bill (see Chapter 6). Proline interrupts helical structure because the imino bond of its ring structure does not allow the polypeptide backbone to form the angles required for α-helical formation.

4. **The answer is A.** The characteristic staining of amyloid arises from fibrils of β-pleated sheet structure perpendicular to the axis of the fiber (thus, B, C, and D are incorrect). The native conformation of a protein is generally the most stable and lowest energy conformation, and the lower its energy state, the more readily a protein folds into its native conformation and the less likely it will assume the insoluble β-pleated sheet structure of amyloid (thus, E is incorrect).

5. **The answer is A.** The protein hydrolyzes ATP, which is a characteristic of the actin fold.

Chapter 8

1. **The answer is B.** In most reactions, the substrate binds to the enzyme before its reaction with the coenzyme occurs. Thus, the substrate may bind but cannot react with the

coenzyme to form the transition state complex. Each coenzyme carries out a single type of reaction, so no other coenzyme can substitute (thus, C is incorrect). The 3-dimensional geometry of the reaction is so specific that functional groups on amino acid side chains cannot substitute (thus, D is incorrect). Free coenzymes are not very reactive because amino acid side chains in the active site are required to activate the coenzyme or the reactants (thus, E is incorrect). However, increasing the supply of vitamins to increase the amount of coenzyme bound to the enzyme can sometimes help.

2. **The answer is D.** The patient was diagnosed with MODY (maturity onset diabetes of the young), caused by this mutation. In glucokinase, binding of glucose normally causes a huge conformational change in the actin fold that creates the binding site for ATP. Although proline and leucine are both nonpolar amino acids, B is incorrect—proline creates kinks in helices and thus would be expected to disturb the large conformational change required (see Chapter 7). In general, binding of the first substrate to an enzyme creates conformational changes that increases the binding of the second substrate or brings functional groups into position for further steps in the reaction. Thus, a mutation need not be in the active site to impair the reaction, and A is incorrect. It would probably take more energy to fold the enzyme into the form required for the transition state complex, and fewer molecules would acquire the energy necessary (thus, C is incorrect). The active site lacks the functional groups required for an alternate mechanism (thus, E is incorrect).

3. **The answer is C.** Enzymes that use histidine to abstract a proton from the substrate in acid-base catalysis are active only over a narrow pH range near neutrality because histidine must be able to accept and donate a proton within this pH range. As the pH decreases to below 6.5, protons will not readily dissociate from histidine. In contrast, lysine is fully protonated at both pH 6.5 and 5.5 (thus, D is incorrect). All intestinal hydrolases (proteases, esterases, glycosidases) use acid-base catalysis to add the elements of water across the bonds (thus, E is incorrect). Usually, the pH must fall much lower before the hydrogen bonding is disrupted and proteins are denatured and lose their tertiary structure (thus, A and B are incorrect).

4. **The answer is A.** The glucose residue from UDP-glucose is being transferred to the alcohol group of another compound. In isomerization reactions, groups are transferred within the same molecule (thus, B is incorrect). There is no cleavage or synthesis of carbon-carbon bonds (thus, C and D are incorrect). Oxidation reduction has not occurred because no hydrogens or oxygen atoms have been removed or added in the conversion of substrate to product.

5. **The answer is C.** Transfer of a carbohydrate residue from one molecule to another is a glycosyltransferase reaction. Kinases transfer phosphate groups, dehydrogenases transfer electrons as hydrogen atoms or hydride ions, transaminases transfer amino groups, and isomerases transfer atoms within the same molecule.

Chapter 9

1. **The answer is B.** The rate of the reaction is directly proportional to the proportion of enzyme molecules containing bound substrate. Thus, it is at 50% of its maximal rate when 50% of the molecules contain bound substrate (A, C, and D are incorrect). The rate of the reaction is directly proportional to the amount of enzyme present, which is incorporated into the term V_{max} ($V_{max} = k$ [total enzme])(thus, E is incorrect).

2. **The answer is A.** The patient's enzyme has a lower K_m than the normal enzyme and therefore requires a lower glucose concentration to reach $\frac{1}{2} V_{max}$. Thus, the mutation may have increased the affinity of the enzyme for glucose, but it has greatly decreased the subsequent steps of the reaction leading to formation of the transition state complex, and thus V_{max} is much slower. The difference in V_{max} is so great that the patient's enzyme is much slower whether you are above or below its K_m for glucose. You can test this by substituting 2 mM glucose and 4 mM glucose into the Michaelis-Menten equation of $v = V_{max} S/(K_m + S)$ for the patient's enzyme and for the normal enzyme. The values are 0.0095 and 0.0129 for the patient's enzyme versus 23.2 and 37.2 for the normal enzyme, respectively (thus, B and C are incorrect). At near saturating glucose concentrations, both enzymes will be near V_{max}, which is equal to k_{cat} times the enzyme concentration. Thus, it will take nearly 500 times as much of the patient's enzyme to achieve the normal rate (93 ÷ 0.2), and C is incorrect. E is incorrect because rates change most as you decrease substrate concentration below the K_m. Thus, the enzyme with the highest K_m will show the largest changes in rate.

3. **The answer is B.** Ethanol has a structure very similar to that of methanol (a structural analog) and thus would be expected to compete with methanol at its substrate binding site. This inhibition is competitive with respect to methanol, and therefore V_{max} for methanol would not be altered, and ethanol inhibition could be overcome by high concentrations of methanol (thus, A, C, and D are incorrect). E is illogical because the substrate methanol stays in the same binding site as it is converted to its product, formaldehyde.

4. **The answer is C.** Allosteric enzymes generally have more than one subunit, each of which contains a binding site for the substrate. As the substrate binds to one site, it changes the conformation of one or more of the other subunits (cooperativity in substrate binding). Thus, plots of velocity versus substrate concentration are usually S-shaped, rather than the rectangular hyperbola of Michaelis-Menten

kinetics (thus, B is incorrect). Generally, a compound binding in the catalytic site cannot be an activator (thus, D is incorrect). Most allosteric inhibitors are reversibly bound at either allosteric sites or the catalytic site, because they must be released from the enzyme when the concentration of activator changes (thus, E is incorrect).

5. **The answer is C.** The most effective regulation should be a "feed-forward" type of regulation in which the toxin activates the pathway. One of the most common ways this occurs is through the toxin acting to increase the amount of enzyme by increasing transcription of its gene. A and B describe mechanisms of feed-back regulation in which the end-product of the pathway decreases its own rate of synthesis, and are therefore incorrect. D is incorrect because a high K_m for the toxin might prevent the enzyme from working effectively at low toxin concentrations, although it would allow the enzyme to respond to increases of toxin concentration. It would do little good for the toxin to allosterically activate any enzyme but the rate-limiting enzyme (thus, E is incorrect).

Chapter 10

1. **The answer is D.** Phosphatidylserine, the only lipid with a net negative charge at neutral pH, is located in the inner leaflet, where it contributes to the more negatively charged intracellular side of the membrane. The membrane is composed principally of phospholipids and cholesterol (thus, A is incorrect). Phospholipids are amphipathic (contain polar and nonpolar ends; see Chapter 5), with their polar head groups extending into the aqueous medium inside and outside of the cell. The fatty acyl groups of the two layers face each other on the inside of the bilayer, and the polar oligosaccharides groups of glycoproteins and glycolipids extend into the aqueous medium (thus, B, C, and E are incorrect).

2. **The answer is E.** The transmembrane regions are α-helices with hydrophobic amino acid side chains binding to membrane lipids. The hydrophobic interactions hinder their extraction (thus, A and D are incorrect). Because they are not easily extracted, they are classified as integral proteins (thus, B is incorrect). The carboxy and amino terminals of transmembrane proteins extend into the aqueous intracellular and extracellular medium, and thus need to contain many hydrophilic residues (thus, C is incorrect).

3. **The answer is A.** Most of fuel oxidation and ATP generation occur in the mitochondrion. Although some may also occur in the cytosol, the amount is much smaller in most cells.

4. **The answer is A.** Na^+, K^+-ATPase has the highest energy requirements of these transport processes, with hydrolysis of one ATP for every 2 Na^+ ions transported. Neither facilitative transport of glucose (carrier-mediated diffusion) nor passive diffusion requires energy (thus, B and C are incorrect). Ligand-gated channels do require ATP for opening, but because the open channels allow the entry of many molecules, the energy requirement is not as large as active transport.

5. **The answer is C.** Members of the Rho family regulate the direction of actin assembly and its attachments to other cellular proteins. Ras is involved principally in regulating gene expression, Ran in nuclear transport, Rab in vesicle assembly and fusion and Arf in formation of coatomer-coated vesicles (thus, A, B, D, and E are incorrect).

Chapter 11

1. **The answer is C.** Each chemical messenger has a specific protein receptor in a target cell that will generally bind only that messenger, and only that cell responds to the message. Only endocrine messengers reach their target cells through the blood (thus, A is incorrect). Many chemical messengers have paracrine actions. Messengers are secreted by only one type of cell (thus, B is incorrect). Many messengers bind to extracellular domains of plasma membrane receptors, and do not enter the cells (thus, D is incorrect). No chemical messengers are metabolized to intracellular second messengers (thus, E is incorrect).

2. **The answer is D.** Only lipophilic chemical messengers are able to diffuse into cells and bind to transcription factor receptors. Because they are water-insoluble, they must be transported in the blood bound to a protein. Cytokines, polypeptide hormones, and small molecule neurotransmitters are not lipophilic (thus, A and B are incorrect). Because they work through regulation of gene transcription, their effects are relatively slow (thus, C is incorrect). Like all messengers, they are secreted in response to a specific stimulus (thus, E is incorrect).

3. **The answer is D.** Parathyroid hormone is a polypeptide hormone and thus must bind to a plasma membrane receptor instead of an intracellular receptor (thus, A and B are incorrect). Hormones that bind to plasma membrane receptors do not need to enter the cell to transmit their signals (thus, C is incorrect). Heptahelical receptors work through heterotrimeric G proteins that have an α subunit, and tyrosine kinase receptors work through monomeric G proteins that have no subunits (thus, D is correct and E is incorrect).

4. **The answer is C.** Gαs normally activates adenylyl cyclase to generate cAMP in response to parathyroid hormone. Because the patient has end-organ unresponsiveness, he must have a deficiency in the signaling pathway (thus, A is incorrect) and cAMP would be decreased. Decreased GTPase activity would increase binding to adenylyl cyclase, and increase responsiveness (thus, B is incorrect). Neither IP_3 nor phosphatidylinositol 3,4,5-trisphosphate are involved in signal transduction by the Gαs subunit.

5. **The answer is A.** Proteins that have SH2 domains bind to a site containing a certain sequence of amino acids and a phosphotyrosine residue. They do not recognize phospho-serine residues (thus, E is incorrect). Pleckstrin homology domains recognize PI-3,4,5 trisphosphate.

Chapter 12

1. **The answer is D.** The complementary strand must run in the opposite direction, so the 5′ end must base pair with the G at the 3′ end of the given strand. Therefore, the 5′ end of the complementary strand must be C. G would then base pair to C, A to T, and T to A. B is incorrect because the bases do not base pair with each other with the sequences indicated, C is incorrect because U is not found in DNA, and E is incorrect because it has the wrong polarity (the 5′ T in answer E would not base pair with the 3′-G in the given sequence).

2. **The answer is C.** The RNA strand must be complementary to the DNA strand, and A in DNA pairs with U in RNA, whereas T in DNA base pairs with A in RNA, G in DNA base pairs with C in RNA, and C in DNA will base pair with G in RNA. A and E are incorrect because they contain T, which is found in DNA, not RNA. B is incorrect because the base pairing rules are broken when the strands are aligned in anti-parallel fashion. D is incorrect because the polarity of the strand is incorrect (If one were to switch the 5′ and 3′ ends, the answer would be correct.).

3. **The answer is D.** The phosphate is in an ester bond to two ribose groups, generating the phosphodiester bond. None of the other interactions is correct.

4. **The answer is E.** There are four possible bases at each position in the molecule, so as a total there are 4^8 possibilities. This comes out to 65,536 possible DNA sequences for a molecule that is only 8 bases long.

5. **The answer is B.** The backbone is composed of the phosphates and deoxyribose in phosphodiester linkages. The bases are internal to the backbone, base-paired to bases in the complementary strand, and forming stacking interactions within the helix.

Chapter 13

1. **The answer is B.** The 3′ to 5′ exonuclease activity is required for proofreading (check the base just inserted, and if it is incorrect, remove it), and reverse transcriptase does not have this activity, whereas pol δ does. Both reverse transcriptase and pol δ synthesize DNA in the 5′ to 3′ directions (all DNA polymerases do this), and both follow standard Watson-Crick base-pairing rules (A with T or U, G with C). Neither polymerase can synthesize DNA in the wrong direction (3′ to 5′) or insert inosine into a growing DNA chain. Thus, the only difference between the two polymerases is answer B.

2. **The answer is D.** In 50 seconds, each replication origin will have synthesized 100 kilobases of DNA (50 in each direction). Because there are 10 origins, 10 times 100 will yield the 1,000 kilobases needed to replicate the DNA. The first origin would be 50 kilobases from one end; then the remaining nine origins would each be 100 kilobases apart.

3. **The answer is E.** The role of the primer is to provide a free 3′-OH group for DNA polymerase to add the next nucleotide and form a phosphodiester bond. When DNA repair occurs, one of the remaining bases in the DNA will have a free 3′-OH, which DNA polymerase I will use to begin extension of the DNA.

4. **The answer is A.** Helicase aids in unwinding DNA strands, along with DNA gyrase, so that the replication fork can keep moving. The 3′ to 5′ exonuclease activity is required for proofreading by DNA polymerases, DNA ligase connects a 3′-OH with an adjacent 5′-phosphate, Primase lays down the RNA primer, and AP endonuclease looks for apurinic or apyrimidinic sites (without a purine or pyrimidine base, respectively) to remove them from the DNA strand.

5. **The answer is B.** Xeroderma pigmentosum is a set of diseases all related to an inability to repair thymine dimers, leading to an inability to excise UV-damaged DNA. It does not affect bypass polymerases, which can synthesize across the damaged region, sometimes making mutations in its path. The primase gene, or mismatch repair, is not involved in excising thymine dimers. Proofreading ability of DNA polymerases is likewise not involved in this process.

Chapter 14

1. **The answer is B.** The transcript that is produced is copied from the DNA template strand, which must be of the opposite orientation from the transcript. So the 5′ end of the template strand should base pair with the 3′ end of the transcript, or the G. Thus, CGTACGGAT would base-pair with the transcript, and would represent the template strand.

2. **The answer is A.** Amanda weighs 50 kg, and if 1 mg per kg body weight is the LD_{50}, then for Amanda 5 mg of toxin would bring her to the LD_{50}. Because one mushroom contains 7 mg of the toxin, ingesting just one mushroom could be a fatal event.

3. **The answer is C.** Enhancer sequences can be thousands of bases away from the basal promoter and still stimulate transcription of the gene. This is accomplished by looping of the DNA so that the protein binding to the enhancer

sequence (transactivators) can also bind to proteins bound to the promoter (coactivators). A promoter proximal element is a DNA sequence nearby the promoter that can bind transcription factors that aid in recruiting RNA polymerase to the promoter region.

4. **The answer is D.** Both prokaryotes and eukaryotes require RNA polymerase binding to an upstream promoter element. Answer A only applies to eukaryotes; prokaryote mRNA is not capped, nor does it contain a poly A tail. Prokaryotes have no nucleus; thus, the 5′ end of an mRNA is immediately available for ribosomes binding and initiation of translation (answer B is thus incorrect). Answer C is incorrect overall; RNA synthesis, like DNA synthesis, is always in the 5′ to 3′ direction. Answer E is incorrect because introns are present only in eukaryotic genes.

5. **The answer is B.** The nontemplate strand should be the message identical strand (with the exception of U for T), and complementary to the template strand. Thus, the sequence of RNA from that stretch of nontemplate strand should be AGCUCACUG (identical to the nontemplate, or coding strand, and complementary to the template strand).

Chapter 15

1. **The answer is A.** It is important to note that the question is asking about prokaryotic mechanisms. In prokaryotes, there is no nucleus (so E cannot be a correct answer), and translation begins before transcription is terminated (coupled translation-transcription, so B is incorrect). Thus, before the ribosome can move from one codon to the next (translocation), or the protein synthesis machinery terminates (via termination factors), the initiating tRNA must bind and align with the mRNA to initiate translation, indicating that answer A is the first step that must occur of the choices listed.

2. **The answer is C.** Because the extract contains all normal components, the cys-tRNA charged with alanine will compete with cys-tRNA charged with cysteine for binding to the cysteine codons. Thus, the protein will have some alanines put in the place of cysteine, leading to a deficiency of cysteine residues. Answer A is incorrect because the tRNA recognizes the cysteine codon, not the alanine codon. Answer B is incorrect because of the competition mentioned above.

3. **The answer is C.** There are 64 triplet codes, and only 20 amino acids, so some amino acids have more than one codon that codes for them. The other answers do not address this issue.

4. **The answer is B.** The KDEL sequence signals receptors in the Golgi apparatus to return proteins to the ER. None of the other modifications listed signal an ER home for the protein.

5. **The answer is D.** Because each codon is three bases long, there are four possible bases that can fill each codon position (A, T, C, or G). That means there are 4 times 4 times 4 possible combinations of bases, for a total of 64 codons. There are fewer than 64 aminoacyl tRNA synthetases because of one tRNA recognizing more than one codon due to wobbling (thus A is incorrect). Not all bases participate in wobbling (G can base-pair with U, and C, A, or U can base-pair with I, but those are the only combinations possible), and only one reading frame is used for each message produced (thus, B and C are incorrect). The rate of protein synthesis is not dependent on the number of codons, but rather on how rapidly the components required to synthesize proteins can be brought to the ribosomes, and how much RNA is present to be translated.

Chapter 16

1. **The answer is E.** Many prokaryotic genes are organized into operons, in which one polycistronic mRNA contains the translational start and stop sites for a number of related genes. Although each gene within the mRNA can be read from a different reading frame, the reading frame is always consistent within each gene (thus, A is incorrect). Redundancy in codon/tRNA interactions has nothing to do with multiple cistrons within an mRNA (thus, B is incorrect). Operator sequences are in DNA and initiate transcription, not translation (C is incorrect). Alternative splicing only occurs in eukaryotes (which have introns), not prokaryotes (D is incorrect).

2. **The answer is D.** To transcribe the lac operon, the repressor protein (*lac* I gene product) must bind allolactose and leave the operator region, and the cAMP-CRP complex must bind to the promoter for RNA polymerase to bind. Of the choices offered, only raising cAMP levels can allow transcription of the operon when both lactose and glucose are high. Raising cAMP, even though glucose is present, will allow the cAMP-CRP complex to bind and recruit RNA polymerase. Answers that call for mutations in the repressor (answers A and E) will not affect binding of cAMP-CRP. Mutations in the DNA (answers B and C) do not allow CRP binding in the absence of cAMP.

3. **The answer is A.** The repressor will bind to the operator and block transcription of all genes in the operon unless prevented by the inducer allolactose. If the repressor has lost its affinity for the inducer, it cannot dissociate from the operator and the genes in the operon will not be expressed (thus, E is incorrect). If the repressor has lost its affinity for the operator (answer B), then the operon would be constitutively expressed. Because the question states that there is a mutation in the I (repressor) gene, answer D is incorrect, and mutations in the I gene do not affect trans-acting factors from binding to the promoter, although the only other one for the lac operon is the CRP.

4. **The answer is B.** The sequence, if read 5′ to 3′, is identical to the complementary sequence read 5′ to 3′. None of the other sequences fits this pattern.

5. **The answer is A.** All DNA binding proteins contain an α-helix that binds to the major groove in DNA. These proteins do not recognize RNA molecules (hence, B is incorrect), nor do they form bonds between the peptide backbone and the DNA backbone (thus, C is incorrect; if this were correct, how could there be any specificity in protein binding to DNA?). Only zinc fingers contain zinc, and dimers are formed by hydrogen bonding—not by disulfide linkages.

Chapter 17

1. **The answer is B.** All DNA fragments are negatively charged and will migrate toward the positive charge. The only difference between the fragments is their size, and the smaller fragments will move faster than the larger fragments because of their ability to squeeze through the gel at a faster rate.

2. **The answer is E.** The enzyme recognizes six bases, and the probability that the correct base is in each position is 1 in 4, so the overall probability is $(1/4)^6$, or one in 4,096 bases.

3. **The answer is B.** The Sanger technique requires both deoxyribonucleotides and dideoxyribonucleotides, and a template DNA. It does not use Taq polymerase (which is for PCR), nor does it need reverse transcriptase (which is required for producing DNA from RNA).

4. **The answer is C.** Ethidium bromide is a dye that intercalates between the stacked bases of DNA and can be visualized by UV light. As the gel is run the smaller fragments migrate farther in the gel (thus, A is incorrect), and the DNA migrates towards the positive charge (due to the negative charges on the phosphate backbone; thus, B is incorrect). When a huge molecule such as human DNA is cut with any endonuclease, many bands will be generated (not just three), and DNA is not denatured before it is run on the gel (thus, D and E are incorrect). When doing a Southern blot, it is denatured after transfer to the filter paper.

5. **The answer is C.** A Northern blot allows one to determine which genes are being transcribed in a tissue at the time of mRNA isolation. The mRNA is run on a gel, transferred to filter paper, and then analyzed with a probe. If albumin is being transcribed, then a probe for albumin should give a positive result in the Northern blot. A library screening will not indicate whether a particular gene is being transcribed, nor will a Southern blot. Those techniques only allow one to determine that the gene is present in the genome. A Western blot analyzes protein content, not mRNA content. Analysis of VNTR's does not provide information as to whether a gene is transcribed.

Chapter 18

1. **The answer is C.** The *ras* oncogene has a point mutation in codon 12 (position 35 of the DNA chain) in which T replaces G. This changes the codon from one that specifies glycine to that of valine. Thus, there is a single amino acid change in the proto-oncogene (a valine for a glycine) that changes *ras* to an oncogene.

2. **The answer is C.** Ras, when oncogenic, has lost its GTPase activity and, thus, remains active for a longer time. A is wrong because GAP proteins activate the GTPase activity of Ras, and this mutation would make Ras less active. cAMP does not directly interact with Ras (thus, B is incorrect), and if Ras could no longer bind GTP, it would not be active (hence, D is also incorrect). Ras is not phosphorylated by the MAP kinase (E is incorrect).

3. **The answer is B.** Retroviral oncogenes were originally obtained from genes on a host chromosome. All retroviruses do not contain oncogenes (thus A is incorrect), proto-oncogenes are found in host cells, not viruses (thus C is incorrect), the oncogenes that lead to human disease are very similar to those that are mutated in animals (thus D is incorrect), and oncogenes are a misexpressed or mutated version of normal cellular genes, not viral genes (thus E is incorrect).

4. **The answer is D.** When p53 increases in response to DNA damage, it acts as a transcription factor and induces the transcription of p21, which blocks phosphorylation of Rb Rb then stays bound to transcription factor E2F, and E2F cannot induce the genes required for the G1 to S transition. p53 does not induce transcription of either cyclin D or cdk4 (thus, A and B are incorrect), nor does p53 bind to E2F (C is incorrect), nor does p53 contain kinase activity (E is incorrect).

5. **The answer is B.** Tumor suppressor genes balance cell growth and quiescence. When not expressed (a loss-of-function mutation), the balance shifts to cell proliferation and tumorigenesis (thus, A is incorrect). Answer C is incorrect because tumor suppressor genes do not act on viral genes, D is incorrect because tumor suppressor genes are not specifically targeted to just one aspect of the cell cycle, and E is incorrect because a loss of expression of tumor suppressor genes leads to tumor formation, not expression of these genes.

Chapter 19

1. **The answer is E.** Both of the high-energy phosphate bonds in ATP are located between phosphate groups (both the α and β phosphates, and the β and γ phosphates). The phosphate bond between the α-phosphate and ribose (or adenosine) is not a high-energy bond (thus, A and B are incorrect). There is no phosphate between the ribose and adenine, or two hydroxyl groups in the ribose ring; therefore, answers C and D are incorrect.

2. **The answer is C.** The change in enthalpy, ΔH, is the total amount of heat that can be released in a reaction. The first law of thermodynamics states that the total energy of a system remains constant, and the second law of thermodynamics states that the universe tends toward a state of disorder (thus, A and B are incorrect). D is incorrect because the $\Delta G^{\circ\prime}$ is the standard free energy change measured at 25°C and a pH of 7. E is incorrect because a high-energy bond releases more than about 7 kcal/mole of heat when it is hydrolyzed. The definition of high-energy bond is based on the hydrolysis of one of the high-energy bonds of ATP.

3. **The answer is A.** The concentration of the substrates and products influence the direction of a reaction. B is incorrect because reactions with a positive free energy, at 1 M concentrations of substrate and product, will proceed in the reverse direction. C is incorrect because substrate and product concentration do influence the free energy of a reaction. D is incorrect because the free energy must be considered (in addition to the substrate and product concentration) to determine the direction of a reaction. E is false; an enzyme's efficiency does not influence the direction of a reaction.

4. **The answer is C.** A heart attack results in decreased pumping of blood, and thus a decreased oxygen supply to the heart (hence, A is incorrect). The lack of oxygen leads to a lack of ATP (thus, B is incorrect) because of an inability to perform oxidative phosphorylation. The lack of ATP impairs the working of the Na^+K^+ ATPase, which pumps sodium out of the cell in exchange for potassium. Therefore, intracellular levels of sodium will increase as Na^+ enters the cell through other transport mechanisms (thus, E is incorrect). The high intracellular sodium concentration then blocks the functioning of the Na^+/H^+ antiporter (which sends protons out of the cell in exchange for sodium. Because intracellular sodium is high, the driving force for this reaction is lost), which leads to increased intracellular H^+, or a lower intracellular pH (thus, C is correct). The intracellular pH also increases because of glycolysis in the absence of oxygen, which produces lactic acid. The loss of the sodium gradient, coupled with the lack of ATP, leads to increased calcium in the cell (thus, D is incorrect) because of an inability to pump calcium out.

5. **The answer is C.** NAD^+ accepts two electrons as hydride ions to form NADH (thus, A and B are incorrect). Answers D and E are incorrect because FAD can accept two single electrons from separate atoms, together with protons, or can accept a pair of electrons.

Chapter 20

1. **The answer is E.** The α-ketoacid dehydrogenase complex uses thiamine pyrophosphate, lipoic acid, FAD, NAD^+, and CoASH. Of these, only lipoate is used by no other enzyme and is unique to the α-ketoacid dehydrogenase complexes. Many dehydrogenases use NAD^+ as a coenzyme (such as malate dehydrogenase) or FAD (such as succinate dehydrogenase) (thus, A and B are incorrect). C is incorrect because GDP is not a coenzyme for α-ketoacid dehydrogenase complexes. D is incorrect because H_2O is not a coenzyme.

2. **The answer is B.** Thiamine pyrophosphate is the coenzyme for the α-ketoglutarate dehydrogenase and pyruvate dehydrogenase complexes. With these complexes inactive, pyruvic acid and α-ketoglutaric acid accumulate and dissociate to generate the anion and H^+. As α-ketoglutarate is not listed as an answer, the only possible answer is pyruvate.

3. **The answer is A.** Succinate dehydrogenase is the only TCA cycle enzyme located in the inner mitochondrial membrane. The other enzymes are in the mitochondrial matrix. B is incorrect because succinate dehydrogenase is not regulated by NADH. C is incorrect because α-ketoglutarate dehydrogenase also contains a bound FAD (the difference is that the FAD(2H) in α-ketoglutarate dehydrogenase donates its electrons to NAD^+, whereas the FAD(2H) in succinate dehydrogenase directly donates its electrons to the electron transfer chain). D is incorrect because both succinate dehydrogenase and aconitase have Fe-S centers. E is incorrect because succinate dehydrogenase is not regulated by a kinase. Kinases regulate enzymes by phosphorylation (e.g., the regulation of pyruvate dehydrogenase occurs through reversible phosphorylation).

4. **The answer is E.** NADH decreases during exercise to generate energy for the exercise (if it were increased, it would inhibit the cycle and slow it down), thus, the NADH/NAD^+ ratio is decreased, and the lack of NADH activates flux through isocitrate dehydrogenase, α-ketoglutarate dehydrogenase, and malate dehydrogenase. Isocitrate dehydrogenase is inhibited by NADH, so A is not correct. Fumarase is not regulated, thus B is incorrect. The four carbon intermediates of the cycle are regenerated during each turn of the cycle, so their concentration does not decrease (thus, C is incorrect). Product inhibition of citrate synthase would slow the cycle and not generate more energy, hence, D is incorrect.

5. **The answer is D.** Pantothenate is the vitamin precursor of coenzyme A. Niacin is the vitamin precursor of NAD, and riboflavin is the vitamin precursor of FAD and FMN. Vitamins A and C are used with only minor modifications, if any.

Chapter 21

1. **The answer is B.** For a component to be in the oxidized state, it must have donated, or never received, electrons. Complex II will metabolize succinate to produce fumarate

(generating FAD(2H)), but no succinate is available in this experiment. Thus, complex II never sees any electrons and is always in an oxidized state. The substrate malate is oxidized to oxaloacetate, generating NADH, which donates electrons to complex I of the electron transfer chain. These electrons are transferred to coenzyme Q, which donates electrons to complex III, to cytochrome C, and then to complex IV. Cyanide will block the transfer of electrons from complex IV to oxygen, so all previous complexes containing electrons will be backed up, and the electrons will be "stuck" in the complexes, making these components reduced. Thus, answers A and C through E must be incorrect.

2. **The answer is D.** The proton motive force consists of two components, a ΔpH, and a $\Delta\psi$ (electrical component). The addition of valinomycin and potassium will destroy the electrical component, but not the pH component. Thus, the proton motive force will decrease but will still be greater than zero. Thus, the other answers are all incorrect.

3. **The answer is D.** Dinitrophenol equilibrates the proton concentration across the inner mitochondrial membrane, thereby destroying the proton motive force. Thus, none of the other answers is correct.

4. A is correct because a deficiency of Fe-S centers in the electron transport chain would impair the transfer of electrons down the chain and reduce ATP production by oxidative phosphorylation. B is incorrect because the decreased production of water from the electron transport chain is not of sufficient magnitude to cause her to become dehydrated. C is incorrect because iron does not form a chelate with NADH and FAD(2H). D is incorrect because iron is not a cofactor for α-ketoglutarate dehydrogenase. E is incorrect because iron does not accompany the protons that make up the proton gradient.

5. B is correct because NADH would not be reoxidized as efficiently by the electron transport chain, and the NADH/NAD$^+$ ratio would increase. (A) is incorrect because ATP would not be produced at a high rate. Therefore, ADP would build up and the ATP:ADP ratio would be low. C is incorrect because OXPHOS diseases can be caused by mutations in nuclear or mitochondrial DNA, and, not all oxphos proteins are encoded by the X chromosome. D is incorrect because, depending on the nature of the mutation, the activity of complex II of the electron transport chain might be normal or decreased, but there is no reason to expect increased activity. E is incorrect because the integrity of the inner mitochondrial membrane would not necessarily be affected. It could be, but this would not be expected for all patients with OXPHOS disorders.

Chapter 22

1. **The answer is B.** The major roles of glycolysis are to generate energy and to produce precursors for other biosyn-

thetic pathways. Gluconeogenesis is the pathway that generates glucose (thus, A is incorrect), FAD(2H) is produced in the mitochondria by a variety of reactions, but not glycolysis (therefore, C is incorrect), glycogen synthesis occurs under conditions in which glycolysis is inhibited (D is incorrect), and glycolysis does not hydrolyze ATP to generate heat (that is nonshivering thermogenesis; hence E is incorrect).

2. **The answer is D.** By starting with glyceraldehyde 3-phosphate, the energy-requiring steps of glycolysis are bypassed. This, as glyceraldehyde 3-phosphate is converted to pyruvate, two molecules of ATP will be produced (at the phosphoglycerate kinase and pyruvate kinase steps), and one molecule of NADH will be produced (at the glyceraldehyde 3-phosphate dehydrogenase step).

3. **The answer is H.** Glucose-1-phosphate is isomerized to glucose-6-phosphate, which then enters glycolysis. This skips the hexokinase step, which uses 1 ATP. Thus, starting from glucose-1-phosphate one would get the normal 2 ATP and 2 NADH produced, but with one less ATP used, for a total yield of 3 ATP and 2 NADH.

4. **The answer is B.** The pathway consumes 2 ATP at the beginning of the pathway and produces 4 ATP at the end of the pathway for each molecule of glucose. Therefore, the net energy production is 2 ATP for each molecule of glucose. Glycolysis synthesizes ATP through substrate-level phosphorylation, not oxidative phosphorylation (thus, A is incorrect) and synthesizes two molecules of pyruvate in the process (hence, D is incorrect). The pathway is cytosolic (thus, D is incorrect), and the rate-limiting step is the one catalyzed by PFK-1 (thus, C is incorrect).

5. **The answer is D.** Each mole of glucose produces 2 moles of pyruvate, 2 moles of ATP, and 2 moles of NADH during glycolysis. As each pyruvate is converted to acetyl CoA, 1 NADH is produced. Each acetyl CoA enters the TCA cycle to produce 1 GTP, 3 NADH, and 1 FAD(2H). Therefore, the oxidation of 1 mole of glucose would yield a total of 2 ATP and 2 NADH from glycolytic reactions; 2 NADH from the conversion of 2 moles of pyruvate to 2 acetyl CoA; and 6 NADH, 2 GTP, and 2 FAD(2H) from the oxidation of 2 moles of acetyl CoA in the TCA cycle. Each GTP has the same energy as 1 ATP. Each mitochondrial NADH is oxidized to produce 2.5 ATP. Each cytoplasmic NADH can generate either 1.5 ATP (using the glycerol-phosphate shuttle) or 2.5 ATP (using the malate–aspartate shuttle). Each mitochondrial FAD(2H) is oxidized to produce 1.5 ATP. Therefore, the total ATP yield from the oxidation of 1 mole of glucose is 30 to 32 ATP (30 if the glycerol–phosphate shuttle is used, 32 if the malate–aspartate shuttle is used).

Chapter 23

1. **The answer is D.** The ETF:CoQ oxidoreductase is required to transfer the electrons from the FAD(2H) of the

acyl-CoA dehydrogenase to coenzyme Q. When the oxidoreductase is missing, the electrons cannot be transferred, and the acyl-CoA dehydrogenase cannot continue to oxidize fatty acids because of having a reduced cofactor instead of an oxidized cofactor. During times of fasting, when fatty acids are the primary energy source, no energy will be forthcoming, gluconeogenesis is shut down, and death may result. The lack of this enzyme does not affect the other pathways listed as potential answers.

2. **The answer is C.** An 18-carbon saturated fatty acid would require eight spirals of fatty acid oxidation, which yields 8 NADH, 8 FAD(2H), and 9 AcCoA. As each NADH gives rise to 2.5 ATP, and each FAD(2H) gives rise to 1.5 ATP, the reduced cofactors will give rise to 32 ATP. Each AcCoA gives rise to 10 ATP, for a total of 90 ATP. This then yields 122 ATP, but we must subtract 2 ATP for the activation step, at which two high-energy bonds are broken. Thus, the net yield is 120 ATPs for each molecule of fatty acid oxidized.

3. **The answer is A.** Fatty acid oxidation is initiated by the acyl-CoA dehydrogenase (an oxidation step), followed by hydration of the double bond formed in the first step, followed by the hydroxyacyl-CoA dehydrogenase step (another oxidation), and then attack of the β-carbonyl by CoA, breaking a carbon–carbon bond (the thiolase step).

4. **The answer is D.** A lack of carnitine would lead to an inability to transport fatty acyl CoAs into the mitochondria. This would lead to a decrease in fatty acid oxidation (thus, A is incorrect); a decrease in ketone body production, because fatty acids cannot be oxidized (thus, B is incorrect); a decrease in blood glucose levels because gluconeogenesis is impaired owing to a lack of energy (thus, C is incorrect); and no increase in the levels of very-long-chain fatty acids, because these are initially oxidized in the peroxisomes and do not require carnitine for entry into that organelle (thus, E is incorrect). The ω-oxidation system, which creates dicarboxylic acids, is found in the ER, and as the concentration of fatty acyl CoAs increases in tissues, they are oxidized by this alternative pathway.

5. **The answer is E.** Fatty acids are the MAJOR fuel for the body during prolonged exercise and fasting. A, B, and C are incorrect because glucose would be the major fuel after eating. D is incorrect because, at the start of exercise, muscle glycogen and gluconeogenesis are being used as the major source of fuel.

Chapter 24

1. **The answer is D.** Pyridoxal phosphate is a water-soluble vitamin that is important for amino acid and glycogen metabolism but has no role in protecting against free radical damage. Ascorbate (vitamin C), vitamin E, and β-carotene all can react with free radicals to terminate chain propagation, whereas superoxide dismutase uses the superoxide radical as a substrate and converts it to hydrogen peroxide, and glutathione peroxidase removes hydrogen peroxide from the cell, converting it to water.

2. **The answer is B.** Superoxide dismutase will combine two superoxide radicals to produce hydrogen peroxide and molecular oxygen. None of the other reactions are correct.

3. **The answer is C.** Vitamin E donates an electron and proton to the radical, thereby converting the radical to a stable form (LOO· → LOOH). The vitamin thus prevents the free radical from oxidizing another compound by extracting an H· from that compound and propagating a free radical chain reaction. The radical form of vitamin E generated is relatively stable and actually donates another electron and proton to a second free radical, forming oxidized vitamin E.

4. **The answer is B.** The Fenton reaction is the nonenzymatic donation of an electron from Fe^{+2} to H_2O_2 to produce Fe^{+3}, the hydroxyl radical, and hydroxide ion. Only Fe^{+2} or Cu^{+1} can be used in this reaction; thus, the other answers are incorrect.

5. **The answer is E.** Histones coat nuclear DNA and protect it from radical damage. Mitochondrial DNA lacks histones, such that when radicals are formed the DNA can be easily oxidized. Answers A and B are nonsensical; superoxide dismutase reduces radical concentrations, so the fact that it is present in the mitochondria should help to protect the DNA from damage, not enhance it, and glutathione also protects against radical damage, and if the nucleus lacks it, then one would expect higher levels of nuclear DNA damage, not reduced levels. Reactive oxygen species can diffuse across membranes, so answers C and D are incorrect. Other factors that increase mitochondrial DNA damage relative to nuclear DNA are the proximity of mitochondrial DNA to the membrane and the fact that most radical species are formed from coenzyme Q, which is found within the mitochondria.

Chapter 25

1. **The answer is A.** Acetate is converted to acetyl CoA by other tissues so that it can enter the TCA cycle to generate ATP. B is incorrect because acetaldehyde, not acetate, is toxic to cells. C is incorrect because acetate is excreted by the lung and kidney, and not in the bile. D is incorrect because acetate cannot directly enter the TCA cycle. It must be converted to acetyl CoA first. E is incorrect because alcohol dehydrogenase converts ethanol into acetaldehyde. It does not convert acetate into NADH.

2. **The answer is B.** There is an increase in the $NADH/NAD^+$ ratio because NADH is produced by the conversion of ethanol to acetate. Thus, D is incorrect. The

increased ratio of NADH/NAD$^+$ favors the conversion of gluconeogenic precursors (such as lactate and oxaloacetate) to their reduced counterparts (lactate and malate, respectively), to generate NAD$^+$ for ethanol metabolism. This reduces the concentration of gluconeogenic precursors, and slows down gluconeogenesis (thus, E is incorrect), and can lead to lacticacidosis. A is incorrect because the increase of NADH inhibits fatty acid oxidation. C is incorrect because ketogenesis increases because of the increase of NADH. NADH inhibits key enzymes of the TCA cycle, thereby diverting acetyl CoA from the TCA cycle and toward ketone body synthesis.

3. **The answer is C.** Disulfiram blocks the conversion of acetaldehyde to acetate. The accumulation of acetaldehyde is toxic and causes vomiting and nausea. A and B are incorrect because disulfiram would not interfere with the absorption of ethanol or the first step of its metabolism. D is incorrect because an acetaldehyde inhibitor (such as disulfiram) would inhibit the conversion of ethanol to acetate, not increase the rate of the conversion. E is incorrect because disulfiram does not interfere with the excretion of acetate, nor does acetate accumulation lead to nausea and vomiting.

4. **The answer is E.** An increase in the concentration of CYP2E1 (the MEOS system) would result in an increase of ethanol metabolism and clearance from the blood. Therefore, A is incorrect. An increased rate of acetaldehyde production would result. Therefore, B is incorrect. The increase in CYP2E1 would cause an increase in the probability of producing free radicals; thus, C is incorrect. D is incorrect because hepatic damage would be more likely to occur because an increase of free radical production occurs. E is correct because the increased clearance rate of ethanol from the blood results in a higher alcohol tolerance level.

5. **The answer is E.** Liver cirrhosis is irreversible. It is an end-stage process of liver fibrosis. A, B, C, and D are all consequences of liver disease, but they are all reversible. Therefore, E is the only answer that is correct.

Chapter 26

1. **The answer is D.** Once insulin is injected, glucose transport into the peripheral tissues is enhanced. If the patient does not eat, the normal, fasting level of glucose will drop even further because of the injection of insulin, which increases the movement of glucose into muscle and fat cells. The patient becomes hypoglycemic, as a result of which epinephrine is released from the adrenal medulla. This, in turn, leads to the signs and symptoms associated with high levels of epinephrine in the blood. A and B are incorrect because as glucose levels drop, glucagon is released from the pancreas to raise blood glucose levels, which would alleviate the symptoms. E is incorrect because ketone body production does not produce hypoglycemic symptoms, nor would they be significantly elevated only a few hours after the insulin shock the patient is experiencing.

2. **The answer is B.** When glucagon binds to its receptor, the enzyme adenylate cyclase is eventually activated (through the action of G proteins), which raises cAMP levels in the cell. The cAMP phosphodiesterase opposes this rise in cAMP and hyrolyzes cAMP to 5'-AMP. If the phosphodiesterase is inhibited by caffeine, cAMP levels would stay elevated for an extended period, enhancing the glucagon response. The glucagon response in liver is to export glucose (hence, E is incorrect) and to inhibit glycolysis (thus, D is incorrect). cAMP activates protein kinase A, making answer C incorrect as well. The effect of insulin is to reduce cAMP levels; thus, A is incorrect.

3. **The answer is B.** Insulin release is dependent on an increase in the [ATP]/[ADP] ratio within the pancreatic β cell. In MODY, the mutation in glucokinase results in a less active glucokinase at glucose concentrations that normally stimulate insulin release. Thus, higher concentrations of glucose are required to stimulate glycolysis and the TCA cycle to effectively raise the ratio of ATP to ADP. A is incorrect because cAMP levels are not related to the mechanism of insulin release. C is incorrect because initially transcription is not involved, because insulin release is attributable to exocytosis of preformed insulin in secretory vesicles. D is incorrect because the pancreas will not degrade glycogen under conditions of high blood glucose, and E is incorrect because lacate does not play in role in stimulating insulin release.

4. **The answer is A.** The brain requires glucose because fatty acids cannot readily cross the blood-brain barrier to enter neuronal cells. Thus, glucose production is maintained at an adequate level to allow the brain to continue to burn glucose for its energy needs. The other organs listed as possible answers can switch to the use of alternative fuel sources (lactate, fatty acids, amino acids), and are not as dependent on glucose for their energy requirements as is the brain.

5. **The answer is E.** Muscle does not express glucagon receptors, so they are refractory to glucagons actions. Muscle does, however, contain GTP (made via the TCA cycle), G proteins, protein kinase A, and adenylate cyclase (epinephrine stimulation of muscle cells raises cAMP levels and activates protein kinase A).

Chapter 27

1. **The answer is E.** The GLUT 5 transporter has a much higher affinity for fructose than glucose and is the facilitator of choice for fructose uptake by cells. The other GLUT

transporters will not transport fructose to any significant extent.

2. **The answer is A.** The pancreas produces α-amylase that digests starch in the intestinal lumen. If pancreatic α-amylase cannot enter the lumen because of the pancreatitis, the starch would not be digested to a significant extent (the salivary α-amylase begins the process, but only for the time the food is in the mouth, as the acidic conditions of the stomach destroy the salivary activity). The discomfort arises from the bacteria in the intestine digesting the starch and producing acids and gases. Lactose, sucrose, and maltose are all disaccharides that would be cleaved by the intestinal disaccharidases located on the brush border of the intestinal epithelial cells (thus, B, D, and E are incorrect). These activities might be slightly reduced, as the pancreas would also have difficulty excreting bicarbonate to the intestine, and the low pH of the stomach contents might reduce the activity of these enzymes. However, these enzymes are present in excess and eventually will digest the disaccharides. Fiber cannot be digested by human enzymes, so C is incorrect.

3. **The answer is C.** Insulin is required to stimulate glucose transport into the muscle and fat cells, but not brain, liver, pancreas, or red blood cells. Thus, muscle would be feeling the effects of glucose deprivation, and would be unable to replenish its own glycogen supplies because of the inability to extract blood glucose, even though blood glucose levels would be high.

4. **The answer is E.** Flour contains starch, which will lead to glucose production in the intestine. Milk contains lactose, a disaccharide of glucose and galactose, which will be split by lactase in the small intestine. Sucrose is a disaccharide of glucose and fructose, which is split by sucrase in the small intestine. Thus, glucose, galactose, and fructose will all be available in the lumen of the small intestine for transport through the intestinal epithelial cells and into the circulation.

5. **The answer is A.** Salivary and pancreatic α-amylase will partially digest starch to glucose, but maltose and disaccharides will pass through the intestine and exit with the stool, because of the limited activity of the brush border enzymes. Because the amylase enzymes are working, there will only be normal levels of starch in the stool (thus, B is incorrect). Because not all available glucose is entering the blood, less insulin will be released by the pancreas (thus, E is incorrect), which leads to less glucose uptake by the muscles, and less glycogen production (thus, D is incorrect). Because neither lactose or fructose can be digested to a large extent in the intestinal lumen, it would be difficult to have elevated levels of glucose or fructose in the blood (thus, C is incorrect).

Chapter 28

1. **The answer is B.** Glycogen phosphorylase produces glucose 1-phosphate; the debranching enzyme hydrolyzes branch points, and thus releases free glucose. Ninety percent of the glycogen contains α (1,4) bonds, and only 10% are α (1,6) bonds, so more glucose 1-phosphate will be produced than glucose.

2. **The answer is D.** If, after fasting, the branches were shorter than normal, glycogen phosphorylase must be functional and capable of being activated by glucagons (hence, answers A and B are incorrect). The branching enzyme (amylo 4,6 transferase) is also normal because branch points are present within the glycogen (thus, E is incorrect). Because glycogen is also present, glycogenin is present to build the carbohydrate chains, indicating that (C) is incorrect. If the debranching activity is abnormal (the amylo 1,6 glucosidase), glycogen phosphorylase would break the glycogen down up to four residues from branch points and would then stop. With no debranching activity, the resultant glycogen would contain the normal number of branches, but the branched chains would be shorter than normal.

3. **The answer is C.** The patient has McArdle's disease, a glycogen storage disease caused by a deficiency of muscle glycogen phosphorylase. Because she cannot degrade glycogen to produce energy for muscle contraction, she becomes fatigued more readily than a normal person (thus, A is incorrect), the glycogen levels in her muscle will be higher than normal because of the inability to degrade them (thus, D is incorrect), and her blood lactate levels will be lower because of the lack of glucose for entry into glycolysis. She will, however, draw on the glucose in the circulation for energy; thus, her forearm blood glucose levels will be decreased (indicating that B is incorrect), and because the liver is not affected, blood glucose levels can be maintained by liver gycogenolysis (thus, E is incorrect).

4. **The answer is A.** After ingestion of glucose, insulin levels rise, cAMP levels within the cell drop (thus, E is incorrect), and protein phosphatase I is activated (thus, D is incorrect). Glycogen phosphorylase a is converted to glycogen phosphorylase b by the phosphatase (thus (B) is incorrect), and glycogen synthase is activated by the phosphatase. Red blood cells continue to use glucose at their normal rate; thus, lactate formation will remain the same (making choice C incorrect).

5. **The answer is F.** In the absence of insulin, glucagon-stimulated activities predominate. This leads to the activation of protein kinase A, the phosphorylation and inactivation of glycogen synthase, the phosphorylation and activation of phosphorylase kinase, and the phosphorylation and activation of glycogen phosphorylase.

Chapter 29

1. **The answer is D.** The aldolase B gene has two alleles. One or both may have mutations. Because HFI is reces-

sive, both alleles must be mutated for the disease to be expressed. Examination of the gel shows that the normal gene is cleaved by AhaII to produce a 306-bp restriction fragment. When a mutation creates a new AhaII site within the gene, this 306-bp fragment is cleaved into two fragments of 183 and 123 bp (which together contain 306 bp). The husband and Jill, thus, are carriers. They have one normal allele that produces the 306-bp fragment and one that has an additional AhaII site, which is cleaved to yield the two fragments of 183 and 123 bp. The wife and Jack have the disease. Both of their alleles have the additional AhaII site and produce only 183- and 123-bp fragments.

2. **The answer is C.** This man could be the father of both children. He could provide either a normal gene (which produces a 306-bp AhaII fragment) or a mutant gene (which produces 183- and 123-bp AhaII fragments) to his offspring. This mother could provide only the mutant gene (of which she has two copies). Jill is a carrier. She received the mutant gene from her mother and could have received the normal gene from this man. Jack has the disease. He received one mutant gene from his mother and another from his father.

3. **The answer is C.** Transketolase requires thiamine pyrophosphate as a cofactor, whereas none of the other enzymes listed do. Thus, if an individual has a thiamine deficiency, transketolase activity as isolated from a patient's blood cells will be enhanced by the addition of thiamine; in well-nourished individuals, the addition of thiamine will not enhance transketolase activity.

4. **The answer is B.** Fructose is converted to fructose 1-phosphate by fructokinase, and aldolase B in the liver splits the fructose-1-P into glyceraldehyde and dihydroxyacetone phosphate. Thus, the major regulated step of glycolysis, PFK-1, is bypassed, and PEP is rapidly produced. As the [PEP] increases, pyruvate kinase produces pyruvate. As the glyceraldehyde 3-phosphate dehydrogenase reaction is proceeding rapidly (remember that fructokinase is a high V_{max} enzyme, so there is a lot of substrate proceeding through the glycolytic pathway), the intracellular [NADH]/[NAD$^+$] ratio is high, and the pyruvate produced is converted to lactate to regenerate NAD$^+$. Thus, the pyruvate kinase step is not bypassed (hence, A is incorrect). Neither aldolase B or lactate dehydrogenase are allosterically regulated (thus, C and D are incorrect), and even though the [ATP]/[ADP] ratio is high in the liver under these conditions, the ratio does not affect lactate formation (thus, E is incorrect).

5. **The answer is B.** Reduction of sugar aldehydes to alcohols requires NADPH, which is primarily generated by the pentose phosphate pathway. 6-Phosphogluconate is not a polyol (thus, A is incorrect; 6-phosphogluconate is glucose oxidized at position 1 to form a carboxylic acid); ribitol is not a product of the pentose phosphate pathway (thus, C is incorrect; ribulose 5-phosphate is a product of the pentose

phosphate pathway); the HMP shunt uses glucose 6-phosphate as the starting material, not free glucose as in the sorbitol pathway (hence, D and E are incorrect).

Chapter 30

1. **The answer is B.** Galactose metabolism requires the phosphorylation of galactose to galactose 1-phosphate, which is then converted to UDP-galactose (which is the step defective in the patient), and then epimerized to UDP-glucose. Although the mother cannot convert galactose to lactose because of the enzyme deficiency, she can make UDP-glucose from glucose 6-phosphate, and once she has made UDP-glucose she can epimerize it to form UDP-galactose and can synthesize lactose (thus, answer A is incorrect). However, because of her enzyme deficiency, the mother cannot convert galactose 1-phosphate to UDP-galactose, or UDP-glucose, so the dietary galactose cannot be used for glycogen synthesis or glucose production (thus, C and D are incorrect). After ingesting milk, the galactose levels will be elevated in the serum because of the metabolic block in the cells (hence, E is incorrect).

2. **The answer is D.** Nucleotide sugars, such as UDP-glucose, UDP-galactose, and CMP-sialic acid donate sugars to the growing carbohydrate chain. The other activated sugars listed do not contribute to this synthesis.

3. **The answer is C.** Bilirubin is conjugated with glucuronic acid residues to enhance its solubility. Glucuronic acid is glucose oxidized at position 6; gluconic acid is glucose oxidized at position 1 and is generated by the HMP shunt pathway.

4. **The answer is C.** Glutamine donates the amide nitrogen to fructose 6-phosphate to form glucosamine 6-phosphate. None of the other nitrogen-containing compounds (answers A, B, and D) donate their nitrogen to carbohydrates. Dolichol contains no nitrogens and is the carrier for carbohydrate chain synthesis of N-linked glycoproteins.

5. **The answer is C.** Sandhoff disease is a deficiency of both hexosaminidase A and B activity, caused by the loss of the β subunit. The step at which amino sugars need to be removed from the glycolipids would be defective, such that globoside and GM2 accumulate in this disease. The other answers are incorrect; GM1 does contain an amino sugar, but it is converted to GM2 before the block is apparent.

Chapter 31

1. **The answer is D.** Glycerol gets converted to glycerol 3-phosphate, which is oxidized to form glyceraldehyde 3-phosphate. The glyceraldehydes 3-phosphate formed then follows the gluconeogenic pathway up to glucose. Lactate is converted to pyruvate, which is then carboxylated to form oxaloacetate. The oxaloacetate is decarboxylated to form phosphoenolpyruvate, and then run up through

gluconeogenesis to glucose. As glycerol enters the gluco-neogenic pathway at the glyceraldehyde 3-phosphate step, and lactate at the PEP step, the only compounds in common between these two starting points are the steps from glyceraldehyde 3-phosphate to glucose. Of the choices listed in the question, only glucose 6-phosphate is in that part of the pathway.

2. **The answer is A.** PEPCK converts oxaloacetate to phos-phoenolpyruvate. In combination with pyruvate carboxy-lase, it is used to bypass the pyruvate kinase reaction. Thus, compounds that enter gluconeogenesis between PEP (such as lactate, alanine, or any TCA cycle interme-diate) must use PEPCK to produce PEP. Glycerol enters gluconeogenesis as glyceraldehyde 3-phosphate, bypass-ing the PEPCK step. Galactose is converted to glucose 1-phosphate, then glucose 6-phosphate, also bypassing the PEPCK step. Even-chain fatty acids can only give rise to acetyl-CoA, which cannot be used to synthesize glucose.

3. **The answer is C.** Glucagon counteracts insulin's action, in that it is a catabolic hormone (thus, A is incorrect), and its levels decrease when insulin levels increase (thus, E is incorrect). As insulin levels rise after a meal, glucagon lev-els will decrease, indicating that D is incorrect. The mus-cle lacks glucagon receptors and cannot respond to glucagon; hence, B is incorrect.

4. **The answer is B.** High blood glucose levels signal the release of insulin from the pancreas; glucagons levels either stay the same or slightly decrease.

5. **The answer is D.** The hyperglycemia in an untreated dia-betic creates an osmotic diuresis, which means that exces-sive water is lost through urination. This can lead to a con-traction of blood volume, leading to low blood pressure, and a rapid heartbeat. It also leads to dehydration. The rapid respirations result from an acidosis-induced stimula-tion of the respiratory center of the brain, to reduce the amount of acid in the blood. Ketone bodies have accumu-lated, leading to diabetic ketoacidosis (thus, B is incor-rect). Patients with a hypoglycemic coma (which can be caused by an insulin shock) do not exhibit dehydration, low blood pressure, or rapid respirations; in fact, they sweat profusely because of epinephrine release (thus, C and E are incorrect). Answer A is incorrect because lack of a pancreas would be a fatal condition.

Chapter 32

1. **The answer is B.** Chylomicrons transport dietary lipids, and 80% or more of the chylomicron is triglyceride. All other components are present at less than 10%; hence, all other answers are incorrect.

2. **The answer is D.** High-density lipoproteins transfer apoproteins CII and E to nascent chylomicrons to convert them to mature chylomicrons. Bile salts are required to emulsify dietary lipid, 2-monacylglycerol is a digestion product of pancreatic lipase, lipoprotein lipase digests tri-acylglycerol from mature chylomicrons, and the lym-phatic system delivers the nascent chylomicrons to the bloodstream.

3. **The answer is A.** Both apoB-48 and apoB-100 are derived from the same gene, and from the same mRNA (there is no difference in splicing between the two; thus, B is incor-rect). However, RNA editing introduces a stop codon in the message such that B-48 stops protein synthesis approximately 48% along the message. Thus, proteolytic cleavage is not correct. B-48 is only found in chylomi-crons, and B-100 is only found in VLDL particles.

4. **The answer is B.** The bile salts must be above their criti-cal micelle concentration (the concentration at which the bile salts will form micelles) to form micelles with the components of lipase digestion, fatty acids and 2-monoa-cylglycerol. In the absence of micelle formation, lipid absorption would not occur. The critical micelle concen-tration is independent of triglyceride concentration (hence, A is incorrect). Bile salts do not bind or activate lipase (hence, C and E are incorrect). The absorption of bile salts in the ileum is not related to actual triglyceride digestion (thus, D is incorrect).

5. **The answer is D.** Nascent chylomicrons would be synthe-sized and can only acquire apoprotein CII from HDL (thus, A is incorrect). The chylomicrons would be degraded in part by lipoprotein lipase, leading to chylomi-cron remnant formation. However, the chylomicron rem-nants would remain in circulation because of the lack of apoprotein E. B is incorrect because VLDL particles are not produced immediately after a meal; it is the chylomi-crons that transport dietary triglycerides throughout the body. Because these remnants still contain a fair amount of triglyceride, serum triglyceride levels would be elevated (meaning that C and E are incorrect).

Chapter 33

1. **The answer is A.** Fatty acids, cleaved from the triacyl-glycerols of blood lipoproteins by the action of lipopro-tein lipase, are taken up by adipose cells and react with coenzyme A to form fatty acyl CoA. Glucose is converted by dihydroxyacetone phosphate to glycerol 3-phosphate, which reacts with fatty acyl CoA to form phosphatidic acid (adipose tissue lacks glycerol kinase, so it cannot use glycerol directly; hence, B is incorrect). After inorganic phosphate is released from phosphatidic acid, the result-ing diacylglycerol reacts with another fatty acyl CoA to form a triacylglycerol, which is stored in adipose cells (2-monoacylglycerol is an intermediate of triacylglycerol synthesis only in the intestine; hence, C is incorrect). LPL

action releases fatty acids from triglycerides and is not involved in triglyceride synthesis (thus, D is incorrect), and acetoacetyl CoA is an intermediate in ketone body or cholesterol biosynthesis, but not triglyceride synthesis (thus, E is incorrect).

2. **The answer is D.** The triacylglycerol is degraded by pancreatic lipase, which releases the fatty acids at positions 1 and 3. The fatty acids released are then transported to the cell surface in a bile salt micelle. The only exceptions are short-chain fatty acids (shorter than palmitic acid), which can diffuse to the cell surface and enter the intestinal cell in the absence of micelle formation.

3. **The answer is B.** Dietary carbohydrate is converted to lipid in the liver, and exported via VLDL. Thus, a low-carbohydrate diet would reduce VLDL formation and reduce the hyperlipoproteinemia.

4. **The answer is C.** Sphingosine is derived from the condensation of palimitoyl CoA and serine. It is converted to ceramide through reaction with a fatty acyl CoA, not a UDP-sugar. There is no glycerol in this structure, and cardiolipin is derived from phosphatidic acid and phosphatidylglycerol. All cells synthesize sphingosine; its synthesis is not restricted to neuronal cells.

5. **The answer is E.** When fatty acids are being synthesized, malonyl CoA accumulates, which inhibits carnitinepalmitoyl transferase I. This blocks fatty acid entry into the mitochondrion for oxidation. Many tissues both synthesize and degrade fatty acids (such as liver and muscle; thus, A is incorrect). NADPH blocks the glucose 6-phosphate dehydrogenase reaction, but not fatty acid oxidation (thus, B is incorrect). Insulin has no effect on the synthesis of the enzymes involved in fatty acid degradation (unlike the effect of insulin on the induction of enzymes involved in fatty acid synthesis; thus, C is incorrect). Finally, newly synthesized fatty acids are converted to their CoA derivatives for elongation and desaturation; hence, D is incorrect.

Chapter 34

1. **The answer is B.** The reduction of HMG-CoA to mevalonate is catalyzed by HMG-CoA reductase, which is an integral enzyme in the smooth endoplasmic reticulum. The activity of HMG-CoA reductase is carefully controlled and is the rate-limiting step for de novo cholesterol biosynthesis. The other steps listed, although on the pathway to cholesterol, are not catalyzed by regulated enzymes.

2. **The answer is C.** The squalene monooxygenase reaction uses one of the oxygen atoms of O_2 to form an epoxide at one end of the squalene molecule, which requires NADPH as a cosubstrate of the reaction. All sterols have four fused rings (thus, A is incorrect). Because the epoxide is formed at one end of the squalene molecule, B is incorrect. D is incorrect because NADPH provides the reducing power, not FADH2, and E is incorrect because carbons 1 and 30 remain independent during the cyclization of squalene.

3. **The answer is C.** The presence of chronic hyperglycemia (usually accompanied by high levels of free fatty acids in the blood) causes diffuse multiorgan toxic effects ("glucose toxicity" and "lipotoxicity") to the extent that it raises the risk for a future atherosclerotic event to a level equal to that posed by a history of the patient having already suffered such an event in the past. The other risk factors, in the absence of a previous myocardial infarction, do not require the suggested lower limits for circulating cholesterol levels.

4. **The answer is B.** ApoCIII appears to inhibit the activation of LPL. ApoE acts as a ligand for binding of several lipoproteins to the LDL receptor, the LDL receptor-related protein (LRP), and possibly to a separate apoE receptor. ApoB-48 is required for the normal assembly and secretion of chylomicrons from the small bowel, whereas apoB-100 is required in the liver for the assembly and secretion of VLDL. ApoC-II is the activator of LPL.

5. **The answer is B.** Because chylomicrons contain the most triacylglycerol, they are the least dense of the blood lipoproteins. Because VLDL contains more protein, it is denser than chylomicrons. Because LDL is produced by degradation of the triacylglycerol in VLDL, LDL is denser than VLDL. HDL is the most dense of the blood lipoproteins. It has the most protein and the least triacylglycerol.

Chapter 35

1. **The answer is C.** Most prostaglandins are synthesized from arachidonic acid (cis Δ 5, 8, 11, 14 $C_{20:4}$), which is derived from the essential fatty acid linoleic acid (cis Δ 9, 12 $C_{18:2}$). Glucose, oleic acid, or acetyl CoA cannot give rise to linoleic or arachidonic acid, because mammals cannot introduce double bonds six carbons from the ω end of a fatty acid. Leukotrienes are also derived from arachidonic acid, but they are not precursors of prostaglandins; they follow a different pathway.

2. **The answer is A.** Arachidonic acid is produced from linoleic acid (an essential fatty acid) by a series of elongation and desaturation reactions. Arachidonic acid is stored in membrane phospholipids, released, and oxidized by a cyclooxygenase (which is inhibited by aspirin) in the first step of the biosynthesis of prostaglandins, prostacyclins, and thromboxanes. Leukotrienes require the enzyme lipoxygenase, rather than cyclooxygenase, for their synthesis from arachidonic acid.

3. **The answer is A.** Aspirin leads to the acetylation of COX-1 and COX-2, which inhibits the enzymes. Tylenol contains acetaminophen, which is a competitive inhibitor of both COX-1 and COX-2, but acetaminophen does not covalently attach to the enzymes. Advil contains ibuprofen, which is another competitive inhibitor of the COX enzymes. Vioxx and Celebrex contain inhibitors specific for COX-2, which is the form of cyclooxygenase that is induced during inflammation. Vioxx and Celebrex do not inhibit COX-1 activity.

4. **The answer is C.** Release of TXA2 by platelets at wounds, while enhancing platelet aggregation (see Chapter 45), also induces vasoconstriction to reduce blood flow to the wounded area. TXA2 has no effect on either COX-1 or COX-2 activities, and does induce bronchial constriction, but not bronchial dilation.

5. **The answer is B.** Phospholipase C is activated by a Gq protein, which is coupled to the prostaglandin receptor. Activation of phospholipase C leads to the hydrolysis of phosphatidylinositol bisphosphate (PIP_2) to produce diacylglycerol and inositol tris phosphate (IP_3). The IP_3 leads to the increase in intracellular calcium levels (see Chapter 11). Activation of the protein kinase A pathway, through a G protein and adenylate cyclase, does not lead to a rise in intracellular calcium levels. Protein kinase C is activated by diacylglycerol, one of the products of PIP_2 hydrolysis, but protein kinase C is not involved in the increase in intracellular calcium levels. Phospholipase A2 releases arachidonic acid from phospholipids, but this response is not required when prostaglandins bind to their receptors.

Chapter 36

1. **The answer is B.** The acetone on her breath (which is produced by decarboxylation of acetoacetate; thus, E is incorrect) and the ketones in the urine indicate that the woman is in diabetic ketoacidosis. This is caused by low insulin levels, so her blood glucose levels are high because the glucose is not being taken up by the peripheral tissues (thus, A and C are incorrect). An insulin injection would reduce her blood glucose levels and decrease the release of fatty acids from adipose triglycerides. Consequently, ketone body production would decrease. Glucagon injections would simply exacerbate the woman's current condition (thus, D is incorrect).

2. **The answer is D.** Chylomicrons are blood lipoproteins produced from dietary fat. VLDL are produced mainly from dietary carbohydrate. IDL and LDL are produced from VLDL. HDL does not transport triacylglycerol to the tissues.

3. **The answer is E.** Excess energy is stored as triglyceride; when caloric excess is primarily triglyceride, to synthesize triglyceride, energy is required in activating the fatty acids to their CoA derivatives before condensation with glycerol 3-phosphate. When caloric excess is primarily carbohydrate derived, energy must be used to synthesize the fatty acids from glucose; however, that energy is balanced by the energy obtained when glucose is converted to two molecules of acetyl CoA (2 ATP + 1 NADH). Thus, the amount of triglyceride that would be stored would be similar regardless of the source of the calories.

4. **The answer is B.** Metabolism of ethanol leads to production of NADH in the liver, which will inhibit fatty acid oxidation in the liver. Because the patient has not eaten for 5 days, the insulin/glucagon ratio is low, hormone-sensitive lipase is activated, and fatty acids are being released by the adipocyte and taken up by the muscle and liver. However, because the liver NADH levels are high because of ethanol metabolism, the fatty acids received from the adipocyte are repackaged into triacylglycerol (the high NADH promotes the conversion of dihydroxyacetone-phosphate to glycerol 3-phosphate as well) and secreted from the liver in the form of VLDL. None of the other answers are correct statements.

5. **The answer is A.** The clotting problems are attributable to a lack of vitamin K, a lipid-soluble vitamin. Vitamin K is absorbed from the diet in mixed micelles and packaged with chylomicrons for delivery to the other tissues. Because individuals with abetalipoproteinemia lack the microsomal triglyceride transfer protein and cannot effectively produce chylomicrons, vitamin K deficiency can result. Such patients also cannot produce VLDL, but lipid-soluble vitamin distribution does not depend on VLDL particles, only chylomicrons. The other answers are incorrect statements.

Chapter 37

1. **The answer is C.** Trypsinogen, which is secreted by the intestine, is activated by enteropeptidase, a protein found in the intestine (thus, D is backwards and incorrect). Once trypsin is formed, it will activate all of the other zymogens secreted by the pancreas. Trypsin does not activate pepsinogen (thus, B is incorrect), as pepsinogen is found in the stomach and autocatalyzes its own activation when the pH drops because of acid secretion. Trypsin has no effect on intestinal motility (hence, E is incorrect) and also does not have a much broader base of substrates than any other protease (trypsin cleaves on the carboxy side of basic side chains, lysine and arginine; hence, A is incorrect).

2. **The answer is C.** Leucine can be transported by a number of different amino acid systems. Leucine is an essential amino acid, so the body cannot synthesize it (thus, A is incorrect). If the intestine cannot absorb leucine, then the kidneys do not have a chance to reabsorb it, so B is incorrect. Leucine and isoleucine have different structures and

cannot substitute for each other in all positions within a protein; thus, D is incorrect. Leucine is an important component of proteins, and is required for protein synthesis; hence, E is incorrect.

3. **The answer is D.** Kwashiorkor is a disease that results from eating a calorie-sufficient diet that lacks protein. None of the other answers is correct.

4. **The answer is C.** Pepsinogen, under acidic conditions, autocatalyzes its conversion to pepsin in the stomach. Both enteropeptidase and aminopeptidases are synthesized in active form by the intestine (thus, A and D are incorrect). Enteropeptidase activates trypsinogen (thus, B is incorrect), which then activates proelastase (hence, E is incorrect).

5. **The answer is E.** Because of a lack of protein in the diet, protein synthesis is impaired in the liver (lack of essential amino acids). The liver can still synthesize fatty acids from carbohydrate or fat sources, but VLDL particles cannot be assembled because of a shortage of apoprotein B100. Thus, the fatty acids remain in the liver, leading to a fatty liver. None of the other answers explains this finding.

Chapter 38

1. Infant I has a defect in carbamoyl phosphate synthetase I (CPSI; answer A), and infant IV has a defect in ornithine transcarbamoylase (OTC; answer B). Infants with high ammonia, low arginine, and low citrulline levels must have a defect in a urea cycle enzyme before the step that produces citrulline, i.e., CPSI or OTC. If CPSI is functional and carbamoyl phosphate is produced but cannot be further metabolized, more than the normal amount is diverted to the pathway for pyrimidine synthesis, and the intermediate orotate appears in the urine. Therefore, infant I has a defect in CPSI (citrulline is low and less than the normal amount of orotate is in the urine). Infant IV has an OTC defect; carbamoyl phosphate is produced, but it cannot be converted to citrulline, so citrulline is low, and orotate is present in the urine.

Infants II and V have high levels of citrulline but low levels of arginine. Therefore, they cannot produce arginine from citrulline. Argininosuccinate synthetase or argininosuccinate lyase is defective. The very elevated citrulline levels in infant II suggest that the block is in argininosuccinate synthetase (answer C). In infant V, citrulline levels are more moderately elevated, suggesting that citrulline can be converted to argininosuccinate and that the defect is in argininosuccinate lyase (answer D). Thus, the accumulated intermediates of the urea cycle are distributed between argininosuccinate and citrulline (which can be excreted in the urine). The high levels of arginine and more moderate hyperammonemia in infant III suggest that, in this case, the defect is in arginase (answer E).

2. **The answer is D.** The nitrogens in urea are derived from carbamoyl phosphate and aspartate directly during one turn of the cycle. The nitrogen in the side chain of ornithine is never incorporated into urea, because it stays with ornithine (thus, answers A, B, and C are incorrect). Glutamine does not donate a nitrogen directly during the urea cycle, so answers E and F are also incorrect.

3. **The answer is C.** Glutamate dehydrogenase fixes ammonia into α-ketoglutarate, generating glutamate, in a reversible reaction that also requires NAD(P)H. Alanine-pyruvate aminotransferase catalyzes the transfer of nitrogen from alanine to an α-keto acid acceptor, but does not use ammonia as a substrate. Glutaminase converts glutamine to glutamate and ammonia, but the reaction is not reversible. Arginase splits arginine into urea, and ornithine and argininosuccinate synthetase forms argininosuccinate from citrulline and aspirate. The only other two enzymes that can fix ammonia into an organic compound are carbamoyl phosphate synthetase I and glutamine synthetase.

4. **The answer is C.** Glycogen phosphorylase requires pyridoxal phosphate to break the α1,4 linkages in glycogen. None of the other pathways listed contain an enzyme that requires this cofactor.

5. **The answer is A.** CPS-I is the major regulated step, being activated by N-acetyl-glutamate, the synthesis of which is stimulated by arginine. None of the other urea cycle enzymes is regulated allosterically.

Chapter 39

1. **The answer is A.** Tyrosine is derived from phenylalanine, which requires BH$_4$, but not vitamin B6. Vitamin B6 is required in the synthesis of serine (TA), of alanine (another TA), cysteine (β-elimination, β-addition, γ-elimination), and aspartate (TA).

2. **The answer is E;** the other end products are acetoacetate, acetyl-CoA, fumarate, oxaloacetate, α-ketoglutarate, and pyruvate.

3. **The answer is C.** The classical form of PKU, a deficiency of phenylalanine hydroxylase, will result in elevations of phenylalanine and phenylpyruvate. However, this enzyme is not a choice. In the nonclassical variant of PKU, there is a problem in either synthesizing or regenerating BH$_4$. The enzyme that converts BH$_2$ to BH$_4$ is dihydropteridine reductase.

4. **The answer is B.** The reaction pathway in which methionine goes to cysteine and α-ketobutyrate requires pyridoxal phosphate at two steps: the cystathionine β-synthase reaction and the cystathionase reaction. Phenylalanine to tyrosine requires BH$_4$; propionyl-CoA to succinyl-CoA requires B12; pyruvate to acetyl-CoA requires thiamine pyrophosphate, lipoic acid, NAD, FAD, and coenzyme A; and glucose going to glycogen does not require a cofactor.

5. **The answer is C.** Folic acid is required for the conversion of serine to glycine, and the serine is produced from 3-phosphoglycerate and alanine. Folic acid is not needed to synthesize aspartate (from oxaloacetate by transamination), glutamate (from α-ketoglutarate by transamination), proline (from glutamate by a series of steps that do not require folic acid), or serine (from 3-phosphoglycerate, with no one-carbon metabolism needed).

Chapter 40

1. **The answer is D.** The homocysteine-to-methionine reaction requires N^5-methyl FH_4, serine to glycine requires free FH_4 and generates N^5, N^{10}-methylene FH_4, betaine donates a methyl group to homocysteine to form methionine without the participation of FH_4, and the purine ring requires N^{10}-formyl FH_4 in its biosynthesis.

2. **The answer is B.** Propionic acid is derived from an accumulation of propionyl-CoA. The normal pathway for the degradation of propionyl-CoA is first, a biotin-dependent carboxylation to D-methylmalonyl-CoA, racemization to L-methylmalonyl-CoA, and, then, the B12-dependent rearrangement to succinyl-CoA.

3. **The answer is C.** An inability to hydrolyze dietary protein and release bound B12 would lead to a deficiency. Pancreatic insufficiency would result in a reduction of proteases in the pancreas and a reduced ability to release B12 from protein. Both R-binders and intrinsic factor are required for appropriate B12 absorption; animal protein contains high levels of B12, and glutamic acid is conjugated to folic acid, not to vitamin B12. Folic acid absorption does not affect B12 absorption.

4. **The answer is B.** The only three forms of folate that transfer carbons are the N^5-methyl FH_4 form, the N^5, N^{10}-methylene FH_4 form, and the N^{10}-formyl form. None of the other forms participates in reactions in which the carbon is transferred. The N^5-methyl form transfers the methyl group to form methionine from homocysteine.

5. **The answer is E.** Choline, derived from phosphatidylcholine, is converted to betaine (trimethylglycine). Betaine can donate a methyl group to homocysteine to form methionine plus dimethylglycine. Sarcosine is N-methylglycine, which is formed when excess SAM methylates glycine, but it is not used as a methyl donor in this reaction.

Chapter 41

1. **The answer is A.** Both carbamoyl phosphate synthetase-I and -II use carbon dioxide as the carbon source in the production of carbamoyl phosphate. CPS-I is located in the mitochondria, whereas CPS-II is in the cytoplasm (thus, B is incorrect). CPS-I can fix ammonia; CPS-II requires glutamine as the nitrogen source (thus, C is incorrect).

N-acetyl glutamate activates CPS-I; CPS-II is activated by PRPP (thus, D is incorrect). UMP inhibits CPS-II, but has no effect on CPS-I (thus, E is also incorrect).

2. **The answer is B.** A lack of glucose 6-phosphatase activity (von Gierke's disease) leads to an accumulation of glucose 6-phosphate, which will lead to an increase in ribose 5-phosphate levels, and then an increase in PRPP levels. As PRPP levels rise, purine synthesis will be stimulated, leading to excessive levels of purines in the blood. The degradation of the extra purines leads to uric acid production and gout. A loss of either PRPP synthetase activity or glutamine phosphoribosyl amidotransferase activity would lead to reduced purine synthesis and hypouricemia (thus, answers A and D are incorrect). A lack of glucose 6-phosphate dehydrogenase would hinder ribose 5-phosphate production and, thus, would not lead to excessive purine synthesis. A lack of purine nucleoside phosphorylase would hinder the salvage pathway, leading to an accumulation of nucleosides. Purine nucleoside phosphorylase activity is required to synthesize uric acid, so in the absence of this enzyme, less uric acid would be produced (thus, E is incorrect).

3. **The answer is C.** The enzyme defect in Lesch-Nyhan syndrome involves hypoxanthine-guanine phosphoribosyl transferase (HGPRT). This enzyme converts the free base to a nucleotide, specifically guanine to GMP and hypoxanthine to IMP. Adenine phosphoribosyltransferase (APRT) converts adenine to AMP (thus, A is incorrect). Adenosine kinase converts adenosine to AMP (hence, B is incorrect). There are no enzymes to convert guanosine to GMP or thymine to TMP (thus, D and E are incorrect). Pyrimidine nucleoside phosphorylase will convert thymine to thymidine but not to the nucleotide level. Thymidine kinase converts thymidine to TMP (thus, F is incorrect).

4. **The answer is B.** Allopurinol inhibits the conversion of both hypoxanthine to xanthine and xanthine to uric acid. This occurs because both of those reactions are catalyzed by xanthine oxidase, the target of allopurinol. A is incorrect because AMP is not directly converted to XMP (AMP, when degraded, is deaminated to form IMP, which loses its phosphate to become inosine, which undergoes phosphorolysis to generate hypoxanthine and ribose 1-phosphate). C is incorrect because the inosine to hypoxanthine conversion, catalyzed by nucleoside phosphorylase, is not inhibited by allopurinol. D is incorrect because the conversion of hypoxanthine to xanthine occurs at the free base level, not at the nucleotide level. E is incorrect because GMP is converted first to guanosine (loss of phosphate), the guanosine is converted to guanine and ribose 1-phosphate, and the guanine is then converted to xanthine by guanase.

5. **The answer is B.** If dGTP were to accumulate in cells, the dGTP would bind to the substrate specificity site of ribonucleotide reductase and direct the synthesis of dADP. This would lead to elevations of dATP levels, which would

inhibit the activity or ribonucleotide reductase. The inhibition of ribonucleotide reductase leads to a cessation of cell proliferation, as the supply of deoxyribonucleotides for DNA synthesis become limiting. A is incorrect because ATP would need to bind to the substrate specificity site to direct the synthesis of dCDP. That would not occur under these conditions of elevated dGTP levels. C is incorrect because the enzyme only works on diphosphates; AMP would never be a substrate for this enzyme. D is incorrect because the thioredoxin is always regenerated and does not become rate-limiting for the reductase reaction. E is incorrect because dGTP does not bind to the activity site of the reductase; only ATP (activator) or dATP (inhibitor) are capable of binding to the activity site.

Chapter 42

1. **The answer is D.** High levels of amino acids in the blood stimulate the pancreas to release glucagon (therefore, answers A, C, E, and G are incorrect). Insulin is also released, but the glucagon/insulin ratio is such that the liver still uses the carbons of amino acids to synthesize glucose (thus, A, E, and F are incorrect). However, the insulin levels are high enough to stimulate BCAA uptake into the muscle for oxidation (thus, E, F, G, and H are incorrect).

2. **The answer is C.** The pathway followed is glutamine to glutamate, to glutamate semialdehyde, to ornithine, and then after condensation with carbamoyl phosphate, to citrulline. Aspartate, succinyl COA, serine and fumarate are not a part of this pathway.

3. **The answer is D.** Cortisol is released during fasting and times of stress and signals muscle cells to initiate ubiquitin-mediated protein degradation. The other hormones listed do not have this effect on muscle protein metabolism. Insulin stimulates protein synthesis; glucagon has no effect on muscle, as muscle lacks glucagon receptors. Epinephrine initiates glycogen degradation, but not protein degradation, and glucose is not a signaling molecule for muscle as it can be for the pancreas.

4. **The answer is D.** Glutamine is derived from glutamate, which is formed from α-ketoglutarate. Only isoleucine and valine can give rise to glutamine, because leucine is strictly ketogenic. These amino acids give rise to succinyl CoA, which goes around the TCA cycle to form citrate (after condensing with acetyl CoA), which then forms isocitrate (the correct answer), and the isocitrate is converted to α-ketoglutarate. Urea, pyruvate, phosphoenolpyruvate, and lactate are not required intermediates in the conversion of BCAA carbons to glutamine carbons.

5. **The answer is B.** An individual in sepsis will be catabolic, and protein degradation exceeds protein intake (leading to negative nitrogen balance; thus, A, C, and E are incorrect). The liver is synthesizing glucose from amino acid precur-

sors to raise blood glucose levels for the immune cells and the nervous system (thus, gluconeogenesis is active, and E and F must be incorrect). Fatty acid release and oxidation also has been stimulated to provide an energy source for the liver and skeletal muscle (indicating that C, D, and F are incorrect).

Chapter 43

1. **The answer is E.** A tumor of the adrenal cortex is secreting excessive amounts of cortisol into the blood, which adversely affects glucose tolerance, suppresses pituitary secretion of ACTH, and, through chronic hypercortisolemia, causes the physical changes described in this patient. Uncomplicated non–insulin-dependent and insulin-dependent diabetes mellitus can be eliminated as possible diagnoses because they are not associated with elevated plasma cortisol levels and low plasma ACTH levels. In this patient, hyperglycemia resulted from the diabetogenic effects of chronic hypercortisolemia. An ACTH-secreting tumor of the anterior pituitary gland would cause hypercortisolemia, which, in turn, could adversely affect glucose tolerance, but, in this case, the plasma ACTH levels would have been high, rather than 0 pg/mL. The posterior pituitary gland secretes oxytocin and vasopressin, neither of which influences blood glucose, cortisol, or ACTH levels.

2. **The answer is A.** High blood glucose levels cause a decrease in growth hormone levels in the blood. This fact serves as the basis for the glucose suppression test for growth hormone. B, C, and D all would cause growth hormone levels to increase, whereas E would have no effect on the test.

3. **The answer is B.** When iodine is deficient in the diet, the thyroid does not make normal amounts of T_3 and T_4. Consequently, there is less feedback inhibition of TSH production and release; hence, an increased secretion of TSH would be observed. There is no direct effect on thyroglobulin synthesis (thus, A is incorrect). TRH is released by the hypothalamus to release TSH from the pituitary; a lack of thyroid hormone would increase production of TRH, not decrease it (thus, C is incorrect). An overproduction of thyroid hormone leads to increased heat production and weight loss; lack of thyroid hormone does not lead to these symptoms (thus, D and E are incorrect).

4. **The answer is A.** The woman is experiencing hypothyroidism; TSH is elevated in an attempt to secrete more thyroid hormone, as the existing dose is too low to suppress TSH release.

5. **The answer is C.** If 15% of the radioactive T4 is bound to antibody, the amount of T_4 in 0.1 mL of the patient's serum is 0.015 µg/0.1 mL, or 15 µg/dL (1.0 dL = 100 mL).

Chapter 44

1. **The answer is A.** Increased 2,3-bisphosphoglycerate in the red cell will favor the deoxy conformation of hemoglobin and thus allow more oxygen to be released in the tissues. This is useful because the hemoglobin is not as saturated at high altitudes as at low elevations, because of the lower concentration of oxygen at high altitudes. Answers C and D are incorrect because the red cells do not synthesize proteins. Answer E is incorrect because reducing the blood pH will not aid in oxygen delivery; the Bohr effect works best when tissue pH is lower than the blood pH, to stabilize the deoxy form of hemoglobin. If the pH of both the blood and tissue are the same, the Bohr effect would not be able to occur.

2. **The answer is D.** The boy is suffering from lead poisoning, which interrupts heme synthesis at the ALA-dehydratase and ferrochelatase steps. Without heme, the oxygen-carrying capability of blood is reduced, and the flow of electrons through the electron transfer chain is reduced because of the lack of functional cytochromes. Together, these lead to an inability to generate energy, and fatigue results. A is incorrect because although an iron deficiency would lead to the same symptoms, this would not be expected in the patient because of his daily vitamin uptake. Lead ingestion will not lead to an iron loss. B and C are incorrect because B12 and folate deficiencies will lead to a macrocytic anemia, because of disruption of DNA synthesis. E is incorrect because the ingestion of paint chips is unlikely to lead to a B6 deficiency in a child, particularly one who is taking daily vitamins.

3. **The answer is C.** Turning on a gene that would provide a functional alternative to the β gene would enable the defective β protein to be bypassed. Only the γ chain can do this, but it is normally only found in fetal hemoglobin. The δ chain is also a β replacement globin, but it was not listed as a potential answer. B is incorrect because the β chain is mutated, and it is already being expressed. Unlike the α gene, of which there are two copies per chromosome, there is only one copy of the β gene per chromosome. The other genes listed (answers A, D, and E) are α-chain replacements, and expression of these genes will not alleviate the problem inherent in the β gene.

4. **The answer is D.** The only two types of blood cells that lack nuclei are the mature red blood cell and platelet. Platelets arise from membrane budding from megakaryocytes and are essentially membrane sacs containing the cytoplasmic contents of their precursor cell. All of the other cell types listed contain a nucleus.

5. **The answer is D.** Thalassemias result from an imbalance in the synthesis of α and β chains. Excessive synthesis of α chains results in their precipitation in developing red cells, which often kills the developing cell. The more severely affected child has an α/β ratio of 1 to 5, whereas the less severely affected child has a ratio of 1 to 2.5. When β chains are in excess, they form stable tetramers that bind but do not release oxygen, thus reducing the red cell's ability to deliver oxygen. Thus, this difference in chain ratio makes an important difference in the functioning of the red cell.

Chapter 45

1. **The answer is D.** Under conditions of reduced protein ingestion, essential amino acids are scarce, and the liver reduces protein synthesis, including circulating plasma proteins. The reduction of protein in the plasma results in a lower osmotic pressure, such that excess fluid in the extravascular spaces cannot return to the blood, and remain outside of the circulation, collecting in tissues.

2. **The answer is C.** Warfarin inhibits the reduction of vitamin K epoxide, such that active vitamin K levels decrease. The reduction in active vitamin K levels reduces the γ-carboxylation of clotting factors. In the absence of γ-carboxylation, the clotting factors cannot bind to calcium to form membrane-associated complexes with other clotting factors. Warfarin has no effect on the liver's ability to synthesize the clotting factor (the synthesized factor does not get modified), nor does warfarin specifically inhibit the activation of Factor XIII. The inhibition is more global than just attacking one step in the coagulation cascade. Plasma calcium levels are not altered by warfarin, and protein C activity is actually decreased in the presence of warfarin, because protein C is one of the proteins that is γ-carboxylated in a vitamin K—dependent reaction.

3. **The answer is C.** Activated protein C turns off the clotting cascade; in the absence of protein C, regulation of clotting is impaired, and clots can develop when not required. Mutations in any of the other answers listed would lead to excessive bleeding, because an essential component of the clotting cascade would have been inactivated.

4. **The answer is C.** Classical hemophilia is absence of Factor VIII, which is a necessary cofactor for the activation of Factor X by Factor IXa. Factor II is directly activated by Factor Xa, and Factor IX is directly activated by Factor XIa. Proteins C and S are directly activated by thrombin, Factor IIa.

5. **The answer is B.** Hemophilia B is an inactivating mutation in Factor IX, such that Factor IXa cannot be formed. Factor XIa is formed, but its substrate, Factor IX is defective, and a nonactive protein results.

Chapter 46

1. **The answer is C.** Grapefruit juice contains a component that blocks CYP3A4 activity, which is the cytochrome P450 isozyme, which converts statins to an inactive form. If the degradative enzyme is inhibited, statin levels rise above normal, accelerating their damage of muscle cells.

Grapefruit juice does not affect hepatic uptake of the drug (thus, A is incorrect), nor is it accelerating statin metabolism (thus, B is also incorrect). Although HMG CoA reductase is the target of the statins, grapefruit juice neither upregulates nor downregulates the amount of enzyme present in the cell (therefore, D and E are incorrect).

2. **The answer is D.** Cytochrome P450 enzymes oxidize their substrates, transferring the electrons to molecular oxygen to form water and a hydroxylated product. The enzymes require NADPH (hence, B is incorrect) and are located in the endoplasmic reticulum membrane (thus, A is incorrect). Oxygen does not induce all cytochrome P450 members (although it is a substrate for all these isozymes; C is therefore incorrect), and while these enzymes proceed through a free radical mechanism, the final products are not radicals (indicating that E is incorrect).

3. **The answer is D.** Hepatocellular disease reduces protein synthesis within the liver, which leads to reduced levels of both LCAT and hepatic triglyceride lipase being produced (thus, answers A and C are incorrect). Because LCAT activity is reduced, cholesterol ester formation in circulating particles will be reduced (thus, B is incorrect). Because a diseased liver has trouble synthesizing glucose, fatty acid release from adipocytes is increased to provide energy (thus, E is incorrect). Serum triacylglycerol levels are increased because of the reduced hepatic triglyceride lipase activity; LPL activity is also reduced in liver disease.

4. **The answer is D.** Ethanol induces the CYP2E1 system, which converts acetaminophen to NAPQI, a toxic intermediate. Under normal conditions (non-induced levels of CYP2E1), the conversion of acetaminophen to NAPQI results in low levels of NAPQI being produced, which can easily be detoxified. However, when CYP2E1 is induced, the excessive levels of NAPQI being produced when Tylenol is taken above suggested levels cannot be readily detoxified, and NAPQI binds to proteins and inactivates them, leading to hepatocyte death. The toxicity is not related to blood glucose levels (thus, A and C are incorrect), nor to secretion of VLDL (answer E is therefore incorrect). Ethanol does not inhibit the detoxification of Tylenol, per se, but rather accelerates one of its potential metabolic fates (thus, B is also incorrect).

5. **The answer is C.** The glucokinase regulatory protein regulates glucokinase expression at a posttranscriptional level. A lack of regulatory protein activity results in less glucokinase being present in the cell and a reduced overall rate of glucose phosphorylation by the liver. This results in less circulating glucose being removed by the liver and a longer clearance time for glucose levels to return to fasting levels. A decrease in the glucokinase K_m, or an increase in the V_{max} for glucokinase, would lead to the opposite effect, enhanced glucose phosphorylation by the liver, and an accelerated clearance from the circulation

(thus, A and B are incorrect). The liver does not express hexokinase, so answers D and E are also incorrect.

Chapter 47

1. **The answer is C.** Stretching aids in stimulating blood flow to the muscles, which will enhance oxidative muscle metabolism (by allowing for better oxygen delivery). Stretching, per se, does not stimulate epinephrine release (thus, A is incorrect), nor does it activate glycolysis in either the liver or muscle.

2. **The answer is D.** Triacylglycerol is the largest energy store in the body and, as such, is the predominant fuel in long-term aerobic exercise. During exercise, muscle glycogen is used for bursts of speed but not for long-term energy requirements. Liver glycogen is used to maintain blood glucose levels for use by the nervous system and as a supplement for use by muscle when rapid speed is required; however, it is not designed as a long-term energy source. The brain does not contain significant levels of glycogen, and lactic acid produced by the red blood cells is used as a gluconeogenic precursor by liver, but not as a fuel for muscle.

3. **The answer is D.** Creatine is synthesized from glycine, arginine, and S-adenosyl methionine (thus, intake of dietary creatine is not relevant). In muscle, creatine is converted to creatine phosphate, which is nonenzymatically cyclized to form creatinine (indicating that choice C is incorrect). The amount of creatinine excreted by the kidneys each day depends on body muscle mass but is constant for each individual (thus, if there is an increase in body muscle mass, there would be an increase in creatinine excretion). In kidney failure, the excretion of creatinine into the urine will be low, and an elevation of serum creatinine would be observed.

4. **The answer is E.** Glycine is required for the synthesis of heme (combining with succinyl CoA in the initial step), for the synthesis of purine rings (the entire glycine molecule is incorporated into adenine and guanine), and for creatine, where glycine reacts with arginine in the first step.

5. **The answer is C.** A decrease in the concentration of ATP (which occurs as muscle contracts) stimulates processes that generate ATP. The proton gradient across the inner mitochondrial membrane decreases as protons enter the matrix via the ATPase to synthesize ATP; NADH oxidation by the electron transport chain increases to reestablish the proton gradient; fuel utilization also increases to generate more ATP. Glycogen synthesis is inhibited because of phosphorylation of glycogen synthase as induced by epinephrine. Palmitate is oxidized, and glycolysis increases because of the activation of PFK-1 by AMP. As ATP decreases, AMP rises because of the myokinase reaction (2 ADP yields ATP + AMP).

Chapter 48

1. **The answer is B.** The symptoms exhibited by the patient are caused by excessive release of epinephrine or norepinephrine. Vanillylmandelic acid is also the degradation product of norepinephrine; thus, these hormones are being overproduced. Acetylcholine degradation leads to the formation of acetic acid and choline, which are not observed (thus, A is incorrect). Although DOPA degradation could lead to vanillylmandelic acid production, serotonin degradation does not (it leads to 5-hydroxyindole acetic acid), and the symptoms exhibited by the patient are not consistent with DOPA or serotonin overproduction (thus, C is incorrect). Histamine and melatonin also do not produce the symptoms exhibited by the patient (hence, D and E are incorrect).

2. **The answer is A.** Myelin contains very high levels of cholesterol and cerebrosides, particularly galactosylcerebrosides.

3. **The answer is E.** Myelin basic protein is a basic protein, indicating that it must contain a significant number of lysine and arginine residues. MBP is found on the intracellular side of the myelin membrane, and its role is to compact the membrane by binding to negative charges on both sides of it, thereby reducing the "width" of the membrane. Both Schwann cells and oligodendrocytes synthesize myelin (thus, A is incorrect). MBP is not a transmembrane protein (PLP in the CNS, and Po in the PNS are; thus, B is incorrect), and because MBP is found intracellularly, answers C and D cannot be correct.

4. **The answer is A.** The accumulation of both phytanic acid and very-long-chain fatty acids indicates a problem in peroxisomal fatty acid oxidation, which is where α-oxidation occurs. Lysosomal transport is, therefore, not required for metabolizing these fatty acids (thus, C is incorrect). The finding that palmitate levels are low indicates that β-oxidation is occurring; therefore, B is incorrect. The compounds that accumulate are not mucopolysaccharides, nor is fatty acid elongation required in the metabolism of these compounds (thus, D and E are incorrect).

5. **The answer is D.** Vitamin B6 participates in transamination and decarboxylation reactions (and indirectly in deamination reactions). The one common feature in the synthesis of serotonin, GABA, norepinephrine, and histamine is a decarboxylation of an amino acid, which requires vitamin B6. The other reactions are not required in the biosynthesis of these neurotransmitters

Chapter 49

1. **The answer is E.** Scurvy is caused by a deficiency of vitamin C. Vitamin C is a required cofactor for the hydroxylation of both proline and lysine residues in collagen. The hydroxyproline residues that are formed stabilize the triple helix through the formation of hydrogen bonds with other collagen molecules within the helix. The loss of this stabilizing force greatly reduces the strength of the collagen fibers. The hydroxylation of lysine allows carbohydrates to be attached to collagen, although the role of the carbohydrates is still unknown. Vitamin C is not required for disulfide bond formation, the formation of lysyl crosslinks (that enzyme is lysyl oxidase), secretion of tropocollagen, or the formation of collagen fibrils. Thus, all other choices are incorrect.

2. **The answer is C.** When elastin expands because of outside forces (such as the respiratory muscles causing the lungs to expand with air), hydrophobic regions of elastin are exposed to the aqueous environment, resulting in a decrease in the entropy of water. When the outside force is removed (by relaxation of the respiratory muscles), the driving force for contraction of elastin is an increase in the entropy of water, such that the hydrophobic residues of elastin are again shielded from the environment. The expansion and contraction of elastin does not involve covalent modifications (thus, answers A, B, and E are incorrect), nor does it involve extensive changes in salt bridge formation (thus, D is also incorrect).

3. **The answer is B.** Glycosaminoglycan chains contain negative charges because of the presence of acidic sugars and the sulfated sugars in the molecule. Thus, in their characteristic bottleneck structure, the chains repel each other (therefore, answer A is incorrect) yet also attract positively charged cations and water into the spaces between the chains. The water forms hydrogen bonds with the sugars, and a gel-like space is created. This gel acts as a diffusion sieve for materials that either leave, or enter, this space. Hydroxylation and cross-linking of chains does not occur (thus, answers D and E are incorrect), nor does hydrogen bonding between chains (they are too far apart because of the charge repulsion, but they do form hydrogen bonds with water).

4. **The answer is E.** For cells to migrate, they must free themselves from the extracellular matrix material, which requires remodeling of the matrix components. Because of the unique structural aspects of these components, only a small subset of protease, the metalloproteinases, are capable of doing this. The other answers listed are all components of the matrix, which must be remodeled for cell migration to occur.

5. **The answer is C.** Fibronectin binds to integrins on the cell surface, as well as to various extracellular matrix components (collagen and glycosaminoglycans). This binding fixes the position of the cell within the matrix. Loss of these binding components can lead to undesirable cell movement. Fibronectin plays no role in any of the other functions listed as possible answers.

Patient Index

Note: Page numbers followed by "f" denote figures.

Index

Note: Page numbers followed by "t" dentoe tables; those followed by "f" denote figures.

A

Abetalipoproteinemia
cause of, 605
described, 592
effects of, 605
lipid metabolism in, 592
symptoms of, 592
ABO blood groups, characteristics of, 552, 552t
Absorption, 23–24, 23f
Absorptive state, 22–29. *See also* Fed state
Abzyme(s), defined, 120
ACAT. *See* Acyl-CoA-cholesterol acyl transferase (ACAT)
Acetaldehyde
alcohol-induced hepatitis due to, 466, 467f
in ethanol oxidation, 460f, 461
toxic effects of, 466–467, 467f
free radical damage due to, 466–467, 467f
Acetaminophen
action of, 660f
detoxification of, 848–849, 848f
Acetate, 877
in diet, 372
metabolism of, in ethanol oxidation, 461, 462f
Acetic acid, titration curve for, 46, 47f
Acetoacetate, 33, 33f
from amino acids, 725–728, 725f–727f
structure of, 55f
synthesis of, 431, 431f, 432f
Acetone
odor of, in diabetic ketoacidosis, 559
structure of, 55f
synthesis of, 432f
Acetyl CoA
acetyl group of, 361, 361f
from amino acids, 725–728, 725f–727f
described, 360
high-energy bonds in, 350f
malonyl CoA from, in fatty acid synthesis, 598, 598f, 599f
mevalonic acid from, in cholesterol synthesis, 623, 623f
phenylalanine from, 725, 726f, 727f
precursors of, in TCA cycle, 371–374, 372f, 373f
pyruvate dehydrogenase complex and, 372, 372f
sources of, in TCA cycle, 372, 372f
in TCA cycle, 360
tyrosine from, 725, 726f, 727f
Acetyl CoA carboxylase
reaction catalyzed by, 598, 598f
regulation of, 598, 599f
in liver, in fed state, 671–672, 671f, 672f

Acetyl group
of acetyl CoA, 361, 361f
in TCA cycle, 361, 361f, 362, 362f
Acetylcholine
inactivation of, 895
in neuromuscular junction, reduction of, acetylcholinesterase A in, 866
release of, 185
structure of, 188f
synthesis of, 893–895, 894f
Acetylcholine receptors, at neuromuscular junction, 186f
Acetylcholinesterase A, in acetylcholine level reduction, 866
N-Acetyl-ß-D-glucosamine, 61f
N-Acetylglucosamine 6-phosphate, formation of, 548
N-Acetylglutamate (NAG), allosteric activation of CPSI by, 706, 707f
Acid(s), 41–53, 44–46, 44f, 46t. *See also specific types, e.g.,* Cholic acid
amino. *See* Amino acids
arachidonic, 64, 602, 603f, 654, 656f, 657f
in blood, 46t
carbonic, 48, 48f
carboxylic, 56f
chenocholic, 628–629, 628f, 629f, 631f
cholic, 628–629, 628f, 629f, 631f
from cholesterol, in bile salt synthesis, 628–629, 628f, 629f
deoxycholic, 631f
deoxyribonucleic. *See* Deoxyribonucleic acid (DNA)
dissociation of, 45, 46f
fatty. *See* Fatty acids
folic. *See* Folate
gastric, secretion of, 50
glycocholic, 850t
glycoheno-deoxycholic, 850t
hydrochloric, 50
K, 45
linoleic, 602, 603f
lithocholic, 631f
metabolic, 41, 47–50, 48f, 49f
mevalonic, 623, 623f
nucleic, 207–221
oleic, 64
palmitoleic, 64, 65
pathogenic, 14t
phosphatidic, 64, 64f
phytanic, 430, 430f
production of, in anaerobic glycolysis, 407

strong and weak, 45–46, 46f
sulfuric, 50
Acid anhydride, 56f
Acidemia, lactic, 412–414, 413f, 414f. *See also* Lactic acidemia
Acidic amino acids, 76f, 77t, 78–79, 79f, 80f
Acidosis, lactic
causes of, 413–414, 413f
ethanol metabolism and, 465f, 466
Acquired immunodeficiency syndrome (AIDS)
treatment of, 256
tuberculosis in, 239
virus causing, production of, 254–256, 255f
Actin filaments, of cytoskeleton, 179–180, 179f
Actin fold, in globular proteins, 98f, 99
Activation-transfer coenzymes, 125–127, 126f, 127f
Active transport
cell death and, 357–358, 357f
requirements for, 166–168, 167f
Acylation, fatty, of proteins, 85, 86f
Acyl-chymotrypsin intermediate, hydrolysis of, 123
Acyl-CoA-cholesterol acyl transferase (ACAT), 627, 628f
Acyl-enzyme intermediate, formation of, 121–123
Acylglycerol(s), 64, 64f
Acyltransferase(s), 135
ADA gene. *See* Adenosine deaminase (ADA) gene
Adaptation, gene expression regulation for, 275
Adenine, in DNA, 209, 209f
Adenine nucleotide translocase (ANT), 381
defined, 394
Adenine phosphoribosyltransferase (APRT), 747
Adenoma(s), defined, 208
Adenosine deaminase (ADA) gene, defect of, 312
Adenosine diphosphate (ADP), 4
in glycolysis regulation, 409–412, 410f, 411f
Adenosine monophosphate, cyclic (CAMP), synthesis of
epinephrine in, 153
glucagon in, 153
Adenosine monophosphate (AMP)
in cholesterol regulation, 676–677
cyclic (cAMP)
described, 488
signal transduction with, 488
structure of, 148f
in glycolysis regulation, 409–412, 410f, 411f
levels of, changes in, 412
in PFK-1 regulation, 411, 411f